Tarascon Pocket Pharmacopoeia®

2017 Professional Desk Reference Edition

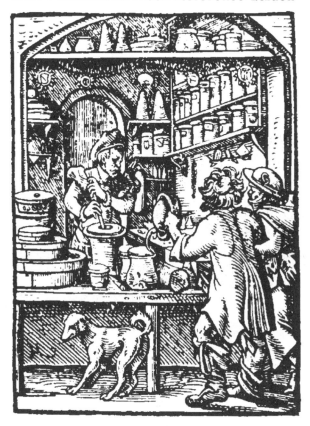

18TH EDITION

"Desire to take medicines ... distinguishes man from animals."
—Sir William Osler

Editor-in-Chief
Richard J. Hamilton, MD, FAAEM, FACMT, FACEP
Professor and Chair, Department of Emergency Medicine
Drexel University College of Medicine
Philadelphia, PA

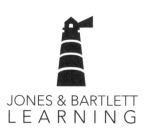

JONES & BARTLETT
LEARNING

World Headquarters
Jones & Bartlett Learning
5 Wall Street
Burlington, MA 01803
978-443-5000
info@jblearning.com
www.jblearning.com

Jones & Bartlett Learning books and products are available through most bookstores and online booksellers. To contact Jones & Bartlett Learning directly, call 800-832-0034, fax 978-443-8000, or visit our website www.jblearning.com.

Production Credits
V.P., Production, Manufacturing, and Content
 Architecture: Paul Belfanti
VP, Executive Publisher: David D. Cella
Executive Acquisitions Editor: Nancy Anastasi Duffy
V.P., Manufacturing and Inventory Control:
 Therese Connell
Manufacturing and Inventory Control Supervisor:
 Amy Bacus

Production Manager: Daniel Stone
Marketing Manager: Lindsay White
Composition: Cenveo
Printing and Binding: Edward Brothers Malloy
Cover Printing: Edward Brothers Malloy

The cover woodcut is *The Apothecary* by Jost Amman, Frankfurt, 1574.

ISSN: 1945-9084
ISBN: 978-1-284-11895-7

6048
Printed in the United States of America
20 19 18 17 16   10 9 8 7 6 5 4 3 2 1

In 2016 we asked you to solve a simple office dilemma that might have you scratching your head. A patient arrives for an office visit and pays a $25 copay. Later the office manager realizes that she overcharged the patient and gives the front desk clerk five one dollar bills to give back to the patient. The unscrupulous front desk clerk keeps $2 and gives the patient $3. So now the patient has paid a $22 copay and the clerk has $2 – where did the other dollar go? The answer is that the confusion is the result of improper accounting created by adding cost ($22 copay) and cash ($2 stolen). In fact, all the cash is accounted for - starting with $25, the office practice has $20, the patient has $3, and the clerk has $2. This is famous puzzle called the missing dollar. Unfortunately, health care today requires us all to understand accounting and find those missing dollars!

This year you need to help the hospital pharmacist with an acetaminophen elixir problem. She has a four ounce cup and a nine ounce cup. She needs to measure out six ounces of elixir. She has only these two cups, plenty of elixir and can fill or dump either cup. What's the fewest number of steps for her to measure six ounces and how would she do it?

CONTENTS

PAGE INDEX FOR TABLES

PREFACE TO THE TARASCON POCKET PHARMACOPOEIA®

The *Tarascon Pocket Pharmacopoeia®* arranges drugs by clinical class with a comprehensive index in the back. Trade names are italicized and capitalized. Drug doses shown in mg/kg are generally intended for children, while fixed doses represent typical adult recommendations. Brackets indicate currently available formulations, although not all pharmacies stock all formulations. The availability of generic, over-the-counter, and scored formulations is mentioned. We have set the disease or indication in red for the pharmaceutical agent. It is meant to function as an aid to find information quickly. Codes are as follows:

▶ **METABOLISM & EXCRETION: L** = primarily liver, **K** = primarily kidney, **LK** = both, but liver > kidney, **KL** = both, but kidney > liver.

♀ Prior FDA system **A** = Safety established using human studies, **B** = Presumed safe based on animal studies, **C** = Uncertain safety; no human studies and animal studies show an adverse effect, **D** = Unsafe - evidence of risk that may in certain clinical circumstances be justifiable, **X** = Highly unsafe - risk of use outweighs any possible benefit. As of June 2015, the FDA no longer uses letter categories to describe pregnancy risk. New drugs do not have a letter category, and letter categories will be gradually removed from product labeling for older drugs. We have developed the Tarascon Safety in Pregnancy Classification System to describe the safety of drugs in pregnancy. We apply this rating system to new drugs and to older drugs when the prior FDA letter is removed from the product label. Our system assigns the following risk category to each trimester of pregnancy (1st/2nd/3rd):

    X: Risk outweighs benefit or contraindicated
    0: Benefit outweighs risk; use in pregnancy as indicated.
    ?: Risk vs. benefit is unclear; consider alternatives.

For example, the Tarascon pregnancy classification of X/X/X for isotretinoin indicates that use is unsafe in all trimesters of pregnancy. The classification of O/O/X for naproxen indicates that use in the third trimester of pregnancy is unsafe. The trimester risk categories may also be followed by a comment. For example, the pregnancy category for asenapine is: ?/?/?R withdrawal and EPS in neonates exposed in 3rd trimester. "**R**" denotes that the drug has a pregnancy exposure registry. Prescribers are encouraged to enroll patients in pregnancy exposure registries; contact information is available in product labeling.

▶ **SAFETY IN LACTATION:** + Generally accepted as safe, **?** Safety unknown or controversial, – Generally regarded as unsafe. Many of our "**+**" listings are from the AAP policy "The Transfer of Drugs and Other Chemicals Into Human Milk" (see www.aap.org) and may differ from those recommended by the manufacturer.

© **DEA CONTROLLED SUBSTANCES: I** = High abuse potential, no accepted use (eg, heroin, marijuana), **II** = High abuse potential and severe dependence liability (eg, morphine, codeine, hydromorphone, cocaine, amphetamines, methylphenidate, secobarbital). Some states require triplicates. **III** = Moderate dependence liability (eg, *Tylenol #3, Vicodin*), **IV** = Limited dependence liability (benzodiazepines, propoxyphene, phentermine), **V** = Limited abuse potential (eg, *Lomotil*).

$ **RELATIVE COST:** Cost codes used are "per month" of maintenance therapy (eg, antihypertensives) or "per course" of short-term therapy (eg, antibiotics). Codes are calculated using average wholesale prices (at press time in US dollars) for the most common indication and route of each drug at a typical adult dosage. For maintenance therapy, costs are calculated based upon a 30-day supply or the quantity that might typically be used in a given month. For short-term therapy (ie, 10 days or less), costs are calculated on a single treatment course. When multiple forms are available (eg, generics), these codes reflect the least expensive generally available product. When drugs don't neatly fit into the classification scheme above, we have assigned codes based upon the relative cost of other similar drugs. *These codes should be used as a rough guide only*, as (1) they reflect cost, not charges, (2) pricing often varies substantially from location to location and time to time, and (3) HMOs, Medicaid, and buying groups often negotiate quite different pricing. Check with your local pharmacy if you have any questions.

Code	Cost
$	< $25
$$	$25 to $49
$$$	$50 to $99
$$$$	$100 to $199
$$$$$	≥ $200

❋ CANADIAN TRADE NAMES: Unique common Canadian trade names not used in the US are listed after a maple leaf symbol. Trade names used in both nations or only in the US are displayed without such notation.

ABBREVIATIONS IN TEXT

AAP	American Academy of Pediatrics	kg	kilogram
ACCP	American College of Chest Physicians	lbs	pounds
ACR	American College of Rheumatology	LFT	liver function test
ACT	activated clotting time	LV	left ventricular
ADHD	attention deficit hyperactivity disorder	LVEF	left ventricular ejection fraction
AHA	American Heart Association	m^2	square meters
Al	aluminum	MAOI	monoamine oxidase inhibitor
ANC	absolute neutrophil count	mcg	microgram
ASA	aspirin	MDI	metered dose inhaler
BP	blood pressure	mEq	milliequivalent
BPH	benign prostatic hyperplasia	mg	milligram
BSA	body surface area	Mg	magnesium
BUN	blood urea nitrogen	MI	myocardial infarction
Ca	calcium	min	minute
CAD	coronary artery disease	mL	milliliter
cap	capsule	mo	months old
cm	centimeter	MRSA	methicillin-resistant *Staphylococcus aureus*
CMV	cytomegalovirus	ng	nanogram
CNS	central nervous system	NHLBI	National Heart, Lung, and Blood Institute
COPD	chronic obstructive pulmonary disease	NPH	neutral protamine hagedorn
CrCl	creatinine clearance	NS	normal saline
CVA	stroke	N/V	nausea/vomiting
CYP	cytochrome P450	NYHA	New York Heart Association
D5W	5% dextrose	OA	osteoarthritis
dL	deciliter	oz	ounces
DM	diabetes mellitus	pc	after meals
DMARD	disease-modifying drug	PO	by mouth
DPI	dry powder inhaler	PR	by rectum
DRESS	drug rash eosinophilia and systemic symptoms	prn	as needed
ECG	electrocardiogram	PTT	partial thromboplastin time
EPS	extrapyramidal symptoms	q	every
ET	endotracheal	RA	rheumatoid arthritis
g	gram	RSV	respiratory syncytial virus
GERD	gastroesophageal reflux disease	SC	subcutaneous
gtts	drops	sec	second
GU	genitourinary	soln	solution
h	hour	supp	suppository
HAART	highly active antiretroviral therapy	susp	suspension
Hb	hemoglobin	tab	tablet
HCTZ	hydrochlorothiazide	TB	tuberculosis
HIT	heparin-induced thrombocytopenia	TCA	tricyclic antidepressant
HSV	herpes simplex virus	TNF	tumor necrosis factor
HTN	hypertension	TPN	total parenteral nutrition
IM	intramuscular	UTI	urinary tract infection
INR	international normalized ratio	wt	weight
IU	international units	y	year
IV	intravenous	yo	years old
JIA	juvenile idiopathic arthritis		

THERAPEUTIC DRUG LEVELS

Drug	Level	Optimal Timing
amikacin peak	20–35 mcg/mL	30 minutes after infusion
amikacin trough	<5 mcg/mL	Just prior to next dose
carbamazepine trough	4–12 mcg/mL	Just prior to next dose
cyclosporine trough	50–300 ng/mL	Just prior to next dose
digoxin	0.8–2.0 ng/mL	Just prior to next dose
ethosuximide trough	40–100 mcg/mL	Just prior to next dose
gentamicin peak	5–10 mcg/mL	30 minutes after infusion
gentamicin trough	<2 mcg/mL	Just prior to next dose
lidocaine	1.5–5 mcg/mL	12–24 hours after start of infusion
lithium trough	0.6–1.2 meq/l	Just prior to first morning dose
NAPA	10–30 mcg/mL	Just prior to next procainamide dose
phenobarbital trough	15–40 mcg/mL	Just prior to next dose
phenytoin trough	10–20 mcg/mL	Just prior to next dose
primidone trough	5–12 mcg/mL	Just prior to next dose
procainamide	4–10 mcg/mL	Just prior to next dose
quinidine	2–5 mcg/mL	Just prior to next dose
theophylline	5–15 mcg/mL	8–12 hours after once daily dose
tobramycin peak	5–10 mcg/mL	30 minutes after infusion
tobramycin trough	<2 mcg/mL	Just prior to next dose
valproate trough (epilepsy)	50–100 mcg/mL	Just prior to next dose
valproate trough (mania)	45–125 mcg/mL	Just prior to next dose
vancomycin trough[1]	10–20 mg/L	Just prior to next dose
zonisamide[2]	10–40 mcg/mL	Just prior to dose

[1]Maintain trough >10 mg/L to avoid resistance; optimal trough for complicated infections is 15–20 mg/L
[2]Ranges not firmly established but supported by clinical trial results

PEDIATRIC DRUGS		Age	2mo	4mo	6mo	9mo	12mo	15mo	2yo	3yo	5yo
		Kg	5	6½	8	9	10	11	13	15	19
		lbs	11	15	17	20	22	24	28	33	42
med	***strength***	***freq***	***teaspoons of liquid per dose*** *(1 tsp = 5 mL)*								
Tylenol (mg)		q4h	80	80	120	120	160	160	200	240	280
Tylenol (tsp)	160/t	q4h	½	½	¾	¾	1	1	1¼	1½	1¾
ibuprofen (mg)		q6h	--	--	75†	75†	100	100	125	150	175
ibuprofen (tsp)	100/t	q6h	--	--	¾t	¾t	1	1	1¼	1½	1¾
amoxicillin or	125/t	bid	1	1¼	1½	1¾	1¾	2	2¼	2¾	3½
Augmentin	200/t	bid	½	¾	1	1	1¼	1¼	1½	1¾	2¼
(not otitis media)	250/t	bid	½	½	¾	¾	1	1	1¼	1¼	1¾
	400/t	bid	¼	½	½	½	¾	¾	¾	1	1
amoxicillin,	200/t	bid	1	1¼	1¾	2	2	2¼	2¾	3	4
(otitis media)‡	250/t	bid	¾	1¼	1½	1½	1¾	1¾	2¼	2½	3¼
	400/t	bid	½	¾	¾	1	1	1¼	1½	1½	2
Augmentin ES‡	600/t	bid	?	½	½	¾	¾	¾	1	1¼	1½
azithromycin*§	100/t	qd	¼†	½†	½	½	½	½	¾	¾	1
(5-day Rx)	200/t	qd	--	¼†	¼	¼	¼	¼	½	½	½
Bactrim/Septra	---	bid	½	¾	1	1	1	1¼	1½	1½	2
cefaclor*	125/t	bid	1	1	1¼	1½	1½	1¾	2	2½	3
"	250/t	bid	½	½	¾	¾	¾	1	1	1¼	1½
cefadroxil	125/t	bid	½	¾	1	1	1¼	1¼	1½	1¾	2¼
"	250/t	bid	¼	½	½	½	¾	¾	¾	1	1
cefdinir	125/t	qd	--	¾†	1	1	1	1¼	1½	1¾	2
Cefixime	100/t	qd	½	½	¾	¾	¾	1	1	1¼	1½
cefprozil*	125/t	bid	--	¾†	1	1	1¼	1½	1½	2	2¼
"	250/t	bid	--	½†	½	½	¾	¾	¾	1	1¼
cefuroxime	125/t	bid	--	¾	¾	1	1	1	1½	1¾	2¼
cephalexin	125/t	qid	--	½	¾	¾	1	1	1¼	1½	1¾
"	250/t	qid	--	¼	¼	½	½	½	¾	¾	1
clarithromycin	125/t	bid	½†	½	½	½	¾	¾	¾	1	1¼
"	250/t	bid	--	--	--	¼	½	½	½	½	¾
dicloxacillin	62½/t	qid	½	¾	1	1	1¼	1¼	1½	1¾	2
nitrofurantoin	25/t	qid	¼	½	½	½	½	¾	¾	¾	1
Pediazole	---	tid	½	½	¾	¾	1	1	1	1¼	1½
penicillin V**	250/t	bid-tid	--	1	1	1	1	1	1	1	1
cetirizine	5/t	qd	--	--	½	½	½	½	½	½	½
Benadryl	12.5/t	q6h	½	½	¾	¾	1	1	1¼	1½	2
prednisolone	15/t	qd	¼	½	½	¾	¾	¾	1	1	1¼
prednisone	5/t	qd	1	1¼	1½	1¾	2	2¼	2½	3	3¾
Robitussin	---	q4h	--	--	¼†	¼†	½	½	¾	¾	1
Tylenol w/ codeine		q4h	--	--	--	--	--	--	--	1	1

* Dose shown is for otitis media only; see dosing in text for alternative indications.

† Dosing at this age/weight not recommended by manufacturer.

‡ AAP now recommends high dose (80-90 mg/kg/d) for all otitis media in children; with Augmentin used as ES only.

§ Give a double dose of azithromycin the first day.

**AHA dosing for streptococcal pharyngitis. Treat for 10 days.

tsp/t = teaspoon; q = every; h = hour; kg = kilogram; Lbs = pounds; ml = mililiter; bid = two times per day; qd = every day; qid = four times per day; tid = three times per day

PEDIATRIC VITAL SIGNS AND INTRAVENOUS DRUGS												
Age		Pre-matr	New-born	2m	4m	6m	9m	12m	15m	2y	3y	5y
Weight	(kg)	2	3½	5	6½	8	9	10	11	13	15	19
	(lbs)	4¼	7½	11	15	17	20	22	24	28	33	42
Maint fluids	(mL/h)	8	14	20	26	32	36	40	42	46	50	58
ET tube	(mm)	2½	3/3½	3½	3½	3½	4	4	4½	4½	4½	5
Defib	(Joules)	4	7	10	13	16	18	20	22	26	30	38
Systolic BP	(high)	70	80	85	90	95	100	103	104	106	109	114
	(low)	40	60	70	70	70	70	70	70	75	75	80
Pulse rate	(high)	145	145	180	180	180	160	160	160	150	150	135
	(low)	100	100	110	110	110	100	100	100	90	90	65
Resp rate	(high)	60	60	50	50	50	46	46	30	30	25	25
	(low)	35	30	30	30	24	24	20	20	20	20	20
adenosine	(mg)	0.2	0.3	0.5	0.6	0.8	0.9	1	1.1	1.3	1.5	1.9
atropine	(mg)	0.1	0.1	0.1	0.13	0.16	0.18	0.2	0.22	0.26	0.30	0.38
Benadryl	(mg)	-	-	5	6½	8	9	10	11	13	15	19
bicarbonate	(meq)	2	3½	5	6½	8	9	10	11	13	15	19
dextrose	(g)	1	2	5	6½	8	9	10	11	13	15	19
epinephrine	(mg)	.02	.04	.05	.07	.08	.09	0.1	0.11	0.13	0.15	0.19
lidocaine	(mg)	2	3½	5	6½	8	9	10	11	13	15	19
morphine	(mg)	0.2	0.3	0.5	0.6	0.8	0.9	1	1.1	1.3	1.5	1.9
mannitol	(g)	2	3½	5	6½	8	9	10	11	13	15	19
naloxone	(mg)	.02	.04	.05	.07	.08	.09	0.1	0.11	0.13	0.15	0.19
diazepam	(mg)	0.6	1	1.5	2	2.5	2.7	3	3.3	3.9	4.5	5
fosphenytoin*	(PE)	40	70	100	130	160	180	200	220	260	300	380
lorazepam	(mg)	0.1	0.2	0.3	0.35	0.4	0.5	0.5	0.6	0.7	0.8	1.0
phenobarb	(mg)	30	60	75	100	125	125	150	175	200	225	275
phenytoin*	(mg)	40	70	100	130	160	180	200	220	260	300	380
ampicillin	(mg)	100	175	250	325	400	450	500	550	650	750	1000
ceftriaxone	(mg)	-	-	250	325	400	450	500	550	650	750	1000
cefotaxime	(mg)	100	175	250	325	400	450	500	550	650	750	1000
gentamicin	(mg)	5	8	12	16	20	22	25	27	32	37	47

*Loading doses; fosphenytoin dosed in "phenytoin equivalents."

CONVERSIONS	Liquid:	Weight:
Temperature:	1 fluid ounce = 30 mL	1 kilogram = 2.2 lbs
F = (1.8) C + 32	1 teaspoon = 5 mL	1 ounce = 30 g
C = (F − 32)/1.8	1 tablespoon = 15 mL	1 grain = 65 mg

INHIBITORS, INDUCERS, AND SUBSTRATES OF CYTOCHROME P450 ISOZYMES

The cytochrome P450 (CYP) inhibitors and inducers below do not necessarily cause clinically important interactions with substrates listed. We exclude *in vitro* data which can be inaccurate. Refer to other resources for more information if an interaction is suspected based on this chart. A drug that inhibits CYP subfamily activity can block the metabolism of substrates by that enzyme, which can lead to substrate accumulation and toxicity. CYP inhibitors are classified by how much they increase the area-under-the-curve (AUC) of a substrate: weak (1.25- to 2-fold), moderate (2- to 5-fold), or strong (≥5 fold). A drug that induces CYP subfamily activity increases substrate metabolism, which can lead to reduced substrate efficacy. CYP inducers are classified by how much they decrease the AUC of a substrate: weak (20 to 50%), moderate (50 to 80%) and strong (>80%). A drug is considered a sensitive substrate if a CYP inhibitor increases the AUC of that drug by ≥ 5-fold. While AUC increases of >50% often do not affect patient response, smaller increases can be important if the drug has a narrow therapeutic range (eg, theophylline, warfarin, cyclosporine). This table may be incomplete since new evidence about drug metabolism is continually being identified.

CYP1A2

Inhibitors. *Strong*: ciprofloxacin, fluvoxamine. ***Moderate:*** methoxalan, mexiletine, oral contraceptives, vemurafenib, zileuton. ***Weak:*** acyclovir, allopurinol, caffeine, cimetidine, deferasirox, disulfiram, echinacea, famotidine, propafenone, propranolol, simeprevir, terbinafine, ticlopidine, verapamil. ***Unclassified:*** amiodarone, atazanavir, citalopram, clarithromycin, estradiol, isoniazid, peginterferon alfa-2a and 2b.

Inducers. *Moderate:* montelukast, phenytoin, smoking. ***Weak:*** omeprazole, phenobarbital. ***Unclassified:*** carbamazepine, charcoal-broiled foods, rifampin, ritonavir, tipranavir-ritonavir.

Substrates. *Sensitive:* caffeine, duloxetine, melatonin, ramelteon, tizanidine. ***Unclassified:*** cetaminophen, amitriptyline, asenapine, bendamustine, cinacalcet, clomipramine, clozapine, cyclobenzaprine, erlotinib, estradiol, fluvoxamine, haloperidol, imipramine, loxapine, mexiletine, mirtazapine, naproxen, olanzapine, ondansetron, pomalidomide, propranolol, rasagiline, riluzole, roflumilast, ropinirole, ropivacaine, R-warfarin, tasimelteon, theophylline, zileuton, zolmitriptan.

CYP2B6

Inhibitors. *Weak:* clopidogrel, prasugrel. ***Unclassified:*** voriconazole.

Inducers. *Moderate:* efavirenz, rifampin. ***Weak:*** isavuconazole, nevirapine, artemether (in *Coartem*). ***Unclassified:*** baicalin (in *Limbrel*), ritonavir.

Substrates. *Sensitive:* bupropion, efavirenz. ***Unclassified:*** cyclophosphamide, ketamine, meperidine, methadone, nevirapine, prasugrel, propofol.

CYP2C8

Inhibitors. *Strong:* clopidogrel, gemfibrozil. ***Moderate:*** deferasirox. ***Weak:*** atazanavir, fluvoxamine, ketoconazole, pazopanib, trimethoprim.

Inducers. *Moderate:* rifampin. ***Unclassified:*** barbiturates, carbamazepine, rifabutin, ritonavir.

Substrates. *Sensitive:* repaglinide. ***Unclassified:*** amiodarone, carbamazepine, dabrafenib, dasabuvir (in *Viekira Pak, Viekira XR*), enzalutamide, iibuprofen, imatinib, isotretinoin, loperamide, montelukast, paclitaxel, pioglitazone, rosiglitazone, selexipag, treprostanil.

(cont.)

INHIBITORS, INDUCERS, AND SUBSTRATES OF CYTOCHROME P450 ISOZYMES (*continued*)

CYP2C9

Inhibitors. *Moderate:* amiodarone, fluconazole, miconazole, oxandrolone. *Weak:* capecitabine, cotrimoxazole, etravirine, fluvastatin, fluvoxamine, metronidazole, oritavancin, tigecycline, voriconazole, zafirlukast. *Unclassified:* cimetidine, fenofibrate, fenofibric acid, fluorouracil, imatinib, isoniazid, leflunomide, ritonavir.

Inducers. *Moderate:* carbamazepine, enzalutamide, rifampin. *Weak:* aprepitant, bosentan, elvitegravir, phenobarbital, St John's wort. *Unclassified:* dabrafenib, rifapentine, ritonavir.

Substrates. *Sensitive:* celecoxib. *Unclassified:* azilsartan, bosentan, chlorpropamide, diclofenac, etravirine, fluoxetine, flurbiprofen, fluvastatin, formoterol, glimepiride, glipizide, glyburide, ibuprofen, irbesartan, lesinurad, losartan, mefenamic acid, meloxicam, montelukast, naproxen, nateglinide, ospemifene, phenytoin, piroxicam, ramelteon, ruxolitinib, sildenafil, tolbutamide, torsemide, vardenafil, voriconazole, S-warfarin, zafirlukast, zileuton.

CYP2C19

Inhibitors. *Strong:* fluconazole, fluvoxamine. *Moderate:* esomeprazole, fluoxetine, moclobemide, omeprazole, voriconazole. *Weak:* armodafinil, carbamazepine, cimetidine, etravirine, felbamate, human growth hormone, ketoconazole, oral contraceptives, oritavancin. *Unclassified* : chloramphenicol, eslicarbazepine, isoniazid, modafinil, oxcarbazepine.

Inducers. *Moderate:* enzalutamide, rifampin. *Unclassified:* efavirenz, ritonavir, St John's wort, tipranavir.

Substrates. *Sensitive:* lansoprazole, omeprazole. *Unclassified:* amitriptyline, bortezomib, brivaracetam, carisoprodol, cilostazol, citalopram, clobazam, clomipramine, clopidogrel, clozapine, cyclophosphamide, desipramine, dexlansoprazole, diazepam, escitalopram, esomeprazole, etravirine, flibanserin, formoterol, imipramine, lacosamide, methadone, moclobamide, nelfinavir, pantoprazole, phenytoin, progesterone, proguanil, propranolol, rabeprazole, sertraline, tofacitinib, voriconazole, R-warfarin.

CYP2D6

Inhibitors. *Strong:* bupropion, fluoxetine, paroxetine, quinidine. *Moderate:* cinacalcet, dronedarone, duloxetine, mirabegron, rolapitant, terbinafine. *Weak:* amiodarone, asenapine, celecoxib, cimetidine, desvenlafaxine, diltiazem, diphenhydramine, echinacea, escitalopram, febuxostat, gefitinib, hydralazine, hydroxychloroquine, imitinib, methadone, oral contraceptives, pazopanib, propafenone, ranitidine, ritonavir, sertraline, telithromycin, venlafaxine, vemurafenib, verapamil. *Unclassified:* abiraterone, chloroquine, clobazam, clomipramine, cobicistat, darunavir-ritonavir, fluphenazine, haloperidol, lorcaserin, lumefantrine (in *Coartem*), metoclopramide, moclobamide, panobinostat, peginterferon alfa-2b, perphenazine, quinine, ranolazine, thioridazine, tipranavir-ritonavir.

Inducers. None known.

Substrates. *Sensitive:* atomoxetine, desipramine, dextromethorphan, metoprolol, nebivolol, perphenazine, tolterodine, venlafaxine. *Unclassified:* amitriptyline, aripiprazole, brexpiprazole, carvedilol, cevimeline, chlorpheniramine, chlorpromazine, clozapine, cinacalcet, clomipramine, codeine*, darifenacin, dihydrocodeine, dolasetron, donepezil, doxepin, duloxetine, fesoterodine, flecainide, fluoxetine, formoterol, galantamine, haloperidol, hydrocodone, iloperidone, imipramine, loratadine, loxapine, maprotiline, methadone, methamphetamine, metoclopramide, meclizine, mexiletine, mirtazapine, morphine,

INHIBITORS, INDUCERS, AND SUBSTRATES OF CYTOCHROME P450 ISOZYMES (*continued*)

nortriptyline, ondansetron, paroxetine, pimozide, primaquine, promethazine, propafenone, propranolol, quetiapine, risperidone, ritonavir, tamoxifen, tamsulosin, tetrabenazine, thioridazine, timolol, tramadol*, trazodone, trimipramine, vortioxetine.

* Metabolism by CYP2D6 required to convert to active analgesic metabolite; analgesia may be impaired by CYP2D6 inhibitors.

CYP3A4

Inhibitors. Strong: clarithromycin, cobicistat, conivaptan, indinavir, itraconazole, ketoconazole, lopinavir-ritonavir, nefazodone, nelfinavir, posaconazole, ritonavir, saquinavir, telithromycin, voriconazole. **Moderate:** aprepitant, atazanavir, ciprofloxacin, crizotinib, darunavir-ritonavir, diltiazem, dronedarone, erythromycin, fluconazole, fosamprenavir, grapefruit juice (variable), imatinib, isavuconazole, netupitant (in *Akynzeo*), verapamil. **Weak:** alprazolam, amiodarone, amlodipine, atorvastatin, bicalutamide, cilostazol, cimetidine, cyclosporine, everolimus, fluoxetine, fluvoxamine, ginko, goldenseal, isoniazid, ivacaftor, lapatinib, lomitapide, nilotinib, oral contraceptives, pazopanib, ranitidine, ranolazine, simeprevir, ticagrelor, tipranavir-ritonavir, zileuton. **Unclassified:** danazol, miconazole, palbociclib, quinine, quinupristin-dalfopristin, sertraline.

Inducers. Strong: carbamazepine, enzalutamide, lumacaftor (in *Orkambi*),mitotane, phenytoin, rifampin, rifapentine, St Johns wort. **Moderate:** bosentan, efavirenz, etravirine, modafinil, nafcillin. **Weak:** aprepitant, armodafinil, clobazam, echinacea, fosamprenavir, lesinurad, oritavancin, pioglitazone, rufinamide. **Unclassified:** artemether (in *Coartem*), barbiturates, bexarotene, dabrafenib, dexamethasone, eslicarbazepine, ethosuximide, griseovulvin, nevirapine, oxcarbazepine, primidone, rifabutin, ritonavir, tocilizumab, vemurafenib.

Substrates. Sensitive: alfentanil, aprepitant, budesonide, buspirone, conivaptan, darifenacin, darunavir, dasatinib, dronedarone, eletriptan, eplerenone, everolimus, felodipine, fluticasone, ibrutinib, indinavir, isavuconazole, ivacaftor, lomitapide, lopinavir (in *Kaletra*), lovastatin, lurasidone, maraviroc, midazolam, nisoldipine, quetiapine, saquinavir, sildenafil, simvastatin, sirolimus, tipranavir, tolvaptan, triazolam, vardenafil. **Unclassified:** alfuzosin, aliskiren, almotriptan, alprazolam, amiodarone, amlodipine, apixaban, apremilast, aripiprazole, armodafinil, artemether (in *Coartem*), atazanavir, atorvastatin, avanafil, axitinib, bedaquiline, bortezomib, bosentan, bosutinib, brentuximab, brexpiprazole, bromocriptine, buprenorphine, cabazitaxel, cabozantinib, carbamazepine, cariprazine, carbamazepine, ceritinib, cevimeline, cilostazol, cinacalcet, cisapride, citalopram, clarithromycin, clobazam, clomipramine, clonazepam, lopidogrel, clozapine, cobicistat, colchicine, corticosteroids, crizotinib, cyclophosphamide, cyclosporine, dabrafenib, daclatasvir, dapsone, desogestrel, desvenlafaxine, dexamethasone, dexlansoprazole, diazepam, dihydroergotamine, diltiazem, disopyramide, docetaxel, dofetilide, dolasetron, domperidone, donepezil, doxorubicin, dutasteride, efavirenz, elbasvir (in *Zepatier*), elvitegravir, enzalutamide, ergotamine, erlotinib, erythromycin, escitalopram, esomeprazole, eszopiclone, ethinyl estradiol, ethosuximide, etoposide, etravirine, exemestane, fentanyl, fesoterodine, finasteride, flibanserin, fosamprenavir, fosaprepitant, galantamine, gefitinib, grazoprevir (in *Zepatier*) guanfacine, haloperidol, hydrocodone, ifosfamide, iloperidone, imatinib, imipramine, irinotecan, isradipine, itraconazole, ivacaftor, ivadrabine, ixabepilone, ketamine, ketoconazole, lansoprazole, lapatinib, letrozole, levonorgestrel, lidocaine, loratadine, loxapine, lumefantrine (in *Coartem*), macitentan, methylergonovine, mifepristone, mirtazapine, odafinil,mometasone, naloxegol, nateglinide, nefazodone, nelfinavir, netupitant (in *Akynzeo*), nevirapine, nicardipine, nifedipine, nilotinib, nimodipine, nintedanib (minor), olaparib, ondansetron, ospemifene, oxybutynin, oxycodone, paclitaxel, panobinostat, pantoprazole, paritaprevir (in *Viekira Pak, Viekira XR*), palbociclib, paricalcitol, pazopanib, pimozide, pioglitazone, pomalidomide, ponatinib, prasugrel, praziquantel quinidine, quinine,

INHIBITORS, INDUCERS, AND SUBSTRATES OF CYTOCHROME P450 ISOZYMES *(continued)*

rabeprazole, ramelteon, ranolazine, regorafenib, repaglinide, rifabutin, rifampin, riociguat, ritonavir, rivaroxaban, roflumilast, romidepsin, ruxolitinib, saxagliptin, sertraline, silodosin, solifenacin, sonidegib, sufentanil, sunitinib, tacrolimus, tadalafil, tamoxifen, tamsulosin, tasimelteon, telithromycin, temsirolimus, testosterone, tiagabine, ticagrelor, tinidazole, tofacitinib, tolterodine, tramadol, trazodone, venetoclax, verapamil, vilazodone, vinblastine, vincristine, vinorelbine, vorapaxar, voriconazole, R-warfarin, zaleplon, ziprasidone, zolpidem, zonisamide.

INHIBITORS, INDUCERS, AND SUBSTRATES OF P-GLYCOPROTEIN

INHIBITORS, INDUCERS, AND SUBSTRATES OF P-GLYCOPROTEIN

The p-glycoprotein (P-gp) inhibitors and inducers listed below do not necessarily cause clinically important interactions with P-gp substrates. We attempt to exclude in vitro data which can be inaccurate. Refer to other resources for more information if an interaction is suspected based on this chart. P-gp is an efflux transporter that pumps drugs out of cells. In the gut, P-gp reduces drug absorption by pumping drugs into the gut lumen. In the kidney, it increases drug excretion by pumping drugs into urine. P-gp inhibitors can increase exposure to P-gp substrates, potentially increasing their risk of toxicity. P-gp inducers can reduce exposure to P-gp substrates, potentially increasing the risk of treatment failure. Some drugs are dual inhibitors of P-gp and CYP3A4 (e.g., clarithromycin, dronedarone, erythromycin, itraconazole, ketoconazole, verapamil), while others are dual inducers of P-gp and CYP3A4 (e.g., carbamazepine, phenytoin, rifampin, St John's wort). Potent P-gp inhibitors are defined here as drugs that increase the area-under-the-curve (AUC) of a P-gp substrate (digoxin or fexofenadine) by ≥1.5-fold. This table may be incomplete since new evidence about drug interactions is continually being indentified.

Inhibitors. *Potent:* amiodarone, clarithromycin, cyclosporine, dronedarone, itraconazole, lapatinib, lopinavir-ritonavir, ranolazine, ritonavir, verapamil. ***Unclassified:*** atorvastatin, azithromycin, captopril, carvedilol, cobicistat, conivaptan, darunavir-ritonavir, diltiazem, dipyridamole, erythromycin, etravirine, everolimus, felodipine, indinavir, isavuconazole, isradipine, ketoconazole, ledipasvir, lomitapide, naproxen, nifedipine, nilotinib, posaconazole, quinidine, saquinavir-ritonavir, simeprevir, telmisartan, ticagrelor.

Inducers: carbamazepine, fosamprenavir, phenytoin, rifampin, St John's wort, tipranavir-ritonavir*. *Tipranavir induces CYP3A4 and P-gp, while ritonavir inhibits both pathways. This makes it difficult to predict the effect of ritonavir-boosted tipranavir on substrates of P-gp.

Substrates: afatinib, aliskiren, ambrisentan, apixaban, boceprevir, ceritinib, clobazam, clopidogrel, colchicine, cyclosporine, dabigatran, dasabuvir (in Viekira Pak), digoxin, diltiazem, docetaxel, dolutegravir, edoxaban, etoposide, everolimus, fexofenadine, fosamprenavir, imatinib, indinavir, lapatinib, ledipasvir (in Harvoni), linagliptin, loperamide, lovastatin, maraviroc, morphine, nadolol, nilotinib, nintedanib, ombitasvir (in Viekira Pak), paclitaxel, paliperidone, paritaprevir (in Viekira Pak), pomalidomide, posaconazole, pravastatin, propranolol, quinidine, ranolazine, rifaximin, ritonavir, rivaroxaban, romidepsin, saquinavir, saxagliptin, silodosin, simeprevir, sirolimus, sitagliptin, sofosbuvir, tacrolimus, tenofovir, tolvaptan, topotecan, vinblastine, vincristine.

CORONARY ARTERY DISEASE 10-YEAR RISK

Framingham model for calculating 10–year risk for coronary artery disease (CAD) in patients without diabetes or clinically evident CAD. Diabetes is considered a CAD risk "equivalent", i.e., the prospective risk of CAD in diabetics is similar to those with established CAD. Automated calculator available at: http://hin.nhlbi.nih.gov/atpiii/calculator.asp?usertype=prof (NCEP, JAMA 2001; 285:2497)

MEN

Age	Points	Age	Points
20–34	-9	55–59	8
35–39	-4	60–64	10
40–44	0	65–69	11
45–49	3	70–74	12
50–54	6	75–79	13

Choles-terol*	Age (years)				
	20–39	40–49	50–59	60–69	70–79
<160	0	0	0	0	0
160–199	4	3	2	1	0
200–239	7	5	3	1	0
240–279	9	6	4	2	1
280+	11	8	5	3	1

Age (years)	20–39	40–49	50–59	60–69	70–79
Nonsmoker	0	0	0	0	0
Smoker	8	5	3	1	1

HDLmg/dL	Points	HDLmg/dL	Points
60+	-1	40–49	1
50–59	0	<40	2

Systolic BP	If Untreated	If Treated
<120mmHg	0	0
120–129 mmHg	0	1
130–139 mmHg	1	2
140–159 mmHg	1	2
160+ mmHg	2	3

Point Total	10–Year Risk	Point Total	10–Year Risk
0	1%	9	5%
1	1%	10	6%
2	1%	11	8%
3	1%	12	10%
4	1%	13	12%
5	2%	14	16%
6	2%	15	20%
7	3%	16	25%
8	4%	17+	30+%

WOMEN

Age	Points	Age	Points
20–34	-7	55–59	8
35–39	-3	60–64	10
40–44	0	65–69	12
45–49	3	70–74	14
50–54	6	75–79	16

Choles-terol*	Age (years)				
	20–39	40–49	50–59	60–69	70–79
<160	0	0	0	0	0
160–199	4	3	2	1	1
200–239	8	6	4	2	1
240–279	11	8	5	3	2
280+	13	10	7	4	2

*Total in mg/dL

Age (years)	20–39	40–49	50–59	60–69	70–79
Nonsmoker	0	0	0	0	0
Smoker	9	7	4	2	1

HDLmg/dL	Points	HDLmg/dL	Points
60+	-1	40–49	1
50–59	0	<40	2

Systolic BP	If Untreated	If Treated
<120 mmHg	0	0
120–129 mmHg	1	3
130–139 mmHg	2	4
140–159 mmHg	3	5
160+ mmHg	4	6

Point Total	10–Year Risk	Point Total	10–Year Risk
<9	<1%	17	5%
9	1%	18	6%
10	1%	19	8%
11	1%	20	11%
12	1%	21	14%
13	2%	22	17%
14	2%	23	22%
15	3%	24	27%
16	4%	25+	30+%

DRUG THERAPY REFERENCE WEBSITES (selected)

Professional societies or governmental agencies with drug therapy guidelines		
AAP	American Academy of Pediatrics	www.aap.org
ACC	American College of Cardiology	www.acc.org
ACCP	American College of Chest Physicians	www.chestnet.org
ACCP	American College of Clinical Pharmacy	www.accp.com
ADA	American Diabetes Association	www.diabetes.org
AHA	American Heart Association	www.heart.org
AHRQ	Agency for Healthcare Research and Quality	www.ahcpr.gov
AIDSinfo	HIV Treatment, Prevention, and Research	www.aidsinfo.nih.gov
AMA	American Medical Association	www.ama-assn.org
APA	American Psychiatric Association	www.psych.org
APA	American Psychological Association	www.apa.org
ASHP	Amer. Society Health-Systems Pharmacists Drug Shortages Resource Center	www.ashp.org/shortages
ATS	American Thoracic Society	www.thoracic.org
CDC	Centers for Disease Control and Prevention	www.cdc.gov
CDC	CDC bioterrorism and radiation exposures	www.bt.cdc.gov
IDSA	Infectious Diseases Society of America	www.idsociety.org
MHA	Malignant Hyperthermia Association	www.mhaus.org

Other therapy reference sites	
Cochrane library	www.cochrane.org
Emergency Contraception Website	www.not-2-late.com
Immunization Action Coalition	www.immunize.org
QTDrug lists	www.crediblemeds.org/
Managing Contraception	www.managingcontraception.com

ANALGESICS

OPIOID EQUIVALENCY[*]

Opioid	PO	IV/SC/IM	Opioid	PO	IV/SC/IM
buprenorphine	n/a	0.3–0.4 mg	meperidine	300 mg	75 mg
butorphanol	n/a	2 mg	methadone	5–15 mg	2.5–10 mg
codeine	130 mg	75 mg	morphine	30 mg	10 mg
fentanyl	?	0.1 mg	nalbuphine	n/a	10 mg
hydrocodone	20 mg	n/a	oxycodone	20 mg	n/a
hydromorphone	7.5 mg	1.5 mg	oxymorphone	10 mg	1 mg
levorphanol	4 mg	2 mg	pentazocine	50 mg	30 mg

[*]Approximate equianalgesic doses as adapted from the 2003 American Pain Society (www.ampainsoc.org) guidelines and the 1992 AHCPR guidelines. n/a = not available. See drug entries themselves for starting doses. Many recommend initially using lower than equivalent doses when switching between different opiods. IV doses should be titrated slowly with appropriate monitoring. All PO doing is with immediate-release preparations. Individualize all dosing, especially in the elderly, children, and in those with chronic pain, opioid naïve, or hepatic/renal insufficiency.

ANALGESICS: Muscle Relaxants

NOTE: May cause drowsiness and/or sedation, which may be enhanced by alcohol and other CNS depressants.

BACLOFEN (✱Lioresal, Lioresal D.S.) ▶K ♀C ▶+ $
  WARNING — Abrupt discontinuation of intrathecal baclofen has been associated with life-threatening sequelae and/or death.
  ADULT — Spasticity related to MS or spinal cord disease/injury: 5 mg PO three times per day for 3 days, 10 mg PO three times per day for 3 days, 15 mg PO three times per day for 3 days, then 20 mg PO three times per day for 3 days. Max dose: 20 mg PO four times per day. Spasticity related to spinal cord disease/injury, unresponsive to oral therapy: Specialized dosing via implantable intrathecal pump.
  PEDS — Spasticity related to spinal cord disease/injury: Specialized dosing via implantable intrathecal pump.
  UNAPPROVED ADULT — Trigeminal neuralgia: 30 to 80 mg/day PO divided three to four times per day. Tardive dyskinesia: 40 to 60 mg/day PO divided three to four times per day. Intractable hiccups: 15 to 45 mg PO divided three times per day.
  UNAPPROVED PEDS — Spasticity age 2 yo or older: 10 to 15 mg/day PO divided q 8 h. Max doses 40 mg/day for age 2 to 7 yo, 60 mg/day for age 8 yo or older.
  FORMS — Generic only: Tabs 10, 20 mg.
  NOTES — Hallucinations and seizures with abrupt withdrawal. Administer with caution if impaired renal function. Efficacy not established for rheumatic disorders, CVA, cerebral palsy, or Parkinson's disease.
  MOA — Skeletal muscle relaxant.
  ADVERSE EFFECTS — Serious: Hallucinations and seizures with abrupt withdrawal. Frequent: Hypotonia, somnolence, dizziness.

CARISOPRODOL (Soma) ▶LK ♀? ▶– ©IV $
  ADULT — Acute musculoskeletal pain: 350 mg PO three to four times per day with meals and at bedtime.
  PEDS — Not approved in children.
  FORMS — Generic/Trade: Tabs 250, 350 mg.
  NOTES — Contraindicated in porphyria, caution in renal or hepatic insufficiency. Abuse potential. Use with caution if addiction-prone. Withdrawal and possible seizures with abrupt discontinuation. Sedative effects can result in impaired driving.
  MOA — Skeletal muscle relaxant.
  ADVERSE EFFECTS — Serious: Idiosyncratic reaction with angioedema, hypotension, and anaphylactoid shock. Frequent: Dizziness and drowsiness.

CHLORZOXAZONE (Parafon Forte DSC, Lorzone, Remular-S) ▶LK ♀C ▶? $
  WARNING — If signs/symptoms of liver dysfunction are observed, discontinue use.
  ADULT — Musculoskeletal pain: Start 500 mg PO three to four times per day, increase prn to 750 mg three to four times per day. After clinical improvement, decrease to 250 mg PO three to four times per day.
  PEDS — Not approved in children.

(cont.)

CHLORZOXAZONE (cont.)

UNAPPROVED PEDS — Musculoskeletal pain: 125 to 500 mg PO three to four times per day or 20 mg/kg/day divided three to four times per day depending on age and wt.

FORMS — Generic/Trade: Tabs 500 mg (Parafon Forte DSC 500 mg tabs, scored). Trade only: Tabs 250 mg (Remular-S), 375, 750 mg (Lorzone).

NOTES — Use with caution in patients with history of drug allergies. Discontinue if allergic drug reactions occur or for signs/symptoms of liver dysfunction. May turn urine orange or purple-red.

MOA — Skeletal muscle relaxant.

ADVERSE EFFECTS — Serious: Hypersensitivity, hepatotoxicity. Frequent: Dizziness and drowsiness.

CYCLOBENZAPRINE (*Amrix, Flexeril, Fexmid*) ▶LK ♀B ▶? $

ADULT — Musculoskeletal pain: 5 to 10 mg PO three times per day up to max dose of 30 mg/day or 15 to 30 mg (extended-release) PO daily. Not recommended in elderly or for use longer than 2 to 3 weeks.

PEDS — Not approved in children.

FORMS — Generic/Trade: Tabs 5, 7.5, 10 mg. Extended-release caps 15, 30 mg ($$$$$).

NOTES — Contraindicated with recent or concomitant MAOI use, immediately post MI, in patients with arrhythmias, conduction disturbances, heart failure, and hyperthyroidism. Not effective for cerebral or spinal cord disease or in children with cerebral palsy. May have similar adverse effects and drug interactions to TCAs. Caution with urinary retention, angle-closure glaucoma, increased intraocular pressure.

MOA — Skeletal muscle relaxant.

ADVERSE EFFECTS — Serious: Arrhythmia. Frequent: Drowsiness, dizziness, dry mouth, blurred vision.

DANTROLENE (*Dantrium, Revonto, Ryanodex*) ▶LK ♀C ▶– $$$$

WARNING — Hepatotoxicity, monitor LFTs. Use the lowest possible effective dose.

ADULT — Chronic spasticity related to spinal cord injury, CVA, cerebral palsy, MS: 25 mg PO daily to start, increase to 25 mg two to four times per day, then by 25 mg up to max of 100 mg two to four times per day if necessary. Maintain each dosage level for 4 to 7 days to determine response. Use the lowest possible effective dose. Malignant hyperthermia: 2.5 mg/kg rapid IV push q 5 to 10 min continuing until symptoms subside or to a max 10 mg/kg/dose (Dantrium, Revonto). Doses of up to 40 mg/kg have been used. Follow with 4 to 8 mg/kg/day PO divided three to four times per day for 1 to 3 days to prevent recurrence. Minimum of 1 mg/kg IV push with additional doses administered if necessary up to a total max dose of 10 mg/kg (Ryanodex). Prevention of malignant hyperthermia in patients at high risk: 2.5 mg/kg over a period of at least 1 min approximately 75 min before surgery (Ryanodex). Additional doses may be given if surgery is prolonged.

PEDS — Chronic spasticity: 0.5 mg/kg PO two times per day to start; increase to 0.5 mg/kg three to four times per day, then by increments of 0.5 mg/kg up to 3 mg/kg two to four times per day. Max dose 100 mg PO four times per day. Malignant hyperthermia: Use adult dose.

UNAPPROVED ADULT — Neuroleptic malignant syndrome, heat stroke: 1 to 3 mg/kg/day PO/IV divided four times per day.

FORMS — Generic/Trade: Caps 25, 50, 100 mg. Trade only: Vials 20 mg (Dantrium, Revonto), 250 mg (Ryanodex).

NOTES — Photosensitization may occur. Warfarin may decrease protein binding of dantrolene and increase dantrolene's effect. Hyperkalemia and cardiovascular collapse have been reported with concomitant calcium channel blockers such as verapamil. The following website may be useful for malignant hyperthermia: www.mhaus.org.

MOA — Skeletal muscle relaxant.

ADVERSE EFFECTS — Serious: Hepatotoxicity. Frequent: Drowsiness, dizziness and weakness.

METAXALONE (*Skelaxin*) ▶LK ♀? ▶? $$$$

ADULT — Musculoskeletal pain: 800 mg PO three to four times per day.

PEDS — Use adult dose for age older than 12 yo.

FORMS — Generic/Trade: Tabs 800 mg, scored. Generic only: Tabs 400 mg.

NOTES — Contraindicated in serious renal or hepatic insufficiency or history of drug-induced hemolytic or other anemia. Beware of hypersensitivity reactions, leukopenia, hemolytic anemia, and jaundice. Monitor LFTs. Coadministration with food, especially a high-fat meal, enhances absorption significantly and may increase CNS depression.

MOA — Skeletal muscle relaxant.

ADVERSE EFFECTS — Serious: Hypersensitivity, jaundice. Frequent: Drowsiness, dizziness, nausea.

METHOCARBAMOL (*Robaxin, Robaxin-750*) ▶LK ♀C ▶? $

ADULT — Musculoskeletal pain, acute relief: 1500 mg PO four times per day or 1000 mg IM/IV three times per day for 48 to 72 h. Maintenance: 1000 mg PO four times per day, 750 mg PO q 4 h, or 1500 mg PO three times per day. Tetanus: Specialized dosing.

PEDS — Tetanus: Specialized dosing.

FORMS — Generic/Trade: Tabs 500, 750 mg. OTC in Canada.

NOTES — Max IV rate of undiluted drug 3 mL/min to avoid syncope, hypotension, and bradycardia. Total parenteral dosage should not exceed 3 g/day for more than 3 consecutive days, except in the treatment of tetanus. Urine may turn brown, black, or green.

MOA — Skeletal muscle relaxant.

ADVERSE EFFECTS — Serious: Syncope, hypotension. Frequent: Drowsiness, dizziness, discolored urine (brown, black, green).

ORPHENADRINE (*Norflex*) ▶LK ♀C ▶? $$

ADULT — Musculoskeletal pain: 100 mg PO two times per day. 60 mg IV/IM two times per day.

(cont.)

ORPHENADRINE (*cont.*)

PEDS — Not approved in children.
UNAPPROVED ADULT — Leg cramps: 100 mg PO at bedtime.
FORMS — Generic only: 100 mg extended-release. OTC in Canada.
NOTES — Contraindicated in glaucoma, pyloric or duodenal obstruction, BPH, and myasthenia gravis. Some products contain sulfites, which may cause allergic reactions. May increase anticholinergic effects of amantadine and decrease therapeutic effects of phenothiazines. Side effects include dry mouth, urinary retention and hesitancy, constipation, headache, and GI upset.
MOA — Skeletal muscle relaxant.
ADVERSE EFFECTS — Serious: Hypersensitivity, syncope. Frequent: Dry mouth, dizziness, constipation.

TIZANIDINE (*Zanaflex*) ▶LK ♀C ▶? $$$$
ADULT — Muscle spasticity due to MS or spinal cord injury: 4 to 8 mg PO q 6 to 8 h prn, max dose 36 mg/day.
PEDS — Not approved in children.
FORMS — Generic/Trade: Tabs 4 mg, scored. Caps 2, 4, 6 mg. Generic only: Tabs 2 mg.
NOTES — Monitor LFTs. Avoid in hepatic or renal insufficiency. Alcohol, oral contraceptives, fluvoxamine, and ciprofloxacin increase tizanidine levels; may cause significant decreases in BP and increased drowsiness and psychomotor impairment. Concurrent antihypertensives may exacerbate hypotension. Dry mouth, somnolence, sedation, asthenia, and dizziness most common side effects.
MOA — Skeletal muscle relaxant.
ADVERSE EFFECTS — Serious: Hypotension, hepatotoxicity. Frequent: Dry mouth, somnolence, asthenia, and dizziness.

ANALGESICS: Non-Opioid Analgesic Combinations

NOTE: Refer to individual components for further information. Carisoprodol and butalbital may be habit-forming; butalbital contraindicated with porphyria. May cause drowsiness and/or sedation, which may be enhanced by alcohol and other CNS depressants. Avoid exceeding 4 g/day of acetaminophen in combination products. Caution people who drink 3 or more alcoholic drinks/day to limit acetaminophen use to 2.5 g/day due to additive liver toxicity.

ASCRIPTIN (acetylsalicylic acid + aluminum hydroxide + magnesium hydroxide + calcium carbonate) ▶ ♀D ▶? $
WARNING — Multiple strengths; see FORMS.
ADULT — Pain: 1 to 2 tabs PO q 4 h.
PEDS — Not approved in children.
FORMS — OTC Trade only: Tabs 325 mg aspirin/50 mg magnesium hydroxide/50 mg Al hydroxide/50 mg Ca carbonate (Ascriptin and Aspir-Mox). 500 mg aspirin/33 mg magnesium hydroxide/33 mg Al hydroxide/237 mg Ca carbonate (Ascriptin Maximum Strength).
NOTES — See NSAIDs—Salicylic Acid subclass warning.
MOA — Anti-inflammatory, analgesic.
ADVERSE EFFECTS — Serious: Hypersensitivity, Reye's syndrome, GI bleeding, nephrotoxicity. Frequent: Nausea, dyspepsia.

BUFFERIN (acetylsalicylic acid + calcium carbonate + magnesium oxide + magnesium carbonate) ▶K ♀ D ▶? $
ADULT — Pain: 1 to 2 tabs/caps PO q 4 h while symptoms persist. Max 12 in 24 h.
PEDS — Not approved in children.
FORMS — OTC Trade only: Tabs/caps 325 mg aspirin/158 mg Ca carbonate/63 mg of magnesium oxide/34 mg of magnesium carbonate. Bufferin ES: 500 mg aspirin/222.3 mg Ca carbonate/88.9 mg of magnesium oxide/55.6 mg of magnesium carbonate.
NOTES — See NSAIDs—Salicylic Acid subclass warning.

MOA — Anti-inflammatory, analgesic.
ADVERSE EFFECTS — Serious: Hypersensitivity, Reye's syndrome, GI bleeding, nephrotoxicity. Frequent: Nausea, dyspepsia.

ESGIC (acetaminophen + butalbital + caffeine) ▶LK ♀C ▶? $
WARNING — Multiple strengths; see FORMS and write specific product on Rx.
ADULT — Tension or muscle contraction headache: 1 to 2 tabs or caps PO q 4 h. Max 6 in 24 h.
PEDS — Not approved in children.
FORMS — Generic only: Tabs/caps, 325 mg acetaminophen/50 mg butalbital/40 mg caffeine. Oral soln 325/50/40 mg per 15 mL. Generic/Trade: Tabs (Esgic Plus) 500/50/40 mg.
MOA — Serious: Hepatotoxicity. Frequent: Drowsiness and dizziness.

EXCEDRIN MIGRAINE (acetaminophen + acetylsalicylic acid + caffeine) ▶LK ♀D ▶? $
ADULT — Migraine headache: 2 tabs/caps/geltabs PO q 6 h while symptoms persist. Max 8 in 24 h.
PEDS — Use adult dose for age 12 or older.
FORMS — OTC Generic/Trade: Tabs/caps/geltabs 250 mg acetaminophen/250 mg aspirin/65 mg caffeine.
NOTES — See NSAIDs—Salicylic Acid subclass warning. Avoid concomitant use of other acetaminophen-containing products.
MOA — Combination analgesic.
ADVERSE EFFECTS — Serious: Hepatotoxicity, hypersensitivity, Reye's syndrome, GI bleeding, nephrotoxicity. Frequent: Dyspepsia, nervousness, insomnia.

FIORICET (acetaminophen + butalbital + caffeine)
▶LK ♀C ▶? $
ADULT — Tension or muscle contraction headache: 1 to 2 tabs PO q 4 h. Max 6 in 24 h.
PEDS — Not approved in children.
FORMS — Generic/Trade: Tabs 325 mg acetaminophen/50 mg butalbital/40 mg caffeine.
MOA — Serious: Hepatotoxicity. Frequent: Drowsiness and dizziness.

GOODY'S EXTRA STRENGTH HEADACHE POWDER (acetaminophen + acetylsalicylic acid + caffeine) ▶LK ♀D ▶? $
ADULT — Headache: Place 1 powder on tongue and follow with liquid, or stir powder into a glass of water or other liquid. Repeat in 4 to 6 h prn. Max 4 powders in 24 h.
PEDS — Use adult dose for age 12 yo or older.
FORMS — OTC trade only: 260 mg acetaminophen/520 mg aspirin/32.5 mg caffeine per powder paper.
NOTES — See NSAIDs—Salicylic Acid subclass warning.
MOA — Combination analgesic.
ADVERSE EFFECTS — Serious: Hepatotoxicity, hypersensitivity, Reye's syndrome, GI bleeding, nephrotoxicity. Frequent: Dyspepsia.

NORGESIC (orphenadrine + acetylsalicylic acid + caffeine) ▶KL ♀D ▶? $$$
WARNING — Multiple strengths; see FORMS and write specific product on Rx.
ADULT — Musculoskeletal pain: Norgesic: 1 to 2 tabs PO three to four times per day. Norgesic Forte: 1 tab PO three to four times per day.
PEDS — Not approved in children.
FORMS — Generic only: Tabs 25 mg orphenadrine/385 mg aspirin/30 mg caffeine (Norgesic). Tabs 50/770/60 mg (Norgesic Forte).
NOTES — See NSAIDs—Salicylic Acid subclass warning.
MOA — Combination analgesic/muscle relaxant.
ADVERSE EFFECTS — Serious: Hypersensitivity, Reye's syndrome, GI bleeding, nephrotoxicity, syncope. Frequent: Dry mouth, dizziness, constipation.

PHRENILIN (acetaminophen + butalbital) ▶LK ♀C ▶? $
WARNING — Multiple strengths; see FORMS and write specific product on Rx.
ADULT — Tension or muscle contraction headache: Phrenilin: 1 to 2 tabs PO q 4 h. Phrenilin Forte: 1 cap PO q 4 h. Max 6 in 24 h.
PEDS — Not approved in children.
FORMS — Generic/Trade: Tabs 325 mg acetaminophen/50 mg butalbital (Phrenilin). Caps, 650/50 mg (Phrenilin Forte).
MOA — Serious: Hepatotoxicity. Frequent: Drowsiness and dizziness.

Sedapap (acetaminophen + butalbital) ▶LK ♀C ▶? $
ADULT — Tension or muscle contraction headache: 1 to 2 tabs PO q 4 h. Max 6 tabs in 24 h.
PEDS — Not approved in children.
FORMS — Generic only: Tabs 650 mg acetaminophen/50 mg butalbital.

MOA — Serious: Hepatotoxicity. Frequent: Drowsiness and dizziness.

SOMA COMPOUND (carisoprodol + acetylsalicylic acid) ▶LK ♀D ▶– ©IV $$$
ADULT — Musculoskeletal pain: 1 to 2 tabs PO four times per day.
PEDS — Not approved in children.
FORMS — Generic only: Tabs 200 mg carisoprodol/325 mg aspirin.
NOTES — See NSAIDs—Salicylic Acid subclass warning. Carisoprodol may be habit-forming. Withdrawal with abrupt discontinuation.
MOA — Combination analgesic/muscle relaxant.
ADVERSE EFFECTS — Serious: Hypersensitivity, Reye's syndrome, GI bleeding, nephrotoxicity. Idiosyncratic reaction with angioedema, hypotension and anaphylactoid shock. Frequent: Dizziness and drowsiness.

FIORINAL (acetylsalicylic acid + butalbital + caffeine, ✱ Tecnal, Trianal) ▶KL ♀D ▶– ©III $$
ADULT — Tension or muscle contraction headache: 1 to 2 tabs PO q 4 h. Max 6 tabs in 24 h.
PEDS — Not approved in children.
FORMS — Generic/Trade: Caps 325 mg aspirin/ 50 mg butalbital/40 mg caffeine.
NOTES — See NSAIDs—Salicylic Acid subclass warning.
MOA — Combination analgesic.
ADVERSE EFFECTS — Serious: Hypersensitivity, Reye's syndrome, GI bleeding, nephrotoxicity. Frequent: Drowsiness and dizziness.

ULTRACET (tramadol + acetaminophen, ✱ Tramacet) ▶KL ♀C ▶– ©IV $$
ADULT — Acute pain: 2 tabs PO q 4 to 6 h prn, (up to 8 tabs/day for no more than 5 days). If CrCl <30 mL/min, increase the dosing interval to 12 h. Consider a similar adjustment in elderly patients and in cirrhosis.
PEDS — Not approved in children.
FORMS — Generic/Trade: Tabs 37.5 mg tramadol/325 mg acetaminophen.
NOTES — Do not use with other acetaminophen-containing drugs due to potential for hepatotoxicity. Contraindicated in acute intoxication with alcohol, hypnotics, centrally acting analgesics, opioids, or psychotropic drugs. Seizures may occur with concurrent antidepressants or with seizure disorder. Use with great caution with MAOIs or in combination with SSRIs due to potential for serotonin syndrome; dose adjustment may be needed. Withdrawal symptoms may occur in patients dependent on opioids or with abrupt discontinuation. Overdose treated with naloxone may increase seizure risk. The most frequent side effects are somnolence and constipation.
MOA — Combination analgesic.
ADVERSE EFFECTS — Serious: Seizures, anaphylactoid reactions, hepatotoxicity. Frequent: Constipation, somnolence.

ANALGESICS: Non-Steroidal Anti-Inflammatories—COX-2 Inhibitors

NOTE: The risk of serious cardiovascular events and GI bleeding may be increased in patients taking long-term, high-dose NSAIDs, COX-2 inhibitors, and non-selective agents. All NSAIDs and COX-2 inhibitors are contraindicated immediately post-CABG surgery. The FDA advises evaluating alternative therapy or using the lowest effective dose of these drugs. Fewer GI side effects than 1st-generation NSAIDs and no effect on platelets, but other NSAID-related side effects (renal dysfunction, fluid retention, CNS) are possible. May cause fluid retention or exacerbate heart failure. May elevate BP or blunt effects of antihypertensives and loop diuretics. Not substitutes for aspirin for cardiovascular prophylaxis due to lack of antiplatelet effects. Monitor INR with warfarin. May increase lithium levels. Caution in aspirin-sensitive asthma. Use around the time of conception appears to increase the risk of miscarriage (use acetaminophen instead).

CELECOXIB (*Celebrex*) ▶L ♀C (D in 3rd trimester) ▶? $$$$$
WARNING — Increases the risk of serious cardiovascular events and GI bleeding. Contraindicated immediately post-CABG surgery.
ADULT — OA, ankylosing spondylitis: 200 mg PO daily or 100 mg PO two times per day. RA: 100 to 200 mg PO two times per day. Familial adenomatous polyposis (FAP), as an adjunct to usual care: 400 mg PO two times per day with food. Acute pain, dysmenorrhea: 400 mg once, then 200 mg PO two times per day. May take an additional 200 mg on day 1.

PEDS — JRA: Give 50 mg PO two times per day for age 2 to 17 yo and wt 10 to 25 kg, give 100 mg PO two times per day for wt greater than 25 kg.
FORMS — Generic/Trade: Caps 50, 100, 200, 400 mg.
NOTES — Contraindicated in sulfonamide allergy. Decrease dose by 50% in hepatic dysfunction. Caps may be opened and sprinkled into 1 teaspoon of applesauce and taken immediately with water. Drugs that inhibit CYP2C9, such as fluconazole, increase concentrations. Lithium concentrations increased.
MOA — Anti-inflammatory, analgesic.
ADVERSE EFFECTS — Serious: Nephrotoxicity, hepatotoxicity, SJS. Frequent: Fluid retention.

ANALGESICS: Non-Steroidal Anti-Inflammatories—Salicylic Acid Derivatives

NOTE: The risk of serious cardiovascular events and GI bleeding may be increased in patients taking long-term, high-dose NSAIDs, both COX-2 inhibitors as well as nonselective agents (excluding aspirin). All NSAIDs and COX-2 inhibitors are contraindicated immediately post-CABG surgery. The FDA advises evaluating alternative therapy or using the lowest effective dose of these drugs. Avoid in aspirin allergy and in children younger than 17 yo with chickenpox or flu due to association with Reye's syndrome. May potentiate warfarin, heparin, valproic acid, methotrexate. Unlike aspirin, derivatives may have less GI toxicity and negligible effects on platelet aggregation and renal prostaglandins. Caution in aspirin-sensitive asthma. Ibuprofen and possibly other NSAIDs may antagonize antiplatelet effects of aspirin if given simultaneously. Use around the time of conception appears to increase the risk of miscarriage (use acetaminophen instead).

ACETYLSALICYLIC ACID (*Ecotrin, Empirin, Halfprin, Bayer, Anacin, ZORprin, aspirin, ✱Asaphen, Entrophen, Novasen*) ▶K ♀D ▶? $
ADULT — Mild to moderate pain, fever: 325 to 650 mg PO/PR q 4 h prn. Acute rheumatic fever: 5 to 8 g/day, initially. RA/OA: 3.2 to 6 g/day in divided doses. Platelet aggregation inhibition: 81 to 325 mg PO daily.
PEDS — Mild to moderate pain, fever: 10 to 15 mg/kg/dose PO q 4 to 6 h not to exceed 60 to 80 mg/kg/day. JRA: 60 to 100 mg/kg/day PO divided q 6 to 8 h. Acute rheumatic fever: 100 mg/kg/day PO/PR for 2 weeks, then 75 mg/kg/day for 4 to 6 weeks. Kawasaki disease: 80 to 100 mg/kg/day divided four times per day PO/PR until fever resolves, then 3 to 5 mg/kg/day PO q am for 7 weeks or longer if there is ECG evidence of coronary artery abnormalities.
UNAPPROVED ADULT — Primary prevention of cardiovascular events (10-year CHD risk more than 6 to 10% based on Framingham risk scoring): 75 to 325 mg PO daily. Post ST-elevation MI: 162 to 325 mg PO on day 1, continue indefinitely at 75 to 162 mg/day. Post non-ST-elevation MI: 162 to 325 mg PO on day 1, continue indefinitely at 75 to 162 mg/day.

Long-term antithrombotic therapy for chronic A-fib/flutter in patients with low to moderate risk of CVA (age younger than 75 yo without risk factors): 325 mg PO daily. Percutaneous coronary intervention pretreatment: Already taking daily aspirin therapy: 75 to 325 mg PO before procedure. Not already taking daily aspirin therapy: 300 to 325 mg PO at least 2 to 24 h before procedure. Post-percutaneous coronary intervention: 325 mg daily in combination with clopidogrel for at least 1 month after bare metal stent placement, at least 3 to 6 months after drug-eluting stent placement; then 75 to 162 mg PO daily indefinitely. Post-percutaneous coronary brachytherapy: 75 to 325 mg daily in combination with clopidogrel indefinitely.
FORMS — Generic/Trade (OTC): Tabs 325, 500 mg; chewable 81 mg; enteric-coated 81, 162 mg (Halfprin), 81, 325, 500 mg (Ecotrin), 650, 975 mg. Trade only: Tabs, controlled-release 650, 800 mg (ZORprin, Rx). Generic only (OTC): Supps 60, 120, 200, 300, 600 mg.
NOTES — Consider discontinuation 1 week prior to surgery (except coronary bypass or in 1st year post-coronary stent implantation) because of the

(cont.)

ACETYLSALICYLIC ACID (cont.)

possibility of postop bleeding. Aspirin intolerance occurs in 4% to 19% of asthmatics. Use caution in liver damage, renal insufficiency, peptic ulcer, or bleeding tendencies. Crush or chew tabs (including enteric-coated products) in 1st dose with acute MI. Higher doses of aspirin (1.3 g/day) have not been shown to be superior to low doses in preventing TIAs and CVAs.

MOA — Anti-inflammatory, antipyretic, analgesic. Inhibits prostaglandin synthesis and platelet aggregation by inactivating the enzyme cyclooxygenase.

ADVERSE EFFECTS — Serious: Hypersensitivity, Reye's syndrome, GI bleeding, nephrotoxicity. Frequent: Nausea, dyspepsia, tinnitus (large doses), dizziness (large doses).

CHOLINE MAGNESIUM TRISALICYLATE (*Trilisate*) ▶K ♀C (D in 3rd trimester) ▶? $$

ADULT — RA/OA: 1500 mg PO two times per day. Mild to moderate pain, fever: 1000 to 1500 mg PO two times per day.

PEDS — RA, mild to moderate pain: 50 mg/kg/day (up to 37 kg) PO divided two times per day.

FORMS — Generic only: Tabs 500, 750, 1000 mg. Soln 500 mg/5 mL.

MOA — Serious: Hypersensitivity, Reye's syndrome, GI bleeding, nephrotoxicity. Frequent: Nausea, dyspepsia.

DIFLUNISAL (*Dolobid*) ▶K ♀C (D in 3rd trimester) ▶– $$$

ADULT — Mild to moderate pain: Initially, 500 mg to 1 g PO, then 250 to 500 mg PO q 8 to 12 h. RA/OA: 500 mg to 1 g PO divided two times per day. Max dose 1.5 g/day.

PEDS — Not approved in children.

FORMS — Generic only: Tabs 500 mg.

NOTES — Do not crush or chew tabs. Increases acetaminophen levels.

MOA — Anti-inflammatory, analgesic.

ADVERSE EFFECTS — Serious: Hypersensitivity, Reye's syndrome, GI bleeding, nephrotoxicity. Frequent: Nausea, dyspepsia.

SALSALATE (*Salflex, Disalcid, Amigesic*) ▶K ♀C (D in 3rd trimester) ▶? $$

ADULT — RA/OA: 3000 mg/day PO divided q 8 to 12 h.

PEDS — Not approved in children.

FORMS — Generic only: Tabs 500, 750 mg, scored.

MOA — Serious: Hypersensitivity, Reye's syndrome, GI bleeding, nephrotoxicity. Frequent: Nausea, dyspepsia.

ANALGESICS—NSAIDs

Salicylic acid derivatives	ASA, diflunisal, salsalate, Trilisate
Propionic acids	flurbiprofen, ibuprofen, ketoprofen, naproxen, oxaprozin
Acetic acids	diclofenac, etodolac, indomethacin, ketorolac, nabumetone, sulindac, tolmetin
Fenamates	meclofenamate
Oxicams	meloxicam, piroxicam
COX-2 inhibitors	celecoxib

Note: If one class fails, consider another.

ANALGESICS: Non-Steroidal Anti-Inflammatories—Other

NOTE: The risk of serious cardiovascular events and GI bleeding may be increased in patients taking long-term, high-dose NSAIDs, both COX-2 inhibitors as well as non-selective agents. All NSAIDs and COX-2 inhibitors are contraindicated immediately post-CABG surgery. The FDA advises evaluating alternative therapy or using the lowest effective dose of these drugs. Chronic use associated with renal insufficiency, gastritis, peptic ulcer disease, GI bleeds. Caution in liver disease. May cause fluid retention or exacerbate heart failure. May elevate BP or blunt effects of antihypertensives and loop diuretics. May increase levels of methotrexate, lithium, phenytoin, digoxin, and cyclosporine. May potentiate warfarin. Caution in aspirin-sensitive asthma. Ibuprofen or other NSAIDs may antagonize antiplatelet effects of aspirin if given simultaneously. Use around the time of conception appears to increase the risk of miscarriage (use acetaminophen instead).

ARTHROTEC (diclofenac + misoprostol) ▶LK ♀X ▶– $$$$$

WARNING — Because of the abortifacient property of the misoprostol component, it is contraindicated in women who are pregnant. Caution in women with childbearing potential; effective contraception is essential.

ADULT — OA: One 50/200 PO three times per day. RA: One 50/200 PO three to four times per day. If intolerant, may use 50/200 or 75/200 PO two times per day.

PEDS — Not approved in children.

(cont.)

ARTHROTEC (*cont.*)

FORMS — Generic/Trade: Tabs 50 mg/200 mcg, 75 mg/200 mcg, diclofenac/misoprostol.

NOTES — Refer to individual components. Abdominal pain and diarrhea may occur. Check LFTs at baseline, within 4 to 8 weeks of initiation, then periodically. Do not crush or chew tabs.

MOA — Anti-inflammatory/mucosalprotectant, analgesic.

ADVERSE EFFECTS — Serious: Fetal death, nephrotoxicity, gastritis, peptic ulcer disease, GI bleeds. Frequent: Diarrhea, abdominal pain, nausea, dyspepsia.

DICLOFENAC (*Voltaren, Voltaren XR, Flector, Zipsor, Cambia, Zorvolex, ✷Voltaren Rapide*) ▶L ♀B (D in 3rd trimester) ▶– $$$

WARNING — Multiple strengths; see FORMS and write specific product on Rx.

ADULT — OA: Immediate- or delayed-release: 50 mg PO two to three times per day or 75 mg two times per day. Extended-release 100 mg PO daily. Gel: Apply 4 g to knees or 2 g to hands four times per day using enclosed dosing card. RA: Immediate- or delayed-release 50 mg PO three to four times per day or 75 mg two times per day. Extended-release 100 mg PO one to two times per day. Ankylosing spondylitis: Immediate- or delayed-release 25 mg PO four times per day and at bedtime. Analgesia and primary dysmenorrhea: Immediate- or delayed-release 50 mg PO three times per day. Acute pain of strains, sprains, or contusions: Apply 1 patch to painful area two times per day. Acute migraine with or without aura: 50 mg single dose (Cambia), mix packet with 30 to 60 mL water.

PEDS — Not approved in children.

UNAPPROVED PEDS — JRA: 2 to 3 mg/kg/day PO.

FORMS — Generic/Trade: Tabs, extended-release (Voltaren XR) 100 mg. Topical gel (Voltaren) 1% 100 g tube. Generic only: Tabs, immediate-release: 25, 50 mg. Generic only: Tabs, delayed-release: 25, 50, 75 mg. Trade only: Patch (Flector) 1.3% diclofenac epolamine. Trade only: Caps, liquid-filled (Zipsor) 25 mg. Caps (Zorvolex) 18, 35 mg. Trade only: Powder for oral soln (Cambia) 50 mg.

NOTES — Check LFTs at baseline, within 4 to 8 weeks of initiation, then periodically. Do not apply patch to damaged or nonintact skin. Wash hands and avoid eye contact when handling the patch. Do not wear patch while bathing or showering.

MOA — Anti-inflammatory, analgesic.

ADVERSE EFFECTS — Serious: Hypersensitivity, GI bleeding, hepato/nephrotoxicity. Frequent: Nausea, dyspepsia, pruritus and dermatitis with patch and gel.

DUEXIS (ibuprofen + famotidine) ▶LK ♀– Avoid NSAID use after 30 weeks gestation. ▶ Ibuprofen and famotidine are present in breast milk in small amounts. Effects on milk production or infant are unknown.

WARNING — Tablets should be swallowed whole. Do not cut, chew, divide, or crush.

ADULT — OA, RA: One 800/26.6 mg ibuprofen/famotidine tablet PO three times per day.

PEDS — Not approved for use in children.

FORMS — Trade only: tabs: 800/26.6 mg ibuprofen/famotidine.

MOA — NSAID/Histamine-2 receptor antagonist combination.

ADVERSE EFFECTS — Serious: Hypersensitivity, GI bleeding, nephrotoxicity, convulsion in renal impairment, interstitial pneumonia, Stevens-Johnson syndrome, rhabdomyolysis. Common: Nausea, dyspepsia, dizziness, headache.

ETODOLAC ▶L ♀C (D in 3rd trimester) ▶– $

WARNING — Multiple strengths; write specific product on Rx.

ADULT — OA: 400 mg PO two to three times per day. 300 mg PO two to three times per day. 200 mg PO three to four times per day. Extended-release 400 to 1200 mg PO daily. Mild to moderate pain: 200 to 400 mg q 6 to 8 h. (Up to 1200 mg/day or if wt 60 kg or less, 20 mg/kg/day.)

PEDS — Not approved in children.

UNAPPROVED ADULT — RA, ankylosing spondylitis: 300 to 400 mg PO two times per day. Tendinitis, bursitis, and acute gout: 300 to 400 mg PO two to four times per day, then taper.

FORMS — Generic only: Caps, immediate-release: 200, 300 mg. Tabs, immediate-release: 400, 500 mg. Tabs, extended-release: 400, 500, 600 mg.

NOTES — Brand name Lodine no longer marketed.

MOA — Anti-inflammatory, analgesic.

ADVERSE EFFECTS — Serious: Hypersensitivity, GI bleeding, nephrotoxicity, toxic epidermal necrolysis. Frequent: Nausea, dyspepsia.

FENOPROFEN (*Nalfon*) ▶L ♀C (D in 3rd trimester) ▶– $$$

WARNING — Appears to represent a greater nephrotoxicity risk than other NSAIDs.

ADULT — RA/OA: 300 to 600 mg PO three to four times per day. Max dose: 3200 mg/day. Mild to moderate pain: 200 mg PO q 4 to 6 h prn.

PEDS — Not approved in children.

FORMS — Generic only: Tabs 600 mg. Trade only: Caps 200, 400 mg.

MOA — Anti-inflammatory, analgesic.

ADVERSE EFFECTS — Serious: Hypersensitivity, GI bleeding, nephrotoxicity. Frequent: Nausea, dyspepsia.

FLURBIPROFEN (*Ansaid*) ▶L ♀B (D in 3rd trimester) ▶+ $$$

ADULT — RA/OA: 200 to 300 mg/day PO divided two to four times per day. Max single dose 100 mg.

PEDS — Not approved in children.

UNAPPROVED ADULT — Ankylosing spondylitis: 150 to 300 mg/day PO divided two to four times per day. Mild to moderate pain: 50 mg PO q 6 h. Primary dysmenorrhea: 50 mg PO daily at onset, discontinue when pain subsides. Tendinitis, bursitis, acute gout, acute migraine: 100 mg PO at onset, then 50 mg PO four times per day, then taper.

UNAPPROVED PEDS — JRA: 4 mg/kg/day PO.

(cont.)

FLURBIPROFEN (*cont.*)

FORMS — Generic/Trade: Tabs, immediate-release 50, 100 mg.

MOA — Serious: Hypersensitivity, GI bleeding, nephrotoxicity. Frequent: Nausea, dyspepsia.

IBUPROFEN (*Motrin, Advil, Nuprin, Rufen, NeoProfen, Caldolor*) ▶L ♀B (D in 3rd trimester) ▶+

ADULT — RA/OA, gout: 200 to 800 mg PO three to four times per day. Mild to moderate pain: 400 mg PO q 4 to 6 h. 400 to 800 mg IV (Caldolor) q 6 h prn. 400 mg IV (Caldolor) q 4 to 6 h or 100 to 200 mg q 4 h prn. Primary dysmenorrhea: 400 mg PO q 4 h prn. Fever: 200 mg PO q 4 to 6 h prn. Migraine pain: 200 to 400 mg PO not to exceed 400 mg in 24 h unless directed by a physician (OTC dosing). Max dose 3.2 g/day.

PEDS — JRA: 30 to 50 mg/kg/day PO divided q 6 h. Max dose 2400 mg/24 h. 20 mg/kg/day may be adequate for milder disease. Analgesic/antipyretic, age older than 6 mo: 5 to 10 mg/kg PO q 6 to 8 h, prn. Max dose 40 mg/kg/day. Patent ductus arteriosus in neonates 32 weeks, gestational age or younger weighing 500 to 1500 g (NeoProfen): Specialized dosing.

FORMS — OTC: Caps/Liqui-Gel caps 200 mg. Tabs 100, 200 mg. Chewable tabs 100 mg. Susp (infant gtts) 50 mg/1.25 mL (with calibrated dropper), 100 mg/5 mL. Rx Generic/Trade: Tabs 400, 600, 800 mg.

NOTES — May antagonize antiplatelet effects of aspirin if given simultaneously. Take aspirin 2 h prior to ibuprofen. Administer IV (Caldolor) over at least 30 min; hydration important.

MOA — Anti-inflammatory/antipyretic, analgesic.

ADVERSE EFFECTS — Serious: Hypersensitivity, GI bleeding, nephrotoxicity. Frequent: Nausea, dyspepsia.

INDOMETHACIN (*Indocin, Indocin SR, Indocin IV*) ▶L ♀B (D in 3rd trimester) ▶+ $

WARNING — Multiple strengths; see FORMS and write specific product on Rx. Use during labor increases risk of fetal and maternal complications: Premature closure of the ductus arteriosus, fetal pulmonary HTN, oligohydramnios, higher rate of postpartum hemorrhage.

ADULT — RA/OA, ankylosing spondylitis: 25 mg PO two to three times per day to start. Increase incrementally to a total daily dose of 150 to 200 mg. Bursitis/tendinitis: 75 to 150 mg/day PO divided three to four times per day. Acute gout: 50 mg PO three times per day until pain tolerable, rapidly taper dose to discontinue. Sustained-release: 75 mg PO one to two times per day.

PEDS — Closure of patent ductus arteriosus in neonates: Initial dose 0.2 mg/kg IV, if additional doses necessary, dose and frequency (q 12 h or q 24 h) based on neonate's age and urine output.

UNAPPROVED ADULT — Primary dysmenorrhea: 25 mg PO three to four times per day. Cluster headache: 75 to 150 mg sustained-release PO daily. Polyhydramnios: 2.2 to 3 mg/kg/day PO based on

maternal wt; premature closure of the ductus arteriosus has been reported. Preterm labor: Initial 50 to 100 mg PO followed by 25 mg PO q 6 to 12 h up to 48 h.

UNAPPROVED PEDS — JRA: 1 to 3 mg/kg/day three to four times per day to start. Increase prn to max dose of 4 mg/kg/day or 200 mg/day, whichever is less.

FORMS — Generic only: Caps, immediate-release 25, 50 mg. Caps, sustained-release 75 mg. Trade only: Supp 50 mg. Oral susp 25 mg/5 mL (237 mL)

NOTES — May aggravate depression or other psychiatric disturbances. Do not crush sustained-release caps.

MOA — Anti-inflammatory, analgesic. Prostaglandin inhibition leads to closure of a patent ductus arteriosus. Tocolytic.

ADVERSE EFFECTS — Serious: Hypersensitivity, GI bleeding, nephrotoxicity. During labor: Premature closure of the ductus arteriosus and fetal pulmonary hypertension, oligohydramnios, postpartum hemorrhage. Frequent: Nausea, dyspepsia, dizziness, drowsiness.

KETOPROFEN (*Orudis, Orudis KT, Actron, Oruvail*) ▶L ♀B (D in 3rd trimester) ▶– $$$

ADULT — RA/OA: 75 mg PO three times per day or 50 mg PO four times per day. Extended-release 200 mg PO daily. Mild to moderate pain, primary dysmenorrhea: 25 to 50 mg PO q 6 to 8 h prn.

PEDS — Not approved in children.

UNAPPROVED PEDS — JRA: 100 to 200 mg/m^2/day PO. Max dose 320 mg/day.

FORMS — Rx Generic only: Caps, extended-release 200 mg. Caps, immediate-release 50, 75 mg.

MOA — Serious: Hypersensitivity, GI bleeding, nephrotoxicity. Frequent: Nausea, dyspepsia.

KETOROLAC (*Toradol*) ▶L ♀C (D in 3rd trimester) ▶+ $

WARNING — Indicated for short-term (up to 5 days) therapy only. Ketorolac is a potent NSAID and can cause serious GI and renal adverse effects. It may also increase the risk of bleeding by inhibiting platelet function. Contraindicated in patients with active peptic ulcer disease, recent GI bleeding or perforation, a history of peptic ulcer disease or GI bleeding, or advanced renal impairment.

ADULT — Moderately severe, acute pain, single-dose treatment: 30 to 60 mg IM or 15 to 30 mg IV. Multiple-dose treatment: 15 to 30 mg IV/IM q 6 h. IV/IM doses are not to exceed 60 mg/day for age 65 yo or older, wt <50 kg, and patients with moderately elevated serum creatinine. Oral continuation therapy: 10 mg PO q 4 to 6 h prn, max dose 40 mg/day. Combined duration IV/IM and PO is not to exceed 5 days.

PEDS — Not approved in children.

UNAPPROVED PEDS — Pain: 0.5 mg/kg/dose IM/IV q 6 h (up to 30 mg q 6 h or 120 mg/day), give 10 mg PO q 6 h prn (up to 40 mg/day) for wt >50 kg.

FORMS — Generic only: Tabs 10 mg.

MOA — Serious: Hypersensitivity, GI bleeding, nephrotoxicity. Frequent: Nausea, dyspepsia.

MECLOFENAMATE ▶L ♀B (D in 3rd trimester) ▶– $$$
ADULT — Mild to moderate pain: 50 mg PO q 4 to 6 h prn. Max dose 400 mg/day. Menorrhagia and primary dysmenorrhea: 100 mg PO three times per day for up to 6 days. RA/OA: 200 to 400 mg/day PO divided three to four times per day.
PEDS — Not approved in children.
UNAPPROVED PEDS — JRA: 3 to 7.5 mg/kg/day PO. Max dose 300 mg/day.
FORMS — Generic only: Caps 50, 100 mg.
NOTES — Reversible autoimmune hemolytic anemia with use for longer than 12 months.
MOA — Anti-inflammatory, analgesic.
ADVERSE EFFECTS — Serious: Hypersensitivity, GI bleeding, nephrotoxicity, autoimmune hemolytic anemia. Frequent: Nausea, dyspepsia.

MEFENAMIC ACID (*Ponstel*, ✻*Ponstan*) ▶L ♀D ▶– $$$$$
ADULT — Mild to moderate pain, primary dysmenorrhea: 500 mg PO initially, then 250 mg PO q 6 h prn for up to 1 week.
PEDS — Use adult dose for age older than 14 yo.
FORMS — Generic/Trade: Caps 250 mg.
MOA — Serious: Hypersensitivity, GI bleeding, nephrotoxicity, autoimmune hemolytic anemia. Frequent: Nausea, dyspepsia.

MELOXICAM (*Mobic*, ✻*Mobicox*) ▶L ♀C (D in 3rd trimester) ▶? $
ADULT — RA/OA: 7.5 mg PO daily. Max dose 15 mg/day.
PEDS — JRA, age 2 yo or older: 0.125 mg/kg PO daily to max of 7.5 mg.
FORMS — Generic/Trade: Tabs 7.5, 15 mg. Generic only: Susp 7.5 mg/5 mL (1.5 mg/mL).
NOTES — Shake susp gently before using. This is not a selective COX-2 inhibitor.
MOA — Anti-inflammatory, analgesic.
ADVERSE EFFECTS — Serious: Hypersensitivity, GI bleeding, nephrotoxicity. Frequent: Nausea, dyspepsia.

NABUMETONE (*Relafen*) ▶L ♀C (D in 3rd trimester) ▶– $$
ADULT — RA/OA: Initial: Two 500 mg tabs (1000 mg) PO daily. May increase to 1500 to 2000 mg PO daily or divided two times per day. Dosages more than 2000 mg/day have not been studied.
PEDS — Not approved in children.
FORMS — Generic only: Tabs 500, 750 mg.
MOA — Serious: Hypersensitivity, GI bleeding, nephrotoxicity, hepatotoxicity, Stevens-Johnson syndrome, erythema multiforme, toxic epidermal necrolysis, eosinophilic pneumonia. Frequent: Nausea, dyspepsia.

NAPROXEN (*Naprosyn, Aleve, Anaprox, EC-Naprosyn, Naprelan, Prevacid NapraPAC*) ▶L ♀B (D in 3rd trimester) ▶+ $$$
WARNING — Multiple strengths; see FORMS and write specific product on Rx.
ADULT — RA/OA, ankylosing spondylitis, pain, dysmenorrhea, acute tendinitis and bursitis, fever: 250 to 500 mg PO two times per day. Delayed-release: 375 to 500 mg PO two times per day (do not crush or chew). Controlled-release: 750 to 1000 mg PO daily. Acute gout: 750 mg PO once, then 250 mg PO q 8 h until the attack subsides. Controlled-release: 1000 to 1500 mg PO once, then 1000 mg PO daily until the attack subsides.
PEDS — JRA: 10 to 20 mg/kg/day PO divided two times per day (up to 1250 mg/24 h). Pain for age older than 2 yo: 5 to 7 mg/kg/dose PO q 8 to 12 h.
UNAPPROVED ADULT — Acute migraine: 750 mg PO once, then 250 to 500 mg PO prn. Migraine prophylaxis, menstrual migraine: 500 mg PO two times per day beginning 1 day prior to onset of menses and ending on last day of period.
FORMS — OTC Generic/Trade (Aleve): Tabs, immediate-release 200 mg. OTC Trade only (Aleve): Caps, Gelcaps, immediate-release 200 mg. Rx Generic/Trade: Tabs, immediate-release (Naprosyn) 250, 375, 500 mg. (Anaprox) 275, 550 mg. Tabs, delayed-release enteric-coated (EC-Naprosyn) 375, 500 mg. Tabs, controlled-release (Naprelan) 375, 500, 750 mg. Susp (Naprosyn) 125 mg/5 mL. Prevacid NapraPAC: 7 lansoprazole 15 mg caps packaged with 14 naproxen tabs 375 mg or 500 mg.
NOTES — All dosing is based on naproxen content; 500 mg naproxen is equivalent to 550 mg naproxen sodium.
MOA — Anti-inflammatory, analgesic.
ADVERSE EFFECTS — Serious: Hypersensitivity, GI bleeding, nephrotoxicity. Frequent: Nausea, dyspepsia.

OXAPROZIN (*Daypro*) ▶L ♀C (D in 3rd trimester) ▶– $$$
ADULT — RA/OA: 1200 mg PO daily. Max dose 1800 mg/day or 26 mg/kg/day, whichever is lower.
PEDS — Not approved in children.
FORMS — Generic/Trade: Tabs 600 mg, trade scored.
MOA — Serious: Hypersensitivity, GI bleeding, nephrotoxicity. Frequent: Nausea, dyspepsia.

PIROXICAM (*Feldene, Fexicam*) ▶L ♀B (D in 3rd trimester) ▶+ $$$
ADULT — RA/OA: 20 mg PO daily or divided two times per day.
PEDS — Not approved in children.
UNAPPROVED ADULT — Primary dysmenorrhea: 20 to 40 mg PO daily for 3 days.
FORMS — Generic/Trade: Caps 10, 20 mg.
MOA — Serious: Hypersensitivity, GI bleeding, nephrotoxicity. Frequent: Nausea, dyspepsia.

SULINDAC (*Clinoril*) ▶L ♀B (D in 3rd trimester) ▶– $
ADULT — RA/OA, ankylosing spondylitis: 150 mg PO two times per day. Bursitis, tendinitis, acute gout: 200 mg PO two times per day, decrease after response. Max dose: 400 mg/day.
PEDS — Not approved in children.
UNAPPROVED PEDS — JRA: 4 mg/kg/day PO divided two times per day.
FORMS — Generic/Trade: Tabs 200 mg. Generic only: Tabs 150 mg.
NOTES — Sulindac-associated pancreatitis and a potentially fatal hypersensitivity syndrome have occurred.

(cont.)

SULINDAC (*cont.*)

MOA — Anti-inflammatory, analgesic.

ADVERSE EFFECTS — Serious: Hypersensitivity, GI bleeding, nephrotoxicity, pancreatitis. Frequent: Nausea, dyspepsia.

TOLMETIN (*Tolectin*) ▶L ♀C (D in 3rd trimester) ▶+ $$$

ADULT — RA/OA: 400 mg PO three times per day to start. Range 600 to 1800 mg/day PO divided three times per day.

PEDS — JRA age 2 yo or older: 20 mg/kg/day PO divided three to four times per day to start. Range 15 to 30 mg/kg/day divided three to four times per day. Max dose 2 g/24 h.

UNAPPROVED PEDS — Pain age 2 yo or older: 5 to 7 mg/kg/dose PO q 6 to 8 h. Max dose 2 g/24 h.

FORMS — Generic only: Tabs 200 (scored), 600 mg. Caps 400 mg.

NOTES — Rare anaphylaxis.

MOA — Anti-inflammatory, analgesic.

ADVERSE EFFECTS — Serious: Hypersensitivity, GI bleeding, nephrotoxicity. Frequent: Nausea, dyspepsia.

VIMOVO (**naproxen + esomeprazole**) ▶L ♀ Avoid NSAID use after 30 weeks gestation. ▶ Naproxen present in breast milk at 1% of serum concentration. Esomeprazole is present in breast milk. Effects on milk production or infant are unknown.

WARNING — Do not crush, split, chew, or dissolve tablets. Must be swallowed whole. Concomitant administration with voriconazole, an inhibitor of CYP2C19 and CYP3A4 may lead to a more than doubling of esomeprazole exposure. Esomeprazole may reduce the efficacy of clopidogrel. Use caution with high-dose methotrexate. Long-term use may cause reduction in vitamin B12 and magnesium levels.

ADULT — OA, RA, ankylosing spondylitis: One 375/20 or 500/20 tab two times per day at least 30 minutes before meals.

PEDS — Not approved for use in children.

FORMS — Trade only: Delayed release tabs 375/20 and 500/20 mg naproxen/esomeprazole.

NOTES — Slower onset of action than other naproxen products. Do not use for initial treatment of acute pain.

MOA — Anti-inflamatory/analagesic and proton pump inhibitor combination.

ADVERSE EFFECTS — Serious: Hypersensitivity, GI bleeding, nephrotoxicity, toxic epidermal necrolysis, Stevens-Johnson syndrome, erythema multiforme, pancreatitis, hepatitis. Frequent: N/V, dyspepsia, headache, dizziness, rash, diarrhea, taste perversion.

ANALGESICS: Opioid Agonist-Antagonists

NOTE: May cause drowsiness and/or sedation, which may be enhanced by alcohol and other CNS depressants. Opioid agonist-antagonists may result in inadequate pain control and/or withdrawal effects in the opioid-dependent. Reserve IM for when alternative routes are not feasible.

BUPRENORPHINE (*Probuphine, Buprenex, Butrans, Subutex*) ▶L ♀C ▶– ©III $ IV, $$$$$ SL

ADULT — Moderate to severe pain: 0.3 to 0.6 mg IM or slow IV, q 6 h prn. Max single dose 0.6 mg. Treatment of opioid dependence: Induction 8 mg SL on day 1, 16 mg SL on day 2. Maintenance: 16 mg SL daily. Can individualize to range of 4 to 24 mg SL daily. Treatment of opioid dependence - Probuphine maintenance (only for patients stable on 8 mg/day or less of transmucosal form): Implant 4 units in the inner aspect of one arm and leave for 6 months then remove. May repeat once in the other arm when orinignal implants removed at 6 months. No experience with treatment beyond 12 months. Moderate to severe chronic pain: 5 to 20 mcg/h patch changed q 7 days.

PEDS — Moderate to severe pain: Age 2 to 12 yo: 2 to 6 mcg/kg/dose IM or slow IV q 4 to 6 h. Max single dose 6 mcg/kg. Patch not approved for use in children.

FORMS — Generic only: SL Tabs 2, 8 mg. Trade only (Butrans): Transdermal patches 5, 10, 20 mcg/h.

NOTES — May cause bradycardia, hypotension, and respiratory depression. Concurrent use with diazepam has resulted in respiratory and cardiovascular collapse. For opioid dependence Subutex is preferred over Suboxone for induction. Suboxone preferred for maintenance. Prescribers must complete training and apply for special DEA number. See www.suboxone.com. Probuphine implants are intended to remain in place for 6 months and then removed. There is no experience with the implants beyond one insertion in each arm (12 months). See PI for instructions on implantation and removal. Once removed, the patient can return to a transmucosal form.

MOA — Opioid agonist-antagonist analgesic.

ADVERSE EFFECTS — Serious: Respiratory depression, hepatitis, hypersensitivity. Frequent: Sedation, dizziness, nausea, headache, constipation.

BUTORPHANOL (*Stadol, Stadol NS*) ▶LK ♀C ▶+ ©IV $$$

WARNING — Approved as a nasal spray in 1991 and has been promoted as a safe treatment for migraine headaches. There have been numerous reports of dependence-addiction and major psychological disturbances. These problems have been documented by the FDA. Stadol NS should be used for patients with infrequent but severe migraine attacks for whom all other common abortive treatments have failed. Experts recommend restriction to no more than 2 bottles (30 sprays) per month in patients who are appropriate candidates for this medication.

ADULT — Pain, including postop pain: 0.5 to 2 mg IV q 3 to 4 h prn. 1 to 4 mg IM q 3 to 4 h prn. Obstetric

(cont.)

BUTORPHANOL (*cont.*)

pain during labor: 1 to 2 mg IV/IM at full term in early labor, repeat after 4 h. Last resort for migraine pain: 1 mg nasal spray (1 spray in 1 nostril). If no pain relief in 60 to 90 min, may give a 2nd spray in the other nostril. Additional doses q 3 to 4 h prn.

PEDS — Not approved in children.

FORMS — Generic only: Nasal spray 1 mg/spray, 2.5 mL bottle (14 to 15 doses/bottle).

NOTES — May increase cardiac workload.

MOA — Opioid agonist-antagonist analgesic.

ADVERSE EFFECTS — Serious: Respiratory depression. Frequent: Sedation, dizziness.

NALBUPHINE (*Nubain*) ▶LK ♀? ▶? $

ADULT — Moderate to severe pain including obstetrical analgesia during labor and delivery: 10 to 20 mg SC/IM/IV q 3 to 6 h prn. Max dose 160 mg/day.

PEDS — Not approved in children.

MOA — Serious: Respiratory depression. Frequent: Sedation, dizziness, nausea.

PENTAZOCINE (*Talwin NX*) ▶LK ♀C ▶? ©IV $$$

WARNING — The oral form (Talwin NX) may cause fatal reactions if injected.

ADULT — Moderate to severe pain: Talwin: 30 mg IM/IV q 3 to 4 h prn, max dose 360 mg/day. Talwin NX: 1 tab PO q 3 to 4 h, max 12 tabs/day.

PEDS — Not approved in children.

FORMS — Generic/Trade: Tabs 50 mg with 0.5 mg naloxone, trade scored.

NOTES — Rotate injection sites. Can cause hallucinations, disorientation, and seizures. Concomitant sibutramine may precipitate serotonin syndrome.

MOA — Opioid agonist-antagonist analgesic.

ADVERSE EFFECTS — Serious: Respiratory depression, seizures, hallucinations, hypersensitivity. Frequent: Sedation, dizziness, nausea.

ANALGESICS: Opioid Agonists

FENTANYL TRANSDERMAL DOSE (Dosing based on ongoing morphine requirement)

Morphine* (IV/IM)	Morphine* (PO)	Transdermal fentanyl*
10–22 mg/d	60–134 mg/d	25 mcg/h
23–37 mg/d	135–224 mg/d	50 mcg/h
38–52 mg/d	225–314 mg/d	75 mcg/h
53–67 mg/d	315–404 mg/d	100 mcg/h

*For higher morphine doses, see product insert for transdermal fentanyl equivalencies.

NOTE: May cause life-threatening respiratory depression. May cause drowsiness and/or sedation, which may be enhanced by alcohol and other CNS depressants. Patients with chronic pain may require more frequent and higher dosing. Opioids commonly cause constipation. All opioids are pregnancy class D if used for prolonged periods or in high doses at term.

CODEINE ▶LK ♀C ▶– ©II $

WARNING — Do not use IV in children due to large histamine-release and cardiovascular effects. Use in nursing mothers has led to infant death.

ADULT — Mild to moderate pain: 15 to 60 mg PO/IM/IV/SC q 4 to 6 h. Max dose 360 mg in 24 h. Antitussive: 10 to 20 mg PO q 4 to 6 h prn. Max dose 120 mg in 24 h.

PEDS — Mild to moderate pain in age 1 yo or older: 0.5 to 1 mg/kg PO/SC/IM q 4 to 6 h, max dose 60 mg/dose. Antitussive: For age 2 to 5 yo, give 2.5 to 5 mg PO q 4 to 6 h prn (up to 30 mg/day); for age 6 to 12 yo, give 5 to 10 mg PO q 4 to 6 h prn (up to 60 mg/day).

FORMS — Generic only: Tabs 15, 30, 60 mg. Oral soln: 30 mg/5 mL.

MOA — Opioid agonist analgesic.

ADVERSE EFFECTS — Serious: Respiratory depression/arrest. Frequent: N/V, constipation, sedation.

EMBEDA (morphine + naltrexone) ▶LK ♀C ▶? ©II $$$$$

WARNING — Must be taken whole. Crushing, chewing, or dissolving capsules will alter delivery and can result in overdose and death. Not appropriate for use as an as-needed analgesic. Dose cautiously; may cause life-threatening respiratory depression. Patients who are being converted from other opioids should be monitored closely.

ADULT — Severe pain: Patients who are not opioid tolerant: 20/0.8 mg morphine/naltrexone once daily. Opioid-tolerant patients: 30/1.2 mg morphine/naltrexone daily. Opioid tolerance is the use for 1 week or longer of 60 mg oral morphine daily, 30 mg oral oxycodone daily, 8 mg hydrocodone daily, 25 mg oxymorphone daily, or 25 mcg/h of transdermal fentanyl. Conversion from other oral morphine products can be done on a mg-to-mg of morphine basis administered daily or split into two divided doses.

(cont.)

EMBEDA (*cont.*)

All other scheduled opioids should be discontinued when Embeda is initiated.

PEDS — Not approved in children.

FORMS — Trade only: Extended-release caps: 20/0.8, 30/1.2, 50/2, 60/2.4, 80/3.2, 100/4 mg morphine/naltrexone.

NOTES — May be dosed twice daily in opioid-experienced patients.

MOA — Opioid agonist analgesic. Opioid antagonist included to discourage parenteral abuse.

ADVERSE EFFECTS — Serious: Respiratory depression/arrest. Frequent: N/V, sedation, constipation.

FENTANYL (*Ionsys, Duragesic, Actiq, Fentora, Sublimaze, Abstral, Subsys, Lazanda, Onsolis*) ▶L ♀C ▶+ ©II $ – varies by therapy

WARNING — Duragesic patches, Actiq, Fentora, Abstral, Subsys, and Lazanda are contraindicated in the management of acute or postop pain due to potentially life-threatening respiratory depression in opioid nontolerant patients. Instruct patients and their caregivers that even used patches/lozenges on a stick can be fatal to a child or pet. Dispose via toilet. Actiq and Fentora are not interchangeable. IONSYS: For hospital use only; remove prior to discharge. Can cause life-threatening respiratory depression.

ADULT — Duragesic patches: Chronic pain: 12 to 100 mcg/h patch q 72 h. Titrate dose to the needs of the patient. Some patients require q 48 h dosing. May wear more than 1 patch to achieve the correct analgesic effect. Actiq: Breakthrough cancer pain: 200 to 1600 mcg sucked over 15 min, if 200 mcg ineffective for 6 units use higher strength. Goal is 4 lozenges on a stick/day in conjunction with long-acting opioid. Buccal tab (Fentora) for breakthrough cancer pain: 100 to 800 mcg, titrated to pain relief; may repeat once after 30 min during single episode of breakthrough pain. See prescribing information for dose conversion from transmucosal lozenges. Buccal soluble film (Onsolis) for breakthrough cancer pain: 200 to 1200 mcg, titrated to pain relief; no more than 4 doses/day separated by at least 2 h. Postop analgesia: 50 to 100 mcg IM; repeat in 1 to 2 h prn. SL tab (Abstral) for breakthrough cancer pain: 100 mcg, may repeat once after 30 minutes. Specialized titration. SL spray (Subsys) for breakthrough cancer pain: 100 mcg, may repeat once after 30 minutes. Specialized titration. Nasal spray (Lazanda) for breakthrough cancer pain: 100 mcg. Specialized titration. IONSYS: Acute postop pain: Specialized dosing.

PEDS — Transdermal (Duragesic): Not approved in children younger than 2 yo or in opioid-naive. Use adult dosing for age older than 2 yo. Children converting to a 25 mcg patch should be receiving 45 mg or more oral morphine equivalents/day. Actiq: Not approved for age younger than 16 yo. IONSYS not approved in children. Abstral, Subsys, and Lazanda: Not approved for age younger than 18.

UNAPPROVED ADULT — Analgesia/procedural sedation/labor analgesia: 50 to 100 mcg IV or IM q 1 to 2 h prn.

UNAPPROVED PEDS — Analgesia: 1 to 2 mcg/kg/dose IV/IM q 30 to 60 min prn or continuous IV infusion 1 to 3 mcg/kg/h (not to exceed adult dosing). Procedural sedation: 2 to 3 mcg/kg/dose for age 1 to 3 yo; 1 to 2 mcg/kg/dose for age 3 to 12 yo, 0.5 to 1 mcg/kg/dose (not to exceed adult dosing) for age older than 12 yo, procedural sedation doses may be repeated q 30 to 60 min prn.

FORMS — Generic/Trade: Transdermal patches 12, 25, 50, 75, 100 mcg/h. Actiq lozenges on a stick, berry-flavored 200, 400, 600, 800, 1200, 1600 mcg. Trade only: (Fentora) buccal tab 100, 200, 400, 600, 800 mcg, packs of 4 or 28 tabs. Trade only: (Onsolis) buccal soluble film 200, 400, 600, 800, 1200 mcg in child-resistant, protective foil, packs of 30 films. Trade only: (Abstral) SL tabs 100, 200, 300, 400, 600, 800 mcg, packs of 4 or 32 tabs. Trade only: (Subsys) SL spray 100, 200, 400, 600, 800, 1200, 1600 mcg blister packs in cartons of 10 and 30 (30 only for 1200 and 1600 mcg). Trade only: (Lazanda) nasal spray 100, 400 mcg/spray, 8 sprays/bottle.

NOTES — Do not use patches for acute pain or in opioid-naive patients. Oral transmucosal fentanyl doses of 5 mcg/kg provide effects similar to 0.75 to 1.25 mcg/kg of fentanyl IM. Lozenges on a stick should be sucked, not chewed. Flush lozenge remnants (without stick) down the toilet. For transdermal systems: Apply patch to non-hairy skin. Clip (do not shave) hair if you have to apply to hairy area. Fever or external heat sources may increase fentanyl released from patch. Patch should be removed prior to MRI and reapplied after the test. Dispose of a used patch by folding with the adhesive side of the patch adhering to itself, then flush it down the toilet immediately. Do not cut the patch in half. For Duragesic patches and Actiq lozenges on a stick: Titrate dose as high as necessary to relieve cancer or nonmalignant pain where chronic opioids are necessary. Do not suck, chew, or swallow buccal tab. IONSYS: Apply to intact skin on the chest or upper arm. Each dose, activated by the patient, is delivered over a 10-min period. Remove prior to hospital discharge. Do not allow gel to touch mucous membranes. Dispose using gloves. Keep all forms of fentanyl out of the reach of children or pets. Concomitant use with potent CYP3A4 inhibitors such as ritonavir, ketoconazole, itraconazole, clarithromycin, nelfinavir, and nefazodone may result in an increase in fentanyl plasma concentrations, which could increase or prolong adverse drug effects and may cause potentially fatal respiratory depression. Onsolis is available only through the FOCUS Program and requires prescriber, pharmacy, and patient enrollment. Used films should be discarded into toilet. Abstral, Subsys, and Lazanda: outpatients, prescribers, pharmacies, and distributors must be enrolled in TIRF REMS Access program before patient may receive medication.

(cont.)

FENTANYL (*cont.*)

MOA — Opioid agonist analgesic.

ADVERSE EFFECTS — Serious: Respiratory depression/arrest, chest wall rigidity. Frequent: N/V, constipation, sedation, skin irritation, dental decay with Actiq.

HYDROCODONE (*Zohydro ER*) ▶LK ♀C ▶? ©II

WARNING — Must be taken whole. Crushing, chewing, or dissolving capsules will alter delivery and can result in overdose and death. Not appropriate for use as an as-needed analgesic. Dose cautiously; may cause life-threatening respiratory depression. Patients who are being converted from other opioids should be monitored closely.

ADULT — Severe pain: Patients who are not opioid tolerant: 10 mg q 12 h. Opioid-tolerant patients: Convert from current opioid regimen using available equivalent dose table. Dose can be increased q 3 to 7 days in increments of 10 mg q 12 h (20 mg/day total).

FORMS — Extended-release caps 10, 15, 20, 30, 40, 50 mg.

NOTES — Metabolized primarily by CYP3A4 isoenzyme. Inhibitors of this isoenzyme (erythromycin, ketoconazole, ritonavir) may increase exposure, while inducers (rifampin, carbamazepine, phenytoin) may decrease exposure.

MOA — Opioid agonist analgesic.

ADVERSE EFFECTS — Serious: Respiratory depression/arrest. Frequent: N/V, sedation, constipation.

HYDROMORPHONE (*Dilaudid, Exalgo,* ✚*Hydromorph Contin*) ▶L ♀C ▶? ©II $$

ADULT — Moderate to severe pain: 2 to 4 mg PO q 4 to 6 h. Initial dose (opioid-naive): 0.5 to 2 mg SC/IM or slow IV q 4 to 6 h prn. 3 mg PR q 6 to 8 h. Controlled-release tabs: 8 to 64 mg daily.

PEDS — Not approved in children.

UNAPPROVED PEDS — Pain age 12 yo or younger: 0.03 to 0.08 mg/kg PO q 4 to 6 h prn. 0.015 mg/kg/dose IV q 4 to 6 h prn, use adult dose for older than 12 yo.

FORMS — Generic/Trade: Tabs 2, 4, 8 mg (8 mg trade scored). Oral soln 5 mg/5 mL. Controlled-release tabs (Exalgo): 8, 12, 16, 32 mg.

NOTES — In opioid-naive patients, consider an initial dose of 0.5 mg or less IM/SC/IV. SC/IM/IV doses after initial dose should be individualized. May be given by slow IV injection over 2 to 5 min. Titrate dose as high as necessary to relieve cancer or nonmalignant pain where chronic opioids are necessary. 1.5 mg IV = 7.5 mg PO. Exalgo intended for opioid-tolerant patients only.

MOA — Opioid agonist analgesic.

ADVERSE EFFECTS — Serious: Respiratory depression/arrest. Frequent: N/V, constipation, sedation.

LEVORPHANOL (*Levo-Dromoran*) ▶L ♀C ▶? ©II $$$$

ADULT — Moderate to severe pain: 2 mg PO q 6 to 8 h prn. Increase to 4 mg if necessary.

PEDS — Not approved in children.

FORMS — Generic only: Tabs 2 mg, scored.

MEPERIDINE (*Demerol, pethidine*) ▶LK ♀C but + ▶+ ©II $$

ADULT — Moderate to severe pain: 50 to 150 mg IM/SC/PO q 3 to 4 h prn. OB analgesia: When pains become regular, 50 to 100 mg IM/SC q 1 to 3 h. May also be given slow IV diluted to 10 mg/mL, or by continuous IV infusion diluted to 1 mg/mL.

PEDS — Moderate to severe pain: 1 to 1.8 mg/kg IM/SC/PO or slow IV (see adult dosing) up to adult dose, q 3 to 4 h prn.

FORMS — Generic/Trade: Tabs 50 (trade scored), 100 mg. Generic only: Syrup 50 mg/5 mL.

NOTES — Avoid in renal insufficiency and in elderly due to risk of metabolite accumulation and increased risk of CNS disturbance and seizures. Multiple drug interactions including MAOIs and SSRIs. Poor oral absorption/efficacy. 75 mg meperidine IV/IM/SC = 300 mg meperidine PO. Take syrup with ½ glass (4 oz) water. Due to the risk of seizures at high doses, meperidine is not a good choice for treatment of chronic pain. Not recommended in children.

MOA — Opioid agonist analgesic.

ADVERSE EFFECTS — Serious: Respiratory depression/arrest, seizures, anaphylaxis. Frequent: N/V, constipation, sedation.

METHADONE (*Diskets, Dolophine, Methadose,* ✚*Metadol*) ▶L ♀C ▶? ©II $

WARNING — High doses (mean approximately 200 mg/day) have been inconclusively associated with arrhythmia (torsades de pointes), particularly in those with preexisting risk factors. Caution in opioid-naive patients. Elimination half-life (8 to 59 h) far longer than its duration of analgesic action (4 to 8 h); monitor for respiratory depression and titrate accordingly. Use caution with escalating doses.

ADULT — Severe pain in opioid-tolerant patients: Initial dose is 2.5 mg IM/SC/PO q 8 to 12 h prn. Titrate up by 2.5 mg per dose q 5 to 7 days as necessary to relieve cancer or nonmalignant pain where chronic opioids are necessary. May start as high as 10 mg per dose if opioid-dependent patient and dosing is managed by experienced practitioner using an opioid conversion formula. Opioid dependence: Typical dose to prevent withdrawal is 20 mg PO daily but must be managed by an experienced practitioner. Treatment longer than 3 weeks is maintenance and only permitted in approved treatment programs. Opioid-naive patients: Not recommended as 1st-line treatment of acute pain, mild chronic pain, postoperative pain, or as a prn medication.

PEDS — Not approved in children.

UNAPPROVED PEDS — Pain age 12 yo or younger: 0.7 mg/kg/24 h divided q 4 to 6 h PO/SC/IM/IV prn. Max 10 mg/dose.

FORMS — Generic/Trade: Tabs 5, 10 mg. Dispersible tabs 40 mg (for opioid dependence only). Oral concentrate (Intensol): 10 mg/mL. Generic only: Oral soln 5, 10 mg/5 mL.

NOTES — Titrate to relieve cancer or nonmalignant pain where chronic opioids are necessary. Avoid

(cont.)

METHADONE (*cont.*)

doses > 200 mg/day due to high adverse event rates. Every 8 to 12 h dosing may decrease the risk of drug accumulation and overdose. Treatment for opioid dependence longer than 3 weeks is maintenance and only permitted in approved treatment programs. Drug interactions leading to decreased methadone levels with enzyme-inducing HIV drugs (eg, efavirenz, nevirapine) and other potent inducers such as rifampin. Monitor for opiate withdrawal symptoms and increase methadone if necessary. Rapid metabolizers may require more frequent daily dosing.

MOA — Opioid agonist analgesic.

ADVERSE EFFECTS — Serious: Respiratory depression/cardiorespiratory arrest, dependence, withdrawal, seizures, bradycardia. Frequent: N/V, constipation, sedation, dry mouth, urinary retention, rash.

MORPHINE (*MS Contin, Kadian, Avinza, Roxanol, Oramorph SR, MSIR, DepoDur, ✚Statex, M.O.S., Doloral, M-Eslon*) ▶LK ♀C ▶+ ©ll varies by therapy

WARNING — Multiple strengths; see FORMS and write specific product on Rx. Drinking alcohol while taking Avinza may result in a rapid release of a potentially fatal dose of morphine.

ADULT — Moderate to severe pain: 10 to 30 mg PO q 4 h (immediate-release tabs, or oral soln). Controlled-release (MS Contin, Oramorph SR): 30 mg PO q 8 to 12 h. (Kadian): 20 mg PO q 12 to 24 h. Extended-release caps (Avinza): 30 mg PO daily. 10 mg q 4 h IM/SC. 2.5 to 15 mg/70 kg IV over 4 to 5 min. 10 to 20 mg PR q 4 h. Pain with major surgery (DepoDur): 10 to 15 mg once epidurally at the lumbar level prior to surgery (max dose 20 mg), or 10 mg epidurally after clamping of the umbilical cord with cesarean section.

PEDS — Moderate to severe pain: 0.1 to 0.2 mg/kg up to 15 mg IM/SC/IV q 2 to 4 h.

UNAPPROVED PEDS — Moderate to severe pain: 0.2 to 0.5 mg/kg/dose PO (immediate-release) q 4 to 6 h. 0.3 to 0.6 mg/kg/dose PO (controlled-release) q 12 h.

FORMS — Generic only: Tabs, immediate-release 15, 30 mg ($). Oral soln 10 mg/5 mL, 20 mg/5 mL, 20 mg/mL (concentrate). Rectal supps 5, 10, 20, 30 mg. Generic/Trade: Controlled-release tabs (MS Contin) 15, 30, 60, 100, 200 mg ($$$$). Controlled-release caps (Kadian) 10, 20, 30, 50, 60, 80, 100 mg ($$$$$). Extended-release caps (Avinza) 30, 45, 60, 75, 90, 120 mg. Trade only: Controlled-release caps (Kadian) 40, 200 mg.

NOTES — Titrate dose as high as necessary to relieve cancer or nonmalignant pain where chronic opioids are necessary. The active metabolites may accumulate in hepatic/renal insufficiency and the elderly leading to increased analgesic and sedative effects. Do not break, chew, or crush MS Contin or Oramorph SR. Kadian and Avinza caps may be opened and sprinkled in applesauce for easier administration; however, the pellets should not be crushed or chewed. Doses more than 1600 mg/day of Avinza contain a potentially nephrotoxic quantity of fumaric acid. Do not mix DepoDur with other medications; do not administer any other medications into epidural space for for at least 48 h. Severe opiate overdose with respiratory depression has occurred with intrathecal leakage of DepoDur.

MOA — Opioid agonist analgesic.

ADVERSE EFFECTS — Serious: Respiratory depression/arrest. Frequent: N/V, constipation, sedation, hypotension.

OXYCODONE (*Roxicodone, OxyContin, Percolone, OxyIR, OxyFAST, Oxecta, ✚Endocodone, Supeudol, OxyNEO*) ▶L ♀B ▶– ©ll varies by therapy

WARNING — Do not prescribe OxyContin tabs on a prn basis. 80 mg tabs for use in opioid-tolerant patients only. Multiple strengths; see FORMS and write specific product on Rx. Do not break, chew, or crush controlled-release preparations.

ADULT — Moderate to severe pain: 5 mg PO q 4 to 6 h prn. Controlled-release tabs: 10 to 40 mg PO q 12 h (no supporting data for shorter dosing intervals for controlled-release tabs).

PEDS — Not approved in children.

UNAPPROVED PEDS — Pain age 12 yo or younger: 0.05 to 0.3 mg/kg/dose q 4 to 6 h PO prn to max of 10 mg/dose.

FORMS — Generic only: Immediate-release: Tabs 5, 10, 20 mg. Caps 5 mg. Oral soln 5 mg/5 mL. Generic/Trade: Tab 15, 30 mg. Oral concentrate 20 mg/mL. Trade only: Immediate-release abuse-deterrent tabs (Oxecta): 5, 7.5 mg. Controlled-release tabs 10, 15, 20, 30, 40, 60, 80 mg ($$$$$).

NOTES — Titrate dose as high as necessary to relieve cancer or nonmalignant pain where chronic opioids are necessary.

MOA — Opioid agonist analgesic.

ADVERSE EFFECTS — Serious: Respiratory depression/arrest. Frequent: N/V, constipation, sedation.

OXYMORPHONE (*Opana, Opana ER*) ▶L ♀C ▶? ©ll $$$$$

WARNING — Do not break, chew, dissolve, or crush extended-release tabs due to a rapid release and absorption of a potentially fatal dose of oxymorphone.

ADULT — Moderate to severe pain: 10 to 20 mg PO q 4 to 6 h (immediate-release) or 5 mg q 12 h (extended-release) 1 h before or 2 h after meals. Titrate q 3 to 7 days until adequate pain relief. 1 to 1.5 mg IM/SC q 4 to 6 h prn. 0.5 mg IV initial dose in healthy patients then q 4 to 6 h prn, increase dose until pain adequately controlled.

PEDS — Not approved in children.

FORMS — Generic/Trade: Immediate-release (IR) tabs 5, 10 mg. Extended-release tabs (ER) 5, 7.5, 10, 15, 20, 30, 40 mg. Trade only: Injection 1 mg/mL.

NOTES — Contraindicated in moderate to severe hepatic dysfunction. Decrease dose in elderly and with CrCl <50 mL/min. Avoid alcohol.

MOA — Opioid agonist analgesic.

ADVERSE EFFECTS — Serious: Respiratory depression/arrest. Frequent: N/V, constipation, sedation.

ANALGESICS: Opioid Analgesic Combinations

NOTE: Refer to individual components for further information. May cause drowsiness and/or sedation, which may be enhanced by alcohol and other CNS depressants. Opioids, carisoprodol, and butalbital may be habit-forming. Avoid exceeding 4 g/day of acetaminophen in combination products. Caution people who drink 3 or more alcoholic drinks/day to limit acetaminophen use to 2.5 g/day due to additive liver toxicity. Opioids commonly cause constipation; concurrent laxatives are recommended. All opioids are pregnancy class D if used for prolonged periods or in high doses at term.

ANEXSIA (hydrocodone + acetaminophen) ▶LK ♀C ▶– ©II $
WARNING — Multiple strengths; see FORMS and write specific product on Rx.
ADULT — Moderate pain: 1 tab PO q 4 to 6 h prn.
PEDS — Not approved in children.
FORMS — Generic only: Tabs 5/325, 7.5/325, 10/325 mg hydrocodone/mg acetaminophen, scored.

CAPITAL WITH CODEINE SUSPENSION (acetaminophen + codeine) ▶LK ♀C ▶? ©V $
ADULT — Moderate pain: 15 mL PO q 4 h prn.
PEDS — Moderate pain: Give 5 mL PO q 4 to 6 h prn for age 3 to 6 yo, give 10 mL PO q 4 to 6 h prn for age 7 to 12 yo, use adult dose for age older than 12 yo.
FORMS — Generic only: Soln 120 mg/5 mL, 12 mg/5 mL (APAP/Codeine). Trade only: Susp 120 mg/5 mL, 12 mg/5 mL (APAP/Codeine).

COMBUNOX (oxycodone + ibuprofen) ▶L ♀C (D in 3rd trimester) ▶? ©II $$$
ADULT — Moderate to severe pain: 1 tab PO q 6 h prn for no more than 7 days. Max dose 4 tabs/24 h.
PEDS — Moderate to severe pain for age 14 yo or older: Use adult dose.
FORMS — Generic only: Tabs 5 mg oxycodone/400 mg ibuprofen.
NOTES — For short-term (no more than 7 days) management of pain. See NSAIDs—Other subclass warning and individual components.
MOA — Combination analgesic.
ADVERSE EFFECTS — Serious: Respiratory depression/arrest, hypersensitivity, GI bleeding, nephrotoxicity. Frequent: N/V, constipation, dyspepsia, sedation.

EMPIRIN WITH CODEINE (acetylsalicylic acid + codeine, ✱ *292 tab*) ▶LK ♀D ▶– ©III $
WARNING — Multiple strengths; see FORMS and write specific product on Rx.
ADULT — Moderate pain: 1 to 2 tabs PO q 4 h prn.
PEDS — Not approved in children.
FORMS — Generic/Trade: No US formulation available. Tabs 325/30, 325/60 mg aspirin/mg codeine

FIORICET WITH CODEINE (acetaminophen + butalbital + caffeine + codeine) ▶LK ♀C ▶– ©III $$$
ADULT — Moderate pain: 1 to 2 caps PO q 4 h prn, max dose 6 caps/day.
PEDS — Not approved in children.
FORMS — Generic/Trade: Caps 325 mg acetaminophen/50 mg butalbital/40 mg caffeine/30 mg codeine.

FIORINAL WITH CODEINE (acetylsalicylic acid + butalbital + caffeine + codeine, ✱ *Fiorinal C-1/4, Fiorinal C-1/2, Trianal C-1/4, Trianal C-1/2*) ▶LK ♀ D ▶– ©III $$$
ADULT — Moderate pain: 1 to 2 caps PO q 4 h prn, max dose 6 caps/day.
PEDS — Not approved in children.
FORMS — Generic/Trade: Caps 325 mg aspirin/50 mg butalbital/40 mg caffeine/30 mg codeine.

IBUDONE REPREXAIN (hydrocodone + ibuprofen) ▶LK ♀– ▶? ©II $$
ADULT — Moderate pain: 1 tab PO q 4 to 6 h prn, max dose 5 tabs/day.
PEDS — Not approved in children.
FORMS — Generic/Trade: Tabs 2.5/200, 5/200, 10/200 mg hydrocodone/ibuprofen.
NOTES — See NSAIDs—Other subclass warning.
MOA — Combination analgesic.
ADVERSE EFFECTS — Serious: Respiratory depression/arrest, hypersensitivity, GI bleeding, nephrotoxicity. Frequent: N/V, constipation, dyspepsia, sedation.

LORCET (hydrocodone + acetaminophen) ▶LK ♀C ▶– ©II $$
WARNING — Multiple strengths; see FORMS and write specific product on Rx.
ADULT — Moderate pain: 1 to 2 caps (5/325) PO q 4 to 6 h prn, max dose 8 caps/day. 1 tab PO q 4 to 6 h prn (7.5/325 and 10/325), max dose 6 tabs/day.
PEDS — Not approved in children.
FORMS — Gene

LORTAB (hydrocodone + acetaminophen) ▶LK ♀C ▶– ©II $
WARNING — Multiple strengths; see FORMS and write specific product on Rx.
ADULT — Moderate pain: 1 to 2 tabs 2.5/325 and 5/325 PO q 4 to 6 h prn, max dose 8 tabs/day. 1 tab 7.5/325 and 10/325 PO q 4 to 6 h prn, max dose 5 tabs/day.
PEDS — Not approved in children.
FORMS — Generic/Trade: Lortab 5/325 (scored), Lortab 7.5/325 (trade scored), Lortab 10/325 mg hydrocodone/mg acetaminophen. Generic only: Tabs 2.5/325 mg.
MOA — Serious: Respiratory depression/arrest, hepatotoxicity. Frequent: N/V, constipation, sedation.
ADVERSE EFFECTS — TAB003

MERSYNDOL WITH CODEINE (acetaminophen + codeine + doxylamine) ▶LK ♀C ▶? $
ADULT — Canada only. Headaches, cold symptoms, muscle aches, neuralgia: 1 to 2 tabs PO q 4 to 6 h prn. Max 12 tabs/24 h.

(cont.)

MERSYNDOL WITH CODEINE (*cont.*)

PEDS — Not approved in children.

FORMS — Canada trade only: OTC tab 325 mg acetaminophen/8 mg codeine phosphate/5 mg doxylamine.

NOTES — May be habit-forming. Hepatotoxicity may be increased with acetaminophen overdose and may be enhanced with concomitant chronic alcohol ingestion.

MOA — Combination analgesic.

ADVERSE EFFECTS — See components.

NORCO (hydrocodone + acetaminophen) ▶L ♀C ▶? ©II $$

WARNING — Multiple strengths; see FORMS and write specific product on Rx.

ADULT — Moderate to severe pain: 1 to 2 tabs PO q 4 to 6 h prn (5/325), max dose 12 tabs/day. 1 tab (7.5/325 and 10/325) PO q 4 to 6 h prn, max dose 8 and 6 tabs/day, respectively.

PEDS — Not approved in children.

FORMS — Generic/Trade: Tabs 5/325, 7.5/325, 10/325 mg hydrocodone/acetaminophen, scored. Generic only: Soln 7.5/325 mg per 15 mL.

PERCOCET (oxycodone + acetaminophen, ✷ *Percocet-Demi, Oxycocet, Endocet*) ▶L ♀C ▶– ©II $

WARNING — Multiple strengths; see FORMS and write specific product on Rx.

ADULT — Moderate to severe pain: 1 to 2 tabs PO q 4 to 6 h prn (2.5/325 and 5/325 mg). 1 tab PO q 4 to 6 h prn (7.5/325 and 10/325 mg).

PEDS — Not approved in children.

FORMS — Generic/Trade: Oxycodone/acetaminophen tabs 2.5/325, 5/325, 7.5/325, 10/325 mg. Trade only: (Primlev) tabs 2.5/300, 5/300, 7.5/300, 10/300 mg. Generic only: 10/325 mg.

PERCODAN (oxycodone + **acetylsalicylic acid**, ✷ *Oxycodan*) ▶LK ♀D ▶– ©II $$

ADULT — Moderate to severe pain: 1 tab PO q 6 h prn.

PEDS — Not approved in children.

FORMS — Generic/Trade: Tabs 4.88/325 mg oxycodone/aspirin (trade scored).

ROXICET (oxycodone + acetaminophen) ▶L ♀C ▶– ©II $

WARNING — Multiple strengths; see FORMS and write specific product on Rx.

ADULT — Moderate to severe pain: 1 tab PO q 6 h prn. Oral soln: 5 mL PO q 6 h prn.

PEDS — Not approved in children.

FORMS — Generic/Trade: Tabs 5/325 mg. Caps/caplets 5/325 mg. Soln 5/325 per 5 mL, mg oxycodone/acetaminophen.

SOMA COMPOUND WITH CODEINE (carisoprodol + acetylsalicylic acid + codeine) ▶L ♀D ▶– ©III $$$$

ADULT — Moderate to severe musculoskeletal pain: 1 to 2 tabs PO four times per day prn.

PEDS — Not approved in children.

FORMS — Generic only: Tabs 200 mg carisoprodol/325 mg aspirin/16 mg codeine.

NOTES — Refer to individual components. Withdrawal with abrupt discontinuation.

MOA — Combination analgesic.

ADVERSE EFFECTS — Serious: Respiratory depression/arrest, hypersensitivity, Reye's syndrome, GI bleeding, nephrotoxicity, idiosyncratic reaction with angioedema, hypotension, and anaphylactoid shock. Frequent: N/V, dyspepsia, constipation, sedation.

SYNALGOS-DC (dihydrocodeine + acetylsalicylic acid + caffeine) ▶L ♀C ▶– ©III $$$

WARNING — Case reports of prolonged erections when taken concomitantly with sildenafil.

ADULT — Moderate to severe pain: 2 caps PO q 4 h prn.

PEDS — Not approved in children.

FORMS — Generic/Trade: Caps 16 mg dihydrocodeine/356.4 mg aspirin/30 mg caffeine.

NOTES — Most common use is dental pain. Refer to individual components.

MOA — Combination analgesic.

ADVERSE EFFECTS — Serious: Respiratory depression/arrest. Frequent: N/V, constipation, sedation.

TYLENOL WITH CODEINE (codeine + acetaminophen, ✷ *Tylenol #1, Tylenol #2, Tylenol #3, Tylenol #4, Atasol 8, Atasol 15, Atasol 30*) ▶LK ♀C ▶? ©III $

WARNING — Multiple strengths; see FORMS and write specific product on Rx.

ADULT — Moderate pain: 1 to 2 tabs PO q 4 h prn.

PEDS — Moderate pain: Elixir: Give 5 mL q 4 to 6 h prn for age 3 to 6 yo, give 10 mL q 4 to 6 h prn for age 7 to 12 yo, use adult dose for age older than 12 yo.

FORMS — Generic only: Tabs Tylenol #2 (15/300). Tylenol with Codeine Elixir/Susp/Soln 12/120 per 5 mL, mg codeine/mg acetaminophen. Generic/Trade: Tabs Tylenol #3 (30/300), Tylenol #4 (60/300).

VICODIN (hydrocodone + acetaminophen) ▶LK ♀C ▶? ©II $$$

WARNING — Multiple strengths; see FORMS and write specific product on Rx.

ADULT — Moderate pain: 5/300 mg (max dose 8 tabs/day) and 7.5/300 mg (max dose of 6 tabs/day): 1 to 2 tabs PO q 4 to 6 h prn. 10/300 mg: 1 tab PO q 4 to 6 h prn (max of 6 tabs/day).

PEDS — Not approved in children.

FORMS — Generic/Trade: Tabs Vicodin (5/300), Vicodin ES (7.5/300), Vicodin HP (10/300), mg hydrocodone/mg acetaminophen, scored.

VICOPROFEN (hydrocodone + ibuprofen) ▶LK ♀– ▶? ©II $$

ADULT — Moderate pain: 1 tab PO q 4 to 6 h prn, max dose 5 tabs/day.

PEDS — Not approved in children.

FORMS — Generic/Trade: Tabs 7.5/200 mg hydrocodone/ibuprofen. Generic only: Tabs 2.5/200, 5/200, 10/200 mg.

NOTES — See NSAIDs—Other subclass warning.

MOA — Combination analgesic.

ADVERSE EFFECTS — Serious: Respiratory depression/arrest, hypersensitivity, GI bleeding, nephrotoxicity. Frequent: N/V, constipation, dyspepsia, sedation.

XODOL (hydrocodone + acetaminophen) ▶LK ♀C ▶–
©II $$$
ADULT — Moderate pain: 1 tab PO q 4 to 6 h prn, max
6 doses/day.
PEDS — Not approved in children.

FORMS — Generic/Trade: Tabs 5/300, 7.5/300,
10/300 mg hydrocodone/acetaminophen.
MOA — Serious: Respiratory depression/arrest, hep-
atotoxicity. Frequent: N/V, constipation, sedation.
ADVERSE EFFECTS — TAB003

ANALGESICS: Opioid Antagonists

NOTE: May result in withdrawal in the opioid-dependent, including life-threatening withdrawal if administered to
neonates born to opioid-dependent mothers. Rare pulmonary edema, cardiovascular instability, hypotension, HTN,
ventricular tachycardia, and ventricular fibrillation have been reported in connection with opioid reversal.

NALOXONE (*Narcan, Evzio*) ▶LK ♀B ▶? $
ADULT — Management of opioid overdose: 0.4 to 2
mg IV. May repeat IV at 2 to 3 min intervals up to
10 mg. Use IM/SC/ET if IV not available. IV infu-
sion: 2 mg in 500 mL D5W or NS (0.004 mg/mL);
titrate according to response. Partial postop opioid
reversal: 0.1 to 0.2 mg IV at 2 to 3 min intervals;
repeat IM doses may be required at 1 to 2 h inter-
vals. Nasal spray dosage form: give 4 mg (1 spray)
every 2-3 minutes until patient responds or medical
assistance arrives.
PEDS — Management of opioid overdose: 0.01 mg/
kg IV. Give a subsequent dose of 0.1 mg/kg if inad-
equate response. Use IM/SC/ET if IV not available.
Partial postop opioid reversal: 0.005 to 0.01 mg IV
at 2 to 3 min intervals. Nasal spray dosage form:

give 4 mg (1 spray) every 2-3 min until patient
responds or medical assistance arrives.
FORMS — Trade only: solution for injection: 0.4 mg/
mL or 1 mg/mL 10 mL multiple-dose vials. Ampules
for injection: 0.02 mg/mL 2 mL ampule (box of 10),
0.4 mg/mL 1 mL ampule (box of 10), 1 mg/mL 2
mL ampule (box of 10). Nasal spray: 4 mg/0.1 mL,
two blister packages of one dose each. Autoinjector
(Evzio): 0.4 mg/injection, carton of 2.
NOTES — Watch patients for re-emergence of opioid
effects.
MOA — Opioid antagonist.
ADVERSE EFFECTS — Serious: Pulmonary edema,
cardiovascular instability, hypo/hypertension, ven-
tricular tachycardia and fibrillation, opioid with-
drawal. Frequent: Nausea and tachycardia.

ANALGESICS: Other Analgesics

ACETAMINOPHEN (*Tylenol, Panadol, Tempra, Ofirmev,
paracetamol, ✽Abenol, Atasol, Pediatrix*) ▶LK ♀B
▶+ $
ADULT — Analgesic/antipyretic: 325 to 1000 mg PO q
4 to 6 h prn. 650 mg PR q 4 to 6 h prn. Max dose 4 g/
day. OA: Extended-release: 2 caps PO q 8 h around
the clock. Max dose 6 caps/day.
PEDS — Analgesic/antipyretic: 10 to 15 mg/kg q 4 to
6 h PO/PR prn. Max 5 doses/day.
UNAPPROVED ADULT — OA: 1000 mg PO four times
per day.
FORMS — OTC: Tabs 325, 500, 650 mg. Chewable
tabs 80 mg. Orally disintegrating tabs 80, 160 mg.
Caps/gelcaps 500 mg. Extended-release caplets
650 mg. Liquid 160 mg/5 mL, 500 mg/15 mL. Supps
80, 120, 325, 650 mg.
NOTES — Risk of hepatotoxicity with chronic use,
especially in alcoholics. Caution in those who drink
three or more drinks/day. Rectal administration may
produce lower/less reliable plasma levels.
MOA — Analgesic/antipyretic.
ADVERSE EFFECTS — Serious: Hepatotoxicity.
Frequent: None.
CANNIBIS SATIVA L. EXTRACT (✽*Sativex*) ▶LK ♀X
▶– $$$$
ADULT — Canada only. Adjunctive treatment for the
symptomatic relief of neuropathic pain in multiple
sclerosis: Start 1 spray q 4 h (max four times per
day), and titrate upward as tolerated. Limited expe-
rience with more than 12 sprays/day.
PEDS — Not approved in children.

FORMS — Canada Trade only: Buccal spray, 27 mg/
mL delta-9-tetrahydrocannabinol and 25 mg/mL
cannabidiol, delivers 100 mcL per actuation; 5.5
mL vials containing up to 51 actuations per vial.
NOTES — Contraindicated in pregnancy, childbear-
ing potential without birth control, history of psy-
chosis, serious heart disease. Contains ethanol.
Use cautiously if history of substance abuse.
MOA — Acts at cannabinoid receptors in the CNS and
peripheral tissues to mediate cannabinoid-induced
analgesia.
ADVERSE EFFECTS — Serious: orthostatic hypoten-
sion, syncope. Frequent: Administration site irrita-
tion, headache, depression, dizziness.
CLONIDINE—EPIDURAL (*Duraclon*) ▶LK ♀C ▶– $$$$$
WARNING — Not recommended for obstetrical, post-
partum, or perioperative pain management due to
hypotension and bradycardia. Abrupt discontinua-
tion may result in a rapid BP rise.
ADULT — Severe cancer pain in combination with
opioids: Specialized epidural dosing.
PEDS — Severe cancer pain in combination with opi-
oids: Specialized epidural dosing.
NOTES — Bradycardia and hypotension common.
May be exacerbated by beta-blockers, certain cal-
cium channel blockers, and digoxin.
MOA — Central analgesic - prevents pain signal
transmission to the brain.
ADVERSE EFFECTS — Serious: Bradycardia, hypoten-
sion. Frequent: Hypotension, sedation, dry mouth.

MIDOL TEEN FORMULA (acetaminophen + pamabrom)
▶LK ♀B ▶+ $
ADULT — Menstrual cramps: 2 caps PO q 4 to 6 h.
PEDS — Use adult dose for age older than 12 yo.
FORMS — Generic/Trade OTC: Caps 325 mg acetaminophen/25 mg pamabrom (diuretic).
NOTES — Hepatotoxicity with chronic use, especially in alcoholics.
MOA — Analgesic/diuretic.
ADVERSE EFFECTS — Serious: Hepatotoxicity. Frequent: None.

TAPENTADOL (*Nucynta, Nucynta ER*) ▶LK ♀C ▶– ©II $$$$
WARNING — Abuse potential.
ADULT — Moderate to severe acute pain: Immediate-release: 50 to 100 mg PO q 4 to 6 h prn. Max dose 600 mg/day. If moderate hepatic impairment, decrease dose to 50 mg PO q 8 h. Moderate to severe chronic pain: Extended-release: 50 to 250 mg PO twice daily. Start at 50 mg PO twice daily if patient not currently taking opioids. Do not use in severe renal or hepatic impairment.
PEDS — Not approved in children younger than 18 yo.
FORMS — Trade only: Immediate-release ($$$$): Tabs 50, 75, 100 mg. Extended-release ($$$$$): Tabs 50, 100, 150, 200, 250 mg.
NOTES — When switching from immediate-release to extended-release form, use same total daily dose. Contraindicated in acute intoxication with alcohol, hypnotics, centrally acting analgesics, opioids, or psychotropic drugs and with respiratory depression. Use with caution in patients with known seizure disorders. Seizures and/or serotonin syndrome may occur with concurrent antidepressants, triptans, linezolid, lithium, St. John's wort.
MOA — Opioid agonist/norepinephrine reuptake inhibitor.
ADVERSE EFFECTS — Serious: Seizures, anaphylactoid reactions, respiratory depression. Frequent: Nausea, dizziness, vomiting, somnolence.

TRAMADOL (*Ultram, Ultram ER, Ryzolt, ConZip, Rybix ODT,* ✲*Zytram XL, Tridural, Ralivia, Durela*) ▶KL ♀C ▶– ©IV $$$
ADULT — Moderate to moderately severe pain: 50 to 100 mg PO q 4 to 6 h prn. Max dose 400 mg/day. If older than 75 yo, use less than 300 mg/day PO in divided doses. If CrCl <30 mL/min, increase the dosing interval to 12 h. If cirrhosis, decrease dose

to 50 mg PO q 12 h. Chronic pain, extended-release: 100 to 300 mg PO daily. Do not use if CrCl <30 mL/min or with severe hepatic dysfunction.
PEDS — Not approved in children younger than 16 yo.
FORMS — Generic/Trade: Tabs, immediate-release 50 mg. Extended-release tabs 100, 200, 300 mg. Trade only: (ConZip) Extended-release caps 100, 150, 200, 300 mg. (Rybix) ODT 50 mg.
NOTES — Contraindicated in acute intoxication with alcohol, hypnotics, centrally acting analgesics, opioids, or psychotropic drugs. Seizures and/or serotonin syndrome may occur with concurrent antidepressants, triptans, linezolid, lithium, St. John's wort, or enzyme-inducing drugs such as ketoconazole and erythromycin; use with caution and adjust dose. Withdrawal symptoms may occur in patients dependent on opioids or with abrupt discontinuation. Overdose treated with naloxone may increase seizures. Carbamazepine decreases tramadol levels. The most frequent side effects are nausea and constipation. ER tabs cannot be crushed, chewed, or split.
MOA — Opioid agonist/norepinephrine and serotonin reuptake inhibitor.
ADVERSE EFFECTS — Serious: Seizures, anaphylactoid reactions. Frequent: Constipation, nausea, somnolence.

ZICONOTIDE (*Prialt*) ▶Plasma ♀C ▶? $$$$$
WARNING — Severe psychiatric and neurologic impairment may occur. Monitor for mood changes, hallucinations, or cognitive changes. Contraindicated if history of psychosis.
ADULT — Severe intractable chronic pain: Specialized intrathecal dosing.
PEDS — Not approved in children younger than 16 yo.
NOTES — Contraindicated in patients with history of psychosis, uncontrolled bleeding, spinal canal obstruction or infection at the infusion site. Does not prevent opioid withdrawal; gradually taper while instituting ziconotide therapy. Monitor CK periodically.
MOA — Blocks N-type calcium channels on nociceptive afferent nerves.
ADVERSE EFFECTS — Serious: Hallucinations, cognitive impairment, meningitis, myopathy, rhabdomyolysis and renal failure. Frequent: Dizziness, nausea, confusion, headache, somnolence, nystagmus, asthenia, pain, increased serum CK levels.

ANESTHESIA

ANESTHESIA: Anesthetics and Sedatives

ALFENTANIL (*Alfenta*) ▶L ♀C ▶? ©II $

WARNING — Titrate according to lean body weight, physical status, underlying pathological condition, use of other drugs, and type/duration of surgical procedure and anesthesia.

ADULT — For analgesia during general anesthesia: with spontaneous breathing/assisted ventilation:Induction of analgesia: 8 to 20 mcg/kg; maintenance: 3 to 5 mcg/kg every 5 to 20 min or 0.5 to 1 mcg/kg/min (total dose up to 8 to 40 mcg/kg), with assisted or controlled ventilation by incremental injection: Induction of analgesia: 20 to 50 mcg/kg; maintenance: 5 to 15 mcg/kg every 5 to 20 min (total dose up to 75 mcg/kg), with assisted or controlled ventilation with continuous infusion: Induction of analgesia: 50 to 75 mcg/kg; maintenance 0.5 to 3 mcg/kg/min (average rate 1 to 1.5 mcg/kg/min) with nitrous oxide/oxygen (total dose depends on duration). Induction of general anesthesia: Induction: 130 to 245 mcg/kg; maintenance: 0.5 to 1.5 mcg/kg/min or use general anesthetic (total dose depends on duration). Monitored anesthesia care: Induction: 3 to 8 mcg/kg; maintenance: 3 to 5 mcg/kg every 5 to 20 min or 0.25 to 1 mcg/kg/min (total dose: 3 to 40 mcg/kg)

PEDS — Not approved in children younger than 12 yo.

UNAPPROVED ADULT — General anesthesia greater than 45 minutes: Induction: 130 to 245 mcg/kg IV once; maintenance: 0.5 to 1.5 mcg/kg/min. General anesthesia continuous infusion greater than 45 minutes: Induction: 50-75 mcg/kg; maintenance: 0.5 to 3 mcg/kg/min. General anesthesia adjunct incremental injection less than 30 minutes: Induction: 3 to 5 mcg/kg every 5 to 20 minutes; maintenance: 0.5-1 mcg/kg/min. General anesthesia incremental injection 30-60 minutes duration: Induction: 5 to 15 mcg/kg every 5 to 20 minutes; maintenance: 5 to 15 mcg/kg every 5-20 minutes. Monitored anesthesia care adjunct: 3 to 5 mcg/kg every 5 to 20 minutes. Conscious sedation: 5 to 7 mcg/kg bolus followed by 2 to 3 mcg/kg doses every 10 to 15min

MOA — Mu opioid receptor agonist

ADVERSE EFFECTS — Serious: Respiratory depression, hypotension, bradycardia, chest wall rigidity, increased intracranial pressure, opiate dependence, hypersensitivity. Frequent: Sedation, N/V.

DESFLURANE (*Suprane*) ▶Respiratory ♀B ▶+ Varies

ADULT — General anesthetic gas: Specialized dosing.

PEDS — Not recommended for induction due to high rate of laryngospasm.

NOTES — Minimum alveolar concentration (MAC) 6.0%. Known trigger of malignant hyperthermia; see www.mhaus.org.

MOA — CNS depressant

ADVERSE EFFECTS — Serious: Apnea, malignant hyperthermia. Frequent: Recovery N/V.

DEXMEDETOMIDINE (*Precedex*) ▶LK ♀C ▶? $$$$$

ADULT — ICU sedation less than 24 h: Load 1 mcg/kg over 10 min followed by infusion 0.6 mcg/kg/h (ranges from 0.2 to 1.0 mcg/kg/h) titrated to desired sedation endpoint. Procedural sedation: Load 1 mcg/kg over 10 min followed by infusion of 0.6 mcg/kg/h titrated up or down to clinical effect in range of 0.2 to 1 mcg/kg/h depending on procedure and patient (0.7 mcg/kg/h for fiberoptic intubation). Reduce dose in impaired hepatic function and geriatric patients.

PEDS — Not recommended age younger than 18 yo.

NOTES — Alpha-2-adrenergic agonist with sedative properties. Beware of bradycardia and hypotension. Avoid in advanced heart block.

MOA — Alpha-2 adrenergic agonist with sedative properties.

ADVERSE EFFECTS — Serious: Bradycardia, heart block, hypotension. Frequent: Sedation.

ETOMIDATE (*Amidate*) ▶L ♀C ▶? $

ADULT — Anesthesia induction/rapid-sequence intubation: 0.3 to 0.6 mg/kg IV.

PEDS — Age younger than 10 yo: Not approved. Age 10 yo or older: Use adult dosing.

UNAPPROVED PEDS — Anesthesia induction/rapid-sequence intubation: 0.3 mg/kg IV.

NOTES — Adrenocortical suppression, but rarely of clinical significance.

MOA — Nonbarbiturate hypnotic without analgesic properties.

ADVERSE EFFECTS — Serious: Respiratory depression, hypotension, adrenal suppression. Frequent: Myoclonus, N/V.

ISOFLURANE (*Forane*) ▶Respiratory ♀C ▶? Varies

ADULT — General anesthetic gas: Specialized dosing.

PEDS — General anesthetic gas: Specialized dosing.

NOTES — Minimum alveolar concentration (MAC) 1.15%. Known trigger of malignant hyperthermia; see www.mhaus.org.

MOA — CNS depressant

ADVERSE EFFECTS — Serious: Apnea, malignant hyperthermia. Frequent: Recovery N/V.

KETAMINE (*Ketalar*) ▶L ♀C ▶? ©III $

WARNING — Postanesthetic emergence reactions up to 24 h later manifested as dreamlike state, vivid imagery, hallucinations, and delirium reported in about 12% of cases. Incidence reduced when (1) age less than 15 yo or greater than 65 yo, (2) concomitant use of benzodiazepines, lower dose, or used as induction agent only (because of use of post-intubation sedation).

ADULT — Induction of anesthesia: Adult: 1 to 2 mg/kg IV over 1 to 2 min (produces 5 to 10 min dissociative state) or 6.5 to 13 mg/kg IM (produces 10 to 20 min dissociative state).

PEDS — Age over 16 yo: same as adult.

(cont.)

KETAMINE (cont.)

UNAPPROVED ADULT — Dissociative sedation: 1 to 2 mg/kg IV over 1-2 min (sedation lasting 10-20 min) repeat 0.5 mg/kg doses every 5 to 15 min may be given; 4 to 5 mg/kg IM (sedation lasting 15-30 min) repeat 2-4 mg/kg IM can be given if needed after 10 to 15 min. Analgesia adjunct subdissociative dose: 0.01 to 0.5 mg/kg in conjunction with opioid analgesia.

UNAPPROVED PEDS — Dissociative sedation: Age older than 3 mo: 1 to 2 mg/kg IV (produces 5 to 10 min dissociative state) over 1 to 2 min or 4 to 5 mg/kg IM (produces 10 to 20 min dissociative state). Not approved for age younger than 3 mo.

FORMS — Generic/Trade: 10, 50, 100 mg/mL.

NOTES — Recent evidence suggests ketamine is not contraindicated in patients with head injuries. However, avoid if CAD or severe HTN. Concurrent administration of atropine no longer recommended. Consider prohylactic ondansetron to reduce vomiting and prophylactic midazolam (0.3 mg/kg) to reduce recovery reactions.

MOA — NMDA receptor antagonist which produces dissociative state.

ADVERSE EFFECTS — Serious: Laryngospasm, hallucinatory emergence reactions, hypersalivation. Frequent: Nystagmus, hypertension, tachycardia, N/V, muscular hypertonicity, myoclonus.

METHOHEXITAL (Brevital) ▶L ♀B ▶? ©IV $$

ADULT — Anesthesia induction: 1 to 2.0 mg/kg IV, duration 5 min, followed by 0.25-1 mg/kg IV every 4-7 min prn.

PEDS — Anesthesia induction: 6.6 to 10 mg/kg IM or 25 mg/kg PR.

UNAPPROVED PEDS — Sedation for diagnostic imaging: 25 mg/kg PR.

MOA — Serious: Respiratory depression, hypotension, bronchospasm. Frequent: Respiratory depression, hypotension.

MIDAZOLAM (Versed) ▶LK ♀D ▶– ©IV $

WARNING — Beware of respiratory depression/apnea. Administer with appropriate monitoring.

ADULT — Sedation/anxiolysis: 0.07 to 0.08 mg/kg IM (5 mg in average adult); or 1 mg IV slowly q 2 to 3 min up to 5 mg. Anesthesia induction: 0.3 to 0.35 mg/kg IV over 20 to 30 sec.

PEDS — Sedation/anxiolysis: Oral route 0.25 to 1 mg/kg (0.5 mg/kg most effective) to max 20 mg PO, IM route 0.1 to 0.15 mg/kg IM. IV route initial dose 0.05 to 0.1 mg/kg IV, then titrated to max 0.6 mg/kg for age 6 mo to 5 yo, initial dose 0.025 to 0.05 mg/kg IV, then titrated to max 0.4 mg/kg for age 6 to 12 yo.

UNAPPROVED PEDS — Sedation/anxiolysis: Intranasal 0.2 to 0.4 mg/kg. Rectal: 0.25 to 0.5 mg/kg PR. Status epilepticus: Load 0.15 mg/kg IV followed by infusion 1 mcg/kg/min and titrate dose upward q 5 min prn.

FORMS — Generic only: Injection 1 mg/mL, 5 mg/mL. Oral liquid 2 mg/mL.

NOTES — Use lower doses in the elderly, chronically ill, and those receiving concurrent CNS depressants.

MOA — Short-acting benzodiazepine sedative.

ADVERSE EFFECTS — Serious: Respiratory depression. Frequent: Sedation.

NITROUS OXIDE (Entonox) ▶Respiratory ♀– ▶? Varies

ADULT — General anesthetic gas: Specialized dosing.

PEDS — General anesthetic gas: Specialized dosing.

NOTES — Always maintain at least 20% oxygen administration.

MOA — CNS depressant

ADVERSE EFFECTS — Serious: Apnea, malignant hyperthermia, pressure accumulation (middle ear, bowel obstruction, pneumothorax), abuse dependence. Frequent: Recovery N/V.

PENTOBARBITAL (Nembutal) ▶LK ♀D ▶? ©II $$$$$

ADULT — Rarely used; other drugs preferred. Hypnotic: 150 to 200 mg IM or 100 mg IV at a rate of 50 mg/min, max dose is 500 mg.

PEDS — FDA approved for active seizing, but other agents preferred.

UNAPPROVED PEDS — Procedural sedation: 1 to 6 mg/kg IV, adjusted in increments of 1 to 2 mg/kg to desired effect, or 2 to 6 mg/kg IM, max 100 mg. Do not exceed 50 mg/min.

MOA — Serious: Respiratory depression, blood dyscrasias, anemia, thrombocytopenia, Stevens-Johnson syndrome, angioedema, dependence, withdrawal reactions. Frequent: Drowsiness, fatigue, N/V bradycardia, paradoxical CNS excitation.

PROPOFOL (Diprivan) ▶L ♀B ▶– $

WARNING — Beware of respiratory depression/apnea. Administer with appropriate monitoring.

ADULT — Anesthesia (age younger than 55 yo): 40 mg IV q 10 sec until induction onset (typical 2 to 2.5 mg/kg). Follow with maintenance infusion generally 100 to 200 mcg/kg/min. Lower doses in elderly or for sedation. ICU ventilator sedation: Infusion 5 to 50 mcg/kg/min.

PEDS — Anesthesia age 3 yo or older: 2.5 to 3.5 mg/kg IV over 20 to 30 sec, followed with infusion 125 to 300 mcg/kg/min. Not recommended if age younger than 3 yo or for prolonged ICU use.

UNAPPROVED ADULT — Deep sedation: 1 mg/kg IV over 20 to 30 sec. Repeat 0.5 mg/kg IV prn. Intubation adjunct: 2.0 to 2.5 mg/kg IV.

UNAPPROVED PEDS — Deep sedation: 1 mg/kg IV (max 40 mg) over 20 to 30 sec. Repeat 0.5 mg/kg (max 20 mg) IV prn.

NOTES — Avoid with egg or soy allergies. Prolonged infusions may lead to hypertriglyceridemia. Injection pain can be treated or pretreated with lidocaine 40 to 50 mg IV.

MOA — Nonbarbiturate hypnotic without analgesic properties.

ADVERSE EFFECTS — Serious: Respiratory depression, hypotension, hypersensitivity. Frequent: Injection site pain, sedation.

REMIFENTANIL (Ultiva) ▶L ♀C ▶? ©II $$

ADULT — General anesthesia: Induction: 0.5 to 1 mcg/kg/min; maintenance 0.05 to 2 mcg/kg/min. Monitored Anesthesia Care Single Dose: 1 mcg/kg over 30-60 seconds; maintenance: 0.025 to 0.2 mcg/kg/min.

(cont.)

REMIFENTANIL (*cont.*)

PEDS — General Anesthesia Maintenance: (with concurrent inhaled agent administration): 0.05 to 1.3 mcg/kg/min.

MOA — Serious: Respiratory depression, hypotension, bradycardia, chest wall rigidity, opiate dependence, hypersensitivity. Frequent: Sedation, N/V.

SEVOFLURANE (*Ultane, ✽Sevorane*) ▶Respiratory/L ♀ B ▶? Varies

ADULT — General anesthetic gas: Specialized dosing.

PEDS — General anesthetic gas: Specialized dosing.

NOTES — Minimum alveolar concentration (MAC) 2.05%. Known trigger of malignant hyperthermia; see www.mhaus.org.

MOA — CNS depressant

ADVERSE EFFECTS — Serious: Apnea, malignant hyperthermia. Frequent: Recovery N/V.

SUFENTANIL (*Sufenta*) ▶L ♀C ▶? ©ll $$

ADULT — General anesthesia: Induction: 8 to 30 mcg/kg IV; maintenance 0.5 to 10 mcg/kg IV. Conscious sedation: Loading dose: 0.1 to 0.5 mcg/kg; maintenance infusion 0.005 to 0.01 mcg/kg/min

PEDS — General anesthesia: Induction: 8 to 30 mcg/kg IV; maintenance 0.5 to 10 mcg/kg IV. Conscious sedation: Loading dose: 0.1 to 0.5 mcg/kg; maintenance infusion 0.005 to 0.01 mcg/kg/min.

MOA — Serious: Respiratory depression, hypotension, bradycardia, chest wall rigidity, opiate dependence, hypersensitivity. Frequent: Sedation, N/V.

ANESTHESIA: Local Anesthetics

NOTE: Risk of chondrolysis in patients receiving intra-articular infusions of local anesthetics following arthroscopic and other surgical procedures.

ARTICAINE (*Septocaine, Zorcaine*) ▶LK ♀C ▶? $

ADULT — Dental local anesthesia: 4% injection up to 7 mg/kg total dose.

PEDS — Dental local anesthesia age 4 yo or older: 4% injection up to 7 mg/kg total dose.

FORMS — 4% (includes epinephrine 1:100,000).

NOTES — Do not exceed 7 mg/kg total dose.

MOA — Amide local anesthetic.

ADVERSE EFFECTS — Serious: Seizures, cardiovascular depression, bradycardia, hypersensitivity, methemoglobinemia. Frequent: None.

BUPIVACAINE (*Marcaine, Sensorcaine*) ▶LK ♀C ▶? $

ADULT — Local anesthesia, nerve block: 0.25% injection. Up to 2.5 mg/kg without epinephrine and up 3.0 mg/kg with epinephrine.

PEDS — Not recommended in children younger than 12 yo.

FORMS — 0.25%, 0.5%, 0.75%, all with or without epinephrine.

NOTES — Onset 5 min, duration 2 to 4 h (longer with epi). Amide group.

MOA — Amide local anesthetic.

ADVERSE EFFECTS — Serious: Seizures, cardiovascular depression, bradycardia, hypersensitivity, methemoglobinemia. Frequent: None.

BUPIVACAINE LIPOSOME (*Exparel*) ▶L– - ♀C ▶– $$$$$

ADULT — Bunionectomy: Infiltrate 7 mL of Exparel into the tissues surrounding the osteotomy and 1 mL into the subcutaneous tissue for a total of 8 mL (106 mg). Hemorrhoidectomy: Dilute 20 mL (266 mg) of Exparel with 10 mL of saline, for a total of 30 mL, and divide the mixture into six 5 mL aliquots. Perform the anal block by visualizing the anal sphincter as a clock face and slowly infiltrating one aliquot to each of the even numbers. Do not inject other local anesthetics into the same site or inject through wet antiseptic on the skin. Dosing forms do not have pharmacologic bioequivalence to plain bupivacaine.

PEDS — Not approved for use age younger than 18 yo.

FORMS — 10, 20 mL single-use vial, 1.3% (13.3 mg/mL).

MOA — Suspension of multivesicular liposomes containing bupivacaine that provides up to 72 hours of pain control.

ADVERSE EFFECTS — Significant systemic absorption with CNS and cardiovascular effects. Hypersensitivity. Intra-articular injections have resulted in chondrolysis. Caution for increase drug effect in hepatic and/or renal impairment as it is metabolized by the liver and cleared by the kidneys.

CHLOROPROCAINE (*Nesacaine*) ▶LK ♀C ▶? $

ADULT — Epidural anesthesia: 2.0-3.0% 18-24 mL will provide 30-60 min of surgical anesthesia. Infiltration and peripheral nerve block: 0.5-40 mL of 1%-3% chloroprocaine.

PEDS — Same as adult, age3 yo or older.

FORMS — 1, 2, 3%.

NOTES — Max local dose: 11 mg/kg.

MOA — Ester local anesthetic

ADVERSE EFFECTS — Serious: Seizures, cardiovascular depression, bradycardia, hypersensitivity, methemoglobinemia. Frequent: None.

***EMLA* (prilocaine—topical + lidocaine—topical)** ▶LK ♀B ▶? $$

ADULT — Topical anesthesia for minor dermal procedures (eg, IV cannulation, venipuncture): Apply 2.5 g over 20 to 25 cm² area or 1 disc at least 1 h prior to procedure; for major dermal procedures (ie, skin grafting/harvesting), apply 2 g/10 cm² area at least 2 h prior to procedure.

PEDS — Prior to circumcision in infants older than 37 weeks' gestation: Apply a max dose 1 g over max of 10 cm². Topical anesthesia: Children age 1 to 3 mo or less than 5 kg: Apply a max 1 g dose over max of 10 cm²; age 4 to 12 mo and more than 5 kg: Apply max 2 g dose over a max of 20 cm². Age 1 to 6 yo and more than 10 kg: Apply max dose 10 g over max of

(cont.)

EMLA (*cont.*)

100 cm². Age 7 to 12 yo and more than 20 kg: Apply max dose 20 g over max of 200 cm².

FORMS — Generic/Trade: Cream (2.5% lidocaine + 2.5% prilocaine) 5, 30 g.

NOTES — Cover cream with an occlusive dressing. Do not use in children younger than 12 mo if child is receiving treatment with methemoglobin-inducing agents. Do not use on open wounds. Patients with glucose-6-phosphate deficiencies are more susceptible to methemoglobinemia. Use caution with amiodarone, bretylium, sotalol, dofetilide; possible additive cardiac effects. Dermal analgesia increases for up to 3 h under occlusive dressings and persists for 1 to 2 h after removal.

MOA — Anesthetic.

ADVERSE EFFECTS — Frequent: None. Severe: CNS effects, tachycardia, bronchospasm, hypotension.

LIDOCAINE—LOCAL ANESTHETIC (*Xylocaine*) ▶LK ♀B ▶? $

ADULT — Without epinephrine: Max dose 4.5 mg/kg not to exceed 300 mg. With epinephrine: Max dose 7 mg/kg not to exceed 500 mg. Dose for regional block varies by region.

PEDS — Same as adult.

FORMS — 0.5, 1, 1.5, 2%. With epi: 0.5, 1, 1.5, 2%.

NOTES — Onset within 2 min, duration 30 to 60 min (longer with epi). Amide group. Use "cardiac lidocaine" (ie, IV formulation) for Bier blocks at max dose of 3 mg/kg so that neither epinephrine nor methylparaben are injected IV.

MOA — Amide local anesthetic.

ADVERSE EFFECTS — Serious: Seizures, cardiovascular depression, bradycardia, hypersensitivity, methemoglobinemia. Frequent: None.

MEPIVACAINE (*Carbocaine, Polocaine*) ▶LK ♀C ▶? $

ADULT — Nerve block: 1 to 2% injection. Onset 3 to 5 min, duration 45 to 90 min. Amide group. Max local dose 5 to 6 mg/kg.

PEDS — Nerve block: 1 to 2% injection. Use less than 2% concentration if age younger than 3 yo or wt less than 30 pounds. Max local dose 5 to 6 mg/kg.

FORMS — 1, 1.5, 2, 3%.

NOTES — Onset 3 to 5 min, duration 45 to 90 min. Amide group. Max local dose 5 to 6 mg/kg.

MOA — Amide local anesthetic.

ADVERSE EFFECTS — Serious: Seizures, cardiovascular depression, bradycardia, hypersensitivity, methemoglobinemia, nephrotoxicity. Frequent: None.

Oraqix (prilocaine + lidocaine—local anesthetic) ▶LK ♀B ▶? $

ADULT — Local anesthetic gel applied to periodontal pockets using blunt-tipped applicator: 4% injection. The maximum recommended dose of Oraqix at one treatment session is 5 cartridges, i.e., 8.5 g gel. Must be used with special blunt-tipped applicator.

PEDS — Not approved in children.

FORMS — Gel 2.5% + 2.5% with applicator.

NOTES — Do not exceed max dose for lidocaine or prilocaine.

MOA — Amide local anesthetic combination.

ADVERSE EFFECTS — Serious: Seizures, cardiovascular depression, bradycardia, hypersensitivity, methemoglobinemia. Frequent: None.

PRILOCAINE (*Citanest*) ▶LK ♀B ▶? $

ADULT — Nerve block and dental procedures: 4% injection. Maximum local dose is 5 mg/kg without epinephrine and 7 mg/kg with epinephrine.

PEDS — Nerve block and dental procedures, age older than 9 mo: 4% injection. If younger than 5 yo, maximum local dose is 3 to 4 mg/kg (with or without epinephrine). If 5 yo or older, maximum local dose is 5 mg/kg without epinephrine and 7 mg/kg with epinephrine.

FORMS — 4%, 4% with epinephrine.

NOTES — Contraindicated if younger than 6 to 9 mo. If younger than 5 yo, max local dose is 3 to 4 mg/kg (with or without epinephrine). If 5 yo or older, max local dose is 5 mg/kg without epinephrine and 7 mg/kg with epinephrine.

MOA — Amide local anesthetic

ADVERSE EFFECTS — Serious: Seizures, cardiovascular depression, bradycardia, hypersensitivity, methemoglobinemia. Frequent: None.

PROCAINE (*Novocain*) ▶Plasma ♀C ▶? $

ADULT — Local and regional anesthesia: 1 to 2% injection. Spinal anesthesia: 10%.

PEDS — Local and regional anesthesia: 1 to 2% injection. Spinal anesthesia: 10%.

FORMS — 1, 2, 10%.

NOTES — Trade name is included only for reference; Novocaine brand was discontinued.

MOA — Ester local anesthetic

ADVERSE EFFECTS — Serious: Seizures, cardiovascular depression, bradycardia, hypersensitivity, methemoglobinemia. Frequent: None.

ROPIVACAINE (*Naropin*) ▶LK ♀B ▶? $

WARNING — Inadvertent intravascular injection may result in arrhythmia or cardiac arrest.

ADULT — Local and regional anesthesia: 0.2 to 1% injection.

PEDS — Not approved in children.

FORMS — 0.2, 0.5, 0.75, 1%.

MOA — Amide local anesthetic

ADVERSE EFFECTS — Serious: Seizures, cardiovascular depression, bradycardia, hypersensitivity, methemoglobinemia. Frequent: None.

TETRACAINE (*Pontocaine*, ✢*amethocaine*) ▶Plasma ♀C ▶? $

ADULT — Spinal anesthesia.

PEDS — Not approved in children.

FORMS — Injection: 1%.

MOA — Ester local anesthetic

ADVERSE EFFECTS — Serious: Seizures, cardiovascular depression, bradycardia, hypersensitivity, methemoglobinemia. Frequent: None.

ANESTHESIA: Neuromuscular Blockade Reversal Agents

NOTE: Should be administered only by those skilled in airway management and respiratory support

NEOSTIGMINE (*Bloxiverz*) ▶L ♀C ▶? $$$$
ADULT — Reversal of nondepolarizing neuromuscular blocking agents: 0.03 to 0.07 mg/kg slow IV (preceded by atropine or glycopyrrolate). Max 0.07 mg/kg or 5 mg, whichever is less.
PEDS — Reversal of nondepolarizing neuromuscular blocking agents: Use adult dosing.
MOA — Reversible cholinesterase inhibitor.
ADVERSE EFFECTS — Serious: Cholinergic toxicity, respiratory paralysis, bronchospasm, arrhythmias, cardiac arrest, seizures. Frequent: N/V, diarrhea, abdominal cramping, dizziness, headache, muscle cramps/weakness, fasciculations, hypersalivation, increased bronchial secretions, miosis.

SUGAMMEDEX (*Bridion*) ▶ renal excretion of unchanged drug ♀ 0/0/0 no data on pregnant women but no evidence of teratogenecity in animals; reduced efficacy of hormonal contraceptives for one week after administration ▶? $$$$$
WARNING — Anyphylaxis with hypotension requiring pressors and bradycardia resuting in cardiac arrest have been reported.

ADULT — Rapid reversal of rocuronium (within 3 minutes): 16 mg/kg reverses a single dose of 1.2 mg/kg of rocuronium. Reversal of rocuronium and vecuronium: 4 mg/kg is recommended if spontaneous recovery of the twitch response has reached 1 to 2 post-tetanic counts (PTC) and there are no twitch responses to train-of-four (TOF) stimulation. 2 mg/kg is recommended if spontaneous recovery has reached the reappearance of the second twitch in response to TOF stimulation.
PEDS — Not approved for use age less than 18 yo.
MOA — Forms a complex with the neuromuscular blocking agents rocuronium and vecuronium and reduces the amount of neuromuscular blocking agent available to bind to nicotinic cholinergic receptors in the neuromuscular junction
ADVERSE EFFECTS — Serious: anaphylaxis, bradycardia, hypotension, and cardiac arrest. Common: hypotension, nausea, pruritis, and urticaria
SIDE EFFECTS — Increase in coagulation parameters.

ANESTHESIA: Neuromuscular Blockers

NOTE: Should be administered only by those skilled in airway management and respiratory support.

ATRACURIUM (*Tracrium*) ▶Plasma ♀C ▶? $
ADULT — Neuromuscular blockade: induction 0.4 to 0.5 mg/kg IV; maintenance 0.08 to 0.1 mg/kg every 15 to 25 min prn.
PEDS — Paralysis age 2 yo or older same as adult dose.
NOTES — Duration 15 to 30 min. Hoffman degradation.
MOA — Nondepolarizing skeletal muscle relaxant.
ADVERSE EFFECTS — Serious: Apnea, bronchospasm, hypersensitivity. Frequent: Apnea, rash.

CISATRACURIUM (*Nimbex*) ▶Plasma ♀B ▶? $
ADULT — Paralysis: Induction 0.15 to 0.2 mg/kg IV; maintenance 0.03 mg/kg IV every 20 min prn.
PEDS — Paralysis: Induction 0.1 mg/kg IV over 5 to 10 sec; maintenance 0.03 mg/kg IV every 20 min prn.
NOTES — Duration 30 to 60 min. Hoffman degradation.
MOA — Nondepolarizing skeletal muscle relaxant.
ADVERSE EFFECTS — Serious: Apnea, bradycardia, bronchospasm. Frequent: Apnea.

PANCURONIUM (*Pavulon*) ▶LK ♀C ▶? $
ADULT — Paralysis: 0.04 to 0.1 mg/kg IV.
PEDS — Paralysis (beyond neonatal age): 0.04 to 0.1 mg/kg IV.
NOTES — Duration 45 min. Decrease dose if renal disease.

MOA — Nondepolarizing skeletal muscle relaxant.
ADVERSE EFFECTS — Serious: Apnea, hypersensitivity, bronchospasm. Frequent: Apnea, tachycardia.

ROCURONIUM (*Zemuron*) ▶L ♀B ▶? $$
ADULT — Rapid-sequence intubation: 0.6 to 1.2 mg/kg IV. Paralysis: induction: 0.6 mg/kg IV; maintenance: 0.1 to 0.2 mg/kg IV prn. Continuous infusion: 10 to 12 mcg/kg/min; first verify spontaneous recovery from bolus dose.
PEDS — Same as adult, adjusted for anesthestic technique and age. Approved in age older than 3 months.
NOTES — Duration 30 min. Decrease dose if severe liver disease.
MOA — Nondepolarizing skeletal muscle relaxant.
ADVERSE EFFECTS — Serious: Apnea, bronchospasm. Frequent: Apnea.

SUCCINYLCHOLINE (*Anectine, Quelicin*) ▶Plasma ♀C ▶? $
ADULT — Paralysis : 0.6 to 1.1 mg/kg IV or up to 3–4 mg/kg IM (maximum 150 mg).
PEDS — Paralysis age younger than 5 yo: 2 mg/kg IV. Paralysis age 5 yo or older: 1 mg/kg IV.
UNAPPROVED ADULT — Rapid sequence intubation paralysis: 1 to 2 mg/kg IV.
NOTES — Possible profound bradyarrythmias and hypotension most commonly with repeated administrationa and in children. Avoid in hyperkalemia,

(cont.)

SUCCINYLCHOLINE (*cont.*)

myopathies, eye injuries, rhabdomyolysis, subacute burn, syndromes of denervated or disused musculature (eg, paralysis from spinal cord injury or major CVA), and in those receiving quinidine, cardiac glycosides, or with suspected cardiac glycoside toxicity. If immediate cardiac arrest and ET tube is in correct place and no tension pneumothorax evident, strongly consider empiric treatment for hyperkalemia. Succinylcholine can trigger malignant hyperthermia; see www.mhaus.org.

MOA — Ultra-short acting depolarizing skeletal muscle relaxant.

ADVERSE EFFECTS — Serious: Apnea, bradycardia, hyperkalemia, malignant hyperthermia. Frequent: Apnea, fasciculations, muscle pain.

VECURONIUM (*Norcuron*) ▶LK ♀C ▶? $

ADULT — Paralysis: 0.08 to 0.1 mg/kg IV bolus. Continuous infusion: 0.8 to 1.2 mcg/kg/min; first verify spontaneous recovery from bolus dose.

PEDS — Age younger than 7 weeks: Safety has not been established. Age 7 weeks to 1 yo: Moderately more sensitive on a mg/kg dose compared to adults and take 1.5 times longer to recover. Age 1 to 10 yo: May require a slightly higher initial dose and may also require supplementation slightly more often than older patients. Paralysis age 10 yo or older: 0.08 to 0.1 mg/kg IV bolus. Continuous infusion: 0.8 to 1.2 mcg/kg/min; first verify spontaneous recovery from bolus dose.

NOTES — Duration 15 to 30 min. Decrease dose in severe liver disease.

MOA — Nondepolarizing skeletal muscle relaxant.

ADVERSE EFFECTS — Serious: Apnea. Frequent: Apnea.

ANTIMICROBIALS

PROPHYLAXIS FOR BACTERIAL ENDOCARDITIS*

Limited to dental or respiratory tract procedures in patients at highest risk. All regimens are single dose administered 30–60 minutes prior to procedure.	
Standard regimen	Amoxicillin 2 g PO
Unable to take oral meds	Ampicillin 2 g IM/IV; or cefazolin† or ceftriaxone† 1 g IM/IV
Allergic to penicillin	Clindamycin 600 mg PO; or cephalexin† 2 g PO; or azithromycin or clarithromycin 500 mg PO
Allergic to penicillin and unable to take oral meds	Clindamycin 600 mg IM/IV; or cefazolin† or ceftriaxone† 1 g IM/IV
Pediatric drug doses	Pediatric dose should not exceed adult dose. Amoxicillin 50 mg/kg, ampicillin 50 mg/kg, azithromycin 15 mg/kg, cephalexin† 50 mg/kg, cefazolin† 50 mg/kg, ceftriaxone† 50 mg/kg, clarithromycin 15 mg/kg, clindamycin 20 mg/kg.

*For additional details of the 2007 AHA guidelines, see http://www.heart.org.
†Avoid cephalosporins if prior penicillin-associated anaphylaxis, angioedema, or urticaria.

OVERVIEW OF BACTERIAL PATHOGENS (Selected)

By bacterial class
Gram-Positive Aerobic Cocci: <u>Staphylococci</u>. Coagulase-positive: *S. aureus*. Coagulase-negative: *S. epidermidis, S. lugdunensis, S. saprophyticus*. <u>Streptococci</u>. Alpha-hemolytic: *S. pneumoniae* (pneumococcus), Viridans group. Other: *S. anginosus* group. Beta-hemolytic: *S. pyogenes* (Group A), *S. agalactiae* (Group B). Enterococcus: *E. facium, E. faecalis*.
Gram-Positive Anaerobic Cocci: *Peptostreptococcus*.
Gram-Positive Aerobic/Facultative Anaerobic Bacilli: *Arcanobacterium, Bacillus, Corynebacterium diphtheriae, C. jeikeium, Erysipelothrix rhusiopathiae, Listeria monocytogenes, Nocardia*.
Gram-Positive Anaerobic Bacilli: *Actinomyces, Clostridium botulinum, C. difficile, C. perfringens, C. tetani, Lactobacillus, Propionibacterium acnes*.
Gram-Negative Aerobic Diplococci: *Moraxella catarrhalis, Neisseria gonorrhoeae, N. meningitides*.
Gram-Negative Aerobic Coccobacilli: *Haemophilus ducreyi, H. influenzae*.
Gram-Negative Aerobic Bacilli: *Acinterbacter, Bartonella, Bordetella pertussis, Brucella, Burkholderia cepacia, Campylobacter, Francisella tularensis, Helicobacter pylori, Legionella pneumophila, Pseudomonas aeruginosa, Stenotrophomonas maltophilia, Vibrio cholerae, V. parahaemolyticus, V. vulnificus*.
Gram-Negative Facultative Anaerobic Bacilli: *Aeromonas hydrophila, Capnocytophaga, Eikenella corrodens, Kingella kingae, Pasteurella multocida*, <u>Enterobacteriaceae</u>: *Citrobacter, Escherichia coli, Enterobacter, Hafnia, Klebsiella pneumoniae, K. granulomatis, Morganella morganii, Proteus mirabilis, P. vulgaris, Providencia, Salmonella, Serratia, Shigella, Yersinia*.
Gram-Negative Anaerobic Bacilli: *Bacteroides fragilis, Fusobacterium, Prevotella*.
Intracellular Bacteria: *Anaplasma, Chlamydia pneumoniae, C. psittaci, C. trachomatis, Coxiella burnetii, Ehrlichia, Mycoplasma genitalium, M. pneumoniae, Rickettsia prowazekii, R. rickettsii, R. typhi, Ureaplasma urealyticum*.
Spirochetes: *Borrelia burgdorferi, B. miyamotoi, Leptospira, Treponema pallidum*.
Mycobacteria: *M. avium* complex, *M. kansasii, M. leprae, M. tuberculosis*.

(cont.)

OVERVIEW OF BACTERIAL PATHOGENS (Selected) (*continued*)

By bacterial name
Acinetobacter Gram-negative aerobic bacilli
Actinomyces Gram-positive anaerobic bacilli
Aeromonas hydrophila Gram-negative facultative anaerobic bacilli
Anaplasma Intracellular bacteria
Arcanobacterium Gram-positive aerobic/facultative anaerobic bacilli
Bacillus Gram-positive aerobic/facultative anaerobic bacilli
Bacteroides fragilis Gram-negative anaerobic bacilli
Bartonella Gram-negative aerobic bacilli
Bordetella pertussis Gram-negative aerobic bacilli
Borrelia burgdorferi Spirochete
Borrelia miyamotoi Spirochete
Brucella Gram-negative aerobic bacilli
Burkholderia cepacia Gram-negative aerobic bacilli
Campylobacter Gram-negative aerobic bacilli
Capnocytophaga Gram-negative facultative anaerobic bacilli
Chlamydia pneumoniae Intracellular bacteria
Chlamydia psittaci Intracellular bacteria
Chlamydia trachomatis Intracellular bacteria
Citrobacter Gram-negative facultative anaerobic bacilli
Clostridium botulinum Gram-positive anaerobic bacilli
Clostridium difficile Gram-positive anaerobic bacilli
Clostridium perfringens Gram-positive anaerobic bacilli
Clostridium tetani Gram-positive anaerobic bacilli
Corynebacterium diphtheriae Gram-positive aerobic/facultative anaerobic bacilli
Corynebacterium jeikeium Gram-positive aerobic/facultative anaerobic bacilli
Coxiella burnetii Intracellular bacteria
Ehrlichia Intracellular bacteria
Eikenella corrodens Gram-negative facultative anaerobic bacilli
Enterobacter Gram-negative facultative anaerobic bacilli
Enterobacteriaceae Gram-negative facultative anaerobic bacilli
Enterococcus facium Gram-positive aerobic cocci
Enterococcus faecalis Gram-positive aerobic cocci
Erysipelothrix rhusiopathiae Gram-positive aerobic/facultative anaerobic bacilli
Escherichia coli Gram-negative facultative anaerobic bacilli
Francisella tularensis Gram-negative aerobic bacilli
Fusobacterium Gram-negative anaerobic bacilli
Haemophilus ducreyi Gram-negative aerobic coccobacilli
Haemophilus influenzae Gram-negative aerobic coccobacilli
Hafnia Gram-negative facultative anaerobic bacilli
Helicobacter pylori Gram-negative aerobic bacilli
Kingella kingae Gram-negative facultative anaerobic bacilli
Klebsiella granulomatis Gram-negative facultative anaerobic bacilli
Klebsiella pneumoniae Gram-negative facultative anaerobic bacilli
Lactobacillus Gram-positive anaerobic bacilli
Legionella pneumophila Gram-negative aerobic bacilli
Leptospira Spirochete

(cont.)

OVERVIEW OF BACTERIAL PATHOGENS (Selected) (*continued*)

By bacterial name (*continued*)
Listeria monocytogenes **Gram-positive aerobic/facultative anaerobic bacilli**
Moraxella catarrhalis **Gram-negative aerobic diplococci**
Morganella morganii **Gram-negative facultative anaerobic bacilli**
Mycobacterium avium complex **Mycobacteria**
Mycobacterium kansasii **Mycobacteria**
Mycobacterium leprae **Mycobacteria**
Mycobacterium tuberculosis **Mycobacteria**
Myocoplasma pneumoniae **Intracellular bacteria**
Mycoplasma genitalium **Intracellular bacteria**
Neisseria gonorrhoeae **Gram-negative aerobic diplococci**
Neisseria meningitidis **Gram-negative aerobic diplococci**
Nocardia **Gram-positive aerobic/facultative anaerobic bacilli**
Pasteurella multocida **Gram-negative facultative anaerobic bacilli**
Peptostreptococcus **Gram-positive anaerobic cocci**
Pneumococcus (*Streptococcus pneumoniae*) **Gram-positive aerobic cocci**
Prevotella **Gram-negative anaerobic bacilli**
Propionibacterium acnes **Gram-positive anaerobic bacilli**
Proteus mirabilis **Gram-negative facultative anaerobic bacilli**
Proteus vularis **Gram-negative facultative anaerobic bacilli**
Providencia **Gram-negative facultative anaerobic bacilli**
Pseudomonas aeruginosa **Gram-negative aerobic bacilli**
Rickettsia prowazekii **Intracellular bacteria**
Rickettsia rickettsii **Intracellular bacteria**
Rickettsia typhi **Intracellular bacteria**
Salmonella **Gram-negative facultative anaerobic bacilli**
Serratia **Gram-negative facultative anaerobic bacilli**
Shigella **Gram-negative facultative anaerobic bacilli**
Staphylococcus aureus (coagulase-positive) **Gram-positive aerobic cocci**
Staphylococcus epidermidis (coagulase-negative) **Gram-positive aerobic cocci**
Staphylococcus lugdunensis (coagulase-negative) **Gram-positive aerobic cocci**
Staphylococcus saprophyticus (coagulase-negative) **Gram-positive aerobic cocci**
Stenotrophomonas maltophilia **Gram-negative aerobic bacilli**
Streptococcus agalactiae (Group B; beta-hemolytic) **Gram-positive aerobic cocci**
Streptococcus anginosus group **Gram-positive aerobic cocci**
Streptococcus pneumoniae (pneumococcus; alpha-hemolytic) **Gram-positive aerobic cocci**
Streptococcus pyogenes (Group A; beta-hemolytic) **Gram-positive aerobic cocci**
Treponema pallidum **Spirochete**
Ureaplasma urealyticum **Intracellular bacteria**
Vibrio cholerae **Gram-negative aerobic bacilli**
Vibrio parahaemolyticus **Gram-negative aerobic bacilli**
Vibrio vulnificus **Gram-negative aerobic bacilli**
Viridans group *Streptococcus* (alpha-hemolytic) **Gram-positive aerobic cocci**
Yersinia **Gram-negative facultative anaerobic bacilli**

ACUTE BACTERIAL SINUSITIS IN ADULTS AND CHILDREN[a] IDSA TREATMENT RECOMMENDATIONS

Initial therapy: mild to moderate infection and no risk factors for resistance	
Adults: Treat for 5 to 7 days with: 1) Amoxicillin-clavulanate 500 mg/125 mg PO three times per day or 875 mg/125 mg PO two times per day for 5 to 7 days 2) Doxycycline 100 mg PO two times per day or 200 mg PO once daily	Peds: Amoxicillin-clavulanate[a] 45 mg/kg/day PO two times per day for 10 to 14 days

Initial therapy: severe infection, risk factors for resistance,[b] or high endemic rate of invasive, penicillin-nonsusceptible *S. pneumoniae* (≥10%)	
Adults: Treat for 5 to 7 days with: 1) Amoxicillin-clavulanate[c] 2000 mg/125 mg PO two times per day 2) Doxycycline 100 mg PO two times per day or 200 mg PO once daily	Peds: Amoxicillin-clavulanate[a, c] 90 mg/kg/day PO two times per day for 10 to 14 days

Beta-lactam allergy	
Adults: Treat for 5 to 7 days with: 1) Doxycycline 100 mg PO two times per day or 200 mg PO once daily 2) Levofloxacin[d] 500 mg PO once daily 3) Moxifloxacin[d] 400 mg PO once daily	Peds, type 1 hypersensitivity: Levofloxacin[d] 10 to 20 mg/kg/day PO divided q 12 to 24 h for 10 to 14 days Peds, not type 1 hypersensitivity: Clindamycin[e] 30 to 40 mg/kg/day PO three times per day plus cefixime 8 mg/kg/day PO two times per day or cefpodoxime 10 mg/kg/day PO two times per day for 10 to 14 days

Risk factors for antibiotic resistance[b] or failed first-line therapy	
Adults: Treat for 5 to 7 days with: 1) Amoxicillin-clavulanate[c] 2000 mg/125 mg PO two times per day 2) Levofloxacin[d] 500 mg PO once daily 3) Moxifloxacin[d] 400 mg PO once daily	Peds: Treat for 10 to 14 days with: 1) Amoxicillin-clavulanate[c] 90 mg/kg/day PO two times per day 2) Clindamycin[e] 30 to 40 mg/kg/day PO three times per day plus cefixime 8 mg/kg/day PO two times per day or cefpodoxime 10 mg/kg/day PO two times per day 3) Levofloxacin[d] 10 to 20 mg/kg/day PO q 12 to 24 h

Severe infection requiring hospitalization	
Adults: 1) Ampicillin-sulbactam 1.5 to 3 g IV q 6 h 2) Levofloxacin[d] 500 mg PO/IV once daily 3) Moxifloxacin[d] 400 mg PO/IV once daily 4) Ceftriaxone 1 to 2 g IV q 12 to 24 h 5) Cefotaxime 2 g IV q 4 to 6 h	Peds: 1) Ampicillin-sulbactam 200 to 400 mg/kg/day IV q 6 h 2) Ceftriaxone 50 mg/kg/day IV q 12 h 3) Cefotaxime 100 to 200 mg/kg/day IV q 6 h 4) Levofloxacin[d] 10 to 20 mg/kg/day IV q 12 to 24 h

Adapted from *Clin Infect Dis* 2012;54(8):e72-e112. Available online at: http://www.idsociety.org.

ACUTE BACTERIAL SINUSITIS IN ADULTS AND CHILDREN[a] IDSA TREATMENT RECOMMENDATIONS (*continued*)

[a]AAP (*Pediatrics* 2013;132:e262-e280; pediatrics.aappublications.org) recommends amoxicillin 1st-line for uncomplicated acute sinusitis in children if antimicrobial resistance is not suspected. It recommends amoxicillin 45 mg/kg/day PO divided two times per day for mild-moderate sinusitis in children 2 yo or older who do not attend daycare and have not received an antibiotic in the past month. It recommends amoxicillin 80 to 90 mg/kg/day (max 4 g/day) divided two times per day in communities with a high prevalence of nonsusceptible *S. pneumoniae* (at least 10%). Amoxicillin-clavulanate 80 to 90 mg/kg/day (max 4 g/day) PO divided two times per day is an option for moderate-severe sinusitis, and for children younger than 2 yo, attending daycare, or who received an antibiotic in the past month.

[b]Risk factors for antibiotic resistance include attendance at daycare, age younger than 2 yo or older than 65 yo, recent hospitalization, antibiotic use within the past month, or patients who are immunocompromised.

[c]High-dose amoxicillin-clavulanate is recommended for geographic regions with high endemic rates (at least 10%) of invasive penicillin-nonsusceptible *S. pneumoniae*, severe infection (eg, evidence of systemic toxicity with fever of 39° C or higher, and threat of suppurative complications), or risk factors for antibiotic resistance. Use the 14:1 formulation that provides amoxicillin 90 mg/kg/day and clavulanate 6.4 mg/kg/day. If the 14:1 formulation is not available, use the 7:1 formulation with additional amoxicillin. Do not increase the dose of the 4:1 or 7:1 formulation in order to achieve a higher dose of amoxicillin; an excessive clavulanate dose increases the risk of diarrhea.

[d]As of May 2016, FDA advises that, for patients with other treatment options, the risk of serious adverse events exceeds the benefit of treating acute sinusitis with a fluoroquinolone. Therefore, fluoroquinolones should be reserved for patients with acute sinusitis who do not have other treatment options.

[e]Clindamycin resistance in *S. pneumoniae* is common in some areas of the United States.

ANTHRAX: CDC AND AAP PREFERRED REGIMENS

Adults[a]	Children, 1 month of age and older[b]
Post-exposure prophylaxis.[c] Treat for 60 days with:	
Ciprofloxacin 500 mg PO q 12 h OR Doxycycline 100 mg PO q 12 h	Ciprofloxacin 30 mg/kg/day PO divided q 12 h (max 500 mg/dose) OR Doxycycline[g] 4.4 mg/kg/day PO divided q 12 h for wt <45 kg (max 100 mg/dose); 100 mg PO divided q 12 h for wt >45 kg
Cutaneous anthrax without systemic involvement.[c,d] Treat naturally acquired disease for 7 to 10 days; treat bioterrorism-related disease for 60 days with:	
Ciprofloxacin 500 mg PO q 12 h OR Doxycycline 100 mg PO q 12 h OR Levofloxacin 750 mg PO q 24 h OR Moxifloxacin 400 mg PO q 24 h	Ciprofloxacin 30 mg/kg/day PO divided q 12 h (max 500 mg/dose)
Systemic anthrax[d] without meningitis. Treat for at least 2 weeks and until clinically stable with:[e]	
Ciprofloxacin 400 mg IV q 8 h[c] PLUS Clindamycin 900 mg IV q 8 h OR Linezolid[f] 600 mg IV q 12 h	Ciprofloxacin 30 mg/kg/day IV divided q 8 h (max 400 mg/dose)[c] PLUS Clindamycin 40 mg/kg/day IV divided q 8 h (max 900 mg/dose)

(cont.)

ANTHRAX: CDC AND AAP PREFERRED REGIMENS (*continued*)

Systemic anthrax[d] with possible/confirmed meningitis. Treat for 2 to 3 weeks and until clinically stable with:[e]	
Ciprofloxacin 400 mg IV q 8 h PLUS Meropenem 2 g IV q 8 h[c] PLUS Linezolid[f] 600 mg IV q 12 h	Ciprofloxacin 30 mg/kg/day IV divided q 8 h (max 400 mg/dose) PLUS Meropenem 120 mg/kg/day divided q 8 h (max 2 g/dose) PLUS Linezolid[f] 30 mg/kg/day divided q 8 h for age less than 12 yo; divide q 12 h for age 12 yo and older (max 600 mg/dose)

Adapted from *Emerg Infect Dis* [Internet]. 2014 Feb. http://dx.doi.org/10.3201/eid2002.130687 and *Pediatrics* 2014;133(5):e1411 at http://pediatrics.aappublications.org/content/early/2014/04/22/peds. 2014-0563.

[a] For women who are pregnant or breastfeeding, refer to *Emerg Infect Dis* [Internet]. 2014 Feb. http://dx.doi.org/10.3201/eid2002.130611.

[b] Refer to AAP clinical report cited above for dosage regimens to treat infants younger than 1 mo.

[c] Alternatives for penicillin-susceptible strains. Post-exposure prophylaxis or cutaneous anthrax. Adults: amoxicillin 1000 mg PO q 8 h OR penicillin 500 mg PO q 6 h. Children: amoxicillin 75 mg/kg/day PO divided q 8 h (max 1 g/dose) OR penicillin 50 to 75 mg/kg/day divided q 6 to 8 h. Systemic anthrax. Adults: penicillin G 4 million units IV q 4 h OR ampicillin 3 g IV q 6 h. Children: penicillin G 400,000 units/kg/day IV divided q 4 h (max 4 million units/dose).

[d] Systemic anthrax is inhalation, injection, or GI anthrax; cutaneous anthrax with systemic involvement, extensive edema, or lesions of the head or neck; or meningitis. In addition to antibiotics, patients with suspected systemic anthrax should receive an antitoxin from the US Strategic National Stockpile. Three available antitoxins bind the protective antigen on *B. anthracis* lethal and edema toxins. Obiltoxaximab (Anthim) and raxibacumab are monoclonal antibodies, and anthrax immune globulin intravenous (AIGIV; Anthrasil) is human IgG polyclonal antibodies. Recommendations for prioritizing antitoxin use are available at: www.cdc.gov/mmwr/pdf/rr/rr6404.pdf.

[e] For patients exposed to aerosolized spores, provide prophylaxis to complete 60 days of treatment from the onset of illness.

[f] Linezolid can cause myelosuppression; monitor CBC weekly esp. in patients with myelosuppression and for courses longer than 2 weeks.

[g] In children younger than 8 yo, the benefit of preventing anthrax outweighs the risk of permanent tooth staining with doxycycline.

C. DIFFICILE INFECTION (CDI) IN ADULTS: IDSA/SHEA AND ACG TREATMENT RECOMMENDATIONS

Clinical signs	Treatment
Initial episode: mild to moderate	
IDSA: WBC ≤15,000 AND serum creatinine <1.5 times premorbid level ACG: Diarrhea with signs or symptoms not meeting severe or complicated criteria	Metronidazole 500 mg PO q 8 h for 10 to 14 days[a] ACG: If no response to metronidazole in 5 to 7 days, consider vancomycin. If unable to take metronidazole, use vancomycin 125 mg PO q 6 h for 10 days.
Initial episode: severe	
IDSA: WBC ≥15,000 OR serum creatinine ≥1.5 times premorbid level ACG: Serum albumin <3 g/dL plus either: • WBC ≥15,000 • Abdominal tenderness	Vancomycin 125 mg PO q 6 h for 10 to 14 days
Initial episode: severe and complicated	
IDSA: Hypotension or shock, ileus, megacolon ACG: Any of the following attributable to CDI: • ICU admission for CDI • Hypotension ± required use of vasopressors • Fever ≥38.5°C • Ileus or significant abdominal distention • Mental status changes • WBC ≥35,000 or <2000 • Serum lactate >2.2 mmol/L • End organ failure	Vancomycin 500 mg PO/NG q 6 h plus metronidazole 500 mg IV q 8 h IDSA: Consider adding vancomycin 500 mg/100 mL[c] normal saline retention enema q 6 h if complete ileus. ACG: Add vancomycin 500 mg/500 mL[c] normal saline enema q 6 h if complicated CDI with ileus or toxic colon and/or significant abdominal distention.
First recurrent episode	
	Same as initial episode, stratified by severity. IDSA: Use vancomycin if WBC ≥15,000 or serum creatinine is increasing.
Second recurrent episode	
	Vancomycin taper and/or pulsed regimen[d]

Adapted from: *Infect Control Hosp Epidemiol* 2010;31:431. Available online at: http://www.idsociety.org.
Am J Gastroenterol 2013;108:478–98. Available online at: http://gi.org.

[a] ACG recommends 10 days of therapy because that is what clinical trials evaluated.

[b] IDSA: Consider colectomy for severe CDI. ACG: Consult surgeon for complicated CDI. Consider surgery for any of the following attributed to CDI: hypotension requiring vasopressors; clinical signs of sepsis and organ dysfunction; mental status changes; WBC ≥50,000; lactate ≥5 mmol/L; or failure to improve after
5 days on medical therapy.

[c] IDSA recommends diluting vancomycin in 100 mL for administration as enema. ACG recommends diluting vancomycin in a larger volume (500 mL) in order to ensure delivery to ascending and transverse colon.

[d] IDSA taper example: Vancomycin 125 mg PO QID for 10 to 14 days, then 125 mg two times per day for
7 days, then 125 mg once daily for 7 days, then 125 mg every 2 or 3 days for 2 to 8 weeks. ACG proposed pulse regimen: Vancomycin 125 mg PO q 6 h for 10 days, then 125 mg once every 3 days for 10 doses. Note: If there is a third recurrence after a pulsed vancomycin regimen, ACG recommends considering fecal microbiota transplant.

ACUTE OTITIS MEDIA (AOM) IN CHILDREN: AMERICAN ACADEMY OF PEDIATICS

Initial Treatment (immediate or delayed[a])	
First-line	**Alternative for Penicillin Allergy[d]**
Amoxicillin 80 to 90 mg/kg/day PO divided 2 times per day[b] *or* Amoxicillin-clavulanate[c] 90 mg/kg/day PO divided 2 times per day[b]	Cefdinir 14 mg/kg/day PO divided 1 or 2 times per day[b] *or* Cefuroxime 30 mg/kg/day PO divided 2 times per day[b] *or* Cefpodoxime 10 mg/kg/day PO divided 2 times per day[b] *or* Ceftriaxone 50 mg IM/IV once daily for 1 or 3 days
Treatment After First Antibiotic Failure	
If initial treatment was amoxicillin, use amoxicillin-clavulanate[c] 90 mg/kg/day PO divided 2 times per day.[b] If initial treatment was amoxicillin-clavulanate or oral 3rd generation cephalosporin, use ceftriaxone 50 mg IM/IV once daily for 3 days. Consider clindamycin 30 to 40 mg/kg/day PO divided 3 times per day ± 3rd generation cephalosporin if penicillin-resistant *S. pneumoniae* suspected.[b]	
Treatment After Second Antibiotic Failure	
Clindamycin 30 to 40 mg/kg/day PO divided 3 times per day + 3rd generation cephalosporin.[b] Consider tympanocentesis and consult infectious diseases specialist if multidrug-resistant bacteria detected.	

Adapted from *Pediatrics* 2013;131:e964–e999. Available online at: http://pediatrics.aappublications.org.

[a] This applies to uncomplicated AOM in children age 6 mo to 12 yo. Immediate treatment is recommended for children with otorrhea or severe symptoms (moderate to severe pain, pain for ˜48 h, or temperature ˜39°C), and bilateral AOM in children age 6 to 23 mo. Observation for 48 to 72 h before antibiotic therapy is an option for children age 6 to 23 mo with unilateral AOM and mild symptoms (mild pain for <48 h and temperature <39°C), or children 2 yo and older with unilateral/bilateral AOM and mild symptoms. Observation must have mechanism to follow-up and start an antibiotic if symptoms do not improve within 48 to 72 hours. Do not use observation if follow-up is unsure.

[b] Treat for 10 days if age <2 yo or any age with severe symptoms, 7 days for age 2 to 5 yo with mild to moderate symptoms, and 5 to 7 days for age 6 yo or older with mild to moderate symptoms.

[c] Consider in patients who have received amoxicillin in the past 30 days or who have the otitis-conjunctivitis syndrome. Use the 14:1 formulation of amoxicillin-clavulanate that provides amoxicillin 90 mg/kg/day and clavulanate 6.4 mg/kg/day. If the 14:1 formulation is not available, give the 7:1 formulation with additional amoxicillin. Do not increase the dose of a 4:1 or 7:1 formulation to achieve a higher dose of amoxicillin; an excessive clavulanate dose increases the risk of diarrhea.

[d] Cefdinir, cefuroxime, cefpodoxime, and ceftriaxone are highly unlikely to cross-react with penicillin. Excluding patients with a history of a severe reaction, the reaction rate in patients who have not undergone penicillin skin testing is estimated at 0.1%. A drug allergy practice parameter (*Ann Allergy Asthma Immunol* 2010;105:259-73; available at http://www.allergyparameters.org) recommends that a cephalosporin can be given to patients who do not have a history of a severe and/or recent allergic reaction to penicillin. Options for patients with a history of an IgE-mediated reaction to penicillin include substitution of a non-beta-lactam antibiotic, or penicillin or cephalosporin skin testing to evaluate the risk of cephalosporin administration.

SEXUALLY TRANSMITTED DISEASES & VAGINITIS*

Bacterial vaginosis	(1) metronidazole 5 g of 0.75% gel intravaginally daily for 5 days OR 500 mg PO two times per day for 7 days; (2) clindamycin 5 g of 2% cream intravaginally at bedtime for 7 days. Alternative: (1) tinidazole 2 g PO once daily for 2 days OR 1 g PO once daily for 5 days; (2) clindamycin 300 mg PO two times per day for 7 days. Treat all symptomatic pregnant women.
Candidal vaginitis	(1) Intravaginal butoconazole, clotrimazole, miconazole, terconazole, or tioconazole; (2) fluconazole 150 mg PO single dose.
Cervicitis	Treat based on NAAT results for chlamydia and gonorrhea. Presumptively treat at-risk women (age younger than 25 yo; sex partner is new, has other partners, or has STD), esp if follow-up not ensured or NAAT not available. Presumptive regimen: (1) azithromycin 1 g PO single dose; (2) doxycycline 100 mg PO two times per day for 7 days. Presumptively treat for gonorrhea if at-risk or high community prevalence.
Chancroid	(1) azithromycin 1 g PO single dose; (2) ceftriaxone 250 mg IM single dose; (3) ciprofloxacin 500 mg PO two times per day for 3 days; (4) erythromycin base 500 mg PO three times per day for 7 days.
Chlamydia	(1) azithromycin 1 g PO single dose; (2) doxycycline 100 mg PO two times per day for 7 days. Alternative: (1) erythromycin base 500 mg PO four times per day for 7 days; (2) levofloxacin 500 mg PO once daily for 7 days. In pregnancy: azithromycin 1 g PO single dose. Alternative: (1) amoxicillin 500 mg PO three times per day for 7 days. (2) erythromycin base 500 mg PO four times per day for 7 days or 250 mg PO four times per day for 14 days. Repeat NAAT 3 to 4 weeks after treatment in pregnant women.
Lymphogranuloma venereum *(Chlamydia trachomatis)*	(1) doxycycline 100 mg PO two times per day for 21 days. Alternative: erythromycin base 500 mg PO four times per day for 21 days.
Epididymitis, acute	Chlamydia and gonorrhea likely: ceftriaxone 250 mg IM single dose + doxycycline 100 mg PO two times per day for 10 days. Chlamydia-gonorrhea and enteric organisms likely: ceftriaxone 250 mg IM single dose + levofloxacin 500 mg PO once daily for 10 days. Enteric organisms likely: levofloxacin 500 mg PO once daily for 10 days.
Genital herpes, first episode	(1) acyclovir 400 mg PO three times per day for 7 to 10 days; (2) famciclovir 250 mg PO three times per day for 7 to 10 days; (3) valacyclovir 1 g PO two times per day for 7 to 10 days.
Genital herpes, recurrent	(1) acyclovir 400 mg PO three times per day for 5 days; (2) acyclovir 800 mg PO three times per day for 2 days or two times per day for 5 days; (3) famciclovir 125 mg PO two times per day for 5 days; (4) famciclovir 1 g PO two times per day for 1 day; (5) famciclovir 500 mg PO 1st dose, then 250 mg PO two times per day for 2 days; (6) valacyclovir 500 mg PO two times per day for 3 days; (7) valacyclovir 1 g PO daily for 5 days.

(cont.)

SEXUALLY TRANSMITTED DISEASES & VAGINITIS* (*continued*)

Genital herpes, suppressive therapy	(1) acyclovir 400 mg PO two times per day; (2) famciclovir 250 mg PO two times per day; (3) valacyclovir 500 or 1000 mg PO daily. Valacyclovir 500 mg PO daily reduces transmission in patients with 9 or fewer recurrences per year, but other valacyclovir/acyclovir regimens may be more effective for suppression in patients who have 10 or more recurrences per year. <u>Pregnant women with recurrent genital herpes:</u> Start at 36 weeks gestation with (1) acyclovir 400 mg PO three times per day; (2) valacyclovir 500 mg PO two times per day.
Genital herpes, recurrent in HIV infection	(1) acyclovir 400 mg PO three times per day for 5 to 10 days; (2) famciclovir 500 mg PO two times per day for 5 to 10 days; (3) valacyclovir 1 g PO two times per day for 5 to 10 days.
Genital herpes, suppressive therapy in HIV infection	(1) acyclovir 400 to 800 mg PO two or three times per day; (2) famciclovir 500 mg PO two times per day; (3) valacyclovir 500 mg PO two times per day.
Genital warts	<u>External anogenital, patient-applied:</u> (1) imiquimod 3.75% or 5% cream; (2) podofilox 0.5% soln or gel; (3) sinecatechins 15% ointment. <u>External anogenital, provider-administered:</u> (1) cryotherapy with liquid nitrogen or cryoprobe; (2) surgical removal; (3) trichloroacetic or bichloroacetic acid 80% to 90% soln. <u>Urethral meatus:</u> (1) cryotherapy with liquid nitrogen; (2) surgical removal. <u>Vaginal, cervical, or intra-anal:</u> (1) cryotherapy with liquid nitrogen; (2) surgical removal; (3) trichloroacetic or bichloroacetic acid 80% to 90% soln.
Gonorrhea[a]	Ceftriaxone 250 mg IM single dose + azithromycin 1 g PO single dose. <u>For cervix, urethra, and rectum if ceftriaxone is unavailable:</u> cefixime 400 mg PO single dose + azithromycin 1 g PO single dose.[a] <u>Ceftriaxone-allergic:</u> consult infectious disease expert and consider (1) gemifloxacin 320 mg PO single dose + azithromycin 2 g PO single dose; (2) gentamicin 240 mg IM single dose + azithromycin 2 g PO single dose.
Gonorrhea, disseminated	<u>Arthritis/arthritis-dermatitis syndrome:</u> ceftriaxone 1 g IM/IV q 24 h + azithromycin 1 g PO single dose. After substantial improvement, can switch to PO drug based on antimicrobial susceptibility to complete at least 7 days of treatment. Alternative: cefotaxime 1 g IV q 8 h OR ceftizoxime 1 g IV q 8 h + azithromycin 1 g PO single dose. <u>Meningitis, endocarditis:</u> ceftriaxone 1 to 2 g IV q 12 to 24 h + azithromycin 1 g PO single dose. Treat IM/IV for at least 10 to 14 days for meningitis, and at least 4 weeks for endocarditis.
Granuloma inguinale	Azithromycin 1 g PO once weekly or 500 mg PO once daily for at least 3 weeks and until lesions completely healed. See STD guideline for alternative treatment regimens.

a For suspected cephalosporin treatment failure, consult infectious disease specialist, an STD/HIV Prevention Training Center clinical expert (www.nnptc.org), or local/state health department STD program or CDC (phone 404-639-8659). Report suspected treatment failure to health department within 24 hours of diagnosis. When reinfection is likely, retreat with ceftriaxone 250 mg IM + azithromycin 1 g PO. For suspected treatment failure after cefixime-azithromycin regimen: Treat with ceftriaxone 250 mg IM single dose + azithromycin 2 g PO single dose. Obtain test-of-cure 7 to 14 days later, preferably with culture (and susceptibility testing of *N. gonorrhoeae* if isolated) and simultaneous NAAT.

(cont.)

SEXUALLY TRANSMITTED DISEASES & VAGINITIS* (*continued*)

Non-gonococcal urethrits (NGU)	(1) azithromycin 1 g PO single dose; (2) doxycycline 100 mg PO two times per day for 7 days. Alternative: (1) erythromycin base 500 mg PO four times per day for 7 days; (2) levofloxacin 500 mg PO once per day for 7 days. Persistant/recurrent: (1) azithromycin 1 g PO single dose for men who initially received doxycycline; (2) moxifloxacin 400 mg PO once daily for 7 days if azithromycin failed; (3) metronidazoleor tinidazole 2 g PO single dose for heterosexual men in areas of high *T vaginalis* prevalence.
Pelvic inflammatory disease (PID)	Parenteral: (1) cefotetan 2 g IV q 12 h + doxycycline 100 mg IV/PO q 12 h OR cefoxitin 2 g IV q 6 h + doxycycline 100 mg IV/PO q 12 h. After 24 to 48 h of improvement, switch to PO doxycycline to complete 14 days. (2) clindamycin 900 mg IV q 8 h + gentamicin IM/IV 2 mg/kg loading dose, then 1.5 mg/kg q 8 h (can substitute 3 to 5 mg/kg once-daily dosing). After 24 to 48 h of improvement, switch to clindamycin 450 mg PO four times per day or doxycycline 100 mg PO two times per day to complete 14 days. For tubo-ovarian abscess, add clindamycin 450 mg PO four times per day or metronidazole 500 mg PO two times per day to doxycycline to provide anaerobic activity. IM/oral regimen: ceftriaxone 250 mg IM single dose + doxycycline 100 mg PO two times per day ± metronidazole 500 mg PO two times per day for 14 days. Metronidazole is added to provide anaerobic coverage and treat bacterial vaginosis.
Proctitis	Ceftriaxone 250 mg IM single dose + doxycycline 100 mg PO two times per day for 7 days.
Pubic lice	(1) permethrin 1% cream rinse (2) pyrethrins with piperonyl butoxide. Apply to affected areas and wash off after 10 minutes. Alternatives: (1) malathion 0.5% lotion; apply to affected areas and wash off after 8 to 12 h (can be used if treatment failure may be due to resistance); (2) ivermectin 250 mcg/kg PO taken with food; repeat in 2 weeks.
Scabies	(1) permethrin 5% cream applied to body from neck down and washed off after 8 to 14 h; (2) ivermectin 200 mcg/kg PO taken with food; repeat in 2 weeks. Use permethrin for infants and children. Alternative: lindane 1% 1 oz of lotion or 30 g of cream applied to body from neck down and thoroughly washed off after 8 h; not for age less than 10 yo. Crusted scabies: 5% benzyl benzoate or 5% permethrin cream, full-body application daily for 7 days then twice weekly until discharge or cure + ivermectin 200 mcg/kg PO on days 1, 2, 8, 9, and 15. Consider additional doses on days 22 and 29 if severe.
Sexual assault prophylaxis	Ceftriaxone 250 mg IM single dose + metronidazole or tinidazole 2 g PO single dose + azithromycin 1 g PO single dose. Consider HBV and HPV vaccination and HIV prophylaxis when appropriate.
Syphilis, primary, secondary, or early latent, ie, duration less than 1 year	Benzathine penicillin 2.4 million units IM single dose. Penicillin-allergic: doxycycline 100 mg PO two times per day for 14 days if primary or secondary syphilis and 28 days if early latent syphilis. Use skin testing and penicillin desensitization protocol if medication compliance or follow-up cannot be ensured.
Syphilis, late latent or unknown duration	Benzathine penicillin 2.4 million units IM q week for 3 doses. Penicillin-allergic: doxycycline 100 mg PO two times per day for 4 weeks.

(cont.)

SEXUALLY TRANSMITTED DISEASES & VAGINITIS* (*continued*)

Syphilis, tertiary	Benzathine penicillin 2.4 million units IM q week for 3 doses. This regimen is for patients with normal CSF exam; use neurosyphilis regimen if CSF abnormalities. Consult infectious disease specialist for management of penicillin-allergic patients.
Syphilis, neuro and ocular	(1) penicillin G 18 to 24 million units/day continuous IV infusion or 3 to 4 million units IV q 4 h for 10 to 14 days; (2) if compliance can be ensured, consider procaine penicillin 2.4 million units IM daily + probenecid 500 mg PO four times per day, both for 10 to 14 days. Penicillin-allergic: (1) ceftriaxone 2 g IM/IV once daily for 10 to 14 days; (2) skin testing and penicillin desensitization protocol.
Syphilis in pregnancy	Treat with penicillin regimen for stage of syphilis as noted above. For primary, secondary, or early latent syphilis, consider a second dose of benzathine penicillin 2.4 million units IM one week after initial dose. Use skin-testing and penicillin-desensitization protocol if penicillin-allergic.
Trichomoniasis	Metronidazole or tinidazole 2 g PO single dose. Use metronidazole if pregnant. Persistent/recurrent: metronidazole 500 mg PO two times per day for 7 days. Treatment-failure: metronidazole or tinidazole 2 g PO two times per day for 7 days. HIV-infected women: metronidazole 500 mg PO two times per day for 7 days.

*MMWR 2015;64(No. RR-3): 1-137 or www.cdc.gov/std/tg2015/default.htm. Treat sexual partners for all except herpes, candida, and bacterial vaginosis. Refer to the STD guideline for additional alternative regimens.

NAAT = nucleic acid amplification test.

ANTIMICROBIALS: Aminoglycosides

NOTE: See also Dermatology and Ophthalmology. Can cause nephrotoxicity, ototoxicity. Mitochondrial DNA mutations (e.g., m.1555A>G) predispose to aminoglycoside-induced deafness that is permanent and dose-independent.

AMIKACIN ▸K ♀D ▶? $$
WARNING — Nephrotoxicity, ototoxicity.
ADULT — Gram-negative infections: 15 mg/kg/day (up to 1500 mg/day) IM/IV divided q 8 to 12 h.
PEDS — Gram-negative infections: 15 mg/kg/day (up to 1500 mg/day) IM/IV divided q 8 to 12 h. Neonates: 10 mg/kg load, then 7.5 mg/kg IM/IV q 12 h.
UNAPPROVED ADULT — Once-daily dosing: 15 mg/kg IV q 24 h. Once-daily dosing for cystic fibrosis pulmonary exacerbation: 30 to 35 mg/kg IV q 24 h with target peak of 80 to 120 mg/L and trough of less than 10 mg/L. Adjust dose based on levels; use past effective dose if available. TB (2nd-line treatment): 15 mg/kg IM/IV daily or 25 mg/kg three times per week.
UNAPPROVED PEDS — Severe infections: 15 to 22.5 mg/kg/day IV divided q 8 h. Some experts recommend 30 mg/kg/day. Once-daily dosing. Age 1 mo and older: 15 to 20 mg/kg IV q 24 h. Age 8 to 28 days old and wt greater than 2 kg: 17.5 mg/kg IV q 24 h. Age 1 to 7 days old and wt greater than 2 kg: 15 mg/kg IV q 24 h. Once-daily dosing for cystic fibrosis pulmonary exacerbation: 30 to 35 mg/kg IV q 24 h with target peak of 80 to 120 mg/L and trough of less than 10 mg/L. Adjust dose based on levels; use past effective dose if available. TB (2nd-line treatment): 15 to 20 mg/kg IM/IV daily.

NOTES — May enhance effects of neuromuscular blockers and exacerbate myasthenia gravis. Nephrotoxicity risk increased by at least 3 days of treatment, nephrotoxic drugs, contrast dye, hypotension, renal impairment. Individualize dose in renal dysfunction, burn patients. Base dose on average of actual and ideal body wt in obesity. Conventional dosing: Peak 20 to 35 mcg/mL, trough less than 5 mcg/mL. Once-daily dosing: Peak 35 to 60 mcg/mL (if obtained), trough less than 4 mcg/mL.
MOA — Inhibits bacterial protein synthesis by interfering with function of ribosomal 30S subunit. Bactericidal.
ADVERSE EFFECTS — Serious and frequent: Nephrotoxicity (risk increased by at least 3 days of treatment), neuromuscular blockade, exacerbation of myasthenia gravis, cochlear toxicity. Serious and rare: Vestibular toxicity.

GENTAMICIN ▸K ♀D ▶+ $$
WARNING — Nephrotoxicity, ototoxicity.
ADULT — Gram-negative infections: 3 to 5 mg/kg/day IM/IV divided q 8 h.
PEDS — Gram-negative infections: 2.5 mg/kg IM/IV q 12 h for age younger than 1 week old and wt greater than 2 kg; 2 to 2.5 mg/kg IM/IV q 8 h for age 1 week old or older and wt greater than 2 kg.

(cont.)

GENTAMICIN (*cont.*)

UNAPPROVED ADULT — Once-daily dosing for Gram-negative infections: 5 to 7 mg/kg IV q 24 h. Endocarditis: 3 mg/kg/day for synergy with another agent. Give once daily for viridans streptococci, 2 to 3 divided doses for staphylococci (prosthetic valve) or enterococci. Adjust to peak of ~ 3 to 4 mcg/mL and trough <1 mcg/mL. AHA does not recommend for S. aureus native valve endocarditis.

UNAPPROVED PEDS — Once-daily dosing. Age 1 mo and older: 5 to 7 mg/kg IV q 24 h. Age 8 to 28 days old and wt greater than 2 kg: 4 to 5 mg/kg IV q 24 h. Age 1 to 7 days old and wt greater than 2 kg: 4 mg/kg IV q 24 h.

NOTES — May enhance effects of neuromuscular blockers and exacerbate myasthenia gravis. Nephrotoxicity risk increased by at least 3 days of treatment, coadministration of nephrotoxic drugs or contrast dye, hypotension, renal impairment. Individualize dose in renal dysfunction, burn patients. Base dose on average of actual and ideal body wt in obesity. Conventional dosing: Peak 5 to 10 mcg/mL, trough less than 2 mcg/mL. Once-daily dosing: Peak 15 to 20 mcg/mL (if obtained), trough less than 1 mcg/mL.

MOA — Inhibits bacterial protein synthesis by interfering with function of ribosomal 30S subunit. Bactericidal.

ADVERSE EFFECTS — Serious and frequent: Nephrotoxicity (risk increased by at least 3 days of treatment); neuromuscular blockade; exacerbation of myasthenia gravis; cochlear toxicity. Serious and rare: Vestibular toxicity.

STREPTOMYCIN ▶K ♀D ▶+ $$$$$

WARNING — Nephrotoxicity, ototoxicity. Monitor audiometry, renal function, and electrolytes.

ADULT — Combined therapy for TB: 15 mg/kg (up to 1 g) IM/IV daily. 10 mg/kg (up to 750 mg) IM/IV daily if age 60 yo or older.

PEDS — Combined therapy for TB: 20 to 40 mg/kg (up to 1 g) IM daily. See Unapproved Peds for ATS dose.

UNAPPROVED ADULT — Same IM dosing can be given IV. Enterococcal endocarditis: 7.5 mg/kg IV/IM two times per day. Go to www.americanheart.org for further info.

UNAPPROVED PEDS — Combined therapy for TB, ATS recommended dose: 15 to 20 mg/kg IM once daily.

NOTES — Contraindicated in pregnancy. Obtain baseline audiogram, vestibular, and Romberg testing, and renal function. Monitor renal function and vestibular and auditory symptoms monthly. May enhance effects of neuromuscular blockers. Avoid other ototoxic/nephrotoxic drugs. Individualize dose in renal dysfunction. AHA recommends against use for endocarditis if CrCl <50 mL/min.

MOA — Inhibits bacterial protein synthesis by interfering with function of ribosomal 30S subunit. Bactericidal.

ADVERSE EFFECTS — Serious and frequent: Ototoxicity, vestibular toxicity. Serious and rare:

Nephrotoxicity, neuromuscular blockade. Frequent: Circumoral paresthesias immediately after injection.

TOBRAMYCIN (*Bethkis, Kitabis Pak, Tobi*) ▶K ♀D ▶+ $$

WARNING — Nephrotoxicity, ototoxicity.

ADULT — Gram-negative infections: 3 to 5 mg/kg/day IM/IV divided q 8 h. Parenteral for severe cystic fibrosis pulmonary exacerbation: Initial dose of 10 mg/kg/day IV divided q 6 h with target peak of 8 to 12 mcg/mL. Adjust dose based on levels; use past effective dose if available. CF Foundation prefers once-daily dosing; see unapproved adult. Inhaled for cystic fibrosis: 300 mg nebulized or 4 caps inhaled (Tobi Podhaler) two times per day 28 days on, then 28 days off.

PEDS — Gram-negative infections: 2 to 2.5 mg/kg IV q 8 h or 1.5 to 1.9 mg/kg IV q 6 h. Give 4 mg/kg/day divided q 12 h for premature/full-term neonates age 1 to 7 days old. Parenteral for severe cystic fibrosis pulmonary exacerbation: Initial dose of 10 mg/kg/day IV divided q 6 h with target peak of 8 to 12 mcg/mL. Adjust dose based on levels; use past effective dose if available. CF Foundation prefers once-daily dosing; see unapproved peds. Inhaled for cystic fibrosis, age 6 yo or older: 300 mg nebulized or 4 caps inhaled (Tobi Podhaler) two times per day 28 days on, then 28 days off.

UNAPPROVED ADULT — Once-daily dosing: 5 to 7 mg/kg IV q 24 h. Once-daily dosing for cystic fibrosis pulmonary exacerbation: 10 to 12 mg/kg IV q 24 h. with target peak of 20 to 30 mg/L and trough of less than 1 mg/L.

UNAPPROVED PEDS — Once-daily dosing. Age 1 mo and older: 5 to 7 mg/kg IV q 24 h. Age 8 to 28 days old and wt greater than 2 kg: 4 to 5 mg/kg IV q 24 h. Age 1 to 7 days old and wt greater than 2 kg: 4 mg/kg IV q 24 h. Once-daily dosing for cystic fibrosis pulmonary exacerbation: 10 to 12 mg/kg IV q 24 h with target peak of 20 to 30 mg/L and trough of less than 1 mg/L.

FORMS — Generic/Trade (Tobi): 300 mg/5 mL ampules for nebulizer. Trade only: Bethkis 300 mg/4 mL ampules for nebulizer. Tobi Podhaler 28 mg caps for inhalation. Kitabis Pak 300 mg/5 mL ampules and nebulizer.

NOTES — May enhance effects of neuromuscular blockers and exacerbate myasthenia gravis. Nephrotoxicity risk increased by at least 3 days of treatment, nephrotoxic drugs, contrast dye, hypotension, renal impairment. Individualize dose in renal dysfunction, burn patients. Base dose on average of actual and ideal body wt in obesity. Conventional dosing: Peak 5 to 10 mcg/mL, trough <2 mcg/mL. Once-daily dosing: Peak 15 to 20 mcg/mL (if obtained), trough <1 mcg/mL. Nebulized/inhaled tobramycin: Routine monitoring of levels not required. Consider audiograms for patients with or at increased risk of auditory dysfunction. Do not coadminister diuretics including IV mannitol. Tobi Podhaler: Do not place caps in Podhaler until immediately before inhalation. Make sure each cap

(cont.)

TOBRAMYCIN (cont.)

is empty after inhalation. If powder is still in cap, repeat inhalation until empty. Patients taking multiple inhaled drugs should take Tobi Podhaler last.

MOA — Inhibits bacterial protein synthesis by interfering with function of ribosomal 30S subunit. Bactericidal.

ADVERSE EFFECTS — Serious and frequent: Nephrotoxicity (risk increased by at least 3 days of treatment), neuromuscular blockade, exacerbation of myasthenia gravis, ototoxicity. Serious and rare: Vestibular toxicity. Inhaled tobramycin. Serious: Bronchospasm, tinnitus, hearing loss. Frequent: rales, dysphonia, wheezing, epistaxis, decreased FEV1. More cough, dysphonia, dysgeusia with Tobi Podhaler.

ANTIMICROBIALS: Antifungal Agents—Azoles

NOTE: See www.idsociety.org for guidelines on the management of fungal infections. See www.aidsinfo.nih.gov for management of fungal infections in HIV-infected patients.

CLOTRIMAZOLE ▶L ♀C ▶? $$$$

ADULT — Oropharyngeal candidiasis: 1 troche dissolved slowly in mouth 5 times per day for 14 days. Prevention of oropharyngeal candidiasis in immunocompromised patients: 1 troche dissolved slowly in mouth three times per day until end of chemotherapy or high-dose corticosteroids.

PEDS — Oropharyngeal candidiasis, age 3 yo or older: Use adult dose.

FORMS — Generic only: Oral troches 10 mg.

MOA — Alters yeast cell membrane permeability.

ADVERSE EFFECTS — Serious: None. Frequent: Increased transaminase levels.

FLUCONAZOLE (*Diflucan*, *✦CanesOral*) ▶K ♀C for single-dose treatment of vaginal candidiasis, D for all other indications. Possible increased risk of miscarriage; 400 to 800 mg/day linked to birth abnormalities. ▶+ $$$$

ADULT — Vaginal candidiasis: 150 mg PO single dose ($). All other dosing regimens IV/PO. Oropharyngeal candidiasis: 200 mg 1st day, then 100 mg daily for at least 2 weeks. Esophageal candidiasis: 200 mg 1st day, then 100 mg daily (up to 400 mg/day) for at least 3 weeks and continuing for 2 weeks past symptom resolution. Systemic candidiasis: Up to 400 mg daily. Candidal UTI, peritonitis: 50 to 200 mg daily. See UNAPPROVED ADULT for IDSA regimens for Candida infections. Cryptococcal meningitis: 400 mg daily until 10 to 12 weeks after cerebrospinal fluid is culture negative (see UNAPPROVED ADULT for 1st-line regimen). Suppression of cryptococcal meningitis relapse in AIDS: 200 mg daily until immune system reconstitution. Prevention of candidiasis after bone marrow transplant: 400 mg daily starting several days before neutropenia and continuing until ANC greater than 1000 cells/mm³ for 7 days. Tinea versicolor: 400 mg PO single dose or 300 mg PO once weekly for 2 weeks (2 doses total).

PEDS — All dosing regimens IV/PO. Oropharyngeal candidiasis: 6 mg/kg 1st day, then 3 mg/kg daily for at least 2 weeks. Esophageal candidiasis: 6 mg/kg 1st day, then 3 mg/kg daily (up to 12 mg/kg daily) for at least 3 weeks and continuing for 2 weeks past symptom resolution. Systemic candidiasis: 6 to 12 mg/kg daily. See UNAPPROVED PEDS for alternative regimens for Candida infections. Cryptococcal

meningitis: 12 mg/kg on 1st day, then 6 to 12 mg/kg daily until 10 to 12 weeks after cerebrospinal fluid is culture negative. Suppression of cryptococcal meningitis relapse in AIDS: 6 mg/kg daily. Peds/adult dose equivalents: 3 mg/kg peds equivalent to 100 mg adult; 6 mg/kg peds equivalent to 200 mg adult; 12 mg/kg peds equivalent to 400 mg adult; max peds dose is 600 mg/day.

UNAPPROVED ADULT — Onychomycosis, fingernail: 150 to 300 mg PO q week for 3 to 6 months. Onychomycosis, toenail: 150 to 300 mg PO q week for 6 to 12 months. Recurrent vaginal candidiasis: 150 mg PO q 3rd day for 3 doses, then 150 mg PO q week for 6 months. Severe vaginal candidiasis: 150 mg PO for 2 or 3 doses given 3 days apart. Oropharyngeal candidiasis: 100 to 200 mg daily for 7 to 14 days. Esophageal candidiasis: 200 to 400 mg daily for 14 to 21 days. Suppression of recurrent esophageal candidiasis: 100 to 200 mg PO three times weekly. Candidemia: 800 mg 1st day, then 400 mg once a day. Treat for 14 days after 1st negative blood culture and resolution of signs/symptoms. Candida pyelonephritis: 200 to 400 mg (3 to 6 mg/kg) daily for 14 days. Prevention of candidal infections in high-risk neutropenic pts: 400 mg/day during period of risk for neutropenia. Cryptococcal meningitis, IDSA regimen: Amphotericin B preferably in combo with flucytosine for at least 2 weeks (induction), followed by fluconazole 400 mg PO once daily for 8 weeks (consolidation), then chronic suppression with fluconazole 200 mg PO once daily until immune system reconstitution. Treatment/suppression of coccidioidomycosis in HIV infection: 400 mg PO once daily.

UNAPPROVED PEDS — Oropharyngeal candidiasis: 6 mg/kg 1st day, then 3 mg/kg once daily for 7 to 14 days. Esophageal candidiasis: 12 mg/kg 1st day, then 6 mg/kg once daily for 14 to 21 days. Systemic Candida infection: 12 mg/kg on 1st day, then 6 to 12 mg/kg once daily. Cryptococcal meningitis, IDSA regimen: Amphotericin B preferably in combo with flucytosine for 2 weeks (induction), followed by fluconazole 12 mg/kg on 1st day, then 6 to 12 mg/kg (max 800 mg) IV/PO once a day for at least 8 weeks (consolidation), then chronic suppression with lower dose of fluconazole.

(cont.)

FLUCONAZOLE (*cont.*)

FORMS — Generic/Trade: Tabs 50, 100, 150, 200 mg. 150 mg tab in single-dose blister pack. Susp 10, 40 mg/mL (35 mL).

NOTES — Can prolong QT interval and cause torsades. Inhibits CYP2C9 (moderate), CYP2C19 (strong), and CYP3A4 (moderate). Many drug interactions, including increased levels of alfentanil, calcium channel blockers, celecoxib, cyclosporine, fentanyl, flurbiprofen, fluvastatin (limit fluvastatin to 20 mg/day), glyburide, glipizide, losartan, lovastatin, methadone, phenytoin, rifabutin, simvastatin, sirolimus, tacrolimus, theophylline, tofacitinib (reduce tofacitinib to 5 mg once daily), tolbutamide, and increased INR with warfarin. Do not coadminister voriconazole, or drugs that prolong the QT interval and are metabolized by CYP3A4 (eg, erythromycin, pimozide, quinidine). Dosing in renal dysfunction: Give a loading dose ranging from 50 mg to 400 mg to patients with impaired renal function who will receive multiple doses of fluconazole. Reduce maintenance dose by 50% for CrCl 11 to 50 mL/min. Hemodialysis: Give 100% of recommended dose after each dialysis.

MOA — Triazole that inhibits the synthesis of ergosterol (a sterol required for normal fungal cytoplasmic membrane).

ADVERSE EFFECTS — Serious: Hepatotoxicity (rare), anaphylaxis (rare), exfoliative skin disorders (rare). Frequent: Increased transaminase levels. Single-dose for vaginal candidiasis: Headache, nausea, abdominal pain.

ISAVUCONAZONIUM (*Cresemba, isavuconazole*) ▶L glucuronidation ♀C ▶– $$$$$

ADULT — Invasive aspergillosis, mucormycosis: Load with 372 mg isavuconazonium IV/PO q 8 h for 6 doses, then 372 mg IV/PO once daily starting 12 to 24 h after last loading dose. Infuse IV doses over at least 1 h with in-line filter. Isavuconazonium is prodrug of isavuconazole; 372 mg isavuconazonium = 200 mg isavuconazole.

PEDS — Safety and efficacy not established in children.

FORMS — Trade only: Caps 186 mg (100 mg isavuconazole).

NOTES — Isavuconazonium is a prodrug that is converted to isavuconazole. Shortens QTc interval; contraindicated in familial short QT syndrome. Can cause severe hepatic reactions; monitor LFTs. Serious hypersensitivity and skin reactions. May be teratogenic; use in pregnancy is risk vs benefit decision. Isavuconazole inhibits CYP3A4 (moderate) and p-glycoprotein. Contraindicated with strong CYP3A4 inhibitors or inducers (see cytochrome P450 table). Monitor levels of digoxin, cyclosporine, sirolimus, tacrolimus.

MOA — Prodrug rapidly hydrolyzed to isavuconazole, a triazole that inhibits the synthesis of ergosterol (a sterol required for normal fungal cytoplasmic membrane).

ADVERSE EFFECTS — Serious: Hepatotoxicity; infusion reactions; hypersensitivity and severe skin reactions; teratogenicity. Frequent: N/V, diarrhea, constipation, headache, increased LFTs, hypokalemia, dyspnea, cough, peripheral edema, back pain.

ITRACONAZOLE (*Onmel, Sporanox*) ▶L ♀C ▶– $$$$$

WARNING — Strong CYP3A4 inhibitor; can lead to dangerously high levels of some drugs. High levels of some can prolong QT interval (see QT drugs table). Contraindicated with felodipine, disopyramide, dofetilide, dronedarone, eplerenone, ergot alkaloids, irinotecan, lovastatin, lurasidone, PO midazolam, methadone, nisoldipine, pimozide, quinidine, ranolazine, simvastatin, ticagrelor, triazolam. Contraindicated with colchicine if renal/hepatic impairment; fesoterodine if moderate/severe renal/hepatic impairment; telithromycin if severe renal/hepatic impairment; solifenacin if severe renal or moderate/severe hepatic impairment. Negative inotrope (may be additive with calcium channel blockers); reassess treatment if signs/symptoms of heart failure develop. Not for use in ventricular dysfunction (CHF or history of CHF) unless for life-threatening or serious infection. Do not use caps for onychomycosis in patients with left ventricular dysfunction.

ADULT — Cap or tab: Take cap or tab with full meal. Onychomycosis, toenails: 200 mg PO daily for 12 weeks. Onychomycosis "pulse dosing" for fingernails: 200 mg PO two times per day for 1st week of month for 2 months. Test nail specimen to confirm diagnosis before prescribing. Aspergillosis in patients intolerant/refractory to amphotericin, blastomycosis, histoplasmosis: 200 mg cap PO one to two times per day. Treat for at least 3 months. For life-threatening infections, load with 200 mg PO three times per day for 3 days. Oral soln: Swish and swallow in 10 mL increments on empty stomach. Oropharyngeal candidiasis: 200 mg soln PO daily for 1 to 2 weeks. Oropharyngeal candidiasis unresponsive to fluconazole: 100 mg soln PO two times per day. Esophageal candidiasis: 100 to 200 mg soln PO daily for at least 3 weeks and continuing for 2 weeks past symptom resolution.

PEDS — Not approved in children.

UNAPPROVED ADULT — Onychomycosis "pulse dosing" for toenails: 200 mg PO two times per day for 1st week of month for 3 to 4 months. Confirm diagnosis with nail specimen lab testing before prescribing. Prevention of histoplasmosis in HIV infection: 200 mg PO once daily. Treatment/suppression of coccidioidomycosis in HIV infection: 200 mg PO two times per day. Fluconazole-refractory oropharyngeal or esophageal candidiasis: 200 mg PO of oral soln daily for 14 to 21 days for esophageal, up to 28 days for oropharyngeal.

UNAPPROVED PEDS — Oropharyngeal candidiasis, age 5 yo or older: Oral soln 2.5 mg/kg PO two times per day (max 200 to 400 mg/day) for 7 to 14 days. Esophageal candidiasis, age 5 yo or older: Oral soln

(cont.)

ITRACONAZOLE (cont.)

2.5 mg/kg PO two times per day or 5 mg/kg PO once daily for minimum of 14 to 21 days.

FORMS — Trade only: Tabs 200 mg (Onmel). Oral soln 10 mg/mL (Sporanox-150 mL). Generic/Trade: Caps 100 mg.

NOTES — Hepatotoxicity, even during 1st week of therapy. Monitor LFTs if baseline abnormal LFTs or history of drug-induced hepatotoxicity; consider monitoring in all patients. Decreased absorption of itraconazole with antacids, buffered didanosine, H2 blockers, proton pump inhibitors, or achlorhydria. Itraconazole levels reduced by carbamazepine, isoniazid, nevirapine, phenobarbital, phenytoin, rifabutin and rifampin, and potentially efavirenz. Itraconazole strongly inhibits CYP3A4 and P-glycoprotein metabolism of many drugs. May increase adverse effects of trazodone; consider reducing trazodone dose. Caps and oral soln not interchangeable. Oral soln recommended for oropharyngeal or esophageal candidiasis, and may be preferred in serious infections due to greater absorption. Oral soln may not achieve adequate levels in cystic fibrosis patients; consider alternative if no response. Start therapy for onychomycosis on days 1 to 2 of menses in women of childbearing potential and advise against pregnancy until 2 months after therapy ends.

MOA — Triazole that inhibits the synthesis of ergosterol (a sterol required for normal fungal cytoplasmic membrane).

ADVERSE EFFECTS — Serious: Negative inotrope, hepatotoxicity (even early in therapy), hypokalemia (with high doses). Frequent: GI complaints, allergic rash.

KETOCONAZOLE (Nizoral) ▶L ♀C ▶?+ $$$

WARNING — Do not use unless other antifungal drugs are not available or tolerated, and benefit of ketoconazole outweighs risk of hepatotoxicity, adrenal insufficiency, and drug interactions. Hepatotoxicity: Inform patients of risk and monitor. Ketoconazole is a strong CYP3A4 inhibitor and can prolong the QT interval. Contraindicated with disopyramide, dofetilide, dronedarone, methadone, pimozide, ranolazine, and quinidine due to increased risk of QT prolongation/ torsades.

ADULT — Blastomycosis, coccidioidomycosis, histoplasmosis, chromomycosis, paracoccidioidomycosis, in patients who failed or did not tolerate other antifungal drugs: 200 to 400 mg PO daily. Do not use to treat skin or nail infactions due to unacceptable risk of fatal liver failure.

PEDS — Blastomycosis, coccidioidomycosis, histoplasmosis, chromomycosis, paracoccidioidomycosis, in patients age 2 yo or older who failed or did not tolerate other antifungal drugs: 3.3 to 6.6 mg/kg PO daily. Do not use to treat skin or nail infactions due to unacceptable risk of fatal liver failure.

FORMS — Generic only: Tabs 200 mg.

NOTES — Hepatotoxicity; obtain baseline LFTs and monitor ALT weekly. Contraindicated in liver disease.

Adrenal insufficiency with doses of 400 mg/day or greater; monitor adrenal function in patients with adrenal insufficiency, borderline adrenal function, or prolonged periods of stress. Decreased absorption of ketoconazole by antacids, H2 blockers, proton pump inhibitors, buffered didanosine, and achlorhydria. Ketoconazole levels reduced by isoniazid, rifampin, and potentially efavirenz. Do not exceed 200 mg/day of ketoconazole with ritonavir, saquinavir, or Kaletra. Ketoconazole inhibits CYP3A4 metabolism of many drugs and can prolong the QT interval. Contraindicated with alprazolam, colchicine, disopyramide, dofetilide, dronedarone, eplerenone, ergot alkaloids, felodipine, irinotecan, lovastatin, lurasidone, oral midazolam, methadone, nisoldipine, pimozide, ranolazine, salmeterol, simvastatin, quinidine, tolvaptan, triazolam. May increase adverse effects of trazodone; consider lower trazodone dose.

MOA — Triazole that inhibits the synthesis of ergosterol (a sterol required for normal fungal cytoplasmic membrane). Inhibits adrenal function at doses of 400 mg/day or more. Reduces testosterone levels at doses of 800 to 1600 mg/day.

ADVERSE EFFECTS — Serious: Hepatotoxicity (even early in therapy). Adrenal insufficiency at doses of 400 mg/day or greater. Frequent: Dose-dependent N/V.

MICONAZOLE—BUCCAL (Oravig) ▶L ♀C ▶? $$$$$

ADULT — Oropharyngeal candidiasis: Apply 50 mg buccal tab to gums once daily for 14 days. Apply rounded side of tab to upper gum above incisor in the morning after brushing teeth. Hold in place for 30 seconds. Tab can be used if it sticks to cheek, inside of lip, or gum. Apply to new site each day.

PEDS — Not approved in children less than 16 yo; use adult dose for age 16 yo and older . Not recommended for younger children due to potential risk of choking.

FORMS — Trade only: Buccal tabs 50 mg.

NOTES — Contraindicated if hypersensitivity to milk protein concentrate. Increased INR with warfarin. Buccal tab is intended to remain in place until it dissolves. If it falls off within 6 h of application, reposition tab. If it does not stay in place, apply a new tab. If tab is swallowed within 1st 6 h, drink a glass of water and apply a new tab. No action is needed if tab falls off or is swallowed after it has been in place for at least 6 h. Do not chew gum while tab is in place.

MOA — Triazole that inhibits the synthesis of ergosterol (a sterol required for normal fungal cytoplasmic membrane).

ADVERSE EFFECTS — Severe: Hypersensitivity, including anaphylaxis.

POSACONAZOLE (Noxafil, ✷Posanol) ▶Glucuronidation ♀C ▶– $$$$$

ADULT — Prevention of invasive Aspergillus or Candida infection. Susp: 200 mg (5 mL) PO three times per day. Delayed-release tabs: Load with 300 mg PO two times per day on day 1, then 300 mg PO once daily. Injection: Load with 300 mg IV two times

(cont.)

POSACONAZOLE (*cont.*)

per day on day 1, then 300 mg IV once daily. Duration of treatment based on recovery from neutropenia or level of immunosuppression. Susp for oropharyngeal candidiasis: Load with 100 mg (2.5 mL) PO twice on day 1, then 100 mg PO once daily for 13 days. Susp for oropharyngeal candidiasis resistant to itraconazole/fluconazole: 400 mg (10 mL) PO two times per day; duration of therapy based on severity of underlying disease and clinical response. See IDSA regimen in UNAPPROVED adult. Take susp during or within 20 min of full meal or liquid nutritional supplement. Take delayed-release tabs with food. Susp and delayed-release tabs not interchangeable. IV posaconazole: Can give 1st dose by peripheral IV infusion over 30 minutes; infuse additional doses over 90 minutes by central venous line or peripherally-inserted central catheter.

PEDS — Prevention of invasive Aspergillus or Candida infection, age 13 yo or older. Susp: 200 mg (5 mL) susp PO three times per day. Delayed-relese tabs: Load with 300 mg two times per day on day 1, then 300 mg once daily. Susp for oropharyngeal candidiasis, age 13 yo or older: 100 mg (2.5 mL) PO twice on day 1, then 100 mg PO once daily for 13 days. Susp for oropharyngeal candidiasis resistant to itraconazole/fluconazole, age 13 yo or older: 400 mg (10 mL) PO two times per day; duration of therapy based on severity of underlying disease and clinical response. Take susp during or within 20 min of full meal or liquid nutritional supplement. Take delayed-release tabs with food. Delayed-release tabs and susp not interchangeable. IV posaconazole is not approved for use in children.

UNAPPROVED ADULT — Invasive pulmonary aspergillosis: 200 mg susp PO four times per day, then 400 mg PO two times per day when stable. Treat invasive pulmonary aspergillosis for at least 6 to 12 weeks; treat immunosuppressed patients throughout immunosuppression and until lesions resolved. Fluconazole-refractory oropharyngeal candidiasis: 400 mg susp PO two times per day for 3 days, then 400 mg PO once daily for up to 28 days.

FORMS — Trade only: Delayed-release tabs 100 mg. Oral susp 40 mg/mL (105 mL).

NOTES — Consider alternative or monitor for breakthrough fungal infection if patient cannot take susp during or within 20 min of a full meal or liquid nutritional supplement. If meal or liquid supplement not tolerated, consider giving with acidic carbonated drink (eg, ginger ale) or switch to delayed-release tab if indicated. When possible avoid cimetidine or proton pump inhibitor with posaconazole susp, but not delayed-release tabs. Monitor for breakthrough fungal infection if severe vomiting/diarrhea, posaconazole susp is given by NG tube, or proton pump inhibitor or metoclopramide is coadministered with susp. Posaconazole is a strong CYP3A4 inhibitor. Contraindicated with atorvastatin, ergot alkaloids, lovastatin, simvastatin, sirolimus, and CYP3A4 substrates that prolong the QT interval,

including pimozide and quinidine. Correct electrolyte imbalances before starting posaconazole. Monitor for adverse effects of atazanavir, ritonavir, alprazolam, midazolam, triazolam. Consider dosage reduction of vinca alkaloids, calcium channel blockers. Reduce cyclosporine dose by 25% and tacrolimus dose by 66% when posaconazole started; monitor levels of cyclosporine, tacrolimus. Posaconazole levels reduced by efavirenz, rifabutin, and phenytoin; phenytoin and rifabutin levels increased by posaconazole. Do not coadminister unless benefit exceeds risk. Monitor for rifabutin adverse effects. Posaconazole levels reduced by fosamprenavir; monitor for breakthrough fungal infection. Posaconazole oral suspension doses >800 mg/day are unlikely to increase posaconazole exposure. Do not split, crush, or chew delayed-release tabs. Renal impairment: Monitor for breakthrough fungal infection in patients with renal impairment receiving PO posaconazole. Vehicle for IV posaconazole can accumulate in renal impairment; avoid if eGFR <50 mL/min unless benefit exceeds risk of accumulation. If IV posaconazole is used in renal impairment, monitor serum creatinine and consider other treatment if increase occurs.

MOA — Triazole that inhibits the synthesis of ergosterol (a sterol required for normal fungal cytoplasmic membrane).

ADVERSE EFFECTS — Serious: Possible hepatotoxicity. Torsades de pointes possibly related to drug interactions in which CYP3A4 inhibiton by posaconazole increases exposure of CYP 3A4 substrates that prolong QT interval. Repeat peripheral infusion of IV posaconazole can cause infusion site reactions. Frequent: diarrhea, N/V, fever, headache, cough, hypokalemia.

VORICONAZOLE (*Vfend*) ▶L ♀D ▶? $$$$$

ADULT — Invasive aspergillosis, scedosporiosis, fusariosis: 6 mg/kg IV q 12 h for 2 doses, then 4 mg/kg IV q 12 h. Systemic candidiasis: 6 mg/kg IV q 12 h for 2 doses, then 3 to 4 mg/kg IV q 12 h. Treat until at least 14 days past resolution of signs/symptoms or last positive blood culture. Maintenance therapy, aspergillosis or candidiasis: 200 mg PO two times per day. For wt less than 40 kg, reduce to 100 mg PO two times per day. See prescribing information for dosage adjustments for poor response/adverse effects. Esophageal candidiasis: 200 mg PO q 12 h for at least 14 days and 7 days past resolution of signs/symptoms. For wt less than 40 kg, reduce to 100 mg PO two times per day. Dosage adjustment for efavirenz: Voriconazole 400 mg PO two times per day with efavirenz 300 mg (use caps) PO once daily. Take tabs or susp 1 h before or after meals.

PEDS — Use adult dose for age 12 yo or older. See UNAPPROVED PEDS for alternative doses for age 12 to 14 yo and wt less than 50 kg.

UNAPPROVED ADULT — Fluconazole-refractory oropharyngeal or esophageal candidiasis: 200 mg PO two times per day for 14 to 21 days. For wt less than 40 kg, reduce to 100 mg PO two times per day.

(cont.)

VORICONAZOLE (*cont.*)

UNAPPROVED PEDS — Invasive aspergillosis, systemic Candida infection, age 2 to 11 yo: 9 mg/kg IV q 12 h for 2 doses, then 8 mg/kg IV q 12 h. After 1 week and clinical improvement, convert to 9 mg/kg (max 350 mg) PO q 12 h. Adolescents, age 12 to 14 yo: Use pediatric dose if wt less than 50 kg; use adult doses if wt 50 kg or greater. Therapeutic drug monitoring recommended due to variable pharmacokinetics in children.

FORMS — Generic/Trade: Tabs 50, 200 mg (contains lactose). Susp 40 mg/mL (75 mL).

NOTES — Anaphylactoid reactions (IV only). QT interval prolongation; correct electrolytes. Severe skin reactions. Phototoxicity (esp in children) that may increase the risk of squamous cell carcinoma and melanoma; avoid direct sunlight and use protective clothing. Hepatotoxicity (rare); monitor LFTs at baseline, weekly for 1st month, then monthly thereafter. Transient visual disturbances common; advise against hazardous tasks (if vision impaired), night driving, and strong, direct sunlight. Monitor visual (if treated for more than 28 days) and renal function. Monitor pancreatic function if at risk for acute pancreatitis (recent chemotherapy/stem cell transplant). Many drug interactions. Substrate and inhibitor of CYP2C9, 2C19, and 3A4. Do not use with carbamazepine, efavirenz 400 mg/day or more, ergot alkaloids, everolimus, fluconazole, lopinavir-ritonavir (Kaletra), phenobarbital, pimozide, quinidine, rifabutin, rifampin, ritonavir 400 mg two times per day, sirolimus, or St. John's wort. Ritonavir decreases voriconazole levels; avoid coadministration unless benefit exceeds risk. Dosage adjustments for drug interactions with cyclosporine, omeprazole, phenytoin, tacrolimus in prescribing information. Increased INR with warfarin. Could inhibit metabolism of benzodiazepines, calcium channel blockers, fentanyl, ibuprofen, methadone, oxycodone, and statins. When combining voriconazole with oral contraceptives, monitor for adverse effects from increased levels of voriconazole, estrogen, and progestin. Dilute IV to 5 mg/mL or less; max infusion rate is 3 mg/kg/h over 1 to 2 h. Do not infuse IV voriconazole at same time as a blood product/concentrated electrolytes even if given by separate IV lines. IV voriconazole can be infused at the same time as non-concentrated electrolytes/total parenteral nutrition if given by separate lines; give TPN by different port if multi-lumen catheter is used. Vehicle in IV form may accumulate in renal impairment; oral preferred if CrCl <50 mL/min. Mild/moderate cirrhosis (Child-Pugh class A/B): Same loading dose and reduce maintenance dose by 50%. Oral susp stable for 14 days at room temperature.

MOA — Triazole that inhibits the synthesis of ergosterol (a sterol required for normal fungal cytoplasmic membrane).

ADVERSE EFFECTS — Serious: Anaphylactoid reactions (IV only); QT interval prolongation; hepatotoxicity (rare); severe skin reactions; photosensitivity (esp in children) which may increase the risk of squamous cell carcinoma or melanoma; pancreatitis. Frequent: Mild transient visual disturbances, rash, elevated LFTs. Other: Hallucinations, confusion.

ANTIMICROBIALS: Antifungal Agents—Echinocandins

NOTE: See www.idsociety.org for guidelines on the management of fungal infections. See www.aidsinfo.nih.gov for management of fungal infections in HIV-infected patients.

ANIDULAFUNGIN (*Eraxis*) ▶Degraded chemically ♀B ▶? $$$$$

ADULT — Candidemia, other systemic candidal infections: 200 mg IV load on day 1, then 100 mg IV once daily until at least 14 days after last positive culture. Esophageal candidiasis: 100 mg IV load on day 1, then 50 mg IV once daily for at least 14 days, and continuing for at least 7 days after symptoms resolved.

PEDS — Not approved in children.

UNAPPROVED PEDS — Systemic candidal infections, age 1 mo and older: Load with 1.5 to 3 mg/kg IV on day 1, then 0.75 to 1.5 mg/kg IV once daily. IDSA recommends 1.5 mg/kg/day to treat systemic Candida infections in neonates and children.

NOTES — Can cause anaphylaxis. Max infusion rate of 1.1 mg/min to prevent histamine reactions. Diluent contains dehydrated alcohol.

MOA — Echinocandin that blocks the synthesis of glucan, a fungal cell wall polysaccharide.

ADVERSE EFFECTS — Hepatotoxicity (rare). Anaphylaxis, including shock. Histamine reactions (rash, urticaria, flushing pruritus, dyspnea, hypotension) minimized by infusion rate less than 1.1 mg/min. Diarrhea, hypokalemia, N/V.

CASPOFUNGIN (*Cancidas*) ▶KL ♀C ▶? $$$$$

ADULT — Infuse IV over 1 h. Aspergillosis, candidemia, empiric therapy of fungal infection in febrile neutropenia: Load with 70 mg on day 1, then 50 mg once daily. Patients taking rifampin: 70 mg once daily. Consider this dose with other enzyme inducers (eg, carbamazepine, dexamethasone, efavirenz, nevirapine, phenytoin) or if inadequate response to lower dose in febrile neutropenia or aspergillosis. Esophageal candidiasis: 50 mg daily. Duration of therapy in invasive aspergillosis is based on severity, treatment response, and resolution of immunosuppression. Treat candidal infections for at least 14 days after last positive culture. For empiric therapy of febrile neutropenia, treat until neutropenia resolved. If fungal infection confirmed, treat for at least 14 days and continue for at least 7 days after symptoms and neutropenia resolved.

(cont.)

CASPOFUNGIN (*cont.*)

PEDS — Infuse IV over 1 h. Aspergillosis, candidemia, esophageal candidiasis, empiric therapy of fungal infection in febrile neutropenia, 3 mo to 17 yo: Load with 70 mg/m^2 on day 1, then 50 mg/m^2 once daily. Consider increasing daily dose to 70 mg/m^2 up to max of 70 mg once daily if coadministered with enzyme inducers (eg, carbamazepine, dexamethasone, efavirenz, nevirapine, phenytoin, or rifampin) or if inadequate response to lower dose in febrile neutropenia or aspergillosis. Duration of therapy in invasive aspergillosis is based on severity, treatment response, and resolution of immunosuppression. Treat Candida infections for at least 14 days after last positive culture. For empiric therapy of febrile neutropenia, treat until neutropenia resolved. If fungal infection confirmed, treat for at least 14 days and continue for at least 7 days after symptoms and neutropenia resolved. For best pediatric dosing accuracy, use 50 mg vial (5 mg/mL) for dose less than 50 mg and 70 mg vial (7 mg/mL) for dose greater than 50 mg.

NOTES — Abnormal LFTs reported; possible risk of hepatitis. Monitor hepatic function if abnormal LFTs. Cyclosporine increases caspofungin levels and hepatic transaminases; risk of concomitant use unclear. Caspofungin decreases tacrolimus levels. Dosage adjustment in adults with moderate liver dysfunction (Child-Pugh score 7 to 9): 35 mg IV daily (after 70 mg loading dose in invasive aspergillosis).

MOA — Echinocandin that blocks the synthesis of glucan, a fungal cell wall polysaccharide.

ADVERSE EFFECTS — Serious: Anaphylaxis (rare). Abnormal LFTs reported; possible risk of hepatitis. Frequent: Fever, rash, N/V, diarrhea, hypokalemia, phlebitis at injection site. Some infusion reactions (like facial flushing, angioedema, bronchospasm) caused by histamine release.

MICAFUNGIN (*Mycamine*) ▶L, feces ♀C ▶? $$$$$

ADULT — Esophageal candidiasis: 150 mg IV once daily. Candidemia, acute disseminated candidiasis, Candida peritonitis/abscess: 100 mg IV once daily. Prevention of candidal infections in bone marrow transplant patients: 50 mg IV once daily. Infuse over 1 h to reduce histamine reactions with rapid infusion. Flush IV line with NS before infusing micafungin.

PEDS — Esophageal candidiasis, age 4 mo and older: 3 mg/kg IV once daily for wt 30 kg or less; 2.5 mg/kg IV up to 150 mg once daily for wt greater than 30 kg. Candidemia, acute disseminated candidiasis, Candida peritonitis/abscess, age 4 mo and older: 2 mg/kg up to 100 mg IV once daily. Prevention of candidal infections in bone marrow transplant patients, age 4 mo and older: 1 mg/kg up to 50 mg IV once daily. Infuse over 1 h to reduce histamine reactions with rapid infusion. Infuse concentrations greater than 1.5 mg/mL by central catheter. Flush IV line with NS before infusing micafungin.

UNAPPROVED ADULT — Prophylaxis of invasive aspergillosis: 50 mg IV once daily infused over 1 h.

NOTES — Increases levels of sirolimus and nifedipine. Not dialyzed. Protect diluted soln from light. Do not mix with other meds; it may precipitate.

MOA — Echinocandin that blocks the synthesis of glucan, a fungal cell wall polysaccharide.

ADVERSE EFFECTS — Serious: Anaphylaxis/anaphylactoid reactions (rare); renal/hepatic dysfunction; hemolysis/hemolytic anemia. Frequent: Thrombocytopenia, N/V, fever, headache. Histamine-related symptoms (more frequent with rapid infusion): Rash, pruritus, facial swelling, vasodilation. Injection site reactions more common with peripheral infusion.

ANTIMICROBIALS: Antifungal Agents—Polyenes

NOTE: See www.idsociety.org for guidelines on the management of fungal infections. See www.aidsinfo.nih.gov for management of fungal infections in HIV-infected patients.

AMPHOTERICIN B DEOXYCHOLATE ▶Tissues ♀B ▶? $$$$$

WARNING — Do not use IV route for noninvasive fungal infections (oral thrush, vaginal or esophageal candidiasis) in patients with normal neutrophil counts.

ADULT — Life-threatening systemic fungal infections: Test dose 1 mg in 20 mL D5W infused IV over 20 to 30 minutes. Wait 2 to 4 h, and if tolerated start 0.25 mg/kg IV daily. Advance to 0.5 to 1.5 mg/kg/day depending on fungal type. Infuse over 2 to 6 h. Hydrate with 500 mL NS before and after infusion to decrease risk of nephrotoxicity.

PEDS — No remaining FDA-approved indications.

UNAPPROVED ADULT — Alternative regimen, life-threatening systemic fungal infections: 1 mg test dose as part of 1st infusion (no need for separate IV bag); if tolerated continue infusion, giving target dose of 0.5 to 1.5 mg/kg on 1st day. Candidemia: 0.5 to 1 mg/kg IV daily. Treat until 14 days after 1st negative blood culture and resolution of signs/symptoms. Symptomatic Candida cystitis: 0.3 to 0.6 mg/kg IV for 1 to 7 days. Candida pyelonephritis: 0.3 to 0.6 mg/kg IV daily (± flucytosine). Cryptococcal meningitis in HIV infection: 0.7 mg/kg/day IV preferably in combo with flucytosine 25 mg/kg PO q 6 h for 2 weeks. Follow with fluconazole consolidation, then fluconazole chronic suppression until immune reconstitution.

UNAPPROVED PEDS — Systemic life-threatening fungal infections: Test dose 0.1 mg/kg (max of 1 mg) slow IV. Wait 2 to 4 h, and if tolerated start 0.25 mg/kg IV once daily. Advance to 0.5 to 1.5 mg/kg/day depending on fungal type. Infuse over 2 to 6 h. Hydrate with 10 to 15 mL/kg NS before infusion to decrease risk of nephrotoxicity. Alternative dosing

(cont.)

AMPHOTERICIN B DEOXYCHOLATE (*cont.*)

regimen: Give test dose as part of 1st infusion (separate IV bag not needed); if tolerated, continue infusion, giving target dose of 0.5 to 1.5 mg/kg on 1st day. Cryptococcal infection in HIV-infected patients: 0.7 to 1 mg/kg IV once daily; may add flucytosine depending on site and severity of infection.

NOTES — Acute infusion reactions, anaphylaxis, nephrotoxicity, hypokalemia, hypomagnesemia, acidosis, anemia. Monitor renal and hepatic function, CBC, serum electrolytes. Lipid formulations better tolerated, preferred in renal dysfunction.

MOA — Polyene antifungal, Insertion into fungal cytoplasmic membrane increases membrane permeability.

ADVERSE EFFECTS — Serious for IV Fungizone: Anaphylaxis, anemia, nephrotoxicity. Frequent: Acute infusion reactions, nephrotoxicity (hypokalemia, hypomagnesemia, renal tubular acidosis).

AMPHOTERICIN B LIPID FORMULATIONS (*Abelcet, AmBisome*) ▶? ♀B ▶? $$$$$

ADULT — Lipid formulations used primarily in patients refractory/intolerant to amphotericin deoxycholate. Abelcet. Invasive fungal infections: 5 mg/kg/day IV at 2.5 mg/kg/h. Shake infusion bag q 2 h. AmBisome. Infuse IV over 2 h. Empiric therapy of fungal infections in febrile neutropenia: 3 mg/kg/day. Aspergillus, candidal, cryptococcal infections: 3 to 5 mg/kg/day. Visceral leishmaniasis: 3 mg/kg IV on days 1 to 5 and days 14 and 21 for immunocompetent patients; 4 mg/kg IV on days 1 to 5 and days 10, 17, 24, 31, and 38 for immunocompromised patients. Cryptococcal meningitis in HIV infection: 6 mg/kg/day.

PEDS — Lipid formulations used primarily in patients refractory/intolerant to amphotericin deoxycholate. Abelcet. Invasive fungal infections: 5 mg/kg/day IV at 2.5 mg/kg/h. Shake infusion bag q 2 h. AmBisome. Infuse IV over 2 h. Empiric therapy of fungal infections in febrile neutropenia: 3 mg/kg/day. Aspergillus, candidal, cryptococcal infections: 3 to 5 mg/kg/day. Visceral leishmaniasis: 3 mg/kg IV on days 1 to 5 and days 14 and 21 for immunocompetent patients; 4 mg/kg IV on days 1 to 5 and days 10, 17, 24, 31, and 38 for immunocompromised patients. Cryptococcal meningitis in HIV infection: 6 mg/kg/day.

NOTES — Acute infusion reactions, anaphylaxis, nephrotoxicity, hypokalemia, hypomagnesemia, acidosis. Lipid formulations better tolerated than amphotericin deoxycholate, preferred in renal dysfunction. Monitor renal and hepatic function, CBC, electrolytes.

MOA — Polyene antifungal, Insertion into fungal cytoplasmic membrane increases membrane permeability.

ADVERSE EFFECTS — Serious: Anaphylaxis. Frequent: Acute infusion reactions, nephrotoxicity (hypokalemia, hypomagnesemia, renal tubular acidosis). Lipid formulations better tolerated than amphotericin deoxycholate.

ANTIMICROBIALS: Antifungal Agents—Other

NOTE: See www.idsociety.org for guidelines on the management of fungal infections. See www.aidsinfo.nih.gov for management of fungal infections in HIV-infected patients.

FLUCYTOSINE (*Ancobon*) ▶K ♀C Contraindicated in first trimester. ▶– $$$$$

WARNING — Extreme caution in renal or bone marrow impairment. Monitor hematologic, hepatic, renal function in all patients.

ADULT — Candidal/cryptococcal infections: 50 to 150 mg/kg/day PO divided four times per day. Candida UTI: 100 mg/kg/day PO divided four times per day for 7 to 10 days for symptomatic cystitis, for 14 days (± amphotericin deoxycholate) for pyelonephritis. Initial therapy for cryptococcal meningitis: 100 mg/kg/day PO divided four times per day.

PEDS — Not approved in children.

UNAPPROVED PEDS — Candidal/cryptococcal infections: 50 to 150 mg/kg/day PO divided four times per day.

FORMS — Generic/Trade: Caps 250, 500 mg.

NOTES — Flucytosine is given with other antifungal agents. Myelosuppression. Reduce nausea by taking caps a few at a time over 15 min. Monitor flucytosine levels with target peak level 2 h after dose of 30 to 80 mcg/mL. Reduce dose in renal dysfunction. Avoid in children with severe renal dysfunction.

MOA — Deaminated to inhibitor of thymidylate synthetase, which interferes with DNA synthesis.

ADVERSE EFFECTS — Serious: Myelosuppression (frequent); anaphylaxis; hepatic, renal, cardiac and CNS toxicity (all rare). Frequent: N/V, diarrhea, rash.

GRISEOFULVIN ▶Skin ♀ X/?/?. Contraindicated in pregnancy. ▶? $$$$$

ADULT — Tinea: 500 mg PO daily for 4 to 6 weeks for capitis, 2 to 4 weeks for corporis, 4 to 8 weeks for pedis, 4 months for fingernails, 6 months for toenails. Can use 1 g/day for pedis and unguium.

PEDS — Tinea: 11 mg/kg PO daily for 4 to 6 weeks for capitis, 2 to 4 weeks for corporis, 4 to 8 weeks for pedis, 4 months for fingernails, 6 months for toenails.

UNAPPROVED PEDS — Tinea capitis: AAP recommends 10 to 20 mg/kg (max 1 g) PO daily for 4 to 6 weeks, continuing for 2 weeks past symptom resolution. Some infections may require 20 to 25 mg/kg/day or ultramicrosize griseofulvin 5 to 10 mg/kg (max 750 mg) PO daily.

FORMS — Generic only: Susp 125 mg/5 mL (120 mL). Tabs 500 mg.

NOTES — Do not use in liver failure, porphyria. May cause photosensitivity, lupus-like syndrome/exacerbation of lupus. Decreased INR with warfarin, decreased efficacy of oral contraceptives.

(cont.)

GRISEOFULVIN *(cont.)*

Ultramicrosize formulations have greater GI absorption and are available with different strengths and dosing.

MOA — Inhibits fungal mitosis by disrupting mitotic spindle.

ADVERSE EFFECTS — Serious: Photosensitivity, lupus-like syndrome/exacerbation of lupus, increased porphyrins (not for use by patients with porphyria). Frequent: Allergic skin reactions, headache.

GRISEOFULVIN ULTRAMICROSIZE *(Gris-PEG)* ▶Skin ♀X/?/?. Contraindicated in pregnancy. ▶? $$$$$

ADULT — Tinea: 375 mg PO daily for 4 to 6 weeks for capitis, 2 to 4 weeks for corporis, 4 to 8 weeks for pedis, 4 months for fingernails, 6 months for toenails. Can use 750 mg/day for pedis and unguium. Best absorption when given after meal containing fat.

PEDS — Tinea, age 2 yo or older: 7.3 mg/kg PO daily for 4 to 6 weeks for capitis, 2 to 4 weeks for corporis, 4 to 8 weeks for pedis, 4 months for fingernails, 6 months for toenails. Give 125 to 187.5 mg PO daily for 16 to 27 kg. Give 187.5 to 375 mg for wt greater than 27 kg. Tinea capitis: AAP recommends 5 to 15 mg/kg (up to 750 mg) PO daily for 4 to 6 weeks, continuing for 2 weeks past symptom resolution. Best absorption when given after meal containing fat. Can crush tabs, sprinkle onto 1 tablespoon of applesauce, and swallow immediately without chewing.

FORMS — Generic/Trade: Tabs 125, 250 mg.

NOTES — Do not use in liver failure, porphyria. May cause photosensitivity, lupus-like syndrome/exacerbation of lupus. Decreased INR with warfarin, decreased efficacy of oral contraceptives. Microsize formulations, which have lower GI absorption, are available with different strengths and dosing.

MOA — Inhibits fungal mitosis by disrupting mitotic spindle.

ADVERSE EFFECTS — Serious: Photosensitivity, lupus-like syndrome/exacerbation of lupus, increased porphyrins (not for use by patients with porphyria). Frequent: Allergic skin reactions, headache.

NYSTATIN ▶Not absorbed ♀C ▶+ $

ADULT — Thrush: 4 to 6 mL susp PO swish and swallow four times per day. Non-esophageal mucus membrane gastrointestinal candidiasis: 1 to 2 tabs PO 3 times per day.

PEDS — Thrush. Infants: 2 mL/dose PO with 1 mL in each cheek four times per day. Premature and low-wt infants: 0.5 mL PO in each cheek four times per day. Older children: 4 to 6 mL PO swish and swallow four times per day.

FORMS — Generic only: Susp 100,000 units/mL (60, 480 mL). Film-coated tabs 500,000 units.

MOA — Alters fungal cell membrane permeability by binding with sterols.

ADVERSE EFFECTS — Serious: Hypersensitivity, including Stevens-Johnson syndrome. Frequent: N/V, diarrhea, rash.

TERBINAFINE *(Lamisil)* ▶LK ♀B ▶− $$$$$

ADULT — Onychomycosis: 250 mg PO daily for 6 weeks (fingernails) or 12 weeks (toenails).

PEDS — Tinea capitis, age 4 yo or older: Give PO once daily at a dose of 125 mg for wt less than 25 kg, 187.5 mg for wt 25 to 35 kg, 250 mg for wt more than 35 kg. Treat T tonsurans for 2 to 4 weeks, M canis for 4 to 6 weeks.

UNAPPROVED PEDS — Onychomycosis: Give PO once daily at dse of 62.5 mg for wt less than 20 kg, 125 mg for wt 20 to 40 kg, 250 mg for wt greater than 40 kg. Treat for 6 weeks (fingernails) or 12 weeks (toenails).

FORMS — Generic/Trade: Tabs 250 mg. No pediatric formulation; pharmacists can make oral susp.

NOTES — Hepatotoxicity; monitor AST and ALT at baseline. Neutropenia; discontinue if neutrophils ≤1000 cells/mm^3. May rarely cause or exacerbate lupus. Do not use in liver disease or CrCl <50 mL/min. Test nail specimen to confirm diagnosis before prescribing. Inhibits CYP2D6.

MOA — Inhibits squalene epoxidase, an enzyme involved in the synthesis of ergosterol (a sterol required for normal fungal cytoplasmic membrane).

ADVERSE EFFECTS — Serious: Hepatotoxicity, neutropenia, depression, Stevens-Johnson syndrome, toxic epidermal necrolysis, DRESS, taste and smell disturbances (severe, prolonged, or permanent). May rarely cause or exacerbate lupus. Frequent: N/V, rash.

ANTIMICROBIALS: Antimalarials

NOTE: For help treating malaria or getting antimalarials, see www.cdc.gov/malaria or call the "malaria hotline" at CDC. Call 770-488-7788 or 855-856-4713 toll-free Monday-Friday 9 am to 5 pm EST; after hours call 770-488-7100 and ask for the Malaria Branch clinician. Pediatric doses of antimalarials should never exceed adult doses.

CHLOROQUINE *(Aralen)* ▶KL ♀C but +. ▶+ $

WARNING — Review product labeling for precautions and adverse effects before prescribing.

ADULT — Doses as chloroquine phosphate. Malaria prophylaxis, chloroquine-sensitive areas: 500 mg PO q week from 1 to 2 weeks before exposure to 4 weeks after. Malaria treatment, chloroquine-sensitive areas: 1 g PO once, then 500 mg PO at 6, 24, and 48 h. Total dose is 2.5 g. Extraintestinal amebiasis: 1 g PO daily for 2 days, then 500 mg PO daily for 2 to 3 weeks.

PEDS — Doses as chloroquine phosphate. Malaria prophylaxis, chloroquine-sensitive areas: 8.3 mg/kg (up to 500 mg) PO q week from 1 to 2 weeks before exposure to 4 weeks after. Malaria treatment, chloroquine-sensitive areas: 16.7 mg/kg PO once, then 8.3 mg/kg at 6, 24, and 48 h. Do not exceed

(cont.)

CHLOROQUINE (*cont.*)

adult dose. Chloroquine phosphate 8.3 mg/kg is equivalent to chloroquine base 5 mg/kg.

FORMS — Generic only: Tabs 250 mg. Generic/Trade: Tabs 500 mg (500 mg phosphate equivalent to 300 mg base).

NOTES — Can prolong QT interval and cause torsades. Retinopathy with chronic/high doses; eye exams required. May cause seizures (caution advised if epilepsy), ototoxicity (caution advised if hearing loss), myopathy (discontinue if muscle weakness develops), bone marrow toxicity (monitor CBC if long-term use), exacerbation of psoriasis. Concentrates in liver; caution advised if hepatic disease, alcoholism, or hepatotoxic drugs. Antacids reduce absorption; give at least 4 h apart. May increase cyclosporine levels. As little as 1 g can cause fatal overdose in a child. Fatal malaria reported after chloroquine used as malaria prophylaxis in areas with chloroquine resistance; use only in areas without resistance. Other agents are superior for severe chloroquine-sensitive malaria. Maternal antimalarial prophylaxis doesn't harm breastfed infant or protect infant from malaria. Use with primaquine phosphate for treatment of P. vivax or P. ovale.

MOA — Plasmodicidal mechanism of action unknown, may inhibit heme polymerase or interact with DNA.

ADVERSE EFFECTS — Serious: Retinopathy with chronic/high doses; can cause torsades. Fatal malaria in patients receiving chloroquine prophylaxis in areas with chloroquine resistance.

COARTEM (**artemether + lumefantrine**) ▶L ♀C ▶? $$$$

ADULT — Uncomplicated malaria, wt 35 kg or greater: 4 tabs PO two times per day for 3 days. On day 1, give 2nd dose 8 h after 1st dose. Take with food.

PEDS — Uncomplicated malaria, wt greater than 5 kg and age 2 mo or older: Take with food two times per day for 3 days. On day 1, give 2nd dose 8 h after 1st dose. Dose based on wt: 1 tab for 5 to 14 kg; 2 tabs for 15 to 24 kg; 3 tabs for 25 to 34 kg; 4 tabs for 35 kg or greater.

FORMS — Trade only: Tabs, artemether 20 mg + lumefantrine 120 mg. Call 1-855-COARTEM for availability.

NOTES — Can prolong QT interval; avoid using in proarrhythmic conditions or with drugs that prolong QT interval. Monitor ECG if quinine/quinidine or other antimalarial that prolongs QT interval is given soon after Coartem, due to long half-life of lumefantrine. Do not use Coartem and halofantrine within 1 month of each other. Contraindicated with strong CYP3A4 inducers (eg, carbamazepine, phenytoin, rifampin, St. John's wort). May inhibit CYP2D6; avoid with drugs metabolized by CYP2D6 that have cardiac effects and caution with CYP3A4 inhibitors as both interactions may prolong QT interval. Repeat the dose if vomiting occurs within 1 to 2 h; use another antimalarial if 2nd dose is

vomited. Can crush tabs and mix with 1 to 2 tsp water immediately before the dose.

MOA — Artemether and lumefantrine are blood schizonticides.

ADVERSE EFFECTS — Serious: Urticaria/angioedema. Can prolong QT interval. Frequent: Headache, anorexia, dizziness, asthenia in adults. Fever, cough, vomiting, anorexia, headache in children.

MALARONE (**atovaquone + proguanil**) ▶ Feces; LK ♀C ▶? $$$$$

ADULT — Malaria prophylaxis: 1 adult tab PO once daily from 1 to 2 days before exposure until 7 days after. Malaria treatment: 4 adult tabs PO once daily for 3 days. Take with food/milky drink at same time each day. Repeat dose if vomiting within 1 h after the dose. CDC recommends for presumptive self-treatment of malaria (same dose as for treatment, but not for patients currently taking it for prophylaxis).

PEDS — Safety and efficacy established in children with wt 11 kg or greater for prevention, and 5 kg or greater for treatment. Prevention of malaria: Give following dose based on wt PO once daily from 1 to 2 days before exposure until 7 days after: 1 ped tab for 11 to 20 kg; 2 ped tabs for 21 to 30 kg; 3 ped tabs for 31 to 40 kg; 1 adult tab for greater than 40 kg. Treatment of malaria: Give following dose based on wt PO once daily for 3 days: 2 ped tabs for 5 to 8 kg; 3 ped tabs for 9 to 10 kg; 1 adult tab for 11 to 20 kg; 2 adult tabs for 21 to 30 kg; 3 adult tabs for 31 to 40 kg; 4 adult tabs for greater than 40 kg. Take with food or milky drink at same time each day. Repeat dose if vomiting occurs within 1 h after dose.

UNAPPROVED PEDS — CDC doses for prevention of malaria: Give following dose based on wt PO once daily from 1 to 2 days before exposure until 7 days after: ½ ped tab for 5 to 8 kg; ¾ ped tab for 9 to 10 kg. Not advised for infants less than 5 kg.

FORMS — Generic/Trade: Adult tabs atovaquone 250 mg + proguanil 100 mg. Pediatric tabs 62.5 mg + 25 mg.

NOTES — Vomiting common with malaria treatment doses (consider antiemetic). Monitor parasitemia. Atovaquone levels may be decreased by efavirenz (avoid) tetracycline, metoclopramide (use another antiemetic if possible), and rifampin (avoid). Proguanil may increase the INR with warfarin. CDC recommends against use by women breastfeeding infant weighing less than 5 kg. Renal impairment: Avoid for prophylaxis and use cautiously for treatment if CrCl <30 mL/min.

MOA — Atovaquone and proguanil interfere with two different pyrimidine biosynthesis pathways. Atovaquone inhibits parasitic mitochondrial electron transport. A proguanil metabolite, cycloguanil, inhibits dihydrofolate reductase.

ADVERSE EFFECTS — Serious: Hepatitis/increased LFTs, anaphylaxis, Stevens-Johnson syndrome, photosensitivity. Frequent: Vomiting with malaria treatment doses, GI complaints, headache, asthenia, dizziness.

MEFLOQUINE ▶L ♀B ▶? $$

WARNING — Neurologic or psychiatric adverse effects such as dizziness, tinnitus, anxiety, hallucinations, and paranoia may persist.

ADULT — Malaria prophylaxis, chloroquine-resistant areas: 250 mg PO once weekly from 1 week before exposure until 4 weeks after. CDC recommends starting mefloquine prophylaxis at least 2 weeks before exposure. Malaria treatment: 1250 mg PO single dose. Take on full stomach with at least 8 ounces water.

PEDS — Malaria treatment: 20 to 25 mg/kg PO; given in 1 to 2 divided doses 6 to 8 h apart to reduce risk of vomiting. Repeat full dose if vomiting within 30 min after dose; repeat ½ dose if vomiting within 30 to 60 min after dose. Experience limited in infants age younger than 3 mo or wt less than 5 kg. Malaria prophylaxis: Approximately 5 mg/kg PO once weekly starting 1 week before exposure until 4 weeks after. CDC recommends starting mefloquine prophylaxis at least 2 weeks before exposure. Dose according to wt: ½ tab for 20 to 30 kg; ¾ tab for 30 to 45 kg; 1 tab for greater than 45 kg. Experience limited with wt less than 20 kg. Pharmacist can compound small doses. Take on full stomach.

UNAPPROVED ADULT — CDC regimen for malaria: 750 mg PO followed by 500 mg PO 6 to 12 h later, for total of 1250 mg. Quinine + doxycycline/tetracycline/clindamycin or atovaquone-proguanil preferred over mefloquine because of high rate of neuropsychiatric adverse effects with malaria treatment doses of mefloquine.

UNAPPROVED PEDS — Malaria prophylaxis, chloroquine-resistant areas, CDC regimen: Give PO once weekly starting at least 2 weeks before exposure until 4 weeks after at a dose of 5 mg/kg for wt 9 kg or less; ¼ tab for wt greater than 9 to 19 kg; ½ tab for wt greater than 19 to 30 kg; ¾ tab for wt greater than 30 to 45 kg; 1 tab for wt greater than 45 kg. Malaria treatment, wt less than 45 kg: 15 mg/kg PO, then 10 mg/kg PO given 8 to 12 h after 1st dose. Take on full stomach.

FORMS — Generic only: Tabs 250 mg.

NOTES — Cardiac conduction disturbances. Do not use with ziprasidone. Do not give until 12 h after the last dose of quinidine, quinine, or chloroquine; may cause ECG changes and seizures. Contraindicated for prophylaxis if depression (active/recent), generalized anxiety disorder, psychosis, schizophrenia, other major psychiatric disorder, or history of seizures. Consider starting up to 3 weeks before travel to assess tolerability. Tell patients to discontinue if psychiatric symptoms occur during prophylaxis. May cause drowsiness (warn about hazardous tasks). Can crush tabs and mix with a little water, milk, or other liquid. Pharmacists can put small doses into caps to mask bitter taste. Decreases valproate levels. Rifampin decreases mefloquine levels. Maternal use of antimalarial prophylaxis doesn't harm or protect breastfed infant from malaria.

MOA — Acts as blood schizonticide, exact mechanism of action is unknown.

ADVERSE EFFECTS — Serious: Cardiac conduction disturbances including QT prolongation, psychiatric reactions. Frequent: Dizziness, loss of balance, sleep disturbances (especially early in therapy and in women). Early vomiting in children with malaria treatment dose.

PRIMAQUINE ▶L ♀– ▶– $$$

WARNING — Review product labeling for precautions and adverse effects and document normal G6PD level before prescribing.

ADULT — Prevention of relapse, P. vivax/ovale malaria: 30 mg base PO daily for 14 days.

PEDS — Not approved in children.

UNAPPROVED ADULT — Pneumocystis in patients intolerant to trimethoprim-sulfamethoxazole: 30 mg primaquine base PO daily plus clindamycin 600 mg IV q 6 h to 900 mg IV q 8 h or 450 mg PO q 6 h or 600 mg PO q 8 h for 21 days. Primary prophylaxis of P. vivax malaria: 30 mg base PO once daily beginning 1 to 2 days before exposure until 7 days after.

UNAPPROVED PEDS — Prevention of relapse, P. vivax/ovale malaria: 0.5 mg/kg (up to 30 mg) base PO once daily for 14 days. Primary prophylaxis of P. vivax malaria: 0.5 mg/kg (up to 30 mg) base PO once daily beginning 1 to 2 days before exposure until 7 days after.

FORMS — Generic only: Tabs 26.3 mg (equiv to 15 mg base).

NOTES — Causes hemolytic anemia in G6PD deficiency, methemoglobinemia in NADH methemoglobin reductase deficiency. Contraindicated in pregnancy and G6PD deficiency; screen for deficiency before prescribing. Rule out G6PD deficiency in breastfed infant before giving primaquine to mother. Stop primaquine if dark urine or anemia. Avoid in patients with RA or SLE, recent quinacrine use, or use of other bone marrow suppressants. May prolong QT interval.

MOA — Unknown. May affect mitochondrial electron transport chain or pyrimidine synthesis. Active against all forms of malaria; only drug active against latent parasites in liver.

ADVERSE EFFECTS — Serious: Hemolytic anemia with G6PD deficiency, methemoglobinemia with NADH methemoglobin reductase deficiency.

QUININE (*Qualaquin*) ▶L ♀C ▶+? $$$$$

WARNING — FDA has repeatedly warned that the risks of treating nocturnal leg cramps with quinine (an unapproved indication) exceed any potential benefit. Risks include life-threatening hematological reactions, especially thrombocytopenia and hemolytic-uremic syndrome/thrombotic thrombocytopenic purpura (HUS/TTP). HUS/TTP can cause chronic renal impairment.

ADULT — Malaria: 648 mg PO three times per day for 3 days (Africa/South America) or 7 days (Southeast Asia). Also give 7-day course of doxycycline, tetracycline, or clindamycin.

(cont.)

QUININE (*cont.*)

PEDS — Malaria, age 16 yo and older: See ADULT for dose.

UNAPPROVED ADULT — Babesiosis, severe: Clindamycin 300 to 600 mg IV q 6 h + quinine 650 mg PO q 6 to 8 h. Treat for 7 to 10 days. Nocturnal leg cramps: 260 to 325 mg PO at bedtime. FDA warns that risks outweigh benefits for this indication.

UNAPPROVED PEDS — Malaria: 25 to 30 mg/kg/day (up to 2 g/day) PO divided q 8 h for 3 days (Africa/South America) or 7 days (Southeast Asia). Also give 7-day course of doxycycline, tetracycline, or clindamycin. Babesiosis, severe: Clindamycin 7 to 10 mg/kg (max 600 mg) IV q 6 h + quinine 8 mg/kg (max 650 mg) PO q 8 h. Treat for 7 to 10 days.

FORMS — Generic/Trade: Caps 324 mg.

NOTES — Thrombocytopenia, hemolytic uremic syndrome/thrombotic thrombocytopenic purpura, cinchonism, hemolytic anemia with G6PD deficiency, cardiac conduction disturbances, hearing impairment. Contraindicated if prolonged QT interval, optic neuritis, myasthenia gravis, or hypersensitivity to quinine, quinidine, or mefloquine. Can prolong PR/QRS interval; esp if structural heart disease/ pre-existing conduction system abnormalities, elderly with sick sinus syndrome, atrial fibrillation with slow ventricular response, myocardial ischemia, other drugs that prolong PR/QRS interval (flecainide, quinidine). Many drug interactions. Do not use with clarithromycin, erythromycin, rifampin, ritonavir, neuromuscular blockers. May increase digoxin levels. Monitor INR with warfarin. Antacids decrease quinine absorption. Rule out G6PD deficiency in breastfed, at-risk infant before giving quinine to mother. Use in hepatic impairment: No dosage adjustment for mild/moderate (Child-Pugh A/B) impairment, but monitor for adverse effects. Do not use if severe (Child-Pugh C) impairment. Malaria treatment, dosage adjustment for severe chronic renal impairment: 648 mg PO loading dose, then 324 mg PO q 12 h for 7 days.

MOA — Unknown, may have similar mechanism of action as chloroquine.

ADVERSE EFFECTS — Serious: Thrombocytopenia, hemolytic uremic syndrome/thrombotic thrombocytopenic purpura, cinchonism, hemolytic anemia with G6PD deficiency, cardiac conduction disturbances, hearing impairment with high levels, hypoglycemia (especially in pregnant women).

ANTIMICROBIALS: Antimycobacterial Agents

NOTE: Treat active mycobacterial infection with at least 2 drugs. See guidelines at www.thoracic.org/statements/ and www.aidsinfo.nih.gov. Get baseline LFTs, creatinine, and platelet count before treating TB. Evaluate at least monthly for adverse drug reactions. Routine liver and renal function tests not needed unless baseline dysfunction or increased risk of hepatotoxicity.

BEDAQUILINE (*Sirturo*) ▶L ♀B ▶– $$$$$

WARNING — Higher mortality with bedaquiline in a clinical trial; use only if other drugs are ineffective. QT interval prolongation that may be additive with other drugs that prolong QT interval.

ADULT — Pulmonary multi-drug resistant TB: 400 mg PO once daily for 2 weeks, then 200 mg PO 3 times per week for 22 weeks. Take with food. Intended for directly observed therapy in combo with at least 3 drugs active against TB isolate.

PEDS — Safety and efficacy not established in children.

FORMS — Trade only: 100 mg tabs.

NOTES — Can prolong QT interval. Monitor ECG at baseline, at weeks 2, 12, and 24, and if syncope occurs. Monitor electrolytes at baseline (correct if needed) and if QT prolongation detected. Monitor ECG if given with other drugs that prolong QT interval, or patient has history of torsades, congenital long QT syndrome, hypothyroidism and bradyarrhythmias, uncompensated heart failure, or low serum calcium, magnesium, or potassium. Discontinue if significant ventricular arrhythmia or QT interval >500 ms. Increases risk of hepatic adverse events; monitor LFTs and symptoms at baseline, monthly, and as needed. If AST/ALT greater than 3 times ULN, repeat test within 48 h, test for viral hepatitis, and discontinue other hepatotoxic drugs. Discontinue bedaquiline if AST/ALT increase plus total bilirubin greater than 2 times ULN, AST/ALT greater than 8 times ULN, or AST/ALT elevation for longer than 2 weeks. Avoid hepatotoxic drugs and alcohol during treatment. Avoid coadministration of strong CYP3A4 inducers including rifamycins. Avoid giving strong CYP3A4 inhibitors for more than 14 days if possible. Tell patients to swallow tabs whole with water. No dosage adjustment for mild/moderate hepatic impairment; monitor for increase in adverse events if severe hepatic impairment.

MOA — Inhibits mycobacterial ATP-synthase, blocking energy generation in mycobacterium.

ADVERSE EFFECTS — Severe: Increased mortality in a clinical trial, QT interval prolongation, increased risk of hepatic adverse events. Frequent: Nausea, arthralgia, headache, hemoptysis, chest pain.

CLOFAZIMINE ▶feces ♀C ▶? –

ADULT — Leprosy: See www.hrsa.gov/hansensdisease/.

PEDS — Not approved in children.

FORMS — Caps 50 mg. For leprosy, contact National Hansen's Disease Program (phone 800-642-2477).

NOTES — Abdominal pain common; rare reports of splenic infarction, bowel obstruction, and GI bleeding. Pink to brown skin pigmentation that may persist for months to years after discontinuation. Discoloration of urine, body secretions.

MOA — Unknown.

(cont.)

CLOFAZIMINE (*cont.*)

ADVERSE EFFECTS — Serious: Rare reports of splenic infarction, bowel obstruction, and GI bleeding. Frequent: Abdominal pain, discoloration of urine and body secretions, pink to brownish-black skin pigmentation that may persist for months to years.

DAPSONE (*Aczone*) ▶LK ♀C ▶– $$$$

ADULT — Leprosy: 100 mg PO daily with other agents; see www.hrsa.gov/hansensdisease/ for regimens. Acne (Aczone; $$$$$): Apply 5% two times per day; apply 7.5% once daily.

PEDS — Leprosy: 1 mg/kg (up to 100 mg) PO daily with other agents; see www.hrsa.gov/hansens-disease/ for regimens. Acne, 12 to 17 yo (Aczone; $$$$$): Apply 5% two times per day; apply 7.5% once daily.

UNAPPROVED ADULT — Pneumocystis pneumonia prophylaxis: 100 mg PO daily. Pneumocystis pneumonia treatment: 100 mg PO daily with trimethoprim 5 mg/kg PO three times per day for 21 days.

UNAPPROVED PEDS — Pneumocystis pneumonia prophylaxis, age 1 mo or older: 2 mg/kg (up to 100 mg/day) PO once daily or 4 mg/kg/week (up to 200 mg/week) PO once weekly.

FORMS — Generic only: Tabs 25, 100 mg. Trade only (Aczone): Topical gel 5% and 7.5% in 30, 60, 90 g.

NOTES — Oral: Blood dyscrasias, severe allergic skin reactions, sulfone syndrome, hemolysis in G6PD deficiency, hepatotoxicity, neuropathy, photosensitivity, leprosy reactional states. Monitor CBC weekly for 4 weeks, then monthly for 6 months, then twice a year. Monitor LFTs. Test for G6DP deficiency before using if possible. Topical: Methemoglobinemia reported; avoid in congenital or idiopathic methemoglobinemia. Applying benzoyl peroxide after topical dapsone can discolor skin yellow-orange, but it washes off.

MOA — Sulfone that inhibits dihydropteroate synthase and prevents bacterial folic acid synthesis.

ADVERSE EFFECTS — Serious: Blood dyscrasias, allergic skin reactions, sulfone syndrome, hemolysis in G6PD deficiency, hepatotoxicity, neuropathy, photosensitivity, leprosy reactional states. Methemoglobinemia reported with topical dapsone. Frequent: Rash, headache, GI complaints, mononucleosis-like syndrome. Topical, frequent: dryness, pruritus, erythema, scaling.

ETHAMBUTOL (*Myambutol*, *✦Etibi*) ▶LK ♀C but + ▶+ $$$$

ADULT — TB: ATS and CDC recommend 15 to 20 mg/kg PO daily. Dose with whole tabs based on estimated lean body weight: 800 mg PO daily for wt 40 to 55 kg, 1200 mg PO daily for wt 56 to 75 kg, 1600 mg PO daily for wt 76 to 90 kg. Max dose regardless of wt is 1600 mg/day. Consider monitoring blood levels to ensure dose is adequate if weight greater than 90 kg.

PEDS — TB: ATS and CDC recommend 15 to 20 mg/kg (up to 1 g) PO daily. Use cautiously if visual acuity cannot be monitored. Manufacturer recommends against use in children younger than 13 yo.

UNAPPROVED ADULT — Treatment or prevention of recurrent Mycobacterium avium complex disease in HIV infection: 15 mg/kg (up to 1600 mg) PO daily with clarithromycin/azithromycin ± rifabutin.

UNAPPROVED PEDS — Treatment or prevention of recurrent Mycobacterium avium complex disease in HIV infection: 15 mg/kg (up to 900 mg) PO daily with clarithromycin/azithromycin ± rifabutin.

FORMS — Generic/Trade: Tabs 100, 400 mg.

NOTES — Can cause retrobulbar neuritis. Avoid, if possible, in patients with optic neuritis. Test visual acuity and color discrimination at baseline. Ask about visual disturbances monthly. Monitor visual acuity and color discrimination monthly if dose is greater than 15 to 20 mg/kg, duration is longer than 2 months, or renal dysfunction. Advise patients to report any change in vision immediately; do not use in those who cannot report visual symptoms (eg children, unconscious). Do not give aluminum hydroxide antacid until at least 4 h after ethambutol dose. Reduce dose in renal impairment.

MOA — Inhibits arabinosyl transferase enzymes involved in synthesis of mycobacterial cell wall.

ADVERSE EFFECTS — Serious: Retrobulbar neuritis, peripheral neuropathy, anaphylactoid reactions.

ISONIAZID (*INH*, *✦Isotamine*) ▶LK ♀C but + ▶+ $

WARNING — Hepatotoxicity. Obtain baseline LFTs. Monitor LFTs monthly in high-risk patients (HIV, signs/history of liver disease, abnormal LFTs at baseline, pregnancy/postpartum, alcoholism/regular alcohol use, some patients older than 35 yo). Tell all patients to stop isoniazid and call at once if hepatotoxicity symptoms develop. Discontinue if ALT at least 3 times the upper limit of normal with hepatotoxicity symptoms or ALT at least 5 times the upper limit of normal without hepatotoxicity symptoms.

ADULT — TB treatment: 5 mg/kg (up to 300 mg) PO daily or 15 mg/kg (up to 900 mg) two or three times a week. Latent TB: 300 mg PO daily.

PEDS — TB treatment: 10 to 15 mg/kg (up to 300 mg) PO daily. Latent TB: 10 mg/kg (up to 300 mg) PO daily.

UNAPPROVED ADULT — American Thoracic Society regimen, latent TB: 5 mg/kg (up to 300 mg) PO daily for 9 months (6 months adequate if HIV-negative, but less effective than 9 months). Weekly regimen for latent TB: Give once weekly for 12 weeks isoniazid 15 mg/kg PO rounded up to nearest 50 or 100 mg (max 900 mg) + rifapentine 750 mg for wt 32.1 to 50 kg or 900 mg for wt greater than 50 kg. Regimen intended for directly observed therapy; not recommended for HIV-infected patients treated with antiretrovirals, or for use during pregnancy.

UNAPPROVED PEDS — American Thoracic Society regimen, latent TB: 10 to 20 mg/kg (up to 300 mg) PO daily for 9 months. Weekly regimen for latent TB, age 12 yo or older: Give once weekly for 12 weeks isoniazid 15 mg/kg PO rounded up to nearest 50 or 100 mg (max 900 mg) + rifapentine dosed

(cont.)

ISONIAZID (*cont.*)

according to wt. Rifapentine dose is 300 mg for 10 to 14 kg; 450 mg for 14.1 to 25 kg; 600 mg for 25.1 to 32 kg; 750 mg for 32.1 to 50 kg; 900 mg for wt greater than 50 kg. Regimen intended for directly observed therapy; not recommended for HIV-infected patients treated with antiretrovirals or use during pregnancy.

FORMS — Generic only: Tabs 100, 300 mg. Syrup 50 mg/5 mL.

NOTES — To reduce risk of peripheral neuropathy, give pyridoxine 25 to 50 mg daily if alcoholism, diabetes, HIV, uremia, malnutrition, seizure disorder, pregnant/breastfeeding woman, breastfed infant of INH-treated mother. Consider pyridoxine 100 mg daily for patients with peripheral neuropathy. Many drug interactions.

MOA — Inhibits synthesis of mycolic acid, a component of mycobacterial cell walls.

ADVERSE EFFECTS — Serious: Hepatotoxicity, peripheral neuropathy, lupus, pancreatitis; hypersensitivity reactions including toxic epidermal necrolysis and DRESS. Frequent: Increased LFTs, positive ANA.

PYRAZINAMIDE (*PZA, ✦Tebrazid*) ▶LK ♀C ▶? $$$$

WARNING — The ATS and CDC recommend against general use of 2-month regimen of rifampin + pyrazinamide for latent TB due to reports of fatal hepatotoxicity.

ADULT — TB: ATS and CDC recommend 20 to 25 mg/kg PO daily. Dose with whole tabs based on estimated lean body weight: Give 1000 mg PO daily for 40 to 55 kg, 1500 mg daily for 56 to 75 kg, 2000 mg for 76 to 90 kg. Max dose regardless of wt is 2000 mg PO daily. Consider monitoring blood levels to ensure dose is adequate if wt greater than 90 kg.

PEDS — TB: 15 to 30 mg/kg (up to 2000 mg) PO daily.

FORMS — Generic only: Tabs 500 mg.

NOTES — Hepatotoxicity, hyperuricemia (avoid in acute gout). Obtain LFTs at baseline. Monitor periodically in high-risk patients (HIV infection, alcoholism, pregnancy, signs/history of liver disease, abnormal LFTs at baseline). Discontinue if ALT is at least 3 times the upper limit of normal with hepatotoxicity symptoms or ALT is at least 5 times upper limit of normal without hepatotoxicity symptoms. Consider reduced dose in renal dysfunction.

MOA — Unknown.

ADVERSE EFFECTS — Serious: Hepatotoxicity. Frequent: Hyperuricemia, polyarthralgia, myalgia, mild anorexia, nausea.

RIFABUTIN (*Mycobutin*) ▶L ♀B ▶? $$$$$

ADULT — Prevention of disseminated Mycobacterium avium complex disease in AIDS: 300 mg PO daily; can give 150 mg PO two times per day if GI upset. Per HIV guidelines, reduce rifabutin dose for coadministration with cobicistat- or ritonavir-boosted protease inhibitors and unboosted atazanavir: 150 mg PO once daily or 300 mg PO three times per week. For cobicistat- or ritonavir-boosted regimens, monitor antimycobacterial activity and consider therapeutic drug monitoring. Reduce dose for nelfinavir (use nelfinavir 1250 mg PO two times per day), unboosted indinavir (increase indinavir to 1000 mg PO q 8 h): 150 mg PO daily. Avoid unboosted fosamprenavir with rifabutin. Dosage increase for efavirenz: Rifabutin 450 to 600 mg PO daily; use 600 mg PO three times per week if no protease inhibitor in regimen. Use standard rifabutin dose with etravirine (without ritonavir-boosted protease inhibitor) or nevirapine. Avoid rifabutin in patients receiving etravirine with a ritonavir-boosted protease inhibitor. Monitor CBC at least weekly. Consider dosage adjustment based on rifabutin levels for patients receiving antiretroviral drugs.

PEDS — Not approved in children.

UNAPPROVED ADULT — TB or Mycobacterium avium complex disease treatment in AIDS: 300 mg PO daily. Dosage reduction for ritonavir-boosted protease inhibitors: 150 mg PO once daily or 300 mg PO three times per week. For ritonavir-boosted regimens, monitor antimycobacterial activity and consider therapeutic drug monitoring.

UNAPPROVED PEDS — Mycobacterium avium complex disease. Prophylaxis: Give 5 mg/kg (up to 300 mg) PO daily for age younger than 6 yo; give 300 mg PO daily for age 6 yo or older. Treatment: 10 to 20 mg/kg (max 300 mg/day) PO once daily. TB: 10 to 20 mg/kg (up to 300 mg/day) PO once daily.

FORMS — Generic/Trade: Caps 150 mg.

NOTES — Uveitis (with high doses or if metabolism inhibited by other drugs), hepatotoxicity, thrombocytopenia, neutropenia. Obtain CBC and LFTs at baseline. Monitor periodically in high-risk patients (HIV infection, alcoholism, pregnancy, signs/history of liver disease, abnormal LFTs at baseline). May induce liver metabolism of other drugs including oral contraceptives, HIV protease inhibitors, and azole antifungals. Substrate of CYP3A4; azole antifungals, clarithromycin, and HIV protease inhibitors increase rifabutin levels. Urine, body secretion, soft contact lenses may turn orange-brown. Consider dosage reduction for hepatic dysfunction.

MOA — Rifamycin derivative that inhibits bacterial RNA polymerase.

ADVERSE EFFECTS — Serious: Uveitis (with high doses or if metabolism inhibited by other drugs), hepatotoxicity, thrombocytopenia, neutropenia. Frequent: Arthralgia/myalgia; GI upset; increased LFTs; orange-brown discoloration of urine, body secretions, soft contact lenses.

RIFAMATE (**isoniazid + rifampin**) ▶LK ♀C but + ▶+ $$$$$

WARNING — Hepatotoxicity.

ADULT — TB: 2 caps PO daily on empty stomach.

PEDS — Not approved in children under 15 years old; use adult doses for 15 yo and older.

FORMS — Trade only: Caps isoniazid 150 mg + rifampin 300 mg.

NOTES — See components.

MOA — See components.

ADVERSE EFFECTS — See components.

RIFAMPIN (*Rifadin, ✲Rofact*) ▶L ♀C but + ▶+ $$$$
WARNING — The ATS and CDC recommend against general use of 2-month regimen of rifampin + pyrazinamide for latent TB due to reports of fatal hepatotoxicity.
ADULT — TB: 10 mg/kg (up to 600 mg) PO/IV daily. Neisseria meningitidis carriers: 600 mg PO two times per day for 2 days. Take oral doses on empty stomach. IV and PO doses are the same.
PEDS — TB: 10 to 20 mg/kg (up to 600 mg) PO/IV daily. Neisseria meningitidis carriers: Age younger than 1 mo, 5 mg/kg PO two times per day for 2 days; age 1 mo or older, 10 mg/kg (up to 600 mg) PO two times per day for 2 days. Take oral doses on empty stomach. IV and PO doses are the same.
UNAPPROVED ADULT — Prophylaxis of H. influenzae type b infection: 20 mg/kg (up to 600 mg) PO daily for 4 days. Leprosy: 600 mg PO q month with dapsone. ATS regimen for latent TB: 10 mg/kg up to 600 mg PO daily for 4 months. Staphylococcal prosthetic valve endocarditis: 300 mg PO q 8 h in combination with gentamicin plus nafcillin, oxacillin, or vancomycin. Take on empty stomach.
UNAPPROVED PEDS — Prophylaxis of H. influenzae type b infection: Age younger than 1 mo, 10 mg/kg PO daily for 4 days; age 1 mo or older, 20 mg/kg up to 600 mg PO daily for 4 days. Prophylaxis of invasive meningococcal disease: Age younger than 1 mo, 5 mg/kg PO two times per day for 2 days; age 1 mo or older, 10 mg/kg (up to 600 mg) PO two times per day for 2 days. ATS regimen for latent tuberculosis: 10 to 20 mg/kg (up to 600 mg) PO daily for 4 months. Take on empty stomach.
FORMS — Generic/Trade: Caps 150, 300 mg. Pharmacists can make oral susp.
NOTES — Hepatotoxicity, thrombocytopenia. When treating TB, obtain baseline CBC, LFTs. Monitor periodically in high-risk patients (HIV infection, alcoholism, pregnancy, signs/history of liver disease, abnormal LFTs at baseline). Discontinue if ALT is at least 3 times the upper limit of normal with hepatotoxicity symptoms or ALT is at least 5 times the upper limit of normal without hepatotoxicity symptoms. Avoid interruptions in rifampin therapy; rare renal hypersensitivity reactions can occur after resumption. Induces hepatic metabolism of many drugs; check other sources for dosage adjustments before prescribing. If used with rifampin, consider increasing efavirenz to 800 mg once daily at bedtime if wt greater than 60 kg. Do not use rifampin with HIV protease inhibitors, rilpivirine, or cobicistat. Decreased efficacy of oral contraceptives; use nonhormonal method. Decreased INR with warfarin; monitor daily or as needed. Adjust dose for hepatic impairment. Colors urine, body secretions, soft contact lenses red-orange. Give prophylactic vitamin K 10 mg IM single dose to newborns of women taking rifampin. IV rifampin is stable for 4 h after dilution in dextrose 5%.
MOA — Rifamycin derivative that inhibits bacterial RNA polymerase.

ADVERSE EFFECTS — Serious: Hepatotoxicity, thrombocytopenia, exacerbation of porphyria, serious skin reactions (rare). Potential risk of hemorrhagic disease in newborns of women taking rifampin; give vitamin K 10 mg IM x 1 to newborn. Frequent: Rash, pruritus, arthralgia/myalgia; orange-brown discoloration of urine, body secretions, soft contact lenses.
RIFAPENTINE (*Priftin, RPT*) ▶ esterases, feces ♀C ▶? $$$$
ADULT — Active pulmonary TB: 600 mg PO two times per week for 2 months, then once weekly for 4 months. Use only for continuation therapy in selected HIV-negative patients. Latent TB: Give with isoniazid both PO once weekly for 12 weeks. Use wt-based rifapentine dose of 600 mg for 25.1 to 32 kg; 750 mg for 32.1 to 50 kg; 900 mg for greater than 50 kg. Regimen intended for directly observed therapy. Take with food.
PEDS — Active pulmonary TB, age 12 yo and older: 600 mg PO two times per week for 2 months, then once weekly for 4 months. Use for continuation therapy only in selected HIV-negative patients. Latent TB, age 2 yo and older: Give with isoniazid, both PO once weekly for 12 weeks. Use wt-based rifapentine dose of 300 mg for 10 to 14 kg; 450 mg for 14.1 to 25 kg; 600 mg for 25.1 to 32 kg; 750 mg for 32.1 to 50 kg; 900 mg for greater than 50 kg. Regimen intended for directly observed therapy. Take with food.
FORMS — Trade only: Tabs 150 mg.
NOTES — Hepatotoxicity, thrombocytopenia, exacerbation of porphyria. Obtain CBC and LFTs at baseline. Monitor LFTs periodically in high-risk patients (alcoholism, pregnancy, signs/history of liver disease, abnormal LFTs at baseline). Do not use in porphyria. Urine, body secretions, contact lenses, and dentures may turn red-orange. May induce liver metabolism of other drugs including oral contraceptives. Advise women taking hormonal contraceptive to use barrier contraceptive during treatment. Potential risk of postpartum hemorrhage in mother and newborn; monitor prothrombin time in both if maternal exposure to rifapentine in last few weeks of pregnancy. Avoid with protease inhibitors, NNRTIs, and maraviroc.
MOA — Long-acting derivative of rifampin, a rifamycin that inhibits bacterial RNA polymerase.
ADVERSE EFFECTS — Serious: Hepatotoxicity, thrombocytopenia, exacerbation of porphyria, neutropenia (rare). Frequent: Hyperuricemia; rash; conjunctivitis; orange-brown discoloration of urine, body secretions, soft contact lenses.
RIFATER (**isoniazid + rifampin + pyrazinamide**) ▶LK ♀C ▶? $$$$$
WARNING — Hepatotoxicity.
ADULT — TB, initial 2 months of treatment: Take PO on empty stomach once daily at a dose of 4 tabs for wt less than 45 kg; 5 tabs for wt 45 to 54 kg, 6 tabs for wt 55 kg or greater. Additional pyrazinamide tabs required to provide adequate dose for

(cont.)

RIFATER (cont.)

wt greater than 90 kg. Can finish treatment with Rifamate.

PEDS — Ratio of formulation may not be appropriate for children younger than 15 yo.

FORMS — Trade only: Tabs isoniazid 50 mg + rifampin 120 mg + pyrazinamide 300 mg.

NOTES — See components. Do not use in patients with renal dysfunction.

MOA — See components.

ADVERSE EFFECTS — See components.

ANTIMICROBIALS: Antiparasitics

ALBENDAZOLE (Albenza) ▶L ♀C ▶? $$$$$

ADULT — Hydatid disease, neurocysticercosis: 15 mg/kg/day (up to 800 mg/day) PO divided in two doses for wt less than 60 kg; 400 mg PO two times per day for wt 60 kg or greater. Treatment duration varies. Take with food.

PEDS — Hydatid disease, neurocysticercosis: 15 mg/kg/day (up to 800 mg/day) PO divided in two doses for wt less than 60 kg; 400 mg PO two times per day for wt 60 kg or greater. Treatment duration varies. Take with food.

UNAPPROVED ADULT — Hookworm, whipworm, pinworm, roundworm: 400 mg PO single dose. Repeat in 2 weeks for pinworm. Cutaneous larva migrans: 200 mg PO two times per day for 3 days. Giardia: 400 mg PO daily for 5 days. Intestinal/disseminated microsporidiosis in HIV infection (not for ocular or caused by E. bieneusi/V. corneae): 400 mg PO two times per day until CD4 count higher than 200 for more than 6 months after starting antiretrovirals.

UNAPPROVED PEDS — Roundworm, hookworm, pinworm, whipworm: 400 mg PO single dose. Repeat in 2 weeks for pinworm. Cutaneous larva migrans: 200 mg PO two times per day for 3 days. Giardia: 400 mg PO daily for 5 days.

FORMS — Trade only: Tabs 200 mg.

NOTES — Associated with bone marrow suppression (especially if liver disease), increased LFTs (common with long-term use), and hepatotoxicity (rare). Monitor CBC and LFTs before starting and then q 2 weeks; discontinue if significant changes. Consider corticosteroids and anticonvulsants in neurocysticercosis. Consider diagnosis of preexisting neurocysticercosis if patient develops neurologic symptoms soon after albendazole treatment for another indication. Get negative pregnancy test before treatment and warn against getting pregnant until 1 month after treatment. Treat close contacts for pinworms. Can crush/chew tabs and swallow with water.

MOA — Anthelmintic that inhibits the formation of microtubules and causes glucose depletion.

ADVERSE EFFECTS — Serious: Nephrotoxicity, bone marrow suppression, hepatotoxicity (usually with long-term use). Increased LFTs increases risk of liver failure or bone marrow suppression. Frequent: Abnormal LFTs, abdominal pain.

ATOVAQUONE (Mepron) ▶feces ♀C ▶? $$$$$

ADULT — Pneumocystis pneumonia in patients intolerant to trimethoprim-sulfamethoxazole. Treatment: 750 mg PO two times per day for 21 days. Prevention: 1500 mg PO daily. Take with meals.

PEDS — Pneumocystis pneumonia in patients intolerant to trimethoprim-sulfamethoxazole, age 13 yo and older. Treatment: 750 mg PO two times per day for 21 days. Prevention: 1500 mg PO daily. Take with meals.

UNAPPROVED ADULT — Toxoplasmosis in HIV infection. Acute treatment: 1500 mg PO two times per day ± sulfadiazine or pyrimethamine-leucovorin for at least 6 weeks. Chronic maintenance: 750 to 1500 mg PO two times per day ± sulfadiazine or pyrimethamine-leucovorin. Babesiosis, mild to moderate: 750 mg PO q 12 h + azithromycin 500 on day 1, then 250 mg PO once daily. Treat for 7 to 10 days. Consider higher doses of azithromycin for immunocompromised patients. Take atovaquone with meals.

UNAPPROVED PEDS — Prevention of recurrent Pneumocystis pneumonia in HIV infection: 30 mg/kg PO daily for age 1 to 3 mo; 45 mg/kg PO daily for age 4 to 24 mo; 30 mg/kg PO daily for age 25 mo or older. Babesiosis, mild to moderate: 20 mg/kg (max 750 mg) PO q 12 h + azithromycin 10 mg/kg (max 500 mg) on day 1, then 5 mg/kg (max 250 mg). Treat for 7 to 10 days. Consider higher doses of azithromycin for immunocompromised patients. Take atovaquone with meals.

FORMS — Generic/Trade: Susp 750 mg/5 mL (210 mL). Trade only: Foil pouch 750 mg/5 mL (5 mL).

NOTES — Efficacy of atovaquone may be decreased by efavirenz (avoid) rifampin (avoid), rifabutin, or rifapentine.

MOA — Ubiquinone analog that may inhibit nucleic acid and ATP synthesis via effects on mitochondrial electron transport.

ADVERSE EFFECTS — Serious: Hepatotoxicity (rare). Frequent: Rash, nausea, fever, headache, insomnia, increased LFTs.

IVERMECTIN (Stromectol) ▶L ♀C ▶+ $$

ADULT — Strongyloidiasis: 200 mcg/kg PO single dose. Onchocerciasis: 150 mcg/kg PO single dose q 3 to 12 months. Take on empty stomach with water.

PEDS — Strongyloidiasis: 200 mcg/kg PO single dose. Onchocerciasis: 150 mcg/kg PO single dose q 3 to 12 months. Take on empty stomach with water. Safety and efficacy not established in children less than 15 kg.

UNAPPROVED ADULT — Scabies: 200 mcg/kg PO (12 mg for 51 to 65 kg; 15 mg for 66 to 79 kg), repeat dose in 7 to 14 days. Crusted scabies: 200 mcg/kg PO on days 1, 2, 8, 9, and 15; give additional doses on days 22 and 29 for severe infection. Use in combination with full-body application of topical

(cont.)

IVERMECTIN (*cont.*)

permethrin 5% daily for 7 days then twice weekly until cure. Pubic lice: 250 mcg/kg PO repeated in 2 weeks. Cutaneous larva migrans: 200 mcg/kg PO once daily for 1 to 2 days. Roundworm: 150 to 200 mcg/kg PO single dose. Take on empty stomach with water.

UNAPPROVED PEDS — Scabies: 200 mcg/kg PO (3 mg for 15 to 24 kg; 6 mg for 25 to 35 kg; 9 mg for 36 to 50 kg; 12 mg for 51 to 65 kg; 15 mg for 66 to 79 kg), repeated at least 7 days later. Head lice: 200 or 400 mcg/kg PO on days 1 and 8. Cutaneous larva migrans: 200 mcg/kg PO once daily for 1 to 2 days. Roundworm: 150 to 200 mcg/kg PO single dose. Take on empty stomach with water. Not for wt less than 15 kg.

FORMS — Generic/Trade: Tabs 3 mg.

NOTES — Mazzotti and ophthalmic reactions with treatment for onchocerciasis. May need repeat/monthly treatment for strongyloidiasis in immuno-compromised/HIV-infected patients. Increased INRs with warfarin reported rarely.

MOA — Binds to glutamate-gated chloride ion channels in invertebrate nerve and muscle cells; this paralyses and kills parasites.

ADVERSE EFFECTS — Serious: Mazzotti & ophthalmic reactions with treatment for onchocerciasis. Frequent: Nausea.

MEBENDAZOLE (*Emverm*) ▶L ♀C ▶? $$$$$

ADULT — Pinworm: 100 mg PO single dose; repeat in 2 weeks. Roundworm, whipworm, hookworm: 100 mg PO two times per day for 3 days.

PEDS — Pinworm: 100 mg PO single dose; repeat dose in 2 weeks. Roundworm, whipworm, hookworm: 100 mg PO two times per day for 3 days.

UNAPPROVED ADULT — Roundworm, whipworm, hookworm: 500 mg PO single dose.

UNAPPROVED PEDS — Roundworm, whipworm, hookworm: 500 mg PO single dose.

FORMS — Trade only: Chewable tabs 100 mg.

NOTES — Treat close contacts for pinworms. Vermox discontinued from US market in 2011; returned in 2016 as Emverm.

MOA — Anthelmintic that inhibits microtubule formation and causes glucose depletion.

ADVERSE EFFECTS — Serious: Angioedema (rare), seizures (rare). Frequent: Transient GI complaints.

MILTEFOSINE (*Impavido*) ▶L ♀D ▶–

WARNING — Can cause fetal harm; contraindicated during pregnancy. Obtain pregnancy test before use in women of childbearing potential and provide effective contraception during and for 5 months after use.

ADULT — Visceral, cutaneous, or mucosal leishmaniasis: 50 mg PO three times per day for 28 days. Give with food to minimize GI adverse effects.

PEDS — Visceral, cutaneous, or mucosal leishmaniasis, age 12 yo and older: 50 mg PO two times per day for 28 days for wt 30 to 44 kg; 50 mg PO three times per day for 28 days for wt 45 kg or greater. Give with food to minimize GI adverse effects.

UNAPPROVED ADULT — Free-living ameba infection: Contact CDC Emergency Operations Center at 770-488-7100 for suspected Naegleria fowleri, Balamuthia mandrillaris, Acanthamoeba infection.

UNAPPROVED PEDS — Free-living ameba infection: Contact CDC Emergency Operations Center at 770-488-7100 for suspected Naegleria fowleri, Balamuthia mandrillaris, or Acanthamoeba infection.

FORMS — Trade only: Caps 50 mg. Provided on blister cards with 14 caps per card.

NOTES — FDA-approved, but not commercially available in US. Contraindicated in Sjogren-Larsson-Syndrome. Potential reproductive toxicity based on impaired fertility in animal studies. Can increase serum creatinine; monitor renal function weekly and for 4 weeks after use. Can increase transaminases; monitor liver function. Can cause volume depletion due to N/V; encourage fluid intake. Monitor platelet count during use for visceral leishmaniasis due to disease-related risk of thrombocytopenia. Advise women of childbearing potential using oral contraceptives to use an additional or alternative contraceptive if they develop N/V or diarrhea with miltefosine. Avoid breastfeeding during and for 5 months after use.

MOA — Unknown, but anti-leishmaniasis activity may involve interactions with membrane lipids, inhibition of mitochondrial function, and apoptosis-like cell death.

ADVERSE EFFECTS — Serious: Potential reproductive toxicity based on impaired fertility in animal studies. Volume depletion due to vomiting and diarrhea. Stevens-Johnson syndrome. Frequent: N/V, diarrhea, headache, anorexia, dizziness, abdominal pain, pruritus, somnolence, increased transaminases, increased serum creatinine.

NITAZOXANIDE (*Alinia*) ▶L ♀ ?/?/? ▶? $$$$

ADULT — Cryptosporidial or giardial diarrhea: 500 mg PO two times per day with food for 3 days.

PEDS — Cryptosporidial or giardial diarrhea: Give PO two times per day with food for 3 days. Dose is 100 mg for age 1 to 3 yo; 200 mg for age 4 to 11 yo; 500 mg for 12 yo and older. Use susp if younger than 12 yo.

UNAPPROVED ADULT — C. difficile–associated diarrhea: 500 mg PO two times per day for 10 days. Cryptosporidiosis in HIV infection (alternative therapy in addition to concurrent HAART): 500 to 1000 mg PO two times per day with food for 14 days.

FORMS — Trade only: Oral susp 100 mg/5 mL (60 mL). Tabs 500 mg.

NOTES — Turns urine bright yellow. Susp contains 1.5 g sucrose/5 mL. Store susp at room temperature for up to 7 days.

MOA — Antiprotozoal agent that interferes with electron transfer reaction required for anaerobic energy metabolism.

ADVERSE EFFECTS — Mild and transient abdominal pain, diarrhea, vomiting, headache. Discolors urine bright yellow.

PAROMOMYCIN ▸Not absorbed ♀C ▶? $$$$$
ADULT — Intestinal amebiasis: 25 to 35 mg/kg/day PO divided three times per day with or after meals for 5 to 10 days.
PEDS — Intestinal amebiasis: 25 to 35 mg/kg/day PO divided three times per day with or after meals for 5 to 10 days.
UNAPPROVED ADULT — Giardiasis: 500 mg PO three times per day with or after meals for 7 days.
UNAPPROVED PEDS — Giardiasis: 25 to 35 mg/kg/day PO divided three times per day with or after meals for 7 days.
FORMS — Generic only: Caps 250 mg.
NOTES — Nephrotoxicity possible in inflammatory bowel disease due to increased systemic absorption. Not effective for extraintestinal amebiasis.
MOA — Aminoglycoside, inhibits parasitic protein synthesis by interfering with function of ribosomal 30S subunit.
ADVERSE EFFECTS — Serious: Nephrotoxicity possible with systemic absorption in inflammatory bowel disease. Frequent: GI distress.

PENTAMIDINE (*Pentam, NebuPent*) ▸K ♀C ▶– $$$$
ADULT — Pneumocystis pneumonia treatment: 4 mg/kg IM/IV daily for 21 days. Can reduce to 3 mg/kg IM/IV daily if toxicity. IV infused over 60 to 90 min. NebuPent for Pneumocystis pneumonia prevention: 300 mg nebulized q 4 weeks.
PEDS — Pneumocystis pneumonia treatment: 4 mg/kg IM/IV daily for 21 days. NebuPent not approved in children.
UNAPPROVED PEDS — Pneumocystis pneumonia prevention, age 5 yo or older: 300 mg NebuPent nebulized q 4 weeks.
FORMS — Trade only: Aerosol 300 mg.
NOTES — Contraindicated with ziprasidone. Fatalities due to severe hypotension, hypoglycemia, cardiac arrhythmias with IM/IV. Have patient lie down, check BP, and keep resuscitation equipment nearby during IM/IV injection. May cause torsades (IV route only), hyperglycemia, neutropenia, nephrotoxicity, pancreatitis, and hypocalcemia. Monitor BUN, serum creatinine, blood glucose, CBC, LFTs, serum calcium, and ECG. Bronchospasm with inhalation (consider bronchodilator). Reduce IM/IV dose in renal dysfunction.
MOA — Unknown.
ADVERSE EFFECTS — Serious: Fatalities due to severe hypotension, hypoglycemia, cardiac arrhythmias with IM/IV. Extravasation of injection site. Can also cause hyperglycemia, neutropenia (frequent), nephrotoxicity, pancreatitis, torsades (IV route only), & hypocalcemia. Inhaled pentamidine can cause bronchospasm.

PRAZIQUANTEL (*Biltricide*) ▸LK ♀B ▶– $$$$
ADULT — Schistosomiasis: 20 mg/kg PO q 4 to 6 h for 3 doses. Liver flukes: 25 mg/kg PO q 4 to 6 h for 3 doses.
PEDS — Schistosomiasis: 20 mg/kg PO q 4 to 6 h for 3 doses. Liver flukes: 25 mg/kg PO q 4 to 6 h for 3 doses.

UNAPPROVED ADULT — Fish, dog, beef, pork intestinal tapeworms: 10 mg/kg PO single dose.
UNAPPROVED PEDS — Fish, dog, beef, pork intestinal tapeworms: 10 mg/kg PO single dose.
FORMS — Trade only: Tabs 600 mg.
NOTES — Contraindicated in ocular cysticercosis. May cause drowsiness; do not drive or operate machinery for 48 h. Phenytoin, carbamazepine, rifampin (contraindicated), and dexamethasone may lower praziquantel levels enough to cause treatment failure. Albendazole is preferred for neurocysticercosis because it avoids these drug interactions. CYP3A4 inhibitors may increase praziquantel exposure. Take with liquids during a meal. Do not chew tabs. Manufacturer advises against breastfeeding until 72 h after treatment.
MOA — Trematodicide that induces rapid contraction of schistosomes by affecting cell membrane permeability.
ADVERSE EFFECTS — Serious: None. Frequent: Drowsiness.

PYRANTEL (*Pinworm, Pin-X✲ Combantrin*) ▸Not absorbed ♀C ▶? $
ADULT — Pinworm, roundworm: 11 mg/kg (up to 1 g) PO single dose. Repeat in 2 weeks for pinworm.
PEDS — Pinworm, roundworm: 11 mg/kg (up to 1 g) PO single dose. Repeat in 2 weeks for pinworm.
UNAPPROVED ADULT — Hookworm: 11 mg/kg (up to 1 g) PO daily for 3 days.
UNAPPROVED PEDS — Hookworm: 11 mg/kg (up to 1 g) PO daily for 3 days.
FORMS — OTC Trade only (Pin-X): Susp 144 mg/mL (equivalent to 50 mg/mL of pyrantel base) 30, 60 mL. Tabs 720.5 mg (equivalent to 250 mg of pyrantel base).
NOTES — Purging not necessary. Treat close contacts for pinworms.
MOA — Acts as agonist at nicotinic acetylcholine receptors of sensitive nematodes, depolarizing neuromuscular blocker that paralyzes the worm.
ADVERSE EFFECTS — Serious: None. Frequent: None.

PYRIMETHAMINE (*Daraprim*) ▸L ♀C ▶+ $$$$$
ADULT — Toxoplasmosis, immunocompetent patients: 50 to 75 mg PO daily for 1 to 3 weeks, then reduce dose by 50% for 4 to 5 more weeks. Give with leucovorin (10 to 15 mg daily) and sulfadiazine. Reduce initial dose in seizure disorders.
PEDS — Toxoplasmosis: 1 mg/kg/day PO divided two times per day for 2 to 4 days, then reduce by 50% for 1 month. Give with sulfadiazine and leucovorin. Reduce initial dose in seizure disorders.
UNAPPROVED ADULT — See regimen for acute treatment of CNS toxoplasmosis in sulfadiazine entry.
UNAPPROVED PEDS — Acquired toxoplasmosis in HIV: 2 mg/kg (max 50 mg) PO once daily for 3 days, then 1 mg/kg (max 25 mg) PO once daily + sulfadiazine 25 to 50 mg/kg (max 1 to 1.5 g/dose) PO four times per day + leucovorin 10 to 25 mg PO once daily for at least 6 weeks. Suppressive therapy of toxoplasmosis in HIV: 1 mg/kg (max 25 mg) PO once daily + sulfadiazine 85 to 120 mg/kg/day (max 2 to

(cont.)

PYRIMETHAMINE (*cont.*)

4 g/day) PO divided twice daily + leucovorin 5 mg PO once every 3 days.

FORMS — Trade only: Tabs 25 mg.

NOTES — Hemolytic anemia in G6PD deficiency, dose-related folate deficiency, hypersensitivity. Monitor CBC.

MOA — Folic acid antagonist.

ADVERSE EFFECTS — Serious: Hemolytic anemia in G6PD deficiency, dose-related folate deficiency, hypersensitivity.

TINIDAZOLE (*Tindamax*) ▶KL ♀C ▶? $$

WARNING — Metronidazole, a related drug, was carcinogenic in animal studies.

ADULT — Trichomoniasis or giardiasis: 2 g PO single dose. Amebiasis: 2 g PO once daily for 3 days. Bacterial vaginosis: 2 g PO once daily for 2 days or 1 g PO once daily for 5 days. See STD table. Take with food.

PEDS — Giardiasis, age older than 3 yo: 50 mg/kg (up to 2 g) PO single dose. Amebiasis, age older than 3 yo: 50 mg/kg (up to 2 g) PO once daily for 3 days. Take with food.

UNAPPROVED ADULT — Recurrent/persistent urethritis: 2 g PO single dose. See STD table.

FORMS — Generic/Trade: Tabs 250, 500 mg. Pharmacists can compound oral susp.

NOTES — Give iodoquinol/paromomycin after treatment for amebic dysentery or liver abscess. Disulfiram reaction; avoid alcohol until at least 3 days after treatment. Can minimize infant exposure by withholding breastfeeding for 3 days after maternal single dose. May increase levels of cyclosporine, fluorouracil, lithium, phenytoin, tacrolimus. May increase INR with warfarin. Do not give at same time as cholestyramine. For patients undergoing hemodialysis: Give supplemental dose after dialysis session.

MOA — 5-Nitroimidazole derivative with amebicidal, Giardiacidal, and trichomonacidal activity.

ADVERSE EFFECTS — Serious: Seizures, peripheral neuropathy. Frequent: Anorexia, headache, dizziness. May be better tolerated than metronidazole. Transient neutropenia, leukopenia.

ANTIMICROBIALS: Antiviral Agents—Anti-CMV

CIDOFOVIR ▶K ♀C ▶– $$$$$

WARNING — Severe nephrotoxicity. Granulocytopenia: Monitor neutrophil counts.

ADULT — CMV retinitis: 5 mg/kg IV weekly for 2 weeks, then 5 mg/kg every other week. Give probenecid 2 g PO 3 h before and 1 g PO 2 h and 8 h after infusion. Give NS with each infusion.

PEDS — Not approved in children.

NOTES — Fanconi-like syndrome. Stop nephrotoxic drugs at least 1 week before cidofovir. Get serum creatinine, urine protein before each dose. See prescribing information for dosage adjustments based on renal function. Do not use if serum creatinine >1.5 mg/dL, CrCl ≤55 mL/min, or urine protein ≥100 mg/dL (2+). Hold/decrease zidovudine dose by 50% on day cidofovir is given. Tell women to avoid pregnancy until 1 month after and men to use barrier contraceptive until 3 months after cidofovir. Ocular hypotony: Monitor intraocular pressure.

MOA — Selectively inhibits cytomegalovirus DNA polymerase.

ADVERSE EFFECTS — Serious: Nephrotoxicity (also frequent), Fanconi syndrome, neutropenia (also frequent), metabolic acidosis, iritis/uveitis, ocular hypotony. Frequent: Nausea, fever, alopecia, myalgia.

FOSCARNET (*Foscavir*) ▶K ♀C ▶? $$$$$

WARNING — Nephrotoxicity; seizures due to mineral/electrolyte imbalance.

ADULT — Hydrate before infusion. CMV retinitis: 60 mg/kg IV (over 1 h) q 8 h or 90 mg/kg IV (over 1.5 to 2 h) q 12 h for 2 to 3 weeks, then 90 to 120 mg/kg IV daily over 2 h. Acyclovir-resistant HSV infection: 40 mg/kg IV (over 1 h) q 8 to 12 h for 2 to 3 weeks or until healed.

PEDS — Not approved in children. Deposits into teeth and bone of young animals.

NOTES — Granulocytopenia, anemia, vein irritation, genital ulcers (tell patients to wash thoroughly after urinating to prevent). Decreased ionized serum calcium, especially with IV pentamidine. Must use IV pump to avoid rapid administration. Monitor renal function, serum calcium, magnesium, phosphate, potassium. Reduce dose in renal impairment.

MOA — Direct inhibitor of herpesvirus DNA polymerase.

ADVERSE EFFECTS — Serious: Nephrotoxicity (also frequent), neutropenia, genital ulcers. Electrolyte/mineral disorders. Frequent: Headache, fatigue, nausea, fever.

GANCICLOVIR (*Cytovene*) ▶K ♀C ▶– $$$$$

WARNING — Neutropenia, anemia, thrombocytopenia. Do not use if ANC less than 500/mm^3 or platelets less than 25,000/mm^3.

ADULT — CMV retinitis. Induction: 5 mg/kg IV q 12 h for 14 to 21 days. Maintenance: 6 mg/kg IV daily for 5 days/week or 5 mg/kg IV daily. Prevention of CMV disease after organ transplant: 5 mg/kg IV q 12 h for 7 to 14 days, then 6 mg/kg IV daily for 5 days/week. Give IV infusion over 1 h.

PEDS — Safety and efficacy not established in children; potential carcinogenic or reproductive adverse effects.

UNAPPROVED PEDS — CMV retinitis, age older than 3 mo. Induction: 5 mg/kg IV q 12 h for 14 to 21 days. Maintenance: 5 mg/kg IV daily or 6 mg/kg IV daily for 5 days/week. Symptomatic congenital CMV infection: 6 mg/kg IV q 12 h for 6 weeks.

NOTES — Neutropenia (worsened by zidovudine), phlebitis/pain at infusion site, increased seizure

(cont.)

GANCICLOVIR (*cont.*)

risk with imipenem. Monitor CBC, renal function. Reduce dose if CrCl <70 mL/min. Adequate hydration required. Potential teratogen; tell women to avoid pregnancy during use and men to use barrier contraceptive during and for at least 3 months after use. Potential carcinogen; follow guidelines for handling/disposal of cytotoxic agents.
MOA — Inhibits viral DNA synthesis.
ADVERSE EFFECTS — Serious: Myelosuppression (frequent), fever (frequent), hepatic and renal dysfunction, retinal detachment. Frequent: GI complaints, headache, phlebitis at injection site, rash, confusion.

VALGANCICLOVIR (*Valcyte*) ▶K ♀C ▶– $$$$$
WARNING — Myelosuppression may occur at any time. Monitor CBC and platelet count frequently. Do not use if ANC less than 500/mm³, platelets less than 25,000/mm³, hemoglobin less than 8 g/dL.
ADULT — CMV retinitis: 900 mg PO two times per day for 21 days, then 900 mg PO daily. Prevention of CMV disease in high-risk transplant patients: 900 mg PO daily given within 10 days post-transplant until 100 days post-transplant for heart or kidney-pancreas or 200 days for kidney transplant. Give with food.

PEDS — Prevention of CMV disease in high-risk kidney/heart transplant patients age 4 mo and older: Daily dose in mg is 7 × body surface area × CrCl (calculated with modified Schwartz formula). Give PO once daily from within 10 days post-transplant to 100 days post-transplant for heart, 200 days post-transplant for kidney. Max dose of 900 mg/day. Give with food.
FORMS — Generic/Trade: Tabs 450 mg. Oral soln 50 mg/mL.
NOTES — Contraindicated in ganciclovir allergy. Potential teratogen; tell women to avoid pregnancy until 1 month after and men to use barrier contraceptive until at least 3 months after use. CNS toxicity; warn against hazardous tasks. May increase serum creatinine; monitor renal function. Reduce dose if CrCl <60 mL/min. Use ganciclovir instead in hemodialysis patients. Potential drug interactions with didanosine, mycophenolate, zidovudine. Potential carcinogen. Avoid direct contact with broken/crushed tabs; do not intentionally break/crush tabs. Follow guidelines for handling/disposal of cytotoxic agents.
MOA — Prodrug of ganciclovir.
ADVERSE EFFECTS — Similar to ganciclovir.

ANTIMICROBIALS: Antiviral Agents—Anti-Hepatitis B

NOTE: Refer to AASLD guideline at www.aasld.org for management of chronic hepatitis B. For managing hepatitis B reactivation during immunosuppressive therapy, refer to AGA guideline at www.gastro.org.

ADEFOVIR (*Hepsera*) ▶K ♀C ▶– $$$$$
WARNING — Severe acute exacerbation of HBV after discontinuation; nephrotoxicity; emergence of HIV resistance in undiagnosed HIV infection; lactic acidosis/hepatic steatosis.
ADULT — Chronic hepatitis B: 10 mg PO daily.
PEDS — Chronic hepatitis B, age 12 yo or older: 10 mg PO daily.
FORMS — Generic/Trade: Tabs 10 mg.
NOTES — Check HIV status before starting; avoid in HIV-coinfected patients. Nephrotoxic; monitor renal function; avoid other nephrotoxic drugs. See prescribing information for dosage reduction if CrCl <50 mL/min. Adefovir resistance can cause viral load rebound. Consider regimen change if persistent serum HBV DNA >1000 copies/mL during adefovir monotherapy.
MOA — Nucleotide reverse transcriptase inhibitor, similar mechanism of action as NRTIs. Negligible activity against HIV virus at 10 mg dose.
ADVERSE EFFECTS — Serious: Lactic acidosis/hepatic steatosis, nephrotoxicity, exacerbation of hepatitis B after discontinuation; emergence of HIV resistance in undiagnosed HIV infection. Frequent: Asthenia.

ENTECAVIR (*Baraclude*) ▶K ♀C ▶– $$$$$
WARNING — Lactic acidosis with hepatic steatosis. Severe acute exacerbation of hepatitis B can occur after discontinuation; monitor closely for at least 2

months after discontinuation. HBV/HIV-coinfected patients receiving entecavir must also receive fully suppressive antiretroviral regimen.
ADULT — Chronic hepatitis B: 0.5 mg PO once daily if treatment-naive; 1 mg if lamivudine- or telbivudine-resistant, history of viremia despite lamivudine treatment, HIV coinfected, or decompensated liver disease. Take on empty stomach (2 h after last meal and 2 h before next meal).
PEDS — Chronic hepatitis B. Use adult dose for 16 yo and older. Treatment-naïve, age 2 to 15 yo:Give oral soln PO once daily at a dose of 3 mL for 10 to 11 kg; 4 mL for wt greater than 11 to 14 kg; 5 mL for wt greater than 14 to 17 kg; 6 mL for wt greater than 17 to 20 kg; 7 mL for wt greater than 20 to 23 kg; 8 mL for wt greater than 23 to 26 kg; 9 mL for wt greater than 26 to 30 kg; 10 mL or 0.5 mg tab for wt greater than 30 kg. Lamivudine-experienced, age 2 to 15 yo: Give oral soln PO once daily at a dose of 6 mL for 10 to 11 kg; 8 mL for wt greater than 11 to 14 kg; 10 mL for wt greater than 14 to 17 kg; 12 mL for wt greater than 17 to 20 kg; 14 mL for wt greater than 20 to 23 kg; 16 mL for wt greater than 23 to 26 kg; 18 mL for wt greater than 26 to 30 kg; 20 mL or 1 mg tab for wt greater than 30 kg. Age 16 yo or older: 0.5 mg PO once daily if treatment-naive; 1 mg if lamivudine- or telbivudine-resistant, history of viremia despite lamivudine treatment, HIV coinfected, or decompensated liver disease. Take on

(cont.)

ENTECAVIR (*cont.*)

empty stomach (2 h after last meal and 2 h before next meal).

FORMS — Generic/Trade: Tabs 0.5, 1 mg. Trade only: Oral soln 0.05 mg/mL (210 mL).

NOTES — HBV/HIV-coinfected patients receiving entecavir must also receive fully suppressive antiretroviral regimen; screen for HIV before use. Do not mix oral soln with water or other liquid. See product labeling for dosage adjustments for CrCl <50 mL/min or dialysis. Give dose after dialysis sessions.

MOA — Guanosine nucleoside analogue that inhibits hepatitis B polymerase. Partial inhibitor of HIV replication may select for lamivudine-resistance.

ADVERSE EFFECTS — Serious: Lactic acidosis/hepatic steatosis; exacerbation of HBV after discontinuation. Frequent: Headache, fatigue, dizziness, nausea.

TELBIVUDINE (*Tyzeka, ✦Sebivo*) ▶K ♀B ▶− $$$$$

WARNING — Lactic acidosis with hepatic steatosis. Severe acute exacerbation of HBV after discontinuation; monitor closely for at least 2 months after discontinuation.

ADULT — Chronic hepatitis B: 600 mg PO once daily. Refer to product labeling for baseline HBV DNA and ALT treatment criteria for HBeAg-positive and -negative patients. Change regimen if HBV DNA is detectable after 24 weeks of treatment.

PEDS — Chronic hepatitis B, age 16 yo or older: 600 mg PO once daily. Refer to product labeling for baseline HBV DNA and ALT treatment criteria for HBeAg-positive and -negative patients. Change regimen if HBV is detectable after 24 weeks of treatment.

FORMS — Trade only: Tabs 600 mg.

NOTES — Avoid in HIV-coinfected patients. Risk of peripheral neuropathy increased by peginterferon alfa 2a; do not coadminister. No dosage adjustment needed for hepatic dysfunction. Dosage adjustment for renal dysfunction: 600 mg PO q 96 h for ESRD, q 72 h for CrCl less than 30 mL/min but not hemodialysis, q 48 h for CrCl 30 to 49 mL/min. Give dose after hemodialysis session.

MOA — Thymidine nucleoside analogue that inhibits hepatitis B polymerase.

ADVERSE EFFECTS — Serious: Myopathy; peripheral neuropathy (incidence and severity increased by peginterferon alfa 2a; do not coadminister); lactic acidosis/hepatic steatosis. Frequent: Headache, dizziness, fatigue, URI/nasopharyngitis/influenza/flu-like symptoms, cough, abdominal pain, increased CK levels, N/V, dyspepsia, diarrhea.

ANTIMICROBIALS: Antiviral Agents—Anti-Hepatitis C

Hepatitis C Direct-Acting Antiviral Agents

NS5B RNA Polymerase Inhibitors "buvirs"	NS3/4A Protease Inhibitors "previrs"	NS5A Protein Inhibitors "asvirs"
dasabuvir (in *Viekira Pak/XR*) sofosbuvir* (in *Harvoni*)	grazoprevir (in *Zepatier*) paritaprevir (in *Technivie, Viekira Pak/XR*) simeprevir*	daclatasvir* elbasvir (in *Zepatier*) ledipasvir (in *Harvoni*) ombitasvir (in *Technivie, Viekira Pak/XR*) velpatasvir (in *Epclusa*)

*Available as single-drug product, but HCV drugs are not intended for monotherapy.

NOTE: Treatment recommendations for HCV infection can change rapidly; refer to www.hcvguidelines.org for current guidance.

DACLATASVIR (*Daklinza*) ▶L ♀?/?/? ▶? $$$$$

ADULT — Chronic hepatitis C, genotype 1 or 3: 60 mg PO once daily with sofosbuvir 400 mg PO once daily for 12 weeks if no cirrhosis. FDA-approved regimen for genotype 1 or 3 with compensated cirrhosis is not guideline-recommended. Daclatasvir + sofosbuvir + ribavirin also indicated for genotype 1 or 3 with decompensated cirrhosis or genotype 1 or 3 post-liver transplant. Increase daclatasvir to 90 mg/day for moderate CYP3A4 inducers such as efavirenz or etravirine; reduce to 30 mg/day for strong CYP3A4 inhibitors such as ritonavir-boosted atazanavir (see cytochrome P450 table).

PEDS — Safety and efficacy not established in children.

UNAPPROVED ADULT — Genotype 2, no cirrhosis: 60 mg PO once daily + sofosbuvir 400 mg PO once daily for 12 weeks. Genotype 2, compensated cirrhosis (alternative regimen): Daclatasivr + sofosbuvir for 16 to 24 weeks. Genotype 3, compensated cirrhosis: Daclatasvir + sofosbuvir ± wt-based ribavirin (1000 mg/day PO for wt less than 75 kg; 1200 mg/day PO for 75 kg or greater) for 24 weeks. Increase daclatasvir to 90 mg/day for moderate CYP3A4 inducers such as efavirenz or etravirine; reduce to 30 mg/day for strong CYP3A4 inhibitors such as

(cont.)

DACLATASVIR (cont.)

ritonavir-boosted atazanavir (see cytochrome P450 table).

FORMS — Trade only: Tabs 30, 60 mg.

NOTES — Cost of daclatasvir is $25,200/month. Not for monotherapy. For ribavirin-containing regimens, see ribavirin–oral entry about teratogenicity and contraceptive issues that affect female patients and female partners of male patients. Sustained virologic response rate lower if cirrhosis; optimal duration of treatment unclear. Life-threatening bradycardia reported with coadministration of amiodarone with sofosbuvir-daclatasvir; avoid amiodarone if possible. Do not coadminister strong CYP3A4 inducers (carbamazepine, phenytoin, phenobarbital, rifampin, St. John's wort, etc.). Do not coadminister with dabigatran if significant renal impairment. Monitor cyclosporine, digoxin, tacrolimus levels. May increase statin levels; monitor for myopathy and other statin adverse effects.

MOA — NS5A protease inhibitor.

ADVERSE EFFECTS — Frequent: Headache, fatigue, nausea, diarrhea.

EPCLUSA (sofosbuvir + velpatasvir) ▶LK ♀?/?/?. Regimens with ribavirin: X/X/X ▶? $$$$$

ADULT — Chronic hepatitis C, all genotypes, no cirrhosis or compensated cirrhosis (Child-Pugh A): 1 tab PO once daily for 12 weeks. All genotypes, decompensated cirrhosis (Child-Pugh B/C): 1 tab PO once daily plus ribavirin (1000 mg/day PO for less than 75 kg; 1200 mg/day PO for 75 kg or greater) for 12 weeks. Take without regard to meals.

PEDS — Safety and efficacy not established in children.

FORMS — Trade only: Tabs velpatasvir 100 mg + sofosbuvir 400 mg.

NOTES — Cost of Epclusa is $29,900/month. For ribavirin-containing regimens, see ribavirin–oral entry for teratogenicity and contraceptive issues that affect female and male patients. Do not coadminister amiodarone, carbamazepine, efavirenz, phenobarbital, phenytoin, oxcarbazepine, rifabutin, rifampin, rifapentine, St. John's wort, topotecan, tipranavir-ritonavir. Give H2 blockers simultaneously with Epclusa or 12 h later at max dose equivalent to famotidine 80 mg/day. Avoid proton pump inhibitors if possible; if unavoidable, give Epclusa with food 4 hours before omeprazole 20 mg. Separate doses of antacids by at least 4 h. May increase digoxin exposure; monitor digoxin levels. May increase tenofovir disoproxil fumarate (TDF) exposure; monitor for tenofovir adverse effects; avoid coadministering if CrCl <60 mL/min. Consider tenofovir alafenamide instead of TDF in patients receiving ritonavir- or cobicistat-boosted regimens. May increase atorvastatin levels; monitor for myopathy and other adverse effects. Do not exceed rosuvastatin 10 mg/day. No dosage adjustment for hepatic impairment (Child-Pugh A to C). No dosage adjustment for CrCl >30 mL/min; do not use if CrCl <30 mL/min or ESRD.

MOA — Velpatasvir is a HCV NS5A inhibitor; sofosbuvir is a hepatitis C nucleotide analog inhibitor of NS5B RNA polymerase.

ADVERSE EFFECTS — Frequent. Monotherapy: Asthenia, fatigue, headache, nausea, insomnia. Epclusa plus ribavirin: Anemia, fatigue, headache, insomina, diarrhea.

HARVONI (edipasvir + sofosbuvir) ▶Bile, LK ♀?/?/? ▶? $$$$$

ADULT — Chronic hepatitis C. Harvoni dose is 1 tab PO once daily without regard to meals. Genotype 1, treatment-naïve, ± compensated cirrhosis: Harvoni alone for 12 weeks. Can consider 8 weeks if pretreatment HCV RNA <6 million international units/mL and no cirrhosis, HIV infection, African-American, or known IL28B polymorphism CT or TT. Genotype 4, 5, 6, treatment-naïve, ± compensated cirrhosis: Harvoni alone for 12 weeks. Also FDA-approved for genotype 1, 4, 5, 6, treatment-experienced patients; genotype 1 and 4 post-liver transplant; genotype 1 with decompensated cirrhosis.

PEDS — Safety and efficacy not established in children.

FORMS — Trade only: Tabs ledipasvir 90 mg + sofosbuvir 400 mg.

NOTES — Cost of Harvoni is $33,750/month. Do not coadminister amiodarone, carbamazepine, phenobarbital, phenytoin, oxcarbazepine, rifampin, rifapentine, rifabutin, rosuvastatin, simeprevir, St. John's wort, Stribild, or tipranavir-ritonavir. Warn patients that OTC antacids, H2 blockers, and proton pump inhibitors can reduce Harvoni exposure. Give H2 blockers simultaneously with Harvoni or 12 h later at dose equivalent to not more than famotidine 80 mg/day. Give proton pump inhibitor at dose equivalent to not more than omeprazole 20 mg simultaneously with Harvoni on an empty stomach. Separate doses of antacids by at least 4 h. Monitor cyclosporine, digoxin, tacrolimus levels. May increase tenofovir disoproxil fumarate (TDF) exposure; monitor for tenofovir adverse effects; avoid combo if CrCl <60 mL/min. Consider tenofovir alafenamide instead of TDF if Harvoni is coadministered with ritonavir- or cobicistat-boosted protease inhibitor. No dosage adjustment for hepatic impairment (Child-Pugh A to C). No dosage adjustment for CrCl >30 mL/min; do not use if CrCl <30 mL/min or ESRD.

MOA — Ledipasvir is an NS5A protein inhibitor; sofosbuvir is an NS5B RNA polymerase inhibitor.

ADVERSE EFFECTS — Can increase bilirubin, lipase. Frequent: Fatigue, headache, nausea, diarrhea, insomnia.

RIBAVIRIN—ORAL (Rebetol, Copegus, Ribasphere) ▶Cellular, K ♀X ▶– $$$$$

WARNING — Teratogen with extremely long half-life; contraindicated if pregnancy possible in patient/partner. Female patients and female partners of male patients must avoid pregnancy by using 2 forms of birth control during and for 6 months after stopping ribavirin. Obtain pregnancy test at

(cont.)

RIBAVIRIN—ORAL (*cont.*)

baseline and monthly. Hemolytic anemia that may worsen cardiac disease. Assess for underlying heart disease before treatment with ribavirin. Do not use in significant/unstable heart disease. Baseline ECG if preexisting cardiac dysfunction.

ADULT — Combination therapy of chronic hepatitis C: Daily dose of 1000 mg/day PO for wt less than 75 kg, 1200 mg/day PO for wt 75 kg or greater. Divide daily dose of ribavirin two times per day and give with food.

PEDS — Chronic hepatitis C, initial treatment: Patients who start peginterferon plus ribavirin before their 18th birthday should continue with peds doses throughout treatment. Rebetol in combination with peginterferon alfa-2b (PegIntron), age 3 yo and older: For wt less than 47 kg or patients who cannot swallow caps: 15 mg/kg/day of soln PO divided two times per day. Caps: 400 mg two times per day for wt 47 to 59 kg, 400 mg q am and 600 mg q pm for wt 60 to 73 kg, 600 mg two times per day for wt greater than 73 kg. Take PO with food. Treat genotype 1 for 48 weeks, genotypes 2 and 3 for 24 weeks. Copegus tabs in combo with peginterferon alfa-2a (Pegasys), age 5 yo or older: 200 mg twice daily for 23 to 33 kg; 200 mg q am and 400 mg q pm for 34 to 46 kg; 400 mg twice daily for 47 to 59 kg; 400 mg q am and 600 mg q pm for 60 to 74 kg; 600 mg twice daily for 75 kg or more. Treat genotypes 2 and 3 for 24 weeks, other genotypes for 48 weeks. Take PO with food.

UNAPPROVED PEDS — Chronic hepatitis C, age 2 yo and older: Treat for 48 weeks with peginterferon alfa-2b (PegIntron) in combination with ribavirin 15 mg/kg/day PO divided two times per day. The regimen provided here is from guideline for the management of chronic hepatitis C; it may vary from regimens in product labeling.

FORMS — Generic/Trade: Caps 200 mg, Tabs 200 mg. Generic only: Tabs 400, 600 mg. Trade only (Rebetol): Oral soln 40 mg/mL (100 mL).

NOTES — Contraindicated in hemoglobinopathies; autoimmune hepatitis; hepatic decompensation in cirrhotic patients (Child-Pugh score greater than 6 if HCV only; score greater than 5 if HIV coinfected). Get CBC at baseline, weeks 2 and 4, and periodically. Risk of anemia increased if age older than 50 yo or renal dysfunction. Decreased INR with warfarin; monitor INR weekly for 4 weeks after ribavirin started/stopped. May increase risk of lactic acidosis with nucleoside reverse transcriptase inhibitors. Avoid didanosine or zidovudine. Coadministration with azathioprine can cause neutropenia; monitor CBC weekly for 1st month, every other week for next 2 months, then monthly or more frequently if doses are adjusted. Dosage adjustment for renal dysfunction in adults: Give 200 mg alternating with 400 mg every other day for CrCl 30 to 50 mL/min; 200 mg once daily for CrCl <30 mL/min, ESRD, or hemodialysis.

MOA — Oral synthetic nucleoside that interferes with viral nucleic acid synthesis.

ADVERSE EFFECTS — Serious and frequent: Hemolytic anemia (especially if older than 50 yo or if renal dysfunction). Frequent: Therapy with interferon plus ribavirin causes more cough, pruritus, and rash than interferon alone. Serious and rare: Severe acute hypersensitivity during co-therapy with interferon. Impaired growth of children during treatment with peginterferon plus ribavirin, with rebound after discontinuation.

SIMEPREVIR (*Olysio, SMV, ✱Galexos*) ▶L bile ♀?/?/?. Regimens with ribavirin: X/X/X ▶– $$$$$

ADULT — Chronic hepatitis C: Simeprevir dose for use only in combination regimens is 150 mg PO once daily with food. Genotype 1, treatment-naive and -experienced, no cirrhosis (guideline recommended regimen): Simeprevir 150 mg + sofosbuvir 400 mg both PO once daily for 12 weeks. Genotype 1, treatment-naive and -experienced, compensated cirrhosis, without Q80K polymorphism for genotype 1a (guideline alternative regimen): Simeprevir + sofosbuvir ± wt-based ribavirin (1000 mg/day PO for wt less than 75 kg; 1200 mg/day PO for 75 kg or greater) for 24 weeks. HCV treatment guideline no longer recommends FDA-approved regimen of simeprevir + wt-based ribavirin + peginterferon alfa for genotype 1 or 4.

PEDS — Safety and efficacy not established in children.

FORMS — Trade only: Caps 150 mg.

NOTES — Cost of simeprevir is $26,500/month. Not for monotherapy. For ribavirin-containing regimens, see ribavirin—oral entry for teratogenicity and contraceptive issues that affect female and male patients. Hepatic decompensation/failure reported primarily in patients with cirrhosis; monitor LFTs esp if total bilirubin increases by 2.5 x ULN. Higher exposure in East Asians (dosage adjustment not established), leading to more frequent adverse events including rash and photosensitivity. Can cause severe photosensitivity (most common in 1st month); tell patients to use sun protection and limit exposure. Rash (most common in 1st month); discontinue if severe. Contains sulfonamide moiety; risk in sulfa allergy is unclear. Do not coadminister carbamazepine, clarithromycin, cobicistat, cyclosporine, dexamethasone, efavirenz, erythromycin, etravirine, fluconazole, HIV protease inhibitors, itraconazole, ketoconazole, milk thistle, nevirapine, oxcarbazepine, phenobarbital, phenytoin, posaconazole, rifabutin, rifampin, rifapentine, St. John's wort, telithromycin, voriconazole. Monitor digoxin, sirolimus, tacrolimus levels. Simeprevir can increase exposure to calcium channel blockers, some antiarrhythmics, and oral midazolam/triazolam. Reduce initial rosuvastatin dose to 5 mg/day and max dose to 10 mg/day. Use lowest possible dose of atorvastatin, with max dose of 40 mg/day. Use lowest possible dose of most statins. Use

(cont.)

SIMEPREVIR (cont.)

in hepatic impairment: Not recommended for moderate/severe (Child-Pugh B/C) impairment.

MOA — NS3/4A protease inhibitor.

ADVERSE EFFECTS — Serious: Photosensitivity (most common in first month); rash (most common in first month). East Asians have higher simeprevir exposure (dosage adjustment not established), leading to more frequent adverse effects including rash and photosensitivity. Hepatic decompensation/failure reported, primarily in patients with advanced or decompensated cirrhosis. Frequent in combination with ribavirin and peginterferon: Rash (including photosensitivity) pruritus, nausea, mild to moderate hyperbilirubinemia. Frequent in combination with sofosbuvir: Fatigue, nausea, headache.

SOFOSBUVIR (Sovaldi, SOF) ▶LK ♀B Regimens with ribavirin: X ▶? $$$$$

ADULT — Chronic hepatitis C: Dose of sofosbuvir for use only in combination regimens is 400 mg PO once daily without regard to food. HCV treatment guidelines no longer recommend FDA-approved 12-week regimen of sofosbuvir + wt-based ribavirin + peginterferon alfa for genotype 1. See daclatasvir entry for daclatasvir-sofosbuvir regimens. See simeprevir entry for simeprevir-sofosbuvir regimens.

PEDS — Not approved in children.

FORMS — Trade only: Tabs 400 mg.

NOTES — Cost of sofosbuvir is $28,000/month. Not for monotherapy. Do not coadminister amiodarone, carbamazepine, oxcarbazepine, phenobarbital, phenytoin, rifabutin, rifampin, rifapentine, St. John's wort, or tipranavir-ritonavir. Monitor cyclosporine, tacrolimus levels. No dosage adjustment for hepatic impairment (Child-Pugh A to C). No dosage adjustment for CrCl >30 mL/min; do not use if CrCl <30 mL/min or ESRD.

MOA — NS5B RNA polymerase inhibitor. Prodrug is metabolized intracellularly to active form which is incorporated into viral RNA and acts as chain terminator.

ADVERSE EFFECTS — Frequent: Sofosbuvir + ribavirin: fatigue, headache. Sofosbuvir + ribavirin + peginterferon alfa: fatigue, headache, nausea, insomnia, anemia, neutropenia.

TECHNIVIE (ombitasvir-paritaprevir-ritonavir) ▶L ♀X ▶– $$$$$

ADULT — Chronic hepatitis C, genotype 4: 2 tabs PO once daily with breakfast for 12 weeks. Intended for use with ribavirin in patients without cirrhosis. Ribavirin dose is 1000 mg/day for wt less than 75 kg and 1200 mg/day for wt 75 kg or greater PO divided two times per day with food.

PEDS — Safety and efficacy not established in children.

FORMS — Trade only: Tabs ombitasvir 12.5 mg + paritaprevir 75 mg + ritonavir 50 mg.

NOTES — Cost of Technivie is $30,600/month. May cause hepatic decompensation or failure, esp if cirrhosis; not indicated in cirrhosis. Monitor LFTs, esp ALT, at baseline, during 1st month, and then as needed. HIV-coinfected patients should receive antiretroviral treatment to reduce the risk of protease inhibitor resistance. Many drug interactions due in part to strong CYP3A4 inhibition of ritonavir: Always check before prescribing. Do not coadminister alfuzosin, atazanavir, carbamazepine, colchicine in renal/hepatic impairment, dronedarone, efavirenz, ergot alkaloids, ethinyl estradiol (including oral contraceptives, due to increased ALT), lopinavir-ritonavir, lovastatin, lurasidone, PO midazolam, phenobarbital, phenytoin, pimozide, ranolazine, rifampin, rilpivirine, salmeterol, high-dose sildenafil for pulmonary arterial hypertension, simvastatin, St. John's wort, and triazolam. Decrease digoxin dose by 30 to 50% and monitor digoxin levels as needed. Do not coadminister with voriconazole unless benefit justifies risk of voriconazole treatment failure. Reduce quetiapine dose to 1/6 of original dose if Technivie is added; use lowest initial quetiapine dose if added to Technivie. Monitor for antiarrhythmic drug toxicity. Consider alternatives to inhaled/intranasal budesonide/fluticasone. Reduce amlodipine dose by at least 50%; may need dosage reduction for diltiazem, nifedipine, verapamil. May need dosage reduction of candesartan, losartan, valsartan. Use progestin-only or non-hormonal contraceptives during a course of Technivie; can restart contraceptives that contain ethinyl estradiol 2 weeks after stopping Technivie. Refer to ribavirin—oral entry for pregnancy and contraceptive concerns for ribavirin. Max dose of pravastatin is 40 mg/day. Reduce cyclosporine dose to 20% of usual dose and adjust dose based on levels. Hold tacrolimus dose on 1st day of Technivie, then adjust dose based on levels (typical tacrolimus dose is 0.5 mg q 7 days). Reduce hydrocodone dose by 50% and monitor for sedation and respiratory depression. Monitor for sedation with buprenorphine and alprazolam. Monitor for decreased efficacy of omeprazole; do not exceed omeprazole 40 mg/day. Use in hepatic impairment: Contraindicated in moderate or severe (Child-Pugh B or C) impairment.

MOA — Ombitasvir is an NS5A inhibitor. Paritaprevir is an NS3/4A protease inhibitor. Ritonavir boosts paritaprevir exposure via CYP3A4 inhibition.

ADVERSE EFFECTS — Serious: Hypersensitivity including angioedema. Frequent: asthenia, fatigue, nausea, insomnia.

VIEKIRA PAK (ombitasvir + paritaprevir + ritonavir + dasabuvir, Viekira XR, ✽ Holkira Pak) ▶L feces ♀?/?/? ▶? $$$$$

ADULT — Chronic hepatitis C. Viekira Pak regimen is 2 tabs of ombitasvir-paritaprevir-ritonavir PO once q am + 1 tab dasabuvir (250 mg) PO two times per day with a meal. Viekira XR regimen is 3 tabs of dasabuvir-ombitasvir-paritaprevir-ritonavir PO once daily with a meal. Genotype 1a, no cirrhosis: Viekira Pak/XR + ribavirin for 12 weeks. Genotype 1a, compensated cirrhosis (Child-Pugh A): Viekira Pak/XR + ribavirin for 24 weeks. Treatment guidelines consider

(cont.)

VIEKIRA PAK (*cont.*)

this an alternative regimen only for patients who can be monitored closely during the first 4 weeks for changes in liver function. Genotype 1b, with/without compensated cirrhosis (Child-Pugh A): Viekira Pak/XR alone for 12 weeks. Ribavirin dose is 1000 mg/day for wt less than 75 kg and 1200 mg/day for wt 75 kg or greater PO divided two times per day with food. Viekira XR: Do not split, crush, or chew tabs; do not drink alcohol within 4 hours after a dose.

PEDS — Safety and efficacy not established in children.

FORMS — Viekira Pak. Trade only: Tabs ombitasvir 12.5 mg + paritaprevir 75 mg + ritonavir 50 mg plus separate tabs dasabuvir 250 mg. Viekira XR. Trade only: Extended-release tabs: dasabuvir 200 mg + ombitasvir 8.33 mg + paritaprevir 50 mg + ritonavir 33.33 mg.

NOTES — Cost of Viekira Pak or Viekira XR is $33,327/month. May cause hepatic decompensation or failure, esp if cirrhosis. Monitor LFTs, including direct bilirubin, at baseline, during 1st month and then as needed. Many drug interactions due in part to strong CYP3A4 inhibition of ritonavir: Always check before prescribing. Do not coadminister alfuzosin, carbamazepine, colchicine in renal/hepatic impairment, darunavir-ritonavir, dronedarone, efavirenz, ergot alkaloids, ethinyl estradiol (including oral contraceptives, due to increased ALT), gemfibrozil, lopinavir-ritonavir, lovastatin, lurasidone, PO midazolam, phenobarbital, phenytoin, pimozide, ranolazine, rifampin, rilpivirine, salmeterol, high-dose sildenafil for pulmonary arterial hypertension, simvastatin, St. John's wort, and triazolam. Do not coadminister with voriconazole unless benefit justifies risk of voriconazole treatment failure. Monitor for antiarrhythmic drug toxicity. Consider alternatives to inhaled/intranasal budesonide/fluticasone. Reduce amlodipine dose by at least 50%; may need dosage reduction for diltiazem, nifedipine, verapamil. May need to reduce dose of candesartan, losartan, valsartan. When coadministered with Viekira, atazanavir dose is 300 mg PO q am. Use progestin-only or nonhormonal contraceptives during a course of Viekira; can restart contraceptives that contain ethinyl estradiol 2 weeks after discontinuation of Viekira. Refer to ribavirin—oral entry for pregnancy and contraceptive concerns with ribavirin. Patients with HIV coinfection should receive adequate antiretroviral regimen. Do not exceed rosuvastatin 10 mg/day or pravastatin 40 mg/day. Reduce cyclosporine dose to 20% of usual dose and adjust dose based on levels. Hold tacrolimus dose on 1st day of Viekira, then adjust dose based on blood levels (typical tacrolimus dose is 0.5 mg q 7 days). Reduce hydrocodone dose by 50% and monitor for sedation and respiratory depression. Monitor for sedation with buprenorphine and alprazolam. Monitor for decreased efficacy of omeprazole; do not exceed omeprazole 40 mg/day. Reduce quetiapine dose to 1/6 of original dose if Viekira is added; use lowest initial quetiapine dose if added to Viekira. No dosage adjustment for renal impairment, including dialysis. Use in hepatic impairment: Contraindicated in moderate or severe (Child-Pugh B/C) impairment.

MOA — Dasabuvir is an NS5B RNA polymerase inhibitor. Ombitasvir is an NS5A inhibitor. Paritaprevir is an NS3/4A protease inhibitor. Ritonavir boosts paritaprevir exposure via CYP 3A4 inhibition.

ADVERSE EFFECTS — Serious: Anemia when used with ribavirin. Frequent with ribavirin: Fatigue, nausea, pruritus, skin reactions, insomnia, asthenia. Frequent without ribavirin: Nausea, pruritus, insomnia. Frequent in HIV-coinfection: Fatigue, insomnia, nausea, headache, pruritus, cough, irritability, ocular icterus, increased bilirubin.

***ZEPATIER* (elbasvir + grasoprevir)** ▶L ♀?/?/? Regimens with ribavirin: X/X/X ▶? $$$$$

ADULT — Chronic hepatitis C. Zapatier dose is 1 tab PO once daily without regard to meals. Treatment duration and need for ribavirin varies by genotype, NS5A resistance polymorphisms, and treatment experience. Test genotype 1a for NS5A resistance. Genotype 1a, treatment-naive: Zapatier alone for 12 weeks if no resistance; Zapatier + wt-based ribavirin for 16 weeks if baseline resistance. Ribavirin dose is 800 mg/day for wt less than 66 kg; 1000 mg/day for 66 to 80 kg; 1200 mg/day for 81 to 105 kg; 1400 mg/day for wt greater than 105 kg; give PO divided two times per day with food. Genotype 1b and 4, treatment-naive: Zapatier alone for 12 weeks. Also for treatment-experienced genotype 1a, 1b, and 4 (genotype 1a, 1b, 4 who failed peginterferon-ribavirin; genotype 1a or 1b who failed peginterferon-ribavirin-boceprevir/simeprevir/telaprevir).

PEDS — Safety and efficacy not established in children.

FORMS — Trade only: Tabs elbasvir 50 mg + grazoprevir 100 mg.

NOTES — Cost of Zepatier is $21,800/month. Monitor LFTs, including at baseline and week 8. For ribavirin-containing regimens, see ribavirin—oral entry for teratogenicity and contraceptive issues that affect female and male patients.Do not coadminister bosentan, carbamazepine, cobicistat, cyclosporine, efavirenz, etravirine, ketoconazole, modafinil, nafcillin, phenytoin, most HIV protease inhibitors, rifampin, St John's wort. May increase tacrolimus levels. Use lowest possible dose of fluvastatin, lovastatin, simvastatin; do not exceed 20 mg/day of atorvastatin or 10 mg/day of rosuvstatin. Renal/hepatic impairment: No dosage adjustment for renal impairment/dialysis or mild hepatic impairment (Child-Pugh A). Contraindicated in moderate to severe hepatic impairment (Child-Pugh B/C).

MOA — Elbasvir is an NS5A protein inhibitor; grazoprevir is a NS3/4A protease inhibitor.

ADVERSE EFFECTS — Serious: ALT increases (esp. women, Asians, elderly). Frequent: Fatigue, headache, nausea.

ANTIMICROBIALS: Antiviral Agents—Anti-Herpetic

ACYCLOVIR (*Zovirax, Sitavig*) ▶K ♀B ▶+ $

ADULT — Genital herpes: 200 mg PO q 4 h (five times per day) for 10 days for first episode, for 5 days for recurrent episodes. Chronic suppression of genital herpes: 400 mg PO two times per day. See STD table. Zoster: 800 mg PO q 4 h (five times per day) for 7 to 10 days. Chickenpox: 800 mg PO four times per day for 5 days. IV: 5 to 10 mg/kg IV q 8 h, each dose over 1 h. Zoster in immunocompromised patients: 10 mg/kg IV q 8 h for 7 days. Herpes simplex encephalitis: 10 mg/kg IV q 8 h for 10 days. Mucosal/cutaneous herpes simplex in immunocompromised patients: 5 mg/kg IV q 8 h for 7 days. Sitavig for recurrent herpes labialis in immunocompetent adults: Within 1 h of prodromal symptom onset, apply buccal tab once to upper gum above incisor on the side of mouth affected by herpes; then press slightly on upper lip for 30 seconds.

PEDS — Safety and efficacy of PO acyclovir not established in children younger than 2 yo. Chickenpox: 20 mg/kg PO four times per day for 5 days. Use adult dose if wt greater than 40 kg. AAP does not recommend routine treatment of chickenpox with acyclovir, but it should be considered in patients older than 12 yo or with chronic cutaneous or pulmonary disease; chronic salicylate use; or short, intermittent, or inhaled courses of corticosteroid. Possibly also for secondary household cases. Zoster in immunocompromised patients, age younger than 12 yo: 20 mg/kg IV q 8 h for 7 days (see dose in UNAPPROVED PEDS). Herpes simplex encephalitis: 20 mg/kg IV q 8 h for 10 days for age 3 mo to 12 yo (see dose in UNAPPROVED PEDS); adult dose for age 13 yo or older. Neonatal herpes simplex, birth to 3 mo: 10 mg/kg IV q 8 h for 10 days; CDC regimen is 20 mg/kg IV q 8 h for 21 days for disseminated/CNS disease, for 14 days for skin/mucous membranes. Mucosal/cutaneous herpes simplex in immunocompromised patients: 10 mg/kg IV q 8 h for 7 days for age younger than 12 yo, adult dose for 13 yo or older. Treat ASAP after symptom onset. Sitavig buccal tabs are not approved in children, and not recommended for younger children due to potential risk of choking.

UNAPPROVED ADULT — Genital herpes: 400 mg PO three times per day for 7 to 10 days for 1st episode, for 5 days for recurrent episodes, for 5 to 10 days for recurrent episodes in HIV-infected patients. Alternative regimens for recurrent episodes: 800 mg PO two times per day for 5 days or 800 mg PO three times per day for 2 days. Chronic suppression of genital herpes in HIV infection: 400 to 800 mg PO two to three times per day. See STD table. Orolabial herpes: 400 mg PO 5 times a day.

UNAPPROVED PEDS — Zoster, immuno-competent or -compromised: 10 mg/kg IV q 8 h for 7 to 10 days. Varicella, immunocompetent, age 2 yo and older: 10 mg/kg IV q 8 h or 500 mg/m² IV q 8 h for 7 to 10 days. Varicella, immunocompromised: 10 to 15 mg/kg IV q 8 h for age younger than 1 yo (some experts also recommend for age over 1 year old); 500 mg/m² IV q 8 h for age 1 yo and older. Treat for 7 to 10 days. Herpes simplex encephalitis, 3 mo to 12 yo:10 to 15 mg/kg IV q 8 h for 14 to 21 days (FDA-approved dose may have higher nephrotoxicity risk). Monitor renal function and for neurologic adverse events; consider specialist consult for weight-based doses greater than 800 mg or coadministration of nephrotoxic drugs. Suppressive therapy after neonatal herpes simplex, birth to 7 mo: 300 mg/m² PO three times per day for 6 months. Primary herpes gingivostomatitis: 15 mg/kg PO 5 times a day for 7 days. First episode genital herpes: 40 to 80 mg/kg/day PO divided three times per day (max 1.2 g/day) for 7 to 10 days. Use dose in Unapproved Adult for adolescents. Treat ASAP after symptom onset.

FORMS — Generic/Trade: Caps 200 mg. Tabs 400, 800 mg. Susp 200 mg/5 mL. Trade only: Buccal tab (Sitavig-$$$$$) 50 mg.

NOTES — Maintain adequate hydration. Severe drowsiness with acyclovir plus zidovudine. Consider suppressive therapy for patients with at least 6 episodes of genital herpes per year. Reduce dose in renal dysfunction and in elderly. Base IV dose on ideal body wt in obese adults. Sitavig: Contraindicated if hypersensitivity to milk protein concentrate. Buccal tab is intended to remain in place until it dissolves. If it falls off within 6 h of application, reposition tab. If it does not stay in place, apply a new tab. If tab is swallowed within first 6 h, drink a glass of water and apply a new tab. No action is needed if tab falls off or is swallowed after it has been in place for at least 6 h. Do not chew gum while tab is in place.

MOA — Activated by viral thymidine kinase to become an inhibitor of viral DNA polymerase and block viral DNA synthesis.

ADVERSE EFFECTS — Serious: Encephalopathy, extravasation, crystalluria with IV. Frequent: GI distress & headache with PO. Sitavig buccal tabs: Application site irritation (rare).

FAMCICLOVIR (*Famvir*) ▶K ♀B ▶? $$

ADULT — Recurrent genital herpes: 1000 mg PO two times per day for 2 days. Chronic suppression of genital herpes: 250 mg PO two times per day. See STD table. Recurrent herpes labialis: 1500 mg PO single dose. Recurrent orolabial/genital herpes in HIV infection: 500 mg PO two times per day for 7 days. Zoster: 500 mg PO three times per day for 7 days. Treat ASAP after symptom onset.

PEDS — Not approved in children.

UNAPPROVED ADULT — First episode genital herpes: 250 mg PO three times per day for 7 to 10 days. Chronic suppression of genital herpes in HIV infection: 500 mg PO two times per day. See STD table. Chickenpox in young adults: 500 mg PO three times per day for 5 days. Bell's palsy: 750 mg PO three times per day plus prednisone 1 mg/kg PO daily for 7 days. Treat ASAP after symptom onset.

(cont.)

FAMCICLOVIR (*cont.*)

UNAPPROVED PEDS — Chickenpox in adolescents: 500 mg PO three times per day for 5 days. First episode genital herpes in adolescents: Use dose in unapproved adult.

FORMS — Generic/Trade: Tabs 125, 250, 500 mg.

NOTES — Consider suppressive therapy for patients with at least 6 episodes of genital herpes per year. Reduce dose for CrCl <60 mL/min.

MOA — Prodrug of penciclovir. Activated by viral thymidine kinase to become an inhibitor of viral DNA polymerase and block viral DNA synthesis.

ADVERSE EFFECTS — Similar to acyclovir. Frequent: Headache, nausea, diarrhea.

VALACYCLOVIR (*Valtrex*) ▶K ♀B ▶+ $$$$

ADULT — First episode genital herpes: 1 g PO two times per day for 10 days. Recurrent genital herpes: 500 mg PO two times per day for 3 days. Chronic suppression of genital herpes in immunocompetent patients: 1 g PO daily. Can use 500 mg PO daily if 9 or fewer recurrences per year; transmission of genital herpes reduced with use of this regimen by source partner, in conjunction with safer sex practices. Chronic suppression of genital herpes in HIV infection: 500 mg PO two times per day. See STD table. Herpes labialis: 2 g PO q 12 h for 2 doses. Zoster: 1 g PO three times per day for 7 days. Treat ASAP after symptom onset.

PEDS — Herpes labialis, age 12 yo or older: 2 g PO q 12 h for 2 doses. Chickenpox, age 2 to 17 yo: 20 mg/kg (max of 1 g) PO three times per day for 5 days. Treat ASAP after symptom onset.

UNAPPROVED ADULT — Recurrent genital herpes: 1 g PO daily for 5 days. First episode or recurrent genital herpes in HIV+ patients: 1 g PO two times per day for 5 to 14 days. See STD table. Bell's palsy: 1 g PO two times per day plus prednisone 1 mg/kg PO daily for 7 days. Orolabial herpes in immunocompromised patients, including HIV infection: 1 g PO three times per day for 7 days. Chickenpox in young adults: 1 g PO three times per day for 5 days. Treat ASAP after symptom onset. Varicella or herpes zoster post-exposure prophylaxis in HIV: 1 g PO three times per day for 5 to 7 days starting 7 to 10 days after exposure.

UNAPPROVED PEDS — First episode genital herpes in adolescents: Use adult dose. Treat ASAP after symptom onset.

FORMS — Generic/Trade: Tabs 500, 1000 mg.

NOTES — Consider suppressive therapy for patients with at least 6 episodes of genital herpes per year. Maintain adequate hydration. CNS and renal adverse effects more common if elderly or renal impairment; avoid inappropriately high doses in these patients. Reduce dose for CrCl <50 mL/min. Thrombotic thrombocytopenic purpura/hemolytic uremic syndrome at dose of 8 g/day.

MOA — Prodrug of acyclovir, which is activated by viral thymidine kinase to become an inhibitor of viral DNA polymerase and block viral DNA synthesis.

ADVERSE EFFECTS — Similar to acyclovir. CNS (e.g., agitation, hallucinations, confusion, encephalopathy): and renal adverse effects more common if elderly or renal impairment. Serious: Acute renal failure and anuria due to precipitation in renal tubules; may require hemodialysis to remove drug.

ANTIMICROBIALS: Antiviral Agents—Anti-HIV—CCR5 Antagonists

MARAVIROC (*Selzentry, MVC, ✦Celsentri*) ▶LK ♀B ▶– $$$$$

WARNING — Hepatotoxicity with allergic features, including DRESS. May have prodrome of severe rash or systemic allergic reaction. Monitor LFTs at baseline and if rash, allergic reaction, or signs/symptoms of hepatitis. Consider discontinuation if signs/symptoms of hepatitis or increased LFTs with rash or other systemic symptoms. Caution if baseline liver dysfunction or coinfection with hepatitis B/C.

ADULT — Combination therapy for HIV infection: 150 mg PO two times per day with strong CYP3A4 inhibitors (clarithromycin, itraconazole, ketoconazole, most HIV protease inhibitors); 300 mg PO two times per day with drugs that are not strong CYP3A4 inducers/inhibitors (NRTIs, tipranavir-ritonavir, nevirapine, enfuvirtide, raltegravir; rifabutin without a strong CYP3A4 inhibitor or inducer); 600 mg PO two times per day with strong CYP3A4 inducers (efavirenz, etravirine, rifampin, carbamazepine, phenobarbital, phenytoin). Do not give maraviroc with unboosted fosamprenavir. Tropism test before treatment; not for dual/mixed or CXCR4-tropic HIV infection.

PEDS — Not recommended for age younger than 16 yo based on lack of data.

FORMS — Trade only: Tabs 150, 300 mg.

NOTES — Discontinue immediately if signs/symptoms of severe skin or hypersensitivity reaction. May increase risk of myocardial ischemia or MI. Theoretical risk of infection/malignancy due to effects on immune system. Metabolized by CYP3A4; do not use with St. John's wort. Increased risk of postural hypotension in renal impairment. Contraindicated in patients with CrCl <30 mL/min who are taking a strong CYP3A4 inhibitor or inducer. Consider dosage reduction to 150 mg two times per day if postural hypotension occurs in patients with CrCL <30 mL/min.

MOA — CCR5 coreceptor antagonist prevents entry of CCR5-tropic HIV into uninfected CD4 T-cells.

ADVERSE EFFECTS — Serious: Hepatotoxicity with allergic features, including DRESS. Severe skin or hypersensitivity reactions. Immune reconstitution syndrome. May increase risk of myocardial ischemia or MI. May cause postural hypotension, esp in patients with impaired renal function. Frequent: Cough, fever, upper respiratory tract infection, rash, joint symptoms, muscle pain, abdominal pain, dizziness, increased AST.

ANTIMICROBIALS: Antiviral Agents—Anti-HIV—Combinations

***ATRIPLA* (efavirenz + emtricitabine + tenofovir disoproxil fumarate)** ▶KL ♀D ▶– $$$$$
WARNING — Emtricitabine and tenofovir: Potentially fatal lactic acidosis and hepatosteatosis. Severe acute HBV exacerbation after discontinuation in HIV/HBV coinfected patients.
ADULT — HIV infection, alone or in combination with other antiretrovirals:1 tab PO once daily on empty stomach, preferably at bedtime.
PEDS — Consider antihistamine prophylaxis to prevent efavirenz rash before starting Atripla. HIV infection, alone or in combination with other antiretrovirals, age 12 yo or older and wt 40 kg or greater: 1 tab PO once daily on empty stomach, preferably at bedtime.
FORMS — Trade only: Tabs efavirenz 600 mg + emtricitabine 200 mg + tenofovir disoproxil fumarate 300 mg.
NOTES — See components. Not for CrCl <50 mL/min; assess CrCl before treatment. Monitor CrCl, urine glucose, urine protein, serum phosphorus before and during treatment in patients at risk for renal impairment. Do not give Atripla with lamivudine or voriconazole. Efavirenz induces CYP3A4, causing many drug interactions. Coadministration with rifampin: Consider adding 200 mg/day of efavirenz to Atripla if wt 50 kg or greater.
MOA — Emtricitabine and tenofovir are NRTIs that have activity against HBV. Emtricitabine has documented cross-resistance to lamivudine. Efavirenz is an NNRTI.
ADVERSE EFFECTS — Serious: Emtricitabine, tenofovir: Lactic acidosis/hepatic steatosis; severe acute HBV exacerbation after discontinuation in HIV/HBV coinfected patients. Efavirenz: Depression, other psychiatric reactions, convulsions, severe rash, Stevens-Johnson syndrome. See components for other adverse effects.

***COMBIVIR* (lamivudine + zidovudine)** ▶LK ♀C ▶– $$$$$
WARNING — Zidovudine: Bone marrow suppression, myopathy. Lamivudine: Potentially fatal lactic acidosis and hepatosteatosis. Severe acute HBV exacerbation after discontinuation in HIV/HBV coinfected patients.
ADULT — Combination therapy of HIV infection: 1 tab PO two times per day.
PEDS — Combination therapy of HIV infection, wt 30 kg or greater: 1 tab PO two times per day.
FORMS — Generic/Trade: Tabs lamivudine 150 mg + zidovudine 300 mg.
NOTES — See components. Monitor CBC. Not for wt less than 30 kg, CrCl <50 mL/min, hepatic dysfunction, or if dosage adjustment required.
MOA — See components.
ADVERSE EFFECTS — Serious: Lactic acidosis/hepatic steatosis; acute HBV exacerbation after discontinuation of lamivudine in HIV/HBV coinfected patients. See components for other adverse effects.

***COMPLERA* (emtricitabine + rilpivirine + tenofovir disoproxil fumarate)** ▶KL ♀B ▶– $$$$$
WARNING — Tenofovir: Potentially fatal lactic acidosis and hepatosteatosis. Emtricitabine and tenofovir: Severe acute exacerbation of hepatitis B after discontinuation in HIV-HBV coinfected patients coinfected with HIV and hepatitis B.
ADULT — HIV infection, treatment-naive with baseline HIV RNA up to 100,000 copies/mL: 1 tab PO once daily with food. When coadministered with rifabutin, give 1 tab Complera plus 25 mg rilpivirine PO once daily with a meal. Also used to replace a stable regimen in certain virologically-suppressed patients; monitor HIV RNA for virologic failure/rebound after switching to Complera.
PEDS — HIV infection, treatment-naive with baseline HIV RNA up to 100,000 copies/mL, age 12 yo and older and wt 35 kg or greater: 1 tab PO once daily with food. When coadministered with rifabutin, give 1 tab Complera plus 25 mg rilpivirine PO once daily with a meal. Also used to replace a stable regimen in certain virologically-suppressed patients; monitor HIV RNA for virologic failure/rebound after switching to Complera.
FORMS — Trade only: Tabs emtricitabine 200 mg + rilpivirine 25 mg + tenofovir disoproxil fumarate 300 mg.
NOTES — See components. Test for hepatitis B before treatment. Not for CrCl <50 mL/min; assess CrCl before treatment. Monitor CrCl, urine glucose, urine protein, serum phosphorus before and during treatment in patients at risk for renal impairment. Dosage adjustment not required for mild/moderate hepatic impairment (Child-Pugh Class A/B). HIV guidelines recommend Complera for treatment-naive patients with HIV RNA less than 100,000 copies/mL and baseline CD4+ count greater than 200 cells/mm³. Contraindicated with carbamazepine, dexamethasone (more than a single dose), oxcarbazepine, phenobarbital, phenytoin, proton pump inhibitors, rifampin, rifapentine, St. John's wort. Give antacids at least 2 h before or 4 h after Complera. Give H2 blockers at least 12 h before or 4 h after Complera. Monitor for reduced response to methadone. Store in original bottle.
MOA — Emtricitabine is a nucleoside reverse transcriptase inhibitor structurally related to lamivudine; cross-resistance documented. Tenofovir is a nucleotide reverse transcriptase inhibitor. Emtricitabine and tenofovir have activity against hepatitis B. Rilpivirine is a non-nucleoside reverse transcriptase inhibitor. Cross-resistance possible between rilpivirine and other NNRTIs.
ADVERSE EFFECTS — Serious: Emtricitabine, tenofovir: Lactic acidosis/hepatic steatosis; severe acute exacerbation of hepatitis B after discontinuing either drug in patients coinfected with HIV and hepatitis B. Rilpivirine: Depressive disorders (frequent), fat redistribution (causality unclear), immune reconstitution syndrome, hepatotoxicity. See components for other adverse effects.

DESCOVY (emtricitabine + tenofovir alafenamide) ▶K ♀?/?/? R ▶– $$$$$
WARNING — Emtricitabine and tenofovir: Potentially fatal lactic acidosis and hepatosteatosis; severe acute HBV exacerbation after discontinuation in HIV/HBV coinfected patients.
ADULT — Combination therapy for HIV infection: 1 tab PO once daily with other antiretroviral drugs.
PEDS — Combination therapy for HIV infection, age 12 yo and older and wt 35 kg or greater: 1 tab PO once daily with other antiretroviral drugs.
UNAPPROVED ADULT — Insufficient evidence to recommend Descovy for pre-exposure prophylaxis in adults at high risk for sexually-acquired HIV.
FORMS — Trade only: Tabs emtricitablline 200 mg + tenofovir alafenamide 25 mg.
NOTES — See entricitabine component. Do not use in a triple nucleoside regimen. Test for HBV at baseline. Not for patients with CrCl <30 mL/min. Monitor CrCl, urine glucose, urine protein before and during treatment. Discontinue if significant decline in renal function or signs of Fanconi syndrome. Monitor serum phosphorus in patients with chronic kidney disease. May decrease bone mineral density; consider calcium and vitamin D supplements and monitoring BMD in at-risk patients. Do not coadminister rifabutin, rifampin, rifapentine, St. John's wort, tipranavir-ritonavir. Consider alternatives to carbamazepine, oxcarbazepine, phenobarbital, phenytoin.
MOA — Emtricitabine and tenofovir alafenamide (TAF) are NRTIs. Emtricitabine has documented cross-resistance to lamivudine. A lower dose of TAF achieves similar/higher intracellular levels and lower serum levels than tenofovir disoproxil fumarate. Emtricitabine and TAF have activity against HBV, but role of TAF in HBV/HIV coinfection is undefined.
ADVERSE EFFECTS — Serious for emtricitabine and tenofovir alafenamide (TAF): Lactic acidosis/hepatic steatosis; fat redistribution (causality unclear); severe acute HBV exacerbation after discontinuing either drug in HIV/HBV coinfected patients. Serious for TAF: Less bone and renal toxicity than tenofovir disoproxil fumarate. See emtricitabine entry for other adverse effects. Frequent: Nausea, increased LDL cholesterol.

EPZICOM (abacavir + lamivudine, ✲ *Kivexa*) ▶LK ♀C ▶– $$$$$
WARNING — Abacavir: Potentially fatal hypersensitivity reactions. HLA-B*5701 predisposes to hypersensitivity; screen before starting. Abacavir is contraindicated if positive test. Never rechallenge with abacavir after suspected reaction. Abacavir and lamivudine: Lactic acidosis and hepatosteatosis. Lamivudine: Severe acute HBV exacerbation after discontinuation in HIV/HBV coinfected patients.
ADULT — Combination therapy of HIV infection: 1 tab PO daily.

PEDS — Combination therapy of HIV infection, wt 25 kg or greater: 1 tab PO daily.
FORMS — Trade only: Tabs abacavir 600 mg + lamivudine 300 mg.
NOTES — See components. Not for patients with CrCl <50 mL/min, moderate to severe hepatic dysfunction, or if dosage adjustment required.
MOA — See components.
ADVERSE EFFECTS — Serious: Potentially fatal hypersensitivity (abacavir); lactic acidosis/hepatic steatosis (abacavir or lamivudine); acute HBV exacerbation after discontinuation in HIV/HBV coinfected patients (lamivudine). See components for other adverse effects.

GENVOYA (elvitegravir + cobicistat + emtricitabine + tenofovir alafenamide) ▶KL ♀B R ▶– $$$$$
WARNING — Emtricitabine and tenofovir: Potentially fatal lactic acidosis and hepatosteatosis. Severe acute HBV exacerbation after discontinuation in HIV/HBV coinfected patients.
ADULT — HIV infection: 1 tab PO once daily with food. Not for use with other antiretroviral drugs.
PEDS — HIV infection, age 12 yo and older and wt 35 kg or greater: 1 tab PO once daily with food. Not for use with other antiretroviral drugs.
FORMS — Trade only: Tabs elvitegravir 150 mg + cobicistat 150 mg + emtricitabine 200 mg + tenofovir alafenamide 10 mg.
NOTES — See components. Test for HBV before treatment. Monitor CrCl, urine glucose, urine protein before and during treatment. Monitor serum phosphorus in patients with chronic renal disease. Loss of bone mineral density is less than Stribild; assess bone mineral density in patients with a history of pathologic fractures or high osteoporosis risk. Many drug interactions. Cobicistat is a strong CYP 3A4 inhibitor. Contraindicated with alfuzosin, carbamazepine, colchicine in patients with renal/hepatic impairment, ergot alkaloids, lovastatin, oral midazolam, phenobarbital, phenytoin, pimozide, rifabutin, rifampin, rifapentine, salmeterol, high-dose sildenafil for pulmonary hypertension, simvastatin, St. John's wort, triazolam. Do not give >200 mg/day of itraconazole/ketoconazole. Reduce clarithromycin dose by 50% if CrCl is 50 to 60 mL/min. Reduce quetiapine to 1/6 of original dose if Genvoya is added; use lowest initial quetiapine dose if it is added to Genvoya. Monitor INR with warfarin. Reduce dose of colchicine, bosentan, or high-dose tadalafil for pulmonary hypertension. For erectile dysfunction, reduce to max single doses of sildenafil 25 mg in 48 h, vardenafil 2.5 mg in 72 h, tadalafil 10 mg in 72 h. Monitor levels of digoxin, cyclosporine, tacrolimus, sirolimus. Use lowest starting dose of atorvastatin. Separate doses of antacids by at least 2 h. Consider alternatives to dexamethasone, inhaled/intranasal fluticasone, oxcarbazepine, voriconazole. Use in renal/hepatic impairment: Not for CrCl <30 mL/min or severe hepatic impairment (Child-Pugh C).
MOA — Elvitegravir is an integrase strand transfer inhibitor. Cobicistat inhibits CYP3A4; it is included

(cont.)

GENVOYA (*cont.*)

in Genvoya to increase exposure to elvitegravir. Emtricitabine and tenofovir are NRTIs. Entricitabine has documented cross-resistance to lamivudine. A lower dose of tenofovir alafenamide (TAF) achieves similar/higher intracellular levels and lower serum levels than tenofovir disoproxil fumarate. Emtricitabine and TAF have activity against HBV, but role of TAF in HBV/HIV coinfection not defined yet.

ADVERSE EFFECTS — Serious: Fat redistribution (causality unclear); immune reconstitution syndrome. Emtricitabine and tenofovir alafenamide (TAF): Lactic acidosis/hepatic steatosis; severe acute HBV exacerbation after discontinuation in HIV/HBV coinfected patients. TAF: Less bone and renal toxicity than tenofovir disoproxil fumarate (in Stribild). Frequent: Nausea, diarrhea, headache.

ODEFSEY (**emtricitabine + rilpivirine + tenofovir alafenamide**) ▶LK ♀?/?/? R ▶– $$$$$

WARNING — Emtricitabine and tenofovir: Potentially fatal lactic acidosis and hepatosteatosis; severe acute HBV exacerbation after discontinuation in HIV/HBV coinfected patients.

ADULT — HIV infection, treatment-naive with baseline HIV RNA up to 100,000 copies/mL: 1 tab PO once daily with food. Also used to replace a stable regimen in certain virologically-suppressed patients; monitor HIV RNA for virologic failure/rebound after switching to Odefsey.

PEDS — HIV infection, treatment-naive with baseline HIV RNA up to 100,000 copies/mL, age 12 yo and older and wt 35 kg or greater: 1 tab PO once daily with food. Also used to replace a stable regimen in certain virologically-suppressed patients; monitor HIV RNA for virologic failure/rebound after switching to Odefsey.

FORMS — Trade only: Tabs emtricitabine 200 mg + rilpivirine 25 mg + tenofovir alafenamide 25 mg.

NOTES — See components. Test for HBV before treatment. Not for CrCl <30 mL/min. Monitor CrCl, urine glucose, urine protein before and during treatment. HIV guidelines recommend for treatment-naive patients with HIV RNA <100,000 copies/mL and baseline CD4 count >200 cells/mm3. Contraindicated with carbamazepine, dexamethasone (more than a single dose), oxcarbazepine, phenobarbital, phenytoin, proton pump inhibitors, rifampin, rifapentine, St. John's wort. Avoid rifabutin. Give antacids at least 2 h before or 4 h after Odefsey. Give H2 blockers at least 12 h before or 4 h after Odefsey. Monitor for reduced response to methadone. No dosage adjustment for mild-moderate (Child-Pugh A-B) hepatic impairment. Store in original bottle.

MOA — Emtricitabine and tenofovir are NRTIs. Entricitabine has documented cross-resistance to lamivudine. A lower dose of tenofovir alafenamide (TAF) achieves similar/higher intracellular levels and lower serum levels than tenofovir disoproxil fumarate. Emtricitabine and TAF have activity

against HBV, but role of TAF in HBV/HIV coinfection not defined yet. Rilpivirine is a NNRTI with possible cross-resistance to other NNRTIs .

ADVERSE EFFECTS — Serious. Emtricitabine and tenofovir alafenamide (TAF): Lactic acidosis/hepatic steatosis; severe acute HBV exacerbation of after discontinuing either drug in HIV/HBV coinfected patients. Rilpivirine: Depression (frequent); severe skin and hypersensitivity reactions; QT interval prolongation at supratherapeutic doses; hepatotoxicity. TAF: Less bone and renal toxicity than tenofovir disoproxil fumarate. See components for other adverse effects.

STRIBILD (**elvitegravir + cobicistat + emtricitabine + tenofovir disoproxil fumarate**) ▶KL ♀B ▶– $$$$$

WARNING — Tenofovir: Potentially fatal lactic acidosis and hepatosteatosis. Emtricitabine and tenofovir: Severe acute exacerbation of HBV after discontinuation in HIV-HBV coinfected patients.

ADULT — HIV infection: 1 tab PO once daily with food. Not for use with other antiretroviral drugs.

PEDS — Safety and efficacy not established in children.

FORMS — Trade only: Tabs elvitegravir 150 mg + cobicistat 150 mg + emtricitabine 200 mg + tenofovir disoproxil fumarate 300 mg.

NOTES — See components. Test for HBV before treatment. Monitor CrCl, urine glucose, urine protein before and during treatment. Monitor serum phosphorus in patients at risk for renal impairment. Do not start if CrCl <70 mL/min; stop if CrCl declines to <50 mL/min. Many drug interactions. Cobicistat is a strong CYP3A4 inhibitor. Contraindicated with alfuzosin, carbamazepine, colchicine in patients with renal/hepatic impairment, ergot alkaloids, ledipasvir-sofosbuvir, lovastatin, oral midazolam, phenobarbital, phenytoin, pimozide, rifabutin, rifampin, rifapentine, salmeterol, high-dose sildenafil for pulmonary hypertension, simvastatin, St. John's wort, triazolam. Do not give >200 mg/day of itraconazole/ketoconazole. Reduce clarithromycin dose by 50% if CrCl is 50 to 60 mL/min. Reduce quetiapine to 1/6 of original dose if Stribild is added; use lowest initial quetiapine dose if it is added to Stribild. Monitor INR with warfarin. Reduce dose of colchicine, bosentan, or high-dose tadalafil for pulmonary hypertension. For erectile dysfunction, reduce to max single doses of sildenafil 25 mg in 48 h, vardenafil 2.5 mg in 72 h, tadalafil 10 mg in 72 h. Monitor levels of digoxin, cyclosporine, tacrolimus, sirolimus. Use lowest starting dose of atorvastatin. Consider alternatives to dexamethasone, inhaled/intranasal fluticasone, oxcarbazepine, voriconazole. Separate doses of antacids by at least 2 h. Use in renal/hepatic impairment: Not for CrCl <50 mL/min or severe hepatic impairment (Child-Pugh C).

MOA — Elvitegravir is an integrase strand transfer inhibitor. Cobicistat inhibits CYP3A4; it is included in Stribild to increase exposure to elvitegravir. Emtricitabine is a nucleoside reverse transcriptase

(cont.)

STRIBILD (*cont.*)

inhibitor. Tenofovir is a nucleotide reverse transcriptase inhibitor.

ADVERSE EFFECTS — Serious: Lactic acidosis/hepatic steatosis; severe acute exacerbation of hepatitis B; new onset or worsening renal impairment; decreases in bone mineral density; immune reconstitution syndrome. Frequent: nausea, diarrhea.

TRIUMEQ (**abacavir + dolutegravir + lamivudine**) ▶LK ♀C ▶– $$$$$

WARNING — Abacavir: Life-threatening hypersensitivity. HLA-B*5701 predisposes to hypersensitivity; screen before starting abacavir and avoid if positive test. Never rechallenge with abacavir after suspected reaction. Abacavir and lamivudine: Lactic acidosis and hepatosteatosis. Lamivudine: Severe acute HBV exacerbation after discontinuation in HIV-HBV coinfected patients.

ADULT — HIV infection, alone or in combination with other drugs: 1 tab PO once daily without regard to food. Coadministration with carbamazepine, efavirenz, fosamprenavir-ritonavir, tipranavir-ritonavir, or rifampin: Add dolutegravir 50 mg PO at least 12 h after dose of Triumeq. Do not use Triumeq alone in patients with INSTI resistance substitutions or suspected INSTI resistance.

PEDS — Safety and efficacy have not been established in children.

FORMS — Trade only: Tabs abacavir 600 mg + dolutegravir 50 mg + lamivudine 300 mg.

NOTES — See components. Not for patients with CrCl <50 mL/min, hepatic impairment, or if dosage adjustment required. Never restart Triumeq, abacavir, or dolutegravir in patients who discontinued Triumeq because of a hypersensitivity reaction. Increased risk of transaminase elevations in patients with hepatitis B-C coinfection; monitor LFTs before and during therapy. Do not coadminister with carbamazepine, dofetilide, oxcarbazepine, phenobarbital, phenytoin, or St. John's wort. Do not use with etravirine unless coadministered with ritonavir-boosted atazanavir, darunavir, or lopinavir. Give Triumeq 2 h before or 6 h after cation-containing antacid/ laxative, sucralfate, oral calcium/ iron, buffered drugs. Triumeq can be given with PO calcium/iron if they are taken with a meal. May increase metformin exposure; do not exceed metformin 1000 mg/day.

MOA — Dolutegravir is an integrase strand transfer inhibitor. Abacavir and lamivudine are NRTIs. See components for further information.

ADVERSE EFFECTS — Serious: Potentially fatal hypersensitivity (abacavir, dolutegravir); lactic acidosis/hepatic steatosis (abacavir or lamivudine); severe acute HBV exacerbation after discontinuation in HIV/HBV coinfected patients (lamivudine). Frequent: Insomnia, headache, fatigue. See components for other adverse effects.

TRIZIVIR (**abacavir + lamivudine + zidovudine**) ▶LK ♀C ▶– $$$$$

WARNING — Abacavir: Life-threatening hypersensitivity. HLA-B*5701 predisposes to hypersensitivity; screen before starting abacavir and avoid if positive test. Never rechallenge with abacavir after suspected reaction. Abacavir and lamivudine: Lactic acidosis and hepatosteatosis. Lamivudine: Severe acute HBV exacerbation after discontinuation in HIV/HBV coinfected patients. Zidovudine: Bone marrow suppression, myopathy.

ADULT — HIV infection, alone (not a preferred regimen) or in combination with other agents: 1 tab PO two times per day.

PEDS — HIV infection in adolescents 40 kg or greater, alone (not a preferred regimen) or in combination with other agents: 1 tab PO two times per day.

FORMS — Generic/Trade: Tabs abacavir 300 mg + lamivudine 150 mg + zidovudine 300 mg.

NOTES — See components. Monitor CBC. Not for wt less than 40 kg, CrCl <50 mL/min, or if dosage adjustment required.

MOA — See components.

ADVERSE EFFECTS — Serious: Life-threatening hypersensitivity (abacavir); lactic acidosis/hepatosteatosis (abacavir, lamivudine); severe acute HBV exacerbation after discontinuation in HIV/HBV coinfected patients (lamivudine); bone marrow suppression, myopathy (zidovudine). See components for other adverse effects. Frequent: Hypersensitivity, N/V, fever/chills.

TRUVADA (**emtricitabine + tenofovir disoproxil fumarate**) ▶K ♀B ▶– $$$$$

WARNING — Emtricitabine and tenofovir: Potentially fatal lactic acidosis and hepatosteatosis; severe acute exacerbation of HBV after discontinuation in HIV-HBV coinfected patients. Confirm HIV-negative status (including acute HIV infection) before using Truvada for pre-exposure prophylaxis of HIV infection.

ADULT — Combination therapy for HIV infection: 1 tab 200/300 mg PO daily in combination with other antiretroviral drugs. Pre-exposure prophylaxis (PrEP) of HIV in adults at high risk for sexually acquired HIV: 1 tab 200/300 mg PO once daily. Screen for HIV q 3 months in PrEP patients.

PEDS — Combination therapy for HIV infection, wt 17 kg or greater: Give 1 tab PO once daily at a dose of 100/150 mg for wt 17 to less than 22 kg; 133/200 mg for 22 to less than 28 kg; 167/250 mg for 28 to less than 35 kg; 200/300 mg for wt 35 kg or greater.

UNAPPROVED ADULT — Antiviral-resistant chronic HBV in HIV-coinfected patients: 1 tab 200/300 mg PO daily. Pre-exposure prophylaxis (PrEP) of HIV in injection-drug users: 1 tab 200/300 mg PO once daily. Screen for HIV q 3 months in PrEP patients.

FORMS — Trade only (emtricitabine/tenofovir disoproxil fumarate): Tabs 200/300 mg, 167/250 mg, 133/200 mg, 100/150 mg.

(cont.)

TRUVADA (*cont.*)

NOTES — See components. Do not use in a triple nucleoside regimen. Monitor CrCl, urine glucose, urine protein, serum phosphorus before and during treatment in patients with or at risk for renal impairment. Not for HIV-infected patients with CrCl <30 mL/min or hemodialysis, hepatic dysfunction, or if dosage adjustment required. Increase dosing interval to q 48 h if CrCl 30 to 49 mL/min. Do not use for pre-exposure prophylaxis if CrCl <60 mL/min. Use with didanosine cautiously; reduce didanosine dose to 250 mg for adults over 60 kg, monitor for adverse effects and discontinue didanosine if they occur. Dosage adjustment of didanosine unclear if wt less than 60 kg. Give Videx EC + Truvada on empty stomach or with light meal. Give buffered didanosine + Truvada on empty stomach.

Atazanavir and lopinavir-ritonavir increase tenofovir disoproxil fumarate levels; monitor and discontinue Truvada if tenofovir adverse effects. Tenofovir disoproxil fumarate decreases atazanavir levels. If atazanavir is used with Truvada, use 300 mg atazanavir + 100 mg ritonavir. Do not use Truvada with lamivudine, adefovir, or unboosted atazanavir.

MOA — See components.

ADVERSE EFFECTS — Serious: Lactic acidosis/hepatic steatosis (emtricitabine and tenofovir); severe acute exacerbation of hepatitis B after discontinuing either drug in patients coinfected with HIV and hepatitis B. See components for other adverse effects. Frequent adverse effects with Truvada for PrEP: headache, abdominal pain, weight loss. Decrease in bone mineral density with Truvada used for PrEP.

ANTIMICROBIALS: Antiviral Agents—Anti-HIV—Fusion Inhibitors

ENFUVIRTIDE (*Fuzeon, T-20*) ▸Serum ♀B ▶– $$$$$

ADULT — Combination therapy for HIV infection: 90 mg SC two times per day. Rotate injection sites on upper arm, anterior thigh, or abdomen; avoid current injection site reactions.

PEDS — Combination therapy for HIV infection, 6 to 16 yo: 2 mg/kg (up to 90 mg) SC two times per day. Rotate injection sites on upper arm, anterior thigh, or abdomen; avoid current injection site reactions.

FORMS — 30-day kit with vials, diluent, syringes, alcohol wipes. Single-dose vial of 108 mg provides 90 mg enfuvirtide.

NOTES — Increased risk of bacterial pneumonia; monitor for signs and symptoms of pneumonia. Biojector 2000 can cause bruising/hematoma and persistent nerve pain if used near large nerves. Reconstitute with 1.1 mL sterile water for injection.

Allow vial to stand until powder dissolves completely (up to 45 min). Do not shake. Inject 1 mL (90 mg) and discard unused soln.

MOA — Peptide that binds with glycoprotein on HIV viral envelope; prevents fusion of virus with CD4+ cells.

ADVERSE EFFECTS — Serious: Increased risk of bacterial pneumonia, hypersensitivity (may include flu-like symptoms, hypotension, increased LFTs), immune reconstitution syndrome, peripheral neuropathy, pancreatitis. Frequent: Injection site reactions (including induration, cysts, nodules), eosinophilia. Biojector 2000 can cause bruising, hematoma, and persistent nerve pain if used near large nerves. Anticoagulants, hemophilia, or other coagulation disorder may increase risk of post-injection bleeding.

ANTIMICROBIALS: Antiviral Agents—Anti-HIV—Integrase Strand Transfer Inhibitor

DOLUTEGRAVIR (*Tivicay, DTG*) ▸glucuronidation ♀?/?/? R ▶– $$$$$

ADULT — Combination therapy for HIV, integrase strand inhibitor (INSTI)-naïve: 50 mg PO once daily; increase to 50 mg PO two times per day if coadministered with certain CYP3A4 or UGT1A inducers (carbamazepine, efavirenz, fosamprenavir-ritonavir, rifampin, tipranavir-ritonavir). INSTI-experienced with INSTI resistance substitutions or suspected INSTI resistance: 50 mg PO two times per day.

PEDS — Combination therapy for HIV, integrase strand inhibitor (INSTI)-naive: wt 30 kg or greater:35 mg PO once daily (25 mg tab + 10 mg tab) for wt 30 to less than 40 kg; 50 mg PO once daily for wt 40 kg or greater. Adjust dosing interval to two times per day for coadministration of certain CYP3A4 or UGT1A inducers (carbamazepine, efavirenz, fosamprenavir-ritonavir, rifampin, tipranavir-ritonavir).

FORMS — Trade only: Tabs 10, 25, 50 mg.

NOTES — Causes small increase in serum creatinine (mean increase of 0.14 mg/dL) without affecting GFR. Give dolutegravir 2 h before or 6 h after Al/Mg antacid/laxative, sucralfate, PO calcium/iron, buffered drugs. Dolutegravir can be given with PO calcium/iron if taken with a meal. May increase metformin exposure; do not exceed metformin 1000 mg/day. Do not give with etravirine unless coadministered with ritonavir-boosted atazanavir or darunavir, or lopinavir-ritonavir. Coadministration with dofetilide contraindicated. Do not coadminister with oxcarbazepine, phenytoin, phenobarbital, St. John's wort. Not recommended for severe hepatic impairment (Child-Pugh C). No dosage adjustment for renal impairment. Caution advised for INSTI-experienced patients with severe renal impairment due to reduced dolutegravir levels in severe renal impairment.

(cont.)

DOLUTEGRAVIR (*cont.*)

MOA — Prevents HIV propagation by inhibiting HIV-1 integrase, an enzyme required for viral insertion into host genome.

ADVERSE EFFECTS — Serious: Severe hypersensitivity reactions; increased transaminases, esp if coinfected with hepatitis B or C. Frequent: Insomnia, headache.

ELVITEGRAVIR (*Vitekta, EVG*) ▶L glucuronidation ♀B ▶– $$$$$

ADULT — Combination therapy for HIV infection: Give elvitegravir with ritonavir-boosted protease inhibitor regimens listed here and additional antiretroviral drug. Elvitegravir 85 mg + atazanavir-ritonavir 300/100 mg all PO once daily. Elvitegravir 85 mg PO once daily + lopinavir-ritonavir 400/100 mg PO two times per day. Elvitegravir 150 mg PO once daily + darunavir-ritonavir 600/100 mg PO two times per day. Elvitegravir 150 mg PO once daily + fosamprenavir-ritonavir 700/100 mg PO two times per day. Elvitegravir 150 mg PO once daily + tipranvir-ritonavir 500/200 mg PO two times per day. Take elvitegravir with food.

PEDS — Safety and efficacy not established in children.

FORMS — Trade only: Film-coated tabs 85, 150 mg.

NOTES — Do not coadminister with cobicistat, efavirenz, indinavir, nelfinavir, nevirapine, rifampin, rifapentine, saquinavir, Stribild, or St. John's wort. Consider alternatives to carbamazepine, dexamethasone, oxcarbazepine, phenobarbital, or phenytoin. Use an additional or alternative non-hormonal contraceptive. Give didanosine on empty stomach either 1 h before or 2 h after elvitegravir given with food. Separate elvitegravir and antacids by at least 2 h. Reduce rifabutin dose to 150 mg PO every other day or 3 times per week. Adjust bosentan dose. No dosage adjustment for renal impairment or mild to moderate (Child-Pugh Class A/B) hepatic impairment.

MOA — Inhibits HIV-1 integrase, an enzyme required for insertion of virus into host genome. Inhibition of integrase prevents viral propagation.

ADVERSE EFFECTS — Serious: Immune reconstitution syndrome. Frequent: Diarrhea.

RALTEGRAVIR (*Isentress, RAL*) ▶glucuronidation ♀C ▶– $$$$$

WARNING —

ADULT — Combination therapy for HIV infection: 400 mg PO two times per day. Increase to 800 mg PO two times per day if given with rifampin.

PEDS — Combination therapy for HIV infection, 4 weeks of age or older: Film-coated tabs, wt 25 kg or greater: 400 mg PO two times per day. Chew tabs, wt 11 kg or greater: Give PO two times per day at a dose of 75 mg for wt 11 to less than 14 kg; 100 mg for 14 to less than 20 kg; 150 mg for 20 to less than 28 kg; 200 mg for 28 to less than 40 kg; 300 mg for 40 kg or greater. Max dose of chew tabs is 300 mg two times per day. Oral susp, age 4 weeks or older and weight 3 kg to less than 20 kg: Give PO two times per day at a dose of 20 mg for 3 to less than 4 kg; 30 mg for 4 to less than 6 kg; 40 mg for 6 to less than 8 kg; 60 mg for 8 to less than 11 kg; 80 mg for 11 to less than 14 kg; 100 mg for 14 to less than 20 kg. Max dose of oral susp is 100 mg PO two times per day. Pour contents of susp packet into 5 mL of water and mix. Measure dose with syringe and give orally within 30 minutes of mixing. Discard any remaining susp. Wt-based dosing of chew tab and susp is ~6 kg/kg/dose two times per day. Do not substitute chew tabs or oral susp for 400 mg film-coated tabs.

FORMS — Trade only: Film-coated tabs 400 mg. Chewable tabs (contain phenylalanine): 25, 100 mg. Single-use packets of powder for oral susp: 100 mg/5 mL.

NOTES — Myopathy and rhabdomyolysis reported; caution advised if used with drugs that cause myopathy. Can cause severe skin and hypersensitivity reactions including Stevens-Johnson syndrome; stop if signs or symptoms occur. Do not give aluminum/magnesium antacids; use calcium carbonate instead. Do not split or crush 400 mg film-coated tabs.

MOA — Inhibits HIV-1 integrase, an enzyme required for insertion of virus into host genome. Inhibition of integrase prevents viral propagation.

ADVERSE EFFECTS — Serious: Myopathy and rhabdomyolysis (causality unclear). Severe skin and hypersensitivity reactions, including Stevens-Johnson syndrome, toxic epidermal necrolysis, and drug rash with eosinophilia and systemic symptoms (DRESS). Immune reconstitution syndrome. Frequent: Insomnia, headache, increased CPK.

ANTIMICROBIALS: Antiviral Agents—Anti-HIV—Non-Nucleoside Reverse Transcriptase Inhibitors

NOTE: Many serious drug interactions - always check before prescribing!

EFAVIRENZ (*Sustiva, EFV*) ▶L ♀ X/O/O. Risk of neural tube defects in 1st 8 weeks; may use later. R ▶– $$$$$

ADULT — Combination therapy for HIV infection: 600 mg PO once daily. Coadministration with voriconazole: Use voriconazole maintenance dose of 400 mg PO two times per day and reduce efavirenz to 300 mg (use caps) PO once daily. Take on empty stomach, preferably at bedtime.

PEDS — Consider antihistamine prophylaxis to prevent rash before starting. Combination therapy for HIV infection, age 3 mo or older and wt 3.5 kg or greater: Give PO once daily at a dose of 100 mg for 3.5 to less than 5 kg; 150 mg for 5 to less than 7.5 kg; 200 mg

(cont.)

EFAVIRENZ (*cont.*)

for 7.5 to less than 15 kg; 250 mg for 15 to less than 20 kg; 300 mg for 20 to less than 25 kg; 350 mg for 25 to less than 32.5 kg; 400 mg for 32.5 to less than 40 kg; 600 mg for wt 40 kg or greater. Take on empty stomach, preferably at bedtime. Capsule contents can be sprinkled on 1 to 2 teaspoons of food; do not give additional food for 2 h.

FORMS — Trade only: Caps 50, 200 mg. Tabs 600 mg.

NOTES — Psychiatric reactions including suicidiality, CNS symptoms (warn about hazardous tasks), rash (stop treatment if severe), increased cholesterol (monitor). False-positive with Microgenics cannabinoid screening test. Monitor LFTs if given with ritonavir, hepatotoxic drugs, or to patients with hepatitis B/C. Induces CYP3A4. Many drug interactions including decreased levels of anticonvulsants, artemether/lumefantrine (Coartem), atorvastatin, atovaquone/proguanil (Malarone), bupropion, diltiazem, itraconazole, methadone, posaconazole, pravastatin, simvastatin, and probably cyclosporine, ketoconazole, sirolimus, and tacrolimus. Do not give with ergot alkaloids, other NNRTIs, pimozide, simeprevir, St. John's wort, or triazolam. Do not give with atazanavir to treatment-experienced patients. Midazolam contraindicated in labeling; but can use single dose IV cautiously with monitoring for procedural sedation. If used with rifampin, product label recommends increasing efavirenz to 800 mg once daily at bedtime if wt 50 kg or greater; HIV guidelines recommend maintaining dose at 600 mg and monitoring virologic response. High risk of rash when taken with clarithromycin; consider alternative antimicrobial. Potentially teratogenic; get negative pregnancy test before use by women of childbearing potential and recommend barrier contraceptive until 12 weeks after efavirenz is stopped.

MOA — Inhibits HIV reverse transcriptase by different mechanism of action from NRTIs. Cross-resistance possible between efavirenz and nevirapine.

ADVERSE EFFECTS — Serious: Depression and other psychiatric reactions, convulsions, severe rash, Stevens-Johnson syndrome, lipoatrophy, hepatotoxicity (rare), immune reconstitution syndrome. Frequent: Rash (especially in children), CNS symptoms (dizziness, insomnia, vivid dreams, impaired concentration; warn about hazardous tasks).

ETRAVIRINE (*Intelence, ETR*) ▶L ♀B ▶– $$$$$

ADULT — Combination therapy for treatment-resistant HIV: 200 mg PO two times per day after meals.

PEDS — Combination therapy for treatment-resistant HIV, age 6 yo and older: Give PO two times per day after meals at a dose of 100 mg for wt 16 to less than 20 kg; 125 mg for wt 20 to less than 25 kg; 150 mg for wt 25 to less than 30 kg; 200 mg for wt 30 kg or greater.

FORMS — Trade only: Tabs 25, 100, 200 mg.

NOTES — Severe skin reactions, Stevens-Johnson syndrome, hypersensitivity. Induces CYP3A4 and inhibits CYP2C9 and 2C19; substrate of CYP2C9,

2C19, and 3A4. Do not give with unboosted atazanavir, carbamazepine, efavirenz, nevirapine, phenobarbital, phenytoin, rifampin, rifapentine, rilpivirine, ritonavir 600 mg two times per day; ritonavir-boosted tipranavir/fosamprenavir; St. John's wort. Give rifabutin 300 mg once daily with etravirine (without ritonavir-boosted protease inhibitor). Give with dolutegravir only if coadministered with atazanavir-ritonavir, darunavir-ritonavir, or lopinavir-ritonavir. Avoid rifabutin in patients receiving etravirine with a protease inhibitor. Monitor INR with warfarin. May need dosage reduction of fluvastatin or diazepam. Consider alternative to clarithromycin for Mycobacterium avium complex treatment or prevention. Consider monitoring antiarrhythmic blood levels. May reduce exposure to Coartem. Can disperse tabs in water and take immediately if swallowing difficulty. Do not disperse tabs in grapefruit juice, or warm or carbonated drinks.

MOA — Inhibits HIV reverse transcriptase by different mechanism of action from NRTIs.

ADVERSE EFFECTS — Serious: Severe rash (rare) including Stevens-Johnson syndrome, toxic epidermal necrolysis, and DRESS. Immune reconstitution syndrome. Frequent: Mild/moderate rash between weeks 2-4 of therapy; nausea.

NEVIRAPINE (*Viramune, Viramune XR, NVP*) ▶LK ♀C ▶– $$$$$

WARNING — Life-threatening skin reactions, hypersensitivity, and hepatotoxicity. Monitor clinical and lab status intensively during 1st 18 weeks of therapy (risk of rash and/or hepatotoxicity greatest during 1st 6 weeks of therapy) and frequently thereafter. Consider LFTs at baseline, before, and 2 weeks after dose increase, and at least once a month. Rapidly progressive liver failure can occur after only a few weeks of therapy. Stop nevirapine and never rechallenge if clinical hepatitis, severe rash, or rash with constitutional symptoms/increased LFTs. Obtain LFTs if rash occurs. Risk of hepatotoxicity with rash high in women or high CD4 count (women with CD4 count greater than 250 especially high risk, including pregnant women). Do not use if CD4 count greater than 250 in women or greater than 400 in men unless benefit clearly outweighs risk. Elevated LFTs or hepatitis B/C infection at baseline increases risk of hepatotoxicity. Hepatotoxicity not reported after single doses of nevirapine or in children.

ADULT — Combination therapy for HIV infection: 200 mg PO daily for 14 days, then 200 mg PO two times per day or Viramune XR 400 mg PO once daily. Patients maintained on immediate-release tabs can switch directly to Viramune XR. Dose titration reduces risk of rash. If rash develops, do not increase dose until it resolves. If stopped for more than 7 days, restart with initial dose.

PEDS — Combination therapy for HIV infection, age 15 days old or older: 150 mg/m^2 PO once daily for 14 days, then 150 mg/m^2 two times per day (max dose 200 mg two times per day). Dose titration reduces risk of rash. If rash develops, do not increase dose

(cont.)

NEVIRAPINE (*cont.*)

until it resolves. If stopped for more than 7 days, restart with initial dose. Per HIV guidelines, children 8 yo or younger may require up to 200 mg/m^2 PO two times per day (max dose 200 mg two times per day). Viramune XR, age 6 yo and older: 200 mg PO once daily for BSA 0.58 to 0.83 m^2; 300 mg PO once daily for BSA 0.84 to 1.16 m^2; 400 mg PO once daily for BSA 1 or greater. To reduce risk of rash, give immediate-release nevirapine 150 mg/m^2 once daily (max 200 mg/day) for at least 14 days before conversion to Viramune XR. Patients already taking twice-daily, immediate-release nevirapine can switch directly to Viramune XR.

UNAPPROVED ADULT — Combination therapy for HIV infection: 200 mg PO daily for 14 days, then 400 mg PO daily. Prevention of maternal-fetal HIV transmission, maternal dosing: 200 mg PO single dose at onset of labor. Do not add single-dose nevirapine to standard HIV regimens in pregnant women in the US.

UNAPPROVED PEDS — Prevention of maternal-fetal HIV transmission, neonatal dose: 2 mg/kg PO single dose within 3 days of birth.

FORMS — Generic/Trade: Tabs 200 mg. Susp 50 mg/5 mL (240 mL). Extended-release tabs 100, 400 mg.

NOTES — CYP3A4 inducer. May require increased methadone dose. Do not give with atazanavir, ketoconazole, hormonal contraceptives, or St. John's wort. Granulocytopenia more common in children receiving zidovudine and nevirapine. Contraindicated if Child-Pugh Class B/C liver failure. Give supplemental dose of 200 mg after dialysis session. Do not use for post-exposure prophylaxis in HIV-uninfected patients. Do not use in infants who have been exposed to nevirapine as part of maternal-infant prophylaxis. Do not chew, crush, or split Viramune XR tabs.

MOA — Inhibits HIV reverse transcriptase by different mechanism of action from NRTIs. Cross-resistance possible between efavirenz and nevirapine.

ADVERSE EFFECTS — Serious: Life-threatening rash (including Stevens-Johnson syndrome, toxic epidermal necrolysis, exfoliative dermatitis), hypersensitivity, hepatotoxicity. Risk of severe rash and/or hepatotoxicity (they can occur together) is greatest in first 6 weeks of therapy and is especially high in women with CD4 count greater than 250. Rhabdomyolysis can occur with skin reaction or hepatotoxicity. Granulocytopenia more common in children receiving zidovudine and nevirapine. Frequent: Increased LFTs, erythema, pruritus, maculopapular rash, dry desquamation.

RILPIVIRINE (*Edurant, RPV*) ▶L ♀B ▶– $$$$$

ADULT — Combination therapy of HIV infection, treatment-naive with HIV RNA less than or equal to 100,000 copies/mL: 25 mg PO once daily with a meal. Dosage adjustment for rifabutin: Rilpivirine 50 mg PO once daily with a meal.

PEDS — Combination therapy of HIV infection, treatment-naive with HIV RNA ≤100,000 copies/mL, age 12 yo or older and wt 35 kg or greater: 25 mg PO once daily with a meal. Dosage adjustment for rifabutin: Rilpivirine 50 mg PO once daily with a meal.

FORMS — Trade only: Tabs 25 mg.

NOTES — Rilpivirine has higher virologic failure rate than efavirenz in patients with baseline HIV RNA >100,000 copies/mL. Rilpivirine resistance rate is increased if baseline CD4+ count <200 cells/mm^3. Rilpivirine has higher overall treatment resistance, NNRTI cross-resistance, and tenofovir and lamivudine-emtricitabine resistance than efavirenz. Hepatotoxicity/increased LFTs: Monitor LFTs in patients with underlying liver disease or increased LFTs at baseline. Consider monitoring LFTs in all patients. Metabolized by CYP3A4. Contraindicated with carbamazepine, dexamethasone (more than single dose), oxcarbazepine, phenobarbital, phenytoin, proton pump inhibitors, rifampin, rifapentine, St. John's wort. Use cautiously with drugs that cause torsades; supratherapeutic doses of rilpivirine prolonged QT interval. Give antacids at least 2 h before or 4 h after rilpivirine. Give H2 blockers at least 12 h before or 4 h after rilpivirine. Monitor for reduced response to methadone. Store in original bottle to protect from light.

MOA — Inhibits HIV reverse transcriptase by different mechanism of action from NRTIs. Cross-resistance possible between rilpivirine and other NNRTIs.

ADVERSE EFFECTS — Serious: Depressive disorders (frequent), fat redistribution (causality unclear), immune reconstitution syndrome, hepatotoxicity (rare), increased LFTs.

ANTIMICROBIALS: Antiviral Agents—Anti-HIV—Nucleoside/Nucleotide Reverse Transcriptase Inhibitors

NOTE: Can cause lactic acidosis and hepatic steatosis.

ABACAVIR (*Ziagen, ABC*) ▶L ♀C ▶– $$$$$

WARNING — Potentially fatal hypersensitivity (look for fever, rash, GI symptoms, cough, dyspnea, pharyngitis, or other respiratory symptoms). Stop at once and never rechallenge after suspected reaction. Fatal reactions can recur within hours of rechallenge in patients with previously unrecognized reaction. HLA-B*5701 predisposes to hypersensitivity; screen before starting. Abacavir is contraindicated if positive test. Label HLA-B*5701-positive patients as abacavir-allergic in medical record.

ADULT — Combination therapy for HIV infection: 300 mg PO two times per day or 600 mg PO daily. Severe hypersensitivity may be more common with single daily dose.

(cont.)

ABACAVIR (cont.)

PEDS — Combination therapy for HIV infection. Oral soln, age 3 mo or older: 8 mg/kg (up to 300 mg) PO two times per day or 16 mg (up to 600 mg) PO once daily. Do not start therapy with once-daily dose of oral soln; can convert from twice- to once-daily dose of oral soln after 6 months with undetectable viral load and stable CD4 count. Tabs: 150 mg PO two times per day or 300 mg PO once daily for wt 14 to less than 20 kg; 150 mg PO q am and 300 mg PO q pm or 450 mg PO once daily for wt 20 to less than 25 kg; 300 mg PO two times per day or 600 mg PO once daily for wt 25 kg or greater.

FORMS — Generic/Trade: Tabs 300 mg scored. Trade only: Soln 20 mg/mL (240 mL).

NOTES — Unclear risk of MI; minimize modifiable CVD risk factors. Reduce dose for mild hepatic dysfunction (Child-Pugh score 5 to 6): 200 mg (10 mL of oral soln) PO two times per day. Contraindicated if moderate to severe hepatic impairment.

MOA — Reduces HIV replication within infected cells by inhibiting HIV reverse transcriptase.

ADVERSE EFFECTS — Serious: Life-threatening hypersensitivity, lactic acidosis/hepatic steatosis. bone marrow suppression. Unclear risk of MI. Frequent: GI complaints.

DIDANOSINE (*Videx, Videx EC, DDI*) ▶LK ♀B ▶– $$$$$

WARNING — Potentially fatal pancreatitis; avoid other drugs that can cause pancreatitis. Avoid didanosine + stavudine in pregnancy due to reports of fatal lactic acidosis with pancreatitis or hepatic steatosis.

ADULT — Combination therapy for HIV: Videx EC: 250 mg PO daily for wt less than 60 kg. 400 mg PO daily for wt 60 kg or greater. Take on empty stomach. If taken with tenofovir, reduce dose to 200 mg for wt less than 60 kg and 250 mg for 60 kg or greater. Dosage reduction unclear with tenofovir if CrCl <60 mL/min. Give tenofovir + Videx EC on empty stomach or with light meal.

PEDS — Combination therapy for HIV: 100 mg/m² PO two times per day for age 2 weeks to 8 mo (see alternative dose in UNAPPROVED PEDS for age 2 weeks to younger than 3 months). 120 mg/m² PO two times per day for age older than 8 mo (do not exceed adult dose). Videx EC: Give PO once daily 200 mg for wt 20 to 24 kg, 250 mg for wt 25 to 59 kg, 400 mg for wt 60 kg or greater. Take on an empty stomach.

UNAPPROVED PEDS — Combination therapy for HIV infection, 2 weeks to younger than 3 mo: 50 mg/m² PO two times per day. HIV guideline recommends this lower dose to reduce toxicity risk.

FORMS — Generic/Trade: Delayed-release caps (Videx EC): 125, 200, 250, 400 mg. Trade only: Pediatric powder for oral soln (buffered with antacid) 10 mg/mL.

NOTES — Not recommended as part of an initial HIV treatment regimen, primarily because of toxicity. Peripheral neuropathy (use cautiously with other neurotoxic drugs), retinal changes, optic neuritis, retinal depigmentation in children, hyperuricemia. Risk of lactic acidosis, pancreatitis, and peripheral neuropathy increased by stavudine. Diarrhea with buffered powder. See prescribing information for reduced dose if CrCl <60 mL/min. Do not use with allopurinol. Give some medications at least 1 h (indinavir), 2 h (atazanavir, ciprofloxacin, levofloxacin, ofloxacin, itraconazole, ketoconazole, ritonavir, dapsone, tetracyclines), or 4 h (moxifloxacin) before buffered didanosine. Contraindicated with ribavirin due to risk of didanosine toxicity. Methadone may reduce didanosine exposure, esp the buffered oral soln; use Videx EC with methadone and monitor for reduced didanosine efficacy.

MOA — Reduces HIV replication within infected cells by inhibiting HIV reverse transcriptase.

ADVERSE EFFECTS — Serious: Lactic acidosis/hepatic steatosis, symptomatic hyperlactatemia, fatal lactic acidosis with stavudine plus didanosine in pregnant women (avoid concomitant use), retinal toxicity, pancreatitis (frequent; risk increased by stavudine), peripheral neuropathy (frequent; risk increased by stavudine), non-cirrhotic portal hypertension (rare). Frequent: Fever, GI complaints, headache, rash.

EMTRICITABINE (*Emtriva, FTC*) ▶K ♀B ▶– $$$$$

WARNING — Severe acute HBV exacerbation after discontinuation in HIV/HBV coinfected patients. Monitor closely for at least 2 months; consider treating HBV.

ADULT — Combination therapy for HIV infection: 200 mg cap PO daily. Oral soln: 240 mg (24 mL) PO daily.

PEDS — Combination therapy for HIV: Give 3 mg/kg oral soln PO once daily for age birth to 3 mo; 6 mg/kg PO once daily (up to 240 mg) for age older than 3 mo. Give 200 mg cap PO once daily for wt greater than 33 kg.

FORMS — Trade only: Caps 200 mg. Oral soln 10 mg/mL (170 mL).

NOTES — Reduce dose in adults with renal dysfunction. Caps: Give 200 mg PO q 96 h if CrCl <15 mL/min or hemodialysis; 200 mg PO q 72 h if CrCl 15 to 29 mL/min; 200 mg PO q 48 h if CrCl 30 to 49 mL/min. Oral soln: 60 mg q 24 h if CrCl <15 mL/min or hemodialysis; 80 mg q 24 h if CrCl 15 to 29 mL/min; 120 mg q 24 h if CrCl 30 to 49 mL/min; refrigerate oral soln if possible; stable for 3 months at room temp.

MOA — Reduces HIV replication within infected cells by inhibiting HIV reverse transcriptase. Structurally related to lamivudine; cross-resistance documented. Has activity against HBV.

ADVERSE EFFECTS — Serious: Lactic acidosis/hepatic steatosis; severe acute HBV exacerbation after discontinuation in HIV/HBV coinfected patients.. Frequent: Headache, diarrhea, nausea, rash. Other: Hyperpigmentation on palms/soles primarily in non-Caucasians.

LAMIVUDINE (*Epivir, Epivir-HBV, 3TC, ✛Heptovir*) ▶K
♀+/+/+ R ▶– $$$$$
WARNING — Lower dose of lamivudine in Epivir-HBV can cause HIV resistance; test for HIV before prescribing Epivir-HBV. Can cause fatal lactic acidosis and hepatomegaly with steatosis; discontinue if signs of lactic acidosis or hepatotoxicity. Severe acute exacerbation of HBV can occur after discontinuation of lamivudine in HIV-HBV coinfected patients. Monitor closely for at least 2 months after discontinuing lamivudine in such patients; consider treating HBV.
ADULT — Epivir for combination therapy for HIV infection: 300 mg PO daily or 150 mg PO two times per day. Epivir-HBV for chronic hepatitis B: 100 mg PO daily. Use HIV dose for HIV-HBV coinfected patients.
PEDS — Epivir for HIV infection, 3 mo or older: 4 mg/kg (up to 150 mg) PO two times per day or 8 mg/kg (up to 300 mg) once daily. Epivir tabs (preferred for children with wt 14 kg or greater who can swallow tabs): 75 mg two times per day or 150 mg once daily for wt 14 to less than 20 kg; 75 mg q am and 150 mg q pm or 225 mg once daily for wt 20 to less than 25 kg; 150 mg two times per day or 300 mg once daily for 25 kg or greater. Generally avoid once-daily dosing of oral soln in infants and young children; soln may suppress HIV less than tabs due to lower absorption. Consider more frequent viral load monitoring with oral soln. Epivir-HBV for chronic hepatitis B: 3 mg/kg (up to 100 mg) PO daily for age 2 yo or older. Use HIV dose for HIV-HBV coinfected patients.
UNAPPROVED PEDS — Epivir for combination therapy for HIV infection. Infants, age younger than 30 days old: 2 mg/kg PO two times per day.
FORMS — Generic/Trade: Tabs 100, 150 (scored), 300 mg. Oral soln 10 mg/mL. Trade only (Epivir-HBV, Heptovir): Oral soln 5 mg/mL.
NOTES — Lamivudine-resistant HBV reported during lamivudine treatment of HIV in HIV-HBV coinfected patients. Epivir: Pancreatitis in children. Monitor for hepatic decompensation (potentially fatal), neutropenia, and anemia if also receiving interferon for hepatitis C. If hepatic decompensation occurs, consider discontinuing lamivudine, and reducing or discontinuing interferon and/or ribavirin. Do not coadminister with other drugs containing lamivudine or emtricitabine. Dosage adjustment of Epivir for renal failure in adults and adolescents with HIV: 150 mg PO once daily for 30 to 49 mL/min; 150 mg PO first dose, then 100 mg PO once daily for 15 to 29 mL/min; 150 mg first dose, then 50 mg once daily for 5 to 14 mL/min; 50 mg first dose, then 25 mg once daily for <5 mL/min. Dosage adjustment of Epivir-HBV for renal failure in adults and adolescents with chronic hepatitis B: 100 mg PO first dose, then 50 mg once daily for 30 to 49 mL/min; 100 mg PO first dose, then 25 mg PO once daily for 15 to 29 mL/min; 35 mg first dose, then 15 mg once daily for 5 to 14 mL/min; 35 mg first dose, then 10 mg once daily for <5 mL/min.

MOA — Nucleoside analog. Reduces HIV replication within infected cells by inhibiting HIV reverse transcriptase. Reduces hepatitis B replication by inhibiting HBV polymerase.
ADVERSE EFFECTS — Serious: Lactic acidosis/hepatic steatosis; exacerbation of hepatitis B after discontinuation of lamivudine; pancreatitis in children; hepatic decompensation in HCV/HIV coinfected patients. Frequent: Headache, fatigue, nausea, dizziness, nasal symptoms (well-tolerated compared with other NRTIs).

TENOFOVIR DISOPROXIL FUMARATE (*Viread, TDF*) ▶K
♀B ▶– $$$$$
WARNING — Stop tenofovir if hepatomegaly or steatosis occurs, even if LFTs normal. Severe acute exacerbation of hepatitis B can occur after discontinuation of tenofovir in patients coinfected with HIV and hepatitis B. Monitor closely for at least 2 months after discontinuing tenofovir in such patients; consider treating hepatitis B.
ADULT — Combination therapy for HIV; chronic hepatitis B: 300 mg PO daily without regard to food. For adults who cannot swallow tabs, use 7.5 scoops of oral powder once daily. High rate of virologic failure with tenofovir + didanosine + lamivudine for HIV infection; avoid this regimen.
PEDS — Combination therapy of HIV. Oral powder, 2 yo and older: 8 mg/kg PO once daily (max 300 mg/day). Dosing scoop for oral powder delivers 40 mg tenofovir per scoop. Mix powder with 2 to 4 ounces of soft food that doesn't need chewing (applesauce, baby food, yogurt). Use immediately after mixing. Do not mix powder with liquid. Tabs, 2 yo and older and wt 17 kg or greater: Give PO once daily at dose of 150 mg for wt 17 kg to less than 22 kg; 200 mg for wt 22 kg to less than 28 kg; 250 mg for wt 28 kg to less than 35 kg; 300 mg for wt 35 kg or greater. Chronic hepatitis B, age 12 yo and older and wt 35 kg or greater: 300 mg PO daily (7.5 scoops of oral powder for those who cannot swallow tabs) without regard to meals.
FORMS — Trade only: Tabs 150, 200, 250, 300 mg. Oral powder 40 mg tenofovir disoproxil fumarate/1 g scoop of powder, 60 g bottle.
NOTES — Decreased bone mineral density; consider bone mineral density monitoring if history of pathologic fracture or other risk factors for osteoporosis/bone loss. Consider calcium and vitamin D supplement. Tenofovir increases didanosine levels and possibly serious didanosine adverse effects (eg, pancreatitis, lactic acidosis, hyperlactatemia, neuropathy). If atazanavir is used with tenofovir, use 300 mg atazanavir + 100 mg ritonavir PO once daily. Atazanavir and lopinavir-ritonavir increase tenofovir levels; monitor and discontinue tenofovir if adverse effects. Ledipasvir-sofosbuvir increases tenofovir levels; monitor for toxicity; consider alternative HCV or HIV regimen in patients receiving an HIV protease inhibitor/cobicistat. Tenofovir can cause renal impairment including acute renal failure and Fanconi syndrome. Evaluate renal function

(cont.)

TENOFOVIR DISOPROXIL FUMARATE (*cont.*)

in patients who develop bone/extremity pain, fractures, muscle pain/weakness (signs of osteomalacia with proximal renal tubulopathy). Estimate CrCl before starting tenofovir. Avoid tenofovir if current/recent nephrotoxic drug use, including high-dose/multiple NSAIDs. Drugs that reduce renal function or undergo renal elimination (eg, acyclovir, adefovir, ganciclovir) may increase tenofovir levels; do not use with adefovir. Monitor CrCl, urine protein, urine glucose, serum phosphorus if mild renal impairment or at risk for renal impairment. Reduce dose for renal dysfunction: 300 mg once weekly (given after dialysis) for dialysis; 300 mg twice weekly if CrCl 10 to 29 mL/min; 300 mg q 48 h if CrCl 30 to 49 mL/min.

MOA — Nucleotide reverse transcriptase inhibitor. Similar mechanism of action as NRTIs, but does not require phosphorylation step required to activate NRTIs. Reduces HIV replication within infected cells by inhibiting HIV reverse transcriptase. Inhibits hepatitis B virus reverse transcriptase.

ADVERSE EFFECTS — Serious: Lactic acidosis/hepatic steatosis, renal impairment including acute renal failure and Fanconi syndrome, hypophosphatemia. Osteomalacia with proximal renal tubulopathy. Decreased bone mineral density in adults & children; fracture risk unknown. Immune reconstitution syndrome, including autoimmune disorders. Exacerbation of hepatitis B after discontinuation of tenofovir. Reports of syncope, usually with vagal syndrome. Frequent: GI complaints, dizziness.

ZIDOVUDINE (*Retrovir, AZT, ZDV*) ▶LK ♀C ▶– $$$$$
WARNING — Bone marrow suppression, myopathy.
ADULT — Combination therapy of HIV infection: 600 mg/day PO divided two or three times per day. IV dosing: 1 mg/kg IV administered over 1 h 5 to 6

times per day. Prevention of maternal-fetal HIV transmission, maternal dose (after 14 weeks of pregnancy): 600 mg/day PO divided two or three times per day until start of labor. During labor, 2 mg/kg (total body wt) IV over 1 h, then 1 mg/kg/h until delivery.

PEDS — Combination therapy of HIV infection, age 4 weeks or older: Give 24 mg/kg/day divided two or three times per day for wt 4 to 8 kg; give 18 mg/kg/day divided two or three times per day for wt 9 kg to 29 kg; give 600 mg/day divided two or three times per day for wt 30 kg or greater. Alternative dose: 480 mg/m²/day PO divided two or three times per day. Prevention of maternal-fetal HIV transmission, infant dose: 2 mg/kg PO q 6 h from within 12 h of birth until 6 weeks old. Can also give infants 1.5 mg/kg IV over 30 min q 6 h.

FORMS — Generic/Trade: Caps 100 mg. Syrup 50 mg/5 mL (240 mL). Generic only: Tabs 300 mg.

NOTES — Not recommended as part of an initial HIV treatment regimen, primarily because of toxicity. Hematologic toxicity; monitor CBC. Increased bone marrow suppression with ganciclovir or valganciclovir. Granulocytopenia more common in children receiving zidovudine and nevirapine. See prescribing information for dosage adjustments for renal dysfunction or hematologic toxicity.

MOA — Decreases or inhibits HIV replication within infected cells by inhibiting HIV reverse transcriptase.

ADVERSE EFFECTS — Serious: Lactic acidosis/hepatic steatosis, lipoatrophy (possibly), hematologic toxicity, symptomatic myopathy, hepatic decompensation in HCV/HIV coinfected patients. Granulocytopenia more common in children receiving zidovudine and nevirapine. Frequent: GI intolerance, headache, insomnia, asthenia, anorexia.

ANTIMICROBIALS: Antiviral Agents—Anti-HIV—Protease Inhibitors and Boosters

NOTE: Many serious drug interactions: Always check before prescribing. Protease inhibitors and cobicistat inhibit CYP3A4. Contraindicated with alfuzosin, dronedarone, ergot alkaloids, lovastatin, pimozide, rifampin, rifapentine, salmeterol, high-dose sildenafil for pulmonary hypertension, simeprevir, simvastatin, St. John's wort, triazolam. Midazolam contraindicated in labeling; but can use single dose IV cautiously with monitoring for procedural sedation. Monitor INR with warfarin. Avoid inhaled/nasal budesonide/fluticasone with ritonavir/cobicistat if possible; increased corticosteroid levels can cause Cushing's syndrome/ adrenal suppression. Other protease inhibitors may increase budesonide/ fluticasone levels; find alternatives for long-term use. Reduce colchicine dose; do not coadminister colchicine and protease inhibitors in patients with renal or hepatic dysfunction. Adjust dose of bosentan or tadalafil for pulmonary hypertension. Reduce quetiapine dose to 1/6 of original dose if protease inhibitor or cobicistat is added; use lowest initial quetiapine dose if it is added to protease inhibitor or cobicistat. Erectile dysfunction: Single dose of sildenafil 25 mg q 48 h, tadalafil 5 mg (not more than 10 mg) q 72 h, or vardenafil initially 2.5 mg q 72 h. Protease inhibitor class adverse effects include spontaneous bleeding in hemophiliacs, hyperglycemia, hyperlipidemia, immune reconstitution syndrome, and fat redistribution. Coinfection with hepatitis C or other liver disease increases the risk of hepatotoxicity with protease inhibitors; monitor LFTs at least twice in 1st month of therapy, then q 3 months.

ATAZANAVIR (*Reyataz, ATV*) ▶L ♀O/O/O/R Ritonavir-boosted atazanavir is a preferred protease inhibitor in ARV-naive pregnant women; maternal hyperbilirubinemia. ▶– $$$$$

ADULT — Combination therapy for HIV. Therapy-naive patients: Atazanavir 300 mg + ritonavir 100 mg PO both once daily. With efavirenz, therapy-naive: 400 mg + ritonavir 100 mg once daily. Therapy-experienced: 300 mg + ritonavir 100 mg both

(cont.)

ATAZANAVIR (cont.)

once daily. Do not give atazanavir with efavirenz in therapy-experienced patients. Pregnancy or post-partum: Usual dose is 300 mg + 100 mg ritonavir PO once daily; do not use unboosted atazanavir. If given with tenofovir or an H2 blocker in treatment-experienced patients in 2nd or 3rd trimester, give atazanavir 400 mg + ritonavir 100 mg PO once daily. Atazanavir exposure can increase during the 1st 2 months postpartum; monitor for adverse effects. Give atazanavir with food; give 2 h before or 1 h after buffered didanosine.

PEDS — Combination therapy for HIV. Oral powder, age 3 mo or older and wt 5 kg to less than 25 kg: 200 mg atazanavir power (4 packets) with 80 mg ritonavir oral soln PO once daily for wt 5 kg to less than 15 kg; 250 mg atazanavir powder (5 packets) with 80 mg ritonavir oral soln PO once daily for wt 15 to less than 25 kg. Mix power with food or beverage and give ritonavir immediately after. Oral capsules, age 6 yo and older: Give atazanavir-ritonavir PO once daily 150/100 mg for wt 15 to less than 20 kg; 200/100 mg for wt 20 kg to less than 40 kg; 300/100 mg for wt 40 kg or greater. Give atazanavir with food. Do not give to infants younger than 3 mo due to risk of kernicterus.

FORMS — Trade only: Caps 150, 200, 300 mg. Powder packets (contain phenylalanine) 50 mg.

NOTES — Does not appear to increase cholesterol or triglycerides. Asymptomatic increases in indirect bilirubin due to inhibition of UDP-glucuronosyl transferase (UGT); may cause jaundice/scleral icterus. May cause nephrolithiasis/cholelithiasis. Do not use with indinavir; both may increase bilirubin. Do not use with nevirapine. May inhibit irinotecan metabolism. Can prolong PR interval and rare cases of 2nd degree AV block reported; caution advised for patients with AV block or on drugs that prolong PR interval, especially if metabolized by CYP3A4. Monitor ECG with calcium channel blockers; consider reducing diltiazem dose by 50%. Reduce clarithromycin dose by 50%; consider alternative therapy for indications other than Mycobacterium avium complex. Acid required for absorption; acid-suppressing drugs can cause treatment failure. Proton pump inhibitors: In treatment-naive patients do not exceed dose equivalent of omeprazole 20 mg; give PPI 12 h before atazanavir 300 mg + ritonavir 100 mg. Do not use PPIs in treatment-experienced patients. H2 blockers: Give atazanavir 300 mg + ritonavir 100 mg simultaneously with H2 blocker and/or at least 10 h after H2 blocker, with max dose equivalent of famotidine 40 mg two times per day for treatment-naive patients and 20 mg two times per day for treatment-experienced patients. For treatment-experienced patients receiving tenofovir and H2 blocker, give atazanavir 400 mg + ritonavir 100 mg once daily with food. For treatment-experienced pregnant women in 2nd or 3rd trimester receiving tenofovir or H2 blocker, give atazanavir 400 mg + ritonavir 100 mg once

daily. Give atazanavir 2 h before or 1 h after antacids or buffered didanosine. Give atazanavir and delayed-release didanosine at different times. Inhibits CYP1A2, 2C9, and 3A4. Monitor for sedation if buprenorphine given with atazanavir-ritonavir. Use lowest possible dose of rosuvastatin (limit to 10 mg/day) or atorvastatin. Monitor levels of immunosuppressants, TCAs. May need dosage adjustment of carbamazepine, lamotrigine, phenobarbital, or phenytoin with ritonavir-boosted atazanavir. Do not give voriconazole with ritonavir-boosted atazanavir unless necessary; monitor for voriconazole adverse effects and reduced response to voriconazole and ritonavir-boosted atazanavir. Use oral contraceptive with at least 35 mcg ethinyl estradiol with ritonavir-boosted atazanavir. Refer to product labeling for unboosted atazanavir drug interactions. In mild to moderate hepatic impairment (Child-Pugh class B), consider dosage reduction to 300 mg PO daily with food. Do not use in Child-Pugh Class C. Dosage adjustment for hemodialysis: Atazanavir 300 mg + ritonavir 100 mg if treatment-naive; do not use atazanavir during hemodialysis if treatment-experienced.

MOA — Prevents cleavage of protein precursors required for HIV maturation, reproduction, and infection of new cells.

ADVERSE EFFECTS — Serious: Can prolong PR interval; second degree AV block reported rarely; serious skin reactions like Stevens-Johnson syndrome and DRESS; nephrolithiasis, cholelithiasis. Frequent: Increased indirect bilirubin, jaundice/scleral icterus, nausea, rash. Class effects: Hyperglycemia, fat redistribution, spontaneous bleeding in hemophiliacs.

COBICISTAT (Tybost, COBI) ▶L ♀B ▶– $$$$$

ADULT — Combination therapy for HIV: Cobicistat 150 mg + atazanavir 300 mg both PO once daily OR cobicistat 150 mg + darunavir 800 mg both PO once daily. Take cobicistat with food at the same time as atazanavir or darunavir. Dosage adjustment of cobicistat-atazanavir for efavirenz, treatment-naive patients: Cobicistat 150 mg + atazanavir 400 mg both PO once daily with food + efavirenz 600 mg PO once daily on an empty stomach, preferably at bedtime. Do not coadminister cobicistat-atazanavir with efavirenz in treatment-experienced patients.

PEDS — Safety and efficacy not established in children.

FORMS — Trade only: Film-coated tabs 150 mg.

NOTES — Cobicistat decreases CrCl (10 to 12 mL/min for GFR >50 mL/min), but does not affect GFR. Obtain baseline estimated CrCl; monitor renal function if serum creatinine increase is >0.4 mg/dL. Only coadminister with tenofovir if baseline CrCl ≥70 mL/min; obtain baseline urine glucose and protein. Many drug interactions due to cobicistat inhibition of CYP3A4 (strong), CYP2D6, P-glycoprotein, BCRP, and OATP transporters. Refer to CYP isozyme and P-glycoprotein tables. Not interchangeable with ritonavir; do not assume drug interactions are the same. Do not coadminister cobicistat with 2 HIV

(cont.)

COBICISTAT (*cont.*)

protease inhibitors or a protease inhibitor + elvitegravir. Do not coadminister with alfuzosin, avanafil, colchicine in renal/hepatic impairment, carbamazepine, dronedarone, ergot alkaloids, etravirine, fosamprenavir, lopinavir-ritonavir, lovastatin, lurasidone, PO midazolam, phenobarbital, phenytoin, pimozide, ranolazine, rifampin, ritonavir, rivaroxaban, salmeterol, saquinavir, high-dose sildenafil for pulmonary arterial hypertension, simeprevir, simvastatin, Stribild, St. John's wort, tipranavir, or triazolam. Do not coadminister cobicistat-atazanavir with efavirenz (in treatment-experienced patients), indinavir, irinotecan, or nevirapine. Do not coadminister cobicistat-darunavir with efavirenz or nevirapine. Consider alternatives to inhaled/intranasal budesonide/fluticasone, clarithromycin, dexamethasone, erythromycin, oxcarbazepine, telithromycin, or voriconazole (unless benefit justifies risk). Reduce maraviroc dose to 150 mg PO two times per day. Reduce rifabutin dose to 150 mg PO every other day and monitor for neutropenia and uveitis. See colchicine drug interaction table for colchicine dosage reduction. For erectile dysfunction, do not exceed sildenafil 25 mg PO once in 48 h, vardenafil 2.5 mg PO once in 72 h, or tadalafil 10 mg PO once in 72 h. For hormonal contraceptives, consider additional or alternative nonhormonal method. Cobicistat-atazanavir interactions with acid-suppressing drugs: Separate doses of cobicistat-atazanavir from antacids by ≥2 h. Give either simultaneously or ≥10 h after an H2 blocker; do not exceed H2 blocker dose equivalent to famotidine 40 mg two times per day for treatment-naïve, or 20 mg two times per day for treatment-experienced patients. For coadministration of H2 blocker and tenofovir, give cobicistat 150 mg + atazanavir 400 mg both PO once daily. For treatment-naïve patients, give cobicistat-atazanavir at least 12 h after a proton pump inhibitor at a max dose equivalent to omeprazole 20 mg/day; do not coadminister with a proton pump inhibitor in treatment-experienced patients. Dosage adjustment of cobicistat not required for renal impairment or mild to moderate hepatic impairment.

MOA — Strong CYP3A4 inhibitor (mechanism-based) intended to increase exposure to HIV protease inhibitors. Also inhibits renal tubular secretion of creatinine. Cobicistat does not have antiviral activity.

ADVERSE EFFECTS — Serious: Cases of acute renal failure and Fanconi syndrome reported with coadministration of cobicistat and tenofovir. Nephrolithiasis with cobicistat-atazanavir. Frequent: Jaundice, ocular icterus, nausea, rash; increased billirubin, serum amylase, LFTs, urine glucose.

DARUNAVIR (*Prezista, DRV*) ▶L ♀O/O/O. Darunavir-ritonavir is a preferred protease inhibitor regimen for ARV-naive pregnant women. R. ▶– $$$$$

ADULT — Combination therapy for HIV infection. Therapy-naive or experienced with no darunavir resistance substitutions: 800 mg + ritonavir 100 mg PO once daily. Therapy-experienced with at least 1 darunavir resistance substitution: 600 mg + ritonavir 100 mg PO two times per day. Dose in pregnancy: 600 mg + ritonavir 100 mg PO two times per day; may continue 800 mg + ritonavir 100 mg once daily if virologically suppressed and unlikely to tolerate/comply with twice daily dose. NOTE: HIV treatment guideline recommends twice-daily regimen for all pregnant women. Take with food.

PEDS — Combination therapy for HIV infection, age 3 yo or older: Give darunavir PO with food. Treatment-naïve or treatment-experienced without resistance substitutions: Give darunavir + ritonavir both once daily according to wt: Darunavir 35 mg/kg + ritonavir 7 mg/kg for wt 10 to less than 15 kg; darunavir 600 mg + ritonavir 100 mg for wt 15 to less than 30 kg; darunavir 675 mg + ritonavir 100 mg for wt 30 to less than 40 kg; darunavir 800 mg + ritonavir 100 mg for wt 40 kg or greater. Treatment-experienced with at least 1 resistance substitution: Give darunavir + ritonavir both two times per day according to wt: Darunavir 20 mg/kg + ritonavir 7 mg/kg for wt 10 to less than 15 kg; darunavir 375 mg + ritonavir 48 mg for wt 15 to less than 30 kg; darunavir 450 mg + ritonavir 60 mg for wt 30 to less than 40 kg; darunavir 600 mg + ritonavir 100 mg for wt 40 kg or greater.

UNAPPROVED PEDS — Do not give darunavir-ritonavir to children younger than 3 yo; animal studies suggest toxicity in this age group.

FORMS — Trade only: Tabs 75, 150, 600, 800 mg. Susp 100 mg/mL (200 mL).

NOTES — Severe skin reactions, including Stevens-Johnson syndrome. Cross-sensitivity with sulfonamides possible; use caution in sulfonamide-allergic patients. Hepatotoxicity; monitor AST/ALT more frequently (especially during 1st few months of therapy) if patient already has liver dysfunction. Do not give with dronedarone, lopinavir-ritonavir, ranolazine, or saquinavir. Reduce dose of clarithromycin if CrCl <60 mL/min (see clarithromycin entry for details). Do not use with more than 200 mg/day of ketoconazole or itraconazole. Ritonavir decreases voriconazole levels; do not use voriconazole with darunavir-ritonavir unless benefit exceeds risk. May decrease oral contraceptive efficacy; consider additional or alternative method. Give didanosine 1 h before or 2 h after darunavir-ritonavir. Use lowest possible dose of atorvastatin (not more than 20 mg/day), pravastatin, or rosuvastatin.

MOA — Prevents cleavage of protein precursors required for HIV maturation, reproduction, and infection of new cells.

ADVERSE EFFECTS — Severe: Stevens-Johnson syndrome and other severe skin reactions. Hepatotoxicity (esp if hepatitis B/C or baseline elevated transaminases). Frequent: Rash, diarrhea, nausea, headache, nasopharyngitis. Class effects: Hyperglycemia, fat redistribution, lipid abnormalities, spontaneous bleeding in hemophiliacs.

EVOTAZ (atazanavir + cobicistat) ▶L ♀B ▶– $$$$$
ADULT — Combination therapy of HIV: 1 tab PO once daily with food.
PEDS — Safety and efficacy not established in children.
UNAPPROVED ADULT — Coadministration of efavirenz in treatment-naive patients: atazanavir 400 mg + cobicistat 150 mg PO once daily (add atazanavir 100 mg to Evotaz tab). Do not coadminister efavirenz and Evotaz in treatment-experienced patients.
FORMS — Trade only: Tabs atazanavir 300 mg + cobicistat 150 mg.
NOTES — See components. Do not coadminister efavirenz (in treatment-experienced patients), elvitegravir, etravirine, nevirapine, HIV protease inhibitors. See cobicistat and atazanavir entries for more contraindicated drugs and dosage adjustments for drug interactions. Obtain CrCl at baseline; do not use with tenofovir if CrCl <70 mL/min. Not recommended if hepatic impairment, or ESRD with hemodialysis.
MOA — Atazanavir prevents cleavage of protein precursors required for HIV maturation, reproduction, and infection of new cells. Cobicistat is a strong CYP3A4 inhibitor intended to increase HIV protease inhibitor exposure.
ADVERSE EFFECTS — See components for serious events. Frequent: Jaundice, ocular icterus, nausea. Protease inhibitor class effects: Hyperglycemia, fat redistribution, lipid abnormalities, spontaneous bleeding in hemophiliacs.

FOSAMPRENAVIR (*Lexiva, FPV, ✦Telzir*) ▶L ♀C ▶– $$$$$
ADULT — Combination therapy for HIV. Therapy-naive patients (not guideline recommended): Fosamprenavir 1400 mg PO two times per day (without ritonavir) OR fosamprenavir 1400 mg PO once daily + ritonavir 100 to 200 mg PO once daily OR fosamprenavir 700 mg PO + ritonavir 100 mg PO both two times per day. Protease inhibitor-experienced patients: 700 mg fosamprenavir + 100 mg ritonavir PO both two times per day. Do not use once-daily regimen. If once-daily ritonavir-boosted regimen given with efavirenz, increase ritonavir to 300 mg/day; no increase of ritonavir dose needed for two times per day regimen with efavirenz. Give nevirapine with fosamprenavir only if two times per day ritonavir-boosted regimen used. No meal restrictions for tabs; take susp with food. Re-dose if vomiting occurs within 30 min of giving oral susp.
PEDS — Combination therapy for HIV. Fosamprenavir/ritonavir for protease inhibitor-naïve patients 4 weeks or older (guideline recommends against use in treatment-naive children or infants younger than 6 mo), or protease inhibitor–experienced patients, 6 mo or older: Give PO two times per day according to wt: Fosamprenavir 45 mg/kg plus ritonavir 7 mg/kg for wt less than 11 kg; fosamprenavir 30 mg/kg plus ritonavir 3 mg/kg for wt 11 to less than 15 kg; fosamprenavir 23 mg/kg plus ritonavir 3 mg/kg for

wt 15 to less than 20 kg; fosamprenavir 18 mg/kg plus ritonavir 3 mg/kg for wt 20 kg or greater. Do not exceed adult dose of fosamprenavir 700 mg plus ritonavir 100 mg both PO two times per day. For fosamprenavir-ritonavir, can use fosamprenavir tabs if wt 39 kg or greater and ritonavir caps if wt 33 kg or greater. Unboosted fosamprenavir for protease inhibitor–naïve patients, 2 yo and older (not guideline recommended): 30 mg/kg PO two times per day; can give 1400 mg as tabs PO two times per day if wt 47 kg or greater. Fosamprenavir is only for infants born at 38 weeks' gestation or more who have attained postnatal age of 28 days. Do not use once-daily dosing of fosamprenavir in children. Take tabs without regard to meals. Take susp with food. Re-dose if vomiting occurs within 30 min of giving oral susp.
FORMS — Trade only: Tabs 700 mg. Susp 50 mg/mL.
NOTES — Life-threatening skin reactions. Cross-sensitivity with sulfonamides possible; use caution in sulfonamide-allergic patients. Increased cholesterol and triglycerides; monitor lipids. Do not give maraviroc with unboosted fosamprenavir. Use lowest possible dose of atorvastatin (not more than 20 mg/day). Monitor CBC at least weekly if taking rifabutin. Monitor levels of immunosuppressants, TCAs. May need to increase dose of methadone. Can give unboosted fosamprenavir 1400 mg PO once daily with Viekira Pak. Do not use more than 200 mg/day ketoconazole/itraconazole with fosamprenavir + ritonavir; may need to reduce antifungal dose if patient is receiving more than 400 mg/day itraconazole or ketoconazole with unboosted fosamprenavir. Do not use more than 2.5 mg vardenafil q 24 h with unboosted fosamprenavir or q 72 h for fosamprenavir + ritonavir. Do not use hormonal contraceptives. More adverse reactions when fosamprenavir is given with Kaletra; appropriate dose for combination therapy unclear. Mild hepatic dysfunction (Child-Pugh score 5 to 6): 700 mg PO two times per day unboosted (for treatment-naive) or 700 mg PO two times per day plus ritonavir 100 mg PO once daily (for treatment-naive or -experienced). Moderate hepatic dysfunction (Child-Pugh score 7 to 9): 700 mg PO two times per day unboosted (for treatment-naive) or 450 mg PO two times per day plus ritonavir 100 mg PO once daily (for treatment-naive or -experienced). Severe hepatic dysfunction: Fosamprenavir 350 mg PO two times per day unboosted (for treatment-naive) or 300 mg PO two times per day plus ritonavir 100 mg PO once daily (for treatment-naive or -experienced). No dosage adjustments available for peds patients with hepatic dysfunction. Refrigeration not required, but may improve taste of oral susp.
MOA — Prodrug of amprenavir. Prevents cleavage of protein precursors required for HIV maturation, reproduction, and infection of new cells.
ADVERSE EFFECTS — Severe: Life-threatening rash possible. Nephrolithiasis. Frequent: Diarrhea, N/V, headache, rash, pruritus, fatigue. GI intolerance

(cont.)

FOSAMPRENAVIR (*cont.*)

more frequent with once-daily dosing. Class effects: Hyperglycemia, fat redistribution, lipid abnormalities, spontaneous bleeding in hemophiliacs.

INDINAVIR (*Crixivan, IDV*) ▶LK ♀C ▶– $$$$$

ADULT — Combination therapy for HIV infection: 800 mg PO q 8 h between meals with water (at least 48 ounces/day).

PEDS — Not approved in children. Do not use in infants; may cause kernicterus.

UNAPPROVED ADULT — Combination therapy for HIV infection: Indinavir 800 mg PO with ritonavir 100 to 200 mg PO both two times per day; or indinavir 400 mg with ritonavir 400 mg both two times per day; or indinavir 600 mg PO with Kaletra 400/100 mg PO both two times per day. Can be given without regard to meals when given with ritonavir.

UNAPPROVED PEDS — Combination therapy for HIV infection: 350 to 500 mg/m²/dose (max of 800 mg/dose) PO q 8 h for children; 800 mg PO q 8 h between meals with water (at least 48 ounces/day) for adolescents.

FORMS — Trade only: Caps 200, 400 mg.

NOTES — Nephrolithiasis (especially in children), hemolytic anemia, indirect hyperbilirubinemia, possible hepatitis, interstitial nephritis with asymptomatic pyuria. Do not use with atazanavir; both may increase bilirubin. Do not give rivaroxaban with ritonavir-boosted indinavir. Avoid using with carbamazepine if possible. Give indinavir and buffered didanosine 1 h apart on empty stomach. Reduce indinavir dose to 600 mg PO q 8 h when given with ketoconazole or itraconazole 200 mg two times per day. Increase indinavir dose to 1000 mg PO q 8 h when given with efavirenz or nevirapine. Use lowest possible dose of atorvastatin or rosuvastatin. For mild to moderate hepatic cirrhosis, give 600 mg PO q 8 h. Indinavir not recommended in pregnancy because of dramatic reduction in blood levels.

MOA — Prevents cleavage of protein precursors required for HIV maturation, reproduction, and infection of new cells.

ADVERSE EFFECTS — Serious: Nephrolithiasis, hematuria, and sterile leukocyturia (most frequent in children), interstitial nephritis with asymptomatic pyuria, hemolytic anemia. Frequent: GI complaints, headache, asthenia, blurred vision, dizziness, rash, metallic taste, indirect hyperbilirubinemia. Class effects: Hyperglycemia, fat redistribution, lipid abnormalities, spontaneous bleeding in hemophiliacs.

KALETRALPV/R (*lopinavir + ritonavir*) ▶L ♀C ▶– $$$$$

ADULT — Combination therapy for HIV infection: 400/100 mg PO two times per day (tabs or oral soln). Can use 800/200 mg PO once daily in patients with less than 3 lopinavir resistance–associated substitutions. Dosage adjustment for coadministration with efavirenz, nevirapine, fosamprenavir, or nelfinavir: 500/125 mg tabs (use two 200/50 mg + one 100/25 mg tab) or 533/133 mg oral soln (6.5 mL) PO two times per day. No once-daily dosing for

pregnant patients; coadministration with carbamazepine, phenobarbital, phenytoin, efavirenz, nevirapine, fosamprenavir, or nelfinavir; or in patients with 3 or more lopinavir resistance-associated substitutions (L10F/I/R/V, K20M/N/R, L24I, L33F, M36I, I47V, G48V, I54L/T/V, V82A/C/F/S/T, and I84V). See Adult Unapproved for dosage adjustment in 2nd and 3rd trimesters of pregnancy. Give tabs without regard to meals; give oral soln with food.

PEDS — Combination therapy for HIV infection, age 14 days to 6 mo: Lopinavir 300 mg/m² or 16 mg/kg PO two times per day. Propylene glycol in oral soln can cause life-threatening toxicity in infants (especially preterm); do not give oral soln to neonates before postmenstrual age of 42 weeks and postnatal age of at least 14 days. Age 6 mo to 12 yo: Lopinavir 230 mg/m² or 12 mg/kg PO two times per day if wt less than 15 kg; 10 mg/kg PO two times per day if wt 15 to 40 kg. Dosage adjustment for coadministration with efavirenz, nevirapine, fosamprenavir, or nelfinavir: Lopinavir 300 mg/m² PO two times per day or 13 mg/kg PO two times per day for wt less than 15 kg; 11 mg/kg PO two times per day for wt 15 to 45 kg. Do not exceed adult dose. Give tabs without regard to meals; give oral soln with food. Beware of medication errors with oral soln; fatal overdose reported in infant given excessive volume of soln.

UNAPPROVED ADULT — Combination therapy for HIV infection, 2nd and 3rd trimesters of pregnancy: Some experts recommend lopinavir-ritonavir 600 mg-150 mg PO two times per day, esp if protease inhibitor-experienced or baseline viral load >50 copies/mL. Consider monitoring virologic response and lopinavir levels (if available) if dose is not increased in 2nd and 3rd trimester of pregnancy.

FORMS — Trade only (lopinavir-ritonavir): Tabs 200/50 mg, 100/25 mg. Oral soln 80/20 mg/mL (160 mL).

NOTES — Do not confuse Keppra (levetiracetam) with Kaletra. May cause pancreatitis. Ritonavir included in formulation to inhibit metabolism and boost levels of lopinavir. Do not give with rivaroxaban or simeprevir. Increases tenofovir levels; monitor for adverse reactions. Many other drug interactions including decreased efficacy of oral contraceptives. Limit rosuvastatin dose to 10 mg/day; use lowest possible dose of atorvastatin. Ritonavir decreases voriconazole levels; do not give with voriconazole unless benefit exceeds risk. Expected to increase fentanyl exposure. May require higher methadone dose. Reduce dose of clarithromycin if CrCl <60 mL/min (see clarithromycin entry for details). Give buffered didanosine 1 h before or 2 h after Kaletra oral soln. Kaletra tabs can be given at same time as didanosine without food. Do not give Kaletra with tipranavir 500 mg + ritonavir 200 mg both two times per day. Monitor lamotrigine and valproic acid levels. Do not give Kaletra once daily with phenytoin, phenobarbital, or carbamazepine; monitor for reduced phenytoin levels. Oral soln contains

(cont.)

KALETRALPV *(cont.)*

alcohol. Use oral soln within 2 months if stored at room temperature. Tabs do not require refrigeration. Do not crush, cut, or chew tabs.

MOA — Prevents cleavage of protein precursors required for HIV maturation, reproduction, and infection of new cells.

ADVERSE EFFECTS — Serious: Hepatitis, pancreatitis. Increased risk of MI possible with cumulative use of Kaletra. PR and QT interval prolongation reported; caution advised for patients at risk of cardiac conduction abnormalities or coadministration of other drugs that prolong PR or QT interval. Propylene glycol in oral soln can cause life-threatening toxicity in infants (especially preterm). Frequent: GI complaints (more common with once daily regimen), transaminase elevation. Class effects: Hyperglycemia, fat redistribution, lipid abnormalities, spontaneous bleeding in hemophiliacs.

NELFINAVIR *(Viracept, NFV)* ▶L ♀B ▶– $$$$$

ADULT — Combination therapy for HIV infection: 750 mg PO three times per day or 1250 mg PO two times per day with meals. Absorption improved when meal contains at least 500 calories with 11 to 28 g of fat.

PEDS — Combination therapy for HIV infection: 45 to 55 mg/kg PO two times per day or 25 to 35 mg/kg PO three times per day (up to 2500 mg/day) for age 2 yo or older. Take with meals. Absorption improved when meal contains at least 500 calories with 11 to 28 g of fat. Tabs can be dissolved in small amount of water.

FORMS — Trade only: Tabs 250, 625 mg.

NOTES — Diarrhea common. Use lowest possible dose of atorvastatin (not more than 40 mg/day) or rosuvastatin or consider pravastatin/fluvastatin. Decreases efficacy of oral contraceptives. May require higher methadone dose. Do not use with proton pump inhibitors. Give nelfinavir 2 h before or 1 h after buffered didanosine. No dosage adjustment for mild hepatic impairment (Child-Pugh Class A); not recommended for more severe hepatic failure (Child-Pugh B/C).

MOA — Prevents cleavage of protein precursors required for HIV maturation, reproduction, and infection of new cells.

ADVERSE EFFECTS — Frequent: Diarrhea, transaminase elevation. Class effects: Hyperglycemia, fat redistribution, lipid abnormalities, spontaneous bleeding in hemophiliacs.

PREZCOBIX (darunavir + cobicistat) ▶L ♀C ▶ – $$$$$

ADULT — Combination therapy of HIV: 1 tab PO once daily with food. Genotypic testing recommended at baseline, especially for treatment-experienced patients.

PEDS — Safety and efficacy not established in children.

FORMS — Trade only: Tabs darunavir 800 mg + cobicistat 150 mg.

NOTES — See components. See cobicistat entry for list of contraindicated drugs and dosage adjustments for drug interactions. See darunavir entry

for hepatotoxicity and sulfonamide cross-sensitivity concerns. Obtain CrCl at baseline; do not use with tenofovir if CrCl <70 mL/min. Do not coadminister other protease inhibitors or elvitegravir. Not for severe hepatic impairment.

MOA — Darunavir prevents cleavage of protein precursors required for HIV maturation, reproduction, and infection of new cells. Cobicistat is a strong CYP3A4 inhibitor intended to increase HIV protease inhibitor exposure.

ADVERSE EFFECTS — See components for serious events. Frequent: Diarrhea, N/V, rash, headache, abdominal pain. Protease inhibitor class effects: Hyperglycemia, fat redistribution, lipid abnormalities, spontaneous bleeding in hemophiliacs.

RITONAVIR *(Norvir, RTV)* ▶L ♀B ▶– $$$$$

WARNING — Contraindicated with many drugs due to risk of drug interactions.

ADULT — See specific protease inhibitor entries for boosting doses of ritonavir. For initial antiretroviral regimens, HIV guidelines recommend against ritonavir as the sole protease inhibitor (600 mg PO two times per day is poorly tolerated), and prefer ritonavir boosting doses that do not exceed 100 mg/ day. Adult doses of 100 to 400 mg/day PO are used to boost levels of other protease inhibitors. Take ritonavir with food.

PEDS — See specific protease inhibitor entries for boosting doses of ritonavir. HIV treatment guidelines recommend against full-dose ritonavir or ritonavir as the sole protease inhibitor for initial therapy of HIV in children.Give ritonavir with meals. Oral soln contains 43.2% (v/v) alcohol and 26.6% (w/v) propylene glycol. It can cause propylene glycol toxicity in preterm infants; do not give oral soln to neonates before a postmenstrual age of 44 weeks. Medication errors or overdose of oral soln could lead to alcohol/propylene glycol toxicity in infants younger than 6 mo.

FORMS — Trade only: Caps 100 mg, tabs 100 mg. Oral soln 80 mg/mL (240 mL).

NOTES — N/V, pancreatitis, alterations in AST, ALT, GGT, CPK, uric acid. Do not give with quinine or rivaroxaban. Ritonavir decreases voriconazole levels. Do not use ritonavir doses of 400 mg two times per day or greater with voriconazole; use ritonavir 100 mg two times per day with voriconazole only if benefit exceeds risk. Decreases efficacy of combined oral or patch contraceptives; consider alternative. May increase fentanyl levels; monitor for increase in fentanyl effects. Increases methadone dosage requirements. May cause serotonin syndrome with fluoxetine. Can prolong PR interval and rare cases of 2nd or 3rd degree AV block reported; caution advised for patients at risk for conduction problems or taking drugs that prolong PR interval, especially if metabolized by CYP3A4. Reduce clarithromycin dose if CrCl <60 mL/min (see clarithromycin entry for details). Give ritonavir 2.5 h before/ after buffered didanosine. Monitor for increased digoxin levels. Caps and oral soln contain alcohol.

(cont.)

RITONAVIR (*cont.*)

Do not refrigerate oral soln. Try to refrigerate caps, but stable for 30 days at less than 77°F. Tabs do not require refrigeration, but must be taken with food.

MOA — Prevents cleavage of protein precursors required for HIV maturation, reproduction, and infection of new cells.

ADVERSE EFFECTS — Serious: Substantial increase in triglycerides; hepatitis, pancreatitis. Can prolong PR interval; rare cases of second/third degree AV block reported. Frequent: GI complaints, paresthesias, asthenia, taste perversion. Class effects: Hyperglycemia, fat redistribution, lipid abnormalities, spontaneous bleeding in hemophiliacs.

SAQUINAVIR (*Invirase, SQV*) ▶L ♀B ▶– $$$$$

ADULT — Combination therapy for HIV infection. Regimen must contain ritonavir; taken together within 2 h after meals. Antiretroviral treatment-naïve or switching from a regimen containing delavirdine or rilpivirine: saquinavir 500 mg PO two times per day with ritonavir 100 mg PO two times per day for 7 days, then saquinavir 1000 mg PO two times per day with ritonavir 100 mg PO two times per day. Patients switching from another protease inhibitor or NNRTI-based regimen should begin with saquinavir 1000 mg PO two times per day with ritonavir 100 mg PO two times per day. If serious toxicity occurs, do not reduce Invirase dose; efficacy unclear for lower doses.

PEDS — Combination therapy for HIV, age 16 yo or older: Use adult dose. Pediatric dose that is effective without increasing risk of QT/PR interval prolongation has not been established.

FORMS — Trade only: Caps 200 mg. Tabs 500 mg.

NOTES — Can prolong QT (increase more than some other boosted protease inhibitors) and PR interval; rare cases of torsades and 2nd/3rd degree AV block. Get ECG at baseline, on day 10 of therapy, and periodically in at-risk patients. Do not use if baseline QT interval is longer than 450 msec. Discontinue if on-treatment QT interval is longer than 480 msec or interval increases by more than 20 msec over baseline. Get ECG at baseline and 3 to 4 days after coadministration of a drug that prolongs the QT interval. Do not use if refractory hypokalemia/hypomagnesemia, congenital long QT syndrome, complete AV block without pacemaker or at high risk for complete AV block, or severe hepatic impairment. Do not use with Class IA or III anti-arrhythmics, neuroleptics, or antimicrobials that prolong QT interval, trazodone, drugs that both increase saquinavir levels and prolong the QT interval, or if QT interval increases by more than 20 msec after coadministration of a drug that prolongs the QT interval. Monitor if used with other drugs that prolong the PR interval (beta blockers, calcium channel blockers, digoxin, atazanavir). Do not use saquinavir with garlic supplements or tipranavir-ritonavir. Use lowest possible dose of atorvastatin (not more than 20 mg/day) or rosuvastatin. Proton pump inhibitors may increase saquinavir levels. Monitor for

increased digoxin levels. May reduce methadone levels. Reduce dose of clarithromycin if CrCl <60 mL/min (see clarithromycin entry for details).

MOA — Prevents cleavage of protein precursors required for HIV maturation, reproduction, and infection of new cells.

ADVERSE EFFECTS — Frequent: GI complaints, headache, LFT elevation. Class effects: hyperglycemia, fat redistribution, lipid abnormalities, spontaneous bleeding in hemophiliacs.

TIPRANAVIR (*Aptivus, TPV*) ▶Feces ♀C ▶– $$$$$

WARNING — Potentially fatal hepatotoxicity. Monitor clinical status and LFTs frequently. Risk increased by coinfection with hepatitis B/C. Contraindicated in moderate to severe (Child-Pugh B/C) hepatic failure. Intracranial hemorrhage can occur with tipranavir + ritonavir; caution if at risk of bleeding from trauma, surgery, other medical conditions, or receiving antiplatelet agents or anticoagulants.

ADULT — Combination therapy for HIV infection, treatment-experienced patients with resistance to multiple protease inhibitors: 500 mg + ritonavir 200 mg PO both two times per day. Take tipranavir plus ritonavir capsules/soln without regard to meals; take tipranavir plus ritonavir tabs with meals.

PEDS — Combination therapy for HIV infection, treatment-experienced patients with resistance to multiple protease inhibitors, age 2 yo or older: 14 mg/kg with 6 mg/kg ritonavir (375 mg/m² with ritonavir 150 mg/m²) PO two times per day to max of 500 mg with ritonavir 200 mg two times per day. Dosage reduction for toxicity in patients infected with virus that is not resistant to multiple protease inhibitors: 12 mg/kg with 5 mg/kg ritonavir (290 mg/m² with 115 mg/m² ritonavir) PO two times per day. Take tipranavir plus ritonavir capsules/soln without regard to meals; take tipranavir plus ritonavir tabs with meals.

FORMS — Trade only: Caps 250 mg. Oral soln 100 mg/mL (95 mL in unit-of-use amber glass bottle).

NOTES — Contains sulfonamide moiety; potential for cross-sensitivity unknown. Al/magnesium antacids may decrease absorption of tipranavir; separate doses. Contraindicated with CYP3A4 substrates that can cause life-threatening toxicity at high concentrations. Do not use with atorvastatin or etravirine. Monitor levels of immunosuppressants, TCAs. May need higher methadone dose. Ritonavir decreases voriconazole levels; do not give together unless benefit exceeds risk. Do not use tipranavir-ritonavir with Kaletra or saquinavir. Decreases ethinyl estradiol levels; consider nonhormonal contraception. Reduce clarithromycin dose if CrCl <60 mL/min (see clarithromycin entry for details). Caps contain alcohol. Refrigerate bottle of caps before opening. Use caps and oral soln within 60 days of opening container. Oral soln contains 116 international units/mL of vitamin E; advise patients not to take supplemental vitamin E other than a multivitamin.

(cont.)

TIPRANAVIR (cont.)

MOA — Non-peptidic protease inhibitor. Prevents cleavage of protein precursors required for HIV maturation, reproduction, and infection of new cells.
ADVERSE EFFECTS — Serious: Life-threatening hepatotoxicity, intracranial hemorrhage. Frequent: Rash (high rate in women, especially those receiving ethinyl estradiol), diarrhea, N/V, fatigue, headache; increased LFTs, total cholesterol, and triglycerides. Class effects: Hyperglycemia, fat redistribution, lipid abnormalities, spontaneous bleeding in hemophiliacs.

ANTIMICROBIALS: Antiviral Agents—Anti-Influenza

NOTE: Whenever possible, immunization is the preferred method of prophylaxis. Avoid anti-influenza antivirals from 48 hours before until 2 weeks after a dose of live influenza vaccine (FluMist) unless medically necessary. Patients with suspected influenza may have primary/concomitant bacterial pneumonia; antibiotics may be indicated. See table for recommendations to prevent and treat influenza with antiviral drugs.

ANTIVIRAL DRUGS FOR INFLUENZA

ANTIVIRAL DRUGS FOR INFLUENZA	Treatment[a] (Duration of 5 days for oseltamivir/zanamivir)	Prevention[b] (Duration of 7 to 10 days post-exposure)
OSELTAMIVIR (Tamiflu)		
Adults and adolescents age 13 years and older		
	75 mg PO bid	75 mg PO once daily
Children, 1 year of age and older[c]		
Body weight ≤15 kg	30 mg PO bid	30 mg PO once daily
Body weight >15 to 23 kg	45 mg PO bid	45 mg PO once daily
Body weight >23 to 40 kg	60 mg PO bid	60 mg PO once daily
Body weight >40 kg	75 mg PO bid	75 mg PO once daily
Infants, newborn to 11 months of age[c]		
Age 3 to 11 months old[d]	3 mg/kg/dose PO bid	3 mg/kg/dose PO once daily
Age younger than 3 months old[e]	3 mg/kg/dose PO bid	Not for routine prophylaxis in infants <3 months old
ZANAMIVIR (Relenza)[f]		
Adults and children (7 years and older for treatment, 5 years and older for prophylaxis)		
	10 mg (two 5-mg inhalations) bid	10 mg (two 5-mg inhalations) once daily
PERAMIVIR (Rapivab)		
Adults with uncomplicated influenza[g]		
	600 mg IV over 15 to 30 minutes as single dose	

Adapted from http://www.cdc.gov/flu/professionals/antivirals/summary-clinicians.htm. bid = two times per day

(cont.)

ANTIVIRAL DRUGS FOR INFLUENZA (*continued*)

[a]Treatment: Start antivirals as soon as possible (ideally within 2 days of symptom onset); do not wait for lab test confirmation. Starting later may help severe/complicated/hospitalized patients. Consider treating longer if patients remain severely ill after 5 days of treatment, especially if immunosuppressed. Treat patients at high risk of influenza complications: age younger than 2 yo or at least 65 yo; chronic pulmonary, cardiovascular (except hypertension only), renal, hepatic, hematologic, metabolic, neurologic/ neurodevelopment disorders; immunosuppressed or HIV; pregnant or within 2 weeks postpartum; child or adolescent on long-term aspirin; native American/ Alaskan native; morbid obesity; resident of nursing home or chronic care facility.

[b]Prevention: Treat for 10 days after household exposure, and for 7 days after most recent known exposure in other situations. For long-term care facilities and hospitals, treat for a minimum of 14 days and up to 7 days after the most recent case was identified.

[c]If Tamiflu suspension is unavailable, pharmacists can compound 6 mg/mL suspension from package insert recipe. Capsule contents of 30, 45, and 75 mg capsules can be mixed with sweetened liquid. Unit of measure is mL for 10 mL Tamiflu suspension oral dispenser; make sure units of measure in dosing instructions match dosing device provided. Tamiflu is FDA-approved for treatment of influenza in infants 2 weeks of age and older and prevention of influenza in children 1 yo and older.

[d]AAP (pediatrics.aappublications.org/content/early/2016/09/01/peds.2016-2527.full-text.pdf) recommends that infants age 9 to 11 mo receive oseltamivir 3.5 mg/kg/dose PO twice daily for treatment and once daily for prevention. This is based on pharmacokinetic data that suggests a higher dose is needed for adequate oseltamivir exposure in this age group. There is no data to suggest the higher dose is more effective or causes more adverse effects than the usual dose.

[e]This dose is not intended for premature infants who may have increased oseltamivir exposure due to immature renal function.

[f]Zanamivir should not be used by patients with underlying pulmonary disease. Do not use Relenza in a nebulizer or ventilator; lactose in the formulation may clog the device.

[g]IV peramivir is FDA-approved for uncomplicated influenza in adults. Per CDC, there is insufficient data to evaluate the efficacy of IV peramivir in hospitalized patients. CDC recommends PO/NG oseltamivir for influenza in hospitalized patients. In patients who cannot tolerate or absorb PO/NG oseltamivir (due to gastric stasis, malabsorption, or GI bleeding), consider IV peramivir (Age 6 yo and older: 10 mg/kg up to 600 mg IV once daily for at least 5 days) or investigational IV zanamivir. In oseltamivir-resistant influenza, consider IV zanamivir. Contact gskclinicalsupportHD@gsk.com, or call 1-877-626-8019 or 1-866-341-9160 (24 h/day) for availability of IV zanamivir.

AMANTADINE ▸K ♀C ▶? $$$$
ADULT — Influenza A: 100 mg PO two times per day; reduce dose to 100 mg PO daily for age 65 yo or older. The CDC generally recommends against amantadine or rimantadine for treatment or prevention of influenza A in the US due to high levels of resistance. Parkinsonism: 100 mg PO two times per day. Max 400 mg/day divided three to four times per day. Drug-induced extrapyramidal disorders: 100 mg PO two times per day. Max 300 mg/day divided three to four times per day.
PEDS — Safety and efficacy not established in infants age younger than 1 yo. Influenza A, treatment or prophylaxis: 5 mg/kg/day (up to 150 mg/day) PO divided two times per day for age 1 to 9 yo and any child wt less than 40 kg. 100 mg PO two times per day for age 10 yo or older. The CDC generally recommends against amantadine or rimantadine for treatment or prevention of influenza A in the US due to high levels of resistance.
FORMS — Generic only: Caps 100 mg. Tabs 100 mg. Syrup 50 mg/5 mL (480 mL).
NOTES — CNS toxicity, suicide attempts, neuroleptic malignant syndrome with dosage reduction/withdrawal, anticholinergic effects, orthostatic hypotension. Do not stop abruptly in Parkinson's disease. Dosage reduction in adults with renal dysfunction: 200 mg PO once a week for CrCl <15 mL/min or hemodialysis. 200 mg PO 1st day, then 100 mg PO every other day for CrCl 15 to 29 mL/min. 200 mg PO 1st day, then 100 mg PO daily for CrCl 30 to 50 mL/min.

MOA — Appears to prevent viral replication by interfering with the function of the M2 protein in influenza virus. May facilitate dopamine release, and act as an NMDA receptor antagonist.
ADVERSE EFFECTS — Serious: Depression, suicidal ideation, seizures, orthostatic hypotension, neuroleptic malignant syndrome with dosage reduction/ withdrawal (rare). Frequent: Anorexia, nausea, peripheral edema, CNS effects (esp. if elderly, renal dysfunction, seizure disorders, anticholinergics, or psychiatric disorder).

OSELTAMIVIR (*Tamiflu*) ▸LK ♀C, but + ▶? $$$$
ADULT — Influenza A/B, treatment: 75 mg PO two times per day for 5 days starting within 2 days of symptom onset. Prophylaxis: 75 mg PO daily. Start within 2 days of exposure and continue for 10 days. Take with food to improve tolerability.
PEDS — Influenza A/B treatment, age 2 weeks old and older: Give dose two times per day for 5 days starting within 2 days of symptom onset. Dose is 3 mg/kg for age 2 weeks old to 11 mo; 30 mg for age at least 1 yo and wt 15 kg or less; 45 mg for wt 16 to 23 kg; 60 mg for wt 24 to 40 kg; 75 mg for wt greater than 40 kg or age at least 13 yo. Influenza A/B prophylaxis, age 1 yo and older: Give once daily for 10 days starting within 2 days of exposure. Dose is 30 mg for age 1 yo or older and wt 15 kg or less; 45 mg for wt 16 to 23 kg; 60 mg for wt 24 to 40 kg; 75 mg for wt greater than 40 kg or age 13 yo and older. Prophylaxis can continue for up to 6 weeks during community outbreak. Can take with food to improve tolerability.

(cont.)

OSELTAMIVIR (*cont.*)

UNAPPROVED ADULT — Influenza A/B, CDC recommendation for severe, complicated, or hospitalized patients: 75 mg (up to 150 mg per some experts) PO/NG two times per day for 5 days or longer. Note: Absorption of PO/NG oseltamivir may be reduced in patients with gastric stasis, malabsorption, or GI bleeding.

UNAPPROVED PEDS — Influenza treatment, age 9 to 11 mo (AAP recommended regimen): 3.5 mg/kg/dose PO two times per day for 5 days. Influenza prophylaxis, age 9 to 11 mo (AAP-recommended regimen): 3.5 mg/kg/dose PO once daily for 10 days starting within 2 days of exposure. Influenza treatment, premature infants: 2 mg/kg/day PO divided two times per day. Influenza prophylaxis in infants 3 to 11 mo: 3 mg/kg/dose PO once daily for 10 days starting within 2 days of exposure. Due to limited data, prophylaxis is not recommended for infants younger than 3 mo unless the situation is critical. Can take with food to improve tolerability.

FORMS — Trade only: Caps 30, 45, 75 mg. Susp 6 mg/mL (60 mL) with 10 mL dosing device (contains sorbitol). Pharmacist can also compound susp (6 mg/mL).

NOTES — Previously not used in children younger than 1 yo; immature blood–brain barrier could lead to high oseltamivir levels in CNS. Increased INR with warfarin. Post-marketing reports (mostly from Japan) of self-injury and delirium, primarily among children and adolescents; monitor for abnormal behavior. CDC recommends as antiviral of choice for influenza in pregnancy. Dosage adjustment for adults (and possibly children if wt >40 kg) with renal impairment. CrCl 31 to 60 mL/min: 30 mg PO two times per day for treatment; 30 mg PO once daily for prevention. CrCl 10 to 30 mL/min: 30 mg PO once daily for treatment; 30 mg PO every other day for prevention. For hemodialysis/CAPD: 30 mg PO after each hemodialysis session/CAPD exchange; initial dose can be given between dialysis sessions. Susp stable for 10 days at room temperature, 17 days refrigerated.

MOA — Oral neuraminidase inhibitor.

ADVERSE EFFECTS — Serious: Anaphylaxis, erythema multiforme, toxic epidermal necrolysis (these reactions rare). Frequent: N/V, stomach discomfort, headache. Post-marketing reports (mostly from Japan) of self-injury and delirium, primarily among children and adolescents.

PERAMIVIR (*Rapivab*) ▶K ♀C ▶? $$$$$

ADULT — Influenza, uncomplicated:600 mg IV single dose infused over 15 to 30 minutes. Intended for patients who have been ill for not more than 2 days.

PEDS — Safety and efficacy not established in children.

UNAPPROVED ADULT — Influenza, hospitalized patients who cannot tolerate or absorb PO/NG oseltamivir: Per CDC, consider IV peramivir 600 mg IV once daily for at least 5 days.

UNAPPROVED PEDS — Influenza, hospitalized patients who cannot tolerate or absorb PO/NG oseltamivir, age 6 yo and older: Per CDC, consider IV peramivir 10 mg/kg up to 600 mg IV once daily for at least 5 days.

NOTES — Per CDC, there is insufficient data to evaluate the efficacy of IV peramivir in hospitalized patients. In a randomized clinical trial of hospitalized patients with influenza, it did not show significant clinical benefit and was well-tolerated. Dosage reduction for renal dysfunction in adults: 200 mg IV once daily for CrCl 30 to 49 mL/min; 100 mg IV once daily for CrCl 10 to 29 mL/min. For hemodialysis patients, give dose after each dialysis session.

MOA — Neuraminidase inhibitor.

ADVERSE EFFECTS — Serious: Skin reactions, including Stevens-Johnson syndrome. Nuropsychiatric events such as delerium and self-injury are possible. Neutropenia. Frequent: Diarrhea.

RIMANTADINE (*Flumadine*) ▶LK ♀C ▶ $$

ADULT — Prophylaxis/treatment of influenza A: 100 mg PO two times per day. Start treatment within 2 days of symptom onset and continue for 7 days. Reduce dose to 100 mg PO once daily if severe hepatic dysfunction, CrCl <30 mL/min, or age older than 65 yo. The CDC generally recommends against amantadine/rimantadine for treatment/prevention of influenza A in the US due to high levels of resistance.

PEDS — Influenza A prophylaxis: 5 mg/kg (up to 150 mg/day) PO once daily for age 1 to 9 yo; 100 mg PO two times per day for age 10 yo and older. The CDC generally recommends against amantadine/rimantadine for treatment/prevention of influenza A in the US due to high levels of resistance.

UNAPPROVED PEDS — Influenza A treatment: 6.6 mg/kg (up to 150 mg/day) PO divided two times per day for age 1 to 9 yo; 100 mg PO two times per day for age 10 yo and older. Start treatment within 2 days of symptom onset and continue for 7 days. The CDC generally recommends against amantadine/rimantadine for treatment/prevention of influenza A in the US due to high levels of resistance.

FORMS — Generic/Trade: Tabs 100 mg. Pharmacist can compound susp.

MOA — Appears to prevent viral replication by interfering with the function of the M2 protein in influenza virus.

ADVERSE EFFECTS — GI effects similar to amantadine, but less CNS toxicity.

ZANAMIVIR (*Relenza*) ▶K ♀C ▶ $$$

ADULT — Influenza A/B treatment: 2 puffs two times per day for 5 days. Take 2 doses on day 1 at least 2 h apart. Start within 2 days of symptom onset. Influenza A/B prevention: 2 puffs once daily for 10 days, starting within 2 days of exposure.

PEDS — Influenza A/B treatment: 2 puffs two times per day for 5 days for age 7 yo or older. Take 2 doses on day 1 at least 2 h apart. Start within 2 days of symptom onset. Influenza A/B prevention: 2 puffs

(cont.)

ZANAMIVIR (*cont.*)

once daily for 10 days for age 5 yo or older, starting within 2 days of exposure.

UNAPPROVED ADULT — Per CDC, consider investigational IV zanamivir in hospitalized patients with influenza who cannot tolerate or absorb PO/NG oseltamivir, or for severe oseltamivir-resistant influenza. For availability of investigational IV zanamivir, contact gskclinicalsupportHD@gsk.com, 1-877-626-8019 or 1-866-341-9160 (available 24 h/day).

UNAPPROVED PEDS — Per CDC, consider investigational IV zanamivir in hospitalized patients with influenza who cannot tolerate or absorb PO/NG oseltamivir, or for severe oseltamivir-resistant influenza. For availability of investigational IV zanamivir, contact gskclinicalsupportHD@gsk.com,

1-877-626-8019 or 1-866-341-9160 (available 24 h/day).

FORMS — Trade only: Rotadisk inhaler 5 mg/puff (20 puffs).

NOTES — Inhaler contains lactose; contraindicated in patients with milk protein allergy. Do not attempt to use in nebulizer or ventilator; lactose may clog the device. May cause bronchospasm and worsen pulmonary function in asthma or COPD; avoid if underlying airways disease. Stop if bronchospasm/decline in respiratory function. Show patient how to use inhaler.

MOA — Inhaled neuraminidase inhibitor.

ADVERSE EFFECTS — Serious: Bronchospasm in patients with reactive airway disease. Possible abnormal behavior and short-term delerium in children and adolescents; monitor for abnormal behavior. Frequent: Nasal and throat irritation.

ANTIMICROBIALS: Antiviral Agents—Other

INTERFERON ALFA-2B (*Intron A*) ▶K ♀C ▶?+ $$$$$

WARNING — May cause or worsen serious neuropsychiatric, autoimmune, ischemic, and infectious diseases. Frequent clinical and lab monitoring required. Stop interferon if signs/symptoms of these conditions are persistently severe or worsen.

ADULT — Chronic hepatitis B: 5 million units/day or 10 million units three times per week SC/IM for 16 weeks if HBeAg positive. Chronic hepatitis C: 3 million units SC/IM three times per week. Currently recommended hepatitis C treatment regimens (see www.hcvguidelines.org) include peginterferon rather than interferon. Other indications: Condylomata acuminata, AIDS-related Kaposi's sarcoma, hairy-cell leukemia, melanoma, and follicular lymphoma—see prescribing information for specific dose.

PEDS — Chronic hepatitis B: 3 million units/m² three times per week for 1st week, then 6 million units/m² (max 10 million units/dose) SC three times per week for age 1 yo or older. Chronic hepatitis C: Interferon alfa-2b 3 million units/m² SC three times per week for age 3 yo or older with PO ribavirin according to wt. Ribavirin: 200 mg two times per day for wt 25 to 36 kg; 200 mg q am and 400 mg q pm for wt 37 to 49 kg; 400 mg two times per day for wt 50 to 61 kg. Use adult dose for wt greater than 61 kg. If ribavirin contraindicated, use interferon 3 to 5 million units/m² (max 3 million units/dose) SC/IM three times per week.

UNAPPROVED ADULT — Other indications: Superficial bladder tumors, chronic myelogenous leukemia, cutaneous T-cell lymphoma, essential thrombocythemia, non-Hodgkin's lymphoma, and chronic granulocytic leukemia.

FORMS — Trade only: Powder/soln for injection 10, 18, 50 million units/vial. Soln for injection 18, 25 million units/multidose vial.

NOTES — Monitor for depression, suicidal behavior (especially in adolescents), other severe neuropsychiatric effects. Thyroid abnormalities, hepatotoxicity, flu-like symptoms, pulmonary and cardiovascular reactions, retinal damage, neutropenia, thrombocytopenia, hypertriglyceridemia (consider monitoring). Monitor CBC, TSH, LFTs, electrolytes. Dosage adjustments for hematologic toxicity in prescribing information. Increases theophylline levels.

MOA — Interferons enhance phagocytic activity of macrophages and cytotoxicity of lymphocytes, and inhibit viral replication.

ADVERSE EFFECTS — Serious: May cause or worsen serious neuropsychiatric, autoimmune, ischemic, & infectious diseases (including thyroid abnormalities, hepatotoxicity, pulmonary & cardiovascular reactions, retinal damage, neutropenia, thrombocytopenia, hypertriglyceridemia, myelosuppression, psychiatric syndromes). May cause growth impairment in children that may rebound after discontinuation; possible reduction in adult height. Frequent: Flu-like syndrome, anorexia, dizziness, rash, depression.

PALIVIZUMAB (*Synagis*) ▶L ♀C ▶? $$$$$

PEDS — Prevention of respiratory syncytial virus pulmonary disease in high-risk infants: 15 mg/kg IM monthly for max of 5 doses per RSV season; give 1st injection before season starts (November to April in Northern hemisphere). See http://pediatrics.aappublications.org for eligibility criteria. Give a dose ASAP after cardiopulmonary bypass (due to decreased palivizumab levels) even if less than 1 month after last dose.

NOTES — AAP recommends stopping monthly prophylaxis after hospitalization for breakthrough RSV; also recommends against prophylaxis in 2nd year of life (with rare exceptions). Preservative-free; use within 6 h of reconstitution. Not more than 1 mL per injection site. Can interfere with immunologic-based diagnostic tests and viral culture assays for RSV, leading to false-negative diagnostic tests.

(cont.)

PALIVIZUMAB (*cont.*)

MOA — Monoclonal antibody against F glycoprotein on surface of respiratory syncytial virus provides passive immunity against the virus.

ADVERSE EFFECTS — Serious: Acute hypersensitivity reactions (rare); anaphylaxis after re-exposure (rare). Frequent: Fever, rash, increased aminotransferase activity.

PEGINTERFERON ALFA-2A (*Pegasys*) ▶LK ♀C ▶– $$$$$

WARNING — May cause or worsen serious neuropsychiatric, autoimmune, ischemic, and infectious diseases. Frequent clinical and lab monitoring recommended. Discontinue if signs/symptoms of these conditions are persistently severe or worsen.

ADULT — Chronic hepatitis C: Regimens of sofosbuvir or simeprevir plus peginterferon are not recommended. Refer to www.hcvguidelines.org for info on remaining indication, genotypes 2, 3, 5, or 6, with GFR 30 mL/min or less and urgency to treat before kidney transplantation. Hepatitis B: 180 mcg SC in abdomen or thigh once a week for 48 weeks.

PEDS — Chronic hepatitis C, initial treatment, age 5 yo or older: 180 mcg/1.73 m^2 (max dose of 180 mcg) SC in abdomen or thigh once weekly. Give with PO ribavirin (see Ribavirin—Oral entry for dose based on wt). Treat genotypes 2 and 3 for 24 weeks; treat genotypes 1 and 4 for 48 weeks.

UNAPPROVED PEDS — Chronic hepatitis C: Some experts suggest deferring treatment for appropriate patients until they are eligible for interferon-free treatment options.

FORMS — Trade only: 180 mcg/1 mL soln in single-use vial, 180 mcg/0.5 mL prefilled syringe, 180 mcg/0.5 mL, 135 mcg/0.5 mL auto-injector.

NOTES — In combination with ribavirin for chronic hepatitis C, peginterferon is preferred over interferon alfa because of substantially higher response rate. Contraindicated in autoimmune hepatitis; hepatic decompensation in cirrhotic patients (Child-Pugh score greater than 6 if HCV only; score 6 or greater if HIV-coinfected). Growth inhibition in children; risk of reduced adult height unclear. Monitor for depression, suicidal behavior, relapse of drug addiction, or other severe neuropsychiatric effects. Interferons can cause thrombocytopenia, neutropenia, thyroid dysfunction, hyperglycemia, hypoglycemia, cardiovascular events, colitis, pancreatitis, hypersensitivity, flu-like symptoms, pulmonary and ophthalmologic disorders. Risk of severe neutropenia/thrombocytopenia greater in HIV-infected patients. Monitor CBC, blood chemistry. Interferons increase risk of hepatic decompensation in hepatitis C/HIV coinfected patients receiving HAART with NRTI. Monitor LFTs and clinical status; discontinue peginterferon if Child-Pugh score 6 or greater. Exacerbation of hepatitis during treatment of hepatitis B; monitor LFTs more often and consider dosage reduction if ALT flares. Discontinue treatment if ALT increase is progressive despite dosage reduction or if flares accompanied by hepatic decompensation or bilirubin increase.

May increase methadone levels. Use cautiously if CrCl <50 mL/min. Reduce adult dose to 135 mcg SC once weekly for CrCl <30 mL/min, ESRD, or hemodialysis. Dosage adjustments for adverse effects or hepatic dysfunction in prescribing information. Store in refrigerator.

MOA — Interferon alfa-2a that is conjugated to polyethylene glycol to increase duration of action. Interferons enhance phagocytic activity of macrophages and cytotoxicity of lymphocytes, and inhibit viral replication.

ADVERSE EFFECTS — Serious: Alpha interferons may cause or worsen serious neuropsychiatric, autoimmune, ischemic, & infectious diseases (including thyroid dysfunction, hyperglycemia, hypoglycemia, hepatotoxicity, colitis, pulmonary & cardiovascular reactions, neutropenia, thrombocytopenia, hypertriglyceridemia, myelosuppression, psychiatric syndromes, ophthalmologic disorders). Interferons increase risk of hepatic decompensation in hep C/HIV coinfected patients receiving HAART with NRTI. Exacerbation of hepatitis during treatment of hepatitis B. Acute hypersensitivity. Growth inhibition in children; risk of reduced adult height unclear. Frequent: Psychiatric reactions, flu-like syndrome, hematologic toxicity, fatigue, injection site reactions, dizziness, pruritus, dermatitis, headache, alopecia, anorexia.

PEGINTERFERON ALFA-2B (*PegIntron*) ▶K? ♀C ▶– $$$$$

WARNING — May cause or worsen serious neuropsychiatric, autoimmune, ischemic, and infectious diseases. Frequent clinical and lab monitoring recommended. Discontinue if signs/symptoms of these conditions are persistently severe or worsen.

ADULT — Chronic hepatitis C. Regimens of sofosbuvir or simeprevir plus peginterferon are not recommended. Refer to www.hcvguidelines.org for info on the only remaining indication, genotypes 2, 3, 5, or 6, with GFR 30 mL/min or less and urgency to treat before kidney transplantation.

PEDS — Chronic hepatitis C not previously treated with alfa-interferon, age 3 yo or older: 60 mcg/m^2 SC once a week with ribavirin 15 mg/kg/day PO divided two times per day (see Ribavirin—Oral entry for dosing of caps). Treat genotype 1 for 48 weeks. Treat genotype 2 or 3 for 24 weeks.

FORMS — Trade only: 50 mcg/0.5 mL single-use vials.

NOTES — Contraindicated in autoimmune hepatitis; hepatic decompensation in cirrhotic patients (Child-Pugh score greater than 6). Coadministration with ribavirin contraindicated if CrCl <50 mL/min. Monitor for depression, suicidal or homicidal behavior, exacerbation of substance use disorders, other severe neuropsychiatric effects. Thrombocytopenia, neutropenia, thyroid dysfunction, hyperglycemia, cardiovascular events, colitis, pancreatitis, hypersensitivity, flu-like symptoms, pulmonary damage. Monitor CBC, blood chemistry. May increase methadone levels. Dosage adjustments for adverse effects

(cont.)

PEGINTERFERON ALFA-2B (cont.)

in prescribing information. Adult dosage reduction for renal dysfunction: 25% reduction for CrCl 30 to 50 mL/min; 50% reduction for CrCl <30 mL/min including hemodialysis. Peginterferon should be used immediately after reconstitution, but can be refrigerated for up to 24 h.

MOA — Interferon alfa-2b that is conjugated to polyethylene glycol. Binding of alpha interferon to cell surface receptors initiates intracellular events that enhances the phagocytic activity of macrophages and cytotoxicity of lymphocytes, and inhibits viral replication.

ADVERSE EFFECTS — Serious: May cause or worsen serious neuropsychiatric, autoimmune, ischemic, & infectious diseases (including thyroid abnormalities, hepatotoxicity, pulmonary & cardiovascular reactions, stroke, retinal damage, neutropenia, thrombocytopenia, hypertriglyceridemia, myelosuppression, psychiatric syndromes). Impaired growth in children during treatment with peginterferon plus ribavirin, with rebound after discontinuation. Frequent: Flu-like syndrome, anorexia, dizziness, rash, depression.

RIBAVIRIN—INHALED (Virazole) ▶Lung ♀X ▶– $$$$$

WARNING — Beware of sudden pulmonary deterioration with ribavirin. Drug precipitation may cause ventilator dysfunction.

PEDS — Severe respiratory syncytial virus infection: Aerosol 12 to 18 h/day for 3 to 7 days.

NOTES — Minimize exposure to healthcare workers, especially pregnant women.

MOA — Inhaled synthetic nucleoside that interferes with viral nucleic acid synthesis.

ADVERSE EFFECTS — Serious: Sudden pulmonary deterioration, ventilator dysfunction due to drug precipitation.

ANTIMICROBIALS: Carbapenems

NOTE: Carbapenems can dramatically reduce valproic acid levels; use another antibiotic (preferred) or add a supplemental anticonvulsant. Possible cross-sensitivity with other beta-lactams; –associated diarrhea; superinfection.

DORIPENEM (Doribax) ▶K ♀B ▶? $$$$$

ADULT — Complicated intra-abdominal infection: 500 mg IV q 8 h for 5 to 14 days. Complicated UTI or pyelonephritis: 500 mg IV q 8 h for 10 to 14 days. Infuse IV over 1 h.

PEDS — Not approved in children.

NOTES — Do not use for ventilator-associated bacterial pneumonia; doripenem had higher mortality and lower response rate than imipenem in clinical trial. May cause seizures, especially if pre-existing CNS disorder, renal impairment, or doses greater than 1500 mg/day. Dose reduction in renal dysfunction: 250 mg q 12 h for CrCl 10 to 30 mL/min, 250 mg q 8 h for CrCl 30 to 50 mL/min.

MOA — Beta-lactam resistant to hydrolysis by most beta-lactamases, including extended-spectrum beta-lactamases.

ADVERSE EFFECTS — Serious: Cross-sensitivity with other beta-lactams; C. difficile associated diarrhea; superinfection; seizures (esp. if pre-existing CNS disorder, renal impairment, or doses >1500 mg/day). Frequent: Headache, nausea, diarrhea, rash, phlebitis.

ERTAPENEM (Invanz) ▶K ♀B ▶? $$$$$

ADULT — Community-acquired pneumonia, diabetic foot, complicated intra-abdominal, skin, urinary tract, acute pelvic infections: 1 g IM/IV over 30 min q 24 h for up to 14 days for IV, up to 7 days for IM. Prophylaxis, elective colorectal surgery: 1 g IV 1 h before incision.

PEDS — Community-acquired pneumonia, complicated intra-abdominal, skin, urinary tract, acute pelvic infections, 3 mo to 12 yo: 15 mg/kg IV/IM q 12 h (up to 1 g/day). Use adult dose for age 13 yo or older. Infuse IV over 30 min. Can give IV for up to 14 days, IM for up to 7 days.

NOTES — Seizures (especially if renal dysfunction or CNS disorder). Not active against Pseudomonas and Acinetobacter species. IM diluted with lidocaine; contraindicated if allergic to amide-type local anesthetics. For adults with renal dysfunction: 500 mg q 24 h for CrCl <30 mL/min or hemodialysis. Give 150 mg supplemental dose if daily dose given within 6 h before hemodialysis session. Do not dilute in dextrose.

MOA — Beta-lactam resistant to hydrolysis by most beta-lactamases, including extended-spectrum beta-lactamases.

ADVERSE EFFECTS — Serious: Cross-sensitivity with other beta-lactams, C. difficile-associated diarrhea, superinfection, seizures (0.5% of patients). Frequent: Diarrhea, N/V, infusion site reactions. Lidocaine diluent can cause allergy.

MEROPENEM (Merrem IV) ▶K ♀B ▶? $$$$$

ADULT — Complicated intra-abdominal infection: 1 g IV q 8 h. Complicated skin infection: 500 mg IV q 8 h; use 1 g IV q 8 h if P. aeruginosa skin infection.

PEDS — Meningitis, age 3 mo and older: 40 mg/kg IV q 8 h; 2 g IV q 8 h for wt greater than 50 kg. Complicated intra-abdominal infection. Age 3 mo and older: 20 mg/kg IV q 8 h; 1 g IV q 8 h for wt greater than 50 kg. Age 2 weeks to less than 3 months: 20 mg/kg IV q 8 h if gestational age less than 32 weeks; 30 mg/kg IV q 8 h if gestational age 32 weeks and older. Age less than 2 weeks: 20 mg/kg IV q 12 h if gestational age less than 32 weeks; 20 mg/kg IV q 8 h if gestational age 32 weeks and older. Complicated skin infection, age 3 mo and older: 10 mg/kg IV q 8 h; 500 mg IV q 8 h for wt greater than 50 kg. Complicated skin infection caused by P. aeruginosa: 20 mg/kg IV q 8 h up to 1 g IV q 8 h; use 1 g IV q 8 h for wt greater than 50 kg.

(cont.)

MEROPENEM (*cont.*)

UNAPPROVED ADULT — Meningitis: 40 mg/kg (max 2 g) IV q 8 h. Hospital-acquired pneumonia, complicated UTI, malignant otitis externa: 1 g IV q 8 h. Anthrax: See table.

UNAPPROVED PEDS — Anthrax: See table.

NOTES — Seizures; thrombocytopenia in renal dysfunction. May cause motor impairment; tell patients to avoid driving or operating machinery. For adults with renal dysfunction: Give 50% of normal dose q 24 h for CrCl <10 mL/min, 50% of normal dose q 12 h for CrCl 10 to 25 mL/min, normal dose q 12 h for CrCl 26 to 50 mL/min.

MOA — Beta-lactam resistant to hydrolysis by most beta-lactamases, including extended-spectrum beta-lactamases.

ADVERSE EFFECTS — Serious: Cross-sensitivity with other beta-lactams, C. difficile-associated diarrhea, superinfection, seizures, thrombocytopenia in renal dysfunction. Frequent: Diarrhea, headache.

PRIMAXIN (imipenem-cilastatin) ▶K ♀C ▶? $$$$$

ADULT — Pneumonia, sepsis, endocarditis, polymicrobic, intra-abdominal, gynecologic, bone and joint, skin infections. Normal renal function, 70 kg or greater: Mild infection: 250 to 500 mg IV q 6 h; moderate infection: 500 mg IV q 6 to 8 h or 1 g IV q 8 h; severe infection: 500 mg IV q 6 h to 1 g IV q 6 to 8 h. Complicated UTI: 500 mg IV q 6 h. See product labeling for doses in adults wt less than 70 kg. Can give up to 1.5 g/day IM for mild/moderate infections.

PEDS — Pneumonia, sepsis, endocarditis, polymicrobic, intra-abdominal, bone and joint, skin infections: 25 mg/kg IV q 12 h for age younger than 1 week old; 25 mg/kg IV q 8 h for age 1 to 4 weeks old; 25 mg/kg IV q 6 h for age 1 to 3 mo; 15 to 25 mg/kg IV q 6 h for older than 3 mo. Not for children with CNS infections, or wt less than 30 kg with renal dysfunction.

UNAPPROVED ADULT — Malignant otitis externa, empiric therapy for neutropenic fever: 500 mg IV q 6 h.

NOTES — Seizures (especially if given with ganciclovir, elderly with renal dysfunction, or cerebrovascular or seizure disorder). See product labeling for dose if CrCl <70 mL/min. Not for CrCl <5 mL/min unless dialysis started within 48 h.

MOA — Beta-lactam resistant to hydrolysis by most beta-lactamases, including extended-spectrum beta-lactamases. Cilastatin inhibits renal tubular metabolism of imipenem.

ADVERSE EFFECTS — Serious: Cross-sensitivity with other beta-lactams (50% in patients with anaphylaxis to penicillin), C. difficile-associated diarrhea, superinfection. Frequent: Seizures in patients with risk factors (ganciclovir, elderly with renal dysfunction, cerebrovascular or seizure disorder).

ANTIMICROBIALS: Cephalosporins—1st Generation

CEPHALOSPORINS: GENERAL ANTIMICROBIAL SPECTRUM

1st generation	Gram-positive (including *S. aureus*); basic Gram-negative coverage
2nd generation	diminished *S. aureus*, improved Gram-negative coverage compared to 1st generation; some with anaerobic coverage
3rd generation	further diminished *S. aureus*, further improved Gram-negative coverage compared to 1st and 2nd generation; some with pseudomonal coverage & diminished Gram-positive coverage
4th generation	same as 3rd generation plus coverage against *Pseudomonas*
5th generation	Gram-negative coverage similar to 3rd generation; also active against *S. aureus* (including MRSA) and *S. pneumoniae*

NOTE: Cephalosporins are second-line to penicillins for group A strep pharyngitis, can rarely be cross-sensitive with penicillins, and can cause C. difficile associated diarrhea.

CEFADROXIL ▶K ♀B ▶+ $$$

ADULT — Simple UTI: 1 to 2 g/day PO divided one to two times per day. Other UTIs: 1 g PO two times per day. Skin infections: 1 g/day PO divided one to two times per day. Group A strep pharyngitis: 1 g/day PO divided one to two times per day for 10 days.

PEDS — UTIs, skin infections: 30 mg/kg/day PO divided two times per day. Group A streptococcal pharyngitis/tonsillitis, impetigo: 30 mg/kg/day PO divided one to two times per day. Treat pharyngitis for 10 days.

(cont.)

CEFADROXIL *(cont.)*

FORMS — Generic only: Tabs 1 g. Caps 500 mg. Susp 250, 500 mg/5 mL.

NOTES — Dosage adjustment for renal dysfunction in adults: 500 mg PO q 36 h for CrCl <10 mL/min; 500 mg PO q 24 h for CrCl 11 to 25 mL/min; 1 g load then 500 mg PO q 12 h for CrCl 26 to 50 mL/min.

MOA — Beta-lactam antibiotic that inhibits the biosynthesis of cell wall mucopeptide. (Beta-lactam fused to different ring structure from penicillins.)

ADVERSE EFFECTS — Serious: Cross-sensitivity with penicillins, C. difficile-associated diarrhea. Frequent: diarrhea.

CEFAZOLIN ▶K ♀B ▶+ $$

ADULT — Pneumonia; sepsis; endocarditis; skin, bone, and joint; and genital infections. Mild infections due to Gram-positive cocci: 250 to 500 mg IM/IV q 8 h. Moderate/severe infections: 0.5 to 1 g IM/IV q 6 to 8 h. Life-threatening infections: 1 to 1.5 g IV q 6 h. Simple UTI: 1 g IM/IV q 12 h. Pneumococcal pneumonia: 500 mg IM/IV q 12 h. Surgical prophylaxis: 1 g IM/IV 30 to 60 min preop, additional 0.5 to 1 g during surgery longer than 2 h, and 0.5 to 1 g q 6 to 8 h for 24 h postop. Prevention of perinatal group B streptococcal disease: Give to mother 2 g IV at onset of labor/after membrane rupture, then 1 g IV q 8 h until delivery. See table for prophylaxis of bacterial endocarditis.

PEDS — Pneumonia; sepsis; endocarditis; skin, bone, and joint infections. Mild to moderate infections: 25 to 50 mg/kg/day IM/IV divided q 6 to 8 h for age 1 mo or older. Severe infections: 100 mg/kg/day IV divided q 6 to 8 h for age 1 mo or older. See table for prophylaxis of bacterial endocarditis.

NOTES — Dose reduction for renal dysfunction in adults: Usual 1st dose, then 50% of usual dose q 18 to 24 h for CrCl <10 mL/min; 50% of usual dose q 12 h for CrCl 11 to 34 mL/min; usual dose q 8 h for CrCl 35 to 54 mL/min. Dose reduction for renal dysfunction in children: Usual 1st dose, then 10% of usual dose q 24 h for CrCl 5 to 20 mL/min; 25% of usual dose q 12 h for CrCl 20 to 40 mL/min; 60% of usual dose q 12 h for CrCl 40 to 70 mL/min.

MOA — Beta-lactam antibiotic that inhibits the biosynthesis of cell wall mucopeptide. (Beta-lactam fused to different ring structure from penicillins.)

ADVERSE EFFECTS — Serious: Cross-sensitivity with penicillins, C. difficile-associated diarrhea. Frequent: Hypersensitivity.

CEPHALEXIN *(Keflex)* ▶K ♀B ▶? $$

ADULT — Pneumonia, bone, GU infections. Usual dose: 250 to 500 mg PO four times per day. Max: 4 g/day. Group A strep pharyngitis, skin infections, simple UTI: 500 mg PO two times per day. Treat pharyngitis for 10 days. See table for prophylaxis of bacterial endocarditis.

PEDS — Pneumonia, GU, bone, skin infections, group A strep pharyngitis. Usual dose: 25 to 50 mg/kg/day PO in divided doses. Max dose: 100 mg/kg/day. Can give two times per day for strep pharyngitis in children older than 1 yo, skin infections. Group A strep pharyngitis, skin infections, simple UTI in patients older than 15 yo: 500 mg PO two times per day. Treat pharyngitis for 10 days. Not for otitis media, sinusitis.

FORMS — Generic/Trade (Keflex $$$$$): Caps 250, 500, 750 mg. Generic only: Tabs 250, 500 mg. Susp 125, 250 mg/5 mL.

NOTES — Dosage adjustment for renal dysfunction: Max dose of 1 g/day for CrCl 30 to 59 mL/min; 250 mg q 8 to 12 h for CrCl 15 to 29 mL/min; 250 mg q 24 h for CrCl 5 to 14 mL/min and not on dialysis; 250 mg q 12 h for hemodialysis with one dose given after dialysis session on dialysis days; 500 mg q 12 h for CAPD.

MOA — Beta-lactam antibiotic that inhibits the biosynthesis of cell wall mucopeptide. (Beta-lactam fused to different ring structure from penicillins.)

ADVERSE EFFECTS — Serious: Cross-sensitivity with penicillins, C. difficile-associated diarrhea. Frequent: Eosinophilia.

ANTIMICROBIALS: Cephalosporins—2nd Generation

NOTE: Cephalosporins are second-line to penicillins for group A strep pharyngitis, can rarely be cross-sensitive with penicillins, and can cause C. difficile–associated diarrhea.

CEFACLOR *(✻Ceclor)* ▶K ♀B ▶+ $$$$

ADULT — Pneumonia, group A strep pharyngitis, UTI, skin infections: 250 to 500 mg PO three times per day. Treat pharyngitis for 10 days. Extended-release tabs for acute exacerbation of chronic bronchitis ($$$$$): 500 mg PO two times per day for 7 days.

PEDS — Pneumonia, group A streptococcal pharyngitis, UTI, skin infections: 20 to 40 mg/kg/day (up to 1 g/day) PO divided two times per day for pharyngitis, three times per day for other infections. Treat pharyngitis for 10 days.

FORMS — Generic only: Caps 250, 500 mg. Susp 125, 250, 375 mg per 5 mL. Extended-release tabs: 500 mg.

MOA — Beta-lactam antibiotic that inhibits the biosynthesis of cell wall mucopeptide. (Beta-lactam fused to different ring structure from penicillins.)

ADVERSE EFFECTS — Serious: Cross-sensitivity with penicillins, C. difficile-associated diarrhea; serum sickness-like reactions with repeated use. Frequent: Headache.

CEFOTETAN ▶K/Bile ♀B ▶? $$$$$

ADULT — Usual dose: 1 to 2 g IM/IV q 12 h. UTI: 0.5 to 2 g IM/IV q 12 h or 1 to 2 g IM/IV q 24 h. Pneumonia; gynecologic, intra-abdominal, bone and joint infections: 1 to 3 g IM/IV q 12 h. Skin infections: 1 to 2 g IM/IV q 12 h or 2 g IV q 24 h. Surgical prophylaxis: 1 to 2 g IV 30 to 60 min preop. Give after cord clamp for C-section.

(cont.)

CEFOTETAN (*cont.*)

PEDS — Not approved in children.

UNAPPROVED PEDS — Usual dose: 40 to 80 mg/kg/day IV divided q 12 h.

NOTES — Hemolytic anemia (higher risk than other cephalosporins), clotting impairment rarely. Disulfiram-like reaction with alcohol. Dosing reduction in adults with renal dysfunction: Usual dose q 48 h for CrCl <10 mL/min; usual dose q 24 h for CrCl 10 to 30 mL/min.

MOA — Beta-lactam antibiotic that inhibits the biosynthesis of cell wall mucopeptide. (Beta-lactam fused to different ring structure from penicillins.) Cefotetan has MTT side-chain.

ADVERSE EFFECTS — Serious: Cross-sensitivity with penicillins, C. difficile-associated diarrhea, hemolytic anemia, clotting impairment rarely, disulfiram-like reaction with alcohol.

CEFOXITIN ▸K ♀B ▶+ $$$$

ADULT — Pneumonia; UTI; sepsis; intra-abdominal, gynecologic, skin, bone, and joint infections. Uncomplicated: 1 g IV q 6 to 8 h. Moderate to severe: 1 g IV q 4 h or 2 g IV q 6 to 8 h. Infections requiring high doses: 2 g IV q 4 h or 3 g IV q 6 h. Uncontaminated GI surgery, vaginal/abdominal hysterectomy: 2 g IV 30 to 60 min preop, then 2 g IV q 6 h for 24 h. C-section: 2 g IV after cord clamped or 2 g IV q 4 h for 3 doses with 1st dose given after cord clamped.

PEDS — Pneumonia; UTI; sepsis; intra-abdominal, skin, bone, and joint infections: 80 to 160 mg/kg/day (up to 12 g/day) IV divided into 4 to 6 doses for age 3 mo or older. Mild to moderate infections: 80 to 100 mg/kg/day IV divided into 3 to 4 doses. Surgical prophylaxis: 30 to 40 mg/kg IV 30 to 60 min preop; additional doses can be given q 6 h up to 24 h postop.

NOTES — Eosinophilia and increased AST with high doses in children. Dosing reduction in adults with renal dysfunction: Load with 1 to 2 g IV then 0.5 g IV q 24 to 48 h for CrCl <5 mL/min; 0.5 to 1 g IV q 12 to 24 h for CrCl 5 to 9 mL/min; 1 to 2 g IV q 12 to 24 h for CrCl 10 to 29 mL/min; 1 to 2 g IV q 8 to 12 h for CrCl 30 to 50 mL/min. Give 1 to 2 g supplemental dose after each hemodialysis.

MOA — Beta-lactam antibiotic that inhibits the biosynthesis of cell wall mucopeptide. (Beta-lactam fused to different ring structure from penicillins.)

ADVERSE EFFECTS — Serious: Cross-sensitivity with penicillins, C. difficile-associated diarrhea, eosinophilia & increased AST with high doses in children.

CEFPROZIL ▸K ♀B ▶+ $$$$

ADULT — Group A strep pharyngitis: 500 mg PO once daily for 10 days. Sinusitis: 250 to 500 mg PO two times per day. Acute exacerbation of chronic/secondary infection of acute bronchitis: 500 mg PO two times per day. Skin infections: 250 to 500 mg PO two times per day or 500 mg PO once daily.

PEDS — Otitis media: 15 mg/kg/dose PO two times per day. Group A strep pharyngitis: 7.5 mg/kg/dose PO two times per day for 10 days. Sinusitis: 7.5 to 15 mg/kg/dose PO two times per day. Skin infections: 20 mg/kg PO once daily. Use adult dose for age 13 yo or older.

FORMS — Generic only: Tabs 250, 500 mg. Susp 125, 250 mg/5 mL.

NOTES — Give 50% of usual dose at usual interval for CrCl <30 mL/min.

MOA — Beta-lactam antibiotic that inhibits the biosynthesis of cell wall mucopeptide. (Beta-lactam fused to different ring structure from penicillins.)

ADVERSE EFFECTS — Serious: Cross-sensitivity with penicillins, C. difficile-associated diarrhea, may cause serum sickness reaction. Frequent: None.

CEFUROXIME (*Zinacef, Ceftin*) ▸K ♀B ▶? $$$$

ADULT — Uncomplicated pneumonia, simple UTI, skin infections, disseminated gonorrhea: 750 mg IM/IV q 8 h. Bone and joint or severe/complicated infections: 1.5 g IV q 8 h. Sepsis: 1.5 g IV q 6 h to 3 g IV q 8 h. Surgical prophylaxis: 1.5 g IV 30 to 60 min preop, then 750 mg IM/IV q 8 h for prolonged procedures. Open heart surgery: 1.5 g IV q 12 h for 4 doses with 1st dose at induction of anesthesia. Cefuroxime axetil tabs: Group A strep pharyngitis, acute sinusitis: 250 mg PO two times per day for 10 days. Acute exacerbation of chronic/secondary infection of acute bronchitis, skin infections: 250 to 500 mg PO two times per day. Lyme disease: 500 mg PO two times per day for 14 days for early disease, for 28 days for Lyme arthritis. Simple UTI: 125 to 250 mg PO two times per day.

PEDS — Most infections: 50 to 100 mg/kg/day IM/IV divided q 6 to 8 h. Bone and joint infections: 150 mg/kg/day IM/IV divided q 8 h (up to adult dose). Cefuroxime axetil tabs: Group A strep pharyngitis: 125 mg PO two times per day for 10 days. Otitis media, sinusitis: 250 mg PO two times per day for 10 days. Cefuroxime axetil oral susp. Group A strep pharyngitis: 20 mg/kg/day (up to 500 mg/day) PO divided two times per day for 10 days. Otitis media, sinusitis, impetigo: 30 mg/kg/day (up to 1 g/day) PO divided two times per day for 10 days. Use adult dose for age 13 yo or older. For otitis media, AAP recommends 5 to 7 days of therapy for age 6 yo and older with mild to moderate symptoms, 7 days for age 2 to 5 yo with mild to moderate symptoms, and 10 days for age younger than 2 yo and childern with severe symptoms.

UNAPPROVED PEDS — Lyme disease: 30 mg/kg/day PO divided two times per day (max 500 mg/dose) for 14 days for early disease, for 28 days for Lyme arthritis. Community-acquired pneumonia: 150 mg/kg/day IV divided q 8 h.

FORMS — Generic/Trade (Ceftin $$$$$): Tabs 500 mg. Susp 125, 250 mg/5 mL. Generic only: Tabs 250 mg.

NOTES — Dosage reduction for renal dysfunction in adults: Usual dose q 24 h for CrCl 10 to <30 mL/min; usual dose q 48 h for CrCl <10 mL/min with no hemodialysis; usual dose at the end of each dialysis session for hemodialysis. Tabs and susp not bioequivalent on mg:mg basis. Do not crush tabs.

(cont.)

CEFUROXIME (*cont.*)

MOA — Beta-lactam antibiotic that inhibits the bio-synthesis of cell wall mucopeptide. (Beta-lactam fused to different ring structure from penicillins.)

ADVERSE EFFECTS — Serious: Cross-sensitivity with penicillins, C. difficile-associated diarrhea. Frequent: Anemia, eosinophilia.

ANTIMICROBIALS: Cephalosporins—3rd Generation

NOTE: Cephalosporins are 2nd-line to penicillins for group A strep pharyngitis, can rarely be cross-sensitive with penicillins, and can cause C. difficile–associated diarrhea.

CEFDINIR (*Omnicef*) ▶K ♀B ▶? $$$$

ADULT — Community-acquired pneumonia, skin infections: 300 mg PO two times per day for 10 days. Sinusitis: 600 mg PO once daily or 300 mg PO two times per day for 10 days. Group A strep pharyngitis, acute exacerbation of chronic bronchitis: 600 mg PO once daily for 10 days or 300 mg PO two times per day for 5 to 10 days.

PEDS — Group A strep pharyngitis, otitis media: 14 mg/kg/day PO divided two times per day for 5 to 10 days or once daily for 10 days. See tables for management of otitis media and acute sinusitis. Sinusitis: 14 mg/kg/day PO divided once daily or two times per day for 10 days. Skin infections: 14 mg/kg/day PO divided two times per day for 10 days. Use adult dose for age 13 yo or older.

FORMS — Generic only: Caps 300 mg. Susp 125, 250 mg/5 mL.

NOTES — Omnicef brand no longer available. Give iron, multivitamins with iron, or antacids at least 2 h before or after cefdinir. Complexation of cefdinir with iron may turn stools red. Reduce dose for renal dysfunction: 300 mg PO daily for adults with CrCl less than 30 mL/min; 7 mg/kg/day PO once daily up to 300 mg/day for children with CrCl less than 30 mL/min. Hemodialysis: 300 mg or 7 mg/kg PO after hemodialysis, then 300 mg or 7 mg/kg PO q 48 h.

MOA — Beta-lactam antibiotic that inhibits the bio-synthesis of cell wall mucopeptide. (Beta-lactam fused to different ring structure from penicillins.)

ADVERSE EFFECTS — Serious: Cross-sensitivity with penicillins, C. difficile-associated diarrhea. Frequent: Diarrhea.

CEFDITOREN (*Spectracef*) ▶K ♀B ▶? $$$$$

ADULT — Skin infections, group A strep pharyngitis: 200 mg PO two times per day for 10 days. Give 400 mg two times per day for 10 days for acute exacerbation of chronic bronchitis, for 14 days for community-acquired pneumonia. Take with food.

PEDS — Skin infections, group A strep pharyngitis, age 12 yo or older: 200 mg PO two times per day with food for 10 days.

FORMS — Generic/Trade: Tabs 200, 400 mg.

NOTES — Contraindicated if milk protein allergy or carnitine deficiency. Not for long-term use due to potential risk of carnitine deficiency. Do not take with drugs that reduce gastric acid (antacids, H2 blockers, etc.). Dosage adjustment for renal dysfunction: Max 200 mg two times per day if CrCl 30 to 49 mL/min; max 200 mg once daily if CrCl <30 mL/min.

MOA — Beta-lactam antibiotic that inhibits the bio-synthesis of cell wall mucopeptide. (Beta-lactam fused to different ring structure from penicillins.)

ADVERSE EFFECTS — Serious: Cross-sensitivity with penicillins, C. difficile-associated diarrhea. Frequent: N/V, diarrhea.

CEFIXIME (*Suprax*) ▶K/Bile ♀B ▶? $$$$$

ADULT — Simple UTI, pharyngitis, acute bacterial bronchitis, acute exacerbation of chronic bronchitis: 400 mg PO once daily. Gonorrhea (not pharyngeal): 400 mg PO single dose + azithromycin 1 g PO single dose. CDC now considers cefixime an alternative for when ceftriaxone cannot be used. See STD table.

PEDS — Otitis media: 8 mg/kg/day susp/chew tab PO divided one to two times per day. Use only susp/chew tabs for otitis media (better blood levels). Pharyngitis: 8 mg/kg/day PO divided one to two times per day for 10 days. Use adult dose for wt greater than 50 kg (greater than 45 kg for 500 mg/5 mL susp) or age 13 yo or older.

UNAPPROVED PEDS — Febrile UTI (3 to 24 mo): 16 mg/kg PO on 1st day, then 8 mg/kg PO daily to complete 14 days. See table for management of acute sinusitis.

FORMS — Generic/Trade: Susp 100, 200 mg/5 mL. Trade only: Susp 500 mg/5 mL. Chewable tabs 100, 200 mg. Caps 400 mg.

NOTES — Poor activity against S. aureus. Increased INR with warfarin. May increase carbamazepine levels. Susp stable at room temp or refrigerated for 14 days. Reduce dose in renal dysfunction: 75% of usual dose at usual interval for CrCl 21 to 60 mL/min or hemodialysis; 50% of usual dose at usual interval for CrCl <20 mL/min or continuous peritoneal dialysis. Can cause false (+) on urine glucose test using Benedict's or Fehling's solution (Clinitest, etc.); use glucose oxidase test (Clinistix, Tes-Tape, etc.) instead.

MOA — Beta-lactam antibiotic that inhibits the bio-synthesis of cell wall mucopeptide. (Beta-lactam fused to different ring structure from penicillins.)

ADVERSE EFFECTS — Serious: Cross-sensitivity with penicillins, C. difficile-associated diarrhea. Frequent: N/V, diarrhea.

CEFOTAXIME (*Claforan*) ▶KL ♀B ▶+ $$$$

ADULT — Pneumonia, sepsis, GU and gynecologic, skin, intra-abdominal, bone and joint infections. Uncomplicated: 1 g IM/IV q 12 h. Moderate/severe: 1 to 2 g IM/IV q 8 h. Infections usually requiring high doses: 2 g IV q 6 to 8 h. Life-threatening: 2 g IV q 4 h. Meningitis: 2 g IV q 4 to 6 h. Gonorrhea: 0.5 to 1 g IM single dose.

(cont.)

CEFOTAXIME *(cont.)*

PEDS — Pneumonia, sepsis, GU, skin, intra-abdominal, bone/joint, CNS infections. Labeled dose: 50 mg/kg/dose IV q 12 h for age younger than 1 week old; 50 mg/kg/dose IV q 8 h for age 1 to 4 weeks; 50 to 180 mg/kg/day IM/IV divided q 4 to 6 h for age 1 mo to 12 yo. AAP recommends 225 to 300 mg/day IV divided q 6 to 8 h for S. pneumoniae meningitis. Mild to moderate infections: 75 to 100 mg/kg/day IV/IM divided q 6 to 8 h. Severe infections: 150 to 200 mg/kg/day IV/IM divided q 6 to 8 h.

UNAPPROVED ADULT — Disseminated gonorrhea, CDC alternate regimen: 1 g IV q 8 h.

UNAPPROVED PEDS — Neonatal disseminated gonorrhea, gonococcal scalp abscess: 25 mg/kg IV/IM q 12 h for 7 days; treat for 10 to 14 days if meningitis documented.

NOTES — Bolus injection through central venous catheter can cause arrhythmias. Decrease dose by 50% for CrCl <20 mL/min.

MOA — Beta-lactam antibiotic that inhibits the biosynthesis of cell wall mucopeptide. (Beta-lactam fused to different ring structure from penicillins.)

ADVERSE EFFECTS — Serious: Cross-sensitivity with penicillins, C. difficile-associated diarrhea. Frequent: Coombs + anemia, phlebitis.

CEFPODOXIME ▸K ♀B ▸? $$$$

ADULT — Acute exacerbation of chronic bronchitis, acute sinusitis: 200 mg PO two times per day for 10 days. Community-acquired pneumonia: 200 mg PO two times per day for 14 days. Group A strep pharyngitis: 100 mg PO two times per day for 5 to 10 days. Skin infections: 400 mg PO two times per day for 7 to 14 days. Simple UTI: 100 mg PO two times per day for 7 days. Approved for treatment of gonorrhea, but CDC does not recommend. Give tabs with food.

PEDS — 5 mg/kg PO two times per day for 5 days for otitis media, for 5 to 10 days for group A strep pharyngitis, for 10 days for sinusitis. Use adult dose for age 12 yo or older. For otitis media, AAP recommends 5 to 7 days of therapy for age 6 yo and older with mild to moderate symptoms, 7 days for age 2 to 5 yo with mild to moderate symptoms, and 10 days for age younger than 2 yo and children with severe symptoms. See tables for management of acute sinusitis and otitis media.

FORMS — Generic: Tabs 100, 200 mg. Susp 50, 100 mg/5 mL.

NOTES — Do not give antacids within 2 h before/after cefpodoxime. Reduce dose in renal dysfunction: Increase dosing interval to q 24 h for CrCl <30 mL/min. Give 3 times per week after dialysis session for hemodialysis patients. Susp stable for 14 days refrigerated.

MOA — Beta-lactam antibiotic that inhibits the biosynthesis of cell wall mucopeptide. (Beta-lactam fused to different ring structure from penicillins.)

ADVERSE EFFECTS — Serious: Cross-sensitivity with penicillins; C. difficile-associated diarrhea; acute hepatitis, bloody diarrhea, and pulmonary infiltrates (rare). Frequent: Diarrhea.

CEFTAZIDIME *(Fortaz, Tazicef)* ▸K ♀B ▸+ $$$$

ADULT — Simple UTI: 250 mg IM/IV q 12 h. Complicated UTI: 500 mg IM/IV q 8 to 12 h. Uncomplicated pneumonia, mild skin infections: 500 mg to 1 g IM/IV q 8 h. Serious gynecologic, intra-abdominal, bone and joint, life-threatening infections; meningitis; empiric therapy of neutropenic fever: 2 g IV q 8 h. Pseudomonas lung infections in cystic fibrosis: 30 to 50 mg/kg IV q 8 h (up to 6 g/day).

PEDS — Use sodium formulations in children (Fortaz, Tazicef). UTIs; pneumonia; skin, intra-abdominal, bone and joint infections: 100 to 150 mg/kg/day (up to 6 g/day) IV divided q 8 h for age 1 mo to 12 yo. Meningitis: 150 mg/kg/day (up to 6 g/day) IV divided q 8 h for age 1 mo to 12 yo; 30 mg/kg IV q 12 h for age younger than 4 weeks old. Use adult dose and formulations for age 12 yo or older.

UNAPPROVED ADULT — P. aeruginosa osteomyelitis of the foot from nail puncture: 2 g IV q 8 h.

UNAPPROVED PEDS — AAP recommends 50 mg/kg IV q 8 to 12 h for age younger than 1 week and wt greater than 2 kg, q 8 h for age 1 week old or older.

NOTES — High levels in renal dysfunction can cause CNS toxicity. Reduce dose in adults with renal dysfunction: Load with 1 g then 500 mg q 48 h for CrCl <5 mL/min; load with 1 g then 500 mg q 24 h for CrCl 6 to 15 mL/min; 1 g IV q 24 h for CrCl 16 to 30 mL/min; 1 g IV q 12 h for CrCl 31 to 50 mL/min. 1 g IV load in hemodialysis patients, then 1 g IV after hemodialysis sessions.

MOA — Beta-lactam antibiotic that inhibits the biosynthesis of cell wall mucopeptide. (Beta-lactam fused to different ring structure from penicillins.)

ADVERSE EFFECTS — Serious: Cross-sensitivity with penicillins, C. difficile-associated diarrhea, CNS toxicity with high levels (esp in renal dysfunction). Frequent: Coombs + anemia, eosinophilia, increased LFTs.

CEFTIBUTEN *(Cedax)* ▸K ♀B ▸? $$$$$

ADULT — Group A streptococcal pharyngitis, acute exacerbation of chronic bronchitis, otitis media not due to S. pneumoniae: 400 mg PO once daily for 10 days.

PEDS — Group A streptococcal pharyngitis, otitis media not due to S. pneumoniae, age 6 mo or older: 9 mg/kg (up to 400 mg) PO once daily for 10 days. Give susp on empty stomach. See otitis media table. For otitis media, AAP recommends 5 to 7 days of therapy for age 6 yo and older with mild to moderate symptoms, 7 days for age 2 to 5 yo with mild to moderate symptoms, and 10 days for age younger than 2 yo and childern with severe symptoms.

FORMS — Generic/Trade: Caps 400 mg. Susp 180 mg/5 mL. Trade only: Susp 90 mg/5 mL.

NOTES — Poor activity against S. aureus and S. pneumoniae. Susp stable for 14 days refrigerated. Reduce dose in adults with renal dysfunction: 100 mg PO daily for CrCl 5 to 29 mL/min; 200 mg PO once daily for CrCl 30 to 49 mL/min. Reduce dose in children with renal dysfunction: 2.25 mg/kg PO once daily for CrCl 5 to 29 mL/min; 4.5 mg/kg PO

(cont.)

CEFTIBUTEN (*cont.*)

once daily for CrCl 30 to 49 mL/min. Hemodialysis: Adults 400 mg PO and children 9 mg/kg PO after each dialysis session.

MOA — Beta-lactam antibiotic that inhibits the biosynthesis of cell wall mucopeptide. (Beta-lactam fused to different ring structure from penicillins.)

ADVERSE EFFECTS — Serious: Cross-sensitivity with penicillins, C. difficile-associated diarrhea. Frequent: Eosinophilia, nausea.

CEFTRIAXONE (*Rocephin*) ▶K/Bile ♀B ▶+ $

WARNING — Contraindicated in neonates who require or may require IV calcium (including in TPN) due to risk of fatal lung/kidney precipitation of ceftriaxone-calcium. In other patients, do not give ceftriaxone and calcium-containing IV solns simultaneously; sequential administration is acceptable if lines are flushed with a compatible fluid between infusions. Do not dilute with Ringer's/Hartmann's soln or TPN containing calcium.

ADULT — Pneumonia, UTI, pelvic inflammatory disease (hospitalized), sepsis, meningitis, skin, bone and joint, intra-abdominal infections: Usual dose 1 to 2 g IM/IV q 24 h (max 4 g/day divided q 12 h; max 2 g/day in elderly). Gonorrhea 250 mg IM plus azithromycin 1 g PO both single dose. See STD table.

PEDS — Meningitis: 100 mg/kg/day (up to 4 g/day) IV divided q 12 to 24 h. Skin, pneumonia, other serious infections: 50 to 75 mg/kg/day (up to 2 g/day) IM/IV divided q 12 to 24 h. Otitis media: 50 mg/kg (up to 1 g) IM single dose. See otitis media table.

UNAPPROVED ADULT — Lyme disease carditis, meningitis: 2 g IV once daily for 14 days. Chancroid: 250 mg IM single dose. Disseminated gonorrhea: 1 g IM/IV q 24 h. Prophylaxis, invasive meningococcal disease: 250 mg IM single dose.

UNAPPROVED PEDS — Otitis media, if initial antibiotic fails (at 48 to 72 h): 50 mg/kg IM q day for 3 days. Otitis media, initial treatment if penicillin allergy: 50 mg/kg IM q day for 1 or 3 days. See tables for acute sinusitis and otitis media. Lyme disease carditis, meningitis: 50 to 75 mg/kg IM/IV once daily (up to 2 g/day) for 14 days. Prophylaxis, invasive meningococcal disease: Single IM dose of 125 mg for age younger than 16 yo, 250 mg for age 16 yo or older. Gonorrhea: 25 to 50 mg/kg IV/IM (max of 125 mg IM) single dose; use adult regimens in STD table if wt 45 kg or greater. Gonococcal bacteremia/ arthritis: 50 mg/kg (max 1 g) IM/IV once daily for 7 days if wt 45 kg or less; 1 g IM/IV once daily for 7 days if wt greater than 45 kg. Gonococcal ophthalmia neonatorum/gonorrhea prophylaxis in newborn: 25 to 50 mg/kg up to 125 mg IM/IV single dose at birth. Disseminated gonorrhea, infants: 25 to 50 mg/kg/day IM/IV once daily for 7 days; treat for 10 to 14 days if meningitis documented. Typhoid fever: 50 to 75 mg/kg IM/IV once daily for 14 days.

NOTES — Can cause prolonged prothrombin time (due to vitamin K deficiency), biliary sludging/symptoms of gallbladder disease. Do not give to neonates with hyperbilirubinemia. Dilute in 1% lidocaine for IM use. Do not exceed 2 g/day in patients with both hepatic and renal dysfunction.

MOA — Beta-lactam antibiotic that inhibits the biosynthesis of cell wall mucopeptide. (Beta-lactam fused to different ring structure from penicillins.)

ADVERSE EFFECTS — Serious: Cross-sensitivity with penicillins, C. difficile-associated diarrhea, prolonged prothrombin time due to vitamin K deficiency, biliary sludging/symptoms of gallbladder disease, hemolytic anemia. Fatal precipitation with calcium in lungs/kidneys of neonates. Frequent: Eosinophilia.

ANTIMICROBIALS: Cephalosporins—4th Generation

NOTE: Cross-sensitivity with penicillins possible. May cause C. difficile–associated diarrhea.

***AVYCAZ* (ceftazidime-avibactam)** ▶K ♀?/?/? ▶? $$$$$

ADULT — Complicated intra-abdominal infection (in combination with metronidazole), complicated UTI, pyelonephritis: 2.5 g IV q 8 h infused over 2 h. Treat abdominal infections for 5 to 14 days, UTI for 7 to 14 days.

PEDS — Safety and efficacy not established in children.

NOTES — Avycaz 2.5 g = 2 g ceftazidime + 0.5 g avibactam. Contraindicated in patients with a history of serious beta-lactam hypersensitivity. Can cause C. difficile–associated diarrhea. In clinical trial of complicated intra-abdominal infection, Avycaz + metronidazole had lower cure rate than meropenem in patients with moderate renal impairment (CrCl 30 to 50 mL/min), but they received 33% lower dose than currently recommended. Monitor CrCl at least daily in patients with changing renal function and adjust dose as needed. Dosage reduction for renal dysfunction: 1.25 g IV q 8 h for CrCl 31 to 50 mL/min; 0.94 g IV q 12 h for CrCl 16 to 30 mL/min; 0.94 g IV q 24 h for CrCl 6 to 15 mL/min; 0.94 g IV q 48 h for CrCl <5 mL/min. Give after dialysis on hemodialysis days.

MOA — Ceftazidime is a beta-lactam antibiotic (different ring structure than penicillins) that inhibits penicillin-binding proteins involved in the synthesis of bacterial cell wall mucopeptides. Avibactam is a non-beta-lactam beta-lactamase inhibitor that inhibits some extended-spectrum beta-lactamases (TEM, SHV, CTX-M, KPCs, AmpC, and certain oxacillinases).

ADVERSE EFFECTS — Serious: Cross-sensitivity with penicillins (rare); hypersensitivity including anaphylaxis and severe skin reactions; C. difficile-associated diarrhea; CNS toxicity (esp in renal dysfunction); eosinophilia; increased LFTs. Frequent: N/V, constipation, anxiety, abdominal pain, dizziness. Other: Seroconversion to (+) direct Coombs test.

CEFEPIME (*Maxipime*) ▸K ♀B ▸? $$$$
ADULT — Mild, moderate UTI: 0.5 to 1 g IM/IV q 12 h. Severe UTI, skin, complicated intra-abdominal infections: 2 g IV q 12 h. Pneumonia: 1 to 2 g IV q 12 h. Empiric therapy of febrile neutropenia: 2 g IV q 8 h.
PEDS — UTI, skin infections, pneumonia: 50 mg/kg IV q 12 h for wt 40 kg or less. Empiric therapy for febrile neutropenia: 50 mg/kg IV q 8 h for wt 40 kg or less. Do not exceed adult dose.
UNAPPROVED ADULT — P. aeruginosa osteomyelitis of the foot from nail puncture: 2 g IV q 12 h. Meningitis: 2 g IV q 8 h.
UNAPPROVED PEDS — Meningitis, cystic fibrosis, other serious infections: 50 mg/kg IV q 8 h (max of 6 g/day).
NOTES — An FDA safety review did not find higher mortality with cefepime than with other beta-lactams. High levels in renal dysfunction can cause CNS toxicity including seizures; dosing for CrCl <60 mL/min in package insert. Hemodialysis: 1 g on Day 1, the 500 mg q 24 h; 1 g q 24 h for febrile neutropenia. Give doses after dialysis.
MOA — Beta-lactam antibiotic that inhibits the biosynthesis of cell wall mucopeptide. (Beta-lactam fused to different ring structure from penicillins.)
ADVERSE EFFECTS — Serious: Cross-sensitivity with penicillins, C. difficile-associated diarrhea, CNS toxicity (encephalopathy, myoclonus, seizures) due to high levels of cefepime, especially in patients with renal dysfunction. An FDA safety review did not find higher mortality with cefepime than with other beta lactams. Frequent: Coombs + anemia.

ZERBAXA (ceftolozane-tazobactam) ▸K ♀B ▸? $$$$$
ADULT — Complicated intra-abdominal infections (in combination with metronidazole), complicated UTI, pyelonephritis: 1.5 g IV q 8 h infused over 1 h.
PEDS — Safety and efficacy not established in children.
NOTES — Zerbaxa 1.5 g = 1 g ceftolozane + 0.5 g tazobactam. Contraindicated in patients with a history of serious beta-lactam hypersensitivity. Can cause C. difficile–associated diarrhea. In complicated intra-abdominal infections, Zerbaxa + metronidazole had lower cure rates than meropenem in patients who were elderly or had moderate renal impairment (CrCl 30 to 50 mL/min). Monitor CrCl at least daily in patients with changing renal function and adjust dose as needed. Dosage adjustment for renal dysfunction: 750 mg IV q 8 h for CrCl 30 to 50 mL/min; 375 mg IV q 8 h for CrCl 15 to 29 mL/min; single loading dose of 750 mg IV followed by 150 mg IV q 8 h for ESRD or hemodialysis. For hemodialysis patients, give at the earliest possible time after dialysis session ends.
MOA — Ceftolozane is a beta-lactam antibiotic that inhibits penicillin-binding proteins involved in bacterial cell wall synthesis. It is structurally similar to ceftazidime, with a side chain that enhances anti-pseudomonal activity. Tazobactam is a beta-lactamase inhibitor.
ADVERSE EFFECTS — Frequent: Nausea, diarrhea, headache, fever.

ANTIMICROBIALS: Cephalosporins—5th Generation

NOTE: Cephalosporins can be cross-sensitive with penicillins and can cause C. difficile associated diarrhea.

CEFTAROLINE (*Teflaro*) ▸K ♀B ▸? $$$$$
ADULT — Community-acquired pneumonia, skin infections: 600 mg IV q12 h infused over 5 to 60 minutes. Treat pneumonia for 5 to 7 days, skin infections for 5 to 14 days.
PEDS — Community-acquired pneumonia, skin infections. Age 2 mo to less than 2 yo: 8 mg/kg IV q 8 h. Age 2 yo and older: 12 mg/kg IV q 8 h for wt 33 kg or less; 400 mg IV q 8 h or 600 mg IV q 12 h for wt greater than 33 kg. Treat for 5 to 14 days.
NOTES — Direct Coombs' test seroconversion reported; hemolytic anemia is possible. Dosage reduction for renal dysfunction in adults: 400 mg IV q 12 h for CrCl 31 to 50 mL/min; 300 mg IV q 12 h for CrCl 15 to 30 mL/min; 200 mg IV q 12 h for ESRD including hemodialysis.
MOA — Beta-lactam antibiotic that inhibits the biosynthesis of cell wall mucopeptide. (Beta-lactam fused to different ring structure from penicillins).
ADVERSE EFFECTS — Serious: Serious: Cross-sensitivity with penicillins, C. difficile associated diarrhea. Coombs + anemia possible. Frequent: Diarrhea, nausea, rash.

ANTIMICROBIALS: Glycopeptides

DALBAVANCIN (*Dalvance*) ▸K ♀?/?/? ▸? $$$$$
ADULT — Gram-positive skin infections, including MRSA: Single dose of 1500 mg IV infused over 30 minutes or 1000 mg followed 1 week later by 500 mg.
PEDS — Safety and efficacy not established in children.
NOTES — "Red Neck" (or "Red Man") syndrome with rapid IV administration. Dosage adjustment for CrCl <30 mL/min: Single dose of 1125 mg IV infused over 30 minutes or 750 mg IV followed 1 week later by 375 mg if not receiving regular hemodialysis. Not removed by hemodialysis; dosage adjustment not required and can give without regard to timing of hemodialysis session.
MOA — Bacteriocidal lipoglycopeptide derived from teicoplanin that inhibits synthesis of cell wall peptidoglycan polymers.
SIDE EFFECTS — Serious: Anaphylaxis, skin reactions, increased ALT, C. difficile–associated

(cont.)

DALBAVANCIN (*cont.*)

diarrhea. "Red Neck" (or "Red Man") syndrome with rapid IV administration. Frequent: Nausea, headache, diarrhea.

ORITAVANCIN (*Orbactiv*) ▶K feces ♀C ▶? $$$$$

ADULT — Gram-positive skin infections, including MRSA: 1200 mg IV single dose infused over 3 h.

PEDS — Not approved for use in children.

NOTES — Can artificially increase aPTT for up to 120 h, PT and INR up to 12 h, activated clotting time up to 24 h, and D-dimer for up to 72 h. Do not give IV unfractionated heparin for 120 h after oritavancin dose. Can increase warfarin exposure; INR monitoring inaccurate for 12 h after oritavancin dose; coadministration with warfarin is a risk vs. benefit decision. Can cause infusion reactions; slow or hold infusion if reaction develops. Hypersensitivity reactions. Cross-sensitivity with other glycopeptide antibiotics possible; monitor for hypersensitivity symptoms during infusion in patients with a history of glycopeptide allergy. Half-life of oritavancin is approximately 10 days. Risk of osteomyelitis higher with oritavancin than vancomycin in premarketing study; monitor for signs/symptoms of osteomyelitis. Incompatible with NS; flush IV line with D5W only. No dosage adjustment for mild to moderate hepatic or renal impairment.

MOA — Bacteriocidal lipoglycopeptide that is a vancomycin analog; inhibits 3 steps in synthesis of cell wall peptidoglycan polymers.

ADVERSE EFFECTS — Hypersensitivity reactions (median onset of 1.2 days and duration of 2.4 days in clinical trials). Infusion reactions (pruritus, urticaria, flushing). C. difficile-associated diarrhea. Frequent: Headache, N/V, diarrhea, limb and SC abcesses.

TELAVANCIN (*Vibativ*) ▶K ♀C ▶? $$$$$

WARNING — In patients with CrCl ≤50 mL/min treated for hospital-acquired/ventilator-associated pneumonia, mortality was higher with telavancin than vancomycin. Do not use if CrCl ≤50 mL/min unless potential benefit outweighs risk. Nephrotoxic; monitor renal function in all patients. Teratogenic in animal studies. Get serum pregnancy test before use in women of child-bearing potential. Do not use in pregnancy unless potential benefit outweighs risk.

ADULT — Complicated skin infections including MRSA: 10 mg/kg IV once daily for 7 to 14 days. Hospital-acquired/ventilator-associated S. aureus pneumonia (not first-line): 10 mg/kg IV once daily for 7 to 21 days. Infuse over 1 h.

PEDS — Safety and efficacy not established in children.

NOTES — QT interval prolongation; do not use in congenital long QT syndrome, uncompensated heart failure, or severe left ventricular hypertrophy. Caution advised for coadministration with other drugs that prolong QT interval. Interferes with phospholipid-based coagulation tests (PTT, INR, aPTT, activated clotting time, coagulation-based factor X activity assay) for up to 18 h after telavancin dose,

but does not affect coagulation. Coadministration of unfractionated heparin is contraindicated because of interference with aPTT. Draw blood for INR, aPTT, clotting time, and factor Xa right before next telavancin dose or use alternative test unaffected by telavancin. Use IV solution within 4 h when stored at room temp. Nephrotoxicity; monitor renal function at least q 2 to 3 days. Efficacy may be decreased in patients with baseline CrCl ≤50 mL/min. Cyclodextrin vehicle may accumulate in renal dysfunction. Dosage adjustment for renal dysfunction in adults: 7.5 mg/kg IV q 24 h for CrCl 30 to 50 mL/min; 10 mg/kg q 48 h for CrCl 10 to 29 mL/min.

MOA — Bactericidal glycopeptide derivative of vancomycin that inhibits synthesis of cell wall peptidoglycan polymers. May also have other mechanisms of action.

ADVERSE EFFECTS — Serious: Nephrotoxicity (may be increased by NSAIDs, ACE inhibitors, loop diuretics); QT interval prolongation. Frequent: N/V, rash, foamy urine, metallic/soapy taste disturbance. May cause "Red Neck" (or "Red Man") syndrome with rapid IV administration.

VANCOMYCIN (*Vancocin*) ▶K ♀C ▶? $$$$$

ADULT — Severe staph infections (including MRSA), endocarditis: 1 g IV q 12 h, each dose over 1 h or 30 mg/kg/day IV divided q 12 h. Empiric therapy, native valve endocarditis: 15 mg/kg (up to 2 g/day unless levels monitored) IV q 12 h with gentamicin. See table for prophylaxis of bacterial endocarditis. Infuse over 1 h; infuse over 1.5 to 2 h if dose greater than 1 g; slow infusion rate and premedicate with antihistamines to reduce "Red Man" syndrome symptoms. C. difficile–associated diarrhea: 125 mg PO four times per day for 10 days. IV administration ineffective for this indication. See table for management of C. difficile infection in adults, including higher dose of vancomycin plus metronidazole for severe complicated disease. Staphylococcal enterocolitis: 500 to 2000 mg/day PO divided three to four times per day for 7 to 10 days.

PEDS — Severe staph infections (including MRSA), endocarditis: 15 mg/kg IV load, then 10 mg/kg q 12 h for age younger than 1 week; 15 mg/kg IV load, then 10 mg/kg q 8 h for age 1 week to 1 mo; 10 mg/kg IV q 6 h for age older than 1 mo. Infuse over 1 h; infuse over 1.5 to 2 h if dose greater than 1 g; slow infusion rate and premedicate with antihistamines to reduce "Red Man" syndrome symptoms. C. difficile–associated diarrhea: 40 mg/kg/day (up to 2 g/day) PO divided four times per day for 10 days. IV administration ineffective for this indication.

UNAPPROVED ADULT — Usual dose: 15 to 20 mg/kg IV q 8 to 12 h. Consider loading dose of 25 to 30 mg/kg for severe infections. Infuse over 1 h; infuse over 1.5 to 2 h if dose greater than 1 g. Base IV dose on absolute body wt. In obese patients, base initial dose on absolute body wt, then adjust dose based on trough levels. C. difficile–associated diarrhea: 125 mg PO four times per day for 10 to 14 days. See table for management of C. difficile infection

(cont.)

VANCOMYCIN (*cont.*)

in adults, including higher dose of vancomycin plus metronidazole for severe complicated disease. Prevention of perinatal group B streptococcal disease: Give to mother 1 g IV q 12 h from onset of labor/after membrane rupture until delivery.

UNAPPROVED PEDS — Newborns: 10 to 15 mg/kg IV q 8 to 12 h for age younger than 1 week; 10 to 15 mg/kg IV q 6 to 8 h for age 1 week and older. Bacterial meningitis: 60 mg/kg/day IV divided q 6 h. Nonmeningeal pneumococcal infections: 40 to 45 mg/kg/day IV divided q 6 h.

FORMS — Generic/Trade: Caps 125, 250 mg. Pharmacist can compound oral liquid from IV formulation.

NOTES — Maintain trough higher than 10 mg/L in all patients to avoid development of resistance; optimal trough for complicated infections is 15 to 20 mg/L. Draw trough just before the next dose after steady state is reached (usually after 4th dose). Monitoring of peak levels no longer recommended. "Red Man" syndrome with rapid IV administration (slow infusion rate and premedicate with antihistamine to reduce), vein irritation with IV extravasation, reversible neutropenia, ototoxicity, or nephrotoxicity rarely. Enhanced effects of neuromuscular blockers. Use caution with other ototoxic/nephrotoxic drugs. Piperacillin-tazobactam may increase the risk of acute kidney injury; monitor renal function if coadministered. Individualize dose if renal dysfunction. Oral vancomycin poorly absorbed; do not use for extraluminal infections.

MOA — Bactericidal glycopeptide that inhibits synthesis of cell wall peptidoglycan polymers. May also have other mechanisms of action.

ADVERSE EFFECTS — Serious: Reversible neutropenia, ototoxicity (rare and reversible with monotherapy) or nephrotoxicity (rare; risk may be increased by high doses, poor renal function, old age, or nephrotoxic drug), superinfection, IgE-mediated hypersensitivity (rare). Can cause C. difficile-associated diarrhea. Frequent: "Red Man" syndrome with rapid IV administration due to non-IgE-mediated histamine release, vein irritation with IV extravasation.

ANTIMICROBIALS: Macrolides

AZITHROMYCIN (*Zithromax, Zmax*) ▶L ♀B ▶? $$

ADULT — Community-acquired pneumonia including Legionella, inpatient: 500 mg IV over 1 h daily for at least 2 days, then 500 mg PO daily for 7 to 10 days total. Pelvic inflammatory disease: 500 mg IV daily for 1 to 2 days, then 250 mg PO daily to complete 7 days. Oral for acute exacerbation of chronic bronchitis, community-acquired pneumonia, group A streptococcal pharyngitis (2nd line to penicillin), skin infections: 500 mg PO on 1st day, then 250 mg PO daily for 4 days. Acute sinusitis, alternative for acute exacerbation of chronic bronchitis: 500 mg PO daily for 3 days. Zmax for community-acquired pneumonia, acute sinusitis: 2 g PO single dose (contents of full bottle) on empty stomach. Azithromycin is a poor option for acute sinusitis due to pneumococcal and H. influenzae resistance; see acute sinusitis treatment table for alternatives. Chlamydia (including pregnancy), chancroid: 1 g PO single dose. Gonorrhea: See STD table. Prevention of disseminated Mycobacterium avium complex disease: 1200 mg PO once per week.

PEDS — Azithromycin is a poor option for otitis media and acute sinusitis due to pneumococcal and H. influenzae resistance; see otitis media and acute sinusitis treatment tables for alternatives. Oral for otitis media, community-acquired pneumonia: 10 mg/kg up to 500 mg PO on 1st day, then 5 mg/kg up to 250 mg PO daily for 4 days. Acute sinusitis: 10 mg/kg PO daily for 3 days. Zmax for community-acquired pneumonia, acute sinusitis: 60 mg/kg (max 2 g) PO single dose on empty stomach for age 6 mo or older; give adult dose of 2 g for wt 34 kg or greater. Otitis media: 30 mg/kg PO single dose or 10 mg/kg PO daily for 3 days. Group A streptococcal pharyngitis (2nd line to penicillin): 12 mg/kg up to 500 mg PO daily for 5 days. Take susp on empty stomach.

UNAPPROVED ADULT — See table for prophylaxis of bacterial endocarditis. Nongonococcal urethritis: 1 g PO single dose. See STD table for recurrent/persistent urethritis. Campylobacter gastroenteritis: 500 mg PO daily for 3 days. For HIV-infected patients, treat mild/moderate disease for 7 to 10 days (not for bacteremia in HIV-infected patients). Traveler's diarrhea: 500 mg PO on 1st day, then 250 mg PO daily for 4 days; or 1 g PO single dose. Mycobacterium avium complex disease in AIDS, treatment: 500 mg PO daily (use at least 2 drugs for active infection). Pertussis treatment/postexposure prophylaxis: 500 mg PO on 1st day, then 250 mg PO daily for 4 days. Cholera: 1 g PO single dose (use this regimen in pregnancy).

UNAPPROVED PEDS — Prevention of disseminated Mycobacterium avium complex disease: 20 mg/kg PO once per week not to exceed adult dose. Mycobacterium avium complex disease treatment: 5 mg/kg PO daily (use at least 2 drugs for active infection). Cystic fibrosis patients colonized with P. aeruginosa, age 6 yo and older: 250 mg three days per week for 24 weeks for wt less than 40 kg, 500 mg PO three days per week for 24 weeks for wt 40 kg or greater. Chlamydia trachomatis: 1 g PO single dose for age younger than 8 yo and wt greater than 44 kg, and for age 8 yo or older for any wt. Chlamydia infant pneumonia: 20 mg/kg PO once daily for 3 days. Pertussis treatment/postexposure prophylaxis: 10 mg/kg PO once daily for 5 days for infants younger than 6 mo; 10 mg/kg (max 500 mg) PO single dose on day 1, then 5 mg/kg (up

(cont.)

AZITHROMYCIN (*cont.*)

to 250 mg) PO once daily for 4 days for age 6 mo or older. See table for bacterial endocarditis prophylaxis. Traveler's diarrhea: 5 to 10 mg/kg PO single dose. Cholera: 20 mg/kg up to 1 g PO single dose.

FORMS — Generic/Trade: Tabs 250, 500, 600 mg. Susp 100, 200 mg/5 mL. Packet 1000 mg. Z-Pak: #6, 250 mg tab. Tri-Pak: #3, 500 mg tab. Trade only: Extended-release oral susp (Zmax): 2 g in 60 mL single-dose bottle.

NOTES — Severe allergic/skin reactions rarely, IV site reactions, hearing loss with prolonged use, hepatotoxicity, exacerbation of myasthenia gravis. Can prolong QT interval and cause torsades. Consider risk vs benefit in at-risk patients: those with history of QT interval prolongation or torsades, uncompensated heart failure, ongoing proarrhythmic conditions such as uncorrected hypokalemia or hypomagnesemia, clinically significant bradycardia, or coadministration of Class IA or III antiarrhythmic drug. Azithromycin had additive dose-dependent QT interval prolongation with chloroquine. Does not inhibit CYP enzymes. Do not take at the same time as Al/magnesium antacids (except Zmax which can be taken with antacids). Monitor INR with warfarin. Zmax: Store at room temperature and use within 12 h of reconstitution. Additional treatment required if vomiting occurs within 5 min of dose; consider for vomiting within 1 h of dose; unnecessary for vomiting more than 1 h after dose.

MOA — Inhibits protein synthesis in susceptible organisms by interfering with function of ribosomal 50s subunit. Mechanism of action in cystic fibrosis is unknown; macrolides may inhibit P. aeruginosa virulence factors or reduce inflammation.

ADVERSE EFFECTS — Serious: Allergic/skin reactions including prolonged cases of DRESS (rare), IV site reactions, hearing loss with prolonged use, hepatotoxicity, exacerbation of myasthenia gravis. Frequent: GI complaints, diarrhea, N/V most common with single-dose and 3-day regimens.

CLARITHROMYCIN (*Biaxin*) ▶KL ♀C ▶? $$$

ADULT — Group A streptococcal pharyngitis (2nd-line to penicillin): 250 mg PO two times per day for 10 days. Acute exacerbation of chronic bronchitis (S. pneumoniae/M. catarrhalis), community-acquired pneumonia, skin infections: 250 mg PO two times per day for 7 to 14 days. Acute exacerbation of chronic bronchitis (H. influenzae): 500 mg PO two times per day for 7 to 14 days. H. pylori: See table in GI section. Mycobacterium avium complex disease prevention/treatment: 500 mg PO two times per day. Treat active mycobacterial infections with at least 2 drugs. Acute sinusitis: 500 mg PO two times per day for 14 days. Clarithromycin is a poor option for acute sinusitis due to pneumococcal and H. influenzae resistance; see acute sinusitis treatment table for alternatives.

PEDS — Group A streptococcal pharyngitis (2nd-line to penicillin), community-acquired pneumonia, sinusitis, otitis media, skin infections: 7.5 mg/kg PO two times per day for 10 days. Clarithromycin is a poor option for acute sinusitis and otitis media due to pneumococcal and H. influenzae resistance; see acute sinusitis and otitis media treatment tables for alternatives. Mycobacterium avium complex prevention/treatment: 7.5 mg/kg up to 500 mg PO two times per day. Two or more drugs are needed for the treatment of active mycobacterial infections.

UNAPPROVED ADULT — Pertussis treatment/postexposure prophylaxis: 500 mg PO two times per day for 7 days. Community-acquired pneumonia: 500 mg PO two times per day. See table for prophylaxis of bacterial endocarditis.

UNAPPROVED PEDS — Pertussis treatment/postexposure prophylaxis (age 1 mo or older): 7.5 mg/kg (up to 500 mg) PO two times per day for 7 days. See table for prophylaxis of bacterial endocarditis.

FORMS — Generic/Trade: Tabs 250, 500 mg. Extended-release tabs 500 mg. Susp 125, 250 mg/5 mL.

NOTES — Can cause or exacerbate myasthenia gravis. Can prolong QT interval and cause torsades. Avoid in patients with history of QT prolongation or ventricular arrhythmia, ongoing proarrhythmic conditions such as uncorrected hypokalemia or hypomagnesemia, clinically significant bradycardia, or coadministration of Class IA or Class III antiarrhythmic drugs. Strong CYP3A4 inhibitor. Many drug interactions including increased levels of carbamazepine, cyclosporine, digoxin, disopyramide (monitor ECG), lovastatin (avoid), quetiapine, quinidine (monitor ECG), rifabutin, simvastatin (avoid), tacrolimus, theophylline. Risk of hypotension and acute renal injury with calcium channel blockers, esp nifedipine. Toxicity with ergotamine, dihydroergotamine, or colchicine (reduce colchicine dose; contraindicated if renal/hepatic impairment). Reduce dose of sildenafil, tadalafil, tolterodine, vardenafil. Monitor INR with warfarin. Clarithromycin levels decreased by efavirenz (avoid concomitant use) and nevirapine enough to impair efficacy in Mycobacterium avium complex disease. Reduce clarithromycin dose by 50% if given with atazanavir; consider alternative for indications other than Mycobacterium avium complex. Dosage reduction for renal insufficiency in patients taking ritonavir, lopinavir-ritonavir (Kaletra), or ritonavir-boosted darunavir, fosamprenavir, saquinavir, or tipranavir: Decrease dose by 75% for CrCl <30 mL/min, decrease dose by 50% for CrCl 30 to 60 mL/min. Do not refrigerate susp.

MOA — Inhibits protein synthesis in susceptible organisms by interfering with function of ribosomal 50s subunit.

ADVERSE EFFECTS — Serious: Myasthenia gravis. Rare arrhythmias in patients with prolonged QT. Increased mortality reported 1 year after 2-week course of clarithromycin for prevention of cardiovascular mortality in patients with stable CHD. Frequent: Diarrhea, metallic taste.

ERYTHROMYCIN BASE (*Ery-Tab, PCE, ✳Eryc*) ▶L ♀B ▶+ $$$$

ADULT — Respiratory, skin infections: 250 to 500 mg PO four times per day or 333 mg PO three times per day. Pertussis, treatment/postexposure prophylaxis: 500 mg PO q 6 h for 14 days. S. aureus skin infections: 250 mg PO q 6 h or 500 mg PO q 12 h. Secondary prevention of rheumatic fever: 250 mg PO two times per day. Chlamydia in pregnancy, nongonococcal urethritis: 500 mg PO four times per day for 7 days. Alternative for chlamydia in pregnancy if high dose not tolerated: 250 mg PO four times per day for 14 days. Erythrasma: 250 mg PO three times per day for 21 days. Legionnaires' disease: 2 g/day PO in divided doses for 14 to 21 days.

PEDS — Usual dose: 30 to 50 mg/kg/day PO divided four times per day for 10 days. Can double dose for severe infections. Pertussis: 40 to 50 mg/kg/day PO divided four times per day for 14 days (azithromycin preferred for age younger than 1 mo due to risk of hypertrophic pyloric stenosis with erythromycin). Chlamydia: 50 mg/kg/day PO divided four times per day for 14 days for wt less than 45 kg.

UNAPPROVED ADULT — Chancroid: 500 mg PO three times per day for 7 days. Campylobacter gastroenteritis: 500 mg PO two times per day for 5 days.

FORMS — Generic only: Tabs 250, 500 mg. Delayed-release caps 250 mg. Trade only: Delayed-release tabs (Ery-Tab, PCE) 250, 333, 500 mg.

NOTES — Can prolong QT interval and cause torsades. Avoid if QT interval prolonged, uncorrected hypokalemia or hypomagnesemia, clinically significant bradycardia, or coadministration of Class IA or III antiarrhythmic drug. Incidence of sudden death may be increased when erythromycin is combined with potent CYP3A4 inhibitors. Exacerbation of myasthenia gravis. Hypertrophic pyloric stenosis in infants primarily younger than 1 mo. CYP3A4 and 1A2 inhibitor. Many drug interactions including increased levels of carbamazepine, cyclosporine, digoxin, tacrolimus, theophylline, some benzodiazepines and statins (avoid simvastatin and lovastatin). Monitor INR with warfarin.

MOA — Inhibits protein synthesis in susceptible organisms by interfering with function of ribosomal 50s subunit.

ADVERSE EFFECTS — Serious: Arrhythmias in patients with prolonged QT (rare), aggravation of myasthenia gravis, hypertrophic pyloric stenosis in infants primarily younger than 1 month old. Incidence of sudden death may be increased when erythromycin is combined with potent CYP 3A4 inhibitors. Frequent: N/V, diarrhea.

ERYTHROMYCIN ETHYL SUCCINATE (*EES, EryPed*) ▶L ♀B ▶+ $

ADULT — Usual dose: 400 mg PO four times per day. Nongonococcal urethritis: 800 mg PO four times per day for 7 days. Chlamydia in pregnancy: 800 mg PO four times per day for 7 days or 400 mg PO four times per day for 14 days if high dose not tolerated. Secondary prevention of rheumatic fever: 400 mg PO two times per day. Legionnaires' disease: 3.2 g/day PO in divided doses for 14 to 21 days.

PEDS — Usual dose: 30 to 50 mg/kg/day PO divided four times per day. Max dose: 100 mg/kg/day. Group A streptococcal pharyngitis: 40 mg/kg/day (up to 1 g/day) PO divided two to four times per day for 10 days. Secondary prevention of rheumatic fever: 400 mg PO two times per day. Pertussis: 40 to 50 mg/kg/day (up to 2 g/day) PO divided four times per day for 14 days.

FORMS — Generic/Trade: Tabs 400 mg. Trade only: Susp 200, 400 mg/5 mL.

NOTES — Can prolong QT interval and cause torsades. Avoid if QT interval prolonged, uncorrected hypokalemia or hypomagnesemia, clinically significant bradycardia, or coadministration of Class IA or III antiarrhythmic drug. Incidence of sudden death may be increased when erythromycin is combined with potent CYP3A4 inhibitors. May aggravate myasthenia gravis. Hypertrophic pyloric stenosis primarily in infants younger than 1 mo. CYP3A4 and 1A2 inhibitor. Many drug interactions including increased levels of carbamazepine, cyclosporine, digoxin, tacrolimus, theophylline, some benzodiazepines and statins (avoid simvastatin and lovastatin). Monitor INR with warfarin.

MOA — Inhibits protein synthesis in susceptible organisms by interfering with function of ribosomal 50s subunit.

ADVERSE EFFECTS — Serious: Arrhythmias in patients with prolonged QT (rare), aggravation of myasthenia gravis, hypertrophic pyloric stenosis primarily in infants younger than 1 month old. Coadministration of strong CYP 3A4 inhibitor with erythromycin may increase risk of sudden death. Frequent: N/V, diarrhea.

ERYTHROMYCIN LACTOBIONATE (*Erythrocin IV*) ▶L ♀B ▶+ $$$$$

ADULT — For severe infections/PO not possible: 15 to 20 mg/kg/day (up to 4 g/day) IV divided q 6 h. Legionella pneumonia: 4 g/day IV divided q 6 h.

PEDS — For severe infections/PO not possible: 15 to 20 mg/kg/day (up to 4 g/day) IV divided q 6 h.

UNAPPROVED PEDS — 20 to 50 mg/kg/day IV divided q 6 h.

NOTES — Dilute and give slowly to minimize venous irritation. Reversible hearing loss (increased risk in elderly given 4 g or more per day), allergic reactions, exacerbation of myasthenia gravis. Can prolong QT interval and cause torsades. Avoid if QT interval prolonged, uncorrected hypokalemia or hypomagnesemia, clinically significant bradycardia, or coadministration of Class IA or III antiarrhythmic drug. Incidence of sudden death may be increased when erythromycin is combined with potent CYP3A4 inhibitors. Hypertrophic pyloric stenosis primarily in infants younger than 1 mo. CYP3A4 and 1A2 inhibitor. Many drug interactions including increased levels of carbamazepine, cyclosporine, digoxin, disopyramide, tacrolimus, theophylline, some

(cont.)

ERYTHROMYCIN LACTOBIONATE (*cont.*)

benzodiazepines and statins (avoid simvastatin and lovastatin). Monitor INR with warfarin.

MOA — Inhibits protein synthesis in susceptible organisms by interfering with function of ribosomal 50s subunit.

ADVERSE EFFECTS — Serious: Arrhythmias in patients with prolonged QT (rare), aggravation of myasthenia gravis, hypertrophic pyloric stenosis primarily in infants younger than 1 month old, reversible hearing loss with high doses (increased risk in elderly given 4 g/day or more), allergic reactions, venous irritation. Incidence of sudden death may be increased when erythromycin is combined with potent CYP3A4 inhibitors. Frequent: N/V, diarrhea.

FIDAXOMICIN (*Dificid*) ▶minimal absorption ♀B ▶? $$$$$

ADULT — C. difficile–associated diarrhea: 200 mg PO two times per day for 10 days.

PEDS — Safety and efficacy not established in children.

FORMS — Trade only: 200 mg tabs.

NOTES — Not for systemic infections. Only treats C. difficile–associated diarrhea.

MOA — Poorly absorbed macrolide that inhibits RNA synthesis by RNA polymerases. Bacteriocidal against C difficile.

ADVERSE EFFECTS — Serious: GI bleeding; acute hypersensitivity reactions (possible cross-reactivity with other macrolides). Frequent: N/V, abdominal pain.

ANTIMICROBIALS: Penicillins—1st Generation—Natural

PENICILLINS — GENERAL ANTIMICROBIAL SPECTRUM

1st generation	Most streptococci; oral anaerobic coverage
2nd generation	Most streptococci; *S. aureus* (but not MRSA)
3rd generation	Most streptococci; basic Gram-negative coverage
4th generation	*Pseudomonas*

NOTE: Anaphylaxis occurs rarely with penicillins; cross-sensitivity with cephalosporins is possible.

BENZATHINE PENICILLIN (*Bicillin L-A*) ▶K ♀B ▶? $$$

WARNING — Not for IV administration, which can cause cardiorespiratory arrest and death.

ADULT — Group A streptococcal pharyngitis: 1.2 million units IM single dose. Secondary prevention of rheumatic fever: 1.2 million units IM q month (q 3 weeks for high-risk patients) or 600,000 units IM q 2 weeks. Primary, secondary, early latent syphilis: 2.4 million units IM single dose. Tertiary (with normal CSF exam), late latent syphilis: 2.4 million units IM q week for 3 doses.

PEDS — Group A streptococcal pharyngitis (AHA regimen): 600,000 units IM for wt 27 kg or less; 1.2 million units IM for wt greater than 27 kg. Secondary prevention of rheumatic fever: 600,000 units IM for wt 27 kg or less; 1.2 million units IM for wt greater than 27 kg; give q month (q 3 weeks for high-risk patients). Primary, secondary, early latent syphilis: 50,000 units/kg (up to 2.4 million units) IM single dose. Late latent syphilis: 50,000 units/kg (up to 2.4 million units) IM for 3 weekly doses.

UNAPPROVED ADULT — Prophylaxis of diphtheria/ treatment of carriers: 1.2 million units IM single dose.

UNAPPROVED PEDS — Prophylaxis of diphtheria/ treatment of carriers: 1.2 million units IM single dose for wt 30 kg or greater; 600,000 units IM single dose for wt less than 30 kg.

FORMS — Trade only: For IM use, 600,000 units/mL; 1, 2, 4 mL syringes.

NOTES — Do not give IV. Doses last 2 to 4 weeks. Not for neurosyphilis. IM injection less painful if warmed to room temp before giving.

MOA — Beta-lactam antibiotic that inhibits the biosynthesis of cell wall mucopeptide.

ADVERSE EFFECTS — Serious: Anaphylaxis (rare), cross-sensitivity with cephalosporins, transient CNS reactions (Hoigne's syndrome), Coombs + hemolytic anemia. Frequent: Allergy.

BICILLIN C-R (procaine penicillin + benzathine penicillin) ▶K ♀B ▶? $$$$

WARNING — Not for IV administration, which can cause cardiorespiratory arrest and death.

ADULT — Scarlet fever; erysipelas; upper respiratory, skin, and soft-tissue infections due to group A strep: 2.4 million units IM single dose. Pneumococcal infections other than meningitis: 1.2 million units IM q 2 to 3 days until temperature normal for 48 h. Not for treatment of syphilis. Give deep IM into upper, outer quadrant of buttock or anterolateral thigh.

(cont.)

BICILLIN C-R (*cont.*)

PEDS — Scarlet fever; erysipelas; upper respiratory, skin, and soft-tissue infections due to group A strep: 600,000 units IM for wt less than 13.6 kg; 900,000 to 1.2 million units IM for wt 13.6 to 27 kg; 2.4 million units IM for wt greater than 27 kg. Pneumococcal infections other than meningitis: 600,000 units IM q 2 to 3 days until temperature normal for 48 h. Not for treatment of syphilis. Give deep IM into upper, outer quadrant of buttock or anterolateral thigh. Midlateral aspect of thigh may be preferred in neonates, infants, small children.

FORMS — Trade only: For IM use 300/300 and 450/150 (Peds) thousand units/mL procaine/benzathine penicillin (600,000 units/mL); 2 mL syringe.

NOTES — Contraindicated if allergic to procaine. Do not give IV. Do not inject into or near an artery or nerve. Do not substitute Bicillin CR for Bicillin LA in treatment of syphilis.

MOA — Beta-lactam antibiotic that inhibits the biosynthesis of cell wall mucopeptide.

ADVERSE EFFECTS — Serious: Anaphylaxis (rare), cross-sensitivity with cephalosporins, Coombs + hemolytic anemia. Frequent: Allergy.

PENICILLIN G ▶K ♀B ▶? $$$$

ADULT — Penicillin-sensitive pneumococcal pneumonia: 8 to 12 million units/day IV divided q 4 to 6 h. Penicillin-sensitive pneumococcal meningitis: 24 million units/day IV divided q 2 to 4 h. Empiric therapy, native valve endocarditis: 20 million units/day IV continuous infusion or divided q 4 h plus nafcillin/oxacillin and gentamicin. Neurosyphilis, ocular syphilis: 18 to 24 million units/day continuous IV infusion or 3 to 4 million units IV q 4 h for 10 to 14 days. Anthrax: See table.

PEDS — Mild to moderate infections: 25,000 to 50,000 units/kg/day IV divided q 6 h. Severe infections including pneumococcal and meningococcal meningitis: 250,000 to 400,000 units/kg/day IV divided q 4 to 6 h. Neonates age younger than 1 week and wt greater than 2 kg: 25,000 to 50,000 units/kg IV q 8 h. Neonates age 1 week or older and wt greater than 2 kg: 25,000 to 50,000 units/kg IV q 6 h. Group B streptococcal meningitis: 250,000 to 450,000 units/kg/day IV divided q 8 h for age 1 week or younger; 450,000 to 500,000 units/kg/day IV divided q 4 to 6 h for age older than 1 week. Congenital syphilis: 50,000 units/kg/dose IV q 12 h during 1st 7 days of life, then q 8 h thereafter to complete 10 days. Congenital syphilis or neurosyphilis: 50,000 units/kg IV q 4 to 6 h for 10 days for age older than 1 mo. Anthrax: See table.

UNAPPROVED ADULT — Prevention of perinatal group B streptococcal disease: Give to mother 5 million units IV at onset of labor/after membrane rupture, then 2.5 to 3 million units IV q 4 h until delivery. Diphtheria: 100,000 to 150,000 units/kg/day IV divided q 6 h for 14 days.

UNAPPROVED PEDS — Diphtheria: 100,000 to 150,000 units/kg/day IV divided q 6 h for 14 days.

NOTES — Reduce dose in renal dysfunction.

MOA — Beta-lactam antibiotic that inhibits the biosynthesis of cell wall mucopeptide.

ADVERSE EFFECTS — Serious: Anaphylaxis (rare); cross-sensitivity with cephalosporins; hematologic and renal toxicity, and seizures with doses greater than 20 million units/day; Coombs + hemolytic anemia. Frequent: Allergy.

PENICILLIN V ▶K ♀B ▶? $

ADULT — Usual dose: 250 to 500 mg PO four times per day. Group A streptococcal pharyngitis, AHA regimen: 500 mg PO two or three times per day for 10 days. Secondary prevention of rheumatic fever: 250 mg PO two times per day. Vincent's infection: 250 mg PO q 6 to 8 h. Anthrax: See table.

PEDS — Usual dose: 25 to 50 mg/kg/day PO divided three to four times per day. Use adult dose for age 12 yo or older. AHA dosing for Group A streptococcal pharyngitis, AHA regimen: 250 mg (for wt 27 kg or less) or 500 mg (wt greater than 27 kg) PO two or three times per day for 10 days. Secondary prevention of rheumatic fever: 250 mg PO two times per day. Anthrax: See table.

UNAPPROVED PEDS — Prevention of pneumococcal infections in functional/anatomic asplenia: 125 mg PO two times per day for age younger than 3 yo; 250 mg PO two times per day for age 3 yo or older.

FORMS — Generic only: Tabs 250, 500 mg. Oral soln 125, 250 mg/5 mL.

NOTES — Oral soln stable in refrigerator for 14 days.

MOA — Beta-lactam antibiotic that inhibits the biosynthesis of cell wall mucopeptide.

ADVERSE EFFECTS — Serious: Anaphylaxis (rare), cross-sensitivity with cephalosporins, Coombs + hemolytic anemia. Frequent: Allergy.

PROCAINE PENICILLIN ▶K ♀B ▶? $$$$$

WARNING — Not for IV administration.

ADULT — Pneumococcal and streptococcal infections, Vincent's infection, erysipeloid: 0.6 to 1 million units IM daily. Neurosyphilis: 2.4 million units IM daily plus probenecid 500 mg PO q 6 h, both for 10 to 14 days.

PEDS — Pneumococcal and streptococcal infections, Vincent's infection, erysipeloid, for wt less than 27 kg: 300,000 units IM daily. AAP dose for mild to moderate infections, age older than 1 mo: 25,000 to 50,000 units/kg/day IM divided one to two times per day. Congenital syphilis: 50,000 units/kg IM once daily for 10 days.

FORMS — Generic: For IM use, 600,000 units/mL; 1, 2 mL syringes.

NOTES — Peak 4 h, lasts 24 h. Contraindicated if procaine allergy; skin test if allergy suspected. Transient CNS reactions with high doses.

MOA — Beta-lactam antibiotic that inhibits the biosynthesis of cell wall mucopeptide.

ADVERSE EFFECTS — Serious: Anaphylaxis (rare), cross-sensitivity with cephalosporins, transient CNS reactions (Hoigne's syndrome), Coombs + hemolytic anemia. Frequent: Allergy.

ANTIMICROBIALS: Penicillins—2nd Generation—Penicillinase-Resistant

NOTE: Anaphylaxis occurs rarely with penicillins; cross-sensitivity with cephalosporins is possible.

DICLOXACILLIN ▶KL ♀B ▶? $$
ADULT — Usual dose: 250 to 500 mg PO four times per day. Take on empty stomach.
PEDS — Mild to moderate upper respiratory, skin and soft-tissue infections: 12.5 mg/kg/day PO divided four times per day for age older than 1 mo. Pneumonia, disseminated infections: 25 mg/kg/day PO divided four times per day for age older than 1 mo. Follow-up therapy after IV antibiotics for staph osteomyelitis: 50 to 100 mg/kg/day PO divided four times per day. Use adult dose for wt 40 kg or greater. Give on empty stomach.
FORMS — Generic only: Caps 250, 500 mg.
NOTES — Increased INR with warfarin.
MOA — Beta-lactam antibiotic that inhibits the biosynthesis of cell wall mucopeptide. Penicillinase-resistant penicillins are resistant to hydrolysis by the beta-lactamase, penicillinase.
ADVERSE EFFECTS — Serious: Anaphylaxis (rare), cross-sensitivity with cephalosporins.

NAFCILLIN ▶L ♀B ▶? $$$$$
ADULT — Staph infections, usual dose: 500 mg IM q 4 to 6 h or 500 to 2000 mg IV q 4 h. Osteomyelitis: 1 to 2 g IV q 4 h. Empiric therapy, native valve endocarditis: 2 g IV q 4 h plus penicillin/ampicillin and gentamicin.
PEDS — Staph infections, usual dose: 25 mg/kg IM two times per day for pediatric patients who weigh less than 40 kg; give 10 mg/kg for neonates.
UNAPPROVED PEDS — Mild to moderate infections: 50 to 100 mg/kg/day IM/IV divided q 6 h. Severe infections: 100 to 200 mg/kg/day IM/IV divided q 4 to 6 h. Neonates, wt greater than 2 kg: 25 mg/kg IM/IV q 8 h for age younger than 1 week old; 25 to 35 mg/kg IM/IV q 6 h for age 1 week or older.

NOTES — Reversible neutropenia with prolonged use. Decreased INR with warfarin. Decreased cyclosporine levels.
MOA — Beta-lactam antibiotic that inhibits the biosynthesis of cell wall mucopeptide. Penicillinase-resistant penicillins are resistant to hydrolysis by the beta-lactamase, penicillinase.
ADVERSE EFFECTS — Serious: Anaphylaxis (rare), cross-sensitivity with cephalosporins, extravasation, hypokalemia with dose of 200 mg/kg/day or greater. Frequent: Reversible neutropenia with duration of therapy longer than 21 days, eosinophilia.

OXACILLIN ▶KL ♀B ▶? $$$$$
ADULT — Staph infections: 250 mg to 2 g IM/IV q 4 to 6 h. Osteomyelitis: 1.5 to 2 g IV q 4 h. Empiric therapy, native valve endocarditis: 2 g IV q 4 h with penicillin/ampicillin and gentamicin.
PEDS — Mild to moderate infections: 100 to 150 mg/kg/day IM/IV divided q 6 h. Severe infections: 150 to 200 mg/kg/day IM/IV divided q 4 to 6 h. Use adult dose for wt 40 kg or greater. Newborns, wt greater than 2 kg: 25 to 50 mg/kg IV q 8 h for age younger than 1 week old, increasing to q 6 h for age 1 week or older.
NOTES — Hepatic dysfunction possible with doses greater than 12 g/day; monitor LFTs.
MOA — Beta-lactam antibiotic that inhibits the biosynthesis of cell wall mucopeptide. Penicillinase-resistant penicillins are resistant to hydrolysis by the beta-lactamase, penicillinase.
ADVERSE EFFECTS — Serious: Anaphylaxis (rare), cross-sensitivity with cephalosporins, hepatic dysfunction possible with doses greater then 12 g/day. Frequent: Eosinophilia.

ANTIMICROBIALS: Penicillins—3rd Generation—Aminopenicillins

NOTE: Anaphylaxis occurs rarely with penicillins; cross-sensitivity with cephalosporins is possible. —associated diarrhea. High risk of rash in patients with mononucleosis or taking allopurinol.

AMOXICILLIN (*Amoxil, Moxatag*) ▶K ♀B ▶+ $
ADULT — ENT, skin, genitourinary infections: 250 to 500 mg PO three times per day or 500 to 875 mg PO two times per day. See table for management of acute sinusitis. Pneumonia: 500 mg PO three times per day or 875 mg PO two times per day. Group A streptococcal pharyngitis, AHA regimen: 1 g PO once daily or 500 mg two times per day for 10 days. Group A streptococcal pharyngitis/tonsillitis, for age 12 yo or older: 775 mg ER tab (Moxatag) PO once daily for 10 days. Do not chew/crush Moxatag tabs. H. pylori: See table in GI section. See table for prophylaxis of bacterial endocarditis.
PEDS — ENT, skin, GU infections: 20 to 40 mg/kg/day PO divided three times per day or 25 to 45 mg/kg/day PO divided two times per day. See tables for management of acute sinusitis and otitis media. Pneumonia: 40 mg/kg/day PO divided three times

per day or 45 mg/kg/day PO divided two times per day. Infants, age younger than 3 mo: 30 mg/kg/day PO divided q 12 h. Group A streptococcal pharyngitis, AHA regimen: Treat for 10 days with 50 mg/kg up to 1 g PO once daily; alternate is 25 mg/kg up to 500 mg PO two times per day. Group A streptococcal pharyngitis/tonsillitis, for age 12 yo or older: 775 mg ER tab (Moxatag) PO once daily for 10 days. Do not chew/crush Moxatag tabs. See table for prophylaxis of bacterial endocarditis.
UNAPPROVED ADULT — High-dose for community-acquired pneumonia: 1 g PO three times per day. Lyme disease: 500 mg PO three times per day for 14 days for early disease, for 28 days for Lyme arthritis. Chlamydia in pregnancy (CDC alternative regimen): 500 mg PO three times per day for 7 days. See tables for STDs and anthrax.

(cont.)

AMOXICILLIN (*cont.*)

UNAPPROVED PEDS — High dose for otitis media, acute sinusitis, community-acquired pneumonia: 80 to 90 mg/kg/day (max of 4 g/day) PO divided two times per day. Treat pneumonia for up to 10 days, sinusitis for 10 to 14 days. Treat otitis media for 5 to 7 days if age 6 yo and older with mild to moderate symptoms, 7 days if age 2 to 5 yo with mild to moderate symptoms, and 10 days if age younger than 2 yo and children with severe symptoms. See otitis media and sinusitis tables. Lyme disease: 50 mg/kg/day (up to 1500 mg/day) PO divided three times per day for 14 days for early disease, for 28 days for Lyme arthritis. Anthrax: See table.

FORMS — Generic only: Caps 250, 500 mg. Tabs 500, 875 mg. Chewable tabs 125, 200, 250, 400 mg. Susp 125, 250 mg/5 mL. Susp 200, 400 mg/5 mL. Trade only: Extended-release tabs (Moxatag) 775 mg.

NOTES — Reduce dose in adults with renal dysfunction: Give 250 to 500 mg PO daily for CrCl <10 mL/min or hemodialysis; 250 to 500 mg PO two times per day for CrCl 10 to 30 mL/min. Do not use 875 mg tab for CrCl <30 mL/min. Give additional dose during and at end of dialysis. Oral susp and infant gtts stable for 14 days at room temperature or in the refrigerator.

MOA — Beta-lactam antibiotic that inhibits the biosynthesis of cell wall mucopeptide. Aminopenicillins are more active than natural penicillins against gram-negative cocci and Enterobacteriaceae.

ADVERSE EFFECTS — Serious: Anaphylaxis (rare), cross-sensitivity with cephalosporins. Frequent: Rash (nonallergic in patients with mononucleosis, chronic myelogenous leukemia, or allopurinol therapy), diarrhea.

AMPICILLIN ▶K ♀B ▶? $$$$$

ADULT — Usual dose: 1 to 2 g IV q 4 to 6 h or 250 to 500 mg PO four times per day. Sepsis, meningitis: 150 to 200 mg/kg/day IV divided q 3 to 4 h. Empiric therapy, native valve endocarditis: 12 g/day IV continuous infusion or divided q 4 h plus nafcillin/oxacillin and gentamicin. See table for prophylaxis of bacterial endocarditis.

PEDS — AAP recommendations: Mild to moderate infections: 100 to 150 mg/kg/day IM/IV divided q 6 h or 50 to 100 mg/kg/day PO divided four times per day. Severe infections: 200 to 400 mg/kg/day IM/IV divided q 6 h. Newborns, wt greater than 2 kg: 25 to 50 mg/kg IV given q 8 h for age younger than 1 week old, increase to q 6 h for age 1 week or older. Use adult doses for wt 40 kg or greater. Group B streptococcal meningitis: 200 to 300 mg/kg/day IV divided q 8 h for age 7 days or younger; 300 mg/kg/day divided q 6 h for age older than 7 days. Give with gentamicin initially. See table for prophylaxis of bacterial endocarditis.

UNAPPROVED ADULT — Prevention of neonatal group B streptococcal disease: Give to mother 2 g IV at onset of labor/after membrane rupture, then 1 g IV q 4 h until delivery.

FORMS — Generic only: Caps 250, 500 mg. Susp 125, 250 mg/5 mL.

NOTES — IV ampicillin, dosage reduction for renal impairment: Consider dosing interval of q 6 to 8 h for CrCl 30 to 50 mL/min (some experts do not recommend dosage reduction for CrCl >30 mL/min); dosing interval of q8 to 12 h for CrCl 10 to 30 mL/min; dosing interval of q 12 to 24 h for CrCl <10 mL/min. Give dose after hemodialysis.

MOA — Beta-lactam antibiotic that inhibits the biosynthesis of cell wall mucopeptide. Aminopenicillins are more active than natural penicillins against gram-negative cocci and Enterobacteriaceae.

ADVERSE EFFECTS — Serious: Anaphylaxis (rare), cross-sensitivity with cephalosporins, C. difficile-associated diarrhea. Frequent: Nonallergic rash in patients with mononucleosis, chronic myelogenous leukemia, or allopurinol therapy; eosinophilia; diarrhea (especially with PO).

AUGMENTIN (amoxicillin-clavulanate, *Augmentin ES-600, Augmentin XR,* ✱ *Clavulin*) ▶K ♀B ▶? $$$

ADULT — Pneumonia, otitis media, sinusitis, skin infections, UTIs: Usual dose 500 mg PO two times per day or 250 mg PO three times per day. More severe infections: 875 mg PO two times per day or 500 mg PO three times per day. Augmentin XR: 2 tabs PO q 12 h with meals for 10 days for acute sinusitis, give 7 to 10 days for community-acquired pneumonia. See table for management of acute sinusitis.

PEDS — 200, 400 mg chewables and 200, 400 mg/5 mL susp for two times per day administration. Pneumonia, otitis media, sinusitis: 45 mg/kg/day PO divided two times per day. Less severe infections such as skin, UTIs: 25 mg/kg/day PO divided two times per day. 125, 250 mg chewables and 125, 250 mg/5 mL susp for three times per day administration. Pneumonia, otitis media, sinusitis: 40 mg/kg/day PO divided three times per day. Less severe infections such as skin, UTIs: 20 mg/kg/day PO divided three times per day. Use 125 mg/5 mL susp and give 30 mg/kg PO q 12 h for age younger than 3 mo. Give adult dose for wt 40 kg or greater. Augmentin ES-600 susp for age 3 mo or older and wt less than 40 kg. Recurrent/ persistent otitis media with risk factors (antibiotics for otitis media in past 3 months and either in daycare or age 2 yo or younger): 90 mg/kg/day PO divided two times per day with food for 10 days. See tables for acute sinusitis and otitis media.

UNAPPROVED ADULT — Treatment of infected dog/cat bite: 875 mg PO two times per day or 500 mg PO three times per day, duration of treatment based on response. See table for management of acute sinusitis.

UNAPPROVED PEDS — See tables for acute sinusitis and otitis media. High dose for community-acquired pneumonia, age older than 3 mo, acute sinusitis, acute otitis media: 90 mg/kg/day (max 4 g/day) PO divided two times per day. Treat pneumonia for up to 10 days, sinusitis for 10 to 14 days. Treat otitis

(cont.)

AUGMENTIN (*cont.*)

media for 5 to 7 days for children 6 yo and older with mild to moderate symptoms, 7 days for children 2 to 5 yo with mild to moderate symptoms, and 10 days for children younger than 2 yo and those with severe symptoms.

FORMS — Generic/Trade (amoxicillin-clavulanate): Tabs 250/125, 500/125, 875/125 mg. Chewables, Susp 200/28.5, 400/57 mg per tab or 5 mL, 250/62.5 mg per 5 mL. (ES) Susp 600/42.9 mg per 5 mL. Extended-release tabs 1000/62.5 mg. Trade only: Susp 125/31.25 per 5 mL, 250/62.5 mg per 5 mL.

NOTES — Diarrhea common (less with twice daily dosing). Do not interchange Augmentin products with different clavulanate content. Do not use 250 mg amoxicillin + 125 mg clavulanate tab in children with wt less than 40 kg. Suspensions stable in refrigerator for 10 days. See prescribing information for dosage reduction of Augmentin tabs if CrCl <30 mL/min. Augmentin XR contraindicated if CrCl <30 mL/min.

MOA — Beta-lactam antibiotic that inhibits the biosynthesis of cell wall mucopeptide. Aminopenicillins are more active than natural penicillins against gram-negative cocci and Enterobacteriaceae. Clavulanate is beta-lactamase inhibitor.

ADVERSE EFFECTS — Serious: Anaphylaxis (rare), cross-sensitivity with cephalosporins, clavulanate-induced cholestatic hepatitis (esp. in elderly men treated for more than 2 weeks). Frequent: Diarrhea (less with bid dosing, incidence related to clavulanate dose), rash (nonallergic in patients with mononucleosis, chronic myelogenous leukemia, or allopurinol therapy).

UNASYN (ampicillin-sulbactam) ▸K ♀B ▶? $$$

ADULT — Skin, intra-abdominal, gynecologic infections: 1.5 to 3 g IM/IV q 6 h. Pelvic inflammatory disease: 3 g IV q 6 h + doxycycline 100 mg PO/IV q 12 h.

PEDS — Skin infections, for age 1 yo or older: 300 mg/kg/day IV divided q 6 h. Use adult dose for wt greater than 40 kg.

UNAPPROVED ADULT — Community-acquired pneumonia: 1.5 to 3 g IM/IV q 6 h with a macrolide or doxycycline.

UNAPPROVED PEDS — AAP regimens. Mild to moderate infections: 100 to 150 mg/kg/day of ampicillin IM/IV divided q 6 h. Severe infections: 200 to 400 mg/kg/day of ampicillin IM/IV divided q 6 h.

NOTES — Can cause hepatic dysfunction/cholestatic jaundice; contraindicated in patients with history of hepatic dysfunction with ampicillin-sulbactam. Dosing for adults with renal impairment: Give usual dose q 24 h for CrCl 5 to 14 mL/min, q 12 h for CrCl 15 to 29 mL/min, q 6 to 8 h for adults with CrCl 30 mL/min or greater.

MOA — Beta-lactam antibiotic that inhibits the biosynthesis of cell wall mucopeptide. Aminopenicillins are more active than natural penicillins against gram-negative cocci and Enterobacteriaceae. Sulbactam is beta-lactamase inhibitor.

ADVERSE EFFECTS — Serious: Anaphylaxis (rare), cross-sensitivity with cephalosporins, C. difficile-associated diarrhea, hepatic dysfunction/cholestatic jaundice. Frequent: Rash (nonallergic in patients with mononucleosis, chronic myelogenous leukemia, or allopurinol therapy), eosinophilia, increased LFTs.

ANTIMICROBIALS: Penicillins—4th Generation—Extended Spectrum

NOTE: Anaphylaxis occurs rarely with penicillins; cross-sensitivity with cephalosporins is possible. Hypokalemia; bleeding and coagulation abnormalities possible especially with renal impairment.

PIPERACILLIN-TAZOBACTAM (*Zosyn*, *✦Tazocin*) ▸K ♀B ▶? $$$$$

ADULT — Appendicitis, peritonitis, skin infections, postpartum endometritis, pelvic inflammatory disease, moderate community-acquired pneumonia: 3.375 g IV q 6 h. Nosocomial pneumonia: 4.5 g IV q 6 h (with aminoglycoside initially and if P. aeruginosa is cultured).

PEDS — Appendicitis/peritonitis: 80 mg/kg of piperacillin IV q 8 h for age 2 to 9 mo; 100 mg/kg of piperacillin IV q 8 h for age older than 9 mo; use adult dose for wt greater than 40 kg.

UNAPPROVED ADULT — Serious infections: 4.5 g IV q 6 h.

UNAPPROVED PEDS — 150 to 300 mg/kg/day of piperacillin IV divided q 6 to 8 h for age younger than 6 mo, 300 to 400 mg/kg/day piperacillin IV divided q 6 to 8 h for age 6 mo or older.

NOTES — May prolong neuromuscular blockade with nondepolarizing muscle relaxants. False-positive result possible with Bio-Rad Laboratories Platelia Aspergillus EIA test. May increase risk of acute kidney injury with vancomycin; monitor renal function during coadministration. May reduce renal excretion of methotrexate; monitor methotrexate levels and toxicity. Reduce dosing in adults with renal impairment: 2.25 g IV q 8 h for CrCl <20 mL/min; 2.25 g IV q 6 h for CrCl 20 to 40 mL/min. Hemodialysis: Max dose of 2.25 g IV q 8 h plus 0.75 g after each dialysis.

MOA — Beta-lactam antibiotic that inhibits the biosynthesis of cell wall mucopeptide. Tazobactam is beta-lactamase inhibitor.

ADVERSE EFFECTS — Serious: Anaphylaxis (rare); cross-sensitivity with cephalosporins; serious skin reactions like Stevens Johnson syndrome, toxic epidermal necrolysis, and DRESS (stop drug if progressive rash); hypokalemia; bleeding and coagulation abnormalities (especially with renal impairment). Frequent: N/V, diarrhea, headache.

ANTIMICROBIALS: Quinolones

NOTE: As of 2016, FDA recommends limiting fluoroquinolone treatment of bronchitis, acute sinusitis, and uncomplicated UTI to patients who lack other treatment options. For these indications, the benefit is generally less than the risk of serious adverse events. These include tendonitis/tendon rupture (risk increased by corticosteroids, age over 60 yo, and organ transplant), exacerbation of myasthenia gravis, QT interval prolongation/ torsades, CNS toxicity (eg, seizures, increased intracranial pressure), peripheral neuropathy, hypersensitivity, -associated diarrhea, and fluoroquinolone-associated disability (FQAD). FQAD is a rare disabling multi-organ reaction with musculoskeletal symptoms (eg, joint/muscle pain, tendonitis), CNS effects (eg, fatigue, insomnia, anxiety) and/or peripheral neuropathy. It has an onset of hours to weeks and may be irreversible.

CIPROFLOXACIN (*Cipro, Cipro XR*) ▶LK ♀C but teratogenicity unlikely ▶?+ $
WARNING — Fluoroquinolones can cause disabling and potentially irreversible reactions in which tendonitis/tendon rupture, peripheral neuropathy, and/or CNS effects may occur together. Stop immediately and do not use fluoroquinolones again if patients experience any of these events. Avoid in patients with myasthenia gravis; may exacerbate muscle weakness. Use for simple UTI, acute exacerbation of chronic bronchitis, or acute sinusitis only if patients have no other treatment options.
ADULT — UTI: 250 to 500 mg PO two times per day or 200 to 400 mg IV q 12 h. Cipro XR for complicated UTI, uncomplicated pyelonephritis: 1000 mg PO once daily for 7 to 14 days. Pneumonia, skin, bone/joint infections: 400 mg IV q 8 to 12 h or 500 to 750 mg PO two times per day. Treat bone/joint infections for 4 to 6 weeks. Chronic bacterial prostatitis: 500 mg PO two times per day for 28 days. Infectious diarrhea: 500 mg PO two times per day for 5 to 7 days. Typhoid fever: 500 mg PO two times per day for 10 days. Nosocomial pneumonia: 400 mg IV q 8 h. Complicated intra-abdominal infection (with metronidazole): 400 mg IV q 12 h, then 500 mg PO two times per day. Empiric therapy of febrile neutropenia: 400 mg IV q 8 h with piperacillin. Plague: 400 mg IV q 8 to 12 h or 500 to 750 mg PO q 12 h for 14 days. Anthrax: See table. Simple UTI in patients with no other treatment options: 250 mg PO two times per day for 3 days or Cipro XR 500 mg PO once daily for 3 days. Acute sinusitis in patients with no other treatment options: 500 mg PO two times per day for 10 days. See acute sinusitis table.
PEDS — Safety and efficacy not established for most indications in children; arthropathy in juvenile animals. Clinical trials in children show no evidence of arthropathy other than transient large-joint arthralgias. In children treated with ciprofloxacin for complicated UTI, musculoskeletal adverse events were mild to moderate in severity and resolved within 1 month. Complicated UTI, pyelonephritis, 1 to 17 yo: 6 to 10 mg/kg IV q 8 h, then 10 to 20 mg/kg PO q 12 h. Max of 400 mg IV or 750 mg PO per dose even for peds patients wt greater than 51 kg. Plague, birth to 17 yo: 10 mg/kg IV q 8 to 12 h or 15 mg/kg (max 500 mg) PO q 8 to 12 h for 10 to 21 days. Anthrax: See table.
UNAPPROVED ADULT — Acute uncomplicated pyelonephritis: 500 mg PO two times per day for 7 days. Chancroid: 500 mg PO two times per day for 3 days. Prophylaxis, high-risk GU surgery: 500 mg PO or 400 mg IV. Prophylaxis, invasive meningococcal disease: 500 mg PO single dose. Traveler's diarrhea (treatment preferred over prophylaxis). Treatment: 500 mg PO two times per day for 1 to 3 days or 750 mg PO single dose. Prophylaxis: 500 mg PO daily for no more than 3 weeks. Infectious diarrhea: 500 mg PO two times per day for 1 to 3 days for Shigella, for 5 to 7 days for non-typhi Salmonella (usually not treated). Malignant otitis externa: 400 mg IV or 750 mg PO q 12 h. TB (2nd-line treatment): 750 to 1500 mg/day IV/PO. Salmonella gastroenteritis in HIV infection: 500 to 750 mg PO two times per day (400 mg IV q 12 h) for 7 to 14 days if CD4 count 200 or greater, for 2 to 6 weeks if CD4 count less than 200. Campylobacter in HIV infection: 500 to 750 mg PO (or 400 mg IV) two times per day for 7 to 10 days for mild/moderate disease, at least 14 days with aminoglycoside for bacteremia.
UNAPPROVED PEDS — Usual dose: 20 to 30 mg/kg/day IV/PO divided q 12 h (max 1.5 g/day PO; max 800 mg/day IV). Acute pulmonary exacerbation of cystic fibrosis: 10 mg/kg/dose IV q 8 h for 7 days, then 20 mg/kg/dose PO q 12 h to complete 10 to 21 days of treatment. TB (2nd-line treatment): 10 to 15 mg/kg PO two times per day (max: 1.5 g/day).
FORMS — Generic/Trade: Tabs 100, 250, 500, 750 mg. Extended-release tabs 500, 1000 mg. Oral susp 250, 500 mg/5 mL.
NOTES — Can prolong QT interval and cause torsades; avoid if known QT interval prolongation, uncorrected electrolyte disorder, or coadministration of drugs that prolong the QT interval. Crystalluria if alkaline urine. Ciprofloxacin inhibits CYP1A2, an enzyme that metabolizes caffeine, clozapine, theophylline, and warfarin. Give ciprofloxacin immediate-release or Cipro XR 2 h before or 6 h after antacids, iron, sucralfate, calcium, zinc, buffered didanosine, or other highly buffered drugs. Can give with meals containing dairy products, but not with yogurt, milk, or calcium-fortified fruit juice alone. Do not give Cipro XR within 2 h of calcium doses greater than 800 mg. Watch for hypoglycemia with glyburide. Do not give oral susp in feeding or nasogastric tube. Cipro XR and immediate-release tabs are not interchangeable. Do not chew microcapsules in oral susp. Do not split, crush, or chew Cipro XR. Dosage reduction for renal impairment in adults. Immediate-release ciprofloxacin: 250 to 500 mg PO q 24 h given after dialysis session for hemodialysis/peritoneal dialysis; 250 to 500 mg PO q 18 h or 200 to 400 mg IV q 18 to 24 h for CrCl 5 to 29 mL/min;

(cont.)

CIPROFLOXACIN (*cont.*)

250 to 500 mg PO q 12 h for CrCl 30 to 50 mL/min. Cipro XR for complicated UTI, acute pyelonephritis: 500 mg PO once daily for CrCl <30 mL/min.

MOA — Inhibits bacterial DNA synthesis by binding with DNA gyrase and topoisomerase IV.

ADVERSE EFFECTS — Serious: Tendon rupture/tendonitis, exacerbation of myasthenia gravis, hypersensitivity, phototoxicity, CNS toxicity, hepatotoxicity, crystalluria if alkaline urine, peripheral neuropathy (rare), QT prolongation/torsades, C. difficile-associated diarrhea, fluoroquinolone-associated disability. Theoretical risk of cartilage toxicity in children, but no clinical evidence of harm other than transient large-joint arthralgias. Musculoskeletal adverse events reported with ciprofloxacin treatment of complicated UTI in peds patients were mild to moderately severe and resolved within 1 month after treatment. Frequent: N/V. More GI, neurologic, and musculoskeletal adverse reactions reported during postexposure prophylaxis of bioterrorism anthrax.

GEMIFLOXACIN (*Factive*) ▶Feces, K ♀C ▶– $$$$$

WARNING — Fluoroquinolones can cause disabling and potentially irreversible reactions in which tendonitis/tendon rupture, peripheral neuropathy, and/or CNS effects may occur together. Stop immediately and do not use fluoroquinolones again if patients experience any of these events. Avoid in patients with myasthenia gravis; may exacerbate muscle weakness. Use for acute exacerbation of chronic bronchitis only if patients have no other treatment options.

ADULT — Community-acquired pneumonia: 320 mg PO daily for 5 to 7 days (7 days for multidrug-resistant S.pneumoniae).Acute exacerbation of chronic bronchitis if no other treatment options: 320 mg PO daily for 5 days.

PEDS — Safety and efficacy not established in children; arthropathy in juvenile animals.

UNAPPROVED ADULT — Gonorrhea in cephalosporin-allergic patient: See STD table.

FORMS — Trade only: Tabs 320 mg.

NOTES — Can prolong QT interval; avoid in patients with QT interval prolongation, uncorrected electrolyte disorders, or coadministration of Class 1A and Class III antiarrhythmics. Maintain fluid intake to prevent crystalluria. Give 2 h before or 3 h after Al/Mg antacids, iron, multivitamins with zinc, buffered didanosine. Give at least 2 h before sucralfate. May increase INR with warfarin. Discontinue if rash develops. Reduce dose for CrCl 40 mL/min or less, hemodialysis, or CAPD: 160 mg PO daily.

MOA — Inhibits bacterial DNA synthesis by binding with DNA gyrase and topoisomerase IV.

ADVERSE EFFECTS — Serious: Tendon rupture/tendonitis, exacerbation of myasthenia gravis, hypersensitivity, phototoxicity, CNS toxicity, peripheral neuropathy (rare), QT prolongation, dysglycemia, fluoroquinolone-associated disability. Frequent: Rash (esp. in women younger than 40 yo or treatment duration more than 7 days).

LEVOFLOXACIN (*Levaquin*) ▶KL ♀C ▶? $$$

WARNING — Fluoroquinolones can cause disabling and potentially irreversible reactions in which tendonitis/tendon rupture, peripheral neuropathy, and/or CNS effects may occur together. Stop immediately and do not use fluoroquinolones again if patients experience any of these events. Avoid in patients with myasthenia gravis; may exacerbate muscle weakness. Use for simple UTI, acute exacerbation of chronic bronchitis, and acute sinusitis only if patients have no other treatment options.

ADULT — IV and PO doses are the same. Community-acquired pneumonia: 750 mg once daily for 5 days or 500 mg once daily for 7 to 14 days. Nosocomial pneumonia: 750 mg once daily for 7 to 14 days. Skin infections: 500 to 750 mg once daily for 7 to 14 days. Complicated UTI or pyelonephritis: 250 mg once daily for 10 days or 750 mg once daily for 5 days. Chronic bacterial prostatitis: 500 mg once daily for 28 days. Plague: 500 mg once daily for 10 to 14 days. Anthrax: See table. Simple UTI in patients with no other treatment options: 250 mg once daily for 3 days. Acute exacerbation of chronic bronchitis in patients with no other treatment options: 500 mg once daily for 7 days. Acute sinusitis in patients with no other treatment options: 750 mg once daily for 5 days or 500 mg once daily for 10 to 14 days. See acute sinusitis table. Take oral soln on empty stomach.

PEDS — IV and PO doses are the same. Anthrax: See table. Plague, age 6 mo and older: Treat for 10 to 14 days with 8 mg/kg (max 250 mg/dose) two times per day if wt less than 50 kg; 500 mg once daily if wt greater than 50 kg. Clinical trials in children show no evidence of arthropathy other than transient large joint arthralgias. Infuse IV doses over 60 min (250 to 500 mg). Take oral soln on empty stomach.

UNAPPROVED ADULT — Legionnaires' disease: 1 g IV/PO on 1st day, then 500 mg IV/PO once daily. Chlamydia, epididymitis: See STD table. TB (2nd-line treatment): 500 to 1000 mg/day IV/PO. Traveler's diarrhea, treatment: 500 mg PO once daily for 1 to 3 days. Infectious diarrhea: 500 mg PO once daily for 1 to 3 days for Shigella, for 5 to 7 days for Salmonella.

UNAPPROVED PEDS — IV and PO doses are the same. Community-acquired pneumonia: 8 to 10 mg/kg two times per day for age 6 mo to 5 yo; 8 to 10 mg/kg/day once daily (max 750 mg once daily) for age 5 to 16 yo. Atypical pneumonia in adolescents with skeletal maturity: 500 mg PO once daily. Infuse IV doses over 60 min (250 to 500 mg). See acute sinusitis table.

FORMS — Trade/Generic: Tabs 250, 500, 750 mg.

NOTES — Can prolong QT interval and cause torsades; avoid if known QT interval prolongation, hypokalemia, or coadministration of Class IA or Class III antiarrhythmic. Give Mg/Al antacids, iron, sucralfate, multivitamins containing zinc, buffered didanosine 2 h before/after PO levofloxacin.

(cont.)

LEVOFLOXACIN (*cont.*)

Increased INR with warfarin. Monitor glucose with antidiabetic agents. Can cause false positive on opiate urine screening immunoassay; may need confirmation test. Dosage adjustment in renal dysfunction is based on dose used in normal renal function. For dose of 750 mg in normal renal function: Give 750 mg q 48 h for CrCl 20 to 49 mL/min; give 750 mg load, then 500 mg q 48 h for CrCl 10 to 19 mL/min, hemodialysis or CAPD. For dose of 500 mg in normal renal function: Give 500 mg load, then 250 mg q 24 h for CrCl 20 to 49 mL/min; give 500 mg load, then 250 mg q 48 h for CrCl 10 to 19 mL/min, hemodialysis or CAPD. For dose of 250 mg in normal renal function: Give 250 mg q 48 h for CrCl 10 to 19 mL/min. Dosage adjustment not necessary for uncomplicated UTI if CrCl is 10 to 19 mL/min.

MOA — Inhibits bacterial DNA synthesis by binding with DNA gyrase and topoisomerase IV.

ADVERSE EFFECTS — Serious: Tendon rupture/tendonitis, exacerbation of myasthenia gravis, hypersensitivity, phototoxicity, CNS toxicity, peripheral neuropathy (rare), QT prolongation/torsades, C. difficile-associated diarrhea, fluoroquinolone-associated disability. Frequent: Headache. Musculoskeletal disorders (arthralgia, arthritis, tendinopathy, gait abnormality) reported in children; safety for treatment duration more than 14 days not established.

MOXIFLOXACIN (*Avelox*) ▸LK ♀C ▶– $$$$

WARNING — Fluoroquinolones can cause disabling and potentially irreversible reactions in which tendonitis/tendon rupture, peripheral neuropathy, and/or CNS effects may occur together. Stop immediately and do not use fluoroquinolones again if patients experience any of these events. Avoid in patients with myasthenia gravis; may exacerbate muscle weakness. Use for acute exacerbation of chronic bronchitis or acute sinusitis only if patients have no other treatment options.

ADULT — IV and PO doses are the same. Complicated intra-abdominal infection:400 mg IV/PO (give IV initially) daily for 5 to 14 days. Community-acquired pneumonia, including penicillin-resistant S. pneumoniae: 400 mg daily for 7 to 14 days. Uncomplicated skin infections: 400 mg daily for 7 days. Complicated skin infections: 400 mg daily for 7 to 21 days. Acute exacerbation of chronic bronchitisif no other treatment options: 400 mg daily for 5 days. Acute sinusitis with no other treatment options: 400 mg daily for 10 days. See acute sinusitis table.

PEDS — Safety and efficacy not established in children; arthropathy in juvenile animals.

UNAPPROVED ADULT — TB (2nd-line treatment): 400 mg IV/PO daily. Anthrax: See table.

UNAPPROVED PEDS — Atypical pneumonia in adolescents with skeletal maturity: 400 mg PO once daily.

FORMS — Generic/Trade: Tabs 400 mg.

NOTES — Can prolong the QT interval and cause torsades; avoid if known QT interval prolongation, proarrhythmic conditions, uncorrected electrolyte disorders, or coadministration of drugs that prolong QT interval. Do not exceed recommended IV dose or infusion rate due to QT prolongation risk. Contraindicated with ziprasidone. Can cause hypo- and hyperglycemia, esp. in elderly diabetics receiving oral hypogycemic drugs or insulin; monitor blood glucose in diabetics and discontinue if hypoglycemic reaction. Give tabs at least 4 h before or 8 h after Al/Mg antacids, iron, multivitamins with zinc, sucralfate, buffered didanosine. Dosage adjustment not required for hepatic insufficiency.

MOA — Inhibits bacterial DNA synthesis by binding with DNA gyrase and topoisomerase IV.

ADVERSE EFFECTS — Serious: Tendon rupture/tendonitis, exacerbation of myasthenia gravis, hypersensitivity, phototoxicity, CNS toxicity, peripheral neuropathy (rare), QT prolongation/torsades, dysglycemia, C. difficile-associated diarrhea, fluoroquinolone-associated disability. Frequent: Nausea, diarrhea.

OFLOXACIN ▸LK ♀C ▶?+ $$$

WARNING — Fluoroquinolones can cause disabling and potentially irreversible reactions in which tendonitis/tendon rupture, peripheral neuropathy, and/or CNS effects may occur together. Stop immediately and do not use fluoroquinolones again if patients experience any of these events. Avoid in patients with myasthenia gravis; may exacerbate muscle weakness. Use for simple UTI, acute exacerbation of chronic bronchitis, or acute sinusitis only if patients have no other treatment options.

ADULT — Acute exacerbation of chronic bronchitis in patients with no other treatment options, community-acquired pneumonia, skin infections: 400 mg PO two times per day for 10 days. Complicated UTI: 200 mg PO two times per day for 10 days. Chronic bacterial prostatitis: 300 mg PO two times per day for 6 weeks. Simple UTI with no other treatment options: 200 mg PO two times per day for 3 days (E. coli, K. pneumoniae) or 7 days (others).

PEDS — Safety and efficacy not established in children; arthropathy in juvenile animals.

UNAPPROVED ADULT — Epididymitis likely due to enteric organisms: 300 mg PO two times per day for 10 days. Traveler's diarrhea, treatment: 300 mg PO two times per day for 1 to 3 days. Infectious diarrhea: 300 mg PO two times per day for 1 to 3 days for Shigella, 5 to 7 days for non-typhi Salmonella (usually not treated). TB (2nd-line treatment): 600 to 800 mg PO daily.

FORMS — Generic only: Tabs 200, 300, 400 mg.

NOTES — May prolong QT interval; avoid in known QT interval prolongation, hypokalemia, or coadministration of Class 1A and Class III antiarrhythmic. Give antacids, iron, sucralfate, multivitamins containing zinc, buffered didanosine 2 h before or after ofloxacin. May decrease metabolism of theophylline,

(cont.)

OFLOXACIN (*cont.*)

increase INR with warfarin. Monitor glucose with antidiabetic agents. Can cause false positive on opiate urine screening immunoassay; may need confirmation test. Reduce dose in renal dysfunction: 50% of usual dose q 24 h for CrCl <20 mL/min; usual dose given q 24 h for CrCl 20 to 50 mL/min.

MOA — Inhibits bacterial DNA synthesis by binding with DNA gyrase and topoisomerase IV.
ADVERSE EFFECTS — Serious: Tendon rupture/tendonitis, exacerbation of myasthenia gravis, hypersensitivity, phototoxicity, CNS toxicity, peripheral neuropathy (rare), QT prolongation, C. difficile-associated diarrhea, fluoroquinolone-associated disability. Frequent: N/V.

ANTIMICROBIALS: Sulfonamides

NOTE: Sulfonamides can cause Stevens-Johnson syndrome; toxic epidermal necrolysis; hepatotoxicity; blood dyscrasias; hemolysis in glucose-6-phosphate dehydrogenase (G6PD) deficiency. Avoid maternal sulfonamides if her breastfed infant is ill, stressed, premature, or has hyperbilirubinemia or G6PD deficiency.

SULFADIAZINE ▸K ♀C ▶+ $$$$$
ADULT — Usual dose: 2 to 4 g PO initially, then 2 to 4 g/day divided into 3 to 6 doses. Secondary prevention of rheumatic fever: 1 g PO daily. Toxoplasmosis treatment: 1 to 1.5 g PO four times per day with pyrimethamine and leucovorin.
PEDS — Not for infants younger than 2 mo, except as adjunct to pyrimethamine for congenital toxoplasmosis. Usual dose: Give 75 mg/kg PO initially, then 150 mg/kg/day up to 6 g/day divided into 4 to 6 doses. Secondary prevention of rheumatic fever, for wt 27 kg or less: 500 mg PO daily. Use adult dose for wt greater than 27 kg.
UNAPPROVED ADULT — CNS toxoplasmosis in AIDS. Acute therapy: For wt less than 60 kg give pyrimethamine 200 mg PO for 1st dose, then 50 mg PO once daily with sulfadiazine 1000 mg PO q 6 h and leucovorin 10 to 25 mg PO once daily (up to 50 mg once daily or two times per day). For wt 60 kg or greater give pyrimethamine 200 mg PO for 1st dose, then 75 mg PO once daily with sulfadiazine 1500 mg PO q 6 h and leucovorin 10 to 25 mg PO once daily (up to 50 mg once daily or two times per day). Treat for at least 6 weeks. Chronic maintenance therapy: Pyrimethamine 25 to 50 mg PO once daily with sulfadiazine 2000 to 4000 mg/day PO divided two to four times per day and leucovorin 10 to 25 mg PO once daily.
UNAPPROVED PEDS — Not for age younger than 2 mo, except as adjunct to pyrimethamine for congenital toxoplasmosis. Acquired toxoplasmosis: 25 to 50 mg/kg (max 1 to 1.5 g/dose) PO four times per day with pyrimethamine and leucovorin for at least 6 weeks. Suppressive therapy of toxoplasmosis in HIV infection: 85 to 120 mg/kg/day (max 2 to 4 g/day) PO divided in 2 doses with pyrimethamine and leucovorin.
FORMS — Generic only: Tabs 500 mg.
NOTES — Maintain fluid intake to prevent crystalluria and stone formation. Reduce dose in renal insufficiency. May increase INR with warfarin. May increase levels of methotrexate, phenytoin.
MOA — Structural analog of PABA that binds with dihydropteroate synthetase and prevents nucleic acid synthesis. Bacteriostatic.
ADVERSE EFFECTS — Serious: Stevens-Johnson syndrome, toxic epidermal necrolysis, hepatotoxicity,

blood dyscrasias, hemolysis in G6PD deficiency, crystalluria and stone formation. Frequent: Rash, N/V, diarrhea, fever.

TRIMETHOPRIM-SULFAMETHOXAZOLE (*Bactrim, cotrimoxazole, Septra, Sulfatrim Pediatric, TMP-SMX*) ▸K ♀C ▶+ $
ADULT — UTI, shigellosis, acute exacerbation of chronic bronchitis: 1 tab PO two times per day, double strength (DS, 160 mg TMP/800 mg SMX). Travelers' diarrhea: 1 DS tab PO two times per day for 5 days. Pneumocystis treatment: 15 to 20 mg/kg/day (based on TMP) IV divided q 6 to 8 h or PO divided three times per day for 21 days total; can use 2 DS tabs PO three times per day for mild to moderate infection. Pneumocystis prophylaxis: 1 DS tab PO daily.
PEDS — UTI, shigellosis, otitis media: 1 mL/kg/day susp PO divided two times per day (up to 20 mL PO two times per day). Use adult dose for wt greater than 40 kg. TMP-SMX is a poor option for otitis media and sinusitis due to high pneumococcus and H. influenzae resistance rates; see otitis media and sinusitis treatment tables for alternatives. Pneumocystis treatment: 15 to 20 mg/kg/day (based on TMP) IV divided q 6 to 8 h or 5 mL susp/8 kg/dose PO q 6 h. Pneumocystis prophylaxis: 150 mg/m²/day (based on TMP) PO divided two times per day on 3 consecutive days each week. Do not use in infants younger than 2 mo; may cause kernicterus.
UNAPPROVED ADULT — Uncomplicated cystitis in women: 1 DS tab PO two times per day for 3 days. Do not use if resistance prevalence greater than 20% or if used for UTI in previous 3 months. Bacterial prostatitis: 1 DS tab PO two times per day for 10 to 14 days for acute, for 1 to 3 months for chronic. Pneumocystis prophylaxis: 1 SS tab PO daily. Primary prevention of toxoplasmosis in AIDS: 1 DS tab PO daily. Pertussis (2nd line to macrolides): 1 DS tab PO two times per day for 14 days. Community-acquired MRSA skin infections: 1 to 2 DS tabs PO two times per day for 5 to 10 days; 2 DS tabs PO two times per day for wt 100 kg or greater or BMI of 40 or greater. MRSA osteomyelitis: 4 mg/kg/dose (based on TMP) PO two times per day with rifampin 600 mg PO once daily. Prevention of spontaneous bacterial peritonitis: 1 DS tab PO once daily for 5 days per week.

(cont.)

TRIMETHOPRIM-SULFAMETHOXAZOLE (*cont.*)

UNAPPROVED PEDS — Community-acquired MRSA skin infections: 1 to 1.5 mL/kg/day PO divided two times per day for 5 to 10 days. Pertussis (2nd line to macrolides): 1 mL/kg/day PO divided two times per day for 14 days.

FORMS — Generic/Trade: Tabs 80 mg TMP/400 mg SMX (SS), 160 mg TMP/800 mg SMX (DS). Susp 40 mg TMP/200 mg SMX per 5 mL. 20 mL susp = 2 SS tabs = 1 DS tab.

NOTES — Not effective for streptococcal pharyngitis. AAP recommends against cotrimoxazole for acute otitis media in children because of high resistance rates. No activity against penicillin-nonsusceptible pneumococci. Bone marrow depression with high IV doses. Significantly increased INR with warfarin; avoid concomitant use if possible. Increases levels of methotrexate, phenytoin. Rifampin reduces TMP-SMX levels. Do not give leucovorin during treatment of pneumocystis pneumonia; may increase treatment failure and mortality. Can cause hyperkalemia (risk increased by high doses of trimethoprim, renal impairment, other drugs that cause hyperkalemia).

Dosing in renal dysfunction: Use 50% of usual dose for CrCl 15 to 30 mL/min. Do not use for CrCl <15 mL/min.

MOA — Sulfonamides (bacteriostatic) are structural analogs of PABA that bind with dihydropteroate synthetase and prevent bacterial folic acid synthesis. Trimethoprim inhibits dihydrofolate reductase, the enzyme after step in folic acid synthesis inhibited by sulfonamides. Trimethoprim acts like a potassium-sparing diuretic, reducing urinary potassium excretion.

ADVERSE EFFECTS — Serious: Stevens-Johnson syndrome, toxic epidermal necrolysis, hepatotoxicity, blood dyscrasias (thrombocytopenia risk possibly increased by thiazide diuretics), hemolysis in G6PD deficiency, hyperkalemia (risk increased by high doses of trimethoprim, renal impairment, or other drugs that cause hyperkalemia); hyponatremia with high doses; hypoglycemia in non-diabetic patients (esp. if renal/hepatic dysfunction, malnutrition, high doses). Bone marrow depression with high IV doses. Frequent: N/V, anorexia, allergic skin reactions, photosensitivity.

ANTIMICROBIALS: Tetracyclines

NOTE: Tetracyclines can cause photosensitivity, pseudotumor cerebri (avoid with isotretinoin), and may increase INR with warfarin. Use caution in renal dysfunction; doxycycline preferred. Generally avoid in children younger than 8 yo due to risk of teeth staining, but benefit of doxycycline for severe infections (e.g., anthrax, Rocky Mountain spotted fever) exceeds potential risk of teeth staining.

DEMECLOCYCLINE ▶K, feces ♀D ▶?+ $$$$

ADULT — Usual dose: 150 mg PO four times per day or 300 mg PO two times per day on empty stomach.

PEDS — Avoid in age younger than 8 yo due to teeth staining. Usual dose: 6.6 to 13.2 mg/kg/day PO given in 2 to 4 divided doses on empty stomach.

UNAPPROVED ADULT — SIADH: 600 to 1200 mg/day PO given in 3 to 4 divided doses.

FORMS — Generic: Tabs 150, 300 mg.

NOTES — Can cause diabetes insipidus, high risk of photosensitivity. Absorption impaired by iron, calcium, Al/Mg antacids. Take with fluids (not milk) to decrease esophageal irritation. SIADH onset of action occurs within 5 to 14 days; do not increase dose more frequently than q 3 to 4 days.

MOA — Inhibits bacterial protein synthesis by binding with ribosomal 30S subunit and blocking addition of amino acids to peptide chain. Active against intracellular bacteria. Bacteriostatic. Blocks action of ADH at level of collecting duct and distal tubule.

ADVERSE EFFECTS — Serious: Pseudotumor cerebri, nephrotoxicity, photosensitivity (high risk), teeth staining in children younger than 8 yo, diabetes insipidus. Frequent: N/V, heartburn, epigastric distress, diarrhea.

DOXYCYCLINE (*Acticlate, Adoxa, Avidoxy, Doryx, Doryx MPC, Doxy, Monodox, Oracea, Vibramycin, ✦Doxycin*) ▶LK ♀D ▶?+ varies by therapy

ADULT — Usual dose: 100 mg PO two times per day on 1st day, then 100 mg/day PO daily or divided two times per day. Severe infections: 100 mg PO two times per day. 100 mg PO two times per day for 5 to 7 days for community-acquired pneumonia; 7 days for Chlamydia or nongonococcal urethritis, 7 to 10 days for community-acquired skin infection. Doryx for chlamydia urethritis/cervicitis: 200 mg PO once daily for 7 days. Doryx MPC: 120 mg PO two times per day on day 1, the 120 mg PO once daily. Consider 120 mg PO two times per day for severe infections. Do not crush or chew; not interchangeable with other formulations. Acne vulgaris: Up to 100 mg PO two times per day. Oracea for inflammatory rosacea (papules and pustules): 40 mg PO once q am on empty stomach. Periodontitis: 20 mg PO two times per day 1 h before breakfast and dinner. Cholera: 300 mg PO single dose. Primary, secondary, early latent syphilis if penicillin-allergic: 100 mg PO two times per day for 14 days. Late latent or tertiary syphilis if penicillin-allergic: 100 mg PO two times per day for 4 weeks. Not for neurosyphilis. Malaria prophylaxis: 100 mg PO daily starting 1 to 2 days before exposure until 4 weeks after. IV: 200 mg on 1st day in 1 to 2 infusions, then 100 to 200 mg/day in 1 to 2 infusions. Anthrax: See table.

PEDS — Usually avoid in age younger than 8 yo due to teeth staining, but benefit for severe infections (e.g., anthrax, Rocky Mountain spotted fever) exceeds potential risk of teeth staining. Severe infections including tickborne rickettsial diseases: 2.2 mg/kg up to 100 mg IV/PO two times per day

DOXYCYCLINE (*cont.*)

for wt less than 45 kg; use adult dose for 45 kg or greater. Treat tickborne rickettisal diseases for a minimum of 5 to 7 days (until clinical improvement and fever resolved for at least 3 days). Treat anaplasmosis for 10 days if Lyme disease suspected. Anthrax:See table. Malaria prophylaxis, age 8 yo and older: 2 mg/kg/day up to 100 mg PO daily starting 1 to 2 days before exposure until 4 weeks after. Most PO and IV doses are equivalent. Doryx MPC. Usual dose, age greater than 8 yo: 5.3 mg/kg/day PO divided two times per day on day 1, then 2.6 mg/kg/day divided once or two times per day for wt less than 45 kg; use adult dose for wt 45 kg or greater. Do not crush or chew; not interchangeable with other formulations.

UNAPPROVED ADULT — See table for management of acute sinusitis. See STD table for granuloma inguinale, lymphogranuloma venereum, pelvic inflammatory disease treatment. Lyme disease: 100 mg PO two times per day for 14 days for early disease, for 28 days for Lyme arthritis. Prevention of Lyme disease in highly endemic area, with deer tick attachment at least 48 h: 200 mg PO single dose with food within 72 h of tick bite. Ehrlichiosis: 100 mg IV/PO two times per day for 7 to 14 days. Malaria, co-therapy with quinine/quinidine: 100 mg IV/PO two times per day for 7 days. Lymphatic filariasis: 100 mg PO two times per day for 8 weeks.

UNAPPROVED PEDS — Community-acquired MRSA skin infections, age 8 yo and older:2 mg/kg/dose PO q 12 h for wt 45 kg or less; 100 mg PO two times per day for wt greater than 45 kg. Treat for 5 to 10 days. Cholera: 2 to 4 mg/kg PO single dose for all ages.

FORMS — Monohydrate salt. Generic/Trade: Caps ($$) 50, 75, 100, 150 mg. Tabs ($$$) 50, 75, 100, 150 mg. Susp (Vibramycin) 25 mg/5 mL. Trade only: Delayed-release caps 40 mg (Oracea $$$$$). Generic: Delayed-release caps 40 mg ($$$$$). Hyclate salt. Tabs: Trade only: 75, 150 mg (Acticlate-$$$$$). Generic only: 20, 100mg. Caps: Generic only: 50 mg. Generic/Trade (Vibramycin): 100 mg. Trade only (Acticlate Cap): 75 mg. Delayed-release tabs: Generic only: 75, 100, 150 mg. Generic/Trade (Doryx $$$$$): 50, 200 mg. Trade only (Doryx MPC $$$$$): 120 mg. Delayed-release caps: Generic only: 75, 100 mg. Calcium salt. Trade only: Syrup (Vibramycin Calcium) 50 mg/5 mL.

NOTES — Photosensitivity, pseudotumor cerebri, increased BUN, painful IV infusion. Do not use Oracea to treat infections; dose is sub-antimicrobial. Risk of teeth staining may be lower than other tetracyclines. Do not give antacids or calcium supplements within 2 h of doxycycline. Barbiturates, carbamazepine, rifampin, and phenytoin may decrease doxycycline levels. Take with fluids to decrease esophageal irritation; can take with food/milk. Can break Doryx tabs and give immediately in a spoonful of applesauce. Do not crush or chew delayed-release pellets in tab. Maternal antimalarial prophylaxis does not harm breastfed infant or protect infant from malaria.

MOA — Inhibits bacterial protein synthesis by binding with ribosomal 30S subunit and blocking addition of amino acids to peptide chain. Active against intracellular bacteria. Bacteriostatic. Subantimicrobial doses have anti-inflammatory effects.

ADVERSE EFFECTS — Serious: Pseudotumor cerebri, Steven-Johnson syndrome, toxic epidermal necrolysis, DRESS, increased BUN, erosive esophagitis if taken lying down, teeth staining in children younger than 8 yo. Frequent: Photosensitivity, vaginitis, painful IV infusion.

MINOCYCLINE (*Minocin, Solodyn*) ▶LK ♀D ▶?+ $$

ADULT — Usual dose: 200 mg IV/PO 1st dose, then 100 mg q 12 h. IV and PO doses are the same. Not more than 400 mg/day IV. Community-acquired MRSA skin infections: 200 mg PO 1st dose, then 100 mg PO two times per day for 5 to 10 days. Solodyn ($$$$$) for inflammatory nonnodular moderate to severe acne: 1 mg/kg PO once daily. Dose is 45 mg for wt 45 to 54 kg, 65 mg for wt 55 to 77 kg, 90 mg for 78 to 102 kg, 115 mg for wt 103 to 125 kg, 135 mg for 126 to 136 kg.

PEDS — Avoid in age younger than 8 yo due to teeth staining. Usual dose: 4 mg/kg PO 1st dose, then 2 mg/kg two times per day. Community-acquired MRSA skin infection: 4 mg/kg PO 1st dose, then 2 mg/kg/dose PO two times per day for 5 to 10 days. Do not exceed adult dose. IV and PO doses are the same. Solodyn ($$$$$) for inflammatory nonnodular moderate to severe acne, age 12 yo or older: Give PO once daily at dose of 45 mg for wt 45 to 54 kg, 65 mg for wt 55 to 77 kg, 90 mg for 78 to 102 kg, 115 mg for wt 103 to 125 kg, 135 mg for 126 to 136 kg.

UNAPPROVED ADULT — Acne vulgaris (traditional dosing, not for Solodyn): 50 mg PO two times per day. RA: 100 mg PO two times per day.

FORMS — Generic/Trade: Caps, Tabs ($) 50, 75, 100 mg. Extended-release tabs ($$$$$) 45, 90, 135 mg. Trade only: Extended-release tabs (Solodyn-$$$$$) 55 , 65, 80, 105, 115 mg.

NOTES — Dizziness, hepatotoxicity, lupus. Do not use Solodyn to treat infections. Do not give antacids or calcium supplements within 2 h of minocycline. Take with fluids (not milk) to decrease esophageal irritation. Do not chew, crush, or split Solodyn.

MOA — Inhibits bacterial protein synthesis by binding with ribosomal 30S subunit and blocking addition of amino acids to peptide chain. Active against intracellular bacteria. Bacteriostatic. Subantimicrobial doses have anti-inflammatory effects.

ADVERSE EFFECTS — Serious: Pseudotumor cerebri, serum sickness, Stevens-Johnson syndrome, drug rash with eosinophilia and systemic symptoms (DRESS), increased BUN, photosensitivity, hepatotoxicity, lupus, hypersensitivity pneumonitis, hyperpigmentation, teeth staining in children younger than 8 yo. Frequent: Dizziness/vestibular toxicity.

TETRACYCLINE ▶LK ♀D ▶?+ $

ADULT — Usual dose: 250 to 500 mg PO four times per day on empty stomach. H. pylori: See table in GI section. Primary, secondary, early latent syphilis if penicillin-allergic: 500 mg PO four times per day for 14 days. Late latent syphilis if penicillin-allergic: 500 mg PO four times per day for 28 days.

PEDS — Avoid in children younger than 8 yo due to teeth staining. Usual dose: 25 to 50 mg/kg/day PO divided in 2 to 4 doses on empty stomach.

UNAPPROVED ADULT — Malaria, co-therapy with quinine: 250 mg PO four times per day for 7 days.

UNAPPROVED PEDS — Avoid in children younger than 8 yo due to teeth staining. Malaria, co-therapy with quinine: 25 mg/kg/day PO divided four times per day for 7 days.

FORMS — Generic only: Caps 250, 500 mg.

NOTES — Increased BUN/hepatotoxicity in patients with renal dysfunction. Do not give antacids or calcium supplements within 2 h of tetracycline. Take with fluids (not milk) to decrease esophageal irritation.

MOA — Inhibits bacterial protein synthesis by binding with ribosomal 30S subunit and blocking addition of amino acids to peptide chain. Active against intracellular bacteria. Bacteriostatic.

ADVERSE EFFECTS — Serious: Pseudotumor cerebri, increased BUN/hepatotoxicity in patients with renal dysfunction, photosensitivity, teeth staining in children younger than 8 yo.

ANTIMICROBIALS: Other Antimicrobials

AZTREONAM (*Azactam, Cayston*) ▶K ♀B ▶+ $$$$$

ADULT — UTI: 500 mg to 1 g IM/IV q 8 to 12 h. Pneumonia, sepsis, skin, intra-abdominal, gynecologic: Moderate infections, 1 to 2 g IM/IV q 8 to 12 h. P. aeruginosa or severe infections, 2 g IV q 6 to 8 h. Use IV route for doses greater than 1 g. Cystic fibrosis respiratory symptoms: 1 vial Cayston nebulized three times per day for 28 days, followed by cycle of 28 days off treatment.

PEDS — Gram-negative infections, usual dose: 30 mg/kg/dose IV q 6 to 8 h. Cystic fibrosis respiratory symptoms, age 7 yo and older: 1 vial Cayston nebulized three times per day for 28 days, followed by cycle of 28 days off treatment.

UNAPPROVED ADULT — Meningitis: 2 g IV q 6 to 8 h.

UNAPPROVED PEDS — P. aeruginosa pulmonary infection in cystic fibrosis: 50 mg/kg/dose IV q 6 to 8 h.

FORMS — Trade only (Cayston): 75 mg/vial with diluent for inhalation.

NOTES — Dosing in adults with renal dysfunction: 1 to 2 g IV load, then 50% of usual dose for CrCl 10 to 30 mL/min; 0.5 to 2 g IV load, then 25% of usual dose for CrCl <10 mL/min. For life-threatening infections, also give 12.5% of initial dose after each hemodialysis. Cayston: Use bronchodilator before each dose (short acting bronchodilator 15 min to 4 h before or long-acting bronchodilator 30 min to 12 h before). Give immediately after reconstitution only with Altera nebulizer. Order of administration is bronchodilator, mucolytic, then Cayston. Stable at room temperature for 28 days.

MOA — Monobactam (monocyclic beta-lactam) that binds only to penicillin-binding proteins in gram-negative organisms.

ADVERSE EFFECTS — Serious: Cross-sensitivity with ceftazidime possible, but unlikely, C. difficile–associated diarrhea. Frequent: Eosinophilia. Cayston for inhalation: Bronchospasm, cough, wheezing, fever.

CHLORAMPHENICOL ▶LK ♀C ▶– $$$$$

WARNING — Serious and fatal blood dyscrasias. Dose-dependent bone marrow suppression common.

ADULT — Typhoid fever, rickettsial infections: 50 mg/kg/day IV divided q 6 h. Up to 75 to 100 mg/kg/day IV for serious infections untreatable with other agents.

PEDS — Severe infections including meningitis: 50 to 100 mg/kg/day IV divided q 6 h. AAP recommends 75 to 100 mg/kg/day for invasive pneumococcal infections only in patients with life-threatening beta-lactam allergy.

NOTES — Monitor CBC q 2 days. Monitor serum levels. Therapeutic peak: 10 to 20 mcg/mL. Trough: 5 to 10 mcg/mL. Use cautiously in acute intermittent porphyria/G6PD deficiency. Gray baby syndrome in preemies and newborns. Barbiturates, rifampin decrease chloramphenicol levels. Chloramphenicol increases barbiturate, phenytoin levels and may increase INR with warfarin. Dosing in adults with hepatic dysfunction: 1 g IV load, then 500 mg q 6 h.

MOA — Inhibits bacterial protein synthesis by interfering with ribosomal 50S subunit. Bacteriostatic/cidal depending on pathogen.

ADVERSE EFFECTS — Serious: Fatal blood dyscrasias, dose-dependent bone marrow suppression common. Gray baby syndrome in preemies and newborns.

CLINDAMYCIN (*Cleocin, ✻Dalacin C*) ▶L ♀B ▶?+ $

WARNING — Can cause C. difficile–associated diarrhea.

ADULT — Serious anaerobic, streptococcal, staph infections: 600 to 900 mg IV q 8 h or 150 to 450 mg PO four times per day. Community-acquired MRSA skin infections: 300 to 450 mg PO three times per day for 5 to 10 days. Complicated MRSA skin infection: 600 mg IV/PO q 8 h for 7 to 14 days. MRSA pneumonia: 600 mg IV/PO q 8 h for 7 to 21 days. MRSA osteomyelitis: 600 mg IV/PO q 8 h. See tables for prophylaxis of bacterial endocarditis and treatment of STDs (pelvic inflammatory disease).

PEDS — Serious anaerobic, streptococcal, staph infections: 20 to 40 mg/kg/day IV divided q 6 to 8 h or 8 to 20 mg/kg/day (as caps) PO divided three to four times per day or 8 to 25 mg/kg/day (as

(cont.)

CLINDAMYCIN (*cont.*)

palmitate oral soln) PO divided three to four times per day. MRSA pneumonia, osteomyelitis, complicated skin infection: 40 mg/kg/day IV divided q 6 to 8 h. Do not use doses that are less than 37.5 mg of oral soln PO three times per day for children with wt less than 11 kg. Infants age younger than 1 mo: 15 to 20 mg/kg/day IV divided three to four times per day. See table for prophylaxis of bacterial endocarditis.

UNAPPROVED ADULT — Bacterial vaginosis: 300 mg PO two times per day for 7 days. Oral/dental infection: 300 mg PO four times per day. Prevention of perinatal group B streptococcal disease: 900 mg IV to mother q 8 h until delivery. CNS toxoplasmosis, AIDS (with leucovorin, pyrimethamine): Acute treatment 600 mg PO/IV q 6 h; secondary prevention 300 to 450 mg PO q 6 to 8 h. AHA dose for group A streptococcal pharyngitis in penicillin-allergic patients: 20 mg/kg/day (max 1.8 g/day) PO divided three times per day for 10 days. Group A streptococcal pharyngitis, repeated culture-positive episodes: 20 mg/kg/day (max 1.8 g/day) PO divided three times per day for 10 days. Malaria, co-therapy with quinine/quinidine: 10 mg/kg base IV loading dose followed by 5 mg/kg IV q 8 h or 20 mg/kg/day base PO divided three times per day to complete 7 days. Anthrax: See table. Babesiosis, severe: See quinine entry.

UNAPPROVED PEDS — Community-acquired MRSA skin infections: 10 to 13 mg/kg/dose PO q 6 to 8 h for 5 to 10 days (max 40 mg/kg/day). AHA dose for group A streptococcal pharyngitis in penicillin-allergic patients: 20 mg/kg/day (max 1.8 g/day) PO divided three times per day for 10 days. Group A streptococcal pharyngitis, repeated culture-positive episodes: 20 to 30 mg/kg/day PO divided q 8 h for 10 days. Otitis media, after failure of initial antibiotic treatment: 30 to 40 mg/kg/day PO divided three times per day plus 3rd-generation cephalosporin. For oral therapy of acute otitis media, AAP recommends 5 to 7 days of therapy for children 6 yo and older with mild to moderate symptoms, 7 days for children 2 to 5 yo with mild to moderate symptoms, and 10 days for children younger than 2 yo and children with severe symptoms. See tables for management of otitis media and acute sinusitis in children. Toxoplasmosis, substitute for sulfadiazine in sulfonamide-intolerant children: 5 to 7.5 mg/kg (up to 600 mg/dose) PO/IV q 6 h + pyrimethamine + leucovorin. Malaria, co-therapy with quinine/quinidine: 10 mg/kg base IV loading dose followed by 5 mg/kg IV q 8 h or 20 mg/kg/day base PO divided three times per day to complete 7 days. Anthrax: See table. Babesiosis, severe: See quinine entry.

FORMS — Generic/Trade: Caps 75, 150, 300 mg. Oral soln 75 mg/5 mL (100 mL).

NOTES — Not for meningitis. Not more than 600 mg/IM injection site. Avoid if lincomycin hypersensitivity. Consider D-test for MRSA inducible resistance.

MOA — Semisynthetic derivative of lincomycin that inhibits RNA-dependent protein synthesis in susceptible organisms by interfering with function of ribosomal 50S subunit. Bacteriostatic.

ADVERSE EFFECTS — Serious: C. difficile-associated diarrhea. Frequent: Diarrhea, allergic reactions. Other: Metallic taste.

COLISTIMETHATE (*Coly-Mycin M Parenteral*) ▶K ♀C ▶? $$$$

ADULT — Gram-negative infections, esp. multidrug-resistant Acinetobacter, E. coli, Klebsiella, P. aeruginosa: 2.5 to 5 mg/kg/day IM/IV divided q 6 to 12 h or IV continuous infusion. Max dose is 5 mg/kg/day (colistin base activity) in patients with normal renal function. Inject IV slowly over 3 to 5 minutes q 12 h. For continuous infusion, inject half of daily dose over 3 to 5 minutes; give remainder as continuous infusion over 22 to 23 h, starting 1 to 2 h after first injection. Base dose on ideal body wt in obesity. Colistin should not be used alone.

PEDS — Gram-negative infections, esp. multidrug-resistant Acinetobacter, E. coli, Klebsiella, P. aeruginosa: 2.5 to 5 mg/kg/day IM/IV divided q 6 to 12 h or IV continuous infusion. Max dose is 5 mg/kg/day (colistin base activity) in patients with normal renal function. Inject IV slowly over 3 to 5 minutes q 12 h. For continuous infusion, inject half of daily dose over 3 to 5 minutes; give remainder as continuous infusion over 22 to 23 h, starting 1 to 2 h after 1st injection. Base dose on ideal body wt in obesity. Colistin should not be used alone.

UNAPPROVED ADULT — Gram-negative infections, alternative dosing regimens: Loading dose of 5 mg/kg IV, then 2.5 mg/kg IV q 12 h. Or consider using a dosing calculator such as http://clincalc.com/Colistin. Cystic fibrosis: Use nebulizer soln promptly after it is made. Storage for longer than 24 h increases the formation of polymyxin E1 which may cause pulmonary toxicity.

FORMS — Generic/Trade: Each vial contains colistimethate sodium equivalent to 150 mg colistin base activity.

NOTES — Each vial contains 150 mg colistin base activity. May enhance neuromuscular junction blockade by aminoglycosides, neuromuscular blockers; extreme caution advised for coadministration. Can cause transient neurologic symptoms that can be relieved by dosage reduction. Dose-dependent, reversible nephrotoxicity. Dosage adjustment in adults with renal dysfunction: 2.5 to 3.8 mg/kg divided into 2 doses per day for CrCl 50 to 79 mL/min; 2.5 mg/kg once daily or divided into 2 doses per day for CrCl 30 to 49 mL/min; 1.5 mg/kg q 36 h for CrCl 10 to 29 mL/min.

MOA — Polypeptide antibiotic that penetrates and disrupts bacterial cell membrane.

ADVERSE EFFECTS — Dose-dependent, reversible nephrotoxicity. Reports of respiratory arrest after IM administration. Transient neurologic symptoms including perioral paresthesia, numbness, vertigo, dizziness, slurred speech, generalized pruritus.

DAPTOMYCIN (*Cubicin*) ▸K ♀B ▸? $$$$$
ADULT — Complicated skin infections (including MRSA): 4 mg/kg IV once daily for 7 to 14 days. S. aureus bacteremia (including MRSA), including right-sided endocarditis: 6 mg/kg IV once daily for at least 2 to 6 weeks. See Adult Unapproved for AHA/IDSA recommended doses. Infuse over 30 min or inject over 2 min.
PEDS — Not approved in children. Avoid use if age less than 12 months; muscle/nervous system adverse effects observed in neonatal dog studies.
UNAPPROVED ADULT — MRSA bacteremia/endocarditis, high-dose regimen: 8 to 10 mg/kg IV once daily. AHA dosing for left-sided methicillin-sensitive S. aureus endocarditis: 8 mg/kg or greater IV once daily for 6 weeks. AHA dosing for enterococcal endocarditis resistant to other agents: 10 to 12 kg/kg IV once daily for 6 weeks or more. AHA recommends infectious diseases consult for daptomycin doses in endocarditis. Vancomycin-resistant MRSA bacteremia: 10 mg/kg IV once daily in combo with another antibiotic. MRSA osteomyelitis: 6 mg/kg IV once daily.
UNAPPROVED PEDS — MRSA bacteremia/endocarditis: 6 to 10 mg/kg IV once daily. MRSA osteomyelitis: 6 mg/kg IV once daily.
NOTES — May cause myopathy (with doses of 6 mg/kg/day or greater), neuropathy, eosinophilic pneumonia (rare), C. difficile–associated diarrhea. Monitor CK levels weekly. Stop if myopathy symptoms and CK more than 5 times upper limit of normal, or no symptoms and CK at least 10 times upper limit of normal. Consider withholding statins during daptomycin treatment. Can falsely elevate PT with certain thromboplastin reagents; minimize effect by drawing PT/INR sample just before daptomycin dose or use another reagent. Not effective for pneumonia (inactivated by surfactant). Reduce dose in adults with CrCl <30 mL/min: 4 mg/kg IV q 48 h for complicated skin infections; 6 mg/kg IV q 48 h for S. aureus bacteremia. Give dose after hemodialysis sessions. Efficacy may be reduced in patients with CrCl <50 mL/min. Reconstituted soln stable for up to 12 h at room temp or 48 h in refrigerator (combined time in vial and IV bag). Do not use in ReadyMed elastomeric infusion pump due to leaching of MBT impurity.
MOA — Cyclic lipopeptide that depolarizes bacterial membrane potential. Inhibition of DNA, RNA, and protein synthesis kills bacteria.
ADVERSE EFFECTS — Serious: Myopathy (with doses of 6 mg/kg/day or greater), neuropathy, eosinophilic pneumonia (rare), C difficile-associated diarrhea. Frequent: Increased CK levels, constipation, nausea, headache, abnormal LFTs, dyspnea.

FOSFOMYCIN (*Monurol*) ▸K ♀B ▸? $$$
ADULT — Simple UTI in women: One 3 g packet PO single dose. Dissolve granules in ½ cup of water.
PEDS — Not approved for age younger than 12 yo.
UNAPPROVED ADULT — Complicated UTI: 3 g PO every 2 to 3 days for 3 to 7 doses (up to 21 days

duration). Chronic prostatitis, due to multi-drug resistant gram-negative bacteria: 3 g PO q 2 to 3 days for 7 to 14 doses.
FORMS — Trade only: 3 g packet of granules.
NOTES — Metoclopramide decreases urinary excretion of fosfomycin. Single dose less effective than ciprofloxacin or TMP-SMX; equivalent to nitrofurantoin.
MOA — Inactivates enolpyruvyl transferase, irreversibly blocking an early step in bacterial cell wall synthesis. Also reduces bacterial adherence to uroepithelial cells. Bactericidal in urine.
ADVERSE EFFECTS — Serious: None. Frequent: Diarrhea.

LINCOMYCIN (*Lincocin*) ▸LK ♀C ▸– $$$$
WARNING — C. difficile–associated diarrhea.
ADULT — Serious Gram-positive infections: 600 mg IM q 12 to 24 h. 600 to 1000 mg IV q 8 to 12 h. Max IV daily dose is 8 g. Infuse IV over at least 1 h at dilution of 1 g/100 mL or more dilute. Reserve for patients who are allergic to or do not respond to penicillins.
PEDS — Serious Gram-positive infections, age older than 1 mo: 10 to 20 mg/kg/day IV divided q 8 to 12 h or 10 mg/kg IM q 12 to 24 h. . Infuse IV over at least 1 h diluted to 1 g/100 mL or more dilute. Reserve for patients who are allergic to or do not respond to penicillins.
NOTES — Do not use in patients with clindamycin hypersensitivity. Monitor hepatic and renal function and CBC during prolonged therapy. Do not coadminister with erythromycin due to potential antagonism. May enhance effects of neuromuscular blockers. Reduce dose by 25% to 30% in patients with severe renal dysfunction and consider monitoring levels.
MOA — Inhibits RNA-dependent protein synthesis in susceptible organisms by interfering with function of ribosomal 50S subunit.
ADVERSE EFFECTS — Serious: C. difficile-associated diarrhea; severe hypersensitivity reactions; Stevens-Johnson syndrome; neutropenia; thrombocytopenia; renal dysfunction. Hypotension/cardiopulmonary arrest possible if IV infusion too rapid. Frequent: No data.

LINEZOLID (*Zyvox*, ✱*Zyvoxam*) ▸Oxidation/K ♀C ▸? $$$$$
ADULT — IV and PO doses are the same. Vancomycin-resistant E. faecium infections: 600 mg IV/PO q 12 h for 14 to 28 days. Pneumonia, complicated skin infections (including MRSA and diabetic foot): 600 mg IV/PO q 12 h for 10 to 14 days. IV infused over 30 to 120 min.
PEDS — Pneumonia, complicated skin infections (including MRSA): 10 mg/kg (up to 600 mg) IV/PO q 8 h for age younger than 12 yo; 600 mg IV/PO q 12 h for age 12 yo or older. Treat for for 10 to 14 days. Vancomycin-resistant E. faecium infections: 10 mg/kg IV/PO q 8 h (up to 600 mg) for age younger than 12 yo; 600 mg IV/PO q 12 h for age 12 yo or older. Treat for 14 to 28 days. Uncomplicated skin

(cont.)

LINEZOLID (*cont.*)

infections: 10 mg/kg PO q 8 h for age younger than 5 yo; 10 mg/kg PO q 12 h for age 5 to 11 yo; 600 mg PO q 12 h for age 12 yo or older. Treat for 10 to 14 days. Preterm infants (less than 34 weeks' gestational age): 10 mg/kg q 12 h, increase to 10 mg/kg q 8 h by 7 days of life. IV infused over 30 to 120 min.

UNAPPROVED ADULT — Community-acquired MRSA skin infection: 600 mg PO two times per day for 5 to 10 days. Anthrax: See table.

UNAPPROVED PEDS — Community-acquired MRSA skin infection: 10 mg/kg (up to 600 mg) PO q 8 h for age younger than 12 yo; 600 mg PO q 12 h for age 12 yo or older. Treat for 5 to 10 days. Anthrax: See table.

FORMS — Generic/Trade: Tabs 600 mg. Susp 100 mg/5 mL.

NOTES — Myelosuppression. Monitor CBC weekly, especially if more than 2 weeks of therapy, pre-existing myelosuppression, other myelosuppressive drugs, or chronic infection treated with other antibiotics. Consider stopping if myelosuppression occurs or worsens. Peripheral and optic neuropathy, primarily in those treated for more than 1 month. Ophthalmic exam recommended for visual changes at any time; monitor visual function in all patients treated for 3 months or longer. In a study comparing linezolid with vancomycin, oxacillin, or dicloxacillin for catheter-related bloodstream infections, mortality was increased in linezolid-treated patients infected only with Gram-negative bacteria. Inhibits MAO; may interact with adrenergic and serotonergic drugs, high-tyramine foods. Limit tyramine to less than 100 mg/meal. Reduce initial dose of dopamine/epinephrine. Serotonin syndrome reported with concomitant administration of serotonergic drugs (SSRIs). Rifampin can reduce linezolid exposure; clinical significance unclear. Hypoglycemia reported in diabetics treated with insulin or oral hypoglycemics. Store susp at room temperature; stable for 21 days. Gently turn bottle over 3 to 5 times before giving a dose; do not shake.

MOA — Oxazolidinone that inhibits bacterial protein synthesis by binding with 50S ribosome (may compete for binding with chloramphenicol). Bacteriostatic.

ADVERSE EFFECTS — Serious: Myelosuppression, reports of serotonin syndrome, peripheral and optic neuropathy (with long-term use; optic neuropathy sometimes progressing to vision loss), lactic acidosis (immediate evaluation if recurrent N/V, unexplained acidosis, low bicarbonate). Hypoglycemia reported in diabetics treated with insulin or oral hypoglycemics. In a study comparing linezolid with vancomycin, oxacillin, dicloxacillin for catheter-related bloodstream infections, mortality was increased in linezolid-treated patients infected only with gram-negative bacteria. Frequent: Thrombocytopenia, N/V, diarrhea. Tooth discoloration (removable with cleaning).

METHENAMINE HIPPURATE (*Hiprex*) ▶KL ♀C ▶? $$$$

ADULT — Long-term suppression of UTI: 1 g PO two times per day.

PEDS — Long-term suppression of UTI: 0.5 to 1 g PO two times per day for 6 to 12 yo; 1 g PO two times per day for older than 12 yo.

FORMS — Generic/Trade: Tabs 1 g.

NOTES — Not for UTI treatment. Contraindicated if renal or severe hepatic impairment, severe dehydration. Acidify urine if Proteus, Pseudomonas infections. Give 1 to 2 g vitamin C PO q 4 h if urine pH greater than 5. Avoid sulfonamides, alkalinizing foods and medications.

MOA — Releases formaldehyde (bactericidal) in acidic urine.

ADVERSE EFFECTS — Frequent: N/V, rash, dysuria.

METRONIDAZOLE (*Flagyl, Flagyl ER, ✳Nidazol*) ▶KL ♀B ▶? – $

WARNING — Carcinogenic in animal studies; avoid unnecessary use.

ADULT — Trichomoniasis: Treat patient and sex partners with 2 g PO single dose (may be used in pregnancy per CDC), 250 mg PO three times per day for 7 days, or 375 mg PO two times per day for 7 days. Flagyl ER for bacterial vaginosis: 750 mg PO daily for 7 days on empty stomach. H. pylori: See table in GI section. Anaerobic bacterial infections: Load 1 g or 15 mg/kg IV, then 500 mg or 7.5 mg/kg IV/PO q 6 to 8 h (up to 4 g/day), each IV dose over 1 h. Prophylaxis, colorectal surgery: 15 mg/kg IV completed 1 h preop, then 7.5 mg/kg IV q 6 h for 2 doses. Acute amebic dysentery: 750 mg PO three times per day for 5 to 10 days. Amebic liver abscess: 500 to 750 mg IV/PO three times per day for 10 days.

PEDS — Amebiasis: 35 to 50 mg/kg/day PO (up to 750 mg/dose) divided three times per day for 10 days.

UNAPPROVED ADULT — Bacterial vaginosis: 500 mg PO two times per day for 7 days. Trichomoniasis (CDC alternative to single dose): 500 mg PO two times per day for 7 days. Pelvic inflammatory disease, recurrent/persistent urethritis: See STD table. C. difficile–associated diarrhea, mild/moderate: 500 mg PO three times per day for 10 to 14 days. C. difficile–associated diarrhea, severe complicated: 500 mg IV q 8 h with PO/PR vancomycin. See table for management of C. difficile infection in adults. Giardia: 250 mg PO three times per day for 5 to 7 days.

UNAPPROVED PEDS — C. difficile–associated diarrhea: 30 mg/kg/day PO divided four times per day for 10 to 14 days (not to exceed adult dose). Trichomoniasis: 5 mg/kg PO three times per day (max 2 g/day) for 7 days. Giardia: 15 mg/kg/day PO divided three times per day for 5 to 7 days. Anaerobic bacterial infections: 30 mg/kg/day IV/PO divided q 6 h, each IV dose over 1 h (up to 4 g/day).

FORMS — Generic/Trade: Tabs 250, 500 mg. Trade only: Caps 375 mg. Extended-release tabs: 750 mg.

(cont.)

METRONIDAZOLE *(cont.)*

NOTES — Peripheral neuropathy (chronic use), seizures, encephalopathy, aseptic meningitis, optic neuropathy. Avoid long-term use. Disulfiram reaction; avoid alcohol until at least 3 days after treatment. Do not give within 2 weeks of disulfiram. Interacts with barbiturates, lithium, phenytoin. Increased INR with warfarin. Darkens urine. Give iodoquinol or paromomycin after treatment for amebic dysentery or liver abscess. Can minimize infant exposure by withholding breastfeeding for 12 to 24 h after maternal single dose. Decrease dose in liver dysfunction.

MOA — Bactericidal agent that is reduced intracellularly to toxic intermediates/free radicals that damage DNA or other macromolecules.

ADVERSE EFFECTS — Serious: Peripheral neuropathy (chronic use), seizures, encephalopathy, aseptic meningitis, optic neuropathy. Frequent: Darkens urine, N/V, diarrhea, metallic aftertaste, disulfiram-like reaction.

NITROFURANTOIN *(Furadantin, Macrodantin, Macrobid)* ▶KL ♀B ▶+? $$

ADULT — Uncomplicated UTI: 50 to 100 mg PO four times per day for 7 days or until 3 days after sterile urine. Long-term suppressive therapy: 50 to 100 mg PO at bedtime. Macrobid for uncomplicated UTI: 100 mg PO two times per day for 7 days. Take nitrofurantoin with food.

PEDS — Uncomplicated UTI: 5 to 7 mg/kg/day PO divided four times per day for 7 days or until 3 days after sterile urine. Long-term suppressive therapy: Doses as low as 1 mg/kg/day PO divided one to two times per day. Macrobid for uncomplicated UTI, age older than 12 yo: 100 mg PO two times per day for 7 days. Take nitrofurantoin with food.

UNAPPROVED ADULT — Uncomplicated cystitis in women: IDSA recommends 100 mg Macrobid PO two times per day for 5 days (avoid if early pyelonephritis suspected).

FORMS — Generic/Trade: Caps (Macrodantin) 25, 50, 100 mg. Caps (Macrobid) 100 mg. Susp (Furadantin) 25 mg/5 mL.

NOTES — Contraindicated if pregnancy 38 weeks or longer, infant age younger than 1 mo, or CrCl <60 mL/min. Per Beers critera, short-term use is acceptable if CrCl ≥30 mL/min. Hemolytic anemia in G6PD deficiency (including susceptible breastfed infants), hepatotoxicity (monitor LFTs periodically), peripheral neuropathy. May turn urine brown. Not for complicated UTI or pyelonephritis.

MOA — Appears to interact with ribosomal proteins and damage bacterial DNA.

ADVERSE EFFECTS — Serious: Pulmonary fibrosis with prolonged use, hepatotoxicity, peripheral neuropathy, hemolytic anemia in G6PD deficiency. Frequent: N/V, allergy, brown discoloration of urine.

RIFAXIMIN *(Xifaxan)* ▶feces ♀X/?/? ▶? $$$$

ADULT — Traveler's diarrhea: 200 mg PO three times per day for 3 days. Prevention of recurrent hepatic encephalopathy ($$$$$): 550 mg PO two times per day. Irritable bowel syndrome with diarrhea: 550 mg PO three times per day for 14 days. Can retreat up to 2 times if recurrence.

PEDS — Traveler's diarrhea, age 12 yo or older: 200 mg PO three times per day for 3 days.

FORMS — Trade only: Tabs 200, 550 mg.

NOTES — Do not use for Traveler's diarrhea with fever/blood in stool or caused by pathogens other than E. coli. Consider alternatives if diarrhea persists for 24 to 48 h or worsens. P-glycoprotein inhibitors (eg cyclosporine; see p-glycoprotein table) can substantially increase rifaximin exposure, esp. if hepatic impairment. Rifaximin exposure may increase in severe hepatic impairment.

MOA — Rifamycin structurally related to rifampin. Inhibits bacterial RNA synthesis by binding with beta-subunit of bacterial DNA-dependent RNA polymerase. Active against entero-toxigenic or aggregative E Coli.

ADVERSE EFFECTS — Serious: None found. Frequent: None found.

SYNERCID *(quinupristin + dalfopristin)* ▶Bile ♀B ▶? $$$$$

ADULT — Complicated staphylococcal/streptococcal skin infections: 7.5 mg/kg IV q 12 h for at least 7 days. Infuse over 1 h.

PEDS — Safety and efficacy not established in children.

UNAPPROVED ADULT — MRSA bacteremia (2nd line): 7.5 mg/kg IV q 8 h.

UNAPPROVED PEDS — Complicated staphylococcal/streptococcal skin infections: 7.5 mg/kg IV q 12 h for at least 7 days. Infuse over 1 h.

NOTES — Indication for vancomycin-resistant E. faecium infections was removed from labeling because efficacy was not demonstrated in clinical trials. Venous irritation (flush with D5W after peripheral infusion; do not use normal saline/heparin), arthralgias/myalgias, hyperbilirubinemia. Infuse by central venous catheter to avoid dose-related vein irritation. CYP3A4 inhibitor. Increases levels of cyclosporine, midazolam, nifedipine, and others.

MOA — Streptogramin fixed-dose combination that inhibits bacterial protein synthesis by binding to different sites of the 50S ribosomal subunit and forming a stable tertiary complex with each other and the ribosome.

ADVERSE EFFECTS — Serious: None. Frequent: Venous irritation after peripheral infusion, arthralgia/myalgia, hyperbilirubinemia.

TEDIZOLID *(Sivextro)* ▶L ♀C ▶? $$$$$

ADULT — Skin infections, including MRSA: 200 mg IV/PO once daily for 6 days. Infuse IV over 1 h.

PEDS — Safety and efficacy not established in children.

FORMS — Trade only: Tabs 200 mg.

NOTES — Consider alternatives in neutropenic patients; not evaluated in neutropenic patients and antibacterial activity reduced in the absence of granulocytes in an animal model. Tedizolid is a weak, reversible MAO inhibitor in vitro. FDA concluded that no restrictions are necessary for

(cont.)

TEDIZOLID (*cont.*)

coadministration with adrenergic or serotonergic drugs and tyramine-rich foods, but phase 3 clinical trials excluded MOA inhibitors, serotonergic drugs, and a high-tyramine diet.

MOA — Oxazolidinone that inhibits bacterial protein synthesis by binding with 50S ribosome. Bacteriostatic.

ADVERSE EFFECTS — Serious: C. difficile-associated diarrhea. Frequent: N/V, diarrhea, headache, dizziness.

TELITHROMYCIN (*Ketek*) ▶LK ♀C ▶? $$$$

WARNING — Contraindicated in myasthenia gravis due to reports of exacerbation, including fatal acute respiratory depression. Warn patients about exacerbation of myasthenia gravis, hepatotoxicity, visual disturbances, and loss of consciousness.

ADULT — Community-acquired pneumonia: 800 mg PO daily for 7 to 10 days. Not for acute sinusitis or acute exacerbation of chronic bronchitis; risks exceed potential benefit.

PEDS — Safety and efficacy not established in children.

FORMS — Trade only: Tabs 300, 400 mg.

NOTES — May prolong QT interval. Avoid in proarrhythmic conditions or with drugs that prolong QT interval. Life-threatening hepatotoxicity. Monitor for signs/symptoms of hepatitis. Contraindicated if history of hepatitis due to any macrolide or telithromycin. Contraindicated in myasthenia gravis. CYP3A4 substrate and strong inhibitor. Contraindicated with pimozide, rifampin, ergot alkaloids. Hold simvastatin, lovastatin, or atorvastatin during course of telithromycin. Consider monitoring INR with warfarin. Give telithromycin and theophylline at least 1 h apart. Monitor for toxicity of digoxin, midazolam, metoprolol. CYP3A4 inducers (ie phenytoin, carbamazepine) could reduce telithromycin levels. Dosage adjustment for CrCl <30 mL/min (including hemodialysis) is 600 mg once daily. On dialysis days, give after hemodialysis session. Dosage adjustment for CrCl <30 mL/min with hepatic dysfunction is 400 mg once daily.

MOA — Ketolide; structure and mechanism of action similar to macrolides. Inhibits protein synthesis in susceptible organisms by interfering with function of ribosomal 50S subunit. Methoxy and ketone groups enhance acid stability and ribosomal binding, and reduce susceptibility to drug efflux pumps.

ADVERSE EFFECTS — Serious: Exacerbation of myasthenia gravis; hepatotoxicity; QT interval prolongation. Frequent: Diarrhea, nausea, dizziness, elevated LFTs. Other: Visual disturbances, esp. difficulty in accommodation (rare; most cases occur after 1st or 2nd dose in women less than 40 yo), transient loss of consciousness.

TIGECYCLINE (*Tygacil*) ▶Bile, K ♀D ▶?+ $$$$$

WARNING — Tigecycline had 0.6% higher mortality rate than comparators in meta-analysis of phase 3 and 4 clinical trials. Use it only when alternatives are not appropriate.

ADULT — Complicated skin infections, complicated intra-abdominal infections, community-acquired pneumonia: 100 mg IV 1st dose, then 50 mg IV q 12 h. Infuse over 30 to 60 min. Not approved for hospital-acquired or ventilator-associated pneumonia (decreased efficacy and higher mortality) or diabetic foot infection (decreased efficacy).

PEDS — Not approved in children unless no alternative. Avoid in children age younger than 8 yo due to permanent teeth staining. Treatment of infections with no alternative: 1.2 mg/kg (max 50 mg) IV q 12 h for age 8 to 11 yo; 50 mg IV q 12 h for age 12 to 17 yo.

NOTES — Caution advised for tigecycline monotherapy of complicated intra-abdominal infection due to intestinal perforation. Discard reconstituted tigecycline if it does not have yellow-orange color. May decrease efficacy of oral contraceptives. Monitor INR with warfarin. Dosage adjustment for severe liver dysfunction (Child-Pugh C): 100 mg IV 1st dose, then 25 mg IV q 12 h.

MOA — Inhibits bacterial protein synthesis by binding with ribosomal 30S subunit and blocking addition of amino acids to peptide chain. Bacteriostatic.

ADVERSE EFFECTS — Serious: Higher mortality than other antibiotics, especially in ventilator-associated pneumonia. Anaphylaxis/anaphylactoid rxns, acute pancreatitis, hepatic dysfunction. Other adverse effects may be similar to tetracyclines (Serious: Pseudotumor cerebri, anti-anabolic effects, photosensitivity, permanent teeth staining in children younger than 8 yo.) Frequent: N/V.

TRIMETHOPRIM (*Primsol,* ✱*Proloprin*) ▶K ♀C ▶– $

ADULT — Uncomplicated UTI: 100 mg PO two times per day or 200 mg PO daily.

PEDS — Otitis media (not for M. catarrhalis), age 2 mo or older: 10 mg/kg/day PO divided two times per day for 10 days for age 6 mo or older. Not a good option for otitis media; see otitis media table for alternatives.

UNAPPROVED ADULT — Prophylaxis of recurrent UTI: 100 mg PO at bedtime. Pneumocystis treatment: 5 mg/kg PO three times per day with dapsone 100 mg PO daily for 21 days.

FORMS — Generic only: Tabs 100 mg. Trade only (Primsol-$$$$): Oral soln 50 mg/5 mL.

NOTES — Contraindicated in megaloblastic anemia due to folate deficiency. Blood dyscrasias. Inhibits metabolism of phenytoin. Can cause hyperkalemia (risk increased by high doses of trimethoprim, renal impairment, or other drugs that cause hyperkalemia). Dosing in adults with renal dysfunction: 50 mg PO q 12 h for CrCl 15 to 30 mL/min. Do not use if CrCl <15 mL/min.

MOA — Folate antagonist; inhibits bacterial dihydrofolate reductase, the enzyme after step in folate synthesis inhibited by sulfonamides.

ADVERSE EFFECTS — Serious: Blood dyscrasias. Frequent: Rash, pruritus.

CARDIOVASCULAR

ACE INHIBITOR DOSING

ACE INHIBITOR	HTN		Heart Failure	
	Initial	*Max/day*	*Initial*	*Max/day*
benazepril (*Lotensin*)	10 mg daily*	80 mg	—	—
captopril (*Capoten*)	25 mg bid/tid	450 mg	6.25 mg tid	450 mg
enalapril (*Vasotec*)	5 mg daily*	40 mg	2.5 mg bid	40 mg
fosinopril (*Monopril*)	10 mg daily*	80 mg	5–10 mg daily	40 mg
lisinopril (*Zestril/Prinivil*)	10 mg daily	80 mg	2.5–5 mg daily	40 mg
moexipril (*Univasc*)	7.5 mg daily*	30 mg	—	—
perindopril (*Aceon*)	4 mg daily*	16 mg	2 mg daily	16 mg
quinapril (*Accupril*)	10–20 mg daily*	80 mg	5 mg bid	40 mg
ramipril (*Altace*)	2.5 mg daily*	20 mg	1.25–2.5 mg bid	10 mg
trandolapril (*Mavik*)	1–2 mg daily*	8 mg	1 mg daily	4 mg

bid = two times per day; tid = three times per day.
Data taken from prescribing information and *Circulation* 2013;128:e240−e327.
* May require bid dosing for 24-h BP control.

BETA-BLOCKER DOSING FOR HEART FAILURE REDUCED EJECTION FRACTION (HFrEF; EF 40% or less)

Beta-blocker	Inital	Max/day
bisoprolol	1.25 mg once daily	10 mg once daily
carvedilol	3.125 mg bid	50 mg bid
carvedilol extended-release	10 mg once daily	80 mg once daily
metoprolol succinate extended-release	12.5 to 25 mg once daily	200 mg once daily

bid = two times per day
Data taken from prescribing information and *Circulation* 2013;128:e240−e327.

CARDIAC PARAMETERS AND FORMULAS

Cardiac output (CO) = heart rate × CVA volume [normal 4 to 8 L/min]

Cardiac index (CI) = CO/BSA [normal 2.8 to 4.2 L/min/m^2]

MAP (mean arterial pressure) = [(SBP − DBP)/3] + DBP [normal 80 to 100 mmHg]

SVR (systemic vascular resistance) = (MAP − CVP) × (80)/CO [normal 800 to 1200 dyne × sec/cm^5]

PVR (pulmonary vasc resisistance) = (PAM − PCWP) × (80)/CO [normal 45 to 120 dyne × sec/cm^5]

QTc = QT/square root of RR [normal 0.38 to 0.42]

Right atrial pressure (central venous pressure) [normal 0 to 8 mmHg]

Pulmonary artery systolic pressure (PAS) [normal 20 to 30 mmHg]

Pulmonary artery diastolic pressure (PAD) [normal 10 to 15 mmHg]

Pulmonary capillary wedge pressure (PCWP) [normal 8 to 12 mmHg (post-MI ~16 mmHg)]

LIPID CHANGE BY CLASS/AGENT[a]

Drug class/agent	LDL-C	HDL-C	TG
Bile acid sequestrants[b]	↓ 15–30%	↑ 3–5%	↑ 0–10%
Cholesterol absorption inhibitor[c]	↓ 18%	↑ 1%	↓ 8%
Fibrates[d]	↓ 5–↑ 20%	↑ 10–20%	↓ 20–50%
Niacin[e]	↓ 5–25%	↑ 15–35%	↓ 20–50%
Omega 3 fatty acids[f]	↓ 6% or ↑144%	↓ 5% or ↑ 7%	↓ 19–44%
PCSK9 inhibitors[g]	↓ 40–72%	↑ 0–10%	↓ 0–17%
Statins[h]	↓ 18–55%	↑ 5–15%	↓ 7–30%

LDL-C = low density lipoprotein cholesterol. HDL-C = high density lipoprotein cholesterol. TG = triglycerides.
[a]Adapted from prescribing information.
[b]Cholestyramine (4–16 g), colestipol (5–20 g), colesevelam (2.6–3.8 g).
[c]Ezetimibe (10 mg). When added to statin therapy, will ↓ LDL-C 25%, ↑ HDL-C 3%, ↓ TG 14% in addition to statin effects.
[d]Fenofibrate (145–200 mg), gemfibrozil (600 mg two times per day).
[e]Extended release nicotinic acid (Niaspan® 1–2 g), immediate release (crystalline) nicotinic acid (1.5–3 g), sustained release nicotinic acid (Slo-Niacin® 1–2 g).
[f]Epanova® (4 g), Lovaza® (4 g), Vascepa® (4 g).
[g]Alirocumab (75, 150 mg/mL), evolocumab (140 mg/mL).
[h]Atorvastatin (10–80 mg), fluvastatin (20–80 mg), lovastatin (20–80 mg), pravastatin (20–80 mg), rosuvastatin (5–40 mg), simvastatin (20–40 mg).

CHOLESTEROL TREATMENT RECOMMENDATIONS (AGE≥21 YEARS)

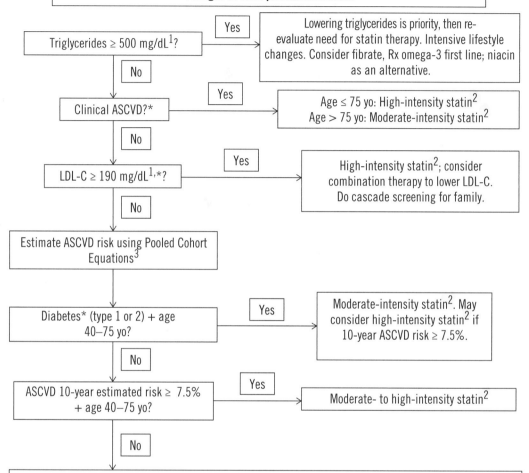

Lifestyle changes should be initiated in all patients; reinforce lifestyle changes at each patient encounter.

Triglycerides ≥ 500 mg/dL[1]? — **Yes** → Lowering triglycerides is priority, then re-evaluate need for statin therapy. Intensive lifestyle changes. Consider fibrate, Rx omega-3 first line; niacin as an alternative.

No ↓

Clinical ASCVD?* — **Yes** → Age ≤ 75 yo: High-intensity statin[2]
Age > 75 yo: Moderate-intensity statin[2]

No ↓

LDL-C ≥ 190 mg/dL[1,*]? — **Yes** → High-intensity statin[2]; consider combination therapy to lower LDL-C. Do cascade screening for family.

No ↓

Estimate ASCVD risk using Pooled Cohort Equations[3]

↓

Diabetes* (type 1 or 2) + age 40–75 yo? — **Yes** → Moderate-intensity statin[2]. May consider high-intensity statin[2] if 10-year ASCVD risk ≥ 7.5%.

No ↓

ASCVD 10-year estimated risk ≥ 7.5% + age 40–75 yo? — **Yes** → Moderate- to high-intensity statin[2]

No ↓

Benefit of statin therapy is less clear.

Recalculate 10-year ASCVD risk every 4–6 years for patients aged 40–75 yo without clinical ASCVD or diabetes + LDL-C 70–189 mg/dL + not receiving statin therapy.

Assess risk factors + 30-year or lifetime ASCVD risk in those 20–59 yo with low 10-year ASCVD risk.

Consider benefits, risks, drug–drug interactions, adverse effects, and patient preferences before initiating statin therapy.

[1]Rule out secondary causes. If non-fasting triglycerides ≥ 500 mg/dL, then a fasting lipid panel is needed.

[2]High-intensity statin = atorvastatin 40, 80 mg; rosuvastatin 20, 40 mg. Moderate-intensity statin is acceptable if patient is not a candidate for high-intensity statin therapy. Moderate-intensity statin = atorvastatin 10, 20 mg; fluvastatin 40 mg twice daily, fluvastatin XL 80 mg; lovastatin 40 mg; pitavastatin 2, 4 mg; pravastatin 40, 80 mg; rosuvastatin 5, 10 mg; simvastatin 20, 40 mg.

[3]Calculator available: http://tools.cardiosource.org/ASCVD-Risk-Estimator/

ASCVD = atherosclerotic cardiovascular disease (includes coronary heart disease, stroke, and peripheral artery disease). LCL-C = low-density lipoprotein cholesterol. Rx = prescription strength.

Adapted from: *J Am Coll Cardiol.* 2014; 63(25_PA), *Circulation.* 2011; 123: 2292–2333.

*Combination of statin and non-statin therapy to lower LDL-C may be appropriate for patients at high-risk for ASCVD. *J Am Coll Cardiol* 2016; 68: 92–125.

HTN THERAPY FOR ADULTS ≥ 18 YEARS OLD[a]

Patient Information		BP Target[a] (mm Hg)	Preferred Therapy	Comments
All patients with CKD (with or without diabetes)	Any age	< 140/90	Start ACEI or ARB; alone or in combination with a CCB or thiazide[b]	
Nonblack (no CKD)	Any age + diabetes	< 140/90	Start ACEI, ARB, CCB, or thiazide; alone or combination[b]	Implement lifestyle interventions; reinforce adherence during patient encounters. Drug treatment strategy based on response and tolerance: Either, titrate first drug to max dose before adding second; add second drug before reaching max dose of first drug; or start with 2 drug classes separately or as fixed dose combinations.[c,d]
Nonblack (no CKD)	Age < 60 yo (no diabetes or CKD)	< 140/90	Start ACEI, ARB, CCB, or thiazide; alone or combination[b]	Implement lifestyle interventions; reinforce adherence during patient encounters. Drug treatment strategy based on response and tolerance: Either, titrate first drug to max dose before adding second; add second drug before reaching max dose of first drug; or start with 2 drug classes separately or as fixed dose combinations.[c,d]
Nonblack (no CKD)	Age ≥ 60 yo (no diabetes or CKD)	< 150/90	Start ACEI, ARB, CCB, or thiazide; alone or combination[b]	Implement lifestyle interventions; reinforce adherence during patient encounters. Drug treatment strategy based on response and tolerance: Either, titrate first drug to max dose before adding second; add second drug before reaching max dose of first drug; or start with 2 drug classes separately or as fixed dose combinations.[c,d]
Black (no CKD)	Any age + diabetes	< 140/90	Start CCB or thiazide; alone or combination[b]	Implement lifestyle interventions; reinforce adherence during patient encounters. Drug treatment strategy based on response and tolerance: Either, titrate first drug to max dose before adding second; add second drug before reaching max dose of first drug; or start with 2 drug classes separately or as fixed dose combinations.[c,d]
Black (no CKD)	Age < 60 yo (no diabetes or CKD)	< 140/90	Start CCB or thiazide; alone or combination[b]	Implement lifestyle interventions; reinforce adherence during patient encounters. Drug treatment strategy based on response and tolerance: Either, titrate first drug to max dose before adding second; add second drug before reaching max dose of first drug; or start with 2 drug classes separately or as fixed dose combinations.[c,d]
Black (no CKD)	Age ≥ 60 yo (no diabetes or CKD)	< 150/90	Start CCB or thiazide; alone or combination[b]	Implement lifestyle interventions; reinforce adherence during patient encounters. Drug treatment strategy based on response and tolerance: Either, titrate first drug to max dose before adding second; add second drug before reaching max dose of first drug; or start with 2 drug classes separately or as fixed dose combinations.[c,d]

[a]These guidelines will be updated in late 2016 or early 2017. The BP targets and treatment recommendations may change based on the results of the SPRINT trial (*N Engl J Med* 2015;373:2103-16.DOI: 10.1056/NEJMoa1511939), which demonstrated fewer fatal and nonfatal major cardiovascular events and death from any cause in patients who were 50 yo or older, at high risk for cardiovascular events, and without diabetes who achieved SBP < 120 mmHg as compared to SBP < 140 mmHg. Patients treated to SBP < 120 mmHg had higher rates of some adverse events (eg, hypotension, syncope, electrolyte abnormalities, acute renal failure).

[b]Do not combine ACEI and ARB therapy.

[c]Consider starting with 2 drugs when SBP is > 160 mmHg and/or DBP is > 100 mmHg, or if SBP is > 20 mmHg above goal and/or DBP is > 10 mmHg above goal. If goal BP is not achieved with 2 drugs, select a 3rd drug from the list. Titrate prn.

[d]If needed, may add another drug (eg, beta-blocker, aldosterone antagonist, others) and/or refer to physician with HTN management expertise.

ACEI = angiotensin converting enzyme inhibitor; ARB = angiotensin-receptor blocker.

CCB = calcium-channel blocker; CKD = chronic kidney disease.

SELECTED DRUGS THAT MAY PROLONG THE QT INTERVAL

alfuzosin	dofetilide*	kinase inhibitors	rocainamide*
amiodarone*	dolasetron	leuprolide	promethazine
anagrelide*	donepezil*	levofloxacin*	propofol*
apomorphine	dronedarone*	lithium	quetiapine
aripiprazole	droperidol*	loperamide*	quinidine*
arsenic trioxide*	eribulin	(excessive doses)	ranolazine*
asenapine	erythromycin*	methadone*	rilpivirin
atazanavir	escitalopram*	mirabegron	risperidone
atomoxetine	ezogabine	mirtazapine	saquinavir
azithromycin*	famotidine	moexipril/HCTZ	sevoflurane*
bedaquiline	felbamate	moxifloxacin*	sotalol*
buprenorphine	fingolimod	nicardipine	tacrolimus
capecitabine	flecainide*	nilotinib	tamoxifen
chloroquine*	fluconazole*	ofloxacin	telithromycin
chlorpromazine*	foscarnet	olanzapine	thioridazine*
cilostazol*	gemifloxacin	ondansetron*	tizanidine
ciprofloxacin*	granisetron	oxytocin	tolterodine
citalopram*	halofantrine*	oxaliplatin*	toremifene
clarithromycin*	haloperidol*	paliperidone	tricyclic antidepressants
clozapine	hydrocodone ER	pentamidine*	vandetanib*
cocaine*	ibutilide*	perflutren lipid	vardenafil
dexmedetomidine	iloperidone	microspheres	venlafaxine
disopyramide*	isradipine	pimozide*	ziprasidone

NOTE: This table may not include all drugs that prolong the QT interval or cause torsades. Risk of drug-induced QT prolongation may be increased in women, elderly, hypokalemia, hypomagnesemia, bradycardia, starvation, CHF, and CNS injuries. Hepatorenal dysfunction and drug interactions can increase the concentration of QT interval-prolonging drugs. Coadministration of QT interval-prolonging drugs can have additive effects. Avoid these (and other) drugs in congenital prolonged QT syndrome (References: prescribing information for individual drugs, www.crediblemeds.org).

*Torsades reported in product labeling/case reports.

HIGH- AND MODERATE-INTENSITY STATIN DOSES

Statin	High-intensity dose (lowers LDL-C at least 50%)	Moderate-intensity dose (lowers LDL-C 30% to 49%)
atorvastatin	40, 80 mg	10, 20 mg
fluvastatin XL	n/a	80 mg
fluvastatin	n/a	40 mg twice daily
lovastatin	n/a	40 mg
pitavastatin	n/a	2, 4 mg
pravastatin	n/a	40, 80 mg
rosuvastatin	20, 40 mg	5, 10 mg
simvastatin	n/a	20, 40 mg

LDL-C = low density lipoprotein cholesterol. Will get ~6% decrease in LDL-C with every doubling of dose.

Adapted from *J Am Coll Cardiol.* 2014; 63(25_PA).

THROMBOLYTIC THERAPY FOR ST-SEGMENT ELEVATION MI (STEMI)

Indications (if high-volume cath lab unavailable)	Clinical history and presentation strongly suggestive of MI within 12 h plus at least 1 of the following: 1 mm ST elevation in at least 2 contiguous leads; new left BBB; or 2 mm ST depression in V1-V4 suggestive of true posterior MI.
Absolute contraindications	Previous intracranial hemorrhage; known cerebral vascular lesion (arteriovenous malformation); known malignant intracranial neoplasm; recent (<3 months) ischemic CVA (except acute ischemic CVA <4.5 h); aortic dissection; active bleeding or bleeding diathesis (excluding menses); significant closed head or facial trauma (<3 months); intracranial or intraspinal surgery (<2 months); severe uncontrolled HTN (unresponsive to emergency therapy); for streptokinase: prior exposure (<6 months).
Relative contraindication	Severe uncontrolled HTN (>180/110 mmHg) on presentation or chronic severe HTN; prior ischemic CVA (>3 months), dementia, other intracranial pathology; traumatic/prolonged (>10 min) cardiopulmonary resuscitation; major surgery (<3 weeks); recent (within 2–4 weeks) internal bleeding; puncture of noncompressible vessel; pregnancy; active peptic ulcer disease; current use of anticoagulants.

Reference: *Circulation* 2013;127:e362-425

CARDIOVASCULAR: ACE Inhibitors

NOTE: See also Antihypertensive Combinations. Contraindicated in pregnancy; with history of angioedema; or with aliskiren in patients with DM. Women of child bearing age should use reliable form of contraception; discontinue ACE inhibitor as soon as pregnancy is detected. In general, avoid combined use with renin-angiotensin system inhibitors (ie, angiotensin receptor blockers, aliskiren); increases risk of renal impairment, hypotension, and hyperkalemia. Patients on diuretics may experience excessive hypotension when ACE inhibitor added to diuretic therapy; to minimize this, decrease dose of diuretic or discontinue diuretic before initiating ACE inhibitor. Hyperkalemia possible, especially if used concomitantly with other drugs that increase K (including K-containing salt substitutes) and in patients with DM or renal impairment. An increase in serum creatinine up to 35% above baseline is acceptable and is not reason to withhold therapy unless hyperkalemia occurs. Concomitant NSAID, including celecoxib, may further deteriorate renal function and decrease antihypertensive effects. Consider intestinal angioedema if abdominal pain (with or without N/V). African Americans and smokers may be at higher risk for angioedema. Concomitant mTOR inhibitor (eg, everolimus, temsirolimus, sirolimus) may increase angioedema risk. Swelling of tongue, glottis, or larynx may result in airway obstruction, especially with history of airway surgery. Increases risk of hypotension with volume depleted or hyponatremic patients. African Americans may need higher dose to achieve adequate response. Renoprotection and decreased cardiovascular morbidity/mortality seen with some ACE inhibitors are most likely a class effect. Anaphylactoid reactions have been reported when ACE inhibitor patients are dialyzed with high-flux membranes (eg, AN69) or undergoing low-density lipoprotein apheresis with dextran sulfate absorption. Nitroid reactions (facial flushing, N/V, hypotension) have been reported with concomitant gold injections. Cholestatic hepatitis or acute liver failure have been reported with ACE inhibitor use; if patient develops jaundice or marked elevations of hepatic enzymes, discontinue ACE inhibitor. Neutropenia or agranulocytosis have been reported with ACE inhibitor use; patients with collagen-vascular disease may be at more risk.

BENAZEPRIL (*Lotensin*) ▶LK ♀X/X/X, Neonatal harm: Potential anuria, hypotension, renal failure, skull hypoplasia, death. ▶ Do not breastfeed while taking an ACE inhibitor. $$
WARNING — Do not use in pregnancy.
ADULT — HTN: Start 10 mg PO daily, usual maintenance dose 20 to 40 mg PO daily or divided two times per day, max 80 mg/day, but added effect not apparent above 40 mg/day. Elderly, renal impairment, or concomitant diuretic therapy: Start 5 mg PO daily.
PEDS — HTN: Start 0.2 mg/kg/day (max 10 mg/day) as monotherapy; doses greater than 0.6 mg/kg/day or 40 mg/day have not been studied. Do not use if age younger than 6 yo or if glomerular filtration rate less than 30 mL/min.
UNAPPROVED ADULT — Renoprotective dosing: 10 mg PO daily. Heart failure: Start 5 mg PO daily, usual 5 to 20 mg/day, max 40 mg/day (in 1 to 2 doses).
FORMS — Generic/Trade: Tabs, unscored 5, 10, 20, 40 mg.
NOTES — Twice-daily dosing may be required for 24 h BP control.
MOA — Inhibits angiotensin-converting enzyme which converts angiotensin I to angiotensin II.
ADVERSE EFFECTS — Serious: Angioedema, hyperkalemia, renal impairment. Frequent: Cough.
CAPTOPRIL (*Capoten*) ▶LK ♀X/X/X, Neonatal harm: Potential anuria, hypotension, renal failure, skull hypoplasia, death. ▶ Do not breastfeed while taking an ACE inhibitor. $$$
WARNING — Do not use in pregnancy.
ADULT — HTN: Start 25 mg PO two to three times per day, usual maintenance dose 25 to 150 mg PO two to three times per day, max 450 mg/day. Elderly, renal impairment, or concomitant diuretic therapy:

Start 6.25 to 12.5 mg PO two to three times per day. Heart failure: Start 6.25 to 12.5 mg PO three times per day, usual 50 to 100 mg PO three times per day, max 450 mg/day. Diabetic nephropathy: 25 mg PO three times per day.
PEDS — Not approved in children.
UNAPPROVED ADULT — Hypertensive urgency: 12.5 to 25 mg PO, repeated once or twice if necessary at intervals of 30 to 60 min.
UNAPPROVED PEDS — Neonates: 0.1 to 0.4 mg/kg/day PO divided q 6 to 8 h. Infants: Initial dose 0.15 to 0.3 mg/kg/dose, titrate to effective dose, max dose 6 mg/kg/day divided one to four times per day. Children: Initial dose 0.3 to 0.5 mg/kg/dose PO q 8 h, titrate to effective dose, max dose 6 mg/kg/day (not to exceed 450 mg/day) divided two to four times per day.
FORMS — Generic only: Tabs, scored 12.5, 25, 50, 100 mg.
NOTES — A captopril soln or susp (1 mg/mL) can be made by dissolving tabs in distilled water or flavored syrup. The soln is stable for 7 days at room temperature.
MOA — Inhibits angiotensin-converting enzyme which converts angiotensin I to angiotensin II.
ADVERSE EFFECTS — Serious: Angioedema, hyperkalemia, renal impairment. Frequent: Cough, rash.
CILAZAPRIL (✱*Inhibace*) ▶LK ♀X/X/X, Neonatal harm: Potential anuria, hypotension, renal failure, skull hypoplasia, death. ▶ Do not breastfeed while taking an ACE inhibitor. $
WARNING — Do not use in pregnancy.
ADULT — Canada only. HTN: Initial dose 2.5 mg PO daily, usual maintenance dose 2.5 to 5 mg daily, max 10 mg daily. Elderly or concomitant diuretic therapy: Initiate 1.25 mg PO daily. Heart failure adjunct: Initially 0.5 mg PO daily, increase to usual

(cont.)

CILAZAPRIL (*cont.*)

maintenance of 1 to 2.5 mg daily. Renal impairment with CrCl 10 to 40 mL/min, initiate 0.5 mg daily, max 2.5 mg/day. CrCl <10 mL/min, 0.25 to 0.5 mg once or twice per week, adjust dose according to BP response.

PEDS — Not approved in children.

FORMS — Generic/Trade: Not available in US. Tabs, scored 1, 2.5, 5 mg.

NOTES — Reduce dose in hepatic/renal impairment.

MOA — Inhibits angiotensin-converting enzyme which converts angiotensin I to angiotensin II.

ADVERSE EFFECTS — Serious: Angioedema, hyperkalemia, renal impairment. Frequent: Cough.

ENALAPRIL (*enalaprilat, Vasotec, Epaned*) ▶LK ♀X/X/X, Neonatal harm: Potential anuria, hypotension, renal failure, skull hypoplasia, death. ▶ Do not breastfeed while taking an ACE inhibitor. $$

WARNING — Do not use in pregnancy.

ADULT — HTN: Start 5 mg PO daily, usual maintenance dose 10 to 40 mg PO daily or divided two times per day, max 40 mg/day. If oral therapy not possible, can use enalaprilat 1.25 mg IV q 6 h over 5 min, and increase up to 5 mg IV q 6 h if needed. Renal impairment or concomitant diuretic therapy: Start 2.5 mg PO daily. Heart failure: Start 2.5 mg PO two times per day, usual dose 10 to 20 mg PO two times per day, max 40 mg/day.

PEDS — HTN, age 1 mo or older: Start 0.08 mg/kg/day, max 5 mg/day; doses greater than 0.58 mg/kg/day or 40 mg/day have not been studied.

UNAPPROVED ADULT — Hypertensive crisis: Enalaprilat 1.25 to 5 mg IV q 6 h. Renoprotective dosing: 10 to 20 mg PO daily.

UNAPPROVED PEDS — HTN: Start 0.1 mg/kg/day PO daily or divided two times per day, titrate to effective dose, max dose 0.5 mg/kg/day; 0.005 to 0.01 mg/kg/dose IV q 8 to 24 h.

FORMS — Generic/Trade: Tabs, scored 2.5, 5 mg, unscored 10, 20 mg. Trade only: Oral Soln 1 mg/mL (Epaned-$$$$$).

NOTES — Twice-daily dosing may be required for 24 h BP control. An enalapril oral susp (0.2 mg/mL) can be made by dissolving one 2.5 mg tab in 12.5 mL sterile water; use immediately. Enalaprilat is the active metabolite of enalapril.

MOA — Inhibits angiotensin-converting enzyme which converts angiotensin I to angiotensin II.

ADVERSE EFFECTS — Serious: Angioedema, hyperkalemia, renal impairment. Frequent: Cough.

FOSINOPRIL ▶LK ♀X/X/X, Neonatal harm: Potential anuria, hypotension, renal failure, skull hypoplasia, death. ▶ Do not breastfeed while taking an ACE inhibitor. $$

WARNING — Do not use in pregnancy.

ADULT — HTN: Start 10 mg PO daily, usual maintenance dose 20 to 40 mg PO daily or divided two times per day, max 80 mg/day, but added effect not apparent above 40 mg/day. Elderly, renal impairment, or concomitant diuretic therapy: Start 5 mg

PO daily. Heart failure: Start 5 to 10 mg PO daily, usual 20 to 40 mg PO daily, max 40 mg/day.

PEDS — HTN, age 6 to 16 yo and wt greater than 50 kg: 5 to 10 mg PO daily.

UNAPPROVED ADULT — Renoprotective dosing: 10 to 20 mg PO daily.

FORMS — Generic only: Tabs, scored 10 mg, unscored 20, 40 mg.

NOTES — Twice-daily dosing may be required for 24 h BP control. Elimination 50% renal, 50% hepatic. Accumulation of drug negligible with impaired renal function. The brand name product (Monopril) is no longer available.

MOA — Inhibits angiotensin-converting enzyme which converts angiotensin I to angiotensin II.

ADVERSE EFFECTS — Serious: Angioedema, hyperkalemia, renal impairment. Frequent: Cough.

LISINOPRIL (*Prinivil, Zestril*) ▶K ♀X/X/X, Neonatal harm: Potential anuria, hypotension, renal failure, skull hypoplasia, death. ▶ Do not breastfeed while taking an ACE inhibitor. $

WARNING — Do not use in pregnancy.

ADULT — HTN: Start 10 mg PO daily, usual maintenance dose 20 to 40 mg PO daily, max 80 mg/day, but added effect not apparent above 40 mg/day. Renal impairment or concomitant diuretic therapy: Start 2.5 to 5 mg PO daily. Heart failure, acute MI: Start 2.5 to 5 mg PO daily, usual 5 to 20 mg PO daily, max 40 mg/day.

PEDS — HTN, age older than 6 yo: 0.07 mg/kg PO daily; 5 mg/day max. Not recommended for age younger than 6 yo or with glomerular filtration rate less than 30 mL/min/1.73 m^2.

UNAPPROVED ADULT — Renoprotective dosing: 10 to 20 mg PO daily.

FORMS — Generic/Trade: Tabs, unscored (Zestril) 2.5, 5, 10, 20, 30, 40 mg. Tabs, scored (Prinivil) 10, 20, 40 mg.

MOA — Inhibits angiotensin-converting enzyme which converts angiotensin I to angiotensin II.

ADVERSE EFFECTS — Serious: Angioedema, hyperkalemia, renal impairment. Frequent: Cough.

MOEXIPRIL (*Univasc*) ▶LK ♀X/X/X, Neonatal harm: Potential anuria, hypotension, renal failure, skull hypoplasia, death. ▶ Do not breastfeed while taking an ACE inhibitor. $$

WARNING — Do not use in pregnancy.

ADULT — HTN: Start 7.5 mg PO daily, usual maintenance dose 7.5 to 30 mg PO daily or divided two times per day, max 30 mg/day. Renal impairment or concomitant diuretic therapy: Start 3.75 mg PO daily; max 15 mg/day with renal impairment.

PEDS — Not approved in children.

FORMS — Generic: Tabs, scored 7.5, 15 mg.

NOTES — Twice daily dosing may be required for 24 h BP control. The brand name product (Univasc) is no longer available.

MOA — Inhibits angiotensin-converting enzyme which converts angiotensin I to angiotensin II.

ADVERSE EFFECTS — Serious: Angioedema, hyperkalemia, renal impairment. Frequent: Cough.

PERINDOPRIL (*Aceon*, *✷Coversyl*) ▶K♀X/X/X, Neonatal harm: Potential anuria, hypotension, renal failure, skull hypoplasia, death. ❱ Do not breastfeed while taking an ACE inhibitor. $$$
WARNING — Do not use in pregnancy.
ADULT — HTN: Start 4 mg PO daily, usual maintenance dose 4 to 8 mg PO daily or divided two times per day, max 16 mg/day. Renal impairment or concomitant diuretic therapy: Start 2 mg PO daily or divided two times per day, max 8 mg/day. Reduction of cardiovascular events in stable CAD: Start 4 mg PO daily for 2 weeks, max 8 mg/day. Elderly (age older than 65 yo): 4 mg PO daily, max 8 mg/day.
PEDS — Not approved in children.
UNAPPROVED ADULT — Heart failure: Start 2 mg PO daily, max dose 16 mg daily. Recurrent CVA prevention: 4 mg PO daily with indapamide.
FORMS — Generic/Trade: Tabs, scored 2, 4, 8 mg.
NOTES — Twice-daily dosing may be required for 24 h BP control.
MOA — Inhibits angiotensin-converting enzyme which converts angiotensin I to angiotensin II.
ADVERSE EFFECTS — Serious: Angioedema, hyperkalemia, renal impairment. Frequent: Cough.

QUINAPRIL (*Accupril*) ▶LK ♀X/X/X, Neonatal harm: Potential anuria, hypotension, renal failure, skull hypoplasia, death. ❱ Do not breastfeed while taking an ACE inhibitor. $$
WARNING — Do not use in pregnancy.
ADULT — HTN: Start 10 to 20 mg PO daily (start 10 mg/day if elderly), usual maintenance dose 20 to 80 mg PO daily or divided two times per day, max 80 mg/day, but added effect not apparent above 40 mg/day. Renal impairment or concomitant diuretic therapy: Start 2.5 to 5 mg PO daily. Heart failure: Start 5 mg PO two times per day, usual maintenance dose 20 to 40 mg/day divided two times per day.
PEDS — Not approved in children.
FORMS — Generic/Trade: Tabs, scored 5 mg, unscored 10, 20, 40 mg.
NOTES — Twice-daily dosing may be required for 24 h BP control.
MOA — Inhibits angiotensin-converting enzyme which converts angiotensin I to angiotensin II.
ADVERSE EFFECTS — Serious: Angioedema, hyperkalemia, renal impairment. Frequent: Cough.

RAMIPRIL (*Altace*) ▶LK ♀X/X/X, Neonatal harm: Potential anuria, hypotension, renal failure, skull hypoplasia, death. ❱ Do not breastfeed while taking an ACE inhibitor. $
WARNING — Do not use in pregnancy.
ADULT — HTN: Start 2.5 mg PO daily, usual maintenance dose 2.5 to 20 mg PO daily or divided two times per day, max 20 mg/day. Renal impairment or concomitant diuretic therapy: Start 1.25 mg PO daily. Heart failure/post-MI: Start 2.5 mg PO two times per day, usual maintenance dose 5 mg PO two times per day. Reduce risk of MI, CVA, death from cardiovascular causes: Start 2.5 mg PO daily for 1 week, then 5 mg daily for 3 weeks, increase as tolerated to maintenance dose 10 mg daily.
PEDS — Not approved in children.
UNAPPROVED ADULT — Renoprotective dosing: Titrate to 10 mg PO daily.
FORMS — Generic/Trade: Caps 1.25, 2.5, 5, 10 mg.
NOTES — Twice-daily dosing may be required for 24 h BP control. Cap contents can be sprinkled on applesauce and eaten or mixed with 120 mL of water or apple juice and swallowed. Mixtures are stable for 24 h at room temperature or 48 h refrigerated. Concomitant insulin or hypoglycemic agents may increase hypoglycemia risk.
MOA — Inhibits angiotensin-converting enzyme which converts angiotensin I to angiotensin II.
ADVERSE EFFECTS — Serious: Angioedema, hepatotoxicity, hyperkalemia, pancreatitis, renal impairment. Frequent: Cough.

TRANDOLAPRIL (*Mavik*) ▶LK ♀X/X/X, Neonatal harm: Potential anuria, hypotension, renal failure, skull hypoplasia, death. ❱ Do not breastfeed while taking an ACE inhibitor. $
WARNING — Do not use in pregnancy.
ADULT — HTN: Start 1 mg PO daily, usual maintenance dose 2 to 4 mg PO daily or divided two times per day, max 8 mg/day, but added effect not apparent above 4 mg/day. Heart failure/post-MI: Start 1 mg PO daily, titrate to target dose 4 mg PO daily. Renal impairment or concomitant diuretic therapy: Start 0.5 mg PO daily.
PEDS — Not approved in children.
FORMS — Generic/Trade: Tabs, scored 1 mg, unscored 2, 4 mg.
NOTES — Twice-daily dosing may be required for 24 h BP control.
MOA — Serious: Angioedema, hyperkalemia, renal impairment. Frequent: Cough.
ADVERSE EFFECTS — TAB013

CARDIOVASCULAR: Aldosterone Antagonists

NOTE: Hyperkalemia possible, especially if used concomitantly with other drugs that increase K (including K-containing salt substitutes) and in patients with heart failure, DM, or renal impairment. Adding an aldosterone antagonist is recommended in select patients with heart failure and reduced LVEF with careful monitoring for preserved renal function and normal K concentration. Serum creatinine should be less than 2.5 mg/dL in men or less than 2.0 mg/dL in women; and K should be less than 5.0 mEq/L.

EPLERENONE (*Inspra*) ▶L ♀B ❱? $$$$
ADULT — HTN: Start 50 mg PO daily; max 50 mg two times per day. HTN and taking concomitant moderate CYP3A inhibitor (eg erythromycin, fluconazole, saquinavir, verapamil): Start 25 mg PO daily; max 25 mg PO two times daily. Heart failure (with

(cont.)

EPLERENONE (*cont.*)

LVEF 40% or less) post MI: Start 25 mg PO daily; titrate to target dose 50 mg daily within 4 weeks, if tolerated. Heart failure (with LVEF 40% or less) post MI and taking concomitant moderate CYP3A inhibitor: Do not exceed 25 mg PO daily.

PEDS — Not approved in children.

UNAPPROVED ADULT — Resistant HTN: 25 to 100 mg PO daily.

FORMS — Generic/trade: Tabs, unscored 25, 50 mg.

NOTES — Contraindicated in all patients with K+ greater than 5.5 mEq/L; CrCl 30 mL/min or less; strong CYP3A4inhibitors (eg, clarithromycin, itraconazole, ketoconazole nefazodone, nelfinavir, ritonavir). Contraindicated in patients treated for HTN with Type 2 DM with microalbuminuria; serum creatinine greater than 2 mg/dL in males or greater than 1.8 mg/dL in females; CrCl < 50 mL/min; or concomitant therapy with K+supplements, K+-sparing diuretics. Measure K+ before initiating, within 1st week, at 1 month after starting treatment or dose adjustment, then prn. Hyperkalemia more common with renal impairment, diabetes, proteinuria, or concomitant ACE inhibitor, ARB, NSAID, or moderate CYP3A inhibitor (eg, erythromycin, fluconazole, saquinavir, verapamil). Measure serum K+and CrCl 3-7 days of initiation of ACE inhibitor, ARB, NSAID, or moderate CYP3A4 inhibitor. Monitor lithium levels with concomitant lithium therapy.

MOA — Blocks the binding of aldosterone to mineralocorticoid receptors.

ADVERSE EFFECTS — Serious: Hyperkalemia, hyponatremia (rare). Frequent: Headache, dizziness.

SPIRONOLACTONE (*Aldactone*) ▶LK ♀D ▶+ $

WARNING — Use only for approved indications. Tumorigen in rats.

ADULT — HTN: 50 to 100 mg PO daily or divided two times per day, increase dose prn after 2 weeks based on serum potassium and BP (usual dose 25 to 50 mg daily according to ASH-ISH guidelines).

Edema (heart failure, hepatic disease, nephrotic syndrome): Start 100 mg PO daily or divided two times per day, maintain for 5 days, increase prn to achieve diuretic response, usual dose range 25 to 200 mg/day. Other diuretics may be needed. Diuretic-induced hypokalemia: 25 to 100 mg PO daily when potassium supplements/sparing regimens inappropriate. Severe heart failure (NYHA III or IV): Start 25 mg PO daily, max 50 mg daily. Primary hyperaldosteronism, maintenance therapy: 100 to 400 mg/day PO until surgery or indefinitely if surgery not an option.

PEDS — Edema: 3.3 mg/kg PO daily or divided two times per day.

UNAPPROVED ADULT — Resistant HTN: 12.5 to 100 mg PO daily. Hirsutism: 50 to 200 mg PO daily, maximal regression of hirsutism in 6 months. Acne: 50 to 200 mg PO daily.

UNAPPROVED PEDS — Edema/HTN: 1 to 3.3 mg/kg/day, PO daily or divided two times per day, max 200 mg/day.

FORMS — Generic/Trade: Tabs, unscored 25 mg, scored 50, 100 mg.

NOTES — May be helpful in patients with resistant hypertension. Contraindicated with anuria, renal insufficiency, hyperkalemia, Addison's disease, or other conditions associated with hyperkalemia. Dosing more frequently than twice daily not necessary. Hyperkalemia more likely with doses 50 mg/day or more and with concomitant ACEIs or K+ supplements. Measure serum K+ and SrCr before initiating, after 1 week, monthly for the 1st 3 months, quarterly for 1 year, then q 6 months after starting treatment or dose adjustment.

MOA — Blocks the binding of aldosterone to mineralocorticoid receptors.

ADVERSE EFFECTS — Serious: Agranulocytosis, hyperkalemia (rare), hypersensitivity, Stevens-Johnson Syndrome. Frequent: Gynecomastia, headache, impotence, irregular menses.

CARDIOVASCULAR: Angiotensin Receptor Blockers (ARBs)

NOTE: See also Antihypertensive Combinations. Contraindicated in pregnancy; or with aliskiren in patients with DM. Women of child bearing age should use reliable form of contraception; discontinue ARB as soon as pregnancy is detected. In general, avoid combined use with renin-angiotensin system inhibitors (i.e. ACE inhibitors, aliskiren); increases risk of renal impairment, hypotension, and hyperkalemia. Hyperkalemia possible, especially if used concomitantly with other drugs that increase K+ (including K+ containing salt substitutes) and in patients with heart failure, DM, or renal impairment. An increase in serum creatinine up to 35% above baseline is acceptable and is not reason to withhold therapy unless hyperkalemia occurs. Concomitant NSAID, including celecoxib, may further deteriorate renal function and decrease antihypertensive effects. May increase lithium levels. Rare cases of angioedema and rhabdomyolysis have been reported with ARBs.

AZILSARTAN (*Edarbi*) ▶L – ♀D ▶? $$$$

WARNING — Do not use in pregnancy.

ADULT — HTN: Start 80 mg daily, max 80 mg daily. Start 40 mg daily with concomitant high-dose diuretic therapy.

FORMS — Trade only: Tabs, unscored 40, 80 mg.

MOA — Blocks binding of angiotensin II to the angiotensin subtype I receptor.

ADVERSE EFFECTS — Serious: angioedema, hyperkalemia, renal impairment.

CANDESARTAN (*Atacand*) ▶K ♀D ▶? $$$

WARNING — Do not use in pregnancy.

ADULT — HTN: Start 16 mg PO daily, max 32 mg/day. Heart failure: (NYHA II–IV and LVEF 40% or less): Start 4 mg PO daily, may double dose q 2 weeks; max 32 mg/day.

(cont.)

CANDESARTAN (cont.)

PEDS — HTN: For age 1 to 5 yo: Start 0.20 mg/kg (oral susp), dose range 0.05 to 0.4 mg/kg/day. For age 6 to 16 yo and wt less than 50 kg: Start 4 to 8 mg/day, range 4 to 16 mg/day. For age 6 to 16 yo, wt greater than 50 kg: Start 8 to 16 mg/day, range 4 to 32 mg/day. Doses higher than 0.4 mg/kg/day (in ages 1 to 5 yo) or 32 mg (ages 6 to 16 yo) have not been studied.

FORMS — Generic/Trade: Tabs 4, 8, 16, 32 mg.

MOA — Blocks binding of angiotensin II to the angiotensin subtype 1 receptor.

ADVERSE EFFECTS — Serious: Hyperkalemia, renal impairment.

EPROSARTAN (Teveten) ▶Fecal excretion ♀D ▶? $$$$

WARNING — Do not use in pregnancy.

ADULT — HTN: Start 600 mg PO daily, max 900 mg/day given daily or divided two times per day.

PEDS — Not approved in children.

FORMS — Generic/Trade: Tabs, unscored 600 mg.

MOA — Blocks binding of angiotensin II to the angiotensin subtype I receptor.

ADVERSE EFFECTS — Serious: Hyperkalemia, renal impairment.

IRBESARTAN (Avapro) ▶L ♀D ▶? $

WARNING — Do not use in pregnancy.

ADULT — HTN: Start 150 mg PO daily, max 300 mg/day. Volume-depleted patients: Start 75 mg PO daily. Type 2 diabetic nephropathy: Start 150 mg PO daily, target dose 300 mg daily.

PEDS — Not approved in children.

FORMS — Generic/Trade: Tabs, unscored 75, 150, 300 mg.

MOA — Blocks binding of angiotensin II to the angiotensin subtype I receptor.

ADVERSE EFFECTS — Serious: Hyperkalemia, renal impairment.

LOSARTAN (Cozaar) ▶L ♀D ▶? $

WARNING — Do not use in pregnancy.

ADULT — HTN: Start 50 mg PO daily, max 100 mg/day given daily or divided two times per day. Volume-depleted patients or history of hepatic impairment: Start 25 mg PO daily. CVA risk reduction in patients with HTN and LV hypertrophy (may not be effective in black patients): Start 50 mg PO daily. If need more BP reduction, add HCTZ 12.5 mg PO daily; then increase losartan to 100 mg/day, then increase HCTZ to 25 mg/day. Type 2 diabetic nephropathy: Start 50 mg PO daily, target dose 100 mg daily.

PEDS — HTN: Start 0.7 mg/kg/day (up to 50 mg), doses greater than 1.4 mg/kg/day or above 100 mg have not been studied. Do not use for age younger than 6 yo or if glomerular filtration rate less than 30 mL/min.

UNAPPROVED ADULT — Heart failure: Start 12.5 mg PO daily, target dose 50 mg daily. Renoprotective dosing: Start 50 mg PO daily, increase to 100 mg daily prn for BP control.

FORMS — Generic/Trade: Tabs, unscored 25, 50, 100 mg.

NOTES — Monitor BP control when adding or discontinuing rifampin, fluconazole, or erythromycin.

MOA — Blocks binding of angiotensin II to the angiotensin subtype 1 receptor.

ADVERSE EFFECTS — Serious: Hyperkalemia, renal impairment, thrombocytopenia (rare).

OLMESARTAN (Benicar, ✸Olmetec) ▶K ♀D ▶? $$$$

WARNING — Do not use in pregnancy.

ADULT — HTN: Start 20 mg PO daily, max 40 mg/day.

PEDS — HTN, 6 to 16 yo, wt 20 to less than 35 kg: Start 10 mg PO daily, max 20 mg/day. Wt 35 kg or more: Start 20 mg PO daily, max 40 mg/day. Contraindicated in children younger than 1 yo.

FORMS — Trade only: Tabs, unscored 5, 20, 40 mg.

NOTES — Take at least 4 h prior to colesevelam. Some patients may develop sprue enteropathy with significant wt loss months to years after starting olmesartan; teach patients to report severe, chronic diarrhea with substantial wt loss; discontinue olmesartan if these symptoms occur.

MOA — Blocks binding of angiotensin II to the angiotensin subtype 1 receptor.

ADVERSE EFFECTS — Serious: Hyperkalemia, renal impairment, sprue enteropathy.

TELMISARTAN (Micardis) ▶L ♀D ▶? $$$$

WARNING — Do not use in pregnancy.

ADULT — HTN: Start 40 mg PO daily, max 80 mg/day. Cardiovascular risk reduction in patients older than 55 yo unable to take ACE inhibitors: Start 80 mg PO daily, max 80 mg/day.

PEDS — Not approved in children.

FORMS — Generic/Trade: Tabs, unscored 20, 40, 80 mg.

NOTES — Swallow tabs whole, do not break or crush. May increase digoxin level.

MOA — Blocks binding of angiotensin II to the angiotensin subtype 1 receptor.

ADVERSE EFFECTS — Serious: Hyperkalemia, renal impairment.

VALSARTAN (Diovan) ▶L ♀D ▶? $$$$

WARNING — Do not use in pregnancy.

ADULT — HTN: Start 80 to 160 mg PO daily, max 320 mg/day. Heart failure: Start 40 mg PO two times per day, target dose 160 mg two times per day; there is no evidence of added benefit when used with adequate dose of ACE inhibitor. Reduce mortality/morbidity post-MI with LV systolic dysfunction/failure: Start 20 mg PO two times per day, increase to 40 mg PO two times per day within 7 days, target dose 160 mg two times per day.

PEDS — HTN: Start 1.3 mg/kg/day (up to 40 mg), max 2.7 mg/kg/day (or 160 mg). Do not use if younger than 6 yo.

UNAPPROVED ADULT — Renoprotective dosing: 80 to 160 mg PO daily.

FORMS — Generic/Trade: Tabs, scored 40 mg, unscored 80, 160, 320 mg.

MOA — Blocks binding of angiotensin II to the angiotensin subtype I receptor.

ADVERSE EFFECTS — Serious: Hyperkalemia, renal impairment.

CARDIOVASCULAR: Antiadrenergic Agents

CLONIDINE—CARDIOLOGY (*Catapres, Catapres-TTS,* ✦*Dixarit*) ▶LK ♀C ▶? $

ADULT — HTN, immediate-release: Start 0.1 mg PO two times per day, may increase by 0.1 mg/day each week, usual maintenance dose 0.2 to 0.6 mg/day in 2 to 3 divided doses, max 2.4 mg/day. HTN, transdermal (Catapres-TTS): Start 0.1 mg/24 h patch q week, titrate to desired effect, max effective dose 0.6 mg/24 h (two 0.3 mg/24 h patches).

PEDS — HTN: Start 5 to 7 mcg/kg/day PO divided q 6 to 12 h, titrate at 5- to 7-day intervals to 5 to 25 mcg/kg/day divided q 6 h; max 0.9 mg/day. Transdermal therapy not recommended in children.

UNAPPROVED ADULT — HTN urgency: Initially 0.1 to 0.2 mg PO, followed by 0.1 mg q 1 h prn up to a total dose of 0.5 to 0.7 mg. Menopausal flushing: 0.1 to 0.4 mg/day PO divided two to three times per day; transdermal applied weekly 0.1 mg/day.

FORMS — Generic/Trade: Tabs, immediate-release, unscored (Catapres) 0.1, 0.2, 0.3 mg. Transdermal weekly patch ($$$$$) 0.1 mg/day (TTS-1), 0.2 mg/day (TTS-2), 0.3 mg/day (TTS-3).

NOTES — The sympatholytic action of clonidine may worsen sinus node dysfunction and atrioventricular block, especially in patients taking other sympatholytic drugs. Monitor for bradycardia when taking concomitant digoxin, nondihydropyridine calcium channel blockers, or beta blockers. Use lower initial dose with renal impairment. Rebound HTN with abrupt discontinuation of tabs, especially at doses that exceed 0.7 mg/day. Taper therapy slowly q 3 to 7 days to avoid rebound HTN. Dispose of used patches carefully, keep away from children. Remove patch before defibrillation, cardioversion, or MRI to avoid skin burns. Transdermal therapy should not be interrupted during the surgical period. Oral therapy should be continued within 4 h of surgery and restarted as soon as possible afterward. May potentiate the CNS depressive effects of alcohol, barbiturates, or other sedating drugs. Concomitant TCAs may reduce the BP-lowering effects. Concomitant neuroleptics may induce or exacerbate orthostatic regulation disturbances (eg, orthostatic hypotension, dizziness, fatigue). With alcoholic delirium, high IV doses of clonidine may increase the arrhythmogenic potential (QT-prolongation, ventricular fibrillation) of high IV doses of haloperidol. Do not crush, chew, or break extended-release tabs. Monitor response and side effects when interchanging between clonidine products; many are not equivalent on mg:mg basis.

MOA — Centrally acting alpha-2 agonist.

ADVERSE EFFECTS — Serious: Rebound hypertension, orthostatic hypotension, depression, bradycardia, syncope. Frequent: Dry mouth, constipation, drowsiness, dizziness, sedation, sexual dysfunction, rash.

DOXAZOSIN (*Cardura, Cardura XL*) ▶L ♀0/0/0; Data in pregnant women are limited and not sufficient to inform a drug-associated risk for major birth defects and miscarriage. ▶ No information available. $$

WARNING — Not 1st-line agent for HTN. Increased risk of heart failure in patients who used doxazosin compared to diuretic in treating HTN.

ADULT — BPH, immediate-release: Start 1 mg PO at bedtime, titrate by doubling the dose over at least 1- to 2-week intervals up to a maximum of 8 mg PO at bedtime. BPH, extended-release (not approved for HTN): Start 4 mg PO q am with breakfast, titrate dose in 3 to 4 weeks to max dose 8 mg PO q am. HTN, immediate-release: Start 1 mg PO at bedtime, max 16 mg/day. Avoid use of doxazosin alone to treat combined HTN and BPH.

PEDS — Not approved in children.

UNAPPROVED ADULT — Promote spontaneous passage of ureteral calculi: 4 mg (XL formulation only) PO daily usually combined with an NSAID, antiemetic, and opioid of choice.

FORMS — Generic/Trade: Tabs, scored 1, 2, 4, 8 mg. Trade only (Cardura XL): Tabs, extended-release, 4, 8 mg.

NOTES — Orthostatic hypotension is common. Bedtime dosing may minimize side effects. Initial 1 mg dose is used to decrease postural hypotension that may occur after the 1st few doses. If therapy is interrupted for several days, restart at the 1 mg dose. Increased risk of hypotension when used with erectile dysfunction medication (eg, sildenafil, tadalafil, vardenafil); use lowest dose of erectile dysfunction medication. Use caution with concomitant strong CYP3A4 inhibitor (eg, clarithromycin, itraconazole, ketoconazole, nefazodone, protease inhibitor, telithromycin, or voriconazole). Intraoperative floppy iris syndrome may occur during cataract surgery, if patient is on or previously taken alpha-1 blocker. Teach men to seek medical attention if erections last longer than 4 h.

MOA — Blocks binding of catecholamines to postsynaptic alpha-1 receptors; decreases urethral resistance.

ADVERSE EFFECTS — Serious: Postural hypotension, heart failure. Frequent: Headache, dizziness, fatigue, nausea, constipation.

GUANFACINE—CARDIOVASCULAR (*Tenex*) ▶K ♀B ▶? $

ADULT — HTN: Start 1 mg PO at bedtime, then may increase by 1 mg at bedtime every 3 to 4 weeks, max 3 mg/day.

PEDS — Not approved in children.

FORMS — Generic/Trade: Tabs, unscored 1, 2 mg.

NOTES — Most of antihypertensive effect is seen at 1 mg/day. Rebound HTN with abrupt discontinuation, taper when discontinuing. Extended-release tabs not indicated for HTN.

MOA — Centrally acting alpha-2 agonist.

ADVERSE EFFECTS — Serious: Syncope, rebound hypertension, hallucinations. Frequent: Sedation, dizziness, dry mouth, constipation, impotence.

METHYLDOPA ►LK ♀B ▶+ $
ADULT — HTN: Start 250 mg PO two to three times per day usual maintenance dose 500 to 3000 mg/day divided two to four times per day, max 3000 mg/day. Hypertensive crisis: 250 to 500 mg IV q 6 h, max 1 g IV q 6 h, max 4000 mg/day.
PEDS — HTN: 10 mg/kg/day PO divided two to four times per day, titrate dose to a max dose 65 mg/kg/day or 3000 mg/day, whichever is less.
FORMS — Generic only: Tabs, unscored 250, 500 mg.
NOTES — May be used to manage BP during pregnancy. IV form has a slow onset of effect and other agents preferred for rapid reduction of BP. Hemolytic anemia possible. The brand name product (Aldomet) is no longer available.
MOA — Stimulates central alpha-adrenergic receptors reducing sympathetic outflow.
ADVERSE EFFECTS — Serious: Hemolytic anemia (rare), LFT abnormalities. Frequent: Sedation, dizziness, dry mouth, constipation, impotence.

PRAZOSIN (*Minipress*) ►L ♀C ▶? $$
WARNING — Not 1st-line agent for HTN. Increased risk of heart failure in patients who used related drug doxazosin compared to diuretic in treating HTN.
ADULT — HTN: Start 1 mg PO two to three times per day, usual maintenance dose 20 mg/day divided two to three times per day, max 40 mg/day, but doses higher than 20 mg/day usually do not increase efficacy.
PEDS — Not approved in children.
UNAPPROVED ADULT — Posttraumatic stress disorder nightmares: Start 1 mg PO bedtime, increase weekly by 1 to 2 mg/day to max dose of 20 mg/day. Doses greater than 10 mg/day are divided early evening and at bedtime.
UNAPPROVED PEDS — HTN: Start 0.005 mg/kg PO single dose; increase slowly prn up to maintenance dose 0.025 to 0.150 mg/kg/day divided q 6 h; max dose 0.4 mg/kg/day.
FORMS — Generic/Trade: Caps 1, 2, 5 mg.
NOTES — Orthostatic hypotension common; to avoid, start with 1 mg at bedtime, and increase dose gradually. Increased risk of hypotension when used with erectile dysfunction medication (eg, sildenafil, tadalafil, vardenafil); use lowest dose of erectile dysfunction medication. Intraoperative floppy iris syndrome may occur during cataract surgery, if patient is on or previously taken alpha-1 blocker.

Teach men to seek medical attention if erections last longer than 4 h.
MOA — Blocks binding of catecholamines to post-synaptic alpha-1 receptors.
ADVERSE EFFECTS — Serious: Postural hypotension, heart failure. Frequent: Headache, dizziness

RESERPINE ►LK ♀C ▶– $$
ADULT — HTN: Start 0.05 to 0.1 mg PO daily or 0.1 mg PO every other day, max dose 0.25 mg/day.
PEDS — Not approved in children.
FORMS — Generic only: Tabs, scored 0.1, 0.25 mg.
NOTES — Should be used in combination with a diuretic to counteract fluid retention and augment BP control. May cause depression at higher doses, avoid use in patients with uncontrolled depression or active peptic ulcer disease.
MOA — Blocks transport of norepinephrine into storage granules.
ADVERSE EFFECTS — Serious: None. Frequent: Nasal stuffiness.

TERAZOSIN ►LK ♀C ▶? $$
WARNING — Not 1st-line for HTN. Increased risk of heart failure in patients who used related drug doxazosin compared to diuretic in treating HTN.
ADULT — HTN: Start 1 mg PO at bedtime, usual effective dose 1 to 5 mg PO daily or divided two times per day, max 20 mg/day. BPH: Start 1 mg PO at bedtime; titrate dose in a stepwise fashion to 2, 5, or 10 mg PO at bedtime to desired effect. Treatment with 10 mg PO at bedtime for 4 to 6 weeks may be needed to assess benefit. Max 20 mg/day.
PEDS — Not approved in children.
FORMS — Generic only: Caps 1, 2, 5, 10 mg.
NOTES — Orthostatic hypotension is common. Bedtime dosing may minimize side effects. Initial 1 mg dose is used to decrease postural hypotension that may occur after the 1st few doses. If therapy is interrupted for several days, restart at the 1 mg dose. Increased risk of hypotension when used with erectile dysfunction medication (eg, sildenafil, tadalafil, vardenafil); use lowest dose of erectile dysfunction medication. Intraoperative floppy iris syndrome may occur during cataract surgery if patient is on or previously taken alpha-1 blocker. The brand name product (Hytrin) is no longer available.
MOA — Blocks binding of catecholamines to post-synaptic alpha-1 receptors, increases urinary flow rate.
ADVERSE EFFECTS — Serious: Postural hypotension, heart failure. Frequent: Headache, dizziness.

CARDIOVASCULAR: Antidysrhythmics/Cardiac Arrest

ADENOSINE (*Adenocard*) ►Plasma ♀C ▶? $
ADULT — PSVT conversion (not A-fib): 6 mg rapid IV and flush, preferably through a central line. If no response after 1 to 2 min then 12 mg. A 3rd dose of 12 mg may be given prn.
PEDS — PSVT conversion wt less than 50 kg: Initial dose 50 to 100 mcg/kg IV, give subsequent doses q

1 to 2 min prn and increase the dose 50 to 100 mcg/kg each time, up to a max single dose of 300 mcg/kg or 12 mg (whichever is less). PST conversion wt 50 kg or greater: Use adult dosage.
NOTES — Half-life is less than 10 sec. Give doses by rapid IV push followed by NS flush. Need higher dose if on theophylline or caffeine, lower dose if on

(cont.)

ADENOSINE (*cont.*)

dipyridamole or carbamazepine. May cause respiratory collapse in patients with asthma, COPD. Use in setting with cardiac resuscitation readily available. Do not use with acute myocardial ischemia, unstable angina, or cardiovascular instability. Do not confuse with adenosine phosphate used for the symptomatic relief of varicose vein complications.
MOA — Blocks cardiac conduction through the AV node.
ADVERSE EFFECTS — Serious: Arrhythmias, heart block, bronchoconstriction, seizures. Frequent: Flushing, chest tightness.

AMIODARONE (*Pacerone, Cordarone*) ▶L ♀X/X/X; Neonatal harm: Potential cardiac, growth, neurodevelopmental, neurological, thyroid effects. ▶ Do not breastfeed while taking amiodarone. $$$$
WARNING — May cause potentially fatal toxicities, including pulmonary toxicity, hepatic injury, and worsened arrhythmia. Only use for adults with life-threatening ventricular arrhythmias when other treatments ineffective or not tolerated.
ADULT — Life-threatening ventricular arrhythmia without cardiac arrest: Load 150 mg IV over 10 min, then 1 mg/min for 6 h, then 0.5 mg/min for 18 h. Mix in D5W. Oral loading dose 800 to 1600 mg PO daily for 1 to 3 weeks, reduce dose to 400 to 800 mg daily for 1 month when arrhythmia is controlled or adverse effects are prominent, then reduce to lowest effective dose, usually 200 to 400 mg daily.
PEDS — Not approved in children.
UNAPPROVED ADULT — Atrial fibrillation (refractory or with accessory pathway): Loading dose 600 to 800 mg PO daily for 7 to 14 days, then 200 to 400 mg daily. Maintain sinus rhythm with A-fib: 100 to 400 mg PO daily. Shock-refractory VF/pulseless VT: 300 mg or 5 mg/kg IV bolus followed by unsynchronized shock, additional 150 mg bolus may be given if serious arrhythmias recur. Stable monomorphic ventricular tachycardia: 150 mg IV over 10 min, repeat q 10 to 15 min prn.
UNAPPROVED PEDS — May cause death or other serious side effects in children (see NOTES); do not use in infants younger than 30 days of age and use only if medically warranted if 30 days of age or older. Ventricular arrhythmia: IV therapy limited data; 5 mg/kg IV over 30 min; followed by 5 mcg/kg/min infusion; increase infusion prn up to max 10 mcg/kg/min or 20 mg/kg/day. Give loading dose in 1 mg/kg aliquots with each aliquot given over 5 to 10 min; do not exceed 30 mg/min.
FORMS — Trade only (Pacerone): Tabs, unscored 100 mg. Generic/Trade: Tabs, scored 200, 400 mg.
NOTES — Proarrhythmic. Contraindicated in cardiogenic shock and in profound/symptomatic bradycardia (whether from AV block or sinus-node dysfunction) in the absence of a functioning pacemaker. Consider inpatient rhythm monitoring during initiation of therapy, especially when treating life-threatening arrhythmias. Consult cardiologist before using with other antiarrhythmic agents. Do not use with iodine allergy. Photosensitivity and skin discoloration (blue/gray color) with oral therapy. Hypo- or hyperthyroidism possible. Monitor LFTs, TFTs, and PFTs. Baseline and regular eye exams. Prompt ophthalmic examination needed with changes in visual acuity or decreased peripheral vision. Most manufacturers of laser refractive devices contraindicate eye laser surgery when taking amiodarone. Long elimination half-life, approximately 26 to 107 days. Drug interactions may persist after discontinuance due to long half-life. May increase levels of substrates of p-glycoprotein and drugs metabolized by CYP 450 enzymes (CYP1A2, CYP2C9, CYP2D6, CYP3A4). Coadministration of fluoroquinolones, macrolides, loratadine, trazodone, azoles, or Class IA and III antiarrhythmic drugs may prolong QTc. Initiating ledipasvir/sofosbuvir or sofosbuvir with simeprevir may cause serious symptomatic bradycardia, some requiring pacemaker insertion; monitor heart rate in patients taking or recently discontinuing amiodarone when starting antiviral treatment. May double or triple phenytoin level. May increase cyclosporine level. May increase digoxin level; discontinue digoxin or reduce dose by 50%. May increase INR with warfarin therapy; reduce warfarin dose by 33 to 50%. Do not use with simvastatin doses greater than 20 mg/day, lovastatin doses greater than 40 mg/day; may increase atorvastatin level (use lower dose); increases risk of myopathy and rhabdomyolysis. Coadministration with clopidogrel may result in ineffective platelet inhibition. Do not use with grapefruit juice. Use cautiously with beta-blockers and calcium channel blockers. Protease inhibitors, cimetidine may increase levels. Give two times per day if intolerable GI effects occur with once daily dosing. IV therapy may cause hypotension and bradycardia in adults. Administer IV infusion using a nonevacuated glass bottle and in-line IV filter. Use central line when concentration exceeds 2 mg/mL. May cause congenital hypothyroidism and hyperthyroidism if given during pregnancy. Avoid use in children younger than 1 mo: IV form contains benzyl alcohol, which may cause gasping syndrome (gasping respirations, hypotension, bradycardia, and cardiovascular collapse). In children 1 mo to 15 yo may cause life-threatening hypotension, bradycardia, and AV block. May adversely affect male reproductive tract development in infants and toddlers from plasticizer exposure from IV tubing; use syringes instead of IV tubing to administer doses to infants and toddlers.
MOA — Prolongs cardiac repolarization (Class III antiarrhythmic properties). Also has sodium channel blockade, beta adrenergic blockade, and calcium channel blockade effects (Class I, II, IV effects).
ADVERSE EFFECTS — Serious: Pulmonary toxicity, thyroid toxicity, bradycardia/heart block, arrhythmias, rhabdomyolysis, blindness, visual impairment, SIADH, hepatotoxicity, acute renal failure, agranulocytosis. Frequent: Hypotension, elevated LFTs, photosensitivity, GI intolerance, corneal microdeposits.

ATROPINE (*AtroPen*) ▸K ♀C ▶– $

ADULT — Bradyarrhythmia/CPR: 0.5 to 1 mg IV q 3 to 5 min, max 0.04 mg/kg (3 mg). Treatment of muscarinic symptoms of insecticide or nerve agent poisonings: Mild symptoms: 1 injection of 2 mg auto-injector pen, 2 additional injections after 10 min may be given in rapid succession if severe symptoms develop. Severe symptoms: 3 injections of 2 mg pen in rapid succession. Administer in mid-lateral thigh. Max 3 injections.

PEDS — CPR: 0.02 mg/kg/dose IV q 5 min for 2 to 3 doses prn (max single dose 0.5 mg); minimum single dose 0.1 mg; max cumulative dose 1 mg. Treatment of muscarinic symptoms of insecticide or nerve agent poisonings: Follow adult dosing instructions, but if wt less than 7 kg use 0.25 mg pen, if wt 7 to 18 kg use 0.5 mg pen, if wt 18 to 41 kg use 1 mg pen, if wt greater than 41 kg use 2 mg pen.

UNAPPROVED ADULT — ET administration prior to IV access: 2 to 2.5 times the recommended IV dose in 10 mL of NS or distilled water.

FORMS — Trade only: Prefilled auto-injector pen: 0.25 mg (yellow), 0.5 mg (blue), 1 mg (dark red), 2 mg (green).

NOTES — Injector should be used by someone who has adequate training in recognizing and treating nerve agent or insecticide intoxication. Seek immediate medical attention after injection(s).

MOA — Blocks acetylcholine activity leading to increased cardiac chronotropic effect.

ADVERSE EFFECTS — Serious: Arrhythmias, tachycardia, paradoxical bradycardia (rare), paralysis (large doses). Frequent: Dry mouth, blurred vision, mydriasis, confusion, palpitations, urinary hesitancy, anhidrosis, constipation, injection site pain.

DIGOXIN (*Lanoxin, Digitek, ✚Toloxin*) ▸KL ♀C ▶+ $

ADULT — Systolic heart failure/rate control of chronic A-fib, age younger than 70 yo: 0.25 mg PO daily; age 70 yo or older: 0.125 mg PO daily; impaired renal function: 0.0625 to 0.125 mg PO daily; titrate based on response. Rapid A-fib: Total loading dose (TLD) 10 to 15 mcg/kg IV/PO, given in 3 divided doses q 6 to 8 h; give ~50% TLD for 1 dose, then ~25% TLD for 2 doses (eg, 70 kg with normal renal function: 0.5 mg, then 0.25 mg q 6 to 8 h for 2 doses). Impaired renal function, 6 to 10 mcg/kg IV/PO TLD, given in 3 divided doses q 6 to 8 h. Titrate to minimum effective dose. Other agents (ie, beta blockers, diltiazem, verapamil) more effective in controlling ventricular rate in A-fib.

PEDS — Heart failure with normal sinus rhythm: IV loading based on age: premature neonate: 15 to 25 mcg/kg; full-term neonate: 20 to 30 mcg/kg; age 1 to 24 mo: 30 to 50 mcg/kg; age 2 to 5 yo: 25 to 35 mcg/kg; age 5 to 10 yo: 15 to 30 mcg/kg; age older than 10 yo: 8 to 12 mcg/kg. Start by administering half of the total loading dose and then reassess in 4 to 8 h to determine need for 2nd half of loading dose. Daily IV maintenance: Use 20 to 30% of actual IV loading dose for premature neonate; use 25 to 35% of actual IV loading dose for age full-term to older than 10 yo; use divided two times per day for age younger than 10 yo. Daily PO maintenance: age 2 to 5 yo: 10 to 15 mcg/kg; age 6 to 10 yo: 7 to 10 mcg/kg; age older than 10 yo: 3 to 5 mcg/kg. Caution: Pediatric doses are in mcg, elixir product is labeled in mg/mL. Atrial fibrillation: Titrate to minimum dose needed to achieve desired ventricular rate without undesirable side effects.

UNAPPROVED ADULT — Reentrant PSVT (after carotid massage, IV adenosine, IV beta-blocker, IV diltiazem): 8 to 15 mcg/kg (based on ideal body wt) IV, give 50% of total dose initially, 25% 4 to 6 h later, and then the final 25% 4 to 6 h later.

FORMS — Generic/Trade: Tabs, scored (Lanoxin, Digitek) 0.125, 0.25 mg. Generic only: Elixir 0.05 mg/mL.

NOTES — Proarrhythmic. Consider patient-specific characteristics (lean/ideal wt, CrCl, age, concomitant disease states, concomitant medications, and factors likely to alter pharmacokinetic/dynamic profile of digoxin) when dosing; see prescribing information for alterations based on wt and renal function. Assess electrolytes, renal function, levels periodically. Elimination prolonged with renal impairment. Maintain normal potassium, magnesium, and calcium levels. Adjust dose based on response and therapeutic serum levels (range from 0.8 to 2 ng/mL); the risk of adverse events increases when the level is more than 1.2 ng/mL. Lower serum trough levels (0.5 to 1 ng/mL) may be appropriate for heart failure; A-fib may need higher levels. Nausea, vomiting, visual disturbances, and cardiac arrhythmias may indicate toxicity. Avoid administering IM due to severe local irritation. Many interactions with other drugs and nutritional supplements. Consider drug interactions before initiating and during digoxin therapy; see prescribing information for complete recommendations. P-glycoprotein inducers or inhibitors may alter digoxin pharmacokinetics. Measure serum digoxin concentrations before initiating a concomitant medication that increases or decreases digoxin level; decrease or increase digoxin dose or change dosing interval based on prescribing information and response. See prescribing information for full information before using in patients with sinus node disease, AV block, accessory AV pathway, certain heart failure disorders with preserved LV function, hypermetabolic states, thyroid disease, beriberi heart disease, or planned cardioversion. Do not use with acute MI or myocarditis. Therapeutic doses may cause ECG changes (PR-interval prolongation, ST-segment depression) and false-positive ST-T changes during exercise testing; these are expected and do not indicate toxicity.

MOA — Slows cardiac conduction through the AV node, increases force of myocardial contraction.

ADVERSE EFFECTS — Serious: Arrhythmias, heart block. Frequent: Dizziness, headache, mental disturbances, N/V, diarrhea.

DIGOXIN IMMUNE FAB (*Digibind, DigiFab*) ▶K ♀C ▶?
$$$$$
ADULT — Digoxin toxicity: Acute ingestion of known amount: 1 vial binds approximately 0.5 mg digoxin. Acute ingestion of unknown amount: 10 vials IV, may repeat once. Toxicity during chronic therapy: 6 vials usually adequate; one formula is: Number vials = (serum dig level in ng/mL) × (kg)/100.
PEDS — Digoxin toxicity: Dose varies. Acute ingestion of known amount: 1 vial binds approximately 0.5 mg digoxin. Acute ingestion of unknown amount: 10 vials IV, may repeat once; monitor for volume overload. Toxicity during chronic therapy: 1 vial usually adequate for infants and small children (less than 20 kg); one formula is: Number vials = (serum dig level in ng/mL) × (kg)/100.
NOTES — After digoxin immune fab infusion, use free digoxin level to guide therapy. Total serum digoxin concentration will be falsely elevated for several days.
MOA — Binds digoxin preventing interaction with sodium pump receptor.
ADVERSE EFFECTS — Serious: Hypersensitivity (rare), hypokalemia.

DISOPYRAMIDE (*Norpace, Norpace CR*) ▶KL ♀C ▶+
$$$
WARNING — Proarrhythmic. Contraindicated in preexisting/congenital QT prolongation, history of torsades de pointes, cardiogenic shock; 2nd/3rd degree heart block without pacemaker. Only use for adults with life-threatening ventricular arrhythmias; increased mortality in patients with non-life-threatening ventricular arrhythmias and structural heart disease (ie, MI, LV dysfunction).
ADULT — Rarely indicated, consult cardiologist. Ventricular arrhythmia: 400 to 800 mg PO daily in divided doses (immediate-release is divided q 6 h, extended-release is divided q 12 h). With cardiomyopathy or possible cardiac decompensation, limit initial dose to 100 mg of immediate-release q 6 to 8 h; do not give a loading dose. With liver disease or moderate renal impairment (CrCl >40 mg/dL): 400 mg/day PO in divided doses. Use immediate-release form when CrCl is less than 40 mg/dL: Give 100 mg q 8 h for CrCl 30 to 40 mg/dL, give 100 mg q 12 h for CrCl 15 to 30 mg/dL, give 100 mg q 24 h for CrCl <15 mg/dL.
PEDS — Ventricular arrhythmia: Divide all doses q 6 h. Younger than 1 yo: 10 to 30 mg/kg/day; age 1 to 4 yo: 10 to 20 mg/kg/day; age 4 to 12 yo:10 to 15 mg/kg/day; age 12 to 18 yo: 6 to 15 mg/kg/day .
UNAPPROVED ADULT — Maintain sinus rhythm with A-fib: 400 to 750 mg/day in divided doses.
FORMS — Generic/Trade: Caps, immediate-release 100, 150 mg. Trade only: Caps, extended-release 100, 150 mg.
NOTES — Proarrhythmic. Consider inpatient rhythm monitoring during initiation of therapy, especially when treating life-threatening arrhythmias. Anticholinergic side effects (dry mouth, constipation, blurred vision, urinary hesitancy) commonly

occur. Reduce dose in patients with CrCl <40 mL/min. Initiate as an outpatient with extreme caution. May start 6 to 12 h after last dose of quinidine, or 3 to 6 h after last dose of procainamide. May start extended-release form 6 h after last dose of immediate-release form.
MOA — Depresses phase 0 depolarization, prolongs cardiac action potential duration (Class 1A).
ADVERSE EFFECTS — Serious: Arrhythmias. Frequent: Dizziness, headache, hypotension, dry mouth, blurred vision, urinary retention, constipation.

DOFETILIDE (*Tikosyn*) ▶KL ♀C ▶– $$$$$
WARNING — Must be initiated or reinitiated in a facility that can provide CrCl calculation, ECG monitoring, and cardiac resuscitation. Monitor on telemetry for a minimum of 3 days.
ADULT — Conversion of A-fib/flutter: Specialized dosing based on CrCl and QTc interval.
PEDS — Not approved in children.
FORMS — Generic/Trade: Caps, 0.125, 0.25, 0.5 mg.
NOTES — Proarrhythmic. Rarely indicated. Contraindicated in acquired/congenital QT prolongation; CrCl <20 mL/min; baseline QTc interval more than 440 msec or more than 500 msec in patients with ventricular conduction abnormalities; or with concomitant HCTZ, verapamil, cimetidine, dolutegravir, ketoconazole, megestrol, prochlorperazine, or trimethoprim. Use with heart rate below 50 bpm has not been studied. Serum K^+, Mg^{++} should be within normal range prior to initiating and during therapy. Monitor K^+ and Mg^{++} (low levels increase risk of arrhythmias). Assess CrCl and QTc prior to 1st dose. Continuously monitor ECG during hospital initiation and adjust dose based on QTc interval. Do not discharge within 12 h after conversion to normal sinus rhythm. Effects may be increased by known CYP3A4 inhibitors and drugs that inhibit renal elimination. Using with phenothiazines, cisapride, TCAs, macrolides, fluoroquinolones may increase QTc.
MOA — Prolongs cardiac repolarization (Class III antiarrhythmic properties).
ADVERSE EFFECTS — Serious: Arrhythmias. Common: Chest pain, headache.

DRONEDARONE (*Multaq*) ▶L ♀X ▶– $$$$$
WARNING — Contraindicated with NYHA Class IV heart failure, symptomatic heart failure with recent decompensation requiring hospitalization, or atrial fibrillation that will not or cannot be cardioverted into normal sinus rhythm. Increases risk of death, stroke, and heart failure in patients with decompensated heart failure or permanent atrial fibrillation.
ADULT — Reduce hospitalization risk for patients with A-fib who are in sinus rhythm and have a history of paroxysmal or persistent A-fib: 400 mg PO two times per day with morning and evening meals.
PEDS — Not approved in children.
FORMS — Trade only: Tabs, unscored 400 mg.
NOTES — Proarrhythmic. Do not use with 2nd or 3rd degree AV block or sick sinus syndrome without functioning pacemaker, bradycardia less than 50

(cont.)

DRONEDARONE (*cont.*)

bpm, QTc Bazett interval greater than 500 ms, liver or lung toxicity related to previous amiodarone use, severe hepatic impairment, pregnancy, lactation, grapefruit juice, drugs or herbals that increase QT interval, Class I or III antiarrhythmic agents, potent inhibitors of CYP3A4 enzyme system (clarithromycin, itraconazole, ketoconazole, nefazodone, ritonavir, voriconazole), or inducers of CYP3A4 enzyme system (carbamazepine, phenytoin, phenobarbital, rifampin, St. John's wort). Correct hypo-/hyperkalemia and hypomagnesemia before giving. Monitor ECG q 3 months; if in A-fib, either stop dronedarone or cardiovert. May initiate or exacerbate heart failure symptoms; teach patients to report symptoms of new or worsening heart failure (eg, wt gain, edema, dyspnea). May be associated with hepatic injury; teach patients to report symptoms of hepatic injury (eg, anorexia, nausea, vomiting, fatigue, malaise, right upper quadrant discomfort, jaundice, dark urine); discontinue if hepatic injury is suspected. Serum creatinine may increase (~0.1 mg/dL) during 1st weeks, but does not reflect change in renal function; reversible when discontinued. Monitor renal function periodically. Give with appropriate antithrombotic therapy. May increase INR when used with warfarin. May increase dabigatran or other P-glycoprotein substrates level. May increase digoxin level; discontinue digoxin or reduce dose by 50%; monitor for digoxin toxicity. Use cautiously with beta-blockers (BB) and calcium channel blockers (CCB); initiate lower doses of BB or CCB; initiate at low dose and monitor ECG. Do not use with more than 10 mg of simvastatin. May increase level of sirolimus, tacrolimus, or CYP3A4 substrates with narrow therapeutic index.

MOA — Has sodium channel blockade, beta-adrenergic blockade, cardiac repolarization, and calcium channel blockade effects (Class I, II, III, IV effects).

ADVERSE EFFECTS — Serious: New/worsening heart failure, bradycardia/heart block, arrhythmias, hepatotoxicity, pulmonary toxicity. Frequent: Abdominal pain, asthenia, diarrhea, nausea.

FLECAINIDE ▶K ♀C ▶– $$$$

WARNING — Proarrhythmic. Increased mortality in patients with non-life-threatening ventricular arrhythmias with history of MI; not recommended for use with chronic atrial fibrillation.

ADULT — Prevention of paroxysmal A-fib/ flutter or PSVT, with symptoms and no structural heart disease: Start 50 mg PO q 12 h, may increase by 50 mg two times per day q 4 days, max 300 mg/day. Life-threatening ventricular arrhythmias without structural heart disease: Start 100 mg PO q 12 h, may increase by 50 mg two times per day q 4 days, max 400 mg/day. With CrCl <35 mL/min: Start 50 mg PO two times per day.

PEDS — Consult pediatric cardiologist.

UNAPPROVED ADULT — Cardioversion of recent onset A-fib: 200 to 300 mg PO single dose. Maintain sinus rhythm with A-fib: 200 to 300 mg/day in divided doses.

FORMS — Generic: Tabs, unscored 50 mg, scored 100, 150 mg.

NOTES — Contraindicated in cardiogenic shock, sick sinus syndrome or significant conduction delay, 2nd/3rd degree heart block or bundle brand block without pacemaker, acquired/congenital QT prolongation, or patients with history of torsades de pointes. Consider inpatient rhythm monitoring during initiation of therapy, especially when treating life-threatening arrhythmias. Use with AV nodal slowing agent (beta-blocker, verapamil, diltiazem) to minimize risk of 1:1 atrial flutter. Reduce dose if QRS widening more than 20% from baseline or if 2nd/3rd degree AV block. Correct hypo-/hyperkalemia before giving. Increases digoxin level 13 to 19%. Consult cardiologist before using with other antiarrhythmic agents. Reduce dose of flecainide 50% when used with amiodarone. Quinidine, cimetidine may increase levels. Use cautiously with disopyramide, verapamil, or impaired hepatic function. Use cautiously with impaired renal function; will take more than 4 days to reach new steady-state level. Target trough level 0.2 to 1 mcg/mL. The brand name product (Tambocor) is no longer available.

MOA — Depresses phase 0 depolarization significantly, slows cardiac conduction significantly (Class 1C).

ADVERSE EFFECTS — Serious: Arrhythmias, depressed conduction/widened QRS at higher heart rates. Frequent: Dizziness, headache, nausea, dyspnea, fatigue, visual disturbances.

IBUTILIDE (*Corvert*) ▶K ♀C ▶? $$$$$

WARNING — Proarrhythmic; only administer by trained personnel with continuous ECG monitoring, capable of identifying and treating acute ventricular arrhythmias. Potentially fatal ventricular arrhythmias may occur with/without QT prolongation and can lead to torsades de pointes.

ADULT — Recent onset A-fib/flutter: Give 0.01 mg/kg over 10 min for wt less than 60 kg, may repeat if no response after 10 min. Give 1 mg (10 mL) IV over 10 min for wt 60 kg or greater, may repeat once if no response after 10 min. Useful in combination with DC cardioversion if DC cardioversion alone is unsuccessful.

PEDS — Not approved in children.

NOTES — Proarrhythmic. Serum K+, Mg++ should be within normal range prior to initiating and during therapy. Monitor K+ and Mg++ (low levels increase risk of arrhythmias). Keep on cardiac monitor at least 4 h. Use with caution, if at all, when QT interval is greater than 500 msec, severe LV dysfunction, or in patients already using class Ia or III antiarrhythmics. Stop infusion when arrhythmia is terminated.

MOA — Prolongs cardiac repolarization (Class III antiarrhythmic properties).

ADVERSE EFFECTS — Serious: Arrhythmias.

ISOPROTERENOL (*Isuprel*) ▶LK ♀C ▶? $$$$$
ADULT — Refractory bradycardia or 3rd degree AV block, bolus method: 0.02 to 0.06 mg IV; infusion method: Dilute 2 mg in 250 mL D5W (8 mcg/mL), a rate of 37.5 mL/h delivers 5 mcg/min. General dose range 2 to 20 mcg/min.
PEDS — Refractory bradycardia or 3rd degree AV block: Dilute 2 mg in 250 mL D5W (8 mcg/mL). Start IV infusion 0.05 mcg/kg/min, increase q 5 to 10 min by 0.1 mcg/kg/min until desired effect or onset of toxicity, max 2 mcg/kg/min. For a 10 kg child, a rate of 8 mL/h delivers 0.1 mcg/kg/min.
MOA — Serious: Arrhythmias, tachycardia. Frequent: Hypertension, palpitations, flushing, sweating, dizziness.
ADVERSE EFFECTS — TAB015,TAB016

LIDOCAINE (*Xylocaine, Xylocard*) ▶LK ♀B ▶? $
ADULT — Ventricular arrhythmia: Load 1 mg/kg IV, then 0.5 mg/kg IV q 8 to 10 min prn to max 3 mg/kg. IV infusion: 4 g in 500 mL D5W (8 mg/mL) at 1 to 4 mg/min.
PEDS — Ventricular arrhythmia: Loading dose 1 mg/kg IV/intraosseous slowly; may repeat for 2 doses 10 to 15 min apart; max 3 to 5 mg/kg in 1 h. ET tube: Use 2 to 2.5 times IV dose. IV infusion: 4 g in 500 mL D5W (8 mg/mL) at 20 to 50 mcg/kg/min. For a 10 kg child a rate of 3 mL/h delivers 40 mcg/kg/min.
UNAPPROVED ADULT — ET administration prior to IV access: 2 to 2.5 times the recommended IV dose in 10 mL of NS or distilled water. Shock refractory VF/pulseless VT: 1 to 1.5 mg/kg IV push once, then 0.5 to 0.75 mg/kg IV push q 5 to 10 min prn to max 3 mg/kg.
NOTES — Reduce infusion in heart failure, liver disease, elderly. Not for routine use after acute MI. Monitor for CNS side effects with prolonged infusions.
MOA — Depresses phase 0 depolarization slightly, shortens cardiac action potential duration (Class 1B).
ADVERSE EFFECTS — Serious: Arrhythmias, hypersensitivity (rare), seizures (rare). Frequent: Hypotension, dizziness, drowsiness.

MEXILETINE (*Mexitil*) ▶L ♀C ▶– $$$$
WARNING — Proarrhythmic. Increased mortality in patients with non-life-threatening ventricular arrhythmias and structural heart disease (ie, MI, LV dysfunction).
ADULT — Rarely indicated, consult cardiologist. Ventricular arrhythmia: Start 200 mg PO q 8 h with food or antacid, max dose 1200 mg/day. Patients responding to q 8 h dosing may be converted to q 12 h dosing with careful monitoring, max 450 mg/dose q 12 h.
PEDS — Not approved in children.
FORMS — Generic only: Caps 150, 200, 250 mg.
NOTES — Patients may require decreased dose with severe liver disease. CNS side effects may limit dose titration. Monitor level when given with phenytoin, rifampin, phenobarbital, cimetidine, fluvoxamine. May increase theophylline level.

MOA — Depresses phase 0 depolarization slightly, shortens cardiac action potential duration (Class 1B).
ADVERSE EFFECTS — Serious: Arrhythmias, blood dyscrasias, pulmonary infiltrates/fibrosis. Frequent: N/V, diarrhea, dizziness, nervousness, headache, blurred vision, tremor, ataxia.

PROCAINAMIDE ▶LK ♀C ▶? $$
WARNING — Proarrhythmic. Increased mortality in patients with non-life-threatening ventricular arrhythmias and structural heart disease (ie, MI, LV dysfunction). Contraindicated with systemic lupus erythematosus. Has been associated with blood dyscrasias.
ADULT — Ventricular arrhythmia: Loading dose: 100 mg IV q 10 min or 20 mg/min (150 mL/h) until QRS widens more than 50%, dysrhythmia suppressed, hypotension, or total of 17 mg/kg or 1000 mg delivered. Infusion: Dilute 2 g in 250 mL D5W (8 mg/mL) run at rate of 15 to 45 mL/h to deliver 2 to 6 mg/min. If rhythm unresponsive, guide therapy by serum procainamide/NAPA levels.
PEDS — Not approved in children.
UNAPPROVED ADULT — Restoration of sinus rhythm in atrial fibrillation with accessory pathway (preexcitation): 100 mg IV q 10 min or 20 mg/min until QRS widens more than 50%, dysrhythmia suppressed, hypotension, or total of 17 mg/kg or 1000 mg delivered.
UNAPPROVED PEDS — Arrhythmia: 2 to 6 mg/kg IV over 5 min, max loading dose 100 mg, repeat loading dose q 5 to 10 min prn up to max 15 mg/kg; 20 to 80 mcg/kg/min IV infusion, max dose 2 g/day. Consult pedi cardiologist or intensivist.
NOTES — Proarrhythmic. Use lower dose or longer dosing interval with liver disease. Use cautiously with renal impairment or failure. Avoid with preexisting peripheral neuropathy. If positive antinuclear antibody (ANA) test develops, weigh risk/benefit of continued therapy. Evaluate complete blood count, including white cell, differential, and platelet counts, weekly for 1st 12 weeks of therapy and periodically afterward, and if patient develops unusual bleeding/bruising or signs of infection. If hematologic disorders are identified, discontinue therapy. The brand-name products (Procan, Pronestyl) are no longer available.
MOA — Depresses phase 0 depolarization, prolongs cardiac action potential duration (Class 1A).
ADVERSE EFFECTS — Serious: Arrhythmias, blood dyscrasias (rare), SLE. Frequent: Hypotension, fever, headache.

PROPAFENONE (*Rythmol, Rythmol SR*) ▶L ♀C ▶? $$
WARNING — Proarrhythmic. Increased mortality in patients with non-life-threatening ventricular arrhythmias and structural heart disease (ie, MI, LV dysfunction).
ADULT — Prevention of paroxysmal A-fib/flutter or PSVT, with symptoms and no structural heart disease; or life-threatening ventricular arrhythmias: Start (immediate-release) 150 mg PO q 8 h; may

(cont.)

PROPAFENONE (*cont.*)

increase after 3 to 4 days to 225 mg PO q 8 h; max 900 mg/day. Prolong time to recurrence of symptomatic A-fib without structural heart disease: 225 mg SR PO q 12 h, may increase after 5 days to 325 mg PO q 12 h, max 425 mg q 12 h.

PEDS — Not approved in children.

UNAPPROVED ADULT — Cardioversion of recent onset A-fib: 600 mg PO single dose. Outpatient prn therapy for recurrent A-fib in highly select patients ("pill-in-the-pocket"): Single dose PO of 450 mg for wt less than 70 kg, 600 mg for wt 70 kg or greater.

FORMS — Generic/Trade: Tabs, immediate-release scored 150, 225 mg. Caps, sustained-release, (SR-$$$$$) 225, 325, 425 mg. Generic only: Tabs, immediate-release, scored 300 mg.

NOTES — Contraindicated with heart failure; cardiogenic shock; SA, AV, or intraventricular disorders of impulse generation or conduction (eg, sick sinus node syndrome, AV block) without pacemaker; hypotension; bradycardia; known Brugada syndrome; bronchospastic disorders and severe COPD; electrolyte imbalance. Use inpatient rhythm monitoring prior to and during therapy; discontinue propafenone if changes are suggestive of Brugada syndrome. Consider using with AV nodal blocking agent (beta-blocker, verapamil, diltiazem) to minimize risk of 1:1 atrial flutter. Reduce dose if QRS widening more than 20% from baseline or if 2nd/3rd degree AV block. Correct hypo-/hyperkalemia and hypomagnesemia before giving. Reduce dose 70 to 80% with impaired hepatic function. Use cautiously with impaired renal function. Poorly metabolized by 10% population; reduce dose and monitor for toxicity. Consult cardiologist before using with other antiarrhythmic agents. Do not use with amiodarone, quinidine, or the combination of CYP3A4 and CYP2D6 inhibitors (or CYP2D6 deficiency). CYP2D6 inhibitors (eg, desipramine, paroxetine, ritonavir, sertraline); CYP3A4 inhibitors (eg, ketoconazole, ritonavir, saquinavir, erythromycin, grapefruit juice); CYP1A2 inhibitors (eg, amiodarone, cigarette smoke); cimetidine; fluoxetine may increase levels. Rifampin reduces level. Orlistat reduces level; taper orlistat withdrawal in patients stabilized on propafenone. May increase digoxin level 35 to 85%. May increase beta-blocker levels. May increase INR when used with warfarin. Concomitant lidocaine increases risk of CNS side effects. Instruct patient to report any changes in OTC, prescription, supplement use, and symptoms that may be associated with altered electrolytes (prolonged/excessive diarrhea, sweating, vomiting, thirst, appetite loss). May affect artificial pacemakers; monitor pacemaker function. May exacerbate myasthenia gravis. Bioavailability of 325 mg SR two times per day is equivalent to 150 mg immediate-release three times per day.

MOA — Depresses phase 0 depolarization significantly, slows cardiac conduction significantly (Class 1C).

ADVERSE EFFECTS — Serious: Agranulocytosis, arrhythmias, heart block. Frequent: Dizziness, headache, nausea, dyspnea, fatigue, blurred vision, metallic taste.

QUINIDINE ▶LK ♀C ▶+ $

WARNING — Proarrhythmic. Associated with QT prolongation and torsades de pointes. Contraindicated with complete AV block or left bundle branch block. Increased mortality in patients with non-life-threatening arrhythmias and structural heart disease (ie, MI, LV dysfunction).

ADULT — Arrhythmia: Gluconate, extended-release: 324 to 648 mg PO q 8 to 12 h; sulfate, immediate-release: 200 to 400 mg PO q 6 to 8 h; sulfate, extended-release: 300 to 600 mg PO q 8 to 12 h. Consider inpatient rhythm and QT monitoring during initiation of therapy. Life-threatening malaria: Load with 10 mg/kg (max 600 mg) IV over 1 to 2 h, then 0.02 mg/kg/min for at least 24 h. Dose given as quinidine gluconate. When parasitemia less than 1% and PO meds tolerated, convert to PO quinine to complete 3 days (Africa/South America) or 7 days (Southeast Asia). Also give doxycycline, tetracycline, or clindamycin.

PEDS — Not approved in children.

UNAPPROVED PEDS — Arrhythmia: Test dose (oral sulfate or IM/IV gluconate) 2 mg/kg (max 200 mg). Sulfate: 15 to 60 mg/kg/day PO divided q 6 h. Life-threatening malaria: Load with 10 mg/kg IV over 1 to 2 h, then 0.02 mg/kg/min for at least 24 h. Dose given as quinidine gluconate. When parasitemia less than 1% and PO meds tolerated, convert to PO quinine to complete 3 days (Africa/South America) or 7 days (Southeast Asia). Also give doxycycline, tetracycline, or clindamycin.

FORMS — Generic only: Gluconate, Tabs ($$$$), extended-release, unscored 324 mg. Sulfate, Tabs ($), scored immediate-release 200, 300 mg, Tabs, extended-release, ($$$$) 300 mg.

NOTES — Proarrhythmic. QRS widening, QT interval prolongation (risk increased by hypokalemia, hypomagnesemia, or bradycardia), hypotension, hypoglycemia. Use cautiously with renal impairment/failure or hepatic disease. Use extreme caution with history of QT prolongation or torsades de pointes. Contraindicated with ziprasidone. Monitor ECG and BP. Drug interactions with some antiarrhythmics, digoxin, phenytoin, phenobarbital, rifampin, verapamil. Do not chew, break, or crush extended-release tabs. Do not use with digitalis toxicity, hypotension, AV/bundle branch block, or myasthenia gravis. Quinidine gluconate 267 mg = quinidine sulfate 200 mg.

MOA — Depresses phase 0 depolarization, prolongs cardiac action potential duration (Class 1A). Unknown antimalarial mechanism.

ADVERSE EFFECTS — Serious: Arrhythmias, syncope (rare), hypersensitivity (rare). Frequent: Diarrhea, hypotension, N/V, cinchonism (disturbed hearing, headaches, visual changes, confusion).

SODIUM BICARBONATE ▶K ♀C ▶? $

ADULT — Cardiac arrest: 1 mEq/kg/dose IV initially, followed by repeat doses up to 0.5 mEq/kg at 10 min intervals during continued arrest. Severe acidosis: 2 to 5 mEq/kg dose IV administered as a 4 to 8 h infusion. Repeat dosing based on lab values.

PEDS — Cardiac arrest, neonates or infants age younger than 2 yo: 1 mEq/kg dose IV slow injection initially, followed by repeat doses up to 1 mEq/kg at 10 min intervals during continued arrest. To avoid intracranial hemorrhage due to hypertonicity, use a 1:1 dilution of 8.4% (1 mEq/mL) sodium bicarbonate and dextrose 5% or use the 4.2% (0.5 mEq/mL) product.

UNAPPROVED ADULT — Prevention of contrast-induced nephropathy: Administer 154 mEq/L soln at 3 mL/kg/h IV for 1 h before contrast, followed by infusion of 1 mL/kg/h for 6 h post procedure. If wt greater than 110 kg then dose based on 110 kg wt.

NOTES — Full correction of bicarbonate deficit should not be attempted during the 1st 24 h. May exacerbate intracellular acidosis.

MOA — Replacement therapy, urinary alkalinization.

ADVERSE EFFECTS — Serious: Hypernatremia (rapid infusion), edema (rapid infusion). Frequent: None.

SOTALOL (*Betapace, Betapace AF, Sotylize, ✷Rylosol*) ▶K ♀B ▶– $$$$

WARNING — Initiate or re-initiate this product in a facility with cardiac resuscitation capacity, continuous ECG, and CrCl monitoring. Do not substitute Betapace for Betapace AF.

ADULT — Ventricular arrhythmia (Sotylize, Betapace): Start 80 mg PO two times per day, Sotylize max 320 mg/day, Betapace max 640 mg/day. A-fib/A-flutter (Sotylize, Betapace AF): Start 80 mg PO two times per day, Sotylize max 160 mg/day, Betapace AF max 640 mg/day. Adjust dose if CrCl <60 mL/min.

PEDS — Not approved in children.

FORMS — Generic/Trade: Tabs, scored 80, 120, 160, 240 mg. Tabs, scored (Betapace AF) 80, 120, 160 mg. Trade only: 5 mg/mL (Sotylize).

NOTES — Proarrhythmic. Caution, higher incidence of torsades de pointes with doses higher than 320 mg/day, in women, or heart failure.

MOA — Prolongs cardiac repolarization (Class III antiarrhythmic properties).

ADVERSE EFFECTS — Serious: Arrhythmias, bradycardia, exacerbation of heart failure.

CARDIOVASCULAR: Antihyperlipidemic Agents—Bile Acid Sequestrants

CHOLESTYRAMINE (*Questran, Questran Light, Prevalite, ✷Olestyr*) ▶Not absorbed ♀C ▶+ $$$$

ADULT — Elevated LDL-C: Start 4 g PO daily to two times per day before meals, usual maintenance 12 to 24 g/day in divided doses two to four times per day before meals, max 24 g/day.

PEDS — Not approved in children.

UNAPPROVED ADULT — Cholestasis-associated pruritus: 4 to 8 g two to three times per day. Diarrhea: 4 to 16 g/day.

UNAPPROVED PEDS — Elevated LDL-C: Start 240 mg/kg/day PO divided three times per day before meals, usual maintenance 8 to 16 g/day divided three times per day.

FORMS — Generic/Trade: Powder for oral susp, 4 g cholestyramine resin/9 g powder (Questran), 4 g cholestyramine resin/5 g powder (Questran Light), 4 g cholestyramine resin/5.5 g powder (Prevalite). Each available in bulk powder and single-dose packets.

NOTES — Administer other drugs at least 2 h before or 4 to 6 h after cholestyramine to avoid decreased absorption of the other agent. May divide up to 6 times per day. Mix powder with 60 to 180 mL of water, milk, fruit juice, or drink. Avoid carbonated liquids for mixing. GI problems common, mainly constipation. May cause elevated triglycerides; do not use when triglycerides exceed 400 mg/dL.

MOA — Binds bile acid in the intestine, preventing their reabsorption.

ADVERSE EFFECTS — Serious: Fecal impaction (rare). Frequent: Constipation.

COLESEVELAM (*Welchol, ✷Lodalis*) ▶Not absorbed ♀B ▶+ $$$$$

ADULT — LDL-C reduction or glycemic control of type 2 DM: 3.75 g once daily or 1.875 g PO two times per day, max 3.75 g/day. Give with meal and 4 to 8 ounces of water, fruit juice, or diet soft drink. 3.75 g is equivalent to 6 tabs; 1.875 g is equivalent to 3 tabs.

PEDS — Hyperlipidemia, 10 yo or older: 3.75 g once daily or 1.875 g PO two times per day, max 3.75 g/day. Give with meal and 4 to 8 ounces of water, fruit juice, or diet soft drink. 3.75 g is equivalent to 6 tabs; 1.875 g is equivalent to 3 tabs.

FORMS — Trade only: Tabs, unscored 625 mg. Powder single-dose packets 3.75 g.

NOTES — Powder packets contain phenylalanine 13.5 mg per colesevelam 1.875 g. GI problems common, mainly constipation. May cause elevation of triglycerides. Do not use with triglycerides greater than 500 mg/dL, or history of bowel obstruction or hypertriglyceridemia-induced pancreatitis. May decrease levels of cyclosporine, glyburide, levothyroxine, oral contraceptives containing ethinyl estradiol and norethindrone, phenytoin, warfarin.

MOA — Binds bile acid in the intestine, preventing their reabsorption.

ADVERSE EFFECTS — Serious: Fecal impaction (rare). Frequent: Constipation, dyspepsia, nausea.

COLESTIPOL (*Colestid, Colestid Flavored*) ▶Not absorbed ♀B ▶+ $$$

ADULT — Elevated LDL-C: Tabs: Start 2 g PO daily to two times per day with full glass of liquid, max 16 g/day. Granules: Start 5 g PO one to two times per

(cont.)

COLESTIPOL (*cont.*)

day, increase by 5 g increments as tolerated at 1- to 2-month intervals, max 30 g/day. Mix granules in at least 90 mL of non-carbonated liquid.

PEDS — Not approved in children.

UNAPPROVED PEDS — 125 to 250 mg/kg/day PO in divided doses two to four times per day, dosing range 10 to 20 g/day.

FORMS — Generic/Trade: Tabs 1 g. Granules for oral susp, 5 g/7.5 g powder. Available in bulk powder and individual packets.

NOTES — Administer other drugs at least 1 h before or 4 to 6 h after colestipol to avoid decreased absorption of the other agent. Swallow tabs whole. GI problems common, mainly constipation. May increase triglycerides; do not use when triglycerides above 400 mg/dL.

MOA — Binds bile acid in the intestine, preventing their reabsorption.

ADVERSE EFFECTS — Serious: Fecal impaction (rare). Frequent: Constipation.

CARDIOVASCULAR: Antihyperlipidemic Agents—Fibrates

NOTE: Contraindicated with active liver disease, gall bladder disease, and/or severe renal impairment (see prescribing information and guidelines for product specific information). Evaluate renal function (SrCr and estimated glomerular filtration rate [eGFR] based on creatinine) at baseline, within 3 months after initiation, q 6 months thereafter. Monitor LFTs (baseline, periodically as indicated). Use in combination with statin therapy is generally discouraged and not proven to reduce risk of CV events beyond stain monotherapy. Increased risk of myopathy and rhabdomyolysis when used with a statin or colchicine. May cause paradoxical decrease in HDL; if severely depressed HDL is detected, discontinue fibrate, monitor HDL until it returns to baseline, and do not restart fibrate. May increase cholesterol excretion into bile, leading to cholelithiasis; if suspected, do gall bladder studies. May increase the effect of warfarin; reduce dose of warfarin; monitor INR. Take either at least 2 h before or 4 h after bile acid sequestrants.

BEZAFIBRATE (✱*Bezalip SR*) ▶K ♀D ▶– $$$

ADULT — Canada only. Hyperlipidemia/hypertriglyceridemia: 200 mg of immediate-release PO two to three times per day, or 400 mg of sustained-release PO q am or q pm with or after food. Reduce dose in renal insufficiency or dialysis. The 400 mg SR tab should not be used if CrCl <60 mL/min or creatinine >1.5 mg/dL.

PEDS — Not approved in children.

FORMS — Canada Trade only: Sustained-release tabs 400 mg.

MOA — Triglyceride reduction — Inhibits lipolysis, decreases FFA uptake, inhibits hepatic VLDL secretion HDL increase – unknown mechanism.

ADVERSE EFFECTS — Serious: Myopathy/rhabdomyolysis (rare), hepatotoxicity (rare), cholelithiasis (rare). Frequent: Epigastric distress, nausea, diarrhea, flatulence.

FENOFIBRATE (*TriCor, Antara, Fenoglide, Lipofen, Triglide, ✱Lipidil Micro, Lipidil Supra, Lipidil EZ*) ▶LK ♀C ▶– $$$

ADULT — Hypertriglyceridemia: Tricor tabs: Start 48 to 145 mg PO daily, max 145 mg/day. Antara: 30 to 90 mg PO daily; max 130 mg daily. Fenoglide: 40 to 120 mg PO daily; max 120 mg daily. Lipofen: 50 to 150 mg PO daily, max 150 mg daily. Triglide: 50 to 160 mg PO daily, max 160 mg daily. Generic tabs: 54 to 160 mg, max 160 mg daily. Generic caps: 67 to 200 mg PO daily, max 200 mg daily. Hypercholesterolemia/mixed dyslipidemia: Tricor tabs: 145 mg PO daily. Antara: 130 mg PO daily. Fenoglide: 120 mg daily. Lipofen: 150 mg daily. Triglide: 160 mg daily. Generic tabs: 160 mg daily. Generic caps: 200 mg PO daily. Renal impairment, elderly: Tricor tabs: Start 48 mg PO daily; Antara: Start 43 mg PO daily; Fenoglide: 40 mg daily/Lipofen: Start 50 mg daily; Triglide: Start 50 mg PO daily; generic tabs: Start 40 to 54 mg PO daily; generic caps 43 mg PO daily.

PEDS — Not approved in children.

FORMS — Generic only: Tabs, unscored 54, 160 mg. Generic caps 67, 134, 200 mg. Generic/Trade: Tabs (TriCor), unscored 48, 145 mg. Caps, (Antara) 30, 90 mg. Tabs (Fenoglide), unscored 40, 120 mg. Trade only: Tabs (Lipofen), unscored 50, 150 mg. Tabs (Triglide), unscored 50, 160 mg.

NOTES — Reduce dose with mild to moderate renal insufficiency (see prescribing information and guidelines for specific information). May consider concomitant therapy with a low- or moderate-intensity statin if the benefits from triglyceride lowering (when 500 mg/dL or more) outweigh the risk of adverse effects. May increase serum creatinine level without changing eGFR. All formulations, except Antara, Tricor, and Triglide, should be taken with food to increase plasma concentrations. Conversion between forms: Generic 200 mg cap with food is equivalent to 145 mg Tricor; Tricor 48 mg and 145 mg replaced micronized Tricor 54 mg and 160 mg. Store Triglide in manufacturer's bottle with desiccant.

MOA — Activates lipoprotein lipase and reduces apoprotein C-III leading to elimination of triglycerides.

ADVERSE EFFECTS — Serious: Tumor (rare), hepatotoxicity (rare), myopathy/rhabdomyolysis (rare), cholelithiasis (rare).

FENOFIBRIC ACID (*Fibricor, Trilipix*) ▶LK ♀C ▶– $$$

ADULT — Hypertriglyceridemia: Fibricor: 35 to 105 mg PO daily, max 105 mg daily. Trilipix: 45 to 135 mg PO daily, max 135 mg daily. Hypercholesterolemia/mixed dyslipidemia: Fibricor: 105 mg PO daily. Trilipix: 135 mg PO daily. Renal impairment: Fibricor: 35 mg PO daily. Trilipix: 45 mg PO daily.

PEDS — Not approved in children.

(cont.)

FENOFIBRIC ACID (*cont.*)

FORMS — Generic/Trade: Caps (Trilipix), delayed-release 45, 135 mg. Trade only: Tabs (Fibricor) 35, 105 mg. Generic only: Tabs 35, 105 mg.

NOTES — May increase serum creatinine level without changing eGFR. Coadministration of immunosuppressant or other potentially nephrotoxic medications may increase the risk of nephrotoxicity.

MOA — Activates lipoprotein lipase and reduces apoprotein C-III leading to elimination of triglycerides.

ADVERSE EFFECTS — Serious: Tumor (rare), hepatotoxicity (rare), myopathy/rhabdomyolysis (rare), cholelithiasis (rare).

GEMFIBROZIL (*Lopid*) ▶LK ♀C ▶? $

ADULT — Hypertriglyceridemia/primary prevention of artery heart disease: 600 mg PO two times per day 30 min before meals.

PEDS — Not approved in children.

FORMS — Generic/Trade: Tabs, scored 600 mg.

NOTES — Contraindicated with dasabuvir, repaglinide, or simvastatin. Do not use with statin; increases risk of myopathy and rhabdomyolysis. Increases exposure to CYP2C8 substrates (eg, dabrafenib, loperamide, montelukast, paclitaxel, pioglitazone, rosiglitazone) and OATP1B1 substrates (eg, atrasentan, bosentan, ezetimibe, glyburide, olmesartan, rifampin, statins, valsartan). Increases warfarin level; reduce warfarin dose; monitor INR. Consider alternative therapy when baseline serum creatinine is greater than 2 mg/dL.

MOA — Activates lipoprotein lipase and reduces apoprotein C-III leading to elimination of triglycerides.

ADVERSE EFFECTS — Serious: Hepatotoxicity (rare), myopathy/rhabdomyolysis (rare), cholelithiasis (rare), angioedema. Frequent: Dyspepsia, abdominal pain, nausea, diarrhea, headache.

CARDIOVASCULAR: Antihyperlipidemic Agents—HMG-CoA Reductase Inhibitors ("Statins") and combinations

NOTE: Each statin has restricted maximum doses that are lower than typical maximum doses when used with certain interacting medications; see prescribing information for complete information. Consider patient characteristics that may modify the decision to use higher-intensity statin therapy, including history of hemorrhagic stroke or Asian descent. Muscle issues: Evaluate muscle symptoms before initiating statin therapy and at each follow-up visit. Measure creatinine kinase before starting statin, if patient at risk for adverse muscle events. Risk of muscle issues increases with advanced age (65 yo or older), female gender, uncontrolled hypothyroidism, low vitamin D level, renal impairment, higher statin doses, history of muscle disorders, and concomitant use of certain medicines (eg, fibrates, niacin 1 gram or more, colchicine, or ranolazine). Teach patients to report promptly unexplained muscle pain, tenderness, or weakness; rule out common causes; discontinue if myopathy diagnosed or suspected. Obtain creatine kinase, TSH, vitamin D level when patient complains of muscle soreness, tenderness, weakness, or pain. With tolerable muscle complaints or asymptomatic creatine kinase increase < 10 times upper limit of normal, continue statin at same or reduced dose; use symptoms to guide continuing/discontinuing statin. With intolerable muscle symptoms with/without creatine kinase elevation, discontinue statin; when asymptomatic, may restart same/different statin at same/lower dose. With rhabdomyolysis, discontinue statin, provide IV hydration; weigh risk/benefit of statin therapy when recovered. Rare reports of immune-mediated necrotizing myopathy. Hepatotoxicity: Rare. Monitor ALT before initiating statin therapy and as clinically indicated thereafter. May initiate, continue, or increase dose of statin with modest LFT elevation (less than 3 times upper limit of normal). Repeat LFTs and rule out other causes with isolated, asymptomatic LFT elevation less than 3 times upper limit of normal. Consider continuing vs. discontinuing statin or reducing statin dose. Discontinue statin with persistent ALT elevations more than 3 times the upper limit of normal or objective evidence of liver injury; seek cause; consider referral to gastroenterologist or hepatologist. Diabetes: Measure A1c before starting statin, if diabetes status unknown. Statins may increase the risk of hyperglycemia and type 2 diabetes in patients with risk factors for diabetes. In 100 individuals treated with statin therapy for 1 year, the risk of diabetes is ~0.1 and ~0.3 excess cases with a moderate-intensity and high-intensity statin respectively. Benefits outweighs risks. Cognition: The 2013 ACC/AHA cholesterol guidelines expert panel did not find evidence that statins adversely affect cognition. If patient complains of confusion or memory impairment while on statin therapy, consider all possible causes, including other drugs (eg, sleep aids, analgesics, OTC antihistamines) and medical conditions (eg, depression, anxiety, sleep apnea) that affect memory.

ATORVASTATIN (*Lipitor*) ▶L ♀X ▶– $

ADULT — Hyperlipidemia/prevention of cardiovascular events: Start 10 mg PO daily, 40 mg daily for LDL-C reduction greater than 45%, increase at intervals of 4 weeks or more to a max of 80 mg/day. Do not give with cyclosporine, tipranavir + ritonavir. Use with caution and lowest dose necessary with lopinavir + ritonavir. Do not exceed 20 mg/day when given with clarithromycin, itraconazole, other protease inhibitors (saquinavir + ritonavir, darunavir + ritonavir, fosamprenavir, or fosamprenavir +

ritonavir). Do not exceed 40 mg/day when given with boceprevir or nelfinavir.

PEDS — Hyperlipidemia, 10 yo or older: Start 10 mg daily, max 20 mg/day. See prescribing information for more information.

FORMS — Generic/Trade: Tabs, unscored 10, 20, 40, 80 mg.

NOTES — Metabolized by CYP3A4 enzyme system. May give any time of day. May increase digoxin level. Take concomitant rifampin at the same time with atorvastatin to avoid reduction of atorvastatin

(cont.)

ATORVASTATIN (*cont.*)

level. May increase levels or norethindrone and ethinyl estradiol. Patients with recent CVA/TIA and no CHD who received atorvastatin 80 mg/day had a higher incidence of hemorrhagic stroke and non-fatal hemorrhagic stroke than placebo group in the post hoc analysis of the SPARCL trial.

MOA — Inhibits 3-hydroxy-3-methyl-glutaryl-coenzyme A (HMG-CoA) reductase which converts HMG-CoA to mevalonate in cholesterol biosynthesis.

ADVERSE EFFECTS — Serious: Hepatotoxicity (rare), myopathy/rhabdomyolysis (rare). Frequent: Headache, dyspepsia.

CADUET (amlodipine + atorvastatin) ▶L ♀X ▶– $$$$$

ADULT — Simultaneous treatment of HTN and hypercholesterolemia: Establish dose using component drugs first. See component drug for other dose restrictions. Dosing interval: Daily.

PEDS — Not approved in children.

FORMS — Generic/Trade: Tabs, 2.5/10, 2.5/20, 2.5/40, 5/10, 5/20, 5/40, 5/80, 10/10, 10/20, 10/40, 10/80 mg.

MOA — See component drugs.

FLUVASTATIN (*Lescol, Lescol XL*) ▶L ♀X ▶– $$$$

ADULT — Hyperlipidemia: Start 20 mg PO at bedtime for LDL-C reduction of less than 25%, 40 to 80 mg at bedtime for LDL-C reduction of 25% or more, max 80 mg/day, give 80 mg daily (Lescol XL) or 40 mg two times per day. Prevention of cardiac events post-percutaneous coronary intervention: 80 mg of extended-release PO daily, max 80 mg daily. Do not exceed 20 mg/day when given with cyclosporine or fluconazole.

PEDS — Hyperlipidemia: Start 20 mg PO at bedtime, max 80 mg daily (XL) or divided two times per day. See prescribing information for more information.

FORMS — Generic/Trade: Caps 20, 40 mg. Trade only: Tabs, extended-release, unscored 80 mg.

NOTES — Mainly metabolized by the CYP2C9, so less potential for drug interactions. Monitor blood sugar levels when given with glyburide and the dose of fluvastatin is changed. Monitor phenytoin levels when given with phenytoin and fluvastatin is initiated or the dose is changed. Monitor INR when given with warfarin and fluvastatin is initiated, discontinued, or the dose is changed.

MOA — Inhibits 3-hydroxy-3-methyl-glutaryl-coenzyme A (HMG-CoA) reductase which converts HMG-CoA to mevalonate in cholesterol biosynthesis.

ADVERSE EFFECTS — Serious: Hepatotoxicity (rare), myopathy/rhabdomyolysis (rare). Frequent: Headache, dyspepsia.

LIPTRUZET (ezetimibe + atorvastatin) ▶L – ♀X ▶– $$$$

ADULT — Hyperlipidemia: Start 10/10 or 10/20 mg PO daily, max 10/80 mg/day. See component drug for other dose restrictions.

PEDS — Not approved in children.

FORMS — Trade only: Tabs, unscored ezetimibe/atorvastatin 10/10, 10/20, 10/40, 10/80 mg.

NOTES — Take either at least 2 h before or 4 h after bile acid sequestrants.

MOA — See compenent drugs.

ADVERSE EFFECTS — See component drugs.

LOVASTATIN (*Altoprev*) ▶L ♀X ▶– $$$

ADULT — Hyperlipidemia/prevention of cardiovascular events: Start 20 mg PO daily with the evening meal, increase at intervals of 4 weeks or more to max 80 mg/day (daily or divided two times per day). Altoprev dosed daily with max dose 60 mg/day. Do not use with clarithromycin, cobicistat-containing products, cyclosporine, erythromycin, gemfibrozil, grapefruit juice, HIV protease inhibitors, itraconazole, ketoconazole, nefazodone, posaconazole, telithromycin, or voriconazole; increases risk of myopathy. Do not exceed 20 mg/day when used with danazol, diltiazem, dronedarone, verapamil, or CrCl <30 mL/min. Do not exceed 40 mg/day when used with amiodarone.

PEDS — Hyperlipidemia, 10 yo or older: Start 10 mg PO q pm, max 40 mg/day. See prescribing information for more information.

FORMS — Generic: Tabs, unscored 10, 20, 40 mg. Trade only: Tabs, extended-release (Altoprev) 20, 40, 60 mg.

NOTES — Metabolized by CYP3A4 enzyme system. The brand name product (Mevacor) is no longer available.

MOA — Inhibits 3-hydroxy-3-methyl-glutaryl-coenzyme A (HMG-CoA) reductase which converts HMG-CoA to mevalonate in cholesterol biosynthesis.

ADVERSE EFFECTS — Serious: Hepatotoxicity (rare), myopathy/rhabdomyolysis (rare). Frequent: Headache, dyspepsia.

PITAVASTATIN (*Livalo*) ▶L – ♀X ▶– $$$$

ADULT — Hyperlipidemia: Start 2 mg PO at bedtime, max 4 mg daily. CrCl 15 to 59 mL/min or end-stage renal disease receiving hemodialysis: Max start 1 mg PO daily, max 2 mg daily. Do not use with cyclosporine. Do not exceed 1 mg/day when given with erythromycin. Do not exceed 2 mg/day when given with rifampin.

PEDS — Not approved in children.

FORMS — Trade only: Tabs 1, 2, 4 mg.

NOTES — Mainly metabolized by CYP2C9.

MOA — Inhibits 3-hydroxy-3-methyl-glutaryl-coenzyme A (HMG-CoA) reductase which converts HMG-CoA to mevalonate in cholesterol biosynthesis.

ADVERSE EFFECTS — Serious: Hepatotoxicity (rare), myopathy/rhabdomyolysis (rare). Frequent: Constipation, diarrhea, myalgia.

PRAVASTATIN (*Pravachol*) ▶L ♀X/X/X; Contraindicated during pregnancy. ▶ Do not breastfeed while taking this medication. $$$

ADULT — Hyperlipidemia/prevention of cardiovascular events: Start 40 mg PO daily, increase at intervals of 4 weeks or more to max 80 mg/day. Renal or hepatic impairment: Start 10 mg PO daily. Do not exceed 20 mg/day when given with cyclosporine. Do not exceed 40 mg/day when given with clarithromycin.

(cont.)

PRAVASTATIN (*cont.*)

PEDS — Hyperlipidemia, 8 to 13 yo: 20 mg PO daily; 14 to 18 yo: 40 mg PO daily. See prescribing information for more information.

FORMS — Generic/Trade: Tabs, unscored 20, 40, 80 mg. Generic: Tabs, unscored 10 mg.

NOTES — Not metabolized substantially by the CYP isoenzyme system, less potential for drug interactions.

MOA — Inhibits 3-hydroxy-3-methyl-glutaryl-coenzyme A (HMG-CoA) reductase, which converts HMG-CoA to mevalonate in cholesterol biosynthesis.

ADVERSE EFFECTS — Serious: Hepatotoxicity (rare), myopathy/rhabdomyolysis (rare). Frequent: Headache, dyspepsia.

ROSUVASTATIN (*Crestor*) ▶L ♀X ▶– $$$$$

ADULT — Hyperlipidemia/slow progression of atherosclerosis/primary prevention of cardiovascular disease: Start 10 to 20 mg daily, may adjust dose after 2 to 4 weeks, max 40 mg/day. Do not start with 40 mg; use 40 mg only when treatment goal not achieved with 20 mg/day. Renal impairment (CrCl <30 mL/min and not on hemodialysis): Start 5 mg PO daily, max 10 mg/day. Asians: Start 5 mg PO daily. When given with atazanavir with or without ritonavir, lopinavir with ritonavir, or simeprevir, do not exceed 10 mg/day. When given with cyclosporine, do not exceed 5 mg/day. Avoid using with gemfibrozil; if used concomitantly, do not exceed 10 mg/day. When given with colchicine, do not exceed 5 mg/day.

PEDS — Heterozygous familial hypercholesterolemia, 8 to 9 yo: 5 to 10 mg PO daily. Heterozygous familial hypercholesterolemia, 10 yo or older: 5 to 20 mg PO daily. Homozygous familial hypercholesterolemia, 7 to 17 yo: 20 mg PO daily. Canada only: May use with age older than 8 yo with homozygous familial hypercholesterolemia.

FORMS — Generic/Trade only: Tabs, unscored 5, 10, 20, 40 mg.

NOTES — Partially metabolized by CYP2C9 enzyme system. Potentiates effects of warfarin; monitor INR. Give aluminum- and magnesium-containing antacids more than 2 h after rosuvastatin. Proteinuria, with unknown clinical significance, reported with 40 mg/day; consider dose reduction when using 40 mg/day with unexplained persistent proteinuria.

MOA — Inhibits 3-hydroxy-3-methyl-glutaryl-coenzyme A (HMG-CoA) reductase which converts HMG-CoA to mevalonate in cholesterol biosynthesis.

ADVERSE EFFECTS — Serious: Hepatotoxicity (rare), myopathy/rhabdomyolysis (rare). Frequent: Myalgia, constipation, nausea, asthenia, abdominal pain, proteinuria (transient), hematuria (transient).

SIMVASTATIN (*Zocor*) ▶L ♀X ▶– $

ADULT — Do not initiate therapy with or titrate to 80 mg/day; only use 80 mg/day in patients who have taken this dose for more than 12 months without evidence of muscle toxicity. Hyperlipidemia: Start 10 to 20 mg PO q pm, max 40 mg/day. Reduce cardiovascular mortality/events in high risk for coronary heart disease event: Start 40 mg PO q pm, max 40 mg/day. Severe renal impairment: Start 5 mg/day, closely monitor. Chinese patients: Do not exceed 20 mg/day with niacin 1 g or more daily. Do not use with clarithromycin, cobicistat-containing products, cyclosporine, danazol, erythromycin, gemfibrozil, grapefruit juice, HIV protease inhibitors, itraconazole, ketoconazole, nefazodone, posaconazole, strong CYP3A4 inhibitors, telithromycin, voriconazole; increases risk of myopathy. Do not exceed 10 mg/day when used with diltiazem, dronedarone, or verapamil. Do not exceed 20 mg/day when used with amiodarone, amlodipine, or ranolazine. Do not exceed 20 mg/day when used with lomitapide; if patient has been on simvastatin 80 mg/day for at least 1 year without muscle toxicity, then do not exceed 40 mg/day when used with lomitapide.

PEDS — Hyperlipidemia, 10 yo or older: Start 10 mg PO q pm, max 40 mg/day. See prescribing information for more information.

FORMS — Generic/Trade: Tabs, unscored 5, 10, 20, 40, 80 mg.

NOTES — May increase INR when given with warfarin.

MOA — Inhibits 3-hydroxy-3-methyl-glutaryl-coenzyme A (HMG-CoA) reductase which converts HMG-CoA to mevalonate in cholesterol biosynthesis.

ADVERSE EFFECTS — Serious: Hepatotoxicity, myopathy/rhabdomyolysis (rare). Frequent: Headache, dyspepsia.

VYTORIN (ezetimibe + simvastatin) ▶L ♀X ▶– $$$$

ADULT — Hyperlipidemia: Start 10/10 or 10/20 mg PO q pm, max 10/40 mg/day. Restrict the use of the 10/80 mg dose to patients who have taken it at least 12 months without muscle toxicity. See simvastatin monograph for other dose restrictions.

PEDS — Not approved in children.

UNAPPROVED ADULT — Reduce risk of CV events in patients with CKD, not on dialysis: 10/20 mg/day.

FORMS — Trade only: Tabs, unscored ezetimibe/simvastatin 10/10, 10/20, 10/40, 10/80 mg.

NOTES — Give at least 2 h before or 4 h after bile acid sequestrant. May increase INR when given with warfarin.

MOA — See component drugs.

ADVERSE EFFECTS — See component drugs.

CARDIOVASCULAR: Antihyperlipidemic Agents—Omega Fatty Acids

NOTE: FDA-approved fish oil. Swallow whole; do not crush, break, or chew. May prolong bleeding time, may potentiate warfarin. Monitor AST/ALT if hepatic impairment. Use caution in patients with known hypersensitivity to fish and/or shellfish.

ICOSAPENT ETHYL (*Vascepa*) ▶L ♀C ▶? $$$$$
ADULT — Adjunct to diet to reduce high triglycerides (500 mg/dL or above): 4 caps PO daily or divided two times per day. Contains EPA.
PEDS — Not approved in children.
FORMS — Trade only: Caps 1 g.
MOA — May reduce hepatic VLDL-TG synthesis and/or secretion; enhances TG clearance from circulating VLDL particles.
ADVERSE EFFECTS — Serious: Hypersensitivity. Frequent: Arthralgia.

OMEGA-3-ACID ETHYL ESTERS (*Omtryg, Lovaza*) ▶L ♀C ▶? $$$$$
ADULT — Adjunct to diet to reduce high triglycerides (500 mg/dL or above): 4 caps PO daily or divided two times per day. Contains EPA + DHA.
PEDS — Not approved in children.
FORMS — Generic/Trade (Lovaza): Caps 1 g. Trade only (Omtryg): Caps 1.2 g.

MOA — May reduce hepatic VLDL-TG synthesis and/or secretion; enhances TG clearance from circulating VLDL particles.
ADVERSE EFFECTS — Serious: Hypersensitivity. Frequent: Belching, dyspepsia, taste changes.

OMEGA-3-CARBOXYLIC ACIDS (*Epanova*) ▶L ♀C ▶? $$$$$
ADULT — Adjunct to diet to reduce high triglycerides (500 mg/dL or above): 2 or 4 caps PO daily. Contains EPA + DHA.
PEDS — Not approved in children.
FORMS — Trade only: Caps 1 g.
MOA — May reduce hepatic VLDL-TG synthesis and/or secretion; enhances TG clearance from circulating VLDL particles.
ADVERSE EFFECTS — Serious: Hypersensitivity. Frequent: abdominal pain, belching, diarrhea, nausea.

CARDIOVASCULAR: Antihyperlipidemic Agents—Other

ALIROCUMAB (*Praluent*) ▶N/A ♀?/?/?; Consider possible risks to fetus before prescribing to pregnant women. ▶ No information available. $$$$$
ADULT — Reduce LDL-C as adjunct to diet and maximally tolerated statin with heterozygous familial hypercholesterolemia or clinical atherosclerotic cardiovascular disease: Start 75 mg SC q 2 weeks; max 150 mg q 2 weeks.
PEDS — Not approved in children.
NOTES — Human monoclonal antibody. Give in abdomen, upper arm, or thigh. Store in a refrigerator at 36-46° F; can be out of refrigeration for no more than 24 h. The prefilled syringe or pen should warm to room temperature for 30-40 min before use. Tell patient that it may take up to 20 sec to inject full dose.
MOA — Increases the number of low-density lipoprotein receptors (LDLR) available to clear LDL by inhibiting the binding of PCSK9 to LDLR.
ADVERSE EFFECTS — Serious: Hypersensitivity reactions. Frequent: Influenza, injection site reactions, nasopharyngitis.

EVOLOCUMAB (*Repatha*) ▶N/A ♀?/?/?; Consider possible risks to fetus before prescribing to pregnant women. ▶ No information available. $$$$$
ADULT — Reduce LDL-C as adjunct to diet and maximally tolerated statin with heterozygous familial hypercholesterolemia or clinical atherosclerotic cardiovascular disease: 140 mg SC every 2 weeks or 420 mg SQ once monthly. Reduce LDL-C as adjunct to diet and other lipid lowering therapies (eg, statins, ezetimibe, LDL apheresis) with homozygous familial hypercholesterolemia: 420 mg SQ once monthly.
PEDS — Not approved in children.
FORMS — Trade only: Single prefilled syringe 140 mg/mL. Multi Dose (x2 Sureclick) prefilled syringe 140 mg/mL. Monthly injection (Pushtronex with on body infusion device) 420 mg/3.5 mL.

NOTES — Human monoclonal antibody. Give in abdomen, upper arm, or thigh. Ideally store in a refrigerator at 36-46° F; can be kept at room temperature (77° F) for up to 30 days. Tell patient that it may take up to 15 seconds to inject full dose.
MOA — Increases the number of low-density lipoprotein receptors (LDLR) available to clear LDL by inhibiting the binding of PCSK9 to LDLR.
ADVERSE EFFECTS — Serious: Hypersensitivity reactions. Frequent: Influenza, injection site reactions, nasopharyngitis.

EZETIMIBE (*Zetia, ✷Ezetrol*) ▶L ♀C ▶? $$$$
WARNING — May increase cyclosporine levels.
ADULT — Hyperlipidemia: 10 mg PO daily alone or in combination with statin or fenofibrate.
PEDS — Not approved in children.
UNAPPROVED PEDS — Hyperlipidemia, 10 yo or older: 10 mg PO daily coadministered with simvastatin.
FORMS — Trade only: Tabs, unscored 10 mg.
NOTES — Take either at least 2 h before or 4 h after bile acid sequestrants. Monitor cyclosporine levels (may increase). When used with statin, monitor LFTs before initiating and as clinically indicated thereafter. Do not use with fibrate other than fenofibrate. Concomitant fenofibrate increases ezetimibe level and may increase risk of cholelithiasis.
MOA — Selectively inhibits small intestine cholesterol absorption.
ADVERSE EFFECTS — Serious: Anaphylaxis, angioedema, cholelithiasis, cholecystitis, myopathy/rhabdomyolysis (rare), pancreatitis, thrombocytopenia. Frequent: Arthralgia, back pain, diarrhea, rash.

LOMITAPIDE (*Juxtapid*) ▶L – ♀X/X/XR; Neonatal harm: Potential teratogen. ▶ Do not breastfeed while taking lomitapide. $$$$$
WARNING — May elevate liver transaminases. Measure ALT, AST, alkaline phosphatase, total bilirubin before starting therapy; measure ALT and

(cont.)

LOMITAPIDE (*cont.*)

AST regularly as recommended. Adjust dose if ALT or AST 3 or more times the upper limit of normal. Discontinue with clinically significant liver toxicity. Increases hepatic steatosis, which may be a risk factor for progressive liver disease, including steatohepatitis and cirrhosis. Only available through restricted Juxtapid REMS program.

ADULT — Only approved in patients with homozygous familial hypercholesterolemia: Start 5 mg PO once daily. May increase as tolerated to 10 mg daily after at least 2 weeks; then to 20 mg daily after at least 4 weeks; then to 40 mg daily after at least 4 weeks; max 60 mg/day. End-stage renal disease on dialysis or with baseline mild hepatic impairment: Do not exceed 40 mg daily. Before initiating therapy, measure ALT, AST, alkaline phosphatase, and total bilirubin; obtain a negative pregnancy test in women of childbearing age and use reliable contraception while taking lomitapide; initiate low-fat diet with less than 20% of energy from fat. Swallow whole; take with water, without food at least 2 h after evening meal. Depletes absorption of fat-soluble vitamins/fatty acids; patient should take daily vitamin E 400 international units and at least linoleic acid 200 mg, alpha-linolenic acid (ALA) 210 mg, eicosapentaenoic acid (EPA) 110 mg, and docosahexaenoic acid (DHA) 80 mg. Do not use with strong or moderate CYP3A4 inhibitors, moderate or severe hepatic impairment, active liver disease, or unexplained persistent abnormal liver function tests. Decrease the lomitapide dose by half when used concomitantly with a weak CYP3A4 inhibitor; do not exceed 30 mg daily of lomitapide with concomitant weak CYP3A4 inhibitors (eg, alprazolam, amiodarone, amlodipine, atorvastatin, bicalutamide, cilostazol, cimetidine, cyclosporine, fluoxetine, fluvoxamine, ginkgo, goldenseal, isoniazid, lapatinib, nilotinib, pazopanib, ranitidine, ranolazine, ticagrelor, zileuton), or 40 mg daily of lomitapide with oral contraceptives. May increase warfarin levels; monitor INR. May increase levels of simvastatin, lovastatin, P-glycoprotein substrates; limit doses of these when used concomitantly with lomitapide. Give bile acid sequestrants at least 4 h before or after lomitapide.

PEDS — Not approved in children.

FORMS — Trade only: Caps 5, 10, 20, 30, 40, 60 mg.

MOA — Decreases the synthesis of chylomicrons and VLDL by inhibiting microsomal triglyceride transfer protein.

ADVERSE EFFECTS — Serious: Diarrhea-related complications (eg volume depletion), hepatotoxicity. Frequent: Abdominal pain, diarrhea, dyspepsia, nausea, vomiting.

MIPOMERSEN (*Kynamro*) ▶tissues ♀–B ▮? $$$$$

WARNING — May elevate liver transaminases. Measure ALT, AST, alkaline phosphatase, total bilirubin before starting therapy; measure ALT and AST regularly as recommended. Hold dose if ALT or AST 3 or more times the upper limit of normal. Discontinue with clinically significant liver toxicity. Increases hepatic steatosis, which may be a risk factor for progressive liver disease, including steatohepatitis and cirrhosis. Only available through restricted Kynamro REMS program.

ADULT — Only approved in patients with homozygous familial hypercholesterolemia: 200 mg subcutaneously once weekly. Before initiating therapy, measure ALT, AST, alkaline phosphatase, and total bilirubin. Do not use as adjunct to LDL apheresis. Do not use with moderate or severe hepatic impairment, active liver disease, or unexplained persistent abnormal liver function tests.

PEDS — Not approved in children.

FORMS — Trade only: Single-use vial or prefilled syringe containing 1 mL of a 200 mg/mL solution.

MOA — Inhibits apolipoprotein B-100 synthesis.

ADVERSE EFFECTS — Serious: Hepatotoxicity. Frequent: flu-like symptoms, headache, injection site reactions, nausea.

CARDIOVASCULAR: Antihypertensive Combinations

ANTIHYPERTENSIVE COMBINATIONS

BY TYPE:	
ACEI + Diuretic	*Accuretic, Capozide,✤ Inhibace Plus, Lotensin HCT, Monopril HCT, Prinzide, Uniretic, Vaseretic, Zestoretic*
ACEI + CCB	*Lotrel, Prestalia, Tarka*
ARB + Beta-blocker	*Byvalson*
ARB + CCB	*Azor, Exforge, Twynsta*
ARB + Diuretic	*Atacand HCT,✤ Atacand Plus, Avalide, Benicar HCT, Diovan HCT, Edarbyclor, Hyzaar, Micardis HCT,✤ Micardis Plus, Teveten HCT*

(cont.)

ANTIHYPERTENSIVE COMBINATIONS (*continued*)

BY TYPE:	
ARB + CCB + Diuretic	*Exforge HCT, Tribenzor*
Beta-blocker + Diuretic	*Corzide, Dutoprol, Inderide, Lopressor HCT, Tenoretic, Ziac*
CCB + Statin	*Caduet*
Direct Renin Inhibitor + Diuretic	♣ *Rasilez HCT, Tekturna HCT*
Diuretic combinations	*Aldactazide, Dyazide, Maxzide,* ♣ *Moduret, Moduretic,* ♣ *Triazide*
Diuretic + Miscellaneous Antihypertensive	*Aldoril, Clorpres, Minizide*

ACEI = ACE Inhibitor ARB = angiotensin receptor blocker CCB = calcium channel blocker **BY NAME:** ***Accuretic*** **(quinapril + HCTZ)**: Generic/Trade: Tabs, scored 10/12.5, 20/12.5, unscored 20/25 mg. ***Aldactazide*** **(spironolactone + HCTZ)**: Generic/Trade: Tabs, unscored 25/25, scored 50/50 mg. **Aldoril (methyldopa + HCTZ)**: Generic: Tabs, unscored 250/15, 250/25 mg. ***Atacand*** **HCT (candesartan + HCTZ,** ♣ ***Atacand Plus*****)**: Generic/Trade: Tab, unscored 16/12.5, 32/12.5, 32/25 mg. ***Avalide*** **(irbesartan + HCTZ)**: Generic/Trade: Tabs, unscored 150/12.5, 300/12.5 mg. ***Azor*** **(amlodipine + olmesartan)**: Trade only: Tabs, unscored 5/20, 5/40, 10/20, 10/40 mg. ***Benicar HCT*** **(olmesartan + HCTZ)**: Trade only: Tabs, unscored 20/12.5, 40/12.5, 40/25 mg. ***Byvalson (valsartan + nebivolol)***: Trade only: Tabs, unscored 80/5 mg. ***Caduet*** **(amlodipine + atorvastatin)**: Generic/Trade: 2.5/10, 2.5/20, 2.5/40, 5/10, 5/20, 5/40, 5/80, 10/10, 10/20, 10/40, 10/80 mg. ***Capozide*** **(captopril + HCTZ)**: Generic only: Tabs, scored 25/15, 25/25, 50/15, 50/25 mg. ***Clorpres*** **(clonidine + chlorthalidone)**: Trade only: Tabs, scored 0.1/15, 0.2/15, 0.3/15 mg. ***Corzide*** **(nadolol + bendroflumethiazide)**: Generic/Trade: Tabs 40/5, 80/5 mg. ***Diovan*** **HCT (valsartan + HCTZ)**: Generic/Trade: Tabs, unscored 80/12.5, 160/12.5, 160/25, 320/12.5, 320/25 mg. ***Dutoprol*** **(metoprolol succinate + HCTZ)**: Trade only: Tabs, unscored 25/12.5, 50/12.5, 100/12.5 mg. ***Dyazide*** **(triamterene + HCTZ)**: Generic/Trade: Caps, (Dyazide) 37.5/25, (generic only) 50/25 mg. ***Edarbyclor*** **(azilsartan + chlorthalidone)**: Trade only: Tabs, unscored 40/12.5, 40/25 mg. ***Exforge*** **(amlodipine + valsartan)**: Generic/Trade only: Tabs, unscored 5/160, 5/320, 10/160, 10/320 mg. ***Exforge HCT*** **(amlodipine + valsartan + HCTZ)**: Generic/Trade only: Tabs, unscored 5/160/12.5, 5/160/25, 10/160/12.5, 10/160/25, 10/320/25 mg. ***Hyzaar*** **(losartan + HCTZ)**: Generic/Trade: Tabs, unscored 50/12.5, 100/12.5, 100/25 mg. ***Inderide*** **(propranolol + HCTZ)**: Generic only: Tabs, scored 40/25, 80/25 mg. ♣ ***Inhibace Plus*** **(cilazapril + HCTZ)**: Trade only: Tabs, scored 5/12.5 mg. ***Lopressor HCT*** **(metoprolol tartrate + HCTZ)**: Generic/Trade: Tabs, scored 50/25, 100/25 mg. Generic: Tabs, scored 100/50 mg. ***Lotensin HCT*** **(benazepril + HCTZ)**: Generic/ Trade: Tabs, scored 5/6.25, 10/12.5, 20/12.5, 20/25 mg. ***Lotrel*** **(amlodipine + benazepril)**: Generic/Trade: Cap, 2.5/10, 5/10, 5/20, 10/20 mg, 5/40, 10/40 mg. ***Maxzide*** **(triamterene + HCTZ,** ♣ **Triazide)**: Generic/Trade: Tabs, scored (Maxzide-25) 37.5/25 (Maxzide) 75/50 mg. ***Micardis HCT*** **(telmisartan + HCTZ,** ♣ ***Micardis Plus*****)**: Generic/Trade: Tabs, unscored 40/12.5, 80/12.5, 80/25 mg. ***Minizide*** **(prazosin + polythiazide)**: Trade only: Caps, 1/0.5, 2/0.5, 5/0.5 mg. ***Moduretic*** **(amiloride + HCTZ,** ♣ ***Moduret*****)**: Generic only: Tabs, scored 5/50 mg. ***Monopril HCT*** **(fosinopril + HCTZ)**: Generic only: Tabs, unscored 10/12.5, scored 20/12.5 mg. ***Prestalia (perindopril + amlodipine)***: Trade: Tabs, unscored 3.5/2.5, 7.5/5 14/10 mg. ***Prinzide*** **(lisinopril + HCTZ)**: Generic/Trade: Tabs, unscored 10/12.5, 20/12.5, 20/25 mg. ***Tarka*** **(trandolapril + verapamil)**: Trade only: Tabs, unscored 2/180, 1/240, 2/240, 4/240 mg. ***Tekturna HCT*** **(aliskiren + HCTZ,** ♣ **Rasilez HCT)**: Trade only: Tabs, unscored 150/12.5, 150/25, 300/12.5, 300/25 mg. ***Tenoretic*** **(atenolol + chlorthalidone)**: Generic/Trade: Tabs, scored 50/25, unscored 100/25 mg. ***Teveten HCT*** **(eprosartan + HCTZ)**: Trade only: Tabs, unscored 600/12.5, 600/25 mg. ***Tribenzor*** **(amlodipine + olmesartan + HCTZ)**: Trade only: Tabs, unscored 5/20/12.5, 5/40/12.5, 5/40/25,10/40/12.5,10/40/25 mg. ***Twynsta*** **(amlodipine + telmisartan)**: Generic/Trade: Tabs,unscored 5/40, 5/80, 10/40, 10/80 mg. ***Uniretic*** **(moexipril + HCTZ)**: Generic/ Trade: Tabs, cored15/12.5, 15/25 mg. Generic: Tabs, scored 7.5/12.5. ***Vaseretic*** **(enalapril + HCTZ)**: Generic/Trade:Tabs, unscored 5/12.5, 10/25 mg. ***Zestoretic*** **(lisinopril HCTZ)**: Generic/Trade: Tabs, unscored10/12.5, 20/12.5, 20/25 mg. ***Ziac*** **(bisoprolol + HCTZ)**: Generic/Trade: Tabs, unscored 2.5/6.25, 5/6.25, 10/6.25 mg.

NOTE: In general, establish dose using component drugs first. See component drugs for metabolism, pregnancy, and lactation.

ACCURETIC **(quinapril + hydrochlorothiazide)** ▶See component drugs ♀See component drugs ◗See component drugs $$

WARNING — Do not use in pregnancy.
ADULT — HTN: Dosing interval: Daily.
PEDS — Not approved in children.
FORMS — Generic/Trade: Tabs, scored 10/12.5, 20/12.5, unscored 20/25 mg.
MOA — See component drugs.

ALDACTAZIDE **(spironolactone + hydrochlorothiazide)** ▶See component drugs ♀See component drugs ◗See component drugs $$

WARNING — Spironolactone is a tumorigen in rats. Use only for approved indications and only if necessary. Should not be used for initial therapy of edema or HTN; these conditions require individualized dosing. Treatment of HTN and edema should be reevaluated as patient's condition warrants.

(cont.)

ALDACTAZIDE (*cont.*)
ADULT — HTN: Dosing interval: Daily to two times per day.
PEDS — Not approved in children.
FORMS — Generic/Trade: Tabs, unscored 25/25 mg. Trade only: Tabs, scored 50/50 mg.
MOA — See component drugs.

ALDORIL (**methyldopa + hydrochlorothiazide**) ▶See component drugs ♀See component drugs ▶See component drugs $$
WARNING — Titrate component drugs first to avoid hypotension.
ADULT — HTN: Dosing interval: two times per day.
PEDS — Not approved in children.
FORMS — Generic only: Tabs, unscored, 250/15, 250/25 mg.
NOTES — The brand name product (Aldoril) is no longer available.
MOA — See component drugs.

ATACAND HCT (**candesartan + hydrochlorothiazide,** ✱ **Atacand Plus**) ▶See component drugs ♀See component drugs ▶See component drugs $$$$
WARNING — Do not use in pregnancy.
ADULT — HTN: Dosing interval: Daily.
PEDS — Not approved in children.
FORMS — Generic/Trade: Tabs, unscored 16/12.5, 32/12.5, 32/25 mg.
MOA — See component drugs.

AVALIDE (**irbesartan + hydrochlorothiazide**) ▶See component drugs ♀See component drugs ▶See component drugs $
WARNING — Do not use in pregnancy.
ADULT — HTN, initial therapy for patients needing multiple medications: Start 150/12.5 mg PO daily, may increase after 1 to 2 weeks, max 300/25 mg daily.
PEDS — Not approved in children.
FORMS — Generic/Trade: Tabs, unscored 150/12.5, 300/12.5 mg.
MOA — See component drugs.

AZOR (**amlodipine + olmesartan**) ▶See component drugs ♀See component drugs ▶See component drugs $$$
WARNING — Do not use in pregnancy.
ADULT — HTN, initial therapy for patients needing multiple medications: Start 5/20 mg PO daily, may increase after 1 to 2 weeks, max 10/40 daily.
PEDS — Not approved in children.
FORMS — Trade only: Tabs, unscored 5/20, 5/40, 10/20, 10/40 mg.
MOA — See component drugs.

BENICAR HCT (**olmesartan + hydrochlorothiazide,** ✱ **Olmetec Plus**) ▶See component drugs ♀See component drugs ▶See component drugs $$$$
WARNING — Do not use in pregnancy.
ADULT — HTN: Dosing interval: Daily.
PEDS — Not approved in children.
FORMS — Trade only: Tabs, unscored 20/12.5, 40/12.5, 40/25 mg.
MOA — See component drugs.

BYVALSON (**valsartan + nebivolol**) ▶♀
WARNING — Do not use in pregnancy.
ADULT — HTN: Dosing interval: Daily.
PEDS — Not approved in children.
FORMS — Trade: Tabs, unscored 80/5 mg.
MOA — See component drugs.
ADVERSE EFFECTS — See component drugs.

CAPOZIDE (**captopril + hydrochlorothiazide**) ▶See component drugs ♀See component drugs ▶See component drugs $$
WARNING — Do not use in pregnancy.
ADULT — HTN: Dosing interval: two to three times per day.
PEDS — Not approved in children.
FORMS — Generic only: Tabs, scored 25/15, 25/25, 50/15, 50/25 mg.
NOTES — The brand name product (Capozide) is no longer available.
MOA — See component drugs.

CLORPRES (**clonidine + chlorthalidone**) ▶See component drugs ♀See component drugs ▶See component drugs $$$$$
ADULT — HTN: Dosing interval: two to three times per day.
PEDS — Not approved in children.
FORMS — Trade only: Tabs, scored 0.1/15, 0.2/15, 0.3/15 mg.
MOA — See component drugs.

CORZIDE (**nadolol + bendroflumethiazide**) ▶See component drugs ♀See component drugs ▶See component drugs $$$
WARNING — Avoid abrupt cessation in coronary heart disease or HTN.
ADULT — HTN: Dosing interval: Daily.
PEDS — Not approved in children.
FORMS — Generic/Trade: Tabs 40/5, 80/5 mg.
MOA — See component drugs.

DIOVAN HCT (**valsartan + hydrochlorothiazide**) ▶See component drugs ♀See component drugs ▶See component drugs $$$$
WARNING — Do not use in pregnancy.
ADULT — HTN, initial therapy for patients needing multiple medications: Start 160/12.5 mg PO daily, may increase after 1 to 2 weeks, max 300/25 mg daily.
PEDS — Not approved in children.
FORMS — Generic/Trade: Tabs, unscored 80/12.5, 160/12.5, 320/12.5, 160/25, 320/25 mg.
MOA — See component drugs.

DUTOPROL (**metoprolol succinate + hydrochlorothiazide**) ▶See component drugs – ♀See component drugs. ▶$
WARNING — Avoid abrupt cessation in coronary heart disease or HTN.
ADULT — HTN: Dosing interval: Daily.
FORMS — Trade only: Tabs, unscored 25/12.5, 50/12.5, 100/12.5.
MOA — See component drugs.
ADVERSE EFFECTS — See component drugs.

DYAZIDE (triamterene + hydrochlorothiazide) ▶See component drugs ♀See component drugs ▶See component drugs $
ADULT — HTN: Dosing interval: Daily.
PEDS — Not approved in children.
FORMS — Generic/Trade: Caps, (Dyazide) 37.5/25 mg. Generic only: Caps, 50/25 mg.
NOTES — Dyazide: Cap 37.5/25 mg same combination as Maxzide-25 tabs.
MOA — See component drugs.
ADVERSE EFFECTS — See component drugs.

EDARBYCLOR (azilsartan + chlorthalidone) ▶See component drugs – See component drugs ♀D ▶? $$$$
WARNING — Do not use in pregnancy.
ADULT — HTN, initial therapy for patients needing multiple medications: Start 40/12.5 PO daily, may increase after 2 to 4 weeks, max 40/25 daily.
FORMS — Trade only: Tabs, unscored 40/12.5, 40/25 mg.
MOA — See component drugs.
ADVERSE EFFECTS — See component drugs.

EXFORGE (amlodipine + valsartan) ▶See component drugs ♀See component drugs ▶See component drugs $$$
WARNING — Do not use in pregnancy.
ADULT — HTN, initial therapy for patients needing multiple medications: Start 5/160 PO daily, may increase after 1 to 2 weeks, max 10/320 daily.
PEDS — Not approved in children.
FORMS — Generic/Trade: Tabs, unscored 5/160, 5/320, 10/160, 10/320 mg.
MOA — See component drugs.

EXFORGE HCT (amlodipine + valsartan + hydrochlorothiazide) ▶See component drugs ♀See component drugs ▶See component drugs $$$$
WARNING — Do not use in pregnancy.
ADULT — HTN, add-on/switch therapy when HTN not adequately controlled on any two of the following classes: calcium channel blockers, angiotensin receptor blockers, and diuretics: Dosing interval: Daily.
PEDS — Not approved in children.
FORMS — Generic/Trade: Tabs, unscored 5/160/12.5, 5/160/25, 10/160/12.5, 10/160/25, 10/320/25 mg.
MOA — See component drugs.

HYZAAR (losartan + hydrochlorothiazide) ▶See component drugs ♀See component drugs ▶See component drugs $$$
WARNING — Do not use in pregnancy.
ADULT — HTN, initial therapy for patients needing multiple medications: Start 50/12.5 mg PO daily, may increase after 2 to 4 weeks, max 100/25 mg daily. CVA risk reduction in HTN and LV hypertrophy (CVA risk reduction may not occur in patients of African descent): Establish dose using component drugs first. Dosing interval: Daily.
PEDS — Not approved in children.
FORMS — Generic/Trade: Tabs, unscored 50/12.5, 100/12.5, 100/25 mg.
MOA — See component drugs.

INDERIDE (propranolol + hydrochlorothiazide) ▶See component drugs ♀See component drugs ▶See component drugs $$$
WARNING — Avoid abrupt cessation in coronary heart disease or HTN.
ADULT — HTN: Dosing interval: Daily to two times per day.
PEDS — Not approved in children.
FORMS — Generic only: Tabs, scored 40/25, 80/25 mg.
NOTES — Do not crush or chew cap contents. Swallow whole. The brand name product (Inderide) is no longer available.
MOA — See component drugs.
ADVERSE EFFECTS — See component drugs.

INHIBACE PLUS (cilazapril + hydrochlorothiazide) ▶See component drugs ♀See component drugs ▶See component drugs $$
WARNING — Do not use in pregnancy.
ADULT — Canada only, HTN: Dosing interval daily.
PEDS — Not approved in children.
FORMS — Trade: Tabs, scored 5/12.5 mg.
MOA — See component drugs.

LOPRESSOR HCT (metoprolol + hydrochlorothiazide) ▶See component drugs ♀See component drugs ▶See component drugs $$$
WARNING — Abrupt cessation in coronary heart disease or HTN.
ADULT — HTN: Dosing interval: Daily to two times per day.
PEDS — Not approved in children.
FORMS — Generic/Trade: Tabs, scored 50/25, 100/25 mg. Generic only: Tabs, scored 100/50 mg.
MOA — See component drugs.

LOTENSIN HCT (benazepril + hydrochlorothiazide) ▶See component drugs ♀See component drugs ▶See component drugs $$$
WARNING — Do not use in pregnancy.
ADULT — HTN: Dosing interval: Daily.
PEDS — Not approved in children.
FORMS — Generic/Trade: Tabs, scored 5/6.25, 10/12.5, 20/12.5, 20/25 mg.
MOA — See component drugs.

LOTREL (amlodipine + benazepril) ▶See component drugs ♀See component drugs ▶See component drugs $$$
WARNING — Do not use in pregnancy.
ADULT — HTN: Dosing interval: Daily.
PEDS — Not approved in children.
FORMS — Generic/Trade: Caps, 2.5/10, 5/10, 5/20, 10/20, 5/40, 10/40 mg.
MOA — See component drugs.

MAXZIDE (triamterene + hydrochlorothiazide, ✦ Triazide) ▶See component drugs ♀See component drugs ▶See component drugs $
ADULT — HTN: Dosing interval: Daily.
PEDS — Not approved in children.
FORMS — Generic/Trade: Tabs, scored 75/50 mg.
MOA — See component drugs.

MAXZIDE-25 (**triamterene + hydrochlorothiazide**) ▶See component drugs ♀See component drugs ▶See component drugs $
ADULT — HTN: Dosing interval: Daily.
PEDS — Not approved in children.
FORMS — Generic/Trade: Tabs, scored 37.5/25 mg.
MOA — See component drugs.

MICARDIS HCT (**telmisartan + hydrochlorothiazide**, ✽ *Micardis Plus*) ▶See component drugs ♀See component drugs ▶See component drugs $$$$
WARNING — Do not use in pregnancy.
ADULT — HTN: Dosing interval: Daily.
PEDS — Not approved in children.
FORMS — Generic/Trade: Tabs, unscored 40/12.5, 80/12.5, 80/25 mg.
NOTES — Swallow tabs whole, do not break or crush. Caution in hepatic insufficiency.
MOA — See component drugs.
ADVERSE EFFECTS — See component drugs.

MINIZIDE (**prazosin + polythiazide**) ▶See component drugs ♀See component drugs ▶See component drugs $$$
ADULT — HTN: Dosing interval: two to three times per day.
PEDS — Not approved in children.
FORMS — Trade only: Caps, 1/0.5, 2/0.5, 5/0.5 mg.
MOA — See component drugs.

MODURETIC (**amiloride + hydrochlorothiazide**, ✽ *Moduret*) ▶See component drugs ♀See component drugs ▶See component drugs $
ADULT — HTN: Dosing interval: Daily. The brand name product (Moduretic) is no longer available.
PEDS — Not approved in children.
FORMS — Generic only: Tabs, scored 5/50 mg.
MOA — See component drugs.

MONOPRIL HCT (**fosinopril + hydrochlorothiazide**) ▶See component drugs ♀See component drugs ▶See component drugs $$
WARNING — Do not use in pregnancy.
ADULT — HTN: Dosing interval: Daily.
PEDS — Not approved in children.
FORMS — Generic only: Tabs, unscored 10/12.5, scored 20/12.5 mg.
NOTES — The brand name product (Monopril HCT) is no longer available.
MOA — See component drugs.

PRESTALIA (**perindopril + amlodipine**) ▶♀▶
WARNING — Do not use in pregnancy.
ADULT — HTN: Start 3.5/2.5 mg PO daily. May adjust dose after 1 to 2 weeks, max 14/10 mg/day.
PEDS — Not approved in children.
FORMS — Trade only: Tabs, unscored 3.5/2.5, 7/5, 14/10 mg.

PRINZIDE (**lisinopril + hydrochlorothiazide**) ▶See component drugs ♀See component drugs ▶See component drugs $
WARNING — Do not use in pregnancy.
ADULT — HTN: Dosing interval: Daily.
PEDS — Not approved in children.

FORMS — Generic/Trade: Tabs, unscored 10/12.5, 20/12.5, 20/25 mg.
MOA — See component drugs.

TARKA (**trandolapril + verapamil**) ▶See component drugs ♀See component drugs ▶See component drugs $$$$
WARNING — Do not use in pregnancy.
ADULT — HTN: Dosing interval: Daily.
PEDS — Not approved in children.
FORMS — Trade only: Tabs, unscored 2/180, 1/240, 2/240, 4/240 mg.
NOTES — Contains extended-release form of verapamil. Do not chew or crush, swallow whole. Hypotension, bradyarrhythmias, and lactic acidosis have occurred in patients receiving concurrent erythromycin or clarithromycin.
MOA — See component drugs.
ADVERSE EFFECTS — See component drugs.

TEKTURNA HCT (**aliskiren + hydrochlorothiazide**, ✽ *Rasilez HCT*) ▶See component drugs ♀See component drugs ▶See component drugs $$$
WARNING — Avoid in pregnancy.
ADULT — HTN, initial therapy for patients needing multiple medications: Start 150/12.5 PO daily, may increase after 2 weeks, max 300/25 daily.
PEDS — Not approved in children.
FORMS — Trade only: Tabs, unscored 150/12.5, 150/25, 300/12.5, 300/25 mg.
MOA — See component drugs.

Tenoretic (**atenolol + chlorthalidone**) ▶See component drugs ♀See component drugs ▶See component drugs $
WARNING — Avoid abrupt cessation in coronary heart disease or HTN.
ADULT — HTN: Dosing interval: Daily.
PEDS — Not approved in children.
FORMS — Generic/Trade: Tabs, scored 50/25, unscored 100/25 mg.
MOA — See component drugs.

TEVETEN HCT (**eprosartan + hydrochlorothiazide**, ✽ *Teveten Plus*) ▶See component drugs ♀See component drugs ▶See component drugs $$$$
WARNING — Do not use in pregnancy.
ADULT — HTN: interval: Daily.
PEDS — Not approved in children.
FORMS — Trade only: Tabs, unscored 600/12.5, 600/25 mg.
MOA — See component drugs.

TRIBENZOR (**amlodipine + olmesartan + hydrochlorothiazide**) ▶See component drugs – ♀▶– $$$$$
WARNING — Do not use in pregnancy.
ADULT — HTN, add-on/switch therapy when HTN not adequately controlled on any two of the following classes: calcium channel blockers, angiotensin receptor blockers, and diuretics: Dosing interval: Daily.
PEDS — Not approved in children.
FORMS — Trade only: Tabs, unscored 5/20/12.5, 5/40/12.5, 5/40/25, 10/40/12.5, 10/40/25 mg.
MOA — See component drugs.

TWYNSTA (amlodipine + telmisartan) ▶See component drugs ♀▶ $$$$
WARNING — Do not use in pregnancy.
ADULT — HTN, initial therapy for patients needing multiple medications: Start 5/40 to 5/80 mg PO daily, may increase after 2 weeks, max 10/80 mg daily. Do not use as initial therapy in patients 75 yo or older or with hepatic impairment.
PEDS — Not approved in children.
FORMS — Generic/Trade: Tabs, unscored 5/40, 5/80, 10/40, 10/80 mg.
MOA — See component drugs.
UNIRETIC (**moexipril + hydrochlorothiazide**) ▶See component drugs ♀See component drugs ▶See component drugs $$
WARNING — Do not use in pregnancy.
ADULT — HTN: Dosing interval: Daily to two times per day.
PEDS — Not approved in children.
FORMS — Generic/Trade: Tabs, scored 15/12.5, 15/25 mg. Generic: Tabs, scored 7.5/12.5.
MOA — See component drugs.
VASERETIC (**enalapril + hydrochlorothiazide**) ▶See component drugs ♀See component drugs ▶See component drugs $$
WARNING — Do not use in pregnancy.

ADULT — HTN: Dosing interval: Daily to two times per day.
PEDS — Not approved in children.
FORMS — Generic/Trade: Tabs, unscored 5/12.5, 10/25 mg.
MOA — See component drugs.
ZESTORETIC (**lisinopril + hydrochlorothiazide**) ▶See component drugs ♀See component drugs ▶See component drugs $$
WARNING — Do not use in pregnancy.
ADULT — HTN: Dosing interval: Daily.
PEDS — Not approved in children.
FORMS — Generic/Trade: Tabs, unscored 10/12.5, 20/12.5, 20/25 mg.
MOA — See component drugs.
ZIAC (**bisoprolol + hydrochlorothiazide**) ▶See component drugs ♀See component drugs ▶See component drugs $$
WARNING — Avoid abrupt cessation in coronary heart disease or HTN.
ADULT — HTN: Dosing interval: Daily.
PEDS — Not approved in children.
FORMS — Generic/Trade: Tabs, unscored 2.5/6.25, 5/6.25, 10/6.25 mg.
MOA — See component drugs.

CARDIOVASCULAR: Antihypertensives—Other

ALISKIREN (*Tekturna,* ✿*Rasilez*) ▶LK ♀D ▶–? $$$$
WARNING — Avoid in pregnancy.
ADULT — HTN: 150 mg PO daily, max 300 mg/day.
PEDS — Not approved in children.
FORMS — Trade only: Tabs, unscored 150, 300 mg.
NOTES — Women of child-bearing age should use reliable form of contraception; discontinue aliskiren as soon as pregnancy is detected. Contraindicated with ACE inhibitors or angiotensin receptor blocks in patients with DM. Avoid use with ACE inhibitors or angiotensin receptor blockers, particularly in patients with <60 mL/min; increases risk of renal impairment, hypotension, and hyperkalemia. Do not use with cyclosporine or itraconazole. Concomitant NSAID, including celecoxib, may further deteriorate renal function (usually reversible) and decrease antihypertensive effects. Hyperkalemia possible, especially if used concomitantly with other drugs that increase K+ (including K+-containing salt substitutes) and in patients with heart failure, DM, or renal impairment. Monitor potassium and renal function periodically. May increase creatine kinase, uric acid levels. Best absorbed on empty stomach; high-fat meals decrease absorption.
MOA — Direct renin inhibitor.
ADVERSE EFFECTS — Serious: Angioedema, hypotension, seizures. Frequent: Diarrhea, cough, dyspepsia, rash, GERD.
FENOLDOPAM (*Corlopam*) ▶LK ♀B ▶? $$$$
ADULT — Severe HTN: Dilute 10 mg in 250 mL D5W (40 mcg/mL), rate at 11 mL/h delivers 0.1 mcg/kg/min for 70 kg adult, titrate q 15 min, usual effective

dose 0.1 to 1.6 mcg/kg/min. Lower initial doses (0.03 to 0.1 mcg/kg/min) associated with less reflex tachycardia.
PEDS — Reduce BP: Start 0.2 mcg/kg/min, increase by up to 0.3 to 0.5 mcg/kg/min q 20 to 30 min. Max infusion 0.8 mcg/kg/min. Administer in hospital by continuous infusion pump; use max 4 h; monitor BP and HR continuously. Refer to prescribing information for dilution instructions and infusion rates.
UNAPPROVED ADULT — Prevention of contrast nephropathy in those at risk (conflicting evidence of efficacy): Start 0.03 mcg/kg/min infusion 60 min prior to dye. Titrate infusion q 15 min up to 0.1 mcg/kg/min if BP tolerates. Maintain infusion (with concurrent saline) up to 4 to 6 h after procedure.
NOTES — Avoid concomitant beta-blocker use due to hypotension. Use cautiously with glaucoma or increased intraocular HTN.
MOA — Stimulates dopamine-1 receptors and alpha-2 receptors causing vasodilation.
ADVERSE EFFECTS — Serious: Hypotension, tachycardia, hypokalemia (rare). Frequent: Headache, flushing, nausea.
HYDRALAZINE (*Apresoline*) ▶LK ♀C ▶+ $$$
ADULT — HTN: Start 10 mg PO two to four times per day for 2 to 4 days, increase to 25 mg two to four times per day, then 50 mg two to four times per day if necessary, max 300 mg/day. Hypertensive emergency: 10 to 20 mg IV; if no IV access, 10 to 50 mg IM. Use lower doses initially and repeat prn to control BP. Preeclampsia/eclampsia: 5 to 10 mg IV

(cont.)

HYDRALAZINE (*cont.*)

initially, followed by 5 to 10 mg IV q 20 to 30 min prn to control BP.

PEDS — Not approved in children.

UNAPPROVED ADULT — Heart failure: Start 10 to 25 mg PO three times per day, target dose 75 mg three times per day, max 100 mg three times per day. Use in combination with isosorbide dinitrate for patients intolerant to ACE inhibitors.

UNAPPROVED PEDS — HTN: Start 0.75 to 1 mg/kg/day PO divided two to four times per day, increase slowly over 3 to 4 weeks up to 7.5 mg/kg/day; initial IV dose 1.7 to 3.5 mg/kg/day divided in 4 to 6 doses. HTN urgency: 0.1 to 0.2 mg/kg IM/IV q 4 to 6 h prn. Max single dose, 25 mg PO and 20 mg IV.

FORMS — Generic only: Tabs, unscored 10, 25, 50, 100 mg.

NOTES — Headache, nausea, dizziness, tachycardia, peripheral edema, systemic lupus erythematosus–like syndrome. Usually used in combination with diuretic and beta-blocker to counter side effects.

MOA — Relaxes peripheral arterial smooth muscle (vasodilation).

ADVERSE EFFECTS — Serious: SLE, angina exacerbation, rash. Frequent: Tachycardia, headache, edema.

MECAMYLAMINE (*Vecamyl*) ▶K – ♀C ▶– $$$$$

ADULT — Moderately severe or severe essential HTN or uncomplicated malignant HTN: Start 2.5 mg PO two times daily, increase as needed by 2.5 mg increments no sooner than q 2 days, usual maintenance dose 25 mg/day divided two to four times.

PEDS — Not approved in children.

FORMS — Trade only: Tabs, unscored 2.5 mg.

NOTES — Do not give with coronary insufficiency, recent AMI, glaucoma, organic pyloric stenosis, renal insufficiency, uremia, antibiotics, or sulfonamides. Orthostatic hypotension common, especially during dosage titration. If taken after eating, may give gradual absorption and smoother control of excessively high BP. Monitor BP standing and supine. Rebound, severe hypertension with sudden drug withdrawal. Discontinue slowly and use other antihypertensives.

MOA — Blocks nerve transmission in sympathetic and parasympathetic ganglia

ADVERSE EFFECTS — Serious: syncope, rebound hypertension, ileus, tremors (rare), choreiform movements (rare). Frequent: postural hypotension, dizziness, sedation, dry mouth, anorexia, N/V, diarrhea, constipation, urinary retention, impotence.

METYROSINE (*Demser*) ▶K ♀C ▶? $$$$$

ADULT — Pheochromocytoma: Start 250 mg PO four times per day, increase by 250 to 500 mg/day prn, max dose 4 g/day.

PEDS — Pheochromocytoma, age older than 12 yo: Use adult dosage.

FORMS — Trade only: Caps 250 mg.

MOA — Decreases excess production of catecholamines by blocking tyrosine hydroxylase, the rate-limiting enzyme of catecholamine synthesis.

ADVERSE EFFECTS — Serious: Crystalluria (rare). Frequent: Sedation, drooling, speech difficulty, tremor, disorientation, diarrhea.

MINOXIDIL ▶K ♀C ▶+ $$

WARNING — Potent vasodilator; may produce serious complications from hypotension and reflex tachycardia. Relatively contraindicated in patients with coronary disease (ie, recent/acute MI, CAD, angina). May increase pulmonary artery pressure. Has been associated with development of pericardial effusion and tamponade; more likely to occur in patients with renal disease.

ADULT — Refractory HTN: Start 2.5 to 5 mg PO daily, increase at no less than 3-day intervals, usual dose 10 to 40 mg daily, max 100 mg/day.

PEDS — Not approved in children younger than 12 yo.

UNAPPROVED PEDS — HTN: Start 0.2 mg/kg PO daily, increase q 3 days prn up to 0.25 to 1 mg/kg/day daily or divided two times per day; max 50 mg/day.

FORMS — Generic only: Tabs, scored 2.5, 10 mg.

NOTES — Usually used in combination with a diuretic and a beta-blocker to counteract side effects. Relatively contraindicated with renal disease, pre-existing pulmonary hypertension, or chronic heart failure not secondary to HTN (drug may increase pulmonary artery pressure).

MOA — Relaxes peripheral arterial smooth muscle (vasodilation).

ADVERSE EFFECTS — Serious: Pericardial effusion (rare), angina exacerbation, heart failure exacerbation. Frequent: Tachycardia, headache, edema, hair growth.

NITROPRUSSIDE (*Nitropress*) ▶RBCs ♀C ▶– $$$$$

WARNING — May cause significant hypotension. Reconstituted soln must be further diluted before use. Cyanide toxicity may occur, especially with high infusion rates (10 mcg/kg/min), hepatic/renal impairment, and prolonged infusions (longer than 3 to 7 days). Protect from light.

ADULT — Hypertensive emergency: 50 mg in 250 mL D5W (200 mcg/mL), start at 0.3 mcg/kg/min (for 70 kg adult give 6 mL/h) via IV infusion, titrate slowly, usual range 0.3 to 10 mcg/kg/min, max 10 mcg/kg/min.

PEDS — Severe HTN: Use adult dosage.

NOTES — Discontinue if inadequate response to 10 mcg/kg/min after 10 min. Cyanide toxicity with high doses, hepatic/renal impairment, and prolonged infusions; check thiocyanate levels. Protect IV infusion minibag from light.

MOA — Relaxes peripheral arterial and venous smooth muscle.

ADVERSE EFFECTS — Serious: Cyanide toxicity (rare), thiocyanate toxicity (rare), methemoglobinemia (rare), severe hypotension. Frequent: N/V, sweating, flushing, weakness.

PHENOXYBENZAMINE (*Dibenzyline*) ▶KL ♀C ▶? $$$$$

ADULT — Pheochromocytoma: Start 10 mg PO two times per day, increase slowly every other day prn, usual dose 20 to 40 mg two to three times per day, max 120 mg/day.

(cont.)

PHENOXYBENZAMINE (*cont.*)
PEDS — Not approved in children.
UNAPPROVED PEDS—Pheochromocytoma: 0.2 mg/kg/day PO daily in divided doses two to three times per day; initial dose no more than 10 mg, increase slowly every other day prn, usual dose 0.4 to 1.2 mg/kg/day.
FORMS — Trade only: Caps 10 mg.
NOTES — Patients should be observed after each dosage increase for symptomatic hypotension and other adverse effects. Do not use for essential HTN.
MOA — Blocks binding of catecholamines to presynaptic and postsynaptic alpha receptors.
ADVERSE EFFECTS — Serious: Hypotension. Frequent: Dizziness, nasal congestion, tachycardia, miosis.
PHENTOLAMINE (*Regitine, ✦Rogitine*) ▶Plasma ♀C ▶? $$$$
ADULT — Diagnosis of pheochromocytoma: 5 mg IV/IM. Rapid IV administration is preferred. An immediate, marked decrease in BP should occur, typically, 60 mmHg SBP and 25 mmHg DBP decrease in 2 min. HTN during pheochromocytoma surgery: 5 mg IV/IM 1 to 2 h preop, 5 mg IV during surgery prn.

PEDS — Diagnosis of pheochromocytoma: 0.05 to 0.1 mg/kg IV/IM, up to 5 mg/dose. Rapid IV administration is preferred. An immediate, marked decrease in BP should occur, typically, 60 mmHg SBP and 25 mmHg DBP decrease in 2 min. HTN during pheochromocytoma surgery: 0.05 to 0.1 mg/kg IV/IM 1 to 2 h preop, repeat q 2 to 4 h prn.
UNAPPROVED ADULT — IV extravasation of catecholamines: 5 to 10 mg in 10 mL NS, inject 1 to 5 mL SC (in divided doses) around extravasation site. Hypertensive crisis: 5 to 15 mg IV.
UNAPPROVED PEDS — IV extravasation of catecholamines, neonates: 2.5 to 5 mg in 10 mL NS, inject 1 mL SC (in divided doses) around extravasation site. Children: Use adult dosage.
NOTES — Weakness, flushing, hypotension; priapism with intracavernous injection. Use within 12 h of extravasation. Distributed to hospital pharmacies at no charge, only for use in life-threatening situations. Call 888-669-6682 for ordering.
MOA — Blocks binding of catecholamines to presynaptic and postsynaptic alpha receptors.
ADVERSE EFFECTS — Serious: Hypotension, tachycardia, arrhythmias. Frequent: Weakness, dizziness, flushing, nasal congestion.

CARDIOVASCULAR: Antiplatelet Drugs

ABCIXIMAB (*ReoPro*) ▶Plasma ♀C ▶? $$$$$
ADULT — Platelet aggregation inhibition, prevention of acute cardiac ischemic events associated with PTCA: 0.25 mg/kg IV bolus over 1 min via separate infusion line 10 to 60 min before procedure, then 0.125 mcg/kg/min up to 10 mcg/min infusion for 12 h. Unstable angina not responding to standard therapy when percutaneous coronary intervention (PCI) is planned within 24 h: 0.25 mg/kg IV bolus over 1 min via separate infusion line, followed by 10 mcg/min IV infusion for 18 to 24 h, concluding 1 h after PCI.
PEDS — Not approved in children.
NOTES — Thrombocytopenia possible. Discontinue abciximab, heparin, and aspirin if uncontrollable bleeding occurs.
MOA — Inhibits platelet aggregation by blocking the effects of fibrinogen and other substances at platelet glycoprotein IIb/IIIa receptors.
ADVERSE EFFECTS — Serious: Bleeding, hypersensitivity (rare), thrombocytopenia (rare). Frequent: Pain.
AGGRENOX (acetylsalicylic acid + dipyridamole) ▶LK ♀D ▶? $$$$$
ADULT — Prevention of CVA after TIA/CVA: 1 cap PO two times per day. Headache is a common adverse effect.
PEDS — Not approved in children.
FORMS — Generic/Trade: Caps 25 mg aspirin/200 mg extended-release dipyridamole.
NOTES — Do not crush or chew capsules. May need supplemental aspirin for prevention of MI. Concomitant anticoagulants, NSAIDs, antiplatelet

agents, fibrinolytics, or anagrelide increase risk of bleeding.
MOA — See component drugs.
ADVERSE EFFECTS — See component drugs.
CANGRELOR (*Kengreal*) ▶degraded chemically ♀C ▶? $$$$$
ADULT — Adjunct to percutaneous coronary intervention (PCI) to reduce thrombotic events, including periprocedural MI, repeat coronary revascularization, and stent thrombosis, in patients who have not been treated with P2Y12 platelet inhibitor and glycoprotein IIb/IIIa inhibitor: Load 30 mcg/kg IV prior to PCI, then IV infusion 4 mcg/kg/min for at least 2 h or duration of procedure, whichever is longer. Use dedicated IV line. Maintain platelet inhibition with oral P2Y12 inhibitor: Give clopidogrel or prasugrel loading dose immediately after discontinuing cangrelor infusion; or give ticagrelor loading dose during cangrelor infusion or immediately after discontinuing infusion.
PEDS — Not approved in children.
NOTES — Do not give clopidogrel or prasugrel during cangrelor infusion.
MOA — Inhibits platelet activation and aggregation by reversibly interacting with the adenosine diphosphate receptor.
ADVERSE EFFECTS — Serious: Bleeding.
CLOPIDOGREL (*Plavix*) ▶LK ♀B ▶? $
WARNING — Requires activation to an active metabolite by the CYP system, mainly CYP2C19. When treated at recommended doses, poor metabolizers have higher cardiovascular event rates after acute coronary syndrome or percutaneous coronary

(cont.)

CLOPIDOGREL (*cont.*)

intervention than patients with normal CYP2C19 function. Tests to determine a patient's CYP2C19 genotype may aid in determining therapeutic strategy. Consider alternative treatment or treatment strategies in patients identified as CYP2C19 poor metabolizers.

ADULT — Reduction of thrombotic events after recent acute MI, recent CVA, established peripheral arterial disease: 75 mg PO daily. Non-ST segment elevation acute coronary syndrome: 300 mg loading dose, then 75 mg PO daily in combination with aspirin PO daily. ST segment elevation MI: Start with/without 300 mg loading dose, then 75 mg PO daily in combination with aspirin, with/without thrombolytic.

PEDS — Not approved in children.

UNAPPROVED ADULT — Medical treatment, without stent, of unstable angina/non-ST segment elevation MI: 300 to 600 mg loading dose, then 75 mg daily in combination with aspirin for at least 1 month and up to 1 year. Medical treatment, without stent and with/without thrombolytics, of ST segment elevation MI: 300 mg loading dose, then 75 mg daily in combination with aspirin for at least 14 days and up to 1 year. When early percutaneous coronary intervention is planned: 600 mg loading dose; consider using 300 mg if patient received thrombolytic within 12 to 24 h, then 150 mg once a day for 6 days, then 75 mg daily for at least 1 year. Post bare-metal stent placement or post drug-eluting stent placement: 75 mg daily in combination with aspirin for at least 1 year (in patients not at high risk for bleeding). Post-percutaneous coronary brachytherapy: 75 mg daily in combination with aspirin for at least 1 year. Acute coronary syndrome with aspirin allergy or reduction of thrombotic events in high-risk patient after TIA: 75 mg PO daily.

FORMS — Generic/Trade: Tabs, unscored 75, 300 mg.

NOTES — Allergic cross-reactivity may occur among thienopyridines (clopidogrel, prasugrel, ticlopidine). Effectiveness is reduced with impaired CYP2C19 function; avoid drugs that are strong or moderate CYP2C19 inhibitors (eg, omeprazole, esomeprazole, cimetidine, etravirine, felbamate, fluconazole, fluoxetine, fluvoxamine, ketoconazole, voriconazole). Contraindicated with active pathologic bleeding (peptic ulcer or intracranial bleed). Prolongs bleeding time. Discontinue use 5 days before elective surgery, except in 1st year post coronary stent implantation; premature discontinuation increases risk of cardiovascular events. Concomitant aspirin, SSRI, or SNRI increases bleeding risk. Cardiovascular (but not CVA) patients may receive additional benefit when given with aspirin. Should not be used with aspirin for primary prevention of cardiovascular events.

MOA — Active metabolite inhibits platelet aggregation by irreversibly blocking the effects of adenosine diphosphate at its platelet receptor.

ADVERSE EFFECTS — Serious: Acute liver failure, anaphylaxis, angioedema, aplastic anemia, agranulocytosis, bleeding, pancreatitis, Stevens-Johnson syndrome, thrombotic thrombocytopenia purpura. Frequent: Pruritus, purpura, diarrhea, rash.

DIPYRIDAMOLE (*Persantine*) ▶L ♀B ▶? $$$

ADULT — Prevention of thromboembolic complications of cardiac valve replacement: 75 to 100 mg PO four times per day in combination with warfarin.

PEDS — Not approved in children younger than 12 yo.

UNAPPROVED ADULT — Platelet aggregation inhibition: 150 to 400 mg/day PO divided three to four times per day.

FORMS — Generic/Trade: Tabs, unscored 25, 50, 75 mg.

NOTES — May cause chest pain when used in CAD.

MOA — Inhibits platelet adhesion by inhibiting phosphodiesterase. Increases coronary blood flow by selective dilation of the coronary arteries.

ADVERSE EFFECTS — Serious: Angioedema, bronchospasm, thrombocytopenia. Frequent: Headache, dizziness, abdominal discomfort, perioperative bleeding (rare).

EPTIFIBATIDE (*Integrilin*) ▶K ♀B ▶? $$$$$

ADULT — Acute coronary syndrome (unstable angina/non-ST segment elevation MI): Load 180 mcg/kg IV bolus, then IV infusion 2 mcg/kg/min for up to 72 h. If percutaneous coronary intervention (PCI) occurs during the infusion, continue infusion for 18 to 24 h after procedure. PCI: Load 180 mcg/kg IV bolus just before procedure, followed by infusion 2 mcg/kg/min and a 2nd 180 mcg/kg IV bolus 10 min after the 1st bolus. Continue infusion for up to 18 to 24 h (minimum 12 h) after the procedure. Renal impairment (CrCl <50 mL/min): No change in bolus dose; decrease infusion to 1 mcg/kg/min. For obese patients (greater than 121 kg): Max bolus dose 22.6 mg; max infusion rate 15 mg/h. Renal impairment and obese: Max bolus dose 22.6 mg; max infusion rate 7.5 mg/h.

PEDS — Not approved in children.

NOTES — Discontinue infusion prior to CABG. Give with aspirin and heparin (unless contraindicated); discontinue heparin after percutaneous coronary intervention. Contraindicated in patients on dialysis, with a history of bleeding diathesis or active abnormal bleeding within past 30 days, severe hypertension (SBP greater than 200 mmHg or DBP greater than 110 mmHg) not controlled on antihypertensive therapy; major surgery within past 6 weeks; stroke within 30 days; or any history of hemorrhagic stroke. Thrombocytopenia possible; monitor platelets. If profound thrombocytopenia occurs or platelets decrease to less than 100,000 mm^3, discontinue eptifibatide and heparin and monitor serial platelet counts, assess for drug-dependent antibodies, and treat as appropriate.

MOA — Inhibits platelet aggregation by blocking the effects of fibrinogen and other substances at platelet glycoprotein IIb/IIIa receptors.

ADVERSE EFFECTS — Serious: Bleeding, thrombocytopenia (rare). Frequent: Pain.

PRASUGREL (*Effient*) ▶LK ♀?/?/?; Consider possible risks to fetus before prescribing to pregnant women. ▶ Consider possible risks to breastfed child before prescribing to the nursing woman. $$$$$

WARNING — May cause significant, fatal bleeding. Do not use with active bleeding or history of TIA or CVA. Generally not recommended for patients 75 yo and older. Do not start in patients likely to need urgent CABG. When possible, discontinue 7 days prior to any surgery. Risk factors for bleeding: Body wt less than 60 kg, propensity to bleed, concomitant medications that increase bleeding risk. Suspect bleeding with hypotension and recent coronary angiography, PCI, CABG, or other surgical procedure. Premature discontinuation increases risk of stent thrombosis, MI, and death.

ADULT — Reduction of thrombotic events, including stent thrombosis, after acute coronary syndrome managed with percutaneous coronary intervention (PCI): 60 mg loading dose, then 10 mg PO daily in combination with aspirin. Wt less than 60 kg: Consider lower maintenance dose, 5 mg PO daily.

PEDS — Not approved in children.

FORMS — Trade only: Tabs, unscored 5, 10 mg.

NOTES — Allergic cross-reactivity may occur among thienopyridines (clopidogrel, prasugrel, ticlopidine). Concomitant warfarin or NSAID increases bleeding risk. Do not break tablet. Dispense and keep prasugrel in original container with desiccant.

MOA — Active metabolite inhibits platelet activation and aggregation by irreversibly blocking the effects of adenosine diphosphate at its platelet receptor.

ADVERSE EFFECTS — Serious: Angioedema, bleeding.

TICAGRELOR (*Brilinta*) ▶L – ♀?/?/?; Consider possible risks to fetus before prescribing to pregnant women. ▶ Do not breastfeed while taking this medication. $$$$$

WARNING — May cause significant, fatal bleeding. Do not use with active bleeding or history of intracranial hemorrhage. Do not start in patients likely to need urgent CABG. When possible, discontinue 5 days prior to any surgery. Suspect bleeding with hypotension and recent coronary angiography, PCI, CABG, or other surgical procedure. If possible, manage bleeding without discontinuing ticagrelor; discontinuation increases risk of cardiovascular events. After the initial dose of aspirin, use with aspirin 75 to 100 mg daily; doses of aspirin greater than 100 mg daily reduce the effectiveness of ticagrelor.

ADULT — Reduction of thrombotic events in patients with acute coronary syndrome (MI or unstable angina) or history of MI: 180 mg loading dose, then 90 mg PO two times daily for first year post-acute coronoary syndrome event, then 60 mg PO two times daily. Give with aspirin; after any initial dose, use with aspirin 75 to 100 mg max per day. After the initial dose of aspirin, do not use more than 100 mg of aspirin daily with ticagrelor.)

PEDS — Not approved in children.

FORMS — Trade only: Tabs, unscored 60, 90 mg.

NOTES — Do not use with strong CYP3A4 inhibitors (eg, clarithromycin, HIV protease inhibitors, itraconazole, ketoconazole, nefazodone, telithromycin, voriconazole), CYP3A4 inducers (eg, carbamazepine, dexamethasone, phenobarbital, phenytoin, rifampin), or severe hepatic impairment. P-glycoprotein inhibitors (eg, cyclosporine) increase ticagrelor levels. Monitor digoxin levels when initiating or changing ticagrelor therapy. Increases risk of statin-related side effects when used concomitantly with more than 40 mg daily of simvastatin or lovastatin.

MOA — Inhibits platelet activation by reversibly interacting with the adenosine diphosphate receptor.

ADVERSE EFFECTS — Serious: Angioedema, bleeding. Frequent: Dyspnea.

TICLOPIDINE ▶L ♀B ▶? $$$$

WARNING — May cause life-threatening neutropenia, agranulocytosis, and thrombotic thrombocytopenia purpura (TTP). During 1st 3 months of treatment, monitor patient clinically and hematologically for neutropenia or TTP; discontinue if evidence is seen.

ADULT — Due to adverse effects, other antiplatelet agents preferred. Platelet aggregation inhibition/reduction of thrombotic CVA: 250 mg PO two times per day with food. Prevention of cardiac stent occlusion: 250 mg PO two times per day in combo with aspirin 325 mg PO daily for up to 30 days post-stent implantation.

PEDS — Not approved in children.

UNAPPROVED ADULT — Prevention of graft occlusion with CABG: 250 mg PO two times per day.

FORMS — Generic: Tabs, unscored 250 mg.

NOTES — Allergic cross-reactivity may occur among thienopyridines (clopidogrel, prasugrel, ticlopidine). Check CBC q 2 weeks during the 1st 3 months of therapy. Neutrophil counts usually return to normal within 1 to 3 weeks following discontinuation. Loading dose 500 mg PO on day 1 may be used for prevention of cardiac stent occlusion. The brand name product (Ticlid) is no longer available.

MOA — Active metabolite inhibits platelet aggregation by irreversibly blocking the effects of adenosine diphosphate at its platelet receptor.

ADVERSE EFFECTS — Serious: Bleeding, thrombocytopenia (rare), neutropenia (rare). Frequent: Diarrhea, nausea, dyspepsia.

TIROFIBAN (*Aggrastat*) ▶K ♀B ▶? $$$$$

ADULT — Non-ST segment elevation acute coronary syndromes: Give 25 mcg/kg within 5 min, then 0.15 mcg/kg/min for up to 18 h. Renal impairment (CrCl 60 mL/min or less): Give 25 mcg/kg within 5 min, then 0.075 mcg/kg/min.

PEDS — Not approved in children.

NOTES — Thrombocytopenia possible. Concomitant aspirin and heparin/enoxaparin use recommended, unless contraindicated. Dose heparin to keep PTT 2 times normal.

MOA — Inhibits platelet aggregation by blocking the effects of fibrinogen and other substances at platelet glycoprotein IIb/IIIa receptors.

ADVERSE EFFECTS — Serious: Bleeding, thrombocytopenia (rare). Frequent: Pain.

VORAPAXAR (*Zontivity*) ▶L ♀B ▶– $$$$$
WARNING — Do not use with active bleeding or history of CVA or stroke.
ADULT — Reduction of thrombotic events in patients with history of MI or with peripheral artery disease: 2.08 mg PO daily.
PEDS — Not approved in children.
FORMS — Trade only: Tabs, unscored 2.08 mg.
NOTES — Avoid use with strong CYP3A4 inhibitors (eg, boceprevir, clarithromycin, conivaptan, indinavir, itraconazole, ketoconazole, nefazodone, nelfinavir, posaconazole, ritonavir, saquinavir, telithromycin) or inducers (eg, carbamazepine, phenytoin, rifampin, St. John's wort). Must be stored in original container with desiccant.
MOA — Irreversibly (due to long half-life) inhibits platelet aggregation by blocking the protease-activated receptor-1 (PAR-1).
ADVERSE EFFECTS — Serious: Bleeding.

CARDIOVASCULAR: Beta-Blockers

NOTE: See also Antihypertensive Combinations. Not first line for HTN (unless concurrent angina, post MI, or heart failure with reduced ejection fraction). Atenolol may be less effective for HTN than other beta-blockers. Nonselective beta-blockers, including carvedilol and labetalol, are contraindicated with asthma; use agents with beta-1 selectivity and monitor cautiously; beta-1 selectivity diminishes at high doses. Contraindicated with acute decompensated heart failure, sick sinus syndrome without pacer, cardiogenic shock, heart block greater than first degree, or severe bradycardia. Agents with intrinsic sympathomimetic activity (eg, pindolol) are contraindicated post acute MI. Abrupt cessation may precipitate angina, MI, arrhythmias, tachycardia, rebound HTN; or with thyrotoxicosis, thyroid storm; discontinue by tapering over 1 to 2 weeks. Do not routinely stop chronic beta-blocker therapy prior to surgery. Discontinue beta-blocker several days before discontinuing concomitant clonidine to minimize the risk of rebound HTN. Some inhalation anesthetics may increase the cardiodepressant effect of beta-blockers. With pheochromocytoma, give beta-blocker only after initiating alpha-blocker; using beta-blocker alone may increase BP due to the attenuation of beta-mediated vasodilatation in skeletal muscle (unopposed alpha stimulation). Patients actively using cocaine should avoid beta-blockers with unopposed alpha-adrenergic vasoconstriction, because this will promote coronary artery vasoconstriction/spasm (carvedilol or labetalol have additional alpha-1-blocking effects and are safer). Concomitant amiodarone, disopyramide, clonidine, digoxin, or nondihydropyridine calcium channel blockers may increase risk of bradycardia. Monitor for heart failure exacerbation and hypotension (particularly orthostatic) when titrating dose. All beta-blockers, except carvedilol, may increase blood glucose or mask tachycardia occurring with hypoglycemia. May aggravate psoriasis or symptoms of arterial insufficiency. Intraoperative floppy iris syndrome may occur during cataract surgery, if patient is on or has previously taken agents with alpha-1 blocking activity.

ACEBUTOLOL (*Sectral*, ✷*Rhotral*) ▶LK ♀B ▶– $$
WARNING — Avoid abrupt cessation in coronary heart disease or HTN.
ADULT — HTN: Start 400 mg PO daily or 200 mg PO two times per day, usual maintenance 400 to 800 mg/day, max 1200 mg/day. Twice-daily dosing appears to be more effective than daily dosing.
PEDS — Not approved in children age younger than 12 yo.
UNAPPROVED ADULT — Angina: Start 200 mg PO two times per day, increase prn up to 800 mg/day.
FORMS — Generic/Trade: Caps 200, 400 mg.
NOTES — Beta-1 receptor selective; has mild intrinsic sympathomimetic activity.
MOA — Blocks binding of catecholamines to beta-1 receptors.
ADVERSE EFFECTS — Serious: Bronchoconstriction (high doses), masks hypoglycemic response and slow recovery, rebound hypertension/angina. Frequent: Bradycardia, fatigue, impotence.

ATENOLOL (*Tenormin*) ▶K ♀D ▶– $
WARNING — Avoid abrupt cessation in coronary heart disease or HTN.
ADULT — Acute MI: 50 to 100 mg PO daily or in divided doses. HTN: Start 25 to 50 mg PO daily or divided two times per day, max 100 mg/day. Renal impairment, elderly: Start 25 mg PO daily, increase prn. Angina: Start 50 mg PO daily or divided two times per day, increase prn to max of 200 mg/day.
PEDS — Not approved in children.
UNAPPROVED ADULT — Reduce perioperative cardiac events (death) in high-risk patients undergoing noncardiac surgery: Start 5 to 10 mg IV prior to anesthesia, then 50 to 100 mg PO daily during hospitalization (max 7 days). Maintain HR between 55 and 65 bpm. Hold dose for HR less than 55 bpm and SBP less than 100 mmHg. Reentrant PSVT associated with ST-elevation MI (after carotid massage, IV adenosine): 2.5 to 5 mg over 2 min to 10 mg max over 10 to 15 min. Rate control of atrial fibrillation/flutter: Start 25 mg PO daily, titrate to desired heart rate.
UNAPPROVED PEDS — HTN: 1 to 1.2 mg/kg/dose PO daily, max 2 mg/kg/day.
FORMS — Generic/Trade: Tabs, unscored 25, 100 mg; scored, 50 mg.
NOTES — Beta-1 receptor selective. Doses greater than 100 mg/day usually do not provide further BP lowering. Risk of hypoglycemia to neonates born to mothers using atenolol at parturition or while

(cont.)

ATENOLOL (*cont.*)

breastfeeding. May be less effective for HTN and lowering CV event risk than other beta-blockers. MOA — Blocks binding of catecholamines to beta-1 receptors. ADVERSE EFFECTS — Serious: Bronchoconstriction (high doses), masks hypoglycemic response and slow recovery, rebound hypertension/angina. Frequent: Bradycardia, fatigue, impotence.

BETAXOLOL (*Kerlone*) ▶LK ♀C ▶? $

WARNING — Avoid abrupt cessation in coronary heart disease or HTN.

ADULT — HTN: Start 5 to 10 mg PO daily, max 20 mg/day. Renal impairment, elderly: Start 5 mg PO daily, increase prn.

PEDS — Not approved in children.

FORMS — Generic/Trade: Tabs, scored 10 mg; unscored 20 mg.

NOTES — Beta-1 receptor selective.

MOA — Blocks binding of catecholamines to beta-1 receptors.

ADVERSE EFFECTS — Serious: Bronchoconstriction (high doses), masks hypoglycemic response and slow recovery, rebound hypertension/angina. Frequent: Bradycardia, fatigue, impotence.

BISOPROLOL (*Zebeta*, *＊Monocor*) ▶LK ♀C ▶? $$

WARNING — Avoid abrupt cessation in coronary heart disease or HTN.

ADULT — HTN: Start 2.5 to 5 mg PO daily, max 20 mg/day. Renal impairment: Start 2.5 mg PO daily, increase prn.

PEDS — Not approved in children.

UNAPPROVED ADULT — Compensated heart failure: Start 1.25 mg PO daily, double dose q 2 weeks as tolerated to goal 10 mg/day. Reduce perioperative cardiac events (death, MI) in high-risk patients undergoing noncardiac surgery: Start 5 mg PO daily, at least 1 week prior to surgery, increase to 10 mg daily to maintain HR less than 60 bpm, continue for 30 days postop. Hold dose for HR less than 50 bpm or SBP less than 100 mmHg.

FORMS — Generic/Trade: Tabs, scored 5 mg; unscored 10 mg.

NOTES — Monitor closely for heart failure exacerbation and hypotension when titrating dose. Avoid in decompensated heart failure (ie NYHA class IV heart failure or pulmonary edema). Stabilize dose of digoxin, diuretics, and ACE inhibitor before starting bisoprolol. Highly beta-1 receptor selective.

MOA — Blocks binding of catecholamines to beta-1 receptors.

ADVERSE EFFECTS — Serious: Bronchoconstriction (high doses), masks hypoglycemic response and slow recovery, rebound hypertension/angina. Frequent: Bradycardia, fatigue, impotence.

CARVEDILOL (*Coreg, Coreg CR*) ▶L ♀C ▶? $$$

WARNING — Avoid abrupt cessation in coronary heart disease or HTN.

ADULT — Heart failure: Immediate-release: Start 3.125 mg PO two times per day, double dose q 2 weeks as tolerated up to max of 25 mg two times

per day (for wt 85 kg or less) or 50 mg two times per day (for wt 85 kg or greater). Heart failure, sustained-release: Start 10 mg PO daily, double dose q 2 weeks as tolerated up to max of 80 mg/day. Reduce cardiovascular risk in post MI with LV dysfunction, immediate-release: Start 3.125 to 6.25 mg PO two times per day, double dose q 3 to 10 days as tolerated to max of 25 mg two times per day. LV dysfunction post MI, sustained-release: Start 10 to 20 mg PO daily, double dose q 3 to 10 days as tolerated to max of 80 mg/day. HTN, immediate-release: Start 6.25 mg PO two times per day, double dose q 7 to 14 days as tolerated to max 50 mg/day. HTN, sustained-release: Start 20 mg PO daily, double dose q 7 to 14 days as tolerated to max 80 mg/day.

PEDS — Not approved in children.

FORMS — Generic/Trade: Tabs, immediate-release, unscored 3.125, 6.25, 12.5, 25 mg. Trade only: Caps, extended-release 10, 20, 40, 80 mg.

NOTES — Alpha-1, beta-1, and beta-2 receptor blocker. Avoid in hepatic impairment. May reversibly elevate LFTs. Amiodarone may increase carvedilol levels. May increase digoxin levels. Reduce the dose with bradycardia (less than 55 bpm). Take with food to decrease orthostatic hypotension. Separate Coreg CR and alcohol (including medications containing alcohol) by at least 2 h. Give Coreg CR in the morning. The contents of Coreg CR may be sprinkled over applesauce and consumed immediately. Dosing conversion from immediate-release to sustained-release: 3.125 mg two times per day = 10 mg CR; 6.25 mg two times per day = 20 mg CR; 12.5 mg two times per day = 40 mg CR; 25 mg two times per day = 80 mg CR.

MOA — Blocks binding of catecholamines to post-synaptic alpha-1, beta-1, and beta-2 receptors.

ADVERSE EFFECTS — Serious: Anaphylaxis, angioedema, bronchoconstriction, masks hypoglycemic response and slow recovery, rebound hypertension/angina. Frequent: Bradycardia, fatigue, impotence, hypotension.

ESMOLOL (*Brevibloc*) ▶K ♀C ▶? $$$$$

ADULT — SVT/HTN emergency: Load 500 mcg/kg over 1 min (dilute 5 g in 500 mL (10 mg/mL) and give 3.5 mL to deliver 35 mg bolus for 70 kg patient) then start infusion 50 to 200 mcg/kg/min (42 mL/h delivers 100 mcg/kg/min for 70 kg patient). If optimal response is not attained, repeat IV load and increase IV infusion to 100 mcg/kg/min for 4 min. If necessary, additional boluses (500 mcg/kg/min over 1 min) may be given followed by IV infusion with increased dose by 50 mcg/kg/min for 4 min. Max IV infusion rate 200 mcg/kg/min.

PEDS — Not approved in children.

UNAPPROVED PEDS — Same schedule as adult except loading dose 100 to 500 mcg/kg IV over 1 min and IV infusion 25 to 100 mcg/kg/min. IV infusions may be increased by 25 to 50 mcg/kg/min q 5 to 10 min. Titrate dose based on response.

NOTES — Hypotension. Beta-1 receptor selective. Half-life is 9 min.

(cont.)

ESMOLOL (*cont.*)

MOA — Blocks binding of catecholamines to beta-1 receptors.

ADVERSE EFFECTS — Serious: Bronchoconstriction (high doses), masks hypoglycemic response and slow recovery, rebound hypertension/angina. Frequent: Bradycardia, fatigue.

LABETALOL (*Trandate*) ▶LK ♀C ▶+ $$$

WARNING — Avoid abrupt cessation in coronary heart disease or HTN.

ADULT — HTN: Start 100 mg PO two times per day, usual maintenance dose 200 to 600 mg two times per day, max 2400 mg/day. HTN emergency: Start 20 mg slow IV injection, then 40 to 80 mg IV q 10 min prn up to 300 mg total cumulative dose or start 0.5 to 2 mg/min IV infusion, adjust rate prn up to total cumulative dose 300 mg.

PEDS — Not approved in children.

UNAPPROVED PEDS — HTN: 4 mg/kg/day PO divided two times per day, increase prn up to 40 mg/kg/day. IV: Start 0.3 to 1 mg/kg/dose (max 20 mg) slow IV injection q 10 min or 0.4 to 1 mg/kg/h IV infusion up to 3 mg/kg/h.

FORMS — Generic/Trade: Tabs, scored 100, 200, 300 mg.

NOTES — Alpha-1, beta-1, and beta-2 receptor blocker. May be used to manage BP during pregnancy. The brand name product (Normodyne) is no longer available.

MOA — Blocks binding of catecholamines to post-synaptic alpha-1, beta-1, and beta-2 receptors.

ADVERSE EFFECTS — Serious: Bronchoconstriction, hepatotoxicity, masks hypoglycemic response and slow recovery, rebound hypertension/angina. Frequent: Bradycardia, fatigue, impotence, hypotension.

METOPROLOL (*Lopressor, Toprol-XL, ✱Betaloc*) ▶L ♀C ▶? $$

WARNING — Avoid abrupt cessation in coronary heart disease or HTN.

ADULT — Acute MI: 50 to 100 mg PO q 12 h; or 5 mg IV q 5 to 15 min up to 15 mg, then start 50 mg PO q 6 h for 48 h, then 100 mg PO two times per day as tolerated. HTN (immediate-release): Start 100 mg PO daily or in divided doses, increase prn up to 450 mg/day; may require multiple daily doses to maintain 24 h BP control. HTN (extended-release): Start 25 to 100 mg PO daily, increase prn q 1 week up to 400 mg/day. Heart failure: Start 12.5 to 25 mg (extended-release) PO daily, double dose q 2 weeks as tolerated up to max 200 mg/day. Angina: Start 50 mg PO two times per day (immediate-release) or 100 mg PO daily (extended-release), increase prn up to 400 mg/day. Immediate-release form is metoprolol tartrate; extended-release form is metoprolol succinate. Take with food.

PEDS — HTN, 6 yo or older: Start 1 mg/kg, max 50 mg/daily. Not recommended for younger than 6 yo.

UNAPPROVED ADULT — Atrial tachyarrhythmia, except with Wolff-Parkinson-White syndrome: 2.5 to 5 mg IV q 2 to 5 min prn to control rapid ventricular response, max 15 mg over 10 to 15 min. Reentrant PSVT (after carotid massage, IV adenosine): 2.5 to 5 mg q 2 to 5 min to 15 mg max over 10 to 15 min. Reduce perioperative cardiac events (death) in high-risk patients undergoing noncardiac surgery: Start 100 mg (extended-release) 2 h prior to anesthesia, then 50 to 100 mg (extended-release) PO daily or 2.5 to 5 mg IV q 6 h during hospitalization (max 7 days). Maintain HR between 55 to 65 bpm. Hold dose for HR less than 55 bpm and SBP less than 100 mmHg. Rate control of atrial fibrillation/flutter: Start 25 mg PO two times per day, titrate to desired heart rate.

FORMS — Generic/Trade: Tabs, immediate release, tartrate, scored 50, 100 mg, extended-release, succinate, 25, 50, 100, 200 mg. Generic only: Tabs, extended-release, tartrate, scored 25 mg.

NOTES — Beta-1 receptor selective. The immediate- and extended-release products may not give same clinical response on mg:mg basis; monitor response and side effects when interchanging between metoprolol products. Do not start high-dose extended-release form in patients undergoing noncardiac surgery. Monitor closely for heart failure exacerbation and hypotension when titrating dose. Stabilize dose of diuretics and ACE inhibitor before starting metoprolol. May need lower doses in elderly and in patients with liver impairment. Extended-release tabs may be broken in half, but do not chew or crush.

MOA — Blocks binding of catecholamines to beta-1 receptors.

ADVERSE EFFECTS — Serious: Bronchoconstriction (high doses), masks hypoglycemic response and slow recovery, rebound hypertension/angina. Frequent: Bradycardia, fatigue, impotence.

NADOLOL (*Corgard*) ▶K ♀C ▶– $$$$

WARNING — Avoid abrupt cessation in coronary heart disease or HTN.

ADULT — HTN: Start 20 to 40 mg PO daily, usual maintenance dose 40 to 80 mg/day, max 320 mg/day. Renal impairment: Start 20 mg PO daily, adjust dosage interval based on severity of renal impairment: For CrCl less than 10 mL/min, give q 40 to 60 h; for CrCl 10 to 30 mL/min, give q 24 to 48 h; for CrCl 31 to 50 mL/min, give q 24 to 36 h. Angina: Start 40 mg PO daily, usual maintenance dose 40 to 80 mg/day, max 240 mg/day.

PEDS — Not approved in children.

UNAPPROVED ADULT — Prevent rebleeding esophageal varices: 40 to 160 mg/day PO. Titrate dose to reduce heart rate to 25% below baseline.

FORMS — Generic/Trade: Tabs, scored 20, 40, 80 mg.

NOTES — Beta-1 and beta-2 receptor blocker.

MOA — Blocks binding of catecholamines to beta-1 and beta-2 receptors.

ADVERSE EFFECTS — Serious: Bronchoconstriction, masks hypoglycemic response and slow recovery, rebound hypertension/angina. Frequent: Bradycardia, fatigue, impotence.

NEBIVOLOL (Bystolic) ▸L ♀C ▶– $$$
WARNING — Avoid abrupt cessation in coronary heart disease or HTN.
ADULT — HTN: Start 5 mg PO daily, max 40 mg/day. Severe renal impairment (CrCl <30 mL/min), moderate hepatic impairment: Start 2.5 mg PO daily, increase cautiously.
PEDS — Not approved in children.
FORMS — Trade only: Tabs, unscored 2.5, 5, 10, 20 mg.
NOTES — Do not use with severe liver impairment.
MOA — At doses of 10 mg or less or for extensive metabolizers: beta-1 receptor selective. At doses greater than 10 mg or poor metazolizers: beta-1 and beta-2 receptor blocker.
ADVERSE EFFECTS — Serious: Bronchoconstriction. Frequent: Dizziness, fatigue, headache.

PINDOLOL ▸K ♀B ▶? $$$
WARNING — Avoid abrupt cessation in coronary heart disease or HTN.
ADULT — HTN: Start 5 mg PO two times per day, usual maintenance dose 10 to 30 mg/day, max 60 mg/day.
PEDS — Not approved in children.
UNAPPROVED ADULT — Angina: 15 to 40 mg/day PO in divided doses three to four times per day.
FORMS — Generic only: Tabs, scored 5, 10 mg.
NOTES — Has intrinsic sympathomimetic activity (partial beta-agonist activity); beta-1 and beta-2 receptor blocker. The brand name product (Visken) is no longer available.
MOA — Blocks binding of catecholamines to beta-1 and beta-2 receptors.
ADVERSE EFFECTS — Serious: Bronchoconstriction, masks hypoglycemic response and slow recovery, rebound hypertension/angina. Frequent: Bradycardia, fatigue, impotence.

PROPRANOLOL (Inderal, Inderal LA, InnoPran XL) ▸L ♀C ▶+ $$
WARNING — Avoid abrupt cessation in coronary heart disease or HTN.
ADULT — HTN: Start 20 to 40 mg PO two times per day, usual maintenance dose 160 to 480 mg/day, max 640 mg/day; extended-release (Inderal LA): Start 60 to 80 mg PO daily, usual maintenance dose 120 to 160 mg/day, max 640 mg/day; extended-release (InnoPran XL): Start 80 mg at bedtime (10 pm), max 120 mg at bedtime. Angina: Start 10 to 20 mg PO three to four times per day, usual maintenance 160 to 240 mg/day, max 320 mg/day; extended-release (Inderal LA): Start 80 mg PO daily, same usual dosage range and max for HTN. Migraine prophylaxis: Start 40 mg PO two times per day or 80 mg PO daily (extended-release), max 240 mg/day. Supraventricular tachycardia or rapid atrial fibrillation/flutter: 10 to 30 mg PO three to four times per day. MI: 180 to 240 mg/day PO in divided doses two to four times per day. Pheochromocytoma surgery: 60 mg PO in divided doses two to three times per day beginning 3 days before surgery, use in combination with an alpha-blocking agent. IV: Reserved for life-threatening arrhythmia, 1 to 3 mg IV, repeat dose in 2 min if needed, additional doses only after 4 h. Not for use in hypertensive emergency. Essential tremor: Start 40 mg PO two times per day, titrate prn to 120 to 320 mg/day.
PEDS — HTN: Start 1 mg/kg/day PO divided two times per day, usual maintenance dose 2 to 4 mg/kg/day PO divided two times per day, max 16 mg/kg/day.
UNAPPROVED ADULT — Prevent rebleeding esophageal varices: 20 to 180 mg PO two times per day. Titrate dose to reduce heart rate to 25% below baseline. Control heart rate with A-fib: 80 to 240 mg/day daily or in divided doses. Thyrotoxicosis: 60 to 80 mg q 4 h; or IV 0.5 to 1 mg over 10 min q 3 h.
UNAPPROVED PEDS — Arrhythmia: 0.01 to 0.1 mg/kg/dose (max 1 mg/dose) by slow IV push. Manufacturer does not recommend IV propranolol in children.
FORMS — Generic/Trade: Caps, extended-release 60, 80, 120, 160 mg. Generic only: Soln 20, 40 mg/5 mL. Tabs, scored 10, 20, 40, 60, 80 mg. Trade only: (InnoPran XL at bedtime) 80, 120 mg.
NOTES — Beta-1 and beta-2 receptor blocker. The immediate, and extended-release products may not give same clinical response on mg:mg basis; monitor response and side effects when interchanging between products. Extended-release caps (Inderal LA) may be opened, and the contents sprinkled on food for administration; cap contents should be swallowed whole without crushing or chewing. InnoPran XL is a chronotherapeutic product; give at bedtime to blunt early morning surge in BP. Acute alcohol use may increase propranolol level; chronic alcohol use may decrease propranolol level.
MOA — Blocks binding of catecholamines to beta-1 and beta-2 receptors.
ADVERSE EFFECTS — Serious: Anaphylaxis, agranulocytosis, bronchoconstriction, masks hypoglycemic response and slows recovery, rebound hypertension/angina, Stevens-Johnson syndrome. Frequent: Bradycardia, fatigue, dizziness, impotence.

TIMOLOL (Blocadren) ▸LK ♀C ▶+ $$$
WARNING — Avoid abrupt cessation in coronary heart disease or HTN.
ADULT — HTN: Start 10 mg PO two times per day, usual maintenance 20 to 40 mg/day, max 60 mg/day. MI: 10 mg PO two times per day, started 1 to 4 weeks post MI. Migraine headaches: Start 10 mg PO two times per day, use 20 mg/day daily or divided two times per day for prophylaxis, increase prn up to max 60 mg/day; stop therapy if satisfactory response not obtained after 6 to 8 weeks of max dose.
PEDS — Not approved in children.
UNAPPROVED ADULT — Angina: 15 to 45 mg/day PO divided three to four times per day.
FORMS — Generic only: Tabs, 5, 10, 20 mg.
NOTES — Beta-1 and beta-2 receptor blocker.
MOA — Blocks binding of catecholamines to beta-1 and beta-2 receptors.
ADVERSE EFFECTS — Serious: Bronchoconstriction, masks hypoglycemic response and slow recovery, rebound hypertension/angina. Frequent: Bradycardia, fatigue, impotence.

CARDIOVASCULAR: Calcium Channel Blockers (CCBs)—Dihydropyridines

NOTE: See also Antihypertensive Combinations. Avoid in decompensated heart failure. Peripheral edema, especially with higher doses. Extended/controlled/sustained-release tabs should be swallowed whole; do not chew or crush. Avoid grapefruit juice, which may enhance effect.

AMLODIPINE (*Norvasc*) ▶L ♀C ▶– $
ADULT — HTN, CAD: Start 5 mg PO daily, max 10 mg/day. Elderly, small, frail, or with hepatic insufficiency: Start 2.5 mg PO daily.
PEDS — HTN (6 to 17 yo): 2.5 to 5 mg PO daily.
UNAPPROVED PEDS — HTN: Start 0.1 to 0.2 mg/kg/day PO daily, max 0.3 mg/kg/day (max 10 mg daily).
FORMS — Generic/Trade: Tabs, unscored 2.5, 5, 10 mg.
NOTES — Do not use with more than 20 mg of simvastatin. Strong or moderate CYP3A4 inhibitors may increase levels and effects of amlodipine. May increase level of cyclosporine or tacrolimus. Monitor for hypotension if given concomitantly with sildenafil. Use cautiously with aortic valve stenosis or severe obstructive coronary artery disease.
MOA — Blocks calcium-dependent contractions in cardiac and peripheral smooth muscle leading to vasodilation.
ADVERSE EFFECTS — Serious: None. Frequent: Peripheral edema, headache, palpitations.

CLEVIDIPINE (*Cleviprex*) ▶KL ♀C ▶? $$$$$
ADULT — HTN: Start 1 to 2 mg/h IV, double dose q 1.5 min as approaches BP goal, then titrate at smaller increments q 5 to 10 min to desired BP, usual maintenance dose 4 to 6 mg/h, max 32 mg/h IV. An increase of 1 to 2 mg/h will decrease SBP approximately 2 to 4 mmHg.
PEDS — Not approved in children.
NOTES — Contraindicated with egg or soy allergy, defective lipid metabolism, or severe aortic stenosis. May exacerbate heart failure.
MOA — Blocks calcium-dependent contractions in cardiac and peripheral smooth muscle leading to vasodilation.
ADVERSE EFFECTS — Serious: Acute renal failure, atrial fib. Frequent: Headache, nausea, vomiting.

FELODIPINE (*Plendil*, ✢*Renedil*) ▶L ♀C ▶? $$
ADULT — HTN: Start 2.5 to 5 mg PO daily, usual maintenance dose 5 to 10 mg/day, max 10 mg/day.
PEDS — Not approved in children.
FORMS — Generic/Trade: Tabs, extended-release, unscored 2.5, 5, 10 mg.
NOTES — Extended-release tab. May increase tacrolimus level. Concomitant CYP3A4 inhibitors (eg ketoconazole, itraconazole, erythromycin, grapefruit juice, cimetidine) may increase felodipine level.
MOA — Blocks calcium-dependent contractions in cardiac and peripheral smooth muscle leading to vasodilation.
ADVERSE EFFECTS — Serious: None. Frequent: Peripheral edema, headache, palpitations.

ISRADIPINE ▶L ♀C ▶? $$$$
ADULT — HTN: Start 2.5 mg PO two times per day, usual maintenance 5 to 10 mg/day, max 20 mg/day divided two times per day (max 10 mg/day in elderly).

PEDS — Not approved in children.
FORMS — Generic only: Immediate-release caps 2.5, 5 mg.
NOTES — The brand name product (DynaCirc) is no longer available.
MOA — Blocks calcium-dependent contractions in cardiac and peripheral smooth muscle leading to vasodilation.
ADVERSE EFFECTS — Serious: Angioedema. Frequent: Peripheral edema, headache, palpitations.

NICARDIPINE (*Cardene, Cardene SR*) ▶L ♀C ▶? $$$
ADULT — HTN: Sustained-release (Cardene SR): Start 30 mg PO two times per day, usual maintenance dose 30 to 60 mg PO two times per day, max 120 mg/day; immediate-release, start 20 mg PO three times per day, usual maintenance dose 20 to 40 mg PO three times per day, max 120 mg/day. Angina: Immediate-release, start 20 mg PO three times per day, usual maintenance dose 20 to 40 mg three times per day. Short-term management of HTN, patient not receiving PO nicardipine: Begin IV infusion at 5 mg/h, titrate infusion rate by 2.5 mg/h q 5 to 15 min prn, max 15 mg/h. Short-term management of HTN, patient receiving PO nicardipine: If using 20 mg PO q 8 h, give 0.5 mg/h IV; if using 30 mg PO q 8 h, give 1.2 mg/h IV; if using 40 mg PO q 8 h, give 2.2 mg/h. When discontinuing IV nicardipine and transitioning to an oral BP regimen: Administer 1st dose of nicardipine PO 1 h prior to discontinuing IV infusion, or initiate BP-lowering agent other than nicardipine upon discontinuation of IV infusion.
PEDS — Not approved in children.
UNAPPROVED PEDS — HTN: 0.5 to 3 mcg/kg/min IV infusion.
FORMS — Generic/Trade: Caps, immediate-release 20, 30 mg. Trade only: Caps, sustained-release 30, 45, 60 mg.
NOTES — Decrease dose if hepatically impaired. Titrate carefully if renally impaired. Use sustained-release caps for HTN only, not for angina. May increase cyclosporine level. Concomitant cimetidine may increase nicardipine level.
MOA — Blocks calcium-dependent contractions in cardiac and peripheral smooth muscle leading to vasodilation.
ADVERSE EFFECTS — Serious: Hypotension. Frequent: Peripheral edema, headache, palpitations.

NIFEDIPINE (*Procardia, Adalat, Procardia XL, Adalat CC, Afeditab CR*, ✢*Adalat XL*) ▶L ♀C ▶– $$
ADULT — HTN: Extended-release: Start 30 to 60 mg PO daily, max 120 mg/day. Angina: Extended-release: Start 30 to 60 mg PO daily, max 120 mg/day; immediate-release: Start 10 mg PO three times per day, usual maintenance dose 10 to 20 mg tid, max 120 mg/day.
PEDS — Not approved in children.

(cont.)

NIFEDIPINE (*cont.*)

UNAPPROVED ADULT — Preterm labor: Loading dose 10 mg PO q 20 to 30 min if contractions persist up to 40 mg within the 1st h. After contractions are controlled, maintenance dose: 10 to 20 mg PO q 4 to 6 h or 60 to 160 mg extended-release PO daily. Duration of treatment has not been established. Promotes spontaneous passage of ureteral calculi: Extended-release, 30 mg PO daily for 10 to 28 days.

UNAPPROVED PEDS — HTN: 0.25 to 0.5 mg/kg/dose PO q 4 to 6 h prn, max 10 mg/dose or 3 mg/kg/day. Doses less than 0.25 mg/kg may be effective.

FORMS — Generic/Trade: Caps 10, 20 mg. Tabs, extended-release (Adalat CC, Afeditab CR, Procardia XL) 30, 60 mg; (Adalat CC, Procardia XL) 90 mg.

NOTES — Do not use immediate-release caps for treating HTN, hypertensive emergencies, or ST-elevation MI. Immediate-release cap should not be chewed and swallowed or given sublingually; may cause excessive hypotension, CVA. Extended-release tabs can be substituted for immediate-release caps at the same dose in patients whose angina is controlled. Extended-release tab has been associated with gastrointestinal obstruction; use extended-release tab cautiously in patients with pre-existing severe gastrointestinal narrowing. Metabolized by the CYP3A4 enzyme system. Use alternative BP-lowering medication when patient on carbamazepine, phenobarbital, phenytoin, rifampin, or St. John's wort; these reduce levels of nifedipine significantly. Concomitant clarithromycin, erythromycin, fluconazole, fluoxetine, grapefruit, HIV protease inhibitors, ketoconazole, itraconazole, or nefazodone increases nifedipine level. Increases tacrolimus level. Avoid grapefruit juice while taking nifedipine. Severe hypotension and/or increased fluid volume requirements may occur when used with beta-blocker for patient who had surgery using high-dose fentanyl anesthesia; when appropriate, discontinue nifedipine at least 36 h prior to surgery that may require high dose fentanyl anesthesia.

MOA — Blocks calcium-dependent contractions in cardiac and peripheral smooth muscle leading to vasodilation. Tocolytic.

ADVERSE EFFECTS — Serious: Hypotension, gastrointestinal obstruction (extended-release tab). Frequent: Peripheral edema, headache, palpitations, flushing.

NISOLDIPINE (*Sular*) ▶L ♀C ▶? $$$$$

ADULT — HTN: Start 17 mg PO daily, may increase by 8.5 mg weekly, max 34 mg/day. Impaired hepatic function, elderly: Start 8.5 mg PO daily, titrate prn.

PEDS — Not approved in children.

FORMS — Generic/Trade: Tabs, extended-release 8.5, 17, 25.5, 34 mg. These replace the former 10, 20, 30, 40 mg tabs. Generic only: Tabs, extended-release 20, 30, 40 mg.

NOTES — Take on an empty stomach. Sular 8.5, 17, 25.5, 34 mg replace 10, 20, 30, 40 mg, respectively.

MOA — Blocks calcium-dependent contractions in cardiac and peripheral smooth muscle leading to vasodilation.

ADVERSE EFFECTS — Serious: None. Frequent: Peripheral edema, headache, palpitations.

CARDIOVASCULAR: Calcium Channel Blockers (CCBs)—Non-Dihydropyridines

NOTE: See also Antihypertensive Combinations. Avoid in decompensated heart failure, 2nd/3rd degree heart block without pacemaker, acute MI and pulmonary congestion, or systolic blood pressure <90 mm Hg systolic.

DILTIAZEM (*Cardizem, Cardizem LA, Cardizem CD, Cartia XT, Dilacor XR, Diltiazem CD, Diltzac, Diltia XT, Matzim LA, Tiazac, Taztia XT*) ▶L ♀C ▶+ $$

ADULT — Atrial fibrillation/flutter, PSVT: 20 mg (0.25 mg/kg) IV bolus over 2 min. If needed and patient tolerated, IV bolus with no hypotension, rebolus 15 min later with 25 mg (0.35 mg/kg). IV infusion: Start 10 mg/h, increase by 5 mg/h (usual range 5 to 15 mg/h). HTN, once a day, extended-release (Cardizem CD, Cartia XT, Dilacor XR, Diltia XT, Taztia XT, Tiazac): Start 120 to 240 mg PO daily, usual maintenance range 240 to 360 mg/day, max 540 mg/day. HTN, once a day, graded extended-release (Cardizem LA): Start 180 to 240 mg, max 540 mg/day. HTN, twice a day, sustained-release (Cardizem SR): Start 60 to 120 mg PO two times per day, max 360 mg/day. Angina, immediate-release: Start 30 mg PO four times per day, max 360 mg/day divided three to four times per day. Angina, extended-release: 120 to 180 mg PO daily, max 540 mg/day. Angina, once a day, graded extended-release (Cardizem LA): Start 180 mg PO daily, doses greater than 360 mg may provide no additional benefit.

PEDS — Not approved in children. Diltiazem injection should be avoided in neonates due to potential toxicity from benzyl alcohol in the injectable product.

UNAPPROVED ADULT — Control heart rate with chronic A-fib: 120 to 360 mg/day daily or in divided doses.

UNAPPROVED PEDS — HTN: Start 1.5 to 2 mg/kg/day PO divided three to four times per day, max 3.5 mg/kg/day.

FORMS — Generic/Trade: Tabs, immediate-release, unscored (Cardizem) 30 mg, scored 60, 90, 120 mg. Caps, extended-release (Cardizem CD, Cartia XT daily) 120, 180, 240, 300, 360 mg, (Diltzac, Taztia XT, Tiazac daily) 120, 180, 240, 300, 360, 420 mg, (Dilacor XR, Diltia XT) 120, 180, 240 mg. Tabs, extended-release (Cardizem LA daily, Matzim LA) 180, 240, 300, 360, 420 mg. Generic only: Caps, extended release (twice daily) 60, 90, 120 mg. Trade only: Tabs, extended-release (Cardizem LA daily) 120 mg.

NOTES — Sinus bradycardia resulting in hospitalization and pacemaker insertion has been reported with concomitant clonidine; monitor heart rate. May

(cont.)

DILTIAZEM (cont.)

increase levels of buspirone, lovastatin, quinidine, simvastatin. Do not use with more than 10 mg of simvastatin or 20 mg of lovastatin. Contents of extended-release caps may be sprinkled over food. Do not chew or crush cap contents. May accumulate with hepatic impairment. Monitor response and side effects when interchanging between diltiazem products; many are not equivalent on mg:mg basis. Cardizem LA is a chronotherapeutic product; give at bedtime to blunt early morning surge in BP.

MOA — Blocks calcium-dependent contractions in cardiac and peripheral smooth muscle leading to vasodilation; slows cardiac conduction through the AV node.

ADVERSE EFFECTS — Serious: Bradycardia, heart block (rare). Frequent: Peripheral edema, headache.

VERAPAMIL (Isoptin SR, Calan, Calan SR, Verelan, Verelan PM) ▸L ♀C ▶– $$

ADULT — SVT: 5 to 10 mg (0.075 to 0.15 mg/kg) IV over 2 min; a 2nd dose of 10 mg IV may be given 15 to 30 min later if needed. PSVT/rate control with atrial fibrillation: 240 to 480 mg/day PO divided three to four times per day. Angina: Start 40 to 80 mg PO three to four times per day, max 480 mg/day; sustained-release(Isoptin SR, Calan SR, Verelan), start 120 to 240 mg PO daily, max 480 mg/day (use twice-daily dosing for doses greater than 240 mg/day with Isoptin SR and Calan SR). HTN: Same as angina (except Verelan PM), start 100 to 200 mg PO at bedtime max 400 mg/day; immediate-release tabs should be avoided in treating HTN.

PEDS — SVT, age 1 to 15 yo: 2 to 5 mg (0.1 to 0.3 mg/kg) IV, max dose 5 mg. Repeat dose once in 30 min if needed, max 2nd dose 10 mg. Immediate-release and sustained-release tabs not approved in children.

FORMS — Generic/Trade: Tabs, immediate-release, scored (Calan) 40, 80, 120 mg. Tabs, sustained-release, unscored (Isoptin SR, Calan SR) 120 mg, scored 180, 240 mg. Caps, sustained-release (Verelan) 120, 180, 240, 360 mg. Caps, extended-release (Verelan PM) 100, 200, 300 mg.

NOTES — Contraindicated in severe LV dysfunction, A-fib/flutter conducted via accessory pathway (ie, Wolff-Parkinson-White). Grapefruit juice may increase level. Do not use with ivabradine. Do not use with more than 10 mg of simvastatin or 20 mg of lovastatin. Hypotension, bradyarrhythmias, and lactic acidosis have been reported with concomitant telithromycin. Sinus bradycardia resulting in hospitalization and pacemaker insertion has been reported with concomitant clonidine; monitor heart rate. May increase digoxin level 50 to 75%. May increase doxorubicin level. May change the level of certain chemotherapeutic agents; may get reduced absorption of verapamil with some chemotherapeutic regimens; see prescribing information for complete list. Scored, sustained-release tabs (Calan SR, Isoptin SR) may be broken and each piece swallowed whole; do not chew or crush. Monitor response and side effects when interchanging between verapamil products; many are not equivalent on mg:mg basis. Contents of sustained-release caps may be sprinkled on food (eg, applesauce). Do not chew or crush cap contents. Use cautiously with impaired renal/hepatic function. Verelan PM is a chronotherapeutic product; give at bedtime to blunt early morning surge in BP.

MOA — Blocks calcium-dependent contractions in cardiac and peripheral smooth muscle leading to vasodilation; slows cardiac conduction through the SA node.

ADVERSE EFFECTS — Serious: Bradycardia, heart block (rare). Frequent: Constipation, headache.

CARDIOVASCULAR: Diuretics—Loop

NOTE: Thiazides are preferred diuretics for HTN. With decreased renal function (CrCl <30 mL/min), loop diuretics may be more effective than thiazides for HTN. Rare hypersensitivity in patients allergic to sulfa-containing drugs, except ethacrynic acid. For diuretics given two times per day, give second dose in mid-afternoon to avoid nocturia.

BUMETANIDE (Bumex, ✦Burinex) ▸K ♀C ▶? $

ADULT — Edema: 0.5 to 2 mg PO daily, repeat doses at 4 to 5 h intervals prn until desired response is attained, max 10 mg/day; 0.5 to 1 mg IV/IM, repeat doses at 2 to 3 h intervals prn until desired response is attained, max 10 mg/day. Dosing for 3 to 4 consecutive days followed by no drug for 1 to 2 days is acceptable. Twice-daily dosing may enhance diuretic effect. IV injections should be over 1 to 2 min. An IV infusion may be used, change bag q 24 h.

PEDS — Not approved in children.

UNAPPROVED PEDS — Edema: 0.015 to 0.1 mg/kg/dose PO/IV/IM daily or every other day, max 0.1 mg/kg/day or 10 mg/day.

FORMS — Generic only: Tabs, scored 0.5, 1, 2 mg.

NOTES — Bumetanide 1 mg is roughly equivalent to furosemide 40 mg. IV administration is preferred when GI absorption is impaired.

MOA — Block chloride reabsorption by inhibiting the $Na^+/K^+/Cl^-$ cotransport system in the thick ascending limb of the loop of Henle.

ADVERSE EFFECTS — Serious: Electrolyte imbalances (hypokalemia, hyponatremia, hypochloremic alkalosis, hypomagnesemia, hypocalcemia, hyperuricemia), dehydration, ototoxicity (rare), skin reactions. Frequent: Dizziness, headache, fatigue, muscle cramps, impotence.

ETHACRYNIC ACID (Edecrin) ▸K ♀B ▶? $$$$$

ADULT — Edema: 0.5 to 1 mg/kg IV, max 100 mg/dose; 25 mg PO daily on day 1, followed by 50 mg PO two times per day on day 2, followed by 100 mg PO in the morning and 50 to 100 mg PO in the evening

(cont.)

ETHACRYNIC ACID (cont.)

depending on the response to the morning dose, max 400 mg/day.

PEDS — Not approved in children.

UNAPPROVED ADULT — HTN: 25 mg PO daily, max 100 mg/day divided two to three times per day.

UNAPPROVED PEDS — Edema: 1 mg/kg IV; 25 mg PO daily, increase slowly by 25 mg increments prn. Ethacrynic acid should not be administered to infants.

FORMS — Trade only: Tabs, scored 25 mg.

NOTES — Ototoxicity possible. Does not contain a sulfonamide group; can be safely used in patients with true sulfa allery. Do not administer SC or IM due to local irritation. IV ethacrynic acid should be reconstituted to a concentration of 50 mg/mL and given slowly by IV infusion over 20 to 30 min. May increase lithium levels.

MOA — Block chloride reabsorption by inhibiting the Na+/K+/Cl- cotransport system in the thick ascending limb of the loop of Henle.

ADVERSE EFFECTS — Serious: Electrolyte imbalances (hypokalemia, hyponatremia, hypochloremic alkalosis, hypomagnesemia, hypocalcemia, hyperuricemia), dehydration, pancreatitis (rare), photosensitivity (rare), ototoxicity (rare). Frequent: Dizziness, headache, fatigue, muscle cramps, impotence.

FUROSEMIDE (Lasix) ▶K ♀C ▶? $

ADULT — HTN: Start 10 to 40 mg PO two times per day, max 600 mg daily. Edema: Start 20 to 80 mg IV/IM/PO, increase dose by 20 to 40 mg in 6 to 8 h until desired response is achieved, max 600 mg/day. Give maintenance dose daily or divided two times per day. IV infusion: 0.05 mg/kg/h, titrate rate to desired response.

PEDS — Edema: 0.5 to 2 mg/kg/dose IV/IM/PO q 6 to 12 h, max 6 mg/kg/dose. IV infusion: 0.05 mg/kg/h, titrate rate to achieve desired response.

UNAPPROVED ADULT — Ascites: 40 mg PO daily in combination with spironolactone; may increase dose after 2 to 3 days if no response.

FORMS — Generic/Trade: Tabs, unscored 20, scored 40, 80 mg. Generic only: Oral soln 10 mg/mL, 40 mg/5 mL.

NOTES — Oral absorption may decrease in acute heart failure exacerbation. Bioequivalence of oral form is 50% of IV dose. Monitor renal function in elderly. Do not use with lithium. Increases risk of ototoxicity when used with other drugs associated with ototoxicity, especially with renal dysfunction. May potentiate renal dysfunction when used with other drugs associated with renal dysfunction. May antagonize the muscle-relaxing effects of tubocurarine. Doses >80 mg/day has been associated with lower total thyroid hormone levels. Ototoxicity is associated with rapid IV administration (more than 4 mg/min).

MOA — Block chloride reabsorption by inhibiting the Na+/K+/Cl- cotransport system in the thick ascending limb of the loop of Henle.

ADVERSE EFFECTS — Serious: Electrolyte imbalances (hypokalemia, hyponatremia, hypochloremic alkalosis, hypomagnesemia, hypocalcemia, hyperuricemia), dehydration, pancreatitis (rare), photosensitivity (rare), hypersensitivity (rare), ototoxicity (rare), dermatologic-hypersensitivity reactions. Frequent: Dizziness, headache, fatigue, muscle cramps, impotence.

TORSEMIDE (Demadex) ▶LK ♀B ▶? $

ADULT — HTN: Start 5 mg PO daily, increase prn q 4 to 6 weeks, max 10 mg daily. Edema: Start 10 to 20 mg IV/PO daily, double dose prn, max 200 mg IV/PO daily. Ascites: 5 to 10 mg IV/PO daily, double dose prn, max 40 mg daily.

PEDS — Not approved in children.

FORMS — Generic/Trade: Tabs, scored 5, 10, 20, 100 mg.

MOA — Block chloride reabsorption by inhibiting the Na+/K+/Cl- cotransport system in the thick ascending limb of the loop of Henle.

ADVERSE EFFECTS — Serious: Electrolyte imbalances (hypokalemia, hyponatremia, hypochloremic alkalosis, hypomagnesemia, hypocalcemia, hyperuricemia), dehydration, pancreatitis (rare), photosensitivity (rare), hypersensitivity (rare). Frequent: Dizziness, headache, fatigue, muscle cramps, impotence.

CARDIOVASCULAR: Diuretics—Potassium-Sparing

NOTE: See also antihypertensive combinations and aldosterone antagonists. May cause hyperkalemia; greater incidence with renal impairment, diabetes, or elderly. Monitor potassium levels before initiating therapy, when adjusting diuretic doses, and with illness that may alter renal function. Use cautiously with other agents that may cause hyperkalemia (ie, ACE inhibitors, ARBs, aliskiren, potassium containing salt substitutes).

AMILORIDE (Midamor) ▶LK ♀B ▶? $$$

WARNING — May cause hyperkalemia.

ADULT — Diuretic-induced hypokalemia: Start 5 mg PO daily, increase prn, max 20 mg/day. Edema/HTN: Start 5 mg PO daily in combination with another diuretic, usually a thiazide for HTN, increase prn, max 20 mg/day. Other diuretics may need to be added when treating edema.

PEDS — Not approved in children.

UNAPPROVED ADULT — Hyperaldosteronism: 10 to 40 mg PO daily. Do not use combination product (Moduretic) for treatment of primary hyperaldosteronism.

UNAPPROVED PEDS — Edema: 0.625 mg/kg daily for children weighing 6 to 20 kg.

FORMS — Generic only: Tabs, unscored 5 mg.

(cont.)

AMILORIDE (*cont.*)

NOTES — Spironolactone is generally preferred for treating primary hyperaldosteronism.

MOA — Block sodium reabsorption and potassium excretion in the distal tubule.

ADVERSE EFFECTS — Serious: Hyperkalemia (rare). Frequent: Headache.

TRIAMTERENE (*Dyrenium*) ▶LK ♀B ▶– $$$

WARNING — May cause hyperkalemia. Incidence is greater with renal impairment, diabetes, or elderly. Monitor potassium frequently, before initiation, when adjusting diuretic doses, and with illness that may alter renal function.

ADULT — Edema (cirrhosis, nephrotic syndrome, heart failure): Start 100 mg PO two times per day, max 300 mg/day. Most patients can be maintained on 100 mg PO daily or every other day after edema is controlled. Other diuretics may be needed.

PEDS — Not approved in children.

UNAPPROVED PEDS — Edema: 4 mg/kg/day divided two times per day after meals, increase to 6 mg/kg/day if needed, max 300 mg/day.

FORMS — Trade only: Caps 50, 100 mg.

NOTES — Combo product with HCTZ (eg Dyazide, Maxzide) available for HTN.

MOA — Block sodium reabsorption and potassium excretion in the distal tubule.

ADVERSE EFFECTS — Serious: Hyperkalemia (rare). Frequent: Headache.

CARDIOVASCULAR: Diuretics—Thiazide Type

NOTE: See also Antihypertensive Combinations. Possible hypersensitivity in sulfa allergy. Should be used for most patients with HTN, alone or combined with other antihypertensive agents. Thiazides are not recommended for gestational HTN. Coadministration with NSAIDs, including selective COX-2 inhibitors, may reduce the antihypertensive, diuretic, and natriuretic effects of thiazides. Thiazide-induced hypokalemia is associated with increased fasting blood glucose and new-onset DM; keep potassium ≥4.0 mg/dL to minimize risk; may use thiazide in combination with oral potassium supplementation, ACE inhibitor, ARB, or potassium-sparing diuretic to maintain K level. Lithium level may increase with concomitant use; monitor lithium level.

CHLOROTHIAZIDE (*Diuril*) ▶L ♀C, D if used in pregnancy-induced HTN ▶+ $

ADULT — HTN: Start 125 to 250 mg PO daily or divided two times per day, max 1000 mg/day divided two times per day. Edema: 500 to 2000 mg PO/IV daily or divided two times per day. Dosing on alternate days or for 3 to 4 consecutive days followed by no drug for 1 to 2 days is acceptable.

PEDS — Edema: Infants: Start 10 to 20 mg/kg/day PO daily or divided two times per day, up to 30 mg/kg/day divided two times per day. Children 6 mo to 2 yo: 10 to 20 mg/kg/day PO daily or divided two times per day, max 375 mg/day. Children 2 to 12 yo: Start 10 to 20 mg/kg/day PO daily or divided two times per day, up to 1 g/day. IV formulation not recommended for infants or children.

FORMS — Trade only: Susp 250 mg/5 mL. Generic only: Tabs, scored 250, 500 mg.

NOTES — Do not administer SC or IM.

MOA — Blocks sodium and chloride reabsorption in the distal tubules.

ADVERSE EFFECTS — Serious: Electrolyte imbalances (hypokalemia, hyponatremia, hypomagnesemia, hypercalcemia, hyperuricemia), pancreatitis (rare), photosensitivity (rare), hypersensitivity (rare). Frequent: Dizziness, headache, fatigue, muscle cramps, impotence.

CHLORTHALIDONE ▶L ♀B, D if used in pregnancy-induced HTN ▶+ $

ADULT — HTN: For generic, start 12.5 to 25 mg PO daily, usual maintenance dose 12.5 to 50 mg/day, max 50 mg/day. Edema: For generic, start 50 to 100 mg PO daily or 100 mg every other day or 100 mg 3 times a week, usual maintenance dose 150 to 200 mg/day, max 200 mg/day.

PEDS — Not approved in children.

UNAPPROVED ADULT — Nephrolithiasis: 25 to 50 mg PO daily.

UNAPPROVED PEDS — Edema: 2 mg/kg PO 3 times a week.

FORMS — Generic only: Tabs, unscored 25, 50 mg.

NOTES — Doses greater than 50 mg/day for HTN have significantly more hypokalemia with no greater antihypertensive effects.

MOA — Blocks sodium and chloride reabsorption in the distal tubules and decreases urinary calcium excretion.

ADVERSE EFFECTS — Serious: Agranulocytosis, aplastic anemia, electrolyte imbalances (hypokalemia, hyponatremia, hypomagnesemia, hypercalcemia, hyperuricemia), pancreatitis (rare), photosensitivity (rare), hypersensitivity (rare), thrombocytopenia. Frequent: Dizziness, headache, fatigue, muscle cramps, impotence.

HYDROCHLOROTHIAZIDE (*HCTZ, Oretic, Microzide*) ▶L ♀B, D if used in pregnancy-induced HTN ▶+ $

ADULT — HTN: Start 12.5 to 25 mg PO daily, usual maintenance dose 25 mg/day, max 50 mg/day. Edema: 25 to 100 mg PO daily or in divided doses or 50 to 100 mg PO every other day or 3 to 5 days/week, max 200 mg/day.

PEDS — Edema: 1 to 2 mg/kg/day PO daily or divided two times per day, max 37.5 mg/day in infants up to 2 yo, max 100 mg/day in children 2 to 12 yo.

UNAPPROVED ADULT — Nephrolithiasis: 50 to 100 mg PO daily.

FORMS — Generic/Trade: Tabs, scored 25, 50 mg. Caps 12.5 mg.

NOTES — Avoid use with hypercalcemia. Doses 50 mg/day or greater may cause hypokalemia with

(cont.)

HYDROCHLOROTHIAZIDE (*cont.*)

little added BP control. Concomitant cyclosporine increases risk of hypercalcemia and gout. Concomitant steroid or ACTH increases risk of hypokalemia. Concomitant diazoxide increases risk of hyperglycemia. May decrease renal excretion of cytotoxic agents (eg cyclophosphamide, methotrexate) and increase myelosuppresive effects.

MOA — Blocks sodium and chloride reabsorption in the distal tubules and decreases urinary calcium excretion.

ADVERSE EFFECTS — Agranulocytosis, aplastic anemia, electrolyte imbalances (hypokalemia, hyponatremia, hypomagnesemia, hypercalcemia, hyperuricemia),acute myopia and secondary acute angle closure glaucoma, pancreatitis (rare), photosensitivity (rare), hypersensitivity (rare), thrombocytopenia. Frequent: Dizziness, headache, fatigue, muscle cramps, impotence.

INDAPAMIDE (✚*Lozide*) ▶L ♀B, D if used in pregnancy-induced HTN ▶? $

ADULT — HTN: Start 1.25 to 2.5 mg PO daily, max 5 mg/day. Edema/heart failure: 2.5 to 5 mg PO q am.

PEDS — Not approved in children.

FORMS — Generic only: Tabs, unscored 1.25, 2.5 mg.

NOTES — The brand name product (Lozol) is no longer available.

MOA — Blocks sodium and chloride reabsorption in the distal tubules.

ADVERSE EFFECTS — Serious: Electrolyte imbalances (hypokalemia, hyponatremia, hypomagnesemia, hypercalcemia, hyperuricemia), pancreatitis (rare), photosensitivity (rare), hypersensitivity (rare). Frequent: Dizziness, headache, fatigue, muscle cramps, impotence.

METHYCLOTHIAZIDE (*Enduron*) ▶L ♀B, D if used in pregnancy-induced HTN ▶? $$$

ADULT — HTN: Start 2.5 mg PO daily, usual maintenance dose 2.5 to 5 mg/day. Edema: Start 2.5 mg PO daily, usual maintenance dose 2.5 to 10 mg/day.

PEDS — Not approved in children.

FORMS — Generic only: Tabs, scored, 5 mg.

MOA — Blocks sodium and chloride reabsorption in the distal tubules.

ADVERSE EFFECTS — Serious: Electrolyte imbalances (hypokalemia, hyponatremia, hypomagnesemia, hypercalcemia, hyperuricemia), pancreatitis (rare), photosensitivity (rare), hypersensitivity (rare). Frequent: Dizziness, headache, fatigue, muscle cramps, impotence.

METOLAZONE ▶L ♀B, D if used in pregnancy-induced HTN ▶? $$$

ADULT — Edema (heart failure, renal disease): 5 to 10 mg PO daily, max 10 mg/day in heart failure, 20 mg/day in renal disease. If used with loop diuretic, start with 2.5 mg PO daily. Reduce to lowest effective dose as edema resolves. May be given every other day as edema resolves.

PEDS — Not approved in children.

UNAPPROVED PEDS — Edema: 0.2 to 0.4 mg/kg/day daily or divided two times per day.

FORMS — Generic: Tabs 2.5, 5, 10 mg.

NOTES — Generally used for diuretic resistance, not HTN. When used with furosemide or other loop diuretics, administer metolazone 30 min before IV loop diuretic. Correct electrolyte imbalances before initiating therapy. Combination diuretic therapy may increase the risk of electrolyte disturbances. The brand name product (Zaroxolyn) is no longer available.

MOA — Blocks sodium and chloride reabsorption in the distal tubules.

ADVERSE EFFECTS — Serious: Electrolyte imbalances (hypokalemia, hyponatremia, hypomagnesemia, hypercalcemia, hyperuricemia), pancreatitis (rare), photosensitivity (rare), hypersensitivity (rare). Frequent: Dizziness, headache, fatigue, muscle cramps, impotence.

CARDIOVASCULAR: Nitrates

NOTE: Avoid if systolic BP below 90 mmHg or below baseline by more than 30 mmHg, severe bradycardia (less than 50 bpm), tachycardia (greater than 100 bpm), or right ventricular infarction. Avoid if patient takes PDE-5 inhibitor (eg, avanafil, sildenafil, tadalafil, vardenafil or guanylate cyclase stimulators (eg, riociguat).

ISOSORBIDE DINITRATE (*Isordil, Dilatrate-SR*) ▶L ♀C ▶? $$$

ADULT — Angina prophylaxis: Start 5 to 20 mg PO three times per day (7 am, noon, and 5 pm), max 40 mg three times per day. Sustained-release (Dilatrate SR): Start 40 mg PO two times per day, max 80 mg PO two times per day (8 am and 2 pm).

PEDS — Not approved in children.

UNAPPROVED ADULT — Heart failure: 10 to 40 mg PO three times per day, max 80 mg three times per day. Use in combination with hydralazine.

FORMS — Generic/Trade: Tabs, scored 5 mg. Trade only: Tabs, scored (Isordil) 40 mg. Caps, extended-release (Dilatrate-SR) 40 mg. Generic only: Tabs, scored 10, 20, 30 mg. Tabs, scored, sustained-release 40 mg.

NOTES — Do not use for acute angina. Extended-release tab may be broken, but do not chew or crush, swallow whole. Allow for a nitrate-free period of 10 to 14 h each day to avoid nitrate tolerance.

MOA — Relaxes cardiac and peripheral smooth muscle (venous greater than arterial).

ADVERSE EFFECTS — Serious: Hypotension, methemoglobinemia (rare). Frequent: Headache, tachycardia, dizziness, flushing.

ISOSORBIDE MONONITRATE ▶L ♀C ▶? $

ADULT — Angina: 20 mg PO two times per day (8 am and 3 pm). Extended-release: Start 30 to 60 mg PO daily, max 240 mg/day.

PEDS — Not approved in children.

(cont.)

ISOSORBIDE MONONITRATE (*cont.*)

FORMS — Generic only: Tabs, 10, 20 mg. Tabs, extended-release, scored 30, 60; unscored 120 mg.

NOTES — Extended-release tab may be broken, but do not chew or crush; swallow whole. Do not use for acute angina. The brand names (Imdur, Ismo, Monoket) are no longer available.

MOA — Relaxes cardiac and peripheral smooth muscle (venous greater than arterial).

ADVERSE EFFECTS — Serious: Hypotension, methemoglobinemia (rare). Frequent: Headache, tachycardia, dizziness, flushing.

NITROGLYCERIN INTRAVENOUS INFUSION ▸L ♀C ▸? $

ADULT — Perioperative HTN, acute MI/heart failure, acute angina: Mix 50 mg in 250 mL D5W (200 mcg/mL), start at 10 to 20 mcg/min IV (3 to 6 mL/h), then titrate upward by 10 to 20 mcg/min q 3 to 5 min until desired effect is achieved.

PEDS — Not approved in children.

UNAPPROVED ADULT — Hypertensive emergency: Start 10 to 20 mcg/min IV infusion, titrate up to 100 mcg/min. Antihypertensive effect is usually evident in 2 to 5 min. Effect may persist for only 3 to 5 min after infusion is stopped.

UNAPPROVED PEDS — IV infusion: Start 0.25 to 0.5 mcg/kg/min, increase by 0.5 to 1 mcg/kg/min q 3 to 5 min prn, max 5 mcg/kg/min.

NOTES — Nitroglycerin migrates into polyvinyl chloride (PVC) tubing. Use lower initial doses (5 mcg/min) with non-PVC tubing. Contraindicated with with pericardial tamponade, restrictive cardiomyopathy, or constrictive pericarditis. Use with caution in inferior/right ventricular MI.

MOA — Relaxes cardiac and peripheral smooth muscle (venous greater than arterial).

ADVERSE EFFECTS — Serious: Hypotension, methemoglobinemia (rare). Frequent: Headache, tachycardia, dizziness, flushing.

NITROGLYCERIN OINTMENT (*Nitro-BID*) ▸L ♀C ▸? $$$

ADULT — Angina prophylaxis: Start 0.5 inch q 8 h applied to nonhairy skin area, maintenance 1 to 2 inch q 8 h, max 4 inch q 4 to 6 h.

PEDS — Not approved in children.

FORMS — Trade only: Oint, 2%, tubes 1, 30, 60 g (Nitro-BID).

NOTES — Do not use for acute angina attack. One inch ointment contains about 15 mg nitroglycerin. Allow for a nitrate-free period of 10 to 14 h each day to avoid nitrate tolerance. Generally change to oral tabs or transdermal patch for long-term therapy.

MOA — Relaxes cardiac and peripheral smooth muscle (venous greater than arterial).

ADVERSE EFFECTS — Serious: Hypotension, methemoglobinemia (rare). Frequent: Headache, tachycardia, dizziness, flushing.

NITROGLYCERIN SPRAY (*Nitrolingual, NitroMist*) ▸L ♀C ▸? $$$$$

ADULT — Acute angina: 1 to 2 sprays under the tongue at the onset of attack, repeat prn, max 3 sprays in 15 min. A dose may be given 5 to 10 min before activities that might provoke angina.

PEDS — Not approved in children.

FORMS — Generic/Trade: Nitrolingual soln, 4.9, 12 g. 0.4 mg/spray (60 or 200 sprays/canister). NitroMist aerosol, 4.1, 8.5 g; 0.4 mg/spray (90 or 200 sprays/canister).

NOTES — AHA guidelines recommend calling 911 if chest pain not relieved or gets worse after using 1 dose of nitroglycerin. May be preferred over SL tabs in patients with dry mouth. Patient can see how much medicine is left in the upright bottle. Nitrolingual: Replace bottle when fluid is below level of center tube; NitroMist: Replace bottle when fluid reaches the bottom of the hole in the side of the container. Before initial use, prime pump: Nitrolingual, spray 5 times into air (away from self and others); NitroMist, spray 10 times into air (away from self and others). Prime at least once q 6 weeks if not used: Nitrolingual spray 1 time into the air (away from self and others); NitroMist spray twice into the air (away from self and others). Do not shake NitroMist before using.

MOA — Relaxes cardiac and peripheral smooth muscle (venous greater than arterial).

ADVERSE EFFECTS — Serious: Hypotension. Frequent: Headache, tingling/mouth burning, tachycardia, dizziness, flushing.

NITROGLYCERIN SUBLINGUAL (*Nitrostat, GONITRO*) ▸L ♀B ▸? $

ADULT — Acute angina, sublingual tabs: 0.4 mg under tongue or between the cheek and gum, repeat dose q 5 min prn up to 3 doses in 15 min. A dose may be given 5 to 10 min before activities that might provoke angina. Acute angina, sublingual powder: 0.4 to 0.8 mg under under tongue, repeat dose q 5 min prn up to 3 packets (1.2 mg total) in 15 min. Angina prophylaxis, sublingual tabs: 0.4 mg under tongue may be given 5 to 10 min before activities that might provoke angina. Angina prophylaxis, sublingual powder: 0.4 to 0.8 mg under tongue may be given 5 to 10 min before activities that might provoke angina.

PEDS — Not approved in children.

FORMS — Trade only: SL tabs, unscored (Nitrostat) 0.3, 0.4, 0.6 mg; in bottles of 100 or package of 4 bottles with 25 tabs each. SL powder packets (GONITRO) 0.4 mg; in boxes of 12, 36, 96 packets each.

NOTES — May produce a burning/tingling sensation when administered, although this should not be used to assess potency. Store in original glass bottle to maintain potency/stability. Traditionally, unused tabs should be discarded 6 months after the original bottle is opened; however, the Nitrostat product is stable for 24 months after the bottle is opened or until the expiration date on the bottle, whichever is earlier. If used rarely, prescribe package with 4 bottles with 25 tabs each.

MOA — Relaxes cardiac and peripheral smooth muscle (venous greater than arterial).

ADVERSE EFFECTS — Serious: Hypotension. Frequent: Headache, tingling/mouth burning, tachycardia, dizziness, flushing.

NITROGLYCERIN SUSTAINED RELEASE ▶L ♀C ▶? $$
ADULT — Angina prophylaxis: Start 2.5 mg PO two to three times per day, then titrate upward prn.
PEDS — Not approved in children.
FORMS — Generic only: Caps, extended-release 2.5, 6.5, 9 mg.
NOTES — Do not use for acute angina attack. Swallow whole; do not chew or crush. Allow for a nitrate-free period of 10 to 14 h each day to avoid nitrate tolerance.
MOA — Relaxes cardiac and peripheral smooth muscle (venous greater than arterial).
ADVERSE EFFECTS — Serious: Hypotension, methemoglobinemia (rare). Frequent: Headache, tachycardia, dizziness, flushing.

NITROGLYCERIN TRANSDERMAL (*Minitran, Nitro-Dur,* ✱*Trinipatch, Transderm-Nitro*) ▶L ♀C ▶? $$
ADULT — Angina prophylaxis: Start with lowest dose and apply 1 patch for 12 to 14 h each day to non-hairy skin.
PEDS — Not approved in children.
FORMS — Generic/Trade: Transdermal system 0.1, 0.2, 0.4, 0.6 mg/h. Trade only: (Nitro-Dur) 0.3, 0.8 mg/h.
NOTES — Do not use for acute angina attack. Allow for a nitrate-free period of 10 to 14 h each day to avoid nitrate tolerance.
MOA — Relaxes cardiac and peripheral smooth muscle (venous greater than arterial).
ADVERSE EFFECTS — Serious: Hypotension, methemoglobinemia (rare). Frequent: Headache, rash, tachycardia, dizziness, drug tolerance, flushing.

CARDIOVASCULAR: Pressors/Inotropes

DOBUTAMINE ▶Plasma ♀D ▶– $
ADULT — Inotropic support in cardiac decompensation (heart failure, cardiogenic shock, surgical procedures): Start 0.5 to 1 mcg/kg/min; titrate based on response; usual dose 2 to 20 mcg/kg/min. Mix 250 mg in 250 mL D5W (1 mg/mL); a rate of 21 mL/h delivers 5 mcg/kg/min for a 70 kg patient; alternatively mix 200 mg in 100 mL D5W (2 mg/mL) set at a rate of 10.5 mL/h, which delivers 5 mcg/kg/min for a 70 kg patient.
PEDS — Not approved in children.
UNAPPROVED ADULT — Refractory septic shock: 2 to 20 mcg/kg/min.
UNAPPROVED PEDS — Use adult dosage. Use lowest effective dose.
NOTES — For short-term use, up to 48 h. Continuously monitor BP and EKG. When possible, monitor pulmonary wedge pressure and cardiac output.
MOA — Stimulates beta-1 receptors (primarily increases cardiac contractility) and stimulates beta-2 receptors (mild peripheral vasodilation).
ADVERSE EFFECTS — Serious: Arrhythmias, tachycardia. Frequent: Hypertension or hypotension.

DOPAMINE ▶Plasma ♀C ▶– $
WARNING — Avoid extravasation; peripheral ischemia, necrosis, gangrene may occur. If extravasation occurs, infiltrate the area as soon as possible with a phentolamine and normal saline solution.
ADULT — Pressor: Start 5 mcg/kg/min, increase prn by 5 to 10 mcg/kg/min increments at 10 min intervals, max 50 mcg/kg/min. Mix 400 mg in 250 mL D5W (1600 mcg/mL); a rate of 13 mL/h, which delivers 5 mcg/kg/min in a 70 kg patient. Alternatively, mix 320 mg in 100 mL D5W (3200 mcg/mL) set at a rate of 6.5 mL/h delivers 5 mcg/kg/min in a 70 kg patient.
PEDS — Not approved in children.
UNAPPROVED ADULT — Symptomatic bradycardia unresponsive to atropine: 5 to 20 mcg/kg/min IV infusion.
UNAPPROVED PEDS — Pressor: Use adult dosage.

NOTES — Doses in mcg/kg/min: 2 to 4 is the traditional renal dose; recent evidence suggests ineffective and active at dopaminergic receptors; 5 to 10 is the cardiac dose: Active at dopaminergic and beta-1 receptors; greater than 10 is active at the dopaminergic, beta-1, and alpha-1 receptors.
MOA — Stimulates beta-1 receptors (increases cardiac contractility and chronotropic effect), stimulates alpha receptors (peripheral vasoconstriction), and stimulates renal dopaminergic receptors (increases renal perfusion).
ADVERSE EFFECTS — Serious: Arrhythmias, tachycardia. Frequent: Hypotension, N/V, palpitations, headache, dyspnea.

EPHEDRINE ▶K ♀C ▶? $
ADULT — Pressor: 10 to 25 mg IV slow injection, with repeat doses q 5 to 10 min prn, max 150 mg/day. Orthostatic hypotension: 25 mg PO daily to four times per day. Bronchospasm: 25 to 50 mg PO q 3 to 4 h prn.
PEDS — Not approved in children.
UNAPPROVED PEDS — Pressor: 3 mg/kg/day SC or IV in 4 to 6 divided doses.
FORMS — Generic only: Caps, 50 mg.
MOA — Stimulates beta-1 receptors (increases cardiac contractility and chronotropic effect), stimulates alpha receptors (peripheral vasoconstriction), stimulates beta-2 receptors (mild peripheral vasodilation).
ADVERSE EFFECTS — Serious: Arrhythmias, tachycardia. Frequent: Hypertension, headache, palpitations, flushing, sweating, dizziness.

EPINEPHRINE (*EpiPen, EpiPen Jr, Adrenalin*) ▶Plasma ♀C ▶– varies by therapy
ADULT — Cardiac arrest: 1 mg (1:10,000 soln) IV, repeat q 3 to 5 min if needed; infusion 1 mg in 250 mL D5W (4 mcg/mL) at rate of 15 to 60 mL/h delivers 1 to 4 mcg/min. Anaphylaxis: 0.3 to 0.5 mg SC/IM (1:1000 soln), may repeat q 5 to 10 min. Acute asthma and hypersensitivity reactions: 0.1 to 0.3 mg of 1:1000 soln SC or IM. Hypersensitivity reactions: 0.01 mg/kg SC autoinjector.

(cont.)

EPINEPHRINE (*cont.*)

PEDS — Cardiac arrest: 0.01 mg/kg IV/intraosseous (max 1 mg/dose) or 0.1 mg/kg ET (max 10 mg/dose), repeat 0.1 to 0.2 mg/kg IV/IO/ET q 3 to 5 min if needed. Neonates: 0.01 to 0.03 mg/kg IV (preferred) or up to 0.1 mg/kg ET, repeat q 3 to 5 min if needed; IV infusion start 0.1 mcg/kg/min, increase in increments of 0.1 mcg/kg/min if needed, max 1 mcg/kg/min. Anaphylaxis, weight > 30 kg: 0.3 to 0.5 mg SC/IM (1:1000 soln), may repeat q 5 to 10 min. Anaphylaxis, weight ≤ 30 kg: 0.01 mg/kg (0.01 mL/kg of 1:1000 injection), up to 0.3 mg (0.3 mL), SC/IM, may repeat q 5 to 10 min. Acute asthma: 0.01 mL/kg (up to 0.5 mL) of 1:1000 soln SC or IM; repeat q 15 min for 3 to 4 doses prn. Hypersensitivity reactions: 0.01 mg/kg SC autoinjector.

UNAPPROVED ADULT — Symptomatic bradycardia unresponsive to atropine: 2 to 10 mcg/min IV infusion. Endotracheal tube administration during cardiac arrest: 2 to 2.5 times the recommended IV dose in 10 mL of NS or distilled water. Shock: 2 to 10 mcg/min increasing to heart rate and blood pressure endpoint. Anaphylactic shock (hypotension in allergic reaction): 0.1 to 0.5 mg IM/SC (1:1000 solution) repeat in 20 min. If hypotension, consider 0.01 to 0.1 mg IV push (1:10,000).

FORMS — Soln for injection: 1:1000 (1 mg/mL in 1 mL amps or 10 mL vial-$). Trade only: EpiPen autoinjector delivers one 0.3 mg (1:1000, 0.3 mL) IM/SC dose. EpiPen Jr. autoinjector delivers one 0.15 mg (1:2000, 0.3 mL) IM/SC dose. 3 mL) EpiPen available in a 2-pack ($$$$$).

NOTES — Cardiac arrest: Adult: Use the 1:10,000 injectable soln for IV use in cardiac arrest (10 mL = 1 mg). Peds: Use 1:10,000 for initial IV dose, then 1:1000 for subsequent dosing or ET doses. Anaphylaxis: Use the 1:1000 injectable soln for SC/IM (0.1 mL = 0.1 mg). Consider EpiPen Jr. in patients weighing less than 30 kg. Directions for Epi-Pen: Remove cap. Place black tip end on thigh and push down to inject. Hold in place for 10 sec. May be injected directly through clothing.

MOA — Stimulates beta-1 receptors (increases cardiac contractility and chronotropic effect), stimulates alpha receptors (peripheral vasoconstriction), stimulates beta-2 receptors (peripheral vasodilation).

ADVERSE EFFECTS — Serious: Arrhythmias, tachycardia. Frequent: Hypertension, headache, palpitations, flushing, sweating, dizziness.

MIDODRINE (✱*Amatine*) ▸LK ♀C ▸? $$$$$

WARNING — May cause significant supine HTN. Contraindicated with severe cardiac disease or persistent/excessive supine HTN.

ADULT — The last daily dose should be no later than 6 pm to avoid supine HTN during sleep. Orthostatic hypotension: Start 10 mg PO three times per day, increase dose prn to max 40 mg/day. Renal impairment: Start 2.5 mg three times per day.

PEDS — Not approved in children.

FORMS — Generic: Tabs, scored 2.5, 5, 10 mg.

NOTES — The last daily dose should be no later than 6 pm to avoid supine HTN during sleep.

MOA — Stimulates alpha receptors (peripheral vasoconstriction).

ADVERSE EFFECTS — Serious: Hypertension. Frequent: Paresthesia, piloerection, pruritus, dysuria, chills.

MILRINONE ▸K ♀C ▸? $$

ADULT — Systolic heart failure (NYHA class III, IV): Load 50 mcg/kg IV over 10 min, then begin IV infusion of 0.375 to 0.75 mcg/kg/min. Renal impairment: Infusion rate for CrCl 5 mL/min or less: 0.2 mcg/kg/min; CrCl 6 to 10 mL/min: 0.23 mcg/kg/min; CrCl 11 to 20 mL/min: 0.28 mcg/kg/min; CrCl 21 to 30 mL/min: 0.33 mcg/kg/min; CrCl 31 to 40 mL/min: 0.38 mcg/kg/min; CrCl 41 to 50 mL/min: 0.43 mcg/kg/min.

PEDS — Not approved in children.

UNAPPROVED PEDS — Inotropic support: Limited data, 50 mcg/kg IV bolus over 10 min, followed by 0.5 to 1 mcg/kg/min IV infusion, titrate to effect within dosing range.

NOTES — The brand name product (Primacor) is no longer available.

MOA — Inhibits phosphodiesterase enzyme leading to increased intracellular cAMP (positive inotropic effect).

ADVERSE EFFECTS — Serious: Arrhythmias. Frequent: None.

NOREPINEPHRINE (*Levophed*) ▸Plasma ♀C ▸? $

WARNING — Tissue ischemia, necrosis, gangrene may occur with extravasation. If extravasation occurs, infiltrate affected area with a soln of phentolamine in NS as soon as possible.

ADULT — Acute hypotension: Start 8 to 12 mcg/min, adjust to maintain BP, average maintenance rate 2 to 4 mcg/min, mix 4 mg in 500 mL D5W (8 mcg/mL); a rate of 22.5 mL/h delivers 3 mcg/min. Ideally through central line.

PEDS — Not approved in children.

UNAPPROVED PEDS — Acute hypotension: Start 0.05 to 0.1 mcg/kg/min IV infusion, titrate to desired effect, max dose 2 mcg/kg/min.

NOTES — Avoid extravasation, do not administer IV push or IM.

MOA — Stimulates beta-1 receptors (increases cardiac contractility and chronotropic effect) and stimulates alpha receptors (peripheral vasoconstriction).

ADVERSE EFFECTS — Serious: Arrhythmias, tissue hypoxia. Frequent: Hypertension, headache.

PHENYLEPHRINE—INTRAVENOUS ▸Plasma ♀C ▸– $

WARNING — Avoid with severe cardiac disease, including CAD and dilated cardiomyopathy. Tissue ischemia, necrosis, gangrene may occur with extravasation. If extravasation occurs, infiltrate affected area with a soln of phentolamine in NS as soon as possible.

ADULT — Mild to moderate hypotension: 0.1 to 0.2 mg slow IV injection, do not exceed 0.5 mg in initial dose, repeat dose prn no less than q 10 to 15 min;

(cont.)

PHENYLEPHRINE—INTRAVENOUS (*cont.*)

1 to 10 mg SC/IM, initial dose should not exceed 5 mg. Infusion for severe hypotension: 20 mg in 250 mL D5W (80 mcg/mL), start 100 to 180 mcg/min (75 to 135 mL/h), usual dose once BP is stabilized 40 to 60 mcg/min.

PEDS — Not approved in children.

UNAPPROVED PEDS — Mild to moderate hypotension: 5 to 20 mcg/kg IV bolus q 10 to 15 min prn; 0.1 to 0.5 mcg/kg/min IV infusion, titrate to desired effect.

NOTES — Avoid SC or IM administration during shock, use IV route to ensure drug absorption.

MOA — Stimulates alpha receptors (peripheral vasoconstriction).

ADVERSE EFFECTS — Serious: Arrhythmias. Frequent: Hypertension, headache, N/V, sweating, dizziness.

VASOPRESSIN (*Vasostrict, ADH, ✦Pressyn AR*) ▶LK ♀C ▶? $$$$$

ADULT — Diabetes insipidus: 5 to 10 units IM/SC two to four times per day prn.

PEDS — Not approved in children.

UNAPPROVED ADULT — Cardiac arrest: 40 units IV; may repeat if no response after 3 min. Septic shock: 0.01 to 0.1 units/min IV infusion, usual dose less than 0.04 units/min. Bleeding esophageal varices: 0.2 to 0.4 units/min initially (max 0.8 units/min).

UNAPPROVED PEDS — Diabetes insipidus: 2.5 to 10 units IM/SC two to four times per day prn. Bleeding esophageal varices: Start 0.002 to 0.005 units/kg/min IV, increase prn to 0.01 units/kg/min. Growth hormone and corticotropin provocative test: 0.3 units/kg IM, max 10 units.

NOTES — Monitor serum sodium. Injectable form may be given intranasally. May cause tissue necrosis with extravasation.

MOA — Promotes water resorption (antidiuretic effect) and smooth muscle contraction; stimulates vasoconstriction of arterioles and capillaries.

ADVERSE EFFECTS — Serious: Angina, arrhythmia, myocardial ischemia, peripheral vasoconstriction, hypersensitivity, anaphylaxis (rare), water intoxication, chronic nephritis, severe vasoconstriction with tissue necrosis (if infusion extravasates). Frequent: Abdominal cramps, dizziness, flatulence, N/V, tremor, sweating, headache.

CARDIOVASCULAR: Pulmonary Arterial Hypertension

AMBRISENTAN (*Letairis, ✦Volibris*) ▶L ♀X ▶– $$$$$

WARNING — Contraindicated with idiopathic pulmonary fibrosis or pregnancy. Women of childbearing age need pregnancy test prior to starting therapy, monthly during treatment, and 1 month after stopping treatment. Prevent pregnancy during treatment and for 1 month after stopping treatment with acceptable methods of contraception. Only available through restricted program; prescribers, pharmacies, female patients must enroll.

ADULT — Pulmonary arterial hypertension: Start 5 mg PO daily; max 10 mg/day. Titrate at 4 week intervals as needed and tolerated. May give with tadalafil to improve exercise ability and decrease disease progression and hospitalizations.

PEDS — Not approved in children.

FORMS — Trade only: Tabs, unscored 5, 10 mg.

NOTES — Monitor hemoglobin at initiation, after 1 month of therapy, then periodically. If pulmonary edema occurs, consider veno-occlusive disease; if confirmed, discontinue therapy. Not recommended with moderate or severe hepatic impairment. Do not exceed 5 mg when given with cyclosporine. May reduce sperm count. Do not split, crush, or chew tablets.

MOA — Endothelin receptor antagonist.

ADVERSE EFFECTS — Serious: Pulmonary veno-occlusive disease. Frequent: Fluid retention, flushing, nasal congestion, peripheral edema, sinusitis.

BOSENTAN (*Tracleer*) ▶L ♀X ▶–? $$$$$

WARNING — Only available through restricted program; prescribers, pharmacies, patients must enroll. Hepatotoxicity; monitor LFTs prior to starting therapy and monthly thereafter. Discontinue bosentan with aminotransferase elevations accompanied by signs/symptoms of liver dysfunction/ injury or increases in bilirubin 2 or more times the upper limit of normal.Contraindicated in pregnancy due to birth defects; women of childbearing age need pregnancy test prior to starting therapy and monthly thereafter. Prevent pregnancy during treatment and for one month after stopping treatment with two reliable methods of contraception, unless the patient had tubal sterilization or uses Copper T 380A IUD or LNg 20 IUS.

ADULT — Pulmonary arterial hypertension: Start 62.5 mg PO two times per day for 4 weeks, increase to 125 mg two times per day maintenance dose. With low body wt (less than 40 kg) and older than 12 yo: 62.5 mg PO two times per day. Stop bosentan more than 36 hr prior to initiating ritonavir; when on ritonavir more than 10 days, give bosentan 62.5 mg PO daily or every other day.

PEDS — Not approved in children.

FORMS — Trade only: Tabs, unscored 62.5, 125 mg.

NOTES — Available only through access program by calling 866-228-3546. Avoid with moderate or severe liver impairment or aminotransferases more than 3 times upper limit of normal prior to initiation. Concomitant glyburide or cyclosporine is contraindicated. Induces metabolism of other drugs (eg, contraceptives, simvastatin, lovastatin, atorvastatin). Do not use with CYP2C9 inhibitor (eg, amiodarone, fluconazole) and strong CYP3A4 inhibitor (eg, ketoconazole, itraconazole, ritonavir) or moderate CYP3A4 inhibitor (eg, erythromycin, fluconazole, diltiazem); will increase levels of bosentan. May decrease warfarin plasma concentration; monitor INR. Rifampin alters bosentan levels; monitor LFTs weekly for 4 weeks, followed by normal monitoring. If pulmonary edema occurs, consider veno-occlusive

(cont.)

BOSENTAN (*cont.***)**

disease; if confirmed, discontinue therapy. Monitor hemoglobin after 1 and 3 months of therapy, then q 3 months. May reduce sperm count.

MOA — Endothelin receptor antagonist.

ADVERSE EFFECTS — Serious: Hepatotoxicity, pulmonary veno-occlusive disease. Frequent: Anemia, fluid retention, flushing, rash.

EPOPROSTENOL (*Flolan, Veletri***)** ▶Plasma ♀B ▶? $$$$$

ADULT — Pulmonary arterial hypertension: Start 2 ng/kg/min IV infusion via central venous catheter. Adjust dose based on response in 1 to 2 ng/kg/min increments at intervals of at least 15 min. Avoid abrupt dose decreases or cessation.

PEDS — Not approved in children.

NOTES — Temporary peripheral IV infusions may be used until central access is established. May potentiate bleeding risk of anticoagulants. May potentiate hypotensive effects of other medications. If pulmonary edema occurs, consider veno-occlusive disease; if confirmed, discontinue therapy.

MOA — Naturally occuring prostaglandin. Dilates pulmonary and sytemic arteries. Inhibits platelet aggregation.

ADVERSE EFFECTS — Serious: Hypotension, may increase risk of bleeding, veno-occlusive disease, sepsis. Frequent: Dizziness, flushing, headache, myalgia, N/V.

ILOPROST (*Ventavis***)** ▶L ♀C ▶? $$$$$

ADULT — Pulmonary arterial hypertension: Start 2.5 mcg/dose by inhalation (as delivered at mouthpiece); if well tolerated, increase to 5 mcg/dose by inhalation (as delivered at mouthpiece). Use 6 to 9 times a day (minimum of 2 h between doses) while awake.

PEDS — Not approved in children.

NOTES — Only administer with I-neb AAD Systems. Each single-use ampule delivers 20 mcg to medication chamber of nebulizer and 2.5 or 5 mcg to the mouthpiece; discard remaining soln after each inhalation. Do not mix with other medications. Avoid contact with skin/eyes or oral ingestion. Monitor vital signs when initiating therapy. Do not initiate therapy if SBP less than 85 mmHg. With Child-Pugh Class B or C hepatic impairment, consider increasing the dosing interval (eg, 3 to 4 h between doses) depending on patient's response at end of dosing interval. May potentiate bleeding risk of anticoagulants. May potentiate hypotensive effects of other medications. Discontinue therapy if pulmonary edema occurs; this may be sign of pulmonary venous hypertension. May induce bronchospasm; carefully monitor patients with COPD, severe asthma, or acute pulmonary infection.

MOA — Prostacyclin analogue. Dilates systemic and pulmonary arteries Inhibits platelet aggregation.

ADVERSE EFFECTS — Serious: Bronchospasm, hepatotoxicity, hypotension, syncope, pneumonia, thrombosis. Frequent: Cough, flushing, headache, hemoptysis, insomnia, myalgia, N/V, tongue pain, trismus.

MACITENTAN (*Opsumit***)** ▶L ♀X ▶– $$$$$

WARNING — Contraindicated with pregnancy. Women of childbearing age need pregnancy test prior to starting therapy, monthly during treatment, and 1 month after stopping treatment. Prevent pregnancy during treatment and for 1 month after stopping treatment with acceptable methods of contraception. Only available through restricted program; prescribers, pharmacies, female patients must enroll.

ADULT — Pulmonary arterial hypertension: 10 mg PO daily.

PEDS — Not approved in children.

FORMS — Trade: Tabs 10 mg.

NOTES — Measure baseline hemoglobin and LFTs; monitor when clinically indicated. If pulmonary edema occurs, consider veno-occlusive disease; if confirmed, discontinue therapy. May reduce sperm count. Avoid concomitant strong CYP3A4 inducers (, rifampin) and strong CYP3A4 inhibitors (eg, ketoconazole, ritonavir). May reduce sperm count.

MOA — Endothelin receptor antagonist.

ADVERSE EFFECTS — Serious: Anemia, angioedema, edema/fluid retention, pulmonary veno-occlusive disease. Frequent: bronchitis, headache, hypotension, influenza, pharyngitis, UTI.

RIOCIGUAT (*Adempas***)** ▶LK ♀X ▶– $$$$$

WARNING — Contraindicated with pregnancy. Women of childbearing age need pregnancy test prior to starting therapy, monthly during treatment, and 1 month after stopping treatment. Prevent pregnancy during treatment and for 1 month after stopping treatment with acceptable methods of contraception. Only available through restricted program; prescribers, pharmacies, female patients must enroll.

ADULT — Pulmonary arterial hypotension: Start 1 mg PO three times daily; may increase by 0.5 mg q 2 weeks as tolerated, max 2.5 mg three times daily. If patient may not tolerate hypotensive effects, start 0.5 mg PO three times daily. Not recommended with CrCl <15 mL/min, dialysis, or severe (Child-Pugh C) hepatic impairment.

PEDS — Not approved in children.

FORMS — Trade: Tabs 0.5, 1, 1.5, 2, 2.5 mg.

NOTES — Contraindicated with nitrates, nitric oxide donors, PDE-5 inhibitors (eg, sildenafil, tadalafil, vardenafil), nonspecific PDE inhibitors (eg, dipyridamole, theophylline). Limited clinical experience with other phosphodiesterase inhibitors (eg, cilostazol, milrinone, roflumilast). Separate from antacid administration by at least 1 h. Concomitant strong CYP and p-glycoprotein/breast cancer resistance protein inhibitors (eg, ketoconazole, itraconazole, ritonavir) increase risk of hypotension; consider initiating 0.5 mg PO three times daily; monitor for hypotension. Smoking reduces plasma concentrations 50 to 60%; if patient smokes, may need more than 2.5 mg PO three times daily; decrease dose if patient stops smoking. If pulmonary edema occurs, consider veno-occlusive

(cont.)

RIOCIGUAT (*cont.***)**

disease; if confirmed, discontinue therapy. May increase bleeding risk.

MOA — Guanylate cyclase stimulator.

ADVERSE EFFECTS — Serious: Anemia, hypotension, may increase risk of bleeding. Frequent: Constipation, diarrhea, dizziness, dyspnea, GERD, headache, N/V.

SELEXIPAG (*Uptravi***)** ▶L ♀?/?/?; Animal reproduction studies showed no clinically relevant effects on embryo fetal development and survival. ▶ Do not breastfeed while taking this medication. $$$$$

ADULT — Pulmonary arterial hypertension: Start 200 mcg PO two times daily, increase by 200 mcg PO two times daily each week to highest tolerated dose, max 1600 mcg PO two times daily. With moderate hepatic impairment (Childs-Pugh class B): Start 200 mcg PO daily, increase by 200 mcg PO daily each week to highest tolerated dose, max 1600 mcg PO daily.

PEDS — Not approved in children.

FORMS — Trade only: Tabs, unscored 200, 400, 600, 800, 1000, 1200, 1400, 1600 mcg.

NOTES — Avoid concomitant strong CYP2C8 inhibitors (eg, gemfibrozil). Avoid with severe hepatic impairment (Childs-Pugh class C). If pulmonary edema occurs, consider veno-occlusive disease.

MOA — Selective prostacyclin receptor (IP receptor) agonist.

ADVERSE EFFECTS — Frequent: Diarrhea,flushing, headache, jaw pain, myalgia, nausea, pain in extremity.

SILDENAFIL—CARDIOVASCULAR (*Revatio***)** ▶LK ♀B ▶ − $$$$

ADULT — Pulmonary arterial hypertension: 5 mg or 20 mg PO three times per day, with doses 4 to 6 h apart; or 2.5 mg or 10 mg IV three times per day.

PEDS — Not approved in children.

FORMS — Generic/Trade: Tabs 20 mg. Trade only: Susp 10 mg/mL.

NOTES — Contraindicated with nitrates or guanylate cyclase stimulators (eg, riociguat). Coadministration is not recommended with ritonavir, potent CYP3A inhibitors, or other phosphodiesterase-5 inhibitors. Concomitant alpha-blockers or amlodipine may potentiate hypotension. Use not recommended for patients with pulmonary veno-occlusive disease or pediatric patients (1 to 17 yo). Sudden vision loss due to nonarteritic ischemic optic neuropathy has been reported. Discontinue with sudden decrease/loss of hearing. Teach patients to seek medical attention for vision loss, hearing loss, or in men if erections last longer than 4 h. Safety and efficacy in treating patients with pulmonary hypertension secondary to sickle cell disease have not been established; may increase risk for vaso-occlusive crisis.

MOA — Selectively inhibits phosphodiesterase-5 resulting in relaxation of pulmonary vascular smooth muscle bed.

ADVERSE EFFECTS — Serious: MI, CVA, hypotension, syncope, cerebral thrombosis, retinal hemorrhage, vision loss (nonarteritic ischemic optic neuropathy). Frequent: Dyspepsia, dyspnea, erythema, epistaxis, flushing, headache, insomnia, rhinitis.

TADALAFIL—CARDIOVASCULAR (*Adcirca***)** ▶L ♀B ▶− $$$$

ADULT — Pulmonary arterial hypertension: 40 mg PO daily, 20 mg if CrCl <80 mL/min or mild to moderate hepatic impairment. Avoid with CrCl <30 mL/min or severe hepatic impairment.

PEDS — Not approved in children.

FORMS — Trade only (Adcirca): Tabs 20 mg.

NOTES — Contraindicated with nitrates or guanylate cyclase stimulators (eg, riociguat). Coadministration is not recommended with potent CYP3A inhibitors (itraconazole, ketoconazole), potent CYP3A inducers (rifampin), or other phosphodiesterase-5 inhibitors. Caution with ritonavir; see prescribing info for specific dose adjustments. Alpha-blockers or alcohol may potentiate hypotension. Use not recommended for patients with pulmonary veno-occlusive disease. Sudden vision loss due to nonarteritic ischemic optic neuropathy has been reported. Retinal artery occlusion has been reported. Discontinue with sudden decrease/loss of hearing. Transient global amnesia. Teach patients to seek medical attention for vision loss, hearing loss, or in men if erections last longer than 4 h.

MOA — Selectively inhibits phosphodiesterase-5 resulting in relaxation of pulmonary vascular smooth muscle bed.

ADVERSE EFFECTS — Serious: Priapism, hypotension, myocardial infarction, vision loss (nonarteritic ischemic optic neuropathy), retinal artery occlusion. Frequent: Headache, flushing, dyspepsia, back pain.

TREPROSTINIL SODIUM—INJECTABLE (*Remodulin***)** ▶KL ♀B ▶? $$$$$

ADULT —Pulmonary arterial hypertension: Continuous SC (preferred) or central IV infusion. Start 1.25 ng/kg/min based on ideal body wt. Reduce to 0.625 ng/kg/min if initial dose not tolerated. Dose based on clinical response and tolerance. Increase by no more than 1.25 ng/kg/min/week in 1st 4 weeks, then increase by no more than 2.5 ng/kg/min/week. Mild to moderate hepatic insufficiency:Start 0.625 ng/kg/min based on ideal body wt; increase cautiously. Not studied with severe hepatic insufficiency. Transitioning from epoprostenol: Must be done in hospital; initiate at 10% epoprostenol dose; gradually increase dose as epoprostenol dose is decreased (see chart in prescribing information).

PEDS — Not approved in children.

NOTES — Avoid abruptly lowering the dose or cessation. Use cautiously in the elderly and those with liver or renal dysfunction. Initiate in setting with personnel and equipment for physiological monitoring and emergency care. Administer by continuous infusion using infusion pump. Patient must have access to backup infusion pump and infusion sets. Must dilute prior to giving IV; use infusion set with in-line filter; see prescribing information for details. May potentiate bleeding risk for patients on

(cont.)

TREPROSTINIL SODIUM—INJECTABLE (cont.)

anticoagulants. May potentiate hypotensive effects of other medications.

MOA — Prostacyclin analogue. Dilates systemic and pulmonary arteries. Inhibits platelet aggregation.

ADVERSE EFFECTS — Serious: Hypotension, may increase risk of bleeding, sepsis (from indwelling central venous catheter). Frequent: Pain at infusion site, local reaction at infusion site, dizziness, headache, diarrhea, nausea, pruritus, jaw pain, vasodilation.

TREPROSTINIL—INHALED SOLUTION (Tyvaso) ▶KL – ♀B ▶? $$$$$

ADULT — Pulmonary arterial hypertension: Start 3 breaths (18 mcg) per treatment session four times per day during waking hours; treatments should be at least 4 h apart; may reduce initial dose to 1 to 2 breaths per treatment session if 3 breaths not tolerated. May increase by 3 breaths q 1 to 2 weeks as tolerated, max 9 breaths (54 mcg) per treatment four times per day.

PEDS — Not approved in children.

FORMS — 1.74 mg in 2.9 mL inhalation soln.

NOTES — Administer undiluted with the Tyvaso Inhalation System. A single breath delivers about 6 mcg treprostinil; discard remaining soln at the end of each day. Do not mix with other medications. Avoid contact with skin/eyes or oral ingestion. Efficacy not established with existing lung disease (asthma, COPD). Monitor patients with acute pulmonary infections for worsening of lung disease and loss of drug effect. May need to adjust doses if CYP2C8 inducers (eg, rifampin) or CYP2C8 inhibitors (eg, gemfibrozil) are added or withdrawn. Use cautiously in the elderly and those with liver or renal dysfunction. Inhibits platelet aggregation and increases risk of bleeding; may potentiate bleeding risk of anticoagulants. May potentiate hypotensive effects of other medications.

MOA — Prostacyclin analogue. Dilates systemic and pulmonary arteries. Inhibits platelet aggregation.

ADVERSE EFFECTS — Serious: Hypotension, may increase risk of bleeding. Frequent: Cough, diarrhea, dizziness, flushing, headache, nausea, pharyngollaryngeal pain.

TREPROSTINIL—ORAL (Orenitram) ▶L ♀C ▶? $$$$$

ADULT — Pulmonary arterial hypertension: Start 0.25 mg PO two times daily; increase by 0.25 to 0.5 mg two times daily or 0.125 mg three times daily q 3 to 4 days as tolerated. Mild liver impairment (Child Pugh Class A) or with strong CYP2C8 inhibitor (ie, gemfibrozil): Start 0.125 mg PO two times daily; increase by 0.125 mg two times daily q 3 to 4 days as tolerated. To transition from intravenous (IV) or subcutaneous (SC) treprostinil, simultaneously decrease IV/SC infusion rate up to 30 ng/kg/min per day and increase the oral treprostinil dose up to 6 mg per day (2 mg TID). To estimate comparable doses between dosage forms: Total daily dose (mg) of oral treprostinil = 0.0072 x injectable dose (ng/kg/min) x weight (kg).

PEDS — Not approved in children.

FORMS — Trade: Extended-release tabs 0.125, 0.25, 1, 2.5 mg.

NOTES — Take with food. Swallow whole; use only intact tablets. Do not abruptly discontinue; taper by 0.5 to 1 mg per day. Avoid use with moderate or severe hepatic impairment. May increase bleeding risk. In patients with diverticulosis, may become lodged in diverticulum. Insoluble shell will be eliminated in feces.

MOA — Prostacyclin analogue. Dilates systemic and pulmonary arteries. Inhibits platelet aggregation.

ADVERSE EFFECTS — Serious: Hypotension, may increase risk of bleeding. Frequent: Diarrhea, headache, nausea.

CARDIOVASCULAR: Thrombolytics

ALTEPLASE (TPA, t-PA, Activase, Cathflo, ✱Activase rt-PA) ▶L ♀C ▶? $$$$$

ADULT — Acute MI, wt 67 kg or less: Give 15 mg IV bolus, then 0.75 mg/kg (max 50 mg) over 30 min, then 0.5 mg/kg (max 35 mg) over the next 60 min; wt greater than 67 kg: Give 15 mg IV bolus, then 50 mg over 30 min, then 35 mg over the next 60 min. Acute ischemic CVA with symptoms 3 h or less: 0.9 mg/kg (max 90 mg); give 10% of total dose as an IV bolus, and the remainder IV over 60 min. Multiple exclusion criteria. Select patients may receive with symptoms 4.5 h or less (age younger than 80 yo, baseline NIHSS score 25 or less, no anticoagulant use, or no combination of prior stroke and diabetes). Acute pulmonary embolism: 100 mg IV over 2 h, then restart heparin when PTT twice normal or less. Occluded central venous access device: 2 mg/mL in catheter for 2 h. May use 2nd dose if needed.

PEDS — Occluded central venous access device: Wt at least 10 kg but less than 30 kg: Dose equal to 110% of the internal lumen volume, not to exceed 2 mg/2 mL. Other uses not approved in children.

NOTES — Must be reconstituted. Soln must be used within 8 h after reconstitution.

MOA — Enhances conversion of plasminogen to plasmin to achieve fibrinolysis.

ADVERSE EFFECTS — Serious: Bleeding, intracranial hemorrhage, hypersensitivity. Frequent: N/V, bleeding, hypotension, fever.

RETEPLASE (Retavase) ▶L ♀C ▶? $$$$$

ADULT — Acute MI: 10 units IV over 2 min; repeat 1 dose in 30 min.

PEDS — Not approved in children.

NOTES — Must be reconstituted with sterile water for injection to 1 mg/mL concentration. Soln must be used within 4 h after reconstitution.

MOA — Enhances conversion of plasminogen to plasmin.

ADVERSE EFFECTS — Serious: Bleeding. Frequent: None.

STREPTOKINASE (*Streptase, Kabikinase*) ▶L ♀C ▶? $$$$$
ADULT — Acute MI: 1.5 million units IV over 60 min. Pulmonary embolism: 250,000 units IV loading dose over 30 min, followed by 100,000 units/h IV infusion for 24 h (maintain infusion for 72 h if concurrent DVT suspected). DVT: 250,000 units IV loading dose over 30 min, followed by 100,000 units/h IV infusion for 24 h. Occluded arteriovenous catheter: 250,000 units instilled into the catheter, remove soln containing 250,000 units of drug from catheter after 2 h using a 5 mL syringe.
PEDS — Not approved in children.
NOTES — Must be reconstituted. Soln must be used within 8 h of reconstitution. Do not shake vial. Do not repeat use in less than 1 year. Do not use with history of severe allergic reaction.

MOA — Enhances conversion of plasminogen to plasmin.
ADVERSE EFFECTS — Serious: Bleeding, hypersensitivity (rare). Frequent: None.

TENECTEPLASE (*TNKase*) ▶L ♀C ▶? $$$$$
ADULT — Acute MI: Single IV bolus dose over 5 sec based on body wt: wt less than 60 kg: 30 mg; wt 60 to 69 kg: 35 mg; wt 70 to 79 kg: 40 mg; wt 80 to 89 kg: 45 mg; wt 90 kg or more: 50 mg.
PEDS — Not approved in children.
NOTES — Must be reconstituted. Soln must be used within 8 h after reconstitution.
MOA — Enhances conversion of plasminogen to plasmin.
ADVERSE EFFECTS — Serious: Bleeding. Frequent: None.

CARDIOVASCULAR: Volume Expanders

ALBUMIN (*Albuminar, Buminate, Albumarc, ✱Plasbumin*) ▶L ♀C ▶? $$$$
ADULT — Shock, burns: 500 mL of 5% soln (50 mg/mL) infused as rapidly as tolerated. Repeat infusion in 30 min if response is inadequate. 25% soln may be used with or without dilution. Undiluted 25% soln should be infused at 1 mL/min to avoid too rapid plasma volume expansion.
PEDS — Shock, burns: 10 to 20 mL/kg IV infusion at 5 to 10 mL/min using 50 mL of 5% soln.
UNAPPROVED PEDS — Shock/hypovolemia: 1 g/kg/dose IV rapid infusion. Hypoproteinemia: 1 g/kg/dose IV infusion over 30 to 120 min.
NOTES — Fever, chills. Monitor for plasma volume overload (dyspnea, fluid in lungs, abnormal increase in BP or CVP). Less likely to cause hypotension than plasma protein fraction, more purified. In treating burns, large volumes of crystalloid solns (0.9% sodium chloride) are used to maintain plasma volume with albumin. Use 5% soln in pediatric hypovolemic patients. Use 25% soln in pediatric patients with volume restrictions.
MOA — Expands plasma volume.
ADVERSE EFFECTS — Serious: Pulmonary edema (rapid infusion), hypersensitivity (rare), bleeding. Frequent: Hypotension (rapid infusion), fever, chills, itching.

DEXTRAN (*Rheomacrodex, Gentran, Macrodex*) ▶K ♀C ▶? $$
ADULT — Shock/hypovolemia: Dextran 40, Dextran 70 and 75, up to 20 mL/kg during the 1st 24 h, up to 10 mL/kg/day thereafter; do not continue for longer than 5 days. The 1st 500 mL may be infused rapidly with CVP monitoring. DVT/PE prophylaxis during surgery: Dextran 40, 50 to 100 g IV infusion the day of surgery, continue for 2 to 3 days postop with 50 g/day. 50 g/day may be given q 2nd or 3rd day thereafter up to 14 days.
PEDS — Total dose should not exceed 20 mL/kg.
UNAPPROVED ADULT — DVT/PE prophylaxis during surgery: Dextran 70 and 75 solns have been used.

Other uses: To improve circulation with sickle cell crisis, prevention of nephrotoxicity with radiographic contrast media, toxemia of late pregnancy.
NOTES — Monitor for plasma volume overload (dyspnea, fluid in lungs, abnormal increase in BP or CVP), and anaphylactoid reactions. May impair platelet function. Less effective than other agents for DVT/PE prevention.
MOA — Expands plasma volume.
ADVERSE EFFECTS — Serious: Pulmonary edema (rapid infusion), anaphylaxis (rare), bleeding. Frequent: Hypotension (rapid infusion), fever, chills, itching.

HETASTARCH (*Hespan, Hextend, Voluven*) ▶K ♀C ▶? $$
WARNING — Do not use in critically ill adult patients, including those with sepsis or in ICU; associated with increased risk of death and renal injury.
ADULT — Shock/hypovolemia: 500 to 1000 mL IV infusion. Hespan, Hextend: Usually should not exceed 20 mL/kg/day (1500 mL for 70 kg). Voluven: do not exceed 50 mL/kg/day (3500 mL for 70 kg). Do not use with renal impairment.
PEDS — Hespan/Hextend: Not approved in children. Voluven: Adapt to patient's needs.
UNAPPROVED PEDS — Shock/hypovolemia: 10 mL/kg/dose; do not exceed 20 mL/kg/day.
NOTES — Monitor for volume overload. Little or no antigenic properties compared to dextran.
MOA — Expands plasma volume.
ADVERSE EFFECTS — Serious: Pulmonary edema (rapid infusion), hypersensitivity (rare), bleeding. Frequent: Hypotension (rapid infusion), fever, chills, itching.

PLASMA PROTEIN FRACTION (*Plasmanate, Protenate, Plasmatein*) ▶L ♀C ▶? $$$$
ADULT — Shock/hypovolemia: Adjust initial rate according to clinical response and BP, but rate should not exceed 10 mL/min. As plasma volume normalizes, infusion rate should not exceed 5 to 8 mL/min. Usual dose 250 to 500 mL. Hypoproteinemia: 1000 to 1500 mL/day IV infusion.

(cont.)

PLASMA PROTEIN FRACTION (*cont.*)

PEDS — Shock/hypovolemia: Initial dose 6.6 to 33 mL/kg infused at a rate of 5 to 10 mL/min.

NOTES — Fever, chills, hypotension with rapid infusion. Monitor for volume overload. Less pure than albumin products.

MOA — Expands plasma volume.

ADVERSE EFFECTS — Serious: Pulmonary edema (rapid infusion), hypersensitivity (rare), bleeding. Frequent: Hypotension (rapid infusion), fever, chills, itching.

CARDIOVASCULAR: Other

***BIDIL* (hydralazine + isosorbide dinitrate)** ▶LK ♀C ▶? $$$$$

ADULT — Heart failure (adjunct to standard therapy in black patients): Start 1 tab PO three times per day, increase as tolerated to max 2 tabs three times per day. May decrease to ½ tab three times per day with intolerable side effects; try to increase dose when side effects subside.

PEDS — Not approved in children.

FORMS — Trade only: Tabs, scored 37.5/20 mg.

NOTES — See component drugs.

MOA — See component drugs.

ADVERSE EFFECTS — See component drugs

CILOSTAZOL (*Pletal*) ▶L ♀C ▶? $$$$

WARNING — Contraindicated in heart failure of any severity due to decreased survival.

ADULT — Intermittent claudication: 100 mg PO two times per day on empty stomach. 50 mg PO two times per day with CYP3A4 inhibitors (eg, ketoconazole, itraconazole, erythromycin, diltiazem) or CYP2C19 inhibitors (eg, omeprazole). Beneficial effect may take up to 12 weeks.

PEDS — Not approved in children.

FORMS — Generic/Trade: Tabs 50, 100 mg.

NOTES — Caution with moderate/severe liver impairment or CrCl <25 mL/min. Give with other antiplatelet therapy (aspirin or clopidogrel) when treating peripheral arterial disease to reduce cardiovascular risk. Grapefruit juice may increase levels and the risk of side effects.

MOA — Inhibits platelet aggregation and causes vasodilation by blocking the effects of phosphodiesterase III enzyme.

ADVERSE EFFECTS — Serious: Heart failure exacerbation, cerebral/pulmonary hemorrhage, Stevens-Johnson syndrome, thrombocytopenia. Frequent: Palpitations, dizziness, nausea, diarrhea, dyspepsia, headache.

***ENTRESTO* (sacubitril + valsartan)** ▶esterases ♀D ▶– $$$$$

WARNING — Do not use in pregnancy.

ADULT — Reduce cardiovascular death and hospitalization for heart failure with chronic heart failure (NYHA Class II to IV) and reduced ejection fraction: Start 49/51 mg PO two times per day, double dose after 2 to 4 weeks as tolerated, target maintenance dose of 97/103 mg PO two times daily. Patients not currently taking ACE inhibitor or angiotensin receptor blocker or previously taking low dose of these agents; severe renal impairment (eGFR <30 mL/min/1.73 m²); moderate hepatic impairment (Child-Pugh B): Start 24/26 mg, PO two times per day, double dose after 2 to 4 weeks as tolerated, target maintenance dose 97/103 mg PO two times daily.

PEDS — Not approved in children.

FORMS — Trade: Tabs, unscored 24/26, 49/51, 97/103 mg.

NOTES — Usually given with other heart failure therapies in place of ACE inhibitor or other angiotensin receptor blocker. If switching from ACE inhibitor, allow 36 h washout period between administration of the drugs. Do not use with severe hepatic impairment. Contraindicated with pregnancy, concomitant ACE inhibitor, concomitant aliskiren in patients with DM, or previous angioedema with ACE inhibitor or angiotensin receptor blocker. Combined use with renin-angiotensin system inhibitors (ie, ACE inhibitors, aliskiren, other angiotensin receptor blocker) increases risk of renal impairment, hypotension, and hyperkalemia. Hyperkalemia possible, especially if used concomitantly with other drugs that increase K⁺ (including K⁺-containing salt substitutes) and in patients with heart failure, DM, or renal impairment. Concomitant NSAID, including celecoxib, may further deteriorate renal function and decrease antihypertensive effects. May increase lithium levels.

MOA — Inhibits neprilysin and blocks binding of angiotensin II to the angiotensin subtype 1 receptor.

ADVERSE EFFECTS — Serious: Angioedema, hypotension, hyperkalemia, renal impairment. Common: Cough, dizziness.

IVABRADINE (*Corlanor*) ▶L ♀? ▶– $$$$$

ADULT — Reduce hospitalization in patients with stable, symptomatic heart failure with ejection fraction less than or equal to 35%, sinus rhythm with heart rate of at least 70 beats per minute, and either maximally tolerated beta-blocker dose or intolerant to beta-blocker: Start 5 mg PO two times per day, titrate based on heart rate, max 15 mg/day. With conduction defect or if bradycardia could lead to hemodynamic compromise, start 2.5 mg PO two times daily.

PEDS — Not approved in children.

FORMS — Trade only: Tabs, unscored 5, 7.5 mg.

NOTES — Fetal toxicity; females should use effective contraception. Contraindicated with strong CYP3A4 inhibitors (eg, azole antifungals, macrolide antibiotics, HIV protease inhibitors, nefazodone); acute decompensated heart failure; BP less than 90/50 mmHg; sick sinus syndrome, sinoatrial block, or 3rd degree AV block without functioning pacemaker; resting heart rate less than 60 bpm prior to treatment; severe hepatic impairment; or pacemaker

(cont.)

IVABRADINE (*cont.*)

dependent. Monitor for atrial fibrillation, brady-cardia. Not recommended with 2nd degree heart block or with demand pacemakers set to at least 60 beats per minute. Avoid concomitant moderate CYP3A4 inhibitors (eg, diltiazem, grapefruit juice, verapamil) or CYP3A4 inducers (eg, phenytoin, rifampin, St. John's wort). Negative chronotropes (eg, amiodarone, beta blockers, digoxin) increase risk of bradycardia; monitor heart rate.

MOA — Slows heart rate by blocking the hyperpo-larization-activated cyclic nucleotide-gated (HCN) channel responsible for the cardiac pacemaker Ic current. Inhibits retinal current Ih.

ADVERSE EFFECTS — Serious: Atrial fibrillation, bradycardia. Frequent: Hypertension, phosphenes.

NESIRITIDE (***Natrecor***) ▶K, Plasma ♀C ▶? $$$$$

ADULT — Hospitalized patients with decompensated heart failure with dyspnea at rest: 2 mcg/kg IV bolus over 1 min, then 0.01 mcg/kg/min IV infusion for up to 48 h. Bolus dose may not be appropriate for patients with SBP less than 110 or with recent use of afterload reducer (eg, nitroglycerin). Do not initiate at higher doses. Limited experience with increased doses: 0.005 mcg/kg/min increments, preceded by 1 mcg/kg bolus, no more frequently than q 3 h up to max infusion dose 0.03 mcg/kg/min. Mix 1.5 mg vial in 250 mL D5W (6 mcg/mL). A bolus of 23.3 mL is 2 mcg/kg for a 70 kg patient, infusion set at rate 7 mL/h delivers 0.01 mcg/kg/min for a 70 kg patient.

PEDS — Not approved in children.

NOTES — Contraindicated with cardiogenic shock or SBP less than 100 mmHg. May increase mortality; meta-analysis showed nonstatistically significant increased risk of death within 30 days post treatment compared with noninotropic control group. Not indicated for outpatient infusion, for scheduled repetitive use, to improve renal function, or to enhance diuresis. Discontinue if dose-related symptomatic hypotension occurs and support BP prn. May restart infusion with dose reduced by 30% (no bolus dose) once BP stabilized. May worsen renal impairment. Do not shake reconstituted vial, and dilute vial prior to administration. Incompatible with most injectable drugs; administer agents using separate IV lines. Do not measure BNP levels while infusing; may measure BNP at least 2 to 6 h after infusion completion.

MOA — Human B-type natriuretic peptide that relaxes cardiac smooth muscle (arterial and venous vasodilation).

ADVERSE EFFECTS — Serious: Arrhythmias, altered kidney function. Frequent: Hypotension, headache, insomnia, dizziness, nausea.

PENTOXIFYLLINE ▶L ♀C ▶? $$$

ADULT — Intermittent claudication: 400 mg PO three times per day with meals. With CNS/GI adverse effects, may decrease to two times per day. CrCl

<30 mL/min: 400 mg PO daily. Beneficial effect may take up to 8 weeks. May be less effective in relieving cramps, tiredness, tightness, and pain during exercise.

PEDS — Not approved in children.

FORMS — Generic: Tabs, extended-release 400 mg.

NOTES — Contraindicated with recent cerebral/retinal bleed. Concomitant anticoagulant, antiplatelet agent, or NSAID increases bleeding risk. Increases theophylline levels. Increases INR with warfarin. Concomitant strong CYP1A2 inhibitors (eg, ciprofloxacin, fluvoxamine) or cimetidine may increase exposure to pentoxifylline. The brand name product (Trental) is no longer available.

MOA — Decreases blood viscosity and improves erythrocyte flexibility.

ADVERSE EFFECTS — None.

RANOLAZINE (***Ranexa***) ▶LK ♀C ▶? $$$$$

ADULT — Chronic angina: 500 mg PO two times per day, increase to 1000 mg PO two times per day prn based on clinical symptoms, max 2000 mg daily. Max 500 mg two times per day, if used with diltiazem, verapamil, or moderate CYP3A4 inhibitors.

PEDS — Not approved in children.

FORMS — Trade only: Tabs, extended-release 500, 1000 mg.

NOTES — Baseline and follow-up ECGs; may prolong QT interval. If CrCl <60 mL/min at baseline, monitor renal function after initiation and periodically; discontinue ranolazine if acute renal failure occurs. Contraindicated with hepatic cirrhosis, potent CYP3A4 inhibitors (eg, clarithromycin, protease inhibitors, itraconazole, ketoconazole, nefazodone), CYP3A4 inducers (eg, carbamazepine, phenobarbital, phenytoin, rifabutin, rifapentine, rifampin, St. John's wort). Limit dose of ranolazine to max 500 mg two times per day with moderate CYP3A inhibitors (eg, diltiazem, erythromycin, fluconazole, grapefruit juice–containing products, verapamil). Limit simvastatin to 20 mg when used with ranolazine. Limit metformin to 1700 mg daily when used with ranolazine 1000 mg two times per day. P-glycoprotein inhibitors (eg, cyclosporine) increase ranolazine levels; titrate ranolazine based on clinical response. Increases levels of CYP3A4 substrates (eg, lovastatin, simvastatin), CYP2D6 substrates (eg, antipsychotic agents, TCAs), OCT2 substrates (eg metformin), cyclosporine, tacrolimus, sirolimus, drugs transported by p-glycoprotein (eg, digoxin); may need dose adjustments. Swallow whole; do not crush, break, or chew. May be less effective in women. Teach patients to report palpitations or fainting spells.

MOA — Unknown; inhibits late sodium current at therapeutic levels. Antianginal and anti-ischemic effects not dependent on HR or BP.

ADVERSE EFFECTS — Serious: Acute renal failure, QT prolongation. Frequent: Constipation, dizziness, headache, nausea.

CONTRAST MEDIA

CONTRAST MEDIA: MRI Contrast—Gadolinium-Based

NOTE: Avoid gadolinium-based contrast agents if severe renal insufficiency (GFR <30 mL/min/1.73 m) due to risk of nephrogenic systemic fibrosis/nephrogenic fibrosing dermopathy. Similarly avoid in acute renal insufficiency of any severity due to hepatorenal syndrome or during the perioperative phase of liver transplant.

GADOBENATE (*MultiHance*) ▶K ♀C ▶? $$$$
  ADULT — Noniodinated, nonionic IV contrast for MRI. Dose 0.1 mmol/kg (0.2 mL/kg) administered as a rapid bolus intravenous injection followed with a saline flush of at least 5 mL.
  PEDS — Not approved in children.
  MOA — Gadolinium-based noniodinated, nonionic IV contrast for MRI.
  ADVERSE EFFECTS — Serious: Hypersensitivity, nephropathy. Frequent: None.

GADOBUTROL (*Gadavist, ✦Gadavist*) ▶K – ♀C ▶? ©V $$$$
  ADULT — 0.1 mL/kg for age 2 yo or older up to max 14 mL.
  PEDS — 0.1 mL/kg for age 2 yo or older.
  NOTES — Formulated at a higher concentration (1 mmol/mL) compared to certain other gadolinium-based contrast agents, resulting in a lower volume of administration.
  MOA — Gadolinium based IV contrast for MRI
  ADVERSE EFFECTS — Serious: Hypersensitivity, nephrogenic systemic fibrosis, dermopathy. Frequent: None

GADODIAMIDE (*Omniscan*) ▶K ♀C ▶? $$$$
  ADULT — Noniodinated, nonionic IV contrast for MRI: Noniodinated IV contrast for MRI: 0.2 mL/kg (0.1 mmol/kg) administered intravenously, at a rate not to exceed 10 mL per 15 sec up to a maximum dose of 26 mL. Administer a 5-mL normal saline flush after the injection.
  PEDS — Noniodinated, nonionic IV contrast for MRI: Age greater than 2 yo: same as adult.
  NOTES — Use caution if renal disease. May falsely lower serum calcium. Not for intrathecal use.
  MOA — Gadolinium-based noniodinated, nonionic IV contrast for MRI.
  ADVERSE EFFECTS — Serious: Hypersensitivity, nephropathy. Frequent: None.

GADOPENTETATE (*Magnevist*) ▶K ♀C ▶? $$$
  ADULT — Noniodinated IV contrast for MRI: 0.2 mL/kg (0.1 mmol/kg) administered intravenously, at a rate not to exceed 10 mL per 15 seconds up to a maximum dose of 26 mL. Administer a 5-mL normal saline flush after the injection.
  PEDS — Noniodinated IV contrast for MRI: Age older than 2 yo: same as adult.
  NOTES — Use caution in sickle cell and renal disease.
  MOA — Gadolinium-based noniodinated IV contrast for MRI.
  ADVERSE EFFECTS — Serious: Black Box Warning for Nephrogenic Systemic Fibrosis in patients with reduced GFR. Serious: Hypersensitivity, nephropathy. Frequent: None.

GADOTERATE MEGLUMINE (*Dotarem*) ▶K ♀–C ▶? $$$$
  ADULT — Gadolinium-based macrocyclic and ionic IV contrast for MRI of the CNS and blood–brain barrier and/or abnormal vascularity: Dose is 0.2 mL/kg (0.1 mmol/kg) IV bolus infused at rate of 2 mL/second.
  PEDS — Age older than 2 yo: 0.2 mL/kg (0.1 mmol/kg) IV bolus infused at rate of 1 to 2 mL/second. Not approved age younger than 2 yo.
  ADVERSE EFFECTS — Hypersensitivity, headache

GADOTERIDOL (*ProHance*) ▶K ♀C ▶? $$$$
  ADULT — Noniodinated, nonionic IV contrast for MRI.
  PEDS — Age older than 2 yo: Noniodinated, nonionic IV contrast for MRI.
  NOTES — Use caution in sickle cell and renal disease.
  MOA — Gadolinium-based noniodinated, nonionic IV contrast for MRI.
  ADVERSE EFFECTS — Serious: Hypersensitivity, nephropathy. Frequent: None.

GADOVERSETAMIDE (*OptiMARK*) ▶K ♀C ▶– $$$$
  ADULT — Noniodinated IV contrast for MRI: bolus peripheral intravenous injection at a dose of 0.2 mL/kg (0.1 mmol/kg) and a rate of 1-2 mL/sec delivered either manually or by power injection (up to 30 mL total dose).
  PEDS — Not approved in children.
  NOTES — Use caution in sickle cell and renal disease.
  MOA — Gadolinium-based noniodinated IV contrast for MRI.
  ADVERSE EFFECTS — Serious: Hypersensitivity, nephropathy. Frequent: None.

CONTRAST MEDIA: MRI Contrast—Other

GA 68 DOTATATE ▶ ♀?/?/? no studies in humans or animals ▶– interrupt breastfeeding and pump and discard breast milk for 12 hours after administration
  WARNING — Handle with appropriate safety measures to minimize radiation exposure. Instruct patients to drink a sufficient amount of water before administration, during the first hours following administration and to void frequently.
  ADULT — Localization of somatostatin receptor positive neuroendocrine tumors (NETs) during PET scan: 2 MBq/kg of body weight (0.054 mCi/kg) up to 200 MBq (5.4 mCi) administered as intravenous bolus injection.
  PEDS — Same as adult.
  FORMS — Single dose kit.

(cont.)

GA 68 DOTATATE (*cont.*)

MOA — Ga 68 dotatate binds to somatostatin receptors in malignant cells.

FERUMOXSIL (*GastroMARK*) ▶L ♀B ▶? $$$$

ADULT — Noniodinated, nonionic, iron-based, oral GI contrast for MRI: 600 mL (105 mg Fe) administered orally at a rate of about 300 mL over 15 minutes (max 900 mL or 157.5 mg Fe). Take after fasting at least 4 hours. Shake bottles for vigorously for 1 min before use.

PEDS — Not approved in children younger than 16 yo.

FORMS — 300 mL bottles

MOA — Noniodinated, nonionic, iron-based, oral GI contrast for MRI.

ADVERSE EFFECTS — Serious: Hypersensitivity. Frequent: Abdominal pain, N/V.

MANGAFODIPIR (*Teslascan*) ▶L ♀– ▶– $$$$

ADULT — Noniodinated IV contrast for MRI.

PEDS — Not approved in children.

NOTES — Contains manganese.

MOA — Non-iodinated IV contrast for MRI.

ADVERSE EFFECTS — Serious: Hypersensitivity. Frequent: Headache.

CONTRAST MEDIA: Radiography Contrast

NOTE: Beware of allergic or anaphylactoid reactions. Avoid IV contrast in renal insufficiency or dehydration. Hold metformin (Glucophage) prior to or at the time of iodinated contrast dye use and for 48 h after procedure. Restart after procedure only if renal function is normal.

BARIUM SULFATE ▶Not absorbed ♀? ▶+ $

ADULT — Noniodinated GI (eg, oral, rectal) contrast: Dosage depends on indication and form, see package insert.

PEDS — Noniodinated GI (eg, oral, rectal) contrast: Dosage depends on indication and form, see package insert.

NOTES — Contraindicated if suspected esophageal, gastric, or intestinal perforation. Use with caution in GI obstruction. May cause abdominal distention, cramping, and constipation with oral use.

MOA — Noniodinated GI contrast.

ADVERSE EFFECTS — Serious: Hypersensitivity, worsening of bowel obstruction. Frequent: Constipation. None.

DIATRIZOATE (*Cystografin, Gastrografin, Hypaque, MD-Gastroview, RenoCal, Reno-DIP, Reno-60, Renografin*) ▶K ♀C ▶? $

ADULT — Iodinated, ionic, high-osmolality IV or GI contrast. Dosage varies based on study and form, see package insert. Oral contrast for abdominal CT: typical dose is 250 mL of solution made by mixing 25 mL of GI formulation (Gastrografin, MD-Gastroview) in one liter of water. Have patient complete drinking 30 minutes prior to study. Avoid use if there is a risk of aspiration.

PEDS — Iodinated, ionic, high-osmolality IV or GI contrast. Dosage varied based on study and age, see package insert.

NOTES — High-osmolality contrast may cause tissue damage if infiltrated/extravasated. IV: Hypaque, Renografin, Reno-DIP, RenoCal. GI: Gastrografin, MD-Gastroview.

MOA — Iodinated, ionic, high-osmolality IV or GI contrast.

ADVERSE EFFECTS — Serious: Hypersensitivity. Frequent: None.

IODIXANOL (*Visipaque*) ▶K ♀B ▶? $$$

ADULT — Iodinated, nonionic, iso-osmolar IV contrast.

PEDS — Iodinated, nonionic, iso-osmolar IV contrast.

NOTES — Not for intrathecal use.

MOA — Iodinated, nonionic, low osmolality IV contrast.

ADVERSE EFFECTS — Serious: Hypersensitivity. Frequent: None.

IOHEXOL (*Omnipaque*) ▶K ♀B ▶? $$$

ADULT — Iodinated, nonionic, low-osmolality IV and oral/body cavity contrast. Dosages vary depending on forms and type of study, see package insert. Oral pass-thru examination of the GI tract: Dosages vary depending on forms, however one example dose would be to mix 50 mL of Omnipaque 350 into one liter of water and have patient drink 500mL one hour prior to study and remainder 30 min prior to study.

PEDS — Iodinated, nonionic, low-osmolality IV and oral/body cavity contrast. Dosages vary based on forms, age, and study, see pacakge insert.

FORMS — Omnipaque 140, 180, 240, 300, 350

MOA — Iodinated, nonionic, low osmolality IV and oral/body cavity contrast.

ADVERSE EFFECTS — Serious: Hypersensitivity. Frequent: None.

IOPAMIDOL (*Isovue*) ▶K ♀? ▶? $$

ADULT — Iodinated, nonionic, low-osmolality IV contrast.

PEDS — Iodinated, nonionic, low-osmolality IV contrast.

MOA — Iodinated, nonionic, low osmolality IV contrast.

ADVERSE EFFECTS — Serious: Hypersensitivity. Frequent: None.

IOPROMIDE (*Ultravist*) ▶K ♀B ▶? $$$

ADULT — Iodinated, nonionic, low-osmolality IV contrast.

PEDS — Iodinated, nonionic, low-osmolality IV contrast.

MOA — Iodinated, nonionic, low osmolality IV contrast.

ADVERSE EFFECTS — Serious: Hypersensitivity. Frequent: None.

IOTHALAMATE (*Conray, ✲Vascoray*) ▶K ♀B ▶– $
ADULT — Iodinated, ionic, high-osmolality IV contrast.
PEDS — Iodinated, ionic, high-osmolality IV contrast.
NOTES — High-osmolality contrast may cause tissue damage if infiltrated/extravasated.
MOA — Iodinated, ionic, high osmolality IV contrast.
ADVERSE EFFECTS — Serious: Hypersensitivity. Frequent: None.

IOVERSOL (*Optiray*) ▶K ♀B ▶? $$
ADULT — Iodinated, nonionic, low-osmolality IV contrast.
PEDS — Iodinated, nonionic, low-osmolality IV contrast.
MOA — Iodinated, nonionic, low osmolality IV contrast.

ADVERSE EFFECTS — Serious: Hypersensitivity. Frequent: None.

IOXAGLATE (*Hexabrix*) ▶K ♀B ▶– $$$
ADULT — Iodinated, ionic, low-osmolality IV contrast.
PEDS — Iodinated, ionic, low-osmolality IV contrast.
MOA — Iodinated, ionic, low osmolality IV contrast.
ADVERSE EFFECTS — Serious: Hypersensitivity. Frequent: None.

IOXILAN (*Oxilan*) ▶K ♀B ▶– $$$
ADULT — Iodinated, nonionic, low-osmolality IV contrast.
PEDS — Iodinated, nonionic, low-osmolality IV contrast.
MOA — Iodinated, nonionic, low osmolality IV contrast.
ADVERSE EFFECTS — Serious: Hypersensitivity. Frequent: None.

CONTRAST MEDIA: Other

INDIGOTINDISULFONATE (*Indigo Carmine*) ▶K ♀C ▶? $
ADULT — Identification of ureteral tears during surgery: 5 mL IV.
PEDS — Identification of ureteral tears during surgery: Use less than the adult dose.
FORMS — Trade only: 40 mg/5 mL vial.
MOA — Blue dye excreted in urine.
ADVERSE EFFECTS — Serious: Hypersensitivity. Frequent: None.

ISOSULFAN BLUE (*Lymphazurin*) ▶LK ♀? ▶? $$$$$
ADULT — Lymphography, identification of lymphatics during cancer surgery: 0.5 to 3 mL SC.
PEDS — Optimal dosing not defined.

FORMS — Trade only: 1% (10 mg/mL) 5 mL vial.
MOA — Blue dye for delineation of lymphatic vessels.
ADVERSE EFFECTS — Serious: Hypersensitivity including anaphylaxis. Frequent: Swelling at injection site.

PENTETATE INDIUM (*Indium DTPA*) ▶K ♀C ▶? $$$$$
ADULT — Radionuclide cisternography.
PEDS — Not approved in children.
FORMS — 1 mCi/mL, 1.5 mL vial.
MOA — Radiopharmaceutical
ADVERSE EFFECTS — Serious: Aseptic meningitis, pyogenic reactions. Frequent: skin reactions, vomiting.

DERMATOLOGY

CORTICOSTEROIDS: TOPICAL

Potency*	Generic	Trade Name**	Forms	Frequency
Low	alclometasone dipropionate	Aclovate	0.05% C/O	bid-tid
Low	clocortolone pivalate	Cloderm	0.1% C	tid
Low	desonide	DesOwen, Desonate, LoKara, Verdeso	0.05% C/L/O/F/G	bid-tid
Low	hydrocortisone	Hytone, others	0.5% C/L/O; 1% C/L/O; 2.5% C/L/O	bid-qid
Low	hydrocortisone acetate	Cortaid, Corticaine	0.5% C/O; 1% C/O/Sp	bid-qid
Medium	betamethasone valerate	Luxiq	0.1% C/L/O; 0.12% F (Luxiq)	qd-bid
Medium	desoximetasone‡	Topicort Topicort LP	0.25% C	bid
Medium	fluocinolone	Synalar, Dermasmoothe FS Scalp Oil	0.01% C/S; 0.025% C/O	bid-qid
Medium	flurandrenolide	Cordran	0.025% C/O; 0.05% C/L/O/T	bid-qid
Medium	fluticasone propionate	Cutivate	0.005% O; 0.05% C/L	daily-bid
Medium	hydrocortisone butyrate	Locoid	0.1% C/O/S	bid-tid
Medium	hydrocortisone valerate	Westcort	0.2% C/O	bid-tid
Medium	mometasone furoate	Elocon	0.1% C/L/O	qd
Medium	triamcinolone‡	Aristocort, Kenalog	0.025% C/L/O; 0.1% C/L/O/S	bid-tid
High	amcinonide	Cyclocort	0.1% C/L/O	bid-tid
High	betamethasone dipropionate‡	Maxivate, others	0.05% C/L/O (non-Diprolene)	qd-bid
High	desoximetasone‡	Topicort	0.05% G; 0.25% C/O	bid
High	diflorasone diacetate‡	Maxiflor	0.05% C/O	bid
High	fluocinonide	Lidex, Vanos	0.1% C	bid-qid
High	halcinonide	Halog	0.1% C/O	bid-tid
High	triamcinolone‡	Aristocort, Kenalog	0.5% C/O	bid-tid

(cont.)

CORTICOSTEROIDS: TOPICAL (*continued*)

Potency*	Generic	Trade Name**	Forms	Frequency
Very high	betamethasone dipropionate‡	Diprolene, Diprolene AF	0.05% C/G/L/O	qd-bid
Very high	clobetasol	Temovate, Cormax, Olux, Temovate E	0.05% C/G/O/L/S/ Sp/F (Olux)	bid
Very high	diflorasone diacetate‡	Psorcon	0.05% C/O	qd-tid
Very high	halobetasol propionate	Ultravate	0.05% C/O	qd-bid

qd = once per day; bid = two times per day; tid = three times per day; qid = four times per day.
*Potency based on vasoconstrictive assays, which may not correlate with efficacy. Not all available.
**Not all brand name products are commercially available, but generic versions are marketed. products are listed, including those lacking potency ratings.
‡These drugs have formulations in more than once potency category.
C, cream; O, ointment; L, lotion; T, tape; F, foam; S, solution; G, gel; Sp, spray

DERMATOLOGY: Acne Preparations

NOTE: For topical agents, wash area prior to application. Wash hands before and after application; avoid eye area.

ACANYA (clindamycin—topical + benzoyl peroxide) ▶K ♀C ▶+ $$$$$
ADULT — Acne: Apply once daily.
PEDS — Not approved in children 12 yo or younger.
FORMS — Trade only: Gel (clindamycin 1.2% + benzoyl peroxide 2.5%) 50 g.
NOTES — Expires 2 months after mixing.
MOA — Antibacterial + drying and sebostatic effects.
ADVERSE EFFECTS — Frequent: Dryness, scaling, erythema, burning, pruritus. Severe: C. difficile-associated diarrhea, anaphylaxis.

ADAPALENE (*Differin*) ▶bile ♀C ▶? $$$$
ADULT — Acne: Apply at bedtime.
PEDS — Not approved in children.
UNAPPROVED PEDS — Acne: Apply at bedtime.
FORMS — OTC: Gel 0.1%. Rx only, Trade/Generic: Cream 0.1% (45 g). Gel 0.3% (45 g). Trade only: Soln 0.1% (59 mL). Generic only: Soln 0.1% (59 mL)
NOTES — During early weeks of therapy, acne exacerbation may occur. May cause erythema, scaling, dryness, pruritus, and burning in up to 40% of patients. Therapeutic results take 8 to 12 weeks.
MOA — Modulates cellular differentiation, inflammation, keratinization.
ADVERSE EFFECTS — Frequent: Dryness, scaling, erythema, burning, pruritus.

AZELAIC ACID (*Azelex, Finacea, Finevin*) ▶K ♀B ▶? $$$$$
ADULT — Acne (Azelex, Finevin): Apply two times per day. Rosacea (Finacea): Apply two times per day.
PEDS — Not approved in children.
UNAPPROVED ADULT — Melasma: Apply two times per day.

UNAPPROVED PEDS — Acne: Apply at bedtime.
FORMS — Trade only: Cream 20%, 30, 50 g (Azelex). Gel 15% 50 g (Finacea). Foam 15% 50g (Finacea).
NOTES — Improvement of acne occurs within 4 weeks. Monitor for hypopigmentation especially in patients with dark complexions. Avoid use of occlusive dressings. Do not apply in eyes and mucous membranes.
MOA — May possess antibacterial activity.
ADVERSE EFFECTS — Frequent: Dryness, scaling, erythema, burning, stinging, tingling, pruritus.

BENZACLIN (clindamycin—topical + benzoyl peroxide) ▶K ♀C ▶+ $$$$$
ADULT — Acne: Apply two times per day.
PEDS — Not approved in children.
UNAPPROVED PEDS — Acne: Apply at bedtime.
FORMS — Generic/Trade: Gel (clindamycin 1% + benzoyl peroxide 5%) 25, 50 g (jar). Trade only: 35 g (pump) and 50 g (pump).
NOTES — Expires 10 weeks after mixing.
MOA — Antibacterial + drying and sebostatic effects.
ADVERSE EFFECTS — Frequent: Dryness, scaling, erythema, burning, pruritus. Severe: C. difficile-associated diarrhea, allergic reactions/hypersensitivity.

BENZAMYCIN (erythromycin—topical + benzoyl peroxide) ▶LK ♀C ▶? $$$
ADULT — Acne: Apply two times per day.
PEDS — Not approved in children.
UNAPPROVED PEDS — Acne: Apply at bedtime.
FORMS — Generic/Trade: Gel (erythromycin 3% + benzoyl peroxide 5%) 23.3, 46.6 g. Trade only: Benzamycin Pak, #60 gel pouches.

(cont.)

BENZAMYCIN (*cont.*)

NOTES — Must be refrigerated, expires 3 months after pharmacy dispensing.

MOA — Antibacterial + drying and sebostatic effects.

ADVERSE EFFECTS — Frequent: Dryness, scaling, erythema, burning, pruritus.

BENZOYL PEROXIDE (*Benzac, Benzagel 10%, Desquam, Clearasil, ✲Solugel*) ▶LK ♀C ▶? $

ADULT — Acne: Cleansers: Wash one to two times per day. Creams/gels/lotion: Apply daily initially, gradually increase to two to three times per day if needed.

PEDS — Not approved in children.

UNAPPROVED PEDS — Acne: Cleansers: Wash one to two times per day. Creams/gels/lotion: Apply daily initially, gradually increase to two to three times per day if needed.

FORMS — OTC and Rx generic: Liquid 2.5, 5, 10%. Bar 5, 10%. Mask 5%. Lotion 4, 5, 8, 10%. Cream 5, 10%. Gel 2.5, 4, 5, 6, 10, 20%. Pad 3, 4, 6, 8, 9%. Other strengths available.

NOTES — If excessive drying or peeling occurs, reduce frequency of application. Use with PABA-containing sunscreens may cause transient skin discoloration. May bleach fabric.

MOA — Antibacterial + drying and sebostatic effects.

ADVERSE EFFECTS — Frequent: Dryness, scaling, erythema, burning, pruritus.

CLINDAMYCIN—TOPICAL (*Cleocin T, Clindagel, Evoclin, ✲Dalacin T*) ▶L ♀B ▶– $$$

ADULT — Acne: Apply daily (Evoclin, Clindagel) or two times per day (Cleocin T).

PEDS — Not approved in children.

UNAPPROVED ADULT — Rosacea: Apply lotion two times per day.

UNAPPROVED PEDS — Acne: Apply two times per day.

FORMS — Generic/Trade: Gel 1% 30, 60 g. Lotion 1% 60 mL. Soln 1% 30, 60 mL. Foam 1% 50, 100 g. Pads 1% 60 ct.

NOTES — Concomitant use with erythromycin may decrease effectiveness. Most common adverse effects are dryness, erythema, burning, peeling, oiliness, and itching. C. difficile–associated diarrhea has been reported with topical use.

MOA — Antibacterial.

ADVERSE EFFECTS — Frequent: Dryness, burning, pruritus. Severe: C. difficile-associated diarrhea.

✲ DIANE-35 (**cyproterone + ethinyl estradiol**) ▶L ♀X ▶– $$

WARNING — Not recommended in women who smoke. Increased risk of thromboembolism, CVA, MI, hepatic neoplasia, and gallbladder disease. Nausea, breast tenderness, and breakthrough bleeding are common, transient side effects. Nighttime dosing may minimize nausea. Effectiveness is reduced by hepatic enzyme-inducing drugs such as certain anticonvulsants and barbiturates, rifampin, rifabutin, griseofulvin, and protease inhibitors. Antibiotics or products that contain St. John's wort may reduce efficacy.

ADULT — Canada only. In women, severe acne unresponsive to oral antibiotics and other treatments, with associated symptoms of androgenization, including seborrhea and mild hirsutism: 1 tab PO daily for 21 consecutive days, stop for 7 days, repeat cycle.

PEDS — Not approved in children.

FORMS — Canada Generic/Trade: Blister pack of 21 tabs 2 mg cyproterone acetate/0.035 mg ethinyl estradiol.

NOTES — Higher thromboembolic risk than other oral contraceptives, therefore only indicated for acne, and not solely for contraception (although effective for the latter). Same warnings, precautions, and contraindications as other oral contraceptives.

MOA — Cyproterone: Potent antiandrogenic, progestogenic and antigonadotrophic activity; blocks androgen receptors and reduces androgen synthesis. Ethinyl estradiol increases levels of sex hormone binding globulin, and decreases circulating plasma levels of androgens. The combination also prevents ovulation and possible conception.

ADVERSE EFFECTS — Serious: DVT/PE, stroke, MI, hepatic neoplasia, gallbladder disease. Frequent: Nausea, breast tenderness, and breakthrough bleeding.

DUAC (**clindamycin—topical + benzoyl peroxide**, ✲ *Clindoxyl*) ▶K ♀C ▶+ $$$$$

ADULT — Acne: Apply at bedtime.

PEDS — Not approved in children.

UNAPPROVED PEDS — Acne: Apply at bedtime.

FORMS — Generic/Trade: Gel (clindamycin 1% + benzoyl peroxide 5%) 45 g.

NOTES — Expires 2 months after pharmacy dispensing.

MOA — Antibacterial + drying and sebostatic effects.

ADVERSE EFFECTS — Frequent: Dryness, scaling, erythema, burning, pruritus. Severe: C. difficile-associated diarrhea, anaphylaxis.

EPIDUO (**adapalene + benzoyl peroxide**, *Epiduo Forte*, ✲ *Tactuo*) ▶bile, K ♀C ▶? $$$$$

ADULT — Acne: Apply daily.

PEDS — Not approved in children younger than 9 yo. Acne: Children 9 yo and older: Apply daily.

FORMS — Trade only: Epiduo, Tactuo Gel (0.1% adapalene + benzoyl peroxide 2.5%) 45 g. Epiduo Forte (0.3% adapalene + benzoyl peroxide 2.5%) 15, 30, 45, 60, 70 g.

NOTES — During early weeks of therapy, acne exacerbation may occur. May cause erythema, scaling, dryness, pruritus, and burning.

MOA — Modulates cellular differentiation, inflammation, keratinization + drying and sebostatic effects.

ADVERSE EFFECTS — Frequent: Erythema, scaling, dryness, stinging, burning.

ERYTHROMYCIN—TOPICAL (*Eryderm, Erycette, Erygel, A/T/S, ✲Sans-Acne, Ery-Sol*) ▶L ♀B ▶? $$

ADULT — Acne: Apply two times per day.

PEDS — Not approved in children.

UNAPPROVED PEDS — Acne: Apply two times per day.

FORMS — Generic/Trade: Soln 2% 60 mL. Pads 2%. Gel 2% 30, 60 g.

(cont.)

ERYTHROMYCIN—TOPICAL (*cont.*)

NOTES — May be more irritating when used with other acne products. Concomitant use with clindamycin may decrease effectiveness.
MOA — Antibacterial.
ADVERSE EFFECTS — Frequent: Dryness, pruritus, erythema, scaling.

ISOTRETINOIN (*Absorica, Amnesteem, Claravis, Sotret, Myorisan, Zenatane, ✤Accutane Roche, Clarus*) ▶LK ♀X ▶– $$$$$
WARNING — Contraindicated in pregnant women or in women who may become pregnant. If used in a woman of childbearing age, patient must have severe, disfiguring acne, be reliable, comply with mandatory contraceptive measures, receive written and oral instructions about hazards of taking during pregnancy, have 2 negative pregnancy tests prior to beginning therapy. Must use 2 forms of effective contraception from 1 month prior until 1 month after discontinuation of therapy, unless absolute abstinence is chosen or patient has undergone a hysterectomy. Men should not father children. May cause depression, suicidal thoughts, and aggressive or violent behavior; monitor for symptoms. Obtain written informed consent. Write prescription for no more than a 1-month supply. Informed consent documents available from the manufacturer.
ADULT — Severe, recalcitrant cystic acne: 0.5 to 2 mg/kg/day PO divided two times per day for 15 to 20 weeks. Typical target dose is 1 mg/kg/day. May repeat 2nd course of therapy after at least 2 months off therapy.
PEDS — Not approved in children.
UNAPPROVED ADULT — Prevention of 2nd primary tumors in patients treated for squamous cell carcinoma of the head and neck: 50 to 100 mg/m²/day PO. Also been used in keratinization disorders.
UNAPPROVED PEDS — Severe, recalcitrant cystic acne: 0.5 to 2 mg/kg/day PO divided two times per day for 15 to 20 weeks. Typical target dose is 1 mg/kg/day. Maintenance therapy for neuroblastoma: 100 to 250 mg/m²/day PO in 2 divided doses.
FORMS — Generic: Caps 10, 20, 40 mg. Generic only: Caps (Absorica) 25, 35 mg. Caps (Sotret, Absorica, Claravis, and Zenatane) 30 mg.
NOTES — Prescription can be for a maximum of a 1-month supply. May cause headache, cheilitis, drying of mucous membranes including eyes, nose, mouth, hair loss, abdominal pain, pyuria, joint and muscle pain/stiffness, conjunctivitis, elevated ESR, and changes in serum lipids and LFTs. Effect on bone loss unknown; use caution in patients predisposed to osteoporosis. In children in whom skeletal growth is not complete, do not exceed the recommended dose for the recommended duration of treatment. Pseudotumor cerebri has occurred during therapy often when used with a tetracycline; avoid concomitant vitamin A, tetracycline, minocycline. May cause corneal opacities, decreased night vision, and inflammatory bowel disease. May

decrease carbamazepine concentrations. Avoid excessive exposure to sunlight.
MOA — Decreases sebaceous gland size and sebum production.
ADVERSE EFFECTS — Frequent: Dryness, burning, pruritus, inflammation, photosensitivity, xerostomia, increased triglycerides, bone pain, arthralgias, myalgias, epistaxis. Severe: Teratogenic, possible depression, aggressive or violent behavior, premature epiphyseal closure, osteoporosis, osteopenia, delayed bone healing, pseudotumor cerebri (more commonly when used with a tetracycle) corneal opacities, hepatitis, back pain, severe skin reactions including Stevens-Johnson syndrome.

ONEXTON (clindamycin—topical + benzoyl peroxide) ▶K ♀C ▶+ $$$$
ADULT — Acne: Apply once daily to the face.
PEDS — Not approved in children younger than 12 yo. In children older than 12 yo, use adult dosing.
FORMS — Trade only: Gel (clindamycin 1.2% + benzoyl peroxide 3.75%) 50 g.
ADVERSE EFFECTS — Frequent: burning, contact dermariris, pruritis, rash. Severe: pseudomembranous colitis.

SALICYLIC ACID (*Akurza, Clearasil Cleanser, Stridex Pads*) ▶not absorbed ♀? ▶? $
ADULT — Acne (OTC): Apply/wash area up to 3 times a day. Removal of excessive keratin in hyperkeratotic disorders (Rx): Apply to affected area at bedtime and cover. Hydrate skin before application.
PEDS — Acne: Apply/wash area up to 3 times a day.
FORMS — OTC Generic/Trade: Pads, Gel, Lotion, Liquid, Mask scrub, 0.5%, 1%, 2%. Rx Trade only (Akurza): Cream 6% 340 g. Lotion 6%, 355 mL.
MOA — Keratolytic.
ADVERSE EFFECTS — Frequent: Irritation, stinging, burning.

SULFACET-R (sulfacetamide—topical + sulfur) ▶K ♀C ▶? $$$
ADULT — Acne, rosacea, seborrheic dermatitis: Apply one to three times per day.
PEDS — Not approved in children.
FORMS — Generic/Trade: Lotions, cleansers, washes.
NOTES — Avoid with sulfa allergy or renal failure.
MOA — Antibacterial.
ADVERSE EFFECTS — Frequent: Local irritation, stinging, burning.

SULFACETAMIDE—TOPICAL (*Klaron*) ▶K ♀C ▶? $$$$
ADULT — Acne: Apply two times per day.
PEDS — Not approved in children.
FORMS — Generic/Trade: Lotion 10% 118 mL.
NOTES — Cross-sensitivity with sulfa or sulfite allergy.
MOA — Antibacterial.
ADVERSE EFFECTS — Frequent: Irritation, stinging, burning. Severe: Stevens-Johnson syndrome, systemic lupus erythematosus.

TAZAROTENE (*Tazorac, Avage, Fabior*) ▶L ♀X ▶? $$$$
ADULT — Acne: Apply 0.1% cream (Tazorac) or foam (Fabior) at bedtime. Palliation of fine facial wrinkles, mottled hyper- and hypopigmentation,

(cont.)

TAZAROTENE (*cont.*)

benign facial lentigines (Avage): Apply at bedtime. Psoriasis: Apply 0.05% cream at bedtime, increase to 0.1% prn.

PEDS — Acne: Apply 1% foam (Fabior) at bedtime.

UNAPPROVED ADULT — Excessive facial oil: Apply 0.1% cream at bedtime.

UNAPPROVED PEDS — Acne: Apply 0.1% cream at bedtime. Psoriasis: Apply 0.05% cream at bedtime.

FORMS — Trade only: Cream (Tazorac) 0.05% and 0.1% 30, 60 g. Foam (Fabior) 0.1% 50, 100 g. Gel 0.05% and 0.1% 30, 100 g. Trade only: Cream (Avage) 0.1% 15, 30 g.

NOTES — Avoid using gel formulation with other medications or cosmetics that are considered drying. In psoriasis, may reduce irritation and improve efficacy by using topical corticosteroid in morning and tazarotene at bedtime. Desquamation, burning, dry skin, erythema, pruritus may occur in up to 30% of patients. May cause photosensitivity.

MOA — Modulates cellular differentiation, keratinization; anti-inflammatory, immunologic activity.

ADVERSE EFFECTS — Frequent: Pruritus, burning, erythema, rash changes in pigmentation. Severe: blister.

TRETINOIN—TOPICAL (*Retin-A, Retin-A Micro, Renova, Retisol-A, Atralin, ✷Stieva-A, Rejuva-A, Vitamin A Acid Cream*) ▶LK ♀C ▶? $$$

ADULT — Acne (Retin A, Retin-A Micro): Apply at bedtime. Wrinkles, hyperpigmentation, tactile roughness (Renova): Apply at bedtime.

PEDS — Not approved in children.

UNAPPROVED ADULT — Used in non-melanoma skin cancer and lamellar ichthyosis, mollusca contagiosa, verrucae plantaris, verrucae planae juvenilis, hyperpigmented lesions in black individuals, ichthyosis vulgaris, and pityriasis rubra pilaris.

FORMS — Generic/Trade: Cream 0.025% 20, 45 g; 0.05% 20, 45 g; 0.1% 20, 45 g. Gel 0.01% 15, 45 g; 0.025% 15, 45 g; 0.05% 45 g . Micro gel 0.04%, 0.1% 20, 45, 50 g pump; 0.08% 50 g pump. Trade only: Renova cream 0.02% 40, 60 g.

NOTES — May induce erythema, peeling. Minimize sun exposure. Concomitant use with sulfur, resorcinol, benzoyl peroxide, or salicylic acid may result in skin irritation. Gel preps are flammable.

MOA — Induces loosening of keratinocytes, inhibits microcomedone formation.

ADVERSE EFFECTS — Frequent: Dryness, erythema, scaling. Severe: Contraindicated in pregnancy.

VELTIN (**clindamycin—topical + tretinoin—topical**) ▶LK ♀C ▶? $$$$$

WARNING — Clindamycin has been reported to cause severe colitis.

ADULT — Acne: Apply at bedtime.

PEDS — Has not been studied in children younger than 12 yo.

FORMS — Trade: Gel clindamycin 1.2% + tretinoin 0.025%, 30, 60 g.

MOA — antibiotic + retinoid

ADVERSE EFFECTS — Frequent: dryness, irritation, exfoliation, erythema, pruritis.

ZIANA (**clindamycin—topical + tretinoin—topical**) ▶LK ♀C ▶? $$$$$

ADULT — Acne: Apply at bedtime.

PEDS — Use adult dose for age 12 yo or older.

FORMS — Trade only: Gel clindamycin 1.2% + tretinoin 0.025% 30, 60 g.

NOTES — May induce erythema, peeling. Minimize sun exposure.

MOA — Induces loosening of keratinocytes, inhibits microcomedone formation, antibacterial.

ADVERSE EFFECTS — Frequent: Dryness, erythema, scaling.

DERMATOLOGY: Actinic Keratosis Preparations

AMINOLEVULINIC ACID (*Levulan Kerastick*) ▶not absorbed ♀C ▶? $$$$$

ADULT — Non-hyperkeratotic actinic keratoses: Apply soln to lesions on scalp or face; expose to special light source 14 to 18 h later.

PEDS — Not approved in children.

FORMS — Trade only: 20% soln, single-use applicator stick.

NOTES — Soln should be applied by healthcare personnel. Advise patients to avoid sunlight during 14 to 18 h period before blue light illumination.

MOA—Photosensitizer as precursor to protoporphyrin.

ADVERSE EFFECTS — Frequent: Scaling, pruritus, hypo- or hyperpigmentation, erosions, stinging, burning.

DICLOFENAC—TOPICAL (*Solaraze, Voltaren, Pennsaid*) ▶L ♀C Category D at 30 weeks gestation and beyond. Avoid use starting at 30 weeks gestation. ▶? $$$

WARNING — Risk of serious cardiovascular and GI events.

ADULT — Actinic/solar keratoses: Apply two times per day to lesions for 60 to 90 days (Solaraze). Osteoarthritis of areas amenable to topical therapy: 2 g (upper extremities) to 4 g (lower extremities) four times per day (Voltaren). 40 gtts to knee(s) four times daily (Pennsaid).

PEDS — Not approved in children.

FORMS — Generic/Trade: Gel 3% (Solaraze) 100 g. Soln 1.5% (Pennsaid) 150 mL. Trade only: Gel 1% (Voltaren) 100 g. Soln 2.0% Pump (Pennsaid) 112 g.

NOTES — Avoid exposure to sun and sunlamps. Use caution in aspirin-sensitive patients. When using for OA (Voltaren), max daily dose 16 g to any single lower extremity joint, 8 g to any single upper extremity joint. Avoid use in setting of aspirin allergy or CABG surgery.

MOA — Inhibits prostaglandins at level of cyclooxygenase.

ADVERSE EFFECTS — Frequent: Rash, abdominal cramps, nausea, indigestion.

FLUOROURACIL—TOPICAL (*5-FU, Tolak, Carac, Efudex, Fluoroplex*) ▶L ♀X ▶− $$$$$
WARNING — Contraindicated in pregnant women or women who plan to get pregnant during therapy. Avoid application to mucous membranes.
ADULT — Actinic or solar keratoses: Apply two times per day to lesions for 2 to 6 weeks or once daily to face, ear or scalp for 4 weeks (Tolak). Superficial basal cell carcinomas: Apply 5% cream/soln two times per day.
PEDS — Not approved in children.
UNAPPROVED ADULT — Condylomata acuminata: 1% soln in 70% ethanol and the 5% cream have been used. Resistant verruca vulgaris alone or in combination with salicylic acid.
UNAPPROVED PEDS — Resistant verruca vulgaris alone or in combination with salicylic acid
FORMS — Trade only: Cream 1% 30 g (Fluoroplex $$$$$). Generic/Trade: Cream 0.5% 30 g (Carac $$$$$). Soln 2%, 5% 10 mL (Efudex $$$$$). Cream 5% 40 g. Cream 4% 40 g (Tolak $$$$).
NOTES — May cause severe irritation and photosensitivity. Contraindicated in women who are or who may become pregnant during therapy. Avoid application to mucous membranes.
MOA — Pyrimidine anti-metabolite that interferes with DNA synthesis.
ADVERSE EFFECTS — Frequent: Dermatitis, pruritic maculopapular rash, alopecia, heartburn, nausea, inflammation along segments of the GI tract, diarrhea. Severe: Myelosuppression, mucositis.

INGENOL (*Picato*) ▶not absorbed ♀C ▶? $$$$$
ADULT — Actinic keratosis on face and scalp: Apply 0.015% gel to affected areas once daily for 3 days.
Actinic keratosis on trunk and extremities: Apply 0.05% gel to affected areas once daily for 2 days.
PEDS — Not approved in children.
FORMS — Trade: Gel 0.015% 0.25 g, 0.05% 0.25 g.
NOTES — Avoid contact with the periocular area. Do not use on more than approximately 25 cm^2 (5 cm × 5 cm) area of contiguous skin.
MOA — Induces cell death by unknown mechanism.
ADVERSE EFFECTS — Frequent: local skin reactions, application site pain, application site pruritus, application site irritation, application site infection, hypersensitivity reactions, contact dermatitis, periorbital edema. Severe: anaphylaxis, reactivation of herpes zoster, vesiculation/pustulation, erosion/ulceration.

METHYL AMINOLEVULINATE (*Metvix, Metvixia*) ▶not absorbed ♀C ▶?
ADULT — Non-hyperkeratotic actinic keratoses of face/scalp: Apply cream 1 mm thick (max 1 g) to lesion and 5 mm surrounding area; cover with dressing for 3 h; remove dressing and cream and perform illumination therapy. Repeat in 7 days.
PEDS — Not approved in children.
FORMS — Trade only: Cream 16.8%, 2 g tube.
NOTES — Use in immunocompetent individuals. Lesion debridement should be performed prior to application of cream. Formulated in peanut and almond oil; has not been tested in patients allergic to peanuts.
MOA — Photosensitizer as precursor to photoactive porphyrin.
ADVERSE EFFECTS — Frequent: Peeling, pruritus, edema, ulceration, bleeding, blisters, stinging, burning, pain, crusting, contact sensitization. Severe: angioedema.

DERMATOLOGY: Antibacterials (Topical)

BACITRACIN—TOPICAL ▶not absorbed ♀C ▶? $
ADULT — Minor cuts, wounds, burns, or skin abrasions: Apply one to three times per day.
PEDS — Not approved in children.
UNAPPROVED PEDS — Minor cuts, wounds, burns, or skin abrasions: Apply one to three times per day.
FORMS — OTC Generic/Trade: Oint 500 units/g 1, 15, 30 g.
NOTES — May cause contact dermatitis or anaphylaxis.
MOA — Antibacterial, inhibit bacterial wall synthesis.
ADVERSE EFFECTS — Frequent: None.

FUSIDIC ACID—TOPICAL (✱*Fucidin*) ▶L ♀? ▶? $
ADULT — Canada only. Skin infections: Apply three to four times per day.
PEDS — Canada only. Skin infections: Apply three to four times per day.
FORMS — Canada trade only: Cream 2% fusidic acid 5, 15, 30 g. Oint 2% sodium fusidate 5, 15, 30 g.
NOTES — Contains lanolin; possible hypersensitivity.
MOA — Antibacterial, interferes with bacterial protein synthesis.
ADVERSE EFFECTS — Serious: Hypersensitivity. Frequent: Mild irritation, pain.

GENTAMICIN—TOPICAL ▶K ♀D ▶? $$$
ADULT — Skin infections: Apply three to four times per day.
PEDS — Skin infections in children older than 1 yo: Apply three to four times per day.
FORMS — Generic only: Oint 0.1% 15, 30 g. Cream 0.1% 15, 30 g.
MOA — Antibacterial, interferes with bacterial protein synthesis.
ADVERSE EFFECTS — Frequent: Neurotoxicity (when applied to large areas), gait instability, ototoxicity, nephrotoxicity.

MAFENIDE (*Sulfamylon*) ▶LK ♀C ▶? $$$
ADULT — Adjunctive treatment of burns: Apply one to two times per day.
PEDS — Adjunctive treatment of burns: Apply one to two times per day.
FORMS — Trade only: Topical soln 50 g packets. Cream 5% 57, 114, 454 g.

(cont.)

MAFENIDE (*cont.*)

NOTES — Can cause metabolic acidosis. Contains sulfonamides.

MOA — Antibacterial, interferes with bacterial folic acid synthesis.

ADVERSE EFFECTS — Frequent: Burning, pain, excoriation.

METRONIDAZOLE—TOPICAL (*Noritate, MetroCream, MetroGel, MetroLotion, ✷Rosasol*) ▶KL ♀B (− in 1st trimester) ▶− $$$$

ADULT — Rosacea: Apply daily (1%) or two times per day (0.75%).

PEDS — Not approved in children.

UNAPPROVED ADULT — A 1% soln prepared from the oral tabs has been used in the treatment of infected decubitus ulcers.

FORMS — Trade only: Cream (Noritate) 1% 60 g. Generic/Trade: Gel (MetroGel) 1% 45, 60 g. Gel 0.75% 45 g. Cream 0.75% 45 g. Lotion (MetroLotion) 0.75% 59 mL.

NOTES — Results usually noted within 3 weeks, with continuing improvement through 9 weeks. Avoid using vaginal prep on face due to irritation because of formulation differences.

MOA — Antibacterial, breakage of bacterial DNA, antiinflammatory.

ADVERSE EFFECTS — Frequent: Dizziness, headache, nausea, diarrhea, anorexia, vomiting.

MUPIROCIN (*Bactroban, Centany*) ▶not absorbed ♀ B ▶? $$

ADULT — Impetigo: Apply three times per day for 3 to 5 days. Infected wounds: Apply three times per day for 10 days. Nasal MRSA eradication: 0.5 g of nasal form only in each nostril two times per day for 5 days.

PEDS — Impetigo (mupirocin cream/ointment): Apply three times per day. Infected wounds: Apply three times per day for 10 days. Nasal form not approved in children younger than 12 yo.

FORMS — Generic/Trade: Oint 2% 22 g. Nasal oint 2% 1 g single-use tubes (for MRSA eradication). Trade only: Cream 2% 15, 30 g.

MOA — Antibacterial; inhibits bacterial protein and RNA synthesis.

ADVERSE EFFECTS — Frequent: Dryness, burning, erythema, stinging, tenderness. Severe: angioedema, anaphylaxis, generalized rash.

NEOSPORIN CREAM (*neomycin—topical + polymyxin—topical + bacitracin—topical*) ▶K ♀C ▶? $

ADULT — Minor cuts, wounds, burns, or skin abrasions: Apply one to three times per day.

PEDS — Not approved in children.

UNAPPROVED PEDS — Minor cuts, wounds, burns, or skin abrasions: Apply one to three times per day.

FORMS — OTC Trade only: neomycin 3.5 mg/g + polymyxin 10,000 units/g; 15 g and unit dose 0.94 g.

NOTES — Neomycin component can cause contact dermatitis.

MOA — Antibacterial.

ADVERSE EFFECTS — Frequent: None.

NEOSPORIN OINTMENT (*bacitracin—topical + neomycin—topical + polymyxin—topical*) ▶K ♀C ▶? $

ADULT — Minor cuts, wounds, burns, or skin abrasions: Apply one to three times per day.

PEDS — Not approved in children.

UNAPPROVED PEDS — Minor cuts, wounds, burns, or skin abrasions: Apply one to three times per day.

FORMS — OTC Generic/Trade: bacitracin 400 units/g + neomycin 3.5 mg/g + polymyxin 5000 units/g 15, 30 g and "to go" 0.9 g packets.

NOTES — Also known as triple antibiotic ointment. Neomycin component can cause contact dermatitis.

MOA — Antibacterial.

ADVERSE EFFECTS — Frequent: None.

POLYSPORIN (*bacitracin—topical + polymyxin—topical, ✷ Polytopic*) ▶K ♀C ▶? $

ADULT — Minor cuts, wounds, burns, or skin abrasions: Apply one to three times per day.

PEDS — Not approved in children.

UNAPPROVED PEDS — Minor cuts, wounds, burns, or skin abrasions: Apply one to three times per day.

FORMS — OTC Trade only: Oint 15, 30 g and unit dose 0.9 g. Powder 10 g.

NOTES — May cause allergic contact dermatitis and rarely contact anaphylaxis.

MOA — Antibacterial.

ADVERSE EFFECTS — May cause allergic contact dermatitis and rarely contact anaphylaxis.

RETAPAMULIN (*Altabax*) ▶not absorbed ♀B ▶? $$$$

ADULT — Impetigo: Apply thin layer (up to 100 cm^2 in total area) two times per day for 5 days.

PEDS — Impetigo (9 mo or older): Apply thin layer (up to 2% total body surface area in pediatric patients) two times per day for 5 days.

FORMS — Trade only: Oint 1% 15, 30 g.

NOTES — Indicated for impetigo caused by methicillin-sensitive S. aureus and Strep. pyogenes. Do not apply to nasal mucosa.

MOA — Antibacterial; inhibits bacterial protein and RNA synthesis.

ADVERSE EFFECTS — Frequent: Skin irritation.

SILVER SULFADIAZINE (*Silvadene, ✷Flamazine*) ▶LK ♀B ▶− $$

ADULT — Burns: Apply one to two times per day.

PEDS — Not approved in children.

UNAPPROVED ADULT — Has been used for pressure ulcers.

UNAPPROVED PEDS — Burns: Apply one to two times per day.

FORMS — Generic/Trade: Cream 1% 20, 50, 85, 400, 1000 g.

NOTES — Avoid in sulfa allergy. Leukopenia, primarily decreased neutrophil count in up to 20% of patients. Significant absorption may occur and serum sulfa concentrations approach therapeutic levels. Avoid in G6PD deficiency. Has been associated with blood dyscrasias including agranulocytosis, aplastic anemia, thrombocytopenia, and hemolytic anemia; dermatologic and allergic reactions, including life-threatening cutaneous reactions such as Stevens-Johnson syndrome, toxic

(cont.)

SILVER SULFADIAZINE (*cont.*)

epidermal necrolysis and exfoliative dermatitis; gastrointestinal reactions; hepatitis and hepatocellular necrosis; CNS reactions; and toxic nephrosis. Use caution in pregnancy nearing term, premature infants, infants 2 mo or younger, and in patients with renal or hepatic dysfunction.

MOA — Sulfonamide antibacterial; acts on bacterial cell wall.

ADVERSE EFFECTS — Frequent: Pruritus, rash. Severe: Erythema multiforme, hemolytic anemia, leukopenia, agranulocytosis, aplastic anemia, interstitial nephritis, hepatitis.

DERMATOLOGY: Antifungals (Topical)

BUTENAFINE (*Lotrimin Ultra, Mentax*) ▶L ♀B ▶? $

ADULT — Treatment of tinea pedis: Apply daily for 4 weeks or two times per day for 7 days. Tinea corporis, tinea versicolor, or tinea cruris: Apply daily for 2 weeks.

PEDS — Not approved in children.

FORMS — Rx Trade only: Cream 1% 15, 30 g (Mentax). OTC Trade only: Cream 1% 12, 24 g (Lotrimin Ultra).

NOTES — Note that different Lotrimin brand name products may contain clotrimazole, miconazole, or butenafine. Most common adverse effects include contact dermatitis, burning, and worsening of condition. If no improvement in 4 weeks, reevaluate diagnosis.

MOA — Antifungal; binds to fungal cell membrane.

ADVERSE EFFECTS — Frequent: Burning, stinging, erythema, irritation.

CICLOPIROX (*Loprox, Loprox TS, Penlac, *Stieprox* shampoo*) ▶K ♀B ▶? $$$$

ADULT — Tinea pedis, tinea cruris, tinea corporis, tinea versicolor, and candidiasis (cream, lotion): Apply two times per day. Onychomycosis of fingernails/toenails (Penlac): Apply daily to affected nails; apply over previous coat; remove with alcohol every 7 days. Seborrheic dermatitis (Loprox shampoo): Shampoo twice weekly for 4 weeks.

PEDS — Onychomycosis of fingernails/toenails in children age 12 yo or older (Penlac): Apply daily to affected nails; apply over previous coat; remove with alcohol q 7 days. Not approved in children younger than 12 yo.

FORMS — Generic/Trade: Shampoo (Loprox) 1% 120 mL. Nail soln (Penlac) 8% 6.6 mL. Generic only: Gel 0.77% 30, 45, 100 g. Cream (Loprox) 0.77% 15, 30, 90 g. Lotion (Loprox TS) 0.77% 30, 60 mL.

NOTES — Clinical improvement of tinea usually occurs within first week. Patients with tinea versicolor usually exhibit clinical and mycological clearing after 2 weeks. If no improvement in 4 weeks, reevaluate diagnosis. Do not get shampoo in eyes. No safety information available in diabetes or immunocompromise. Shampoo may affect hair color in those with light-colored hair. For nail soln, infected portion of each nail should be removed by healthcare professional as frequently as monthly. Oral antifungal therapy is more effective for onychomycosis than Penlac.

MOA — Antifungal; inhibits fungal DNA, RNA, protein synthesis.

ADVERSE EFFECTS — Frequent: Pruritus, erythema, burning.

CLOTRIMAZOLE—TOPICAL (*Lotrimin AF, Mycelex, *Canesten, Clotrimaderm*) ▶L ♀B ▶? $

ADULT — Treatment of tinea pedis, tinea cruris, tinea corporis, tinea versicolor, and cutaneous candidiasis: Apply two times per day.

PEDS — Treatment of tinea pedis, tinea cruris, tinea corporis, tinea versicolor, and cutaneous candidiasis: Apply two times per day.

UNAPPROVED ADULT — Seborrheic dermatitis.

FORMS — Note that different Lotrimin brand name products may contain clotrimazole, miconazole, or butenafine. Rx Generic only: Cream 1% 15, 30, 45 g. Soln 1% 10, 30 mL. OTC Generic/Trade (Lotrimin AF): Cream 1% 12, 24 g.

NOTES — If no improvement in 4 weeks, reevaluate diagnosis.

MOA — Antifungal; alters fungal cell wall permeability.

ADVERSE EFFECTS — Frequent: Burning, irritation, stinging.

ECONAZOLE (*Ecoza*) ▶not absorbed ♀C ▶? $$

ADULT — Treatment of tinea pedis, tinea cruris, tinea corporis, and tinea versicolor: Apply daily. Cutaneous candidiasis: Apply two times per day.

PEDS — Not approved in children.

FORMS — Generic only: Cream 1% 15, 30, 85 g. Trade only: Foam 1% 70 g (Ecoza-$$$$$).

NOTES — Treat candidal infections, tinea cruris, and tinea corporis for 2 weeks and tinea pedis for 1 month to reduce risk of recurrence. May interact with warfarin, monitor INR.

MOA — Antifungal; alters fungal cell wall permeability.

ADVERSE EFFECTS — Frequent: Burning, stinging, pruritus, erythema.

EFINACONAZOLE (*Jublia*) ▶minimal absorption ♀C ▶? $$$$$

ADULT — Onychomycosis of toenail: Apply once daily to affected toenail for 48 weeks.

PEDS — Not approved for use in children.

FORMS — Trade: Soln 1% 4, 8 mL brush applicator.

MOA — Inhibits ergosterol.

ADVERSE EFFECTS — Common: ingrown toenail, application site vesicles and pain.

KETOCONAZOLE—TOPICAL (*Extina, Nizoral, Nizoral AD, Xolegel, *Ketoderm*) ▶L ♀C ▶? $$

ADULT — Shampoo (2%): Tinea versicolor: Apply to affected area, leave on for 5 min, rinse. Cream: Cutaneous candidiasis, tinea corporis, tinea cruris, and tinea versicolor: Apply daily. Seborrheic dermatitis: Apply cream (2%) two times per day for 4 weeks or gel daily for 2 weeks or foam two times per

(cont.)

KETOCONAZOLE—TOPICAL (*cont.*)

day for 4 weeks. Dandruff: Apply shampoo (Nizoral AD 1%) twice a week.

PEDS — Not approved in children younger than 12 yo.

UNAPPROVED ADULT — Seborrheic dermatitis: Apply cream (2%) daily.

UNAPPROVED PEDS — Shampoo (2%): Tinea versicolor: Apply to affected area, leave on for 5 min, rinse. Cream: Cutaneous candidiasis, tinea corporis, tinea cruris, and tinea versicolor: Apply daily. Seborrheic dermatitis: Apply cream (2%) two times per day. Dandruff: Apply shampoo (1%) twice a week.

FORMS — Generic/Trade: Shampoo 2% 120 mL. Generic only: Cream 2% 15, 30, 60 g. Trade only: Shampoo 1% 125, 200 mL (OTC Nizoral AD). Gel 2% 45 g (Xolegel). Foam 2% 50, 100 g (Extina).

NOTES — Treat candidal infections, tinea cruris, tinea corporis, and tinea versicolor for 2 weeks. Treat seborrheic dermatitis for 4 weeks. Treat tinea pedis for 6 weeks.

MOA — Antifungal; alters fungal cell wall permeability.

ADVERSE EFFECTS — Frequent: Burning, stinging, irritation, erythema. Severe: angioedema.

LULICONAZOLE (*Luzu*) ▶minimal absorption ♀C ▶? $$$$$

ADULT — Tinea pedis: Apply once daily for 2 weeks. Tinea cruris, tinea corporis: Apply once daily for 1 week.

PEDS — Not approved for use in children.

FORMS — Trade: 1% cream, 60 g.

MOA — Inhibits ergosterol synthesis

ADVERSE EFFECTS — Common: application site reactions.

MICONAZOLE—TOPICAL (*Micatin, Lotrimin AF, Zeasorb AF*) ▶L ♀+ ▶? $

ADULT — Tinea pedis, tinea cruris, tinea corporis, tinea versicolor, and cutaneous candidiasis: Apply two times per day.

PEDS — Not approved in children.

UNAPPROVED PEDS — Tinea pedis, tinea cruris, tinea corporis, tinea versicolor, and cutaneous candidiasis: Apply two times per day.

FORMS — OTC Generic only: Cream 2% 15, 45 g. OTC Trade only: Powder 2% 70, 160 g. Spray powder 2% 90, 100, 140 g. Spray liquid 2% 90, 105 mL. Gel 2% 24 g.

NOTES — Note that different Lotrimin brand name products may contain clotrimazole, miconazole, or butenafine. Symptomatic relief generally occurs in 2 to 3 days. Treat candida, tinea cruris, tinea corporis for 2 weeks, tinea pedis for 1 month to reduce risk of recurrence.

MOA — Antifungal; alters fungal cell wall permeability.

ADVERSE EFFECTS — Frequent: Rash, pruritus.

NAFTIFINE (*Naftin*) ▶LK ♀B ▶? $$$$$

ADULT — Tinea pedis, tinea cruris, and tinea corporis: Apply daily (cream) or two times per day (gel).

PEDS — Not approved in children.

FORMS — Generic/Trade: Cream 1% 60, 90 g. Cream 2% 45, 60 g. Trade only: Cream 1% Pump 90 g. Gel 1% 40, 60, 90 g. Gel 2% 45, 60 g.

NOTES — If no improvement in 4 weeks, reevaluate diagnosis.

MOA — Antifungal; alters fungal cell wall synthesis.

ADVERSE EFFECTS — Frequent: Burning, stinging, erythema, irritation, pruritus.

NYSTATIN—TOPICAL (*Mycostatin, Nyamyc, ✱Nyaderm*) ▶not absorbed ♀C ▶? $$

ADULT — Cutaneous or mucocutaneous Candida infections: Apply two to three times per day.

PEDS — Cutaneous or mucocutaneous Candida infections: Apply two to three times per day.

FORMS — Generic only: Cream, Oint 100,000 units/g 15, 30 g. Generic/Trade: Powder 100,000 units/g 15, 30, 60 g.

NOTES — Ineffective for dermatophytes/tinea. Dust feet and footwear with powder.

MOA — Antifungal; alters fungal cell wall permeability.

ADVERSE EFFECTS — Frequent: Contact dermatitis, N/V, diarrhea, stomach pain. Severe: Stevens-Johnson syndrome, hypersensitivity.

OXICONAZOLE (*Oxistat, Oxizole*) ▶minimal absorption ♀B ▶? $$$$$

ADULT — Tinea pedis, tinea cruris, and tinea corporis: Apply one to two times per day. Tinea versicolor (cream only): Apply daily.

PEDS — Cream: Tinea pedis, tinea cruris, and tinea corporis: Apply one to two times per day. Tinea versicolor: Apply daily.

FORMS — Generic/Trade : Cream 1% 30, 60, 90 g. Trade only: Lotion 1% 30, 60 mL.

MOA — Antifungal; alters fungal cell wall integrity.

ADVERSE EFFECTS — Frequent: Burning, stinging, erythema, irritation, pruritus, xeroderma.

SERTACONAZOLE (*Ertaczo*) ▶minimal absorption ♀C ▶? $$$$$

ADULT — Tinea pedis: Apply two times per day.

PEDS — Not approved for children younger than 12 yo.

FORMS — Trade only: Cream 2% 60 g.

MOA — Antifungal; alters fungal cell wall integrity.

ADVERSE EFFECTS — Frequent: Burning, dermatitis, dry skin.

TERBINAFINE—TOPICAL (*Lamisil, Lamisil AT*) ▶L ♀B ▶? $

ADULT — Tinea pedis: Apply two times per day. Tinea cruris and tinea corporis: Apply one to two times per day. Tinea versicolor (soln): Apply two times per day.

PEDS — Not approved in children.

UNAPPROVED ADULT — Cutaneous candidiasis. Prevent recolonization of dermatophyte after successful oral treatment of onychomycoses.

UNAPPROVED PEDS — Tinea pedis: Apply two times per day. Tinea cruris and tinea corporis: Apply one to two times per day. Tinea versicolor (soln): Apply two times per day.

FORMS — OTC Generic/Trade (Lamisil AT): Cream 1% 12, 24 g. OTC Trade only: Spray pump soln 1% 30 mL. Gel 1% 6, 12 g.

(cont.)

TERBINAFINE—TOPICAL (cont.)

NOTES — In many patients, improvement noted within 3 to 4 days, but therapy should continue for a minimum of 1 week, maximum of 4 weeks. Topical therapy not effective for nail fungus.

MOA — Fungicidal; alters fungal cell wall synthesis.

ADVERSE EFFECTS — Frequent: Contact dermatitis, burning, irritation, pruritus.

TOLNAFTATE (Tinactin) ▶? ♀? ▶? $

ADULT — Tinea pedis, tinea cruris, tinea corporis, and tinea versicolor: Apply two times per day. Prevention of tinea pedis (powder and aerosol): Apply prn.

PEDS — Tinea pedis, tinea cruris, tinea corporis, and tinea versicolor: Apply two times per day for older than 2 yo. Prevention of tinea pedis (powder and aerosol): Apply prn.

FORMS — OTC Generic/Trade: Cream 1% 15, 30 g. Soln 1% 10 mL. Powder 1% 45 g. OTC Trade only: Gel 1% 15 g. Powder 1% 90 g. Spray powder 1% 100, 133, 150 g. Spray liquid 1% 100, 113 mL.

MOA — Antifungal; inhibits fungal cell growth.

ADVERSE EFFECTS — Frequent: Contact dermatitis, stinging, irritation, pruritus.

DERMATOLOGY: Antiparasitics (Topical)

BENZYL ALCOHOL (Ulesfia) ▶not absorbed ♀B ▶? $$$$

WARNING — Flammable. Wash hands after application.

ADULT — Lice: Apply to dry hair to saturate scalp and hair. Amount depends on hair length. Rinse after 10 min. Reapply in 7 to 10 days.

PEDS — Lice, 6 mo or older: Apply to dry hair to saturate scalp and hair. Rinse after 10 minutes. Reapply in 7 to 10 days, if necessary.

FORMS — Trade only: Lotion 5% 60 mL and in 2-pack with nit comb.

MOA — Asphyxiation.

ADVERSE EFFECTS — Frequent: eye irritation, scalp irritation and anesthesia.

CROTAMITON (Eurax) ▶? ♀C ▶? $$$$$

ADULT — Scabies: Massage cream/lotion into entire body from chin down, repeat 24 h later, bathe 48 h later. Pruritus: Massage into affected areas prn.

PEDS — Not approved in children.

UNAPPROVED PEDS — Scabies: Massage cream/lotion into entire body from chin down, repeat 24 h later, bathe 48 h later. Pruritus: Massage into affected areas prn.

FORMS — Trade only: Cream 10% 60 g. Lotion 10% 60, 480 mL.

NOTES — Advise patients to ensure application under nails. Patients with scabies should change bed linen and clothing in am after second application and bathe 48 h after last application. Consider treating entire family if treating scabies.

MOA — Scabicidal; mechanism of action unknown.

ADVERSE EFFECTS — Frequent: None.

LINDANE ▶L ♀B ▶? $$$$

WARNING — For use only in patients who have failed other agents. Seizures and deaths have been reported with repeat or prolonged use. Use caution with infants, children, elderly, those who weigh less than 50 kg. Contraindicated in premature infants and patients with uncontrolled seizures.

ADULT — Head/crab lice: Lotion: Apply 30 to 60 mL to affected area, wash off after 12 h. Shampoo: Apply 30 to 60 mL, wash off after 4 min. Scabies (lotion): Apply 30 to 60 mL to total body from neck down, wash off after 8 to 12 h.

PEDS — Lindane penetrates human skin and has potential for CNS toxicity. Studies indicate potential toxic effects of topical lindane are greater in young. Max dose for age younger than 6 yo is 30 mL.

FORMS — Generic only: Lotion 1% 60 mL. Shampoo 1% 60 mL.

NOTES — For lice, reapply if living lice noted after 7 days. After shampooing, comb with fine-tooth comb to remove nits. Consider treating entire family if treating scabies.

MOA — Nervous system stimulant lethal to ova and parasites.

ADVERSE EFFECTS — Frequent: None. Severe: CNS side effects—headache, restlessness, seizures, aplastic anemia, arrhythmias, hepatitis, pulmonary edema, hematuria.

MALATHION (Ovide) ▶? ♀B ▶? $$$$

ADULT — Lice: Apply to dry hair, let dry naturally, wash off in 8 to 12 h. Repeat in 7 to 10 days, if lice present.

PEDS — Lice in children 6 yo or older: Apply to dry hair, let dry naturally, wash off in 8 to 12 h. Repeat in 7 to 10 days if lice present.

FORMS — Generic/Trade only: Lotion 0.5% 59 mL.

NOTES — Do not use hair dryer; flammable. Avoid contact with eyes. Use a fine-tooth comb to remove nits and dead lice.

MOA — Pediculicide via cholinesterase inhibition.

ADVERSE EFFECTS — Frequent: None.

PERMETHRIN (Elimite, Acticin, Nix, ✷Kwellada-P) ▶L ♀B ▶? $$

ADULT — Scabies (cream): Massage cream into entire body (avoid mouth, eyes, nose), wash off after 8 to 14 h. 30 g is typical adult dose. Repeat in 7 days. Lice (liquid): Apply to clean, towel-dried hair, saturate hair and scalp, wash off after 10 min.

PEDS — Scabies (cream) age older than 2 mo: Massage cream into entire body (avoid mouth, eyes, nose), wash off after 8 to 14 h. Lice (liquid) in age older than 2 yo: Saturate hair and scalp, wash off after 10 min. Repeat in 7 to 10 days if lice present.

FORMS — Generic/Trade: Cream (Elimite, Acticin) 5% 60 g. OTC Generic/Trade: Liquid creme rinse (Nix) 1% 60 mL.

NOTES — If necessary, may repeat application in 7 days, paying particular attention to under nail beds. Consider treating entire family if treating scabies. Residual itch often lasts for up to 1 month after treatment.

(cont.)

PERMETHRIN *(cont.)*

MOA — Neuronal toxin which paralyzes lice.

ADVERSE EFFECTS — Frequent: Burning, stinging, erythema, numbness, pruritus.

(pyrethrins + piperonyl butoxide, ✱ *R&C*) ▶L ♀C ▶? $

ADULT — Canada only. Lice: Apply shampoo, wash after 10 min. Reapply in 5 to 10 days.

PEDS — Canada only. Lice: Apply shampoo, wash after 10 min. Reapply in 5 to 10 days.

FORMS — OTC Generic/Trade: Shampoo (0.33% pyrethrins, 4% piperonyl butoxide) 60, 120 mL.

NOTES — Use caution if allergic to ragweed. Avoid contact with mucous membranes. A-200 brand name no longer available.

MOA — Neuronal toxin to lice; inhibits pyrethrin metabolism.

ADVERSE EFFECTS — Frequent: Burning, stinging, pruritus.

RID (pyrethrins + piperonyl butoxide) ▶L ♀C ▶? $

ADULT — Lice: Apply shampoo/mousse, wash after 10 min. Reapply in 5 to 10 days prn.

PEDS — Lice: Apply shampoo/mousse, wash after 10 min. Reapply in 5 to 10 days prn.

FORMS — OTC Generic/Trade: Shampoo 60, 120, 240 mL. OTC Trade only: Mousse 5.5 oz.

NOTES — Use caution if allergic to ragweed. Avoid contact with mucous membranes. Available alone or as part of a RID 1-2-3 kit containing shampoo, egg, and nit comb-out gel and home lice-control spray for nonwashable items.

MOA — Neuronal toxin to lice; inhibits pyrethrin metabolism.

ADVERSE EFFECTS — Frequent: Burning, stinging, pruritus.

SPINOSAD (*Natroba*) ▶not absorbed ♀B ▶? $$$$$

ADULT — Lice: Apply to dry hair/scalp to cover. Leave on 10 min then rinse. Retreat if live lice seen after 7 days.

PEDS — 6 mo and older: Lice: Apply to dry hair/scalp to cover. Leave on 10 min then rinse. Retreat if live lice seen after 7 days.

FORMS — Generic/Trade: Topical susp, 0.9%, 120 mL.

MOA — Pediculide which causes hyperexcitation-induced paralysis in lice.

ADVERSE EFFECTS — Frequent: erythema, irritation.

DERMATOLOGY: Antipsoriatics

ACITRETIN (*Soriatane*) ▶L ♀X ▶– $$$$$

WARNING — Contraindicated in pregnancy and avoid pregnancy for 3 years following medication discontinuation. Major human fetal abnormalities have been reported. Females of child-bearing age must avoid alcohol while on medication and for 2 months following therapy since alcohol prolongs elimination of a teratogenic metabolite. Use in reliable females of reproductive potential only if they have severe, unresponsive psoriasis, have received written and oral warnings of the teratogenic potential, are using 2 reliable forms of contraception, and have 2 negative pregnancy tests within 1 week prior to starting therapy. Contraception should start at least 1 month prior to therapy and continue for 3 years following discontinuation. Must have negative monthly pregnancy test during treatment. Therefore, prescribe limited amount and do not allow refill until documented negative pregnancy test. Following discontinuation, repeat pregnancy test q 3 months. It is unknown whether residual acitretin in seminal fluid poses a risk to the fetus while a male patient is taking the drug or after it is discontinued.

ADULT — Severe psoriasis: Initiate at 25 to 50 mg PO daily.

PEDS — Not approved in children.

UNAPPROVED ADULT — Lichen planus: 30 mg/day PO for 4 weeks, then titrate to 10 to 50 mg/day for 12 weeks total. Sjögren-Larsson syndrome: 0.47 mg/kg/day PO. Also used in Darier's disease, palmoplantar pustulosis, nonbullous and bullous ichthyosiform erythroderma, lichen sclerosus et atrophicus of the vulva, palmoplantar lichen nitidus, and chemoprevention for high-risk immunosuppressed patients with history of squamous cell carcinomas of the skin. Pityriasis rubra pilaris: 25 mg to 50 mg PO once daily.

UNAPPROVED PEDS — Has been used in children with lamellar ichthyosis. Pediatric use is not recommended. Adverse effects on bone growth are suspected.

FORMS — Generic/Trade: Caps 10, 17.5, 25 mg.

NOTES — Transient worsening of psoriasis may occur, and full benefit may take 2 to 3 months. Elevated LFTs may occur in one-third of patients; monitor LFTs at 1- to 2-week intervals until stable and then periodically thereafter. Monitor serum lipid concentrations q 1 to 2 weeks until response to drug is established. May decrease tolerance to contact lenses due to dry eyes. Avoid prolonged exposure to sunlight. May cause hair loss. May cause depression. May cause bone changes, especially with use more than 6 months. Many adverse drug reactions.

MOA — Unknown.

ADVERSE EFFECTS — Frequent: Cheilitis, xerostomia, rhinitis, epistaxis, alopecia, skin peeling, pruritus, erythematous rash, rigors, arthralgias, xerophthalmus. Severe: Hepatitis, pancreatitis, pseudotumor cerebri, angioedema, urticaria, capillary leak syndrome.

ANTHRALIN (*Zithranol*) ▶minimal absorption ♀C ▶? $$$$$

ADULT — Scalp psoriasis: Apply shampoo to scalp 3 to 4 times a week. Lather and leave on for 3 to 5 min. Rinse. Psoriasis of skin or scalp: Apply cream once a day. Initially use short contact times (5 to 15 min) and gradually increase to 30 min. Wash off.

PEDS — Not approved in children.

(cont.)

ANTHRALIN (*cont.*)

FORMS — Trade: Shampoo 1% (Zithranol shampoo) 85 g. Cream 1.2% (Zithranol RR cream) 15, 45 g.

NOTES — May cause staining. Avoid contact with fabrics, plastics, and other materials.

MOA — Unknown.

ADVERSE EFFECTS — Frequent: skin irriation, staining, discoloation of skin and fabric.

ANTHRALIN (*Drithocreme*) ▶? ♀C ▶— $$$

ADULT — Chronic psoriasis: Apply daily.

PEDS — Not approved in children.

UNAPPROVED ADULT — Alopecia areata.

UNAPPROVED PEDS — Chronic psoriasis: Apply daily.

FORMS — Trade only: Cream 0.5, 1% 50 g.

NOTES — Short contact periods (ie 15 to 20 min) followed by removal with an appropriate solvent (soap or petrolatum) may be preferred. May stain fabric, skin, or hair.

MOA — Inhibits proliferation of epidermal cells in psoriasis.

ADVERSE EFFECTS — Frequent: Irritation, discoloration of skin and clothing.

CALCIPOTRIENE (*Dovonex, Sorilux*) ▶L ♀C ▶? $$$$

WARNING — Contact dermatitis, including allergic contact dermatitis, has occurred.

ADULT — Moderate plaque psoriasis: Apply two times per day.

PEDS — Not approved in children.

UNAPPROVED ADULT — Has been used for vitiligo and morphea.

UNAPPROVED PEDS — Moderate plaque psoriasis: Apply two times per day. Has been used for vitiligo.

FORMS — Trade only: Oint 0.005% 30, 60, 100 g (Dovonex). Cream 0.005% 30, 60, 100 g (Dovonex). Foam for scalp 0.005% 60, 120 g (Sorilux). Generic/Trade: Scalp soln 0.005% 60 mL.

NOTES — Avoid contact with face. Do not exceed 100 g/week to minimize risk of hypercalcemia, hypercalciuria. Burning, itching, and skin irritation may occur in 10 to 15% of patients.

MOA — Regulates skin cell production and proliferation.

ADVERSE EFFECTS — Frequent: Burning, irritation, drying, rash, worsening of psoriasis, pruritus.

✤ **DOVOBET** (calcipotriol + betamethasone—topical) ▶L ♀D ▶? $$$$$

ADULT — Canada only: Severe scalp psoriasis: Apply once daily for up to 4 weeks. Mild to moderate plaque psoriasis of body: Apply once daily for up to 8 weeks.

PEDS — Not approved for use in children.

FORMS — Rx: Trade: Gel (50 mcg/g calcipotriol and 0.5 mg/g betamethasone) 30g, 60g.

NOTES — Do not use more than 100 g/week due to risk of hypercalcemia. Do not use on more than 30% of body surface area.

MOA — Vitamin D3 analog that inhibits cell proliferation, regulates skin cell production, anti-inflammatory.

ADVERSE EFFECTS — See components.

ENSTILAR (calcipotriene + betamethasone dipropionate) ▶L ♀C ▶— $$$$$

WARNING — Avoid use on face, groin, axillae, under occlusive dressings or if skin atrophy is present

ADULT — Plaque psoriasis: Apply to affected area once daily for up to 4 weeks. Discontinue when control is achieved. Do not use more than 60 g every 4 days.

PEDS — Not approved for use in children younger than 18 years.

FORMS — Foam (0.005% calcipotriene + 0.064% betamethasone dipropionate) 60 g.

NOTES — Flammable. Monitor for hypercalcemia and hypercalciuria. Avoid use on face, groin, axillae, under occlusive dressings or if skin atrophy is present

MOA — See components.

ADVERSE EFFECTS — See components.

IXEKIZUMAB (*Taltz*) ▶proteolysis ♀?/?/? ▶? $$$$$

WARNING — Increased risk of severe infections, including TB. Crohn's disease and ulcerative colitis, including exacerbations, have occurred during clinical trials, monitor these patients closely.

ADULT — Moderate to severe plaque psoriasis: 160 mg SQ at week 0, then 80 mg SQ at weeks 2, 4, 6, 8, 10, and 12, then 80 mg SQ every 4 weeks.

PEDS — Not approved for use in children.

FORMS — Trade only: prefilled autoinjector 80 mg, prefilled syringe 80 mg.

NOTES — Do not give live vaccines.

MOA — Monoclonal antibody that selectively binds with the interleukin 17A cytokine and inhibits interaction with IL-17 receptor.

ADVERSE EFFECTS — Frequent: injection site reactions, nausea, tinea infections. Severe: infections, hypersensitivity reactions.

METHOXSALEN (*8-MOP, Oxsoralen-Ultra, Uvadex*) ▶skin ♀C ▶? $$$$$

WARNING — Should only be prescribed by physicians who have special training. For the treatment of patients with psoriasis, restrict to severe cases. Possibility of ocular damage, aging of the skin, and skin cancer (including melanoma).Women of childbearing potential should avoid becoming pregnant

ADULT — Psoriasis: Dose based on wt (0.4 mg/kg/dose), 1½ to 2 h before ultraviolet light exposure. Specialized dosing of sterile solution for photopheresis (Uvadex).

PEDS — Not approved in children.

FORMS — Generic/Trade: Soft gelcap 10 mg (Oxsoralen-Ultra). Trade only: Hard gelcap 10 mg (8-MOP). Sterile soln for use in photopheresis 20 mcg/mL (Uvadex).

NOTES — Oxsoralen-Ultra (soft gelcap) cannot be interchanged with 8-MOP (hard gelcap) due to significant bioavailability differences and photosensitization onset times. Take with food or milk. Wear ultraviolet light-blocking glasses and avoid sun exposure after ingestion and for remainder of day.

MOA — DNA photodamage and decreased cell proliferation.

(cont.)

METHOXSALEN (*cont.*)

ADVERSE EFFECTS — Frequent: Nausea, pruritus, erythema, nervousness, insomnia. Severe: Depression, skin cancer with prolonged use, cataracts.

***TACLONEX* (calcipotriene + betamethasone—topical) ▶L ♀C ▶? $$$$$**

ADULT — Psoriasis: Apply daily for up to 4 weeks. Max dose 100 g weekly.

PEDS — Psoriasis: Children age 12 to 17 yo: Apply once daily for 4 weeks. Children should not use more than 60 g per week.

FORMS — Calcipotriene 0.005% + betamethasone dipropionate 0.064%. Generic/Trade: Oint 60, 100 g. Trade only: Topical susp (Taclonex) 60, 120 g.

NOTES — Do not exceed 100 g/week due to risk of hypercalcemia. Do not use on more than 30% of body surface area. Do not apply to face, groin, or axillae to avoid irritant dermatitis.

MOA — Vitamin D3 analog that inhibits cell proliferation, regulates skin cell production, anti-inflammatory.

ADVERSE EFFECTS — See calcipotriene and betamethasone.

USTEKINUMAB (*Stelara*) ▶L ♀B ▶? $$$$$

WARNING — Can cause serious infections. Discontinue if serious infection. Caution if high risk of malignancy or a history of malignancy. Theoretical risk of infection from Mycobacterium, Salmonella, and BCG vaccine. Evaluate patients for TB prior to therapy. Risk of reversible posterior leukoencephalopathy syndrome. Live vaccines should not be given to patients receiving injections.

ADULT — Severe plaque psoriasis, active psoriatic arthritis, wt less than or equal to 100 kg: 45 mg SC initially and again 4 weeks later, followed by 45 mg SC q 12 weeks. For wt greater than 100 kg and psoriatic arthritis with moderate to severe plaque psoriasis: 90 mg SC initially and again 4 weeks later, followed by 90 mg SC q 12 weeks.

PEDS — Not approved in children.

FORMS — Trade only: 45 and 90 mg prefilled syringe and vial.

NOTES — After proper training, may be self-administered at home, if appropriate.

MOA — Interleukin 12/23 antagonist.

ADVERSE EFFECTS — Frequent: Headache, fatigue, nasopharyngitis, URI. Severe: Serious infection, malignancy, disseminated TB-reversible posterior leukoencephalopathy syndrome.

DERMATOLOGY: Antivirals (Topical)

ACYCLOVIR—TOPICAL (*Zovirax*) ▶K ♀C ▶? $$$$$

ADULT — Initial episodes of herpes genitalis: Apply ointment q 3 h (6 times per day) for 7 days. Non-life-threatening mucocutaneous herpes simplex in immunocompromised patients: Apply ointment q 3 h (6 times per day) for 7 days. Recurrent herpes labialis: Apply cream 5 times per day for 4 days.

PEDS — Recurrent herpes labialis: Children 12 yo or older: Apply cream 5 times per day for 4 days.

UNAPPROVED PEDS — Initial episodes of herpes genitalis: Apply ointment q 3 h (6 times per day) for 7 days. Non-life-threatening mucocutaneous herpes simplex in immunocompromised patients: Apply ointment q 3 h (6 times per day) for 7 days.

FORMS — Generic/Trade: Oint 5% 5, 15, 30 g. Trade only: Cream 5% 5 g.

NOTES — Use finger cot or rubber glove to apply ointment to avoid dissemination. Burning/stinging may occur in up to 28% of patients. Oral form more effective than topical for herpes genitalis.

MOA — Antiviral; inhibits DNA synthesis and viral replication.

ADVERSE EFFECTS — Frequent: Rash (oint). Skin irritation (cream). Severe: Cutaneous sensitization.

DOCOSANOL (*Abreva*) ▶not absorbed ♀B ▶? $

ADULT — Oral-facial herpes (cold sores): Apply 5 times per day until healed.

PEDS — Oral-facial herpes (cold sores): Use adult dose for age 12 yo or older.

FORMS — OTC Trade only: Cream 10% 2 g.

MOA — Inhibits entry of lipid-enveloped viruses.

ADVERSE EFFECTS — Frequent: Headache, site reaction, rash, pruritus, dry skin, ache.

IMIQUIMOD (*Aldara, Zyclara, ✦Vyloma*) ▶not absorbed ♀C ▶? $$$

ADULT —External genital and perianal warts, 3.75% cream: Apply 3 times a week at bedtime for up to 16 weeks. Wash off after 8 h. Non-hyperkeratotic, non-hypertrophic actinic keratoses on face/scalp in immunocompetent adults, 2.5% or 3.75% cream: Apply to face or scalp (but not both) twice a week for up to 16 weeks (Aldara) or once daily for two 2-week periods separated by a 2-week break (Zyclara). Wash off after 8 h. Primary superficial basal cell carcinoma: Apply 5 times per week for 6 weeks (Aldara). Wash off after 8 h.

PEDS — External genital and perianal warts: Apply 3 times per week at bedtime and wash off after 6 to 10 h for age 12 yo or older (Aldara) or once daily for two 2-week periods separated by a 2-week break (Zyclara).

UNAPPROVED ADULT — Molluscum contagiosum. Apply 3 times per week, wash off after 6 to 10 h.

UNAPPROVED PEDS — Molluscum contagiosum.

FORMS — Generic/Trade: Cream 5% (Aldara) single-use packets. Trade only: Cream 3.75% (Zyclara-$$$$$) single-use packets, box of 28 and 7.5 g pump. Cream 2.5% 7.5 g pump.

NOTES — May weaken condoms and diaphragms. Avoid sexual contact while cream is on when used for genital/perianal warts. Most common adverse effects include erythema, itching, erosion, burning, excoriation, edema, and pain. Discard partially used packets.

MOA — Mechanism unknown but may increase cytokine concentrations.

(cont.)

IMIQUIMOD (*cont.*)

ADVERSE EFFECTS — Frequent: Pruritus, erythema, burning, erosion, edema, flu-like symptoms. Severe: Erythema, erosion, edema, severe local inflammation of the external female genitalia leading to urinary retention.

INTERFERON ALFA-N3 (*Alferon N*) ▶K ♀C ▶– $$$$$
WARNING — Flu-like syndrome, myalgias, alopecia. Contraindicated in egg protein or neomycin allergy.
ADULT — Condylomata acuminata: Inject 0.05 mL into the base of each wart twice a week for a maximum of 8 weeks, and a 0.5 mL maximum dose per session.
PEDS — Not approved in children younger than 18 yo.
FORMS — 1 mL vials
NOTES — Treatment should not be repeated for at least 3 months unless new or enlarging warts.
MOA — Interferons enhance phagocytic activity of macrophages and cytotoxicity of lymphocytes, and inhibit viral replication.
ADVERSE EFFECTS — Serious: Hypersensitivity. Frequent: Flu-like syndrome, myalgias.

PENCICLOVIR (*Denavir*) ▶not absorbed ♀B ▶? $$$$$
ADULT — Recurrent herpes labialis (cold sores): Apply q 2 h while awake for 4 days.
PEDS — Not approved in children.
UNAPPROVED PEDS — Recurrent herpes labialis: Apply q 2 h while awake for 4 days.
FORMS — Trade only: Cream 1% tube 5 g.
NOTES — Start therapy as soon as possible during prodrome. For moderate to severe cases of herpes labialis, systemic treatment with famciclovir or acyclovir may be preferred.
MOA — Antiviral: Inhibits viral DNA synthesis and replication.
ADVERSE EFFECTS — Frequent: Headache, erythema.

PODOFILOX (*Condylox, ✲Condyline, Wartec*) ▶? ♀C ▶? $$$
ADULT — External genital warts (gel and soln) and perianal warts (gel only): Apply two times per day for 3 consecutive days of a week and repeat for up to 4 weeks.
PEDS — Not approved in children.

FORMS — Generic/Trade: Soln 0.5% 3.5 mL. Trade only: Gel 0.5% 3.5 g.
MOA — Unknown.
ADVERSE EFFECTS — Frequent: Inflammation, burning, erosion, pain, pruritus, bleeding.

PODOPHYLLIN (*Podocon-25, Podofin, Podofilm*) ▶? ♀– ▶– $$$
ADULT — Genital wart removal: Initial application: Apply to wart and leave on for 30 to 40 min to determine patient's sensitivity. Thereafter, use minimum contact time necessary (1 to 4 h depending on result). Remove dried podophyllin with alcohol or soap and water.
PEDS — Not approved in children.
FORMS — Not to be dispensed to patients. For hospital/clinic use; not intended for outpatient prescribing. Trade only: Liquid 25% 15 mL.
NOTES — Do not treat large areas or numerous warts all at once. Contraindicated in diabetics, pregnancy, patients using steroids or with poor circulation, and on bleeding warts.
MOA — Arrests mitosis by binding to microtubule spindle.
ADVERSE EFFECTS — Frequent: Pruritus, N/V, abdominal pain, diarrhea. Severe: Hallucination, hepatotoxicity, leukopenia, thrombocytopenia, renal failure.

SINECATECHINS (*Veregen*) ▶minimal absorption ♀C ▶? $$$$$
ADULT — Apply three times per day to external genital and perianal warts for up to 16 weeks.
PEDS — Not approved in children.
FORMS — Trade only: Oint 15% 30 g.
NOTES — Botanical drug product. Contains a partially purified fraction of the water extract of green tea leaves. Do not use on open wounds. Do not use in immunocompromised patients. Generic name used to be kunecatechins.
MOA — Unknown, but thought to be immunomodulatory.
ADVERSE EFFECTS — Frequent: Burning, pain, erythema at application site, erosion, edema, induration, rash.

DERMATOLOGY: Atopic Dermatitis Preparations

NOTE: Long-term safety has not been established. Avoid use in immunocompromised patients and in children younger than 2 yo. Use minimum amount to control symptoms.

PIMECROLIMUS (*Elidel*) ▶L ♀C ▶? $$$$$
WARNING — Use minimum amount, only on involved areas and avoid occlusion.
ADULT — Atopic dermatitis: Apply two times per day.
PEDS — Atopic dermatitis: Apply two times per day for age 2 yo or older.
UNAPPROVED ADULT — Perioral dermatitis, oral lichen planus, intertriginous/facial psoriasis.
FORMS — Trade only: Cream 1% 30, 60, 100 g.
NOTES — Long-term safety unclear.
MOA — Calcineurin inhibitor modulator.

ADVERSE EFFECTS — Frequent: Burning headache, nasopharyngitis, cough, influenza, pyrexia, viral infection.

TACROLIMUS—TOPICAL (*Protopic*) ▶minimal absorption ♀C ▶? $$$$$
WARNING — May be associated with skin cancer or lymphoma. Avoid continuous long-term use. Avoid in children younger than 2 yo.
ADULT — Atopic dermatitis: Apply two times per day.
PEDS — Atopic dermatitis: Apply 0.03% ointment two times per day for age 2 to 15 yo.

(cont.)

TACROLIMUS—TOPICAL (cont.)

UNAPPROVED ADULT — Vitiligo: Apply 0.1% two times per day. Chronic allergic contact dermatitis (eg nickel-induced): Apply 0.1% ointment two times per day.

FORMS — Generic/Trade: Oint 0.03%, 0.1% 30, 60, 100 g.

NOTES — Do not use with an occlusive dressing. Continue treatment for 1 week after clearing of symptoms.

MOA — Topical immunomodulator that suppresses T-cell activation and cytokine release.

ADVERSE EFFECTS — Frequent: Skin burning/tingling, pruritus, flu-like symptoms, erythema, headache, urticaria, acne. Severe: LFT increase, anaphylactoid reaction, angina, angioedema.

DERMATOLOGY: Corticosteroid/Antimicrobial Combinations

CORTISPORIN (neomycin—topical + polymyxin—topical + hydrocortisone—topical) ▶LK ♀C ▶? $$$$

ADULT — Corticosteroid-responsive dermatoses with secondary infection: Apply two to four times per day.

PEDS — Not approved in children.

UNAPPROVED PEDS — Corticosteroid-responsive dermatoses with secondary infection: Apply two to four times per day.

FORMS — Trade only: Cream 7.5 g. Oint (also contains bacitracin) 15 g.

NOTES — Due to concerns about nephrotoxicity and ototoxicity associated with neomycin, do not use over wide areas or for prolonged periods of time.

MOA — Antibacterial + anti-inflammatory.

ADVERSE EFFECTS — Ocular: Frequent: Blurred vision, itching, elevation of intraocular pressure, glaucoma, allergic contact dermatitis (usually due to neomycin component). Severe: Hypersensitivity, anaphylaxis.

✱ FUCIDIN-H (fusidic acid—topical + hydrocortisone—topical) ▶L ♀? ▶? $$

ADULT — Canada only. Atopic dermatitis: Apply three times per day.

PEDS — Canada only. Atopic dermatitis: Apply three times per day for age 3 yo or older.

FORMS — Canada Trade only: Cream (2% fusidic acid, 1% hydrocortisone acetate) 30 g.

NOTES — Not to be used longer than 2 weeks; notify prescriber if improvement not seen after 1 week.

MOA — Antibacterial, interferes with bacterial protein synthesis + anti-inflammatory.

ADVERSE EFFECTS — Serious: Hypersensitivity. Frequent: Mild irritation, flare of dermatitis.

LOTRISONE (clotrimazole—topical + betamethasone—topical, ✱ Lotriderm) ▶L ♀C ▶? $$$

ADULT — Tinea pedis, tinea cruris, and tinea corporis: Apply two times per day.

PEDS — Not approved in children younger than 17 yo.

FORMS — Generic/Trade: Cream (clotrimazole 1% + betamethasone 0.05%) 15, 45 g. Lotion (clotrimazole 1% + betamethasone 0.05%) 30 mL.

NOTES — Treat tinea cruris and tinea corporis for 1 week (no longer than 2 weeks) and tinea pedis for 2 weeks (no longer than 4 weeks). Do not use for diaper dermatitis.

MOA — Antifungal + anti-inflammatory.

ADVERSE EFFECTS — Frequent: Erythema, stinging, blistering, peeling, edema, pruritus, urticaria, irritation, telangiectasia.

MYCOLOG II (nystatin—topical + triamcinolone—topical) ▶L ♀C ▶? $$$$$

ADULT — Cutaneous candidiasis: Apply two times per day.

PEDS — Not approved in children.

UNAPPROVED PEDS — Sometimes used for diaper dermatitis, but not recommended due to risk of adrenal suppression.

FORMS — Generic only: Cream, Oint 15, 30, 60 g.

NOTES — Avoid occlusive dressings.

MOA — Antifungal + anti-inflammatory.

ADVERSE EFFECTS — Frequent: None. Severe: Stevens-Johnson syndrome.

DERMATOLOGY: Corticosteroids (Topical)

NOTE: After long-term use, do not discontinue abruptly; switch to a less potent agent or alternate use of corticosteroids and emollient products. Monitor for hyperglycemia/adrenal suppression if used for long period of time or over a large area of the body, especially in children. Chronic administration may cause skin atrophy and interfere with pediatric growth and development.

ALCLOMETASONE DIPROPIONATE (Aclovate) ▶L ♀C ▶? $$$$

ADULT — Inflammatory and pruritic manifestations of corticosteroid-responsive dermatoses: Apply sparingly two to three times per day.

PEDS — Inflammatory and pruritic manifestations of corticosteroid-responsive dermatoses: Apply sparingly two to three times per day for age 1 yo or older. Safety and efficacy for more than 3 weeks have not been established.

FORMS — Generic/Trade: Ointment, Cream 0.05% 15, 45, 60 g.

MOA — Anti-inflammatory; suppresses DNA synthesis, decreases WBC influx.

ADVERSE EFFECTS — Frequent: Burning, pruritus, dryness, irritation, erythema.

AMCINONIDE (Cyclocort) ▶L ♀C ▶? $$

ADULT — Inflammatory and pruritic manifestations of corticosteroid-responsive dermatoses: Apply sparingly two to three times per day.

(cont.)

AMCINONIDE (cont.)

PEDS — Inflammatory and pruritic manifestations of corticosteroid-responsive dermatoses: Apply sparingly two to three times per day.

FORMS — Generic only: Cream 0.1% 15, 30, 60 g. Ointment 0.1% 60 g. Lotion 0.1% 60 mL.

MOA — Anti-inflammatory; suppresses DNA synthesis, decreases WBC influx.

ADVERSE EFFECTS — Frequent: Burning, pruritus, dryness, irritation, erythema. Severe: Steroid atrophy, hypothalamic axis suppression with higher potency preparations.

AUGMENTED BETAMETHASONE DIPROPIONATE (Diprolene, Diprolene AF, ✸Topilene Glycol) ▶L ♀C ▶? $$$

ADULT — Inflammatory and pruritic manifestations of corticosteroid-responsive dermatoses: Apply sparingly one to two times per day.

PEDS — Not approved younger than 12 yo.

FORMS — Generic/Trade: Diprolene: Ointment 0.05% 15, 50 g. Lotion 0.05% 30, 60 mL. Diprolene AF: Cream 0.05% 15, 50 g. Generic only: Gel 0.05% 15, 50 g.

NOTES — Do not use occlusive dressings. Do not use for longer than 2 consecutive weeks and do not exceed a total dose of 45 to 50 g per week or 50 mL per week of the lotion.

MOA — Anti-inflammatory; suppresses DNA synthesis, decreases WBC influx.

ADVERSE EFFECTS — Frequent: Burning, pruritus, dryness, irritation, erythema. Severe: Steroid atrophy, hypothalamic axis suppression with higher potency preparations.

BETAMETHASONE DIPROPIONATE (Maxivate, ✸Propaderm, TARO-sone) ▶L ♀C ▶? $$$

ADULT — Inflammatory and pruritic manifestations of corticosteroid-responsive dermatoses: Apply sparingly one to two times per day.

PEDS — Inflammatory and pruritic manifestations of corticosteroid-responsive dermatoses: Apply sparingly one to two times per day.

FORMS — Generic only: Ointment, Cream 0.05% 15, 45 g. Lotion 0.05% 60 mL.

NOTES — Do not use occlusive dressings.

MOA — Anti-inflammatory; suppresses DNA synthesis, decreases WBC influx.

ADVERSE EFFECTS — Frequent: Burning, pruritus, dryness, irritation, erythema. Severe: Steroid atrophy, hypothalamic axis suppression with higher potency preparations.

BETAMETHASONE VALERATE (Luxiq, Beta-Val, ✸Betaderm) ▶L ♀C ▶? $$

ADULT — Inflammatory and pruritic manifestations of corticosteroid-responsive dermatoses: Apply sparingly one to two times per day. Dermatoses of scalp: Apply small amount of foam to scalp two times per day.

PEDS — Inflammatory and pruritic manifestations of corticosteroid-responsive dermatoses: Apply sparingly one to two times per day.

FORMS — Generic only: Ointment, Cream 0.1% 15, 45 g. Lotion 0.1% 60 mL. Generic/Trade: Foam (Luxiq) 0.12% 50, 100 g.

MOA — Anti-inflammatory; suppresses DNA synthesis, decreases WBC influx.

ADVERSE EFFECTS — Frequent: Burning, pruritus, dryness, irritation, erythema. Severe: Steroid atrophy, hypothalamic axis suppression with higher potency preparations.

CLOBETASOL (Temovate, Olux, Clobex, Cormax, ✸Dermasone) ▶L ♀C ▶? $$$$

ADULT — Inflammatory and pruritic manifestations of corticosteroid-responsive dermatoses: Apply sparingly two times per day. For scalp apply foam two times per day.

PEDS — Not approved in children.

FORMS — Generic/Trade: Cream, Ointment 0.05% 15, 30, 45, 60 g. Scalp application 0.05% 25, 50 mL. Gel 0.05% 15, 30, 60 g. Foam (Olux) 0.05% 50, 100 g. Lotion (Clobex) 0.05% 60, 120 mL. Shampoo 0.05% 118 mL. Spray 0.05% 60, 125 mL.

NOTES — Adrenal suppression at doses as low as 2 g per day. Do not use occlusive dressings. Do not use for longer than 2 consecutive weeks and do not exceed a total dose of 50 g per week.

MOA — Anti-inflammatory; suppresses DNA synthesis, decreases WBC influx.

ADVERSE EFFECTS — Frequent: Burning, pruritus, dryness, irritation, erythema, alopecia. Severe: Steroid atrophy, hypothalamic axis suppression with higher potency preparations.

CLOCORTOLONE PIVALATE (Cloderm) ▶L ♀C ▶? $$$$$

ADULT — Inflammatory and pruritic manifestations of corticosteroid-responsive dermatoses: Apply sparingly three times per day.

PEDS — Inflammatory and pruritic manifestations of corticosteroid-responsive dermatoses: Apply sparingly three times per day.

FORMS — Generic/Trade: Cream 0.1% 30, 45, 75, 90 g.

MOA — Anti-inflammatory; suppresses DNA synthesis, decreases WBC influx.

ADVERSE EFFECTS — Frequent: Burning, pruritus, dryness, irritation, erythema. Severe: Hypothalamic axis suppression with higher potency preparations.

DESONIDE (DesOwen, Desonate, Tridesilon, Verdeso) ▶L ♀C ▶? $$$$

ADULT — Inflammatory and pruritic manifestations of corticosteroid-responsive dermatoses: Apply sparingly two to three times per day.

PEDS — Inflammatory and pruritic manifestations of corticosteroid-responsive dermatoses: Apply sparingly two to three times per day.

FORMS — Generic/Trade: Cream, Ointment 0.05%, 15, 60 g. Lotion 0.05%, 60, 120 mL. Trade only: Gel (Desonate) 0.05% 60 g, Foam (Verdeso) 0.05%, 100 g.

NOTES — Do not use with occlusive dressings.

MOA — Anti-inflammatory; suppresses DNA synthesis, decreases WBC influx.

ADVERSE EFFECTS — Frequent: Burning, pruritus, dryness, irritation, erythema.

DESOXIMETASONE (*Topicort, Topicort LP, ✦Desoxi*) ▶L ♀C ▶? $$$$
ADULT — Inflammatory and pruritic manifestations of corticosteroid-responsive dermatoses: Apply sparingly two times per day.
PEDS — Safety and efficacy have not been established for Topicort 0.25% ointment. For inflammatory and pruritic manifestations of corticosteroid-responsive dermatoses (cream and gel): Apply 0.05% sparingly two times per day.
FORMS — Generic/Trade: Cream, Gel 0.05% 15, 60 g. Cream, Ointment 0.25% 15, 60, 100 g. Trade only: Spray 0.25% 100 mL.
MOA — Anti-inflammatory; suppresses DNA synthesis, decreases WBC influx.
ADVERSE EFFECTS — Frequent: Burning, pruritus, dryness, irritation, erythema. Severe: Steroid atrophy, hypothalamic axis suppression with higher potency preparations.

DIFLORASONE (*Psorcon E, Maxiflor*) ▶L ♀C ▶? $$$$$
ADULT — Inflammatory and pruritic manifestations of corticosteroid-responsive dermatoses: Apply sparingly one to three times per day.
PEDS — Not approved in children.
FORMS — Generic/Trade: Cream, Ointment 0.05% 15, 30, 60 g.
NOTES — Doses of 30 g/day of diflorasone 0.05% cream for 1 week resulted in adrenal suppression in some psoriasis patients.
MOA — Anti-inflammatory; suppresses DNA synthesis, decreases WBC influx.
ADVERSE EFFECTS — Frequent: Burning, pruritus, dryness, irritation, erythema. Severe: Steroid atrophy, hypothalamic axis suppression with higher potency preparations.

FLUOCINOLONE—TOPICAL (*Synalar, Capex, Derma-Smoothe/FS*) ▶L ♀C ▶? $$$
ADULT — Inflammatory and pruritic manifestations of corticosteroid-responsive dermatoses: Apply sparingly two to three times per day. Psoriasis of the scalp (Derma-Smoothe/FS): Massage into scalp, cover with shower cap, and leave on 4 or more h or overnight and then wash off.
PEDS — Inflammatory and pruritic manifestations of corticosteroid-responsive dermatoses: Apply sparingly two to four times per day. Atopic dermatitis: Moisten skin and apply to affected areas two times per day for up to 4 weeks (Derma-Smoothe/FS).
FORMS — Generic/Trade: Cream, Ointment 0.025% 15, 60, 120 g. Soln 0.01% 60 mL, 90 mL. (Derma-Smoothe/FS): Topical oil 0.01% 120 mL. Generic only: Cream 0.01% 15, 60 g. Trade only (Capex): Shampoo 0.01% 120 mL.
MOA — Anti-inflammatory; suppresses DNA synthesis, decreases WBC influx.
ADVERSE EFFECTS — Frequent: Burning, pruritus, dryness, irritation, erythema. Severe: Hypothalamic axis suppression with higher potency preparations.

FLUOCINONIDE (*Lidex, Lidex-E, Vanos, ✦Lidemol, Topsyn, Tiamol*) ▶L ♀C ▶? $$
ADULT — Inflammatory and pruritic manifestations of corticosteroid-responsive dermatoses: Apply sparingly two to four times per day. Plaque-type psoriasis: Apply 0.1% cream (Vanos) one to two times per day for 2 consecutive weeks only; no more than 60 g per week. Atopic dermatitis: Apply 0.1% cream (Vanos) once a day.
PEDS — Inflammatory and pruritic manifestations of corticosteroid-responsive dermatoses: Apply sparingly two to four times per day.
FORMS — Generic/Trade: Cream, Ointment, Gel 0.05% 15, 30, 60 g. Soln 0.05% 20, 60 mL. Cream (Vanos) 0.1% 30, 60, 120 g .
MOA — Anti-inflammatory by inhibiting production of prostaglandins and leukotrienes; suppresses DNA synthesis, decreases WBC influx.
ADVERSE EFFECTS — Frequent: Burning, pruritus, dryness, irritation, erythema. Severe: Immunosuppression (with more than 2 weeks use), steroid atrophy, hypothalamic axis suppression with higher potency preparations.

FLURANDRENOLIDE (*Cordran, Cordran SP*) ▶L' ♀C ▶? $$$$$
ADULT — Inflammatory and pruritic manifestations of corticosteroid-responsive dermatoses: Apply sparingly two to three times per day.
PEDS — Inflammatory and pruritic manifestations of corticosteroid-responsive dermatoses: Apply sparingly two to three times per day.
FORMS — Trade only: Cream 0.05% 15, 30, 60, 120 g. Ointment 0.05% 60 g. Lotion 0.05% 15, 60, 120 mL. Tape 4 mcg/cm^2.
MOA — Anti-inflammatory; suppresses DNA synthesis, decreases WBC influx.
ADVERSE EFFECTS — Frequent: Burning, pruritus, dryness, irritation, erythema. Severe: Hypothalamic axis suppression with higher potency preparations.

FLUTICASONE—TOPICAL (*Cutivate*) ▶L ♀C ▶? $$
ADULT — Eczema: Apply sparingly one to two times per day. Other inflammatory and pruritic manifestations of corticosteroid-responsive dermatoses: Apply sparingly two times per day.
PEDS — Children older than 3 mo: Eczema: Apply sparingly one to two times per day. Other inflammatory and pruritic manifestations of corticosteroid-responsive dermatoses: Apply sparingly two times per day.
FORMS — Generic/Trade: Cream 0.05% 15, 30, 60 g. Ointment 0.005% 15, 30, 60 g. Lotion 0.05% 60, 120 mL.
NOTES — Do not use with an occlusive dressing.
MOA — Anti-inflammatory; suppresses DNA synthesis, decreases WBC influx.
ADVERSE EFFECTS — Frequent: Burning, pruritus, dryness, irritation, erythema. Severe: Hypothalamic axis suppression with higher potency preparations.

HALCINONIDE (Halog) ▶L ♀C ▶? $$$$$
ADULT — Inflammatory and pruritic manifestations of corticosteroid-responsive dermatoses: Apply sparingly two to three times per day.
PEDS — Inflammatory and pruritic manifestations of corticosteroid-responsive dermatoses: Apply sparingly two to three times per day.
FORMS — Trade only: Cream 0.1% 30, 60, 216 g. Ointment 0.1% 30, 60 g.
MOA — Anti-inflammatory; suppresses DNA synthesis, decreases WBC influx.
ADVERSE EFFECTS — Frequent: Burning, pruritus, dryness, irritation, erythema. Severe: Steroid atrophy, hypothalamic axis suppression with higher potency preparations.

HALOBETASOL PROPIONATE (Ultravate) ▶L ♀C ▶? $$$
ADULT — Inflammatory and pruritic manifestations of corticosteroid-responsive dermatoses: Apply sparingly one to two times per day.
PEDS — Not approved in children.
FORMS — Generic/Trade: Cream, Ointment 0.05% 15, 50 g.
NOTES — Do not use occlusive dressings. Do not use for more than 2 consecutive weeks and do not exceed a total dose of 50 g per week.
MOA — Anti-inflammatory; suppresses DNA synthesis, decreases WBC influx.
ADVERSE EFFECTS — Frequent: Burning, pruritus, dryness, irritation, erythema. Severe: Steroid atrophy, hypothalamic axis suppression with higher potency preparations.

HYDROCORTISONE ACETATE (Cortaid, Corticaine, Cortifoam, Micort-HC Lipocream, ✷Hyderm, Cortamed) ▶L ♀C ▶? $
ADULT — Inflammatory and pruritic manifestations of corticosteroid-responsive dermatoses: Apply sparingly two to four times per day.
PEDS — Inflammatory and pruritic manifestations of corticosteroid-responsive dermatoses: Apply sparingly two to four times per day.
FORMS — OTC Generic/Trade: Ointment 0.5% 15 g. Ointment 1% 15, 30 g. Cream 0.5% 15 g. Cream 1% 15, 30, 60 g. Topical spray 1% 60 mL. Rx Trade only: Cream 2.5% 30 g (Micort-HC Lipocream). Rectal foam 15 g (Cortifoam).
MOA — Anti-inflammatory; suppresses DNA synthesis, decreases WBC influx.
ADVERSE EFFECTS — Frequent: Burning, pruritus, dryness, irritation, erythema.

HYDROCORTISONE BUTYRATE (Locoid, Locoid Lipocream) ▶L ♀C ▶? $$$$
ADULT — Inflammatory and pruritic manifestations of corticosteroid-responsive dermatoses: Apply sparingly two to three times per day. Seborrheic dermatitis (soln only): Apply two to three times per day.
PEDS — Inflammatory and pruritic manifestations of corticosteroid-responsive dermatoses: Apply sparingly two to three times per day. Seborrheic dermatitis (soln only): Apply two to three times per day.

FORMS — Generic/Trade: Cream 0.1% 15, 45, 60 g. Ointment 0.1% 15, 45 g. Soln 0.1% 20, 60 mL. Trade only: Lotion 0.1% 60, 120 mL.
MOA — Anti-inflammatory; suppresses DNA synthesis, decreases WBC influx.
ADVERSE EFFECTS — Frequent: Burning, pruritus, dryness, irritation, erythema. Severe: Hypothalamic axis suppression with higher potency preparations.

HYDROCORTISONE PROBUTATE (Pandel) ▶L ♀C ▶? $$$$
ADULT — Inflammatory and pruritic manifestations of corticosteroid-responsive dermatoses: Apply sparingly one to two times per day.
PEDS — Not approved in children.
FORMS — Trade only: Cream 0.1% 15, 45, 80 g.
MOA — Anti-inflammatory; suppresses DNA synthesis, decreases WBC influx.
ADVERSE EFFECTS — Frequent: Burning, pruritus, dryness, irritation, erythema. Severe: Hypothalamic axis suppression with higher potency preparations.

HYDROCORTISONE VALERATE (Westcort, ✷Hydroval) ▶L ♀C ▶? $$$$
ADULT — Inflammatory and pruritic manifestations of corticosteroid-responsive dermatoses: Apply sparingly two to three times per day.
PEDS — Safety and efficacy of Westcort ointment have not been established in children. Inflammatory and pruritic manifestations of corticosteroid-responsive dermatoses (cream only): Apply sparingly two to three times per day.
FORMS — Generic/Trade: Cream, Ointment 0.2% 15, 45, 60 g.
MOA — Anti-inflammatory; suppresses DNA synthesis, decreases WBC influx.
ADVERSE EFFECTS — Frequent: Burning, pruritus, dryness, irritation, erythema. Severe: Hypothalamic axis suppression with higher potency preparations.

HYDROCORTISONE—TOPICAL (Cortizone, Hycort, Hytone, Tegrin-HC, Dermolate, Synacort, Anusol-HC, ProctoCream HC, ✷Cortoderm, Prevex-HC, Cortate, Emo-Cort) ▶L ♀C ▶? $
ADULT — Inflammatory and pruritic manifestations of corticosteroid-responsive dermatoses: Apply sparingly two to four times per day. External anal itching: Apply cream three to four times per day prn or suppository two times per day or rectal foam one to two times per day.
PEDS — Inflammatory and pruritic manifestations of corticosteroid-responsive dermatoses: Apply sparingly two to four times per day.
FORMS — Products available OTC and Rx depending on labeling. 2.5% preparation available Rx only. Generic/Trade: Ointment 0.5% 30 g. Ointment 1% 15, 20, 30, 60, 454 g. Ointment 2.5% 5, 20, 30, 454 g. Cream 0.5% 30 g. Cream 1% 5, 15, 20, 30, 120 g. Cream 2.5% 5, 20, 30, 454 g. Lotion 1% 120 mL. Lotion 2.5% 60 mL. Anal preparations: Generic/Trade: Cream 2.5% 30 g (Anusol HC, ProctoCream HC). Supp 25 mg (Anusol HC).
MOA — Anti-inflammatory; suppresses DNA synthesis, decreases WBC influx.

(cont.)

HYDROCORTISONE—TOPICAL (*cont.*)

ADVERSE EFFECTS — Frequent: Burning, pruritus, dryness, irritation, erythema.

MOMETASONE—TOPICAL (*Elocon, ✴Elocom*) ▶L ♀C ▶? $$

ADULT — Inflammatory and pruritic manifestations of corticosteroid-responsive dermatoses: Apply sparingly once a day.

PEDS — Inflammatory and pruritic manifestations of corticosteroid-responsive dermatoses: Apply sparingly once a day for age 2 yo or older. Safety and efficacy for more than 3 weeks have not been established.

FORMS — Generic/Trade: Cream, 0.1% 15, 45, 60 g. Ointment 0.1% 15, 45 g. Lotion 0.1% 30, 60 mL.

NOTES — Do not use an occlusive dressing. Not for ophthalmic use.

MOA — Anti-inflammatory; suppresses DNA synthesis, decreases WBC influx.

ADVERSE EFFECTS — Frequent: Burning, pruritus, dryness, irritation, erythema. Severe: Hypothalamic axis suppression with higher potency preparations, skin atrophy.

PREDNICARBATE (*Dermatop*) ▶L ♀C ▶? $$$

ADULT — Inflammatory and pruritic manifestations of corticosteroid-responsive dermatoses: Apply sparingly two times per day.

PEDS — Inflammatory and pruritic manifestations of corticosteroid-responsive dermatoses: Apply sparingly two times per day for age 1 yo or older. Safety and efficacy for more than 3 weeks have not been established.

FORMS — Generic/Trade: Ointment 0.1% 15, 60 g. Cream 0.1% 60 g.

NOTES — Can damage latex (condoms, diaphragms, etc.). Avoid contact with latex.

MOA — Anti-inflammatory; suppresses DNA synthesis, decreases WBC influx.

ADVERSE EFFECTS — Frequent: Burning, pruritus, dryness, irritation, erythema. Severe: Hypothalamic axis suppression with higher potency preparations.

TRIAMCINOLONE—TOPICAL (*Kenalog, Kenalog in Orabase, Trianex, ✴Oracort, Triaderm*) ▶L ♀C ▶? $

ADULT — Inflammatory and pruritic manifestations of corticosteroid-responsive dermatoses: Apply sparingly three to four times per day. Oral paste: Aphthous ulcers: Using finger, apply about 1 cm of paste to oral lesion and a thin film will develop. Apply paste two to three times per day, ideally after meals and at bedtime.

PEDS — Inflammatory and pruritic manifestations of corticosteroid-responsive dermatoses: Apply sparingly three to four times per day.

FORMS — Generic only: Cream, 0.1% 15, 30, 80, 454 g. Cream 0.5% 15 g. Cream 0.025% 15, 80, 454 g. Ointment, 0.1% 15, 80, 454 g. Ointment, 0.5% 15 g, Ointment, 0.025% 15, 80, 454 g. Lotion 0.025% and 0.1% 60 mL. Generic/Trade: Oral paste (in Orabase) 0.1% 5 g. Aerosol topical spray 0.147 mg/g, 63, 100 g. Trade only: Ointment (Trianex) 0.05% 430 g.

MOA — Anti-inflammatory; suppresses DNA synthesis, decreases WBC influx.

ADVERSE EFFECTS — Frequent: Burning, pruritus, dryness, irritation, erythema. Severe: Steroid atrophy, hypothalamic axis suppression with higher potency preparations.

DERMATOLOGY: Hemorrhoid Care

ANALPRAM-HC (hydrocortisone—topical + pramoxine—topical, *Epifoam, Proctofoam HC, Pramosone*) ▶L ♀C ▶? $$$

ADULT — Inflammatory and pruritic manifestations of corticosteroid-responsive dermatoses of the anal region: Apply two to four times per day.

PEDS — Use with caution. Inflammatory and pruritic manifestations of corticosteroid-responsive dermatoses of the anal region: Apply two to four times per day.

FORMS — Generic/Trade: Cream (Analpram-HC 1% hydrocortisone + 1% pramoxine, 2.5% hydrocortisone + 1% pramoxine) 4, 30 g. Trade only: Topical aerosol foam (Proctofoam HC, Epifoam 1% hydrocortisone + 1% pramoxine) 10 g. Lotion (Analpram-HC, Pramosone 2.5% hydrocortisone + 1% pramoxine) 60, 120 mL. Lotion (Pramosone 1% hydrocortisone + 1% pramoxine) 60, 120, 240 mL. Oint (Pramosone 1% hydrocortisone + 1% pramoxine, 2.5% hydrocortisone + 1% pramoxine) 28 g.

MOA — Combination of local anesthetic and anti-inflammatory; suppresses DNA synthesis, decreases WBC influx.

ADVERSE EFFECTS — Frequent: Redness, irritation, pain.

DIBUCAINE (*Nupercainal*) ▶L ♀? ▶? $

ADULT — Hemorrhoids or other anorectal disorders: Apply three to four times per day prn.

PEDS — Not approved in children.

UNAPPROVED PEDS — Hemorrhoids or other anorectal disorders: Apply three to four times per day prn for age older than 2 yo or wt greater than 35 lbs or 15.9 kg.

FORMS — OTC Generic/Trade: Oint 1% 30, 60 g.

NOTES — Do not use if younger than 2 yo or wt less than 35 pounds.

MOA — Anesthetic, anti-inflammatory.

ADVERSE EFFECTS — Frequent: None.

PRAMOXINE—TOPICAL (*Tucks Hemorrhoidal Ointment, Fleet Pain Relief, ProctoFoam NS*) ▶not absorbed ♀+ ▶+ $

ADULT — Hemorrhoids: Apply ointment, pads, or foam up to 5 times per day prn.

PEDS — Not approved in children.

FORMS — OTC Trade only: Oint (Tucks Hemorrhoidal Ointment) 30 g. Pads (Fleet Pain Relief) 100 each. Aerosol foam (ProctoFoam NS) 15 g.

(cont.)

PRAMOXINE—TOPICAL (cont.)

MOA — Anesthetic.
ADVERSE EFFECTS — Frequent: Redness, irritation, swelling, pain.

STARCH (Tucks Suppositories) ▶not absorbed ♀+ ▶+ $
ADULT — Hemorrhoids: 1 suppository PR up to 6 times per day prn or after each bowel movement.
PEDS — Not approved in children.
FORMS — OTC Trade only: Supp (51% topical starch; vegetable oil, tocopheryl acetate) 12, 24 each.

MOA — Lubricant.
ADVERSE EFFECTS — Frequent: None.

WITCH HAZEL (Tucks) ▶? ♀+ ▶+ $
ADULT — Hemorrhoids: Apply to anus/perineum up to 6 times per day prn.
PEDS — Not approved in children.
FORMS — OTC Generic/Trade: Pads 50% 12, 40, 100 ea, generically available in various quantities.
MOA — Astringent.
ADVERSE EFFECTS — Frequent: None.

DERMATOLOGY: Other Dermatologic Agents

ALITRETINOIN (Panretin, ✸Toctino) ▶not absorbed ♀ D ▶− $$$$$
WARNING — May cause fetal harm if significant absorption were to occur. Women of child-bearing age should be advised to avoid becoming pregnant during treatment.
ADULT — Cutaneous lesions of AIDS-related Kaposi's sarcoma: Apply two to four times per day.
PEDS — Not approved in children.
FORMS — Trade only: Gel 0.1% 60 g.
MOA — Binds retinoid receptors to inhibit Kaposi's sarcoma.
ADVERSE EFFECTS — Frequent: Pain, rash, pruritus, paresthesia, edema, dermatitis.

ALUMINUM CHLORIDE (Drysol, Certain Dri) ▶K ♀? ▶? $
ADULT — Hyperhidrosis: Apply at bedtime. For maximum effect, cover area with plastic wrap held in place with tight shirt and wash area following morning. Once excessive sweating stopped, use once or twice a week.
PEDS — Not approved in children.
FORMS — Rx Trade only: Soln 20% 37.5 mL bottle, 35, 60 mL bottle with applicator. OTC Trade only (Certain Dri): Soln 12.5% 36 mL bottle.
NOTES — To prevent irritation, apply to dry area.
MOA — Astringent.
ADVERSE EFFECTS — Frequent: Irritation, burning, prickling.

BECAPLERMIN (Regranex) ▶minimal absorption ♀C ▶? $$$$$
WARNING — Increased rate of mortality due to malignancy in patients who used 3 or more tubes. Use with caution in patients with known malignancy.
ADULT — Diabetic neuropathic ulcers: Apply daily and cover with saline-moistened gauze for 12 h. Rinse after 12 h and cover with saline gauze without medication.
PEDS — Not approved in children.
FORMS — Trade only: Gel 0.01%, 15 g.
NOTES — Length of gel to be applied calculated by size of wound (length × width × 0.6 = amount of gel in inches). If ulcer does not decrease by 30% in size by 10 weeks or complete healing has not occurred by 20 weeks, continued therapy should be reassessed. Ineffective for stasis ulcers and pressure ulcers.
MOA — Recombinant human platelet-derived growth factor, which promotes cellular proliferation and angiogenesis, enhances new granulation tissue, and induces fibroblast proliferation and differentiation.
ADVERSE EFFECTS — Frequent: None Severe: Increased cancer mortality.

BRIMONIDINE—TOPICAL (Mirvaso) ▶L ♀B ▶− $$$$$
WARNING — Caution when combining with antihypertensives, CNS depressants, and MAO inhibitors.
ADULT — Persistent erythema associated with rosacea: Apply once daily to chin, forehead, nose, and each cheek.
PEDS — Not approved in children younger than 18 yo.
FORMS — 0.33% gel, 30, 45 g.
NOTES — Use caution in patients with severe or uncontrolled CV disease. May potentiate vascular insufficiency.
MOA — alpha adrenergic agonist.
ADVERSE EFFECTS — Common: erythema, flushing, pallor, burning, contact dermatitis. Severe: systemic hypersensitivity, systemic effects consistent with the alpha-2 adrenergic agonists

CALAMINE ▶? ♀? ▶? $
ADULT — Itching due to poison ivy/oak/sumac, insect bites, or minor irritation: Apply up to three to four times per day prn.
PEDS — Itching due to poison ivy/oak/sumac, insect bites, or minor irritation: Apply up to three to four times per day prn for age older than 2 yo.
FORMS — OTC Generic only: Lotion 120, 240, 480 mL.
MOA — Astringent.
ADVERSE EFFECTS — Frequent: Dryness.

CAPSAICIN (Zostrix, Zostrix-HP, Qutenza) ▶? ♀? ▶? $
ADULT — Pain due to RA, OA, and neuralgias such as zoster or diabetic neuropathies: Apply to affected area up to three to four times per day. Post herpetic neuralgia: 1 patch (Qutenza) applied for 1 hour in medical office, may repeat every 3 months.
PEDS — Children older than 2 yo: Pain due to RA, OA, and neuralgias such as zoster or diabetic neuropathies: Apply to affected area up to three to four times per day.
UNAPPROVED ADULT — Psoriasis and intractable pruritus, postmastectomy/postamputation neuromas (phantom limb pain), vulvar vestibulitis, apocrine chromhidrosis, and reflex sympathetic dystrophy.
FORMS — Rx: Patch 8% (Qutenza). OTC Generic/Trade: Cream 0.025% 60 g, 0.075% (HP) 60 g. OTC Generic only: Lotion 0.025% 59 mL, 0.075% 59 mL.

(cont.)

CAPSAICIN (*cont.*)

NOTES — Burning occurs in 30% or more of patients but diminishes with continued use. Pain more commonly occurs when applied less than three to four times per day. Wash hands immediately after application.

MOA — Counter-irritant, releases Substance P.

ADVERSE EFFECTS — Frequent: Burning, redness, sensation of warmth.

COAL TAR (*Polytar, Tegrin, Cutar, Tarsum*) ▶? ♀? ▶? $

ADULT — Dandruff, seborrheic dermatitis: Apply shampoo at least twice a week. Psoriasis: Apply to affected areas one to four times per day or use shampoo on affected areas.

PEDS — Children older than 2 yo: Dandruff, seborrheic dermatitis: Apply shampoo at least twice a week. Psoriasis: Apply to affected areas one to four times per day or use shampoo on affected areas.

FORMS — OTC Generic/Trade: Shampoo, cream, ointment, gel, lotion, liquid, oil, soap.

NOTES — May cause photosensitivity for up to 24 h after application.

MOA — Unknown.

ADVERSE EFFECTS — Frequent: folliculitis, skin and hair staining, photosensitivity, contact dermatitis.

DEET (*Off, Cutter, Repel, Ultrathon, n-n-diethyl-m-toluamide*) ▶L ♀+ ▶+ $

ADULT — Mosquito repellant: 10% to 50% q 2 to 6 h. Higher concentration products do not work better, but have a longer duration of action.

PEDS — Up to 30% spray/lotion q 2 to 6 h for age 2 mo or older.

FORMS — OTC Generic/Trade: Spray, lotion, towelette 4.75% to 100%.

NOTES — Duration of action varies by concentration. For example, 23.8% DEET provides approximately 5 h of protection from mosquito bites, 20% DEET provides approximately 4 h of protection, 6.65% DEET provides approximately 2 h of protection and products with 4.75% DEET provides approximately 1.5 h of protection. Apply sunscreen prior to application of DEET-containing products.

MOA — Repels female mosquitos; does not kill them.

ADVERSE EFFECTS — Frequent: Dermatitis.

DEOXYCHOLIC ACID (*Kybella*) ▶not absorbed ♀? ▶? $$$$$

ADULT — Reduction of chin fullness: 0.2 mL injections 1 cm apart until all of planned treatment area have been injected. Up to 50 injections or 10 mL may be injected in a single treatment. Up to 6 treatments may be administered at least 1 month apart.

PEDS — Not approved for use in children younger than 18 yo.

FORMS — Injectable solution.

NOTES — Avoid injecting in proximity to vulnerable anatomic structures. Use with caution in patients taking antiplatelet or anticoagulant therapies, or in those with coagulation abnormalities.

MOA — Cytolytic

ADVERSE EFFECTS — Frequent: hematoma, bruising, dysphagia. Severe: Marginal mandibular nerve (MMN) injury.

DOXEPIN—TOPICAL (*Prudoxin, Zonalon*) ▶L ♀B ▶– $$$$$

ADULT — Pruritus associated with atopic dermatitis, lichen simplex chronicus, eczematous dermatitis: Apply four times per day for up to 8 days.

PEDS — Not approved in children.

FORMS — Trade only: Cream 5% 30, 45 g.

NOTES — Risk of systemic toxicity increased if applied to more than 10% of body. Can cause contact dermatitis.

MOA — Inhibits pre-synaptic uptake of serotonin +/- norepinephrine.

ADVERSE EFFECTS — Frequent: None.

EFLORNITHINE (*Vaniqa*) ▶K ♀C ▶? $$$

ADULT — Reduction of facial hair: Apply to face two times per day at least 8 h apart.

PEDS — Not approved in children.

FORMS — Trade only: Cream 13.9% 30, 45 g.

NOTES — Takes 4 to 8 weeks or more to see an effect.

MOA — Specific, irreversible inhibition of ornithine decarboxylase, reduces length of growing cycle so hair becomes progressively shorter.

ADVERSE EFFECTS — Frequent: Stinging, burning, tingling, erythema, rash.

HYALURONIC ACID (*Bionect, Restylane, Perlane*) ▶? ♀? ▶? $$$

ADULT — Moderate to severe facial wrinkles: Inject into wrinkle/fold (Restylane, Perlane). Protection of dermal ulcers: Apply gel/cream/spray to wound two or three times per day (Bionect).

PEDS — Not approved in children.

FORMS — OTC Trade only: Cream 2% 15, 30 g. Rx Generic/Trade: Soln 3% 30 mL. Gel 4% 30 g. Cream 4% 15, 30, 60 g. Injectable gel 2%.

NOTES — Do not use more than 1.5 mL of injectable form per treatment area. Injectable product contains trace amounts of Gram-positive bacterial proteins; contraindicated if history of anaphylaxis or severe allergy.

MOA — Increases volume under skin to smooth out wrinkle.

ADVERSE EFFECTS — Frequent (injectable product): Bruising, redness, swelling, pain, tenderness, itching. Severe (injectable product): Bacterial infections, anaphylaxis, severe allergic reactions.

IVERMECTIN—TOPICAL (*Sklice, Soolantra*) ▶minimal absorption – ♀C ▶? $$$$$

WARNING — Avoid applying to lips or eyes.

ADULT — Lice (Sklice): Apply lotion to dry hair and scalp. Rinse after 10 min. Single application only. Rosacea (Sooantra): Apply cream to affected area once daily.

PEDS — Not approved in children younger than 6 mo. In children 6 mo and older, use adult dosing (Sklice). Soolantra is not approved for use in children.

FORMS — Trade: Lotion (Sklice) 0.5%, 120 mL. Cream (Soolantra) 1% 30, 45, 60 g.

MOA — Selectively binds glutamate-gated chloride channels, resulting in louse paralysis and death. Unknown in rosacea.

ADVERSE EFFECTS — Frequent: conjunctivitis, ocular hyperemia, eye irritation, dandruff, dry skin, and skin burning sensation.

LACTIC ACID (*Lac-Hydrin, AmLactin, ✤Dermalac*) ▶? ♀? ▶? $$
ADULT — Ichthyosis vulgaris and xerosis (dry, scaly skin): Apply two times per day to affected area.
PEDS — Ichthyosis vulgaris and xerosis (dry, scaly skin) in children older than 2 yo: Apply two times per day to affected area.
FORMS — Trade only: Lotion 12% 150, 360 mL. OTC: Cream 12% 140, 385 g. AmLactin AP is lactic acid (12%) with pramoxine (1%).
NOTES — Frequently causes irritation in nonintact skin. Minimize exposure to sun, artificial sunlight.
MOA — Humectant, reduce corneocyte cohesion.
ADVERSE EFFECTS — Frequent: Stinging, burning.

LIDOCAINE—TOPICAL (*Xylocaine, Lidoderm, Numby Stuff, LMX, Zingo, ✤Maxilene*) ▶LK ♀B ▶+ $ – varies by therapy
WARNING — Contraindicated in allergy to amide-type anesthetics.
ADULT — Topical anesthesia: Apply to affected area prn. Dose varies with anesthetic procedure, degree of anesthesia required, and individual patient response. Postherpetic neuralgia (patch): Apply up to 3 patches to affected area at once for up to 12 h within a 24 h period.
PEDS — Topical anesthesia: Apply to affected area prn. Dose varies with anesthetic procedure, degree of anesthesia required and individual patient response. Max 3 mg/kg/dose, do not repeat dose within 2 h. Intradermal powder injection for venipuncture/IV cannulation, for age 3 to 18 yo (Zingo): 0.5 mg to site 1 to 10 min prior.
UNAPPROVED PEDS — Topical anesthesia prior to venipuncture: Apply 30 min prior to procedure (ELA-Max 4%).
FORMS — For membranes of mouth and pharynx: Spray 10%, Oint 5%, Liquid 5%, Soln 2%, 4%, Dental patch. For urethral use: Jelly 2%. Patch (Lidoderm $$$$$) 5%. Intradermal powder injection system: 0.5 mg (Zingo). OTC Trade only: Liposomal lidocaine 4% (ELA-Max).
NOTES — Apply patches only to intact skin to cover the most painful area. Patches may be cut into smaller sizes with scissors prior to removal of the release liner. Store and dispose out of the reach of children and pets to avoid possible toxicity from ingestion.
MOA — Anesthetic.
ADVERSE EFFECTS — Frequent: Skin irritation. Severe: CNS effects, bradycardia, bronchospasm, hypotension, allergic reactions.

MINOXIDIL—TOPICAL (*Rogaine, Women's Rogaine, Rogaine Extra Strength, Minoxidil for Men*) ▶K ♀C ▶– $
ADULT — Androgenetic alopecia in men or women: 1 mL to dry scalp two times per day (2% soln) or once daily (5% soln).
PEDS — Not approved in children.
UNAPPROVED ADULT — Alopecia areata.
UNAPPROVED PEDS — Alopecia: Apply to dry scalp two times per day.
FORMS — OTC Generic/Trade: Soln 2% 60 mL (Rogaine, Women's Rogaine). Soln 5% 60 mL (Rogaine Extra Strength, Theroxidil Extra Strength—for men only). Foam 5% 60 g (Rogaine Extra Strength).
NOTES — 5% strength for men only. Alcohol content may cause burning and stinging. Evidence of hair growth usually takes at least 4 months. If treatment is stopped, new hair will be shed in a few months.
MOA — Promotes hair growth.
ADVERSE EFFECTS — None.

OATMEAL (*Aveeno*) ▶not absorbed ♀? ▶? $
ADULT — Pruritus from poison ivy/oak, varicella: Apply lotion four times per day prn. Also available in packets to be added to bath.
PEDS — Pruritus from poison ivy/oak, varicella: Apply lotion four times per day prn. Also available in bath packets for tub.
FORMS — OTC Generic/Trade: Lotion. Bath packets.
MOA — Anti-pruritic, lubricating.
ADVERSE EFFECTS — Frequent: None.

PLIAGLIS **(tetracaine—topical + lidocaine—topical)** ▶minimal absorption ♀B ▶? $$
WARNING — Contraindicated in allergy to amide or ester-type anesthetics.
ADULT — Prior to venipuncture, intravenous cannulation, dermal filler injection, laser resurfacing and pulsed-dye laser treatments, other superficial dermatological procedure: Apply 20 to 30 min prior to procedure. Tattoo removal: Apply 60 min prior to procedure.
PEDS — Not approved in children.
FORMS — Generic/Trade: Cream lidocaine 7% + tetracaine 7% (30, 60, 100 g).
NOTES — Remove after the appropriate time interval.
MOA — Topical anesthetic.
ADVERSE EFFECTS — Frequent: Skin irritation, erythema, blanching, rash. Severe: CNS effects, bradycardia, bronchospasm, hypotension.

POLIDOCANOL (*Varithena, Asclera*) ▶minimal absorption ♀C ▶? $$$$
ADULT — Varicose veins: Variable dose injected into varicose vein, depending on size and extent of varicose vein.
PEDS — Not approved for use in children.
FORMS — Trade: Inj soln 0.5 (Asclera only), 1%.
MOA — Sclerosing agent.
ADVERSE EFFECTS — Common: mild, local reactions at site of injection. Severe: anaphylaxis

POLY-L-LACTIC ACID (*Sculptra*) ▶not absorbed ♀? ▶? $$$$$
ADULT — Restoration of facial fat loss due to HIV lipoatrophy: Dose based on degree of correction needed.
PEDS — Not approved in children younger than 18 yo.
MOA — Biocompatible, biodegradable, synthetic polymer.
ADVERSE EFFECTS — Frequent: Bruising, edema, discomfort, hematoma, inflammation, erythema, injection site papule.

PRAMOSONE (pramoxine—topical + hydrocortisone—topical, ✳ *Pramox HC*) ▶not absorbed ♀C ▶? $$$
ADULT — Apply three to four times per day.
PEDS — Apply two to three times per day.
FORMS — Generic/Trade: 1% pramoxine/1% hydrocortisone: Cream 30, 60 g. 1% pramoxine/2.5% hydrocortisone acetate: Cream 30, 60 g. Trade only: 1% pramoxine/1% hydrocortisone: Oint 30 g. Lotion 60, 120, 240 mL. 1% pramoxine/2.5% hydrocortisone acetate: Oint 30 g. Lotion 60, 120 mL.
NOTES — Monitor for hyperglycemia/adrenal suppression if used for long period of time or over a large area of the body, especially in children. Chronic administration may interfere with pediatric growth and development.
MOA — Anti-inflammatory; suppresses DNA synthesis, decreases WBC influx.
ADVERSE EFFECTS — Frequent: Burning, pruritus, dryness, irritation, erythema.

SELENIUM SULFIDE (*Selsun, Exsel, Versel, Tersi*) ▶? ♀C ▶? $
ADULT — Dandruff, seborrheic dermatitis: Massage 5 to 10 mL of shampoo into wet scalp, allow to remain 2 to 3 min, rinse. Apply twice a week for 2 weeks. For maintenance, less frequent administration needed. Tinea versicolor: Apply 2.5% shampoo/lotion to affected area, allow to remain on skin 10 min, rinse. Repeat daily for 7 days.
PEDS — Dandruff, seborrheic dermatitis: Massage 5 to 10 mL of shampoo into wet scalp, allow to remain 2 to 3 min, rinse. Apply twice a week for 2 weeks. For maintenance, less frequent administration needed. Tinea versicolor: Apply 2.5% lotion/shampoo to affected area, allow to remain on skin 10 min, rinse. Repeat daily for 7 days.
FORMS — OTC Generic/Trade: Lotion/Shampoo 1% 120, 210, 240, 325 mL, 2.5% 120 mL. Rx Generic/Trade: Lotion/Shampoo 2.5% 120 mL. Trade only: Foam 2.25% 70 g.
MOA — May inhibit epidermal growth enzymes.
ADVERSE EFFECTS — Frequent: Unusual dryness, oiliness of skin.

SUNSCREEN ▶minimal absorption ♀? ▶+ $
ADULT — Apply at least 2 tablespoons for full-body coverage 30 min before going outdoors. If in the sun between 10 am and 4 pm, reapply sunscreen q 2 h (more often if swimming or sweating).
PEDS — Avoid sun exposure if younger than 6 mo. For age 6 mo or older: Apply at least 2 tablespoons for full-body coverage 30 min before going outdoors. If in the sun between 10 am and 4 pm, reapply sunscreen q 2 h (more often if swimming or sweating). Apply prior to sun exposure.
FORMS — Many formulations available.
NOTES — Sun protection factor (SPF) numbers equal the ratio of doses of ultraviolet radiation (predominantly UVB radiation) that result in sunburn with protection to the doses that result in erythema without protection. SPF 2 equals a 50% block, SPF 15 equals a 93% block, and SPF 45 equals a 98% block.

MOA — Physical block from sun (eg, zinc, titanium oxide); or absorption of high-energy ultraviolet rays and release as lower-energy rays, thereby preventing the skin-damaging ultraviolet rays from reaching the skin (eg, avobenzone).
ADVERSE EFFECTS — Frequent: irritation.

SYNERA (tetracaine—topical + lidocaine—topical) ▶minimal absorption ♀B ▶? $$
WARNING — Contraindicated in allergy to amide or ester-type anesthetics
ADULT — Prior to venipuncture or IV cannulation: Apply for 20 to 30 min prior to procedure. Prior to superficial dermatologic procedure: Apply for 30 min prior to procedure.
PEDS — Children 3 yo or older: Prior to venipuncture or IV cannulation: Apply for 20 to 30 min prior to procedure. Prior to superficial dermatologic procedure: Apply for 30 min prior to procedure.
FORMS — Trade only: Topical patch (lidocaine 70 mg + tetracaine 70 mg).
NOTES — Do not cut patch or remove top cover. Remove before patient undergoes MRI.
MOA — Topical anesthetic.
ADVERSE EFFECTS — Frequent: Skin irritation, erythema, blanching, rash. Severe: CNS effects, bradycardia, bronchospasm, hypotension.

TRI-LUMA (fluocinolone—topical + hydroquinone + tretinoin—topical) ▶minimal absorption ♀C ▶? $$$$
ADULT — Melasma of the face: Apply at bedtime for 4 to 8 weeks.
PEDS — Not approved in children.
FORMS — Trade only: Cream 30 g (fluocinolone 0.01% + hydroquinone 4% + tretinoin 0.05%).
NOTES — Minimize exposure to sunlight. Not intended for melasma maintenance therapy.
MOA — Competitively inhibits melantin precursors, anti-inflammatory.
ADVERSE EFFECTS — Frequent: Erythema, desquamation, burning, dryness, pruritus, acne.

VUSION (miconazole—topical + zinc oxide + white petrolatum) ▶minimal absorption ♀C ▶? $$$$$
ADULT — Not approved in adults.
PEDS — Diaper rash in infants 4 weeks or older: Apply to affected area with each change for 7 days.
FORMS — Trade only: Oint 50 g.
NOTES — Use only in documented cases of candidiasis.
MOA — Antifungal; alters fungal cell wall permeability; barrier.
ADVERSE EFFECTS — Frequent: None.

XERESE (acyclovir—topical + hydrocortisone—topical) ▶minimal absorption ♀B ▶? $$$$$
ADULT — Recurrent herpes labialis: Apply 5 times a day, starting at the first sign of symptoms.
PEDS — Recurrent herpes labialis (6 years or older): Apply 5 times a day, starting at the first signs and symptoms.
MOA — Herpes simplex virus analog DNA polymerase inhibitor
ADVERSE EFFECTS — Frequent: dryness, flaking of skin, burning, tingling. erythema, pigmentation changes, inflammation.

ENDOCRINE AND METABOLIC

A1C REDUCTION IN TYPE 2 DIABETES

Intervention	Expected A1C Reduction with Monotherapy
Alpha-glucosidase inhibitors	0.5–0.8%
DPP-4 inhibitors (Gliptins)	0.5–0.8%
GLP-1 agonists	0.5–1%
Insulin	1.5–3.5%
Lifestyle modifications	1–2%
Meglitinides	0.5–1.5%
Metformin	1–2%
Pramlintide	0.5–1%
Sodium-glucose cotransporter 2 (SGLT2) inhibitors	0.5–1%
Sulfonylureas	1–2%
Thiazolidinediones	0.5–1.4%

References: *Diabetes Care* 2009;32:195. *Diabetes Care* 2015;38:141.

IV SOLUTIONS

Solution	Dextrose	Calories/Liter	Na*	Ca*	Lactate*	Osm*
0.9 NS	0 g/L	0	154	0	0	310
LR	0 g/L	9	130	3	28	273
D5 W	50 g/L	170	0	0	0	253
D5 0.2 NS	50 g/L	170	34	0	0	320
D5 0.45 NS	50 g/L	170	77	0	0	405
D5 0.9 NS	50 g/L	170	154	0	0	560
D5 LR	50 g/L	170	130	2.7	28	527

* All given in mEq/L

CORTICOSTEROIDS

CORTICOSTEROIDS	Approximate Equivalent Dose (mg)	Relative Anti-inflammatory Potency	Relative Mineralocorti-coid Potency	Biological Half-life (h)
betamethasone	0.6–0.75	20–30	0	36–54
cortisone	25	0.8	2	8–12
dexamethasone	0.75	20–30	0	36–54
fludrocortisone	n/a	10	125	18–36
hydrocortisone	20	1	2	8–12
methylprednisolone	4	5	0	18–36
prednisolone	5	4	1	18–36
prednisone	5	4	1	18–36
triamcinolone	4	5	0	12–36

n/a, not available.

DIABETES NUMBERS*

Criteria for diagnosis
Pre-diabetes: Fasting glucose 100–125 mg/dL
A1C 5.7–6.4%
2 h after 75 g oral glucose load: 140–199 mg/dL
Diabetes:[†] A1C ≥ 6.5%
Fasting glucose ≥ 126 mg/dL
Random glucose with symptoms ≥ 200 mg/dL
2 h after 75 g oral glucose load ≥ 200 mg/dL

Self-monitoring glucose goals (non-pregnant adults)
Preprandial: 80–130 mg/dL
Postprandial: < 180 mg/dL

Glucose goals in hospitalized patients
Non-critically ill: 140–180 mg/dL; may individualize based on glycemic control prior to hospitalization and comorbidities.
Critically ill: 140–180 mg/dL; more stringent goals (eg, 110–140 mg/dL) may be considered in select patients if safely achievable without significant hypoglycemia

A1C goal: < 7% for most non-pregnant adults, individualize based on patient-specific factors. Consider A1C < 6.5% if goal can be achieved without significant hypoglycemia or other adverse effects (eg, no cardiovascular disease, long life expectancy, managed with lifestyle modifications). Consider A1C < 8% if history of severe hypoglycemia, advanced microvascular or macrovascular complications, unable to achieve goal despite optimal management, complicated comorbidities, limited life expectancy. A1C goal < 7.5% for pediatric Type 1 diabetes.

Mean glucose levels by A1C:

A1C (%)	Glucose (mg/dL)
6	126
7	154
8	183
9	212
10	240

Estimated average glucose (eAG):
eAG (mg/dL) = (28.7 × 46.7 A1C) − 46.7

(cont.)

DIABETES NUMBERS* (*continued*)

Complications prevention & management:

ASA[‡] (75–162 mg/day) in Type 1 & 2 adults for primary prevention if 10-year cardiovascular risk > 10% (includes most men and women older than 50 yo with at least one other major risk factor of hypertension, smoking, dyslipidemia, albuminuria, or family history of premature ASCVD) and secondary prevention (those with ASCVD) without increased bleeding risk.

ACE inhibitor or **ARB** if hypertensive or albuminuria

Statin: high-intensity therapy in those with established ASCVD or as below in other risk groups. In those age 40 or older with recent acute coronary syndrome and LDL greater than 50 mg/dL, consider adding ezetimibe to moderate-intensity statin if unable to tolerate high-intensity statin therapy.

Statin recommendations for those without established ASCVD:

Age	ASCVD Risk Factors (hypertension, overweight/obesity, smoking, LDL ≥ 100 mg/dL)	Statin Intensity Recommendation
Less than 40 yo	No	None
	Yes	Moderate or high
40 yo or older	No	Moderate
	Yes	High, if 40–75 yo Moderate or high, if older than 75 yo

Immunizations: Annual flu vaccine; hepatitis B vaccine if previously unvaccinated and 19 to 59 yo, consider if age 60 yo or older; pneumococcal vaccine: PPSV23 to all age 2 or older, if age 65 yo or older and unvaccinated give PCV13 then PPSV23 6–12 months later, if age 65 yo or older and previously vaccinated with PPSV23, give PCV13 ≥ 12 months later.

Every visit: Measure BP (goal < 140/90 mm Hg[§]); weight (calculate BMI & provide recommendations if overweight/obese); visual foot exam; review self-monitoring glucose record; review/adjust meds; review self-mgmt skills, dietary needs, and physical activity; smoking cessation counseling.

Twice a year: A1C in those meeting treatment goals with stable glycemia (quarterly if not); dental exam.

Annually: Screening fasting lipid profile (or q 2 years with low-risk lipid values)**; creatinine; spot urinary albumin to creatinine ratio; dilated eye exam (q 2 years if no evidence of retinopathy).

*See recommendations at: care.diabetesjournals.org. References: *Diabetes Care* 2016;39(Suppl 1):S1–104. Glucose values are plasma. ASCVD = atherosclerotic cardiovascular disease.
[†]In the absence of symptoms, confirm diagnosis with glucose testing on subsequent day.
[‡]Avoid ASA if younger than 21 yo due to Reye's Syndrome risk; use if younger than 30 yo has not been studied.
[§]Lower systolic targets (ie, < 130 mmHg) may be considered on a patient-specific basis (eg, albuminuria, younger patients, additional ASCVD risk factors) if treatment goals can be met without excessive treatment burden.
**In those on statin therapy, check a fasting lipid panel as needed to monitor for adherence.

ENDOCRINE AND METABOLIC: Androgens/Anabolic Steroids

NOTE: See OB/GYN section for other hormones.

METHYLTESTOSTERONE (*Android, Methitest, Testred*) ▶L ♀X ▶? ©III $$$$$

ADULT — Advancing inoperable breast cancer in women who are 1 to 5 years postmenopausal: 50 to 200 mg/day PO in divided doses.

PEDS — Delayed puberty in males: 10 mg PO daily for 4 to 6 months.

FORMS — Trade/Generic: Caps 10 mg, Tabs 10 mg.

NOTES — Transdermal or injectable therapy preferred to oral for hypogonadism. Pediatric use by specialists who monitor bone maturation q 6 months. Prolonged high-dose use may cause hepatic adenomas, hepatocellular carcinoma, and peliosis hepatitis. Monitor LFTs. Monitor Hb for polycythemia.

MOA — Steroid with anabolic and androgenic actions.

ADVERSE EFFECTS — Serious: Peliosis hepatitis, liver tumors, cholestatic hepatitis, habituation, heart failure exacerbation, polycythemia. Frequent: Virilization, testicular atrophy, oligospermia, excitation, insomnia, anxiety, depression, paresthesia, altered libido, bladder irritability, menstrual irregularity, gynecomastia, acne, edema, lipid abnormalities.

OXANDROLONE (*Oxandrin*) ▶L ♀X ▶? ©III $$$$$

WARNING — Peliosis hepatitis, liver cell tumors, and lipid changes have occurred secondary to anabolic steroid use.

ADULT — Weight gain promotion following extensive surgery, chronic infection, or severe trauma; in some patients who fail to gain or maintain wt without a physiologic cause; to offset protein catabolism associated with long-term corticosteroid therapy: 2.5 mg/day to 20 mg/day PO divided two to four times per day for 2 to 4 weeks. May repeat therapy intermittently as indicated.

PEDS — Weight gain: Up to 0.1 mg/kg or up to 0.045 mg/pound PO divided two to four times per day for 2 to 4 weeks. May repeat therapy intermittently as indicated.

FORMS — Generic/Trade: Tabs 2.5, 10 mg.

NOTES — Contraindicated in known or suspected prostate/breast cancer. Not shown to enhance athletic ability. Associated with dyslipidemia; monitor lipids. Pediatric use by specialists who monitor bone maturation q 6 months. Long-term use may cause hepatic adenomas, hepatocellular carcinoma, and peliosis hepatitis; monitor LFTs. May increase anticoagulant effects of warfarin.Monitor Hb for polycythemia.

MOA — Steroid with anabolic and androgenic actions.

ADVERSE EFFECTS — Serious: Peliosis hepatitis, liver tumors, cholestatic hepatitis, habituation, heart failure exacerbation, polycythemia. Frequent: Virilization, testicular atrophy, oligospermia, excitation, insomnia, anxiety, depression, paresthesia, altered libido, bladder irritability, menstrual irregularity, gynecomastia, acne, edema, lipid abnormalities.

TESTOSTERONE (*Androderm, AndroGel, Axiron, Aveed, Depo-Testosterone, Striant, Testim, Testopel, Vogelxo, Natesto, ✷Andriol*) ▶L ♀X ▶? ©III varies by therapy

WARNING — Risk of transfer and secondary exposure with topical products. Virilization has been reported in children after secondary exposure to gel. Women and children should avoid contact with skin areas to which gel has been applied. Advise patient to wash hands with soap and water following application and cover area with clothing once gel has dried. Aveed: Serious pulmonary oil microembolism reactions and anaphylaxis reported; observe for 30 min following dose. Aveed only available via restricted program.

ADULT — Hypogonadism in men: Injectable enanthate or cypionate, 50 to 400 mg IM q 2 to 4 weeks. Injectable undecanoate (Aveed): 750 mg IM, repeat in 4 weeks then q 10 weeks thereafter. Testopel: 2 to 6 pellets (150 to 450 mg testosterone) SC q 3 to 6 months. 2 pellets for each 25 mg testosterone propionate required weekly. Transdermal: Androderm: Start 4 mg patch at bedtime to clean, dry area of skin on back, abdomen, upper arms, or thighs. Nonvirilized patients start with 2 mg patch at bedtime. Adjust based on serum testosterone concentrations; see product information. AndroGel 1%: Apply 5 g from gel pack or 4 pumps (5 g gel; 50 mg testosterone) from dispenser daily to clean, dry, intact skin of the shoulders, upper arms, or abdomen. May increase dose to 7.5 to 10 g (100 mg testosterone) after 2 weeks. Androgel 1.62%: Apply 2 pumps (40.5 mg testosterone) from dispenser daily to shoulders or upper arms. Adjust based on serum testosterone concentration q 14 to 28 days. Dose range 1 to 4 pumps daily. Axiron: 60 mg (1 pump of 30 mg to each axilla) once daily. Testim: 1 tube (5 g) daily to the clean, dry intact skin of the shoulders or upper arms. May increase dose to 2 tubes (10 g) after 2 weeks. Vogelxo: Start 50 mg (1 tube, 1 packet, or 4 pumps) once daily; may increase to 100 mg after 2 weeks. Buccal (Striant): 30 mg q 12 h on upper gum above the incisor tooth; alternate sides for each application.

PEDS — Not approved in children.

FORMS — Generic/Trade: Gel 1% 2.5, 5 g packet, 75 g multidose pump (AndroGel 1% 1.25 g gel containing 12.5 mg testosterone per actuation). Gel (Fortesta) 10 mg/actuation. Injection 100, 200 mg/mL (cypionate), 200 mg/mL (ethanate). Trade only: Patch 2, 4 mg/24 h (Androderm). Gel 1.62% (AndroGel 1.62%), 1.25, 2.5 g (package of 30), 75 g multidose pump (AndroGel 1.62% 20.25 mg testosterone/actuation). Gel 1%, 5 g tube (Testim). Gel (Vogelxo): 50 mg tube, 50 mg packet or multi-dose pump: 12.5 mg/actuation. Soln 90 mL multidose pump (Axiron,

(cont.)

TESTOSTERONE *(cont.)*

30 mg/actuation). Nasal Gel (Natesto 5.5 mg/actuation pump) 7.32 g. Pellet 75 mg (Testopel). Buccal: Blister packs: 30 mg (Striant). IM injection (Aveed): 750 mg/3 mL through restricted access program.

NOTES — Wash hands after topical product administration. Do not apply Androderm or AndroGel to scrotum. Apply Axiron only to axilla. Do not apply Testim to the scrotum or abdomen. Do not apply Vogelxo to genitals or abdomen. Do not shower or swim for 5 h after applying AndroGel. Pellet implantation is less flexible for dosage adjustment; therefore, take great care when estimating the amount of testosterone. Confirm diagnosis of hypogonadism with serum testosterone levels on two separate mornings. Safety and efficacy in age-related hypogonadism not established. For testosterone gel form, obtain serum testosterone level 2 weeks after initiation, then increase dose if necessary. Inject IM formulations slowly into gluteal muscle; rare reports of cough or respiratory distress following injection. Prolonged high-dose use of oral forms of testosterone have caused hepatic adenomas, hepatocellular carcinoma, and peliosis hepatitis.

The overall risk of testosterone use on heart disease and the prostate (including prostate cancer) remain uncertain. Monitor prostate exam, PSA, and hemoglobin to detect polycythemia. Advise patient to regularly inspect the gum region where Striant is applied and report any abnormality; refer for dental consultation as appropriate. Injectable forms less expensive than gel or patch. Reports of venous thromboembolism; evaluate for DVT/PE if lower extremity swelling or shortness of breath. Educate patient about possible increased risk of major adverse cardiovascular events; data inconclusive.

MOA — Steroid with anabolic and androgenic actions.

ADVERSE EFFECTS — Serious: Peliosis hepatitis, liver tumors, cholestatic hepatitis, habituation, heart failure exacerbation, polycythemia, venous thromboembolism, serious pulmonary oil microembolism reactions, anaphylaxis. Frequent: Virilization, testicular atrophy, oligospermia, excitation, insomnia, anxiety, depression, paresthesia, altered libido, bladder irritability, menstrual irregularity, gynecomastia, acne, edema, gum or mouth irritation (buccal), transient cough (IM).

ENDOCRINE AND METABOLIC: Bisphosphonates

NOTE: Supplemental Vitamin D and calcium are recommended for osteoporosis prevention and treatment. Osteonecrosis of the jaw has been reported with bisphosphonates; generally associated with tooth extraction and/or local infection with delayed healing. Prior to treatment, consider dental exam and appropriate preventive dentistry, particularly with risk factors (eg, cancer, chemotherapy, angiogenesis inhibitors, corticosteroids, poor oral hygiene). While on bisphosphonate therapy, avoid invasive dental procedures when possible. Severe musculoskeletal pain has been reported; may occur at any time during therapy. Atypical, low-trauma femoral shaft fractures have been reported; evaluate new thigh/groin pain for possible fracture. ASMBR Task Force recommendations (J Bone Miner Res. 2016;31:16-35) are to re-assess risk and consider a 2- to 3-year drug holiday in post-menopausal women after 5 years (oral) or 3 years (IV) for women not at high fracture risk. In women at high fracture risk, treatment continuation for 10 years (oral) or 6 years (IV) should be considered with periodic reevaluation.

ALENDRONATE *(Fosamax, Fosamax Plus D, Binosto, ✚Fosavance)* ▸K ♀C ▶− $

ADULT — Prevention of postmenopausal osteoporosis (Fosamax): 5 mg PO daily or 35 mg PO weekly. Treatment of postmenopausal osteoporosis (Fosamax, Fosamax Plus D, Binosto): 10 mg daily, 70 mg PO weekly, 70 mg/vitamin D3 2800 international units PO weekly, or 70 mg/vitamin D3 5600 international units PO weekly. Treatment of glucocorticoid-induced osteoporosis (Fosamax): 5 mg PO daily in men and women or 10 mg PO daily in postmenopausal women not taking estrogen. Treatment of osteoporosis in men (Fosamax, Fosamax Plus D, Binosto): 10 mg PO daily, 70 mg PO weekly, or 70 mg/vitamin D3 2800 international units PO weekly, or 70 mg/vit D3 5600 international units PO weekly. Paget's disease (Fosamax): 40 mg PO daily for 6 months.

PEDS — Not approved in children.

FORMS — Generic/Trade (Fosamax): Tabs 10, 70 mg. Generic only: Tabs 5, 35, 40 mg; Oral soln 70 mg/75 mL. Trade only: Fosamax Plus D: 70 mg + either 2800 or 5600 units of vitamin D3. Binosto: 70 mg effervescent tab.

NOTES — May cause esophagitis, esophageal ulcers, and esophageal erosions, occasionally with bleeding and rarely followed by esophageal stricture or perforation. Monitor frequently for dysphagia, odynophagia, and retrosternal pain. Not recommended if CrCl <35 mL/min. All products: Take 30 min before first food, beverage, and medication of the day. Remain in upright position for at least 30 min following dose. Fosamax/Fosamax Plus D: Take with a full glass of water only. Binosto: Dissolve in 4 ounces plain water, wait 5 min after effervescence stops, stir then drink.

MOA — Inhibits osteoclast-mediated bone resorption, increases bone mineral density.

ADVERSE EFFECTS — Serious: Esophageal disease (ulcers, erosion, esophagitis, stricture, perforation), gastric/duodenal ulcer, osteonecrosis of the jaw, severe skin reactions. Low-energy femoral shaft and subtrochanteric fractures, asthma exacerbation. Frequent: Headache, musculoskeletal pain, abdominal pain, diarrhea, dizziness, joint swelling, rash, photosensitivity.

ETIDRONATE ▸K ♀C ▶? $$$$$
ADULT — Paget's disease: 5 to 10 mg/kg PO daily for 6 months or 11 to 20 mg/kg daily for 3 months. Heterotopic ossification with hip replacement: 20 mg/kg/day PO for 1 month before and 3 months after surgery. Heterotopic ossification with spinal cord injury: 20 mg/kg/day PO for 2 weeks, then 10 mg/kg/day PO for 10 weeks.
PEDS — Not approved in children.
FORMS — Generic only: Tabs 200, 400 mg.
NOTES — Divide dose if GI discomfort occurs. Avoid in abnormalities of the esophagus that may delay esophageal emptying (eg, stricture). Avoid food, vitamins with minerals, or antacids within 2 h of dose.
MOA — Inhibits osteoclast-mediated bone resorption, blocks growth and mineralization of hydroxyapatite crystals.
ADVERSE EFFECTS — Serious: Esophageal disease (ulcers, esophagitis, perforation), peptic ulcer disease, agranulocytosis, pancytopenia, leukopenia, fractures, osteonecrosis of the jaw, toxic epidermal necrolyisis, asthma exacerbation. Frequent: Headache, gastritis, leg cramps, arthralgia, bone pain.

IBANDRONATE (*Boniva*) ▸K ♀C ▶? $$$$
ADULT — Prevention and treatment of postmenopausal osteoporosis: Oral: 150 mg PO q month. IV: 3 mg IV q 3 months.
PEDS — Not approved in children.
FORMS — Generic/Trade: Tab 150 mg. IV 3 mg.
NOTES — May cause esophagitis. Avoid in abnormalities of the esophagus that may delay esophageal emptying (eg, stricture). Avoid if CrCl <30 mL/min. Oral: Take 1 h before first food/beverage with a full glass of plain water; remain in upright position 1 h after taking. IV: Administer over 15 to 30 sec. Anaphylaxis reported with injection.
MOA — Inhibits osteoclast-mediated bone resorption, increases bone mineral density.
ADVERSE EFFECTS — Serious: Esophageal disease (ulcer, esophagitis), osteonecrosis of the jaw, asthma exacerbation, anaphylaxis (IV), Stevens-Johnson syndrome, erythema multiforme, dermitis bullous. Frequent: Back pain, dyspepsia, diarrhea, myalgia, headache, injection site reaction.

PAMIDRONATE ▸K ♀D ▶? $$$
WARNING — Single dose should not exceed 90 mg due to risk of renal impairment/failure.
ADULT — Hypercalcemia of malignancy, moderate (corrected Ca in the range of 12 to 13.5 mg/dL): 60 to 90 mg IV single dose infused over 2 to 24 h. Hypercalcemia of malignancy, severe (Ca more than 13.5 mg/dL): 90 mg IV single dose infused over 2 to 24 h. Wait at least 7 days before considering retreatment. Paget's disease: 30 mg IV over 4 h daily for 3 days. Osteolytic bone lesions: 90 mg IV over 4 h once a month. Osteolytic bone metastases: 90 mg IV over 2 h q 3 to 4 weeks.
PEDS — Not approved in children.

UNAPPROVED ADULT — Mild hypercalcemia: 30 mg IV single dose over 4 h. Treatment of osteoporosis: 30 mg IV q 3 months. Prevention of bone loss during androgen deprivation treatment for prostate cancer: 60 mg IV q 12 weeks.
NOTES — Fever occurs in more than 20% of patients. Monitor creatinine (prior to each dose), electrolytes, calcium, phosphate, magnesium, and CBC (regularly). Avoid in severe renal impairment and hold dosing if worsening renal function. Longer infusions (more than 2 h) may reduce renal toxicity. Not studied in patients with SCr above 3 mg/dL. Maintain adequate hydration.
MOA — Inhibits osteoclast-mediated bone resorption, decreases serum calcium.
ADVERSE EFFECTS — Serious: Atrial fibrillation, syncope, hypertension, tachycardia, osteonecrosis of the jaw, severe musculoskeletal pain, orbital inflammation, atypical femoral shaft fracture, renal tubular disorders, glomerulonephropathy, adult respiratory distress syndrome, interstitial lung disease. Frequent: Electrolyte depletion (potassium, magnesium, calcium, phosphate), fever, infusion site reaction, bone pain, dyspepsia, anorexia, nausea, diarrhea.

RISEDRONATE (*Actonel, Atelvia*) ▸K ♀C ▶? $$$$$
ADULT — Prevention and treatment of postmenopausal osteoporosis: 5 mg PO daily, 35 mg PO weekly, or 150 mg once a month. Treatment of osteoporosis in men: 35 mg PO weekly. Prevention and treatment of glucocorticoid-induced osteoporosis: 5 mg PO daily. Paget's disease: 30 mg PO daily for 2 months.
PEDS — Not approved in children.
UNAPPROVED ADULT — Prevention and treatment of glucocorticoid-induced osteoporosis: 35 mg PO weekly.
FORMS — Generic/Trade: Tabs 5, 30, 35, 150 mg. Delayed-release tabs (Atelvia) 35 mg.
NOTES — May cause esophagitis, monitor frequently for dysphagia, odynophagia, and retrosternal pain. Remain in upright position for at least 30 min following dose. Take Actonel 30 min before first food, beverage, or medication of the day with a full glass of water only. Take delayed-release (Atelvia) in the morning immediately following breakfast with 4 ounces or more of water only. Avoid in abnormalities of the esophagus that may delay esophageal emptying (eg, stricture).
MOA — Inhibits osteoclast-mediated bone resorption, increases bone mineral density.
ADVERSE EFFECTS — Serious: Esophageal disease (ulcers, erosion, esophagitis, stricture, perforation), gastric/duodenal ulcer, hypersensitivity, Stevens-Johnson syndrome, toxic epidermal necrolysis, asthma exacerbation. Frequent: Headache, musculoskeletal pain, abdominal pain, diarrhea.

ZOLEDRONIC ACID (*Reclast, Zometa, ✲Aclasta*) ▶K ♀D ▶? $$$$$
ADULT — Treatment of postemenopausal osteoporosis and osteoporosis in men (Reclast): 5 mg once yearly IV infusion over 15 min or longer. Prevention of postmenopausal osteoporosis: (Reclast) 5 mg IV infusion q 2 years. Prevention and treatment of glucocorticoid-induced osteoporosis in patients expected to receive glucocorticoids for at least 12 months (Reclast): 5 mg once yearly IV infusion over 15 min or longer. Hypercalcemia of malignancy (corrected Ca at least 12 mg/dL, Zometa): 4 mg single-dose IV infusion over 15 min or longer. Wait at least 7 days before considering retreatment. Paget's disease (Reclast): 5 mg IV single dose. Multiple myeloma and metastatic bone lesions from solid tumors (Zometa): 4 mg (CrCl >60 mL/min), 3.5 mg (CrCl 50 to 60 mL/min), 3.3 mg (CrCl 40 to 49 mL/min), or 3 mg (CrCl 30 to 39 mL/min) IV infusion over 15 min or longer q 3 to 4 weeks.
PEDS — Not approved in children.
UNAPPROVED ADULT — Osteoporosis (Zometa): 4 mg once yearly IV infusion over 15 min or longer. Paget's disease (Zometa; approved in Canada): 5 mg IV single dose. Treatment of hormone-refractory prostate cancer metastatic to bone (Zometa): 4 mg IV q 3 to 4 weeks. Prevention of bone loss during androgen-deprivation treatment for nonmetastatic prostate cancer (Zometa): 4 mg IV q 3 months for 1 year or 4 mg q 12 months. Prevention of bone loss during aromatase inhibitor use in breast cancer (Zometa): 4 mg IV q 6 months. Suppression of breast cancer in combination with adjuvant endocrine therapy (tamoxifen): 4 mg IV q 6 months for 3 years.
FORMS — Generic/Trade: 4 mg/5 mL IV (Zometa), 5 mg/100 mL IV (Reclast)
NOTES — Contraindicated in severe renal impairment (CrCl <35 mL/min) and hold dosing with worsening renal function. Monitor creatinine (before each dose), electrolytes, calcium, phosphate, magnesium, and Hb/HCT (regularly). Avoid single doses higher than 4 mg (Zometa) or higher than 5 mg (Reclast), infusions less than 15 min. Fever occurs in more than 15%. Correct preexisting hypocalcemia before therapy; life-threatening hypocalcemia reported (cardiac arrhythmias, seizures). Maintain adequate hydration for those with hypercalcemia of malignancy, and give 500 mg calcium supplement and vitamin D 400 international units PO daily to those with multiple myeloma or metastatic bone lesions. Acute phase reactions reported (fever, fatigue, bone pain/arthralgias, myalgias, flu-like illness); typically onset is within 3 days and usually resolves within 7 to 14 days.
MOA — A bisphosphonate that inhibits osteoclast-mediated bone resorption, increases bone mineral density, decreases serum calcium.
ADVERSE EFFECTS — Serious: Hypotension, renal impairment, pancytopenia, osteonecrosis of the jaw, osteonecrosis of other bones, severe musculoskeletal pain, atypical femoral shaft fracture, acute phase reaction, bronchospasm, interstitial lung disease, asthma exacerbation, acute phase reaction, hypocalcemia, cardiac arrhythmias, seizures, joint swelling, Stevens-Johnson syndrome, toxic epidermal necrolysis, , ocular inflammation. Frequent: Electrolyte depletion (potassium, magnesium, calcium, phosphate), flu-like symptoms, fever, infusion site reaction, N/V, skeletal pain, arthritis, constipation, diarrhea, conjunctivitis.

ENDOCRINE AND METABOLIC: Corticosteroids

NOTE: See also Dermatology, Ophthalmology.

BETAMETHASONE (*Celestone Soluspan, ✲Betaject*) ▶L ♀C ▶– $$$$$
ADULT — Anti-inflammatory/immunosuppressive: 0.6 to 7.2 mg/day PO divided two to four times per day or up to 9 mg/day IM. 0.25 to 2 mL intra-articular depending on location and size of joint.
PEDS — Dosing guidelines not established.
UNAPPROVED ADULT — Fetal lung maturation, maternal antepartum between 24 and 34 weeks' gestation: 12 mg IM q 24 h for 2 doses.
UNAPPROVED PEDS — Anti-inflammatory/immunosuppressive: 0.0175 to 0.25 mg/kg/day PO divided three to four times per day. Fetal lung maturation, maternal antepartum: 12 mg IM q 24 h for 2 doses.
FORMS — Generic: Syrup 0.6 mg/5 mL.
NOTES — Avoid prolonged use in children due to possible bone growth retardation. If such therapy necessary, monitor growth and development.
MOA — Long-acting glucocorticoid.
ADVERSE EFFECTS — Serious: Hypertension, diabetes, osteoporosis, immunosuppression, impaired wound healing, adrenal suppression, peptic ulcer disease, cataracts. Frequent: Cushingoid state, N/V, weight gain, myopathy, leukocytosis, skin atrophy, edema.

CORTISONE ▶L ♀D ▶– $$$$$
ADULT — Adrenocortical insufficiency: 25 to 300 mg PO daily.
PEDS — Dosing guidelines not established.
UNAPPROVED PEDS — Adrenocortical insufficiency: 0.5 to 0.75 mg/kg/day PO divided q 8 h.
FORMS — Generic only: Tabs 25 mg.
MOA — Short-acting glucocorticoid with mineralocorticoid activity at higher doses.
ADVERSE EFFECTS — Serious: Hypertension, diabetes, osteoporosis, immunosuppression, impaired wound healing, adrenal suppression, peptic ulcer disease, cataracts. Frequent: Cushingoid state, N/V, weight gain, myopathy, leukocytosis, skin atrophy, edema.

DEXAMETHASONE (*DexPak, Dexamethasone Intensol, ✲Dexasone*) ▶L ♀C ▶– $

ADULT — Anti-inflammatory/immunosuppressive: 0.5 to 9 mg/day PO/IV/IM divided two to four times per day. Cerebral edema: 10 to 20 mg IV load, then 4 mg IM q 6 h (off-label IV use common) or 1 to 3 mg PO three times per day. Multiple sclerosis (acute exacerbation): 30 mg/day for 1 week, then 4 to 12 mg every other day for 1 mo.

PEDS — Dosing varies by indication; start 0.02 to 0.3 mg/kg/day divided three to four times per day.

UNAPPROVED ADULT — Initial treatment of immune thrombocytopenic purpura: 40 mg PO daily for 4 days. Fetal lung maturation, maternal antepartum between 24 and 34 weeks' gestation: 6 mg IM q 12 h for 4 doses. Bacterial meningitis (controversial): 0.15 mg/kg IV q 6 h for 2 to 4 days; start 10 to 15 min before the 1st dose of antibiotic. Antiemetic, prophylaxis: 8 mg IV or 12 mg PO prior to chemotherapy; 8 mg PO daily for 2 to 4 days. Antiemetic, treatment: 10 to 20 mg PO/IV q 4 to 6 h.

UNAPPROVED PEDS — Anti-inflammatory/immunosuppressive: 0.08 to 0.3 mg/kg/day PO/IV/IM divided q 6 to 12 h. Croup: 0.6 mg/kg PO/IV/IM for one dose. Bacterial meningitis (controversial): 0.15 mg/kg IV q 6 h for 2 to 4 days; start 10 to 15 min before the 1st dose of antibiotic. Bronchopulmonary dysplasia in preterm infants: 0.5 mg/kg PO/IV divided q 12 h for 3 days, then taper. Acute asthma: Older than 2 yo: 0.6 mg/kg to max 16 mg PO daily for 2 days.

FORMS — Generic only: Tabs 0.5, 0.75, 1.0, 1.5, 2, 4, 6 mg; Elixir 0.5 mg/5 mL; Soln 0.5 mg/5 mL. Trade only: Tabs DexPak 13 day (51 total 1.5 mg tabs for a 13-day taper), DexPak 10 day (35 total 1.5 mg tabs for 10-day taper), DexPak 6 days (21 total 1.5 mg tabs for 6-day taper); Soln Dexamethasone Intensol 1 mg/1 mL (concentrate).

NOTES — Avoid prolonged use in children due to possible bone growth retardation. If such therapy necessary, monitor growth and development.

MOA — Long-acting glucocorticoid.

ADVERSE EFFECTS — Serious: Hypertension, diabetes, osteoporosis, immunosuppression, impaired wound healing, adrenal suppression, peptic ulcer disease, cataracts. Frequent: Cushingoid state, N/V, weight gain, myopathy, leukocytosis, skin atrophy, edema.

FLUDROCORTISONE ▶L ♀C ▶? $

ADULT — Adrenocortical insufficiency/Addison's disease: 0.1 mg PO 3 times a week to 0.2 mg PO daily. Salt-losing adrenogenital syndrome: 0.1 to 0.2 mg PO daily.

PEDS — Not approved in children.

UNAPPROVED ADULT — Orthostatic hypotension: Start 0.1 mg PO daily; increase by 0.1 mg per week if needed to max 1 mg PO daily.

UNAPPROVED PEDS — Adrenocortical insufficiency: 0.05 to 0.2 mg PO daily.

FORMS — Generic only: Tabs 0.1 mg.

NOTES — For primary adrenocortical insufficiency usually given in conjunction with cortisone or hydrocortisone.

MOA — Potent mineralocorticoid with high glucocorticoid activity; primarily used for its mineralocorticoid effects.

ADVERSE EFFECTS — Serious: Hypokalemic alkalosis, hypertension, diabetes, osteoporosis, immunosuppression, impaired wound healing, adrenal suppression, peptic ulcer disease, cataracts. Frequent: Edema, cushingoid state, N/V, weight gain, myopathy, leukocytosis, skin atrophy.

HYDROCORTISONE (*A-Hydrocort, Cortef, Solu-Cortef*) ▶L ♀C ▶– $$$

ADULT — Adrenocortical insufficiency: 20 to 240 mg/day PO divided three to four times per day or 100 to 500 mg IV/IM q 2 to 10 h prn (sodium succinate). Ulcerative colitis: 100 mg retention enema at bedtime (lying on side for 1 h or longer) for 21 days. May use for 2 to 3 months for severe cases; when course extends more than 3 weeks then discontinue gradually by decreasing frequency to every other night for 2 to 3 weeks. Multiple sclerosis acute exacerbation: 800 mg daily then 320 mg every other day for 1 month.

PEDS — Dosing guidelines not established. Prescribing information suggests tailoring doses to the specific disease being treated with a range of initial doses of 0.56 to 8 mg/kg/day IV/PO divided three to four times per day.

UNAPPROVED ADULT — Adrenocortical insufficiency (chronic): 15 to 25 mg/day PO divided two to three times per day with one-half to two-thirds of dose given in am.

UNAPPROVED PEDS — Chronic adrenocortical insufficiency: 0.5 to 0.75 mg/kg/day PO divided q 8 h or 0.25 to 0.35 mg/kg/day IM daily. Acute adrenocortical insufficiency: Infants and young children 1 to 2 mg/kg IV bolus, then 25 to 150 mg/day divided q 6 to 8 h. Older children 1 to 2 mg/kg IV bolus, then 150 to 250 mg/day IV q 6 to 8 h.

FORMS — Generic/Trade: Tabs 5, 10, 20 mg; Enema 100 mg/60 mL.

NOTES — Agent of choice for adrenocortical insufficiency because of mixed glucocorticoid and mineralocorticoid properties at doses more than 100 mg/day.

MOA — Short-acting glucocorticoid with mineralocorticoid activity at higher doses.

ADVERSE EFFECTS — Serious: Hypertension, diabetes, osteoporosis, immunosuppression, impaired wound healing, adrenal suppression, peptic ulcer disease, cataracts. Frequent: Cushingoid state, N/V, weight gain, myopathy, leukocytosis, skin atrophy, edema.

METHYLPREDNISOLONE (*Solu-Medrol, Medrol, Depo-Medrol*) ▶L ♀C ▶– $$

ADULT — Anti-inflammatory/immunosuppressive: Parenteral (Solu-Medrol) 10 to 250 mg IV/IM q 4 h prn. Oral (Medrol) 4 to 48 mg PO daily. Medrol Dosepak tapers 24 to 0 mg PO over 7 days. IM/

(cont.)

METHYLPREDNISOLONE (cont.)

joints (Depo-Medrol) 4 to 120 mg IM q 1 to 2 weeks. Multiple sclerosis flare: 160 mg IV/IM daily for 1 week followed by 64 mg every other day for 1 month. PEDS — Dosing guidelines not established. UNAPPROVED ADULT — Acute asthma exacerbation ("burst" therapy): 40 to 60 mg PO daily or divided two times per day for 3 to 10 days. Acute asthma exacerbation (vomiting or nonadherent): 240 mg IM once. Optic neuritis: 1 g IV daily (or in divided doses) for 3 days, then PO prednisone 1 mg/kg/day for 11 days (followed by a 3-day taper). Multiple sclerosis flare: 1 g IV daily (or in divided doses) for 3 to 5 days. May follow with PO prednisone 1 mg/kg/day for 14 days, then taper off. Spinal cord injury: 30 mg/kg IV over 15 min, followed in 45 min by 5.4 mg/kg/h IV infusion for 23 h (if initiated within 3 h of injury) or for 47 h (if initiated 3 to 8 h after injury). Due to insufficient evidence, routine use in spinal cord injury not recommended. UNAPPROVED PEDS — Anti-inflammatory/immuno-suppressive: 0.5 to 1.7 mg/kg/day PO/IV/IM divided q 6 to 12 h. Spinal cord injury: 30 mg/kg IV over 15 min, followed in 45 min by 5.4 mg/kg/h IV infusion for 23 h. Due to insufficient evidence, routine use in spinal cord injury not recommended. Acute asthma exacerbation ("burst" therapy): 1 to 2 mg/kg/day PO; max 60 mg daily for 3 to 10 days. Acute asthma exacerbation (vomiting or nonadherent): Age younger than 5 yo: 7.5 mg/kg IM once; age 5 to 11 yo: 240 mg IM once; age at least 12: 240 mg IM once. FORMS — Trade only: Tabs 2 mg. Generic/Trade: Tabs 4, 8, 16, 32 mg. Medrol Dosepak (4 mg, 21 tabs). NOTES — Other dosing regimens have been used for MS and optic neuritis. Avoid initial treatment of optic neuritis with oral steroids, as it may increase the risk of new episodes. Contains benzyl alcohol, contraindicated in premature infants and for intrathecal administration. Do not use for traumatic brain injury. MOA — Intermediate-acting glucocorticoid. ADVERSE EFFECTS — Serious: Cardiac arrest or arrhythmia (with IV), hypertension, osteoporosis, immunosuppression, impaired wound healing, adrenal suppression, peptic ulcers, cataracts, postinjection flare, HPA axis suppression. Frequent: Cushingoid state, N/V, weight gain, edema, hyperglycemia, hypokalemia, injection site hypo/hyperpigmentation, myopathy, dermal or subdermal changes, deltoid muscle atrophy with IM injection.

PREDNISOLONE (Pediapred, Orapred ODT, Millipred, Veripred 20) ▶L ♀C ▶+ $$$

ADULT — Anti-inflammatory/immunosuppressive: 5 to 60 mg/day PO; individualize to severity of disease and response. Multiple sclerosis: 200 mg PO daily for 1 week, then 80 mg every other day for 1 month. PEDS — Anti-inflammatory/immunosuppressive: 0.14 to 2 mg/kg/day PO divided three to four times per day (4 to 60 mg/m²/day); individualize to severity of disease and response. Acute asthma: 1 to 2 mg/kg/day daily or divided two times per day for 3 to 10 days. Nephrotic syndrome: 60 mg/m²/day divided three times per day for 4 weeks; then 40 mg/m²/day every other day for 4 weeks. UNAPPROVED ADULT — Acute asthma exacerbation ("burst" therapy): 40 to 60 mg PO daily or divided two times per day for 3 to 10 days. Bell's palsy: prednisolone 25 mg PO twice daily for 10 days or 60 mg PO daily for 5 days, then tapered over 5 days. UNAPPROVED PEDS — Acute asthma exacerbation ("burst" therapy): 1 to 2 mg/kg/day PO; max 60 mg daily for 3 to 10 days. Early active RA: 10 mg/day PO. FORMS — Generic/Trade: Tabs 5 mg. Soln 5 mg/5 mL (Pediapred, raspberry flavor). Orally disintegrating tabs 10, 15, 30 mg (Orapred ODT). Trade only: Soln 10 mg/5 mL (Millipred, grape), 20mg/5 mL (Veripred). Generic only: Syrup 15 mg/5 mL. Soln 15 mg/5 mL, 25mg/5mL. MOA — Intermediate-acting glucocorticoid with mineralocorticoid activity; primarily used for its glucocorticoid effects. ADVERSE EFFECTS — Serious: Hypertension, diabetes, osteoporosis, immunosuppression, impaired wound healing, adrenal suppression, peptic ulcer disease, cataracts. Frequent: Cushingoid state, N/V, weight gain, myopathy, leukocytosis, skin atrophy, edema.

PREDNISONE (Deltasone, Prednisone Intensol, Rayos, ✷Winpred) ▶L ♀C ▶+ $

ADULT — Anti-inflammatory/immunosuppressive: 5 to 60 mg/day PO daily or divided two to four times per day. If using delayed-release tabs (Rayos), start 5 mg PO daily if steroid-naive. PEDS — Dosing guidelines not established. UNAPPROVED ADULT — Acute asthma exacerbation ("burst" therapy): 40 to 60 mg PO daily or divided two times per day for 3 to 10 days. UNAPPROVED PEDS — Anti-inflammatory/immunosuppressive: 0.05 to 2 mg/kg/day divided one to four times per day. Acute asthma exacerbation ("burst" therapy): 1 to 2 mg/kg/day PO; max 60 mg daily for 3 to 10 days. FORMS — Generic only: Tabs 1, 2.5, 5, 10, 20, 50 mg. Soln 5 mg/5 mL. Dosepacks (5 mg tabs: Tapers 30 to 5 mg PO over 6 days or 30 to 10 mg over 12 days), Dosepacks Double Strength (10 mg tabs: Tapers 60 to 10 mg over 6 days, or 60 to 20 mg PO over 12 days) taper packs. Trade only: Delayed-release tabs 1, 2, 5 mg; Soln 5 mg/mL (Prednisone Intensol). NOTES — Conversion to prednisolone may be impaired in liver disease. MOA — Intermediate-acting glucocorticoid with mineralocorticoid activity; primarily used for its glucocorticoid effects. ADVERSE EFFECTS — Serious: Hypertension, diabetes, osteoporosis, immunosuppression, impaired wound healing, adrenal suppression, peptic ulcer disease, cataracts, psychosis, depression. Frequent: Cushingoid state, N/V, weight gain, myopathy, leukocytosis, skin atrophy, edema.

TRIAMCINOLONE (*Aristospan, Kenalog*) ▶L ♀C ▶– $
ADULT — Anti-inflammatory/immunosuppressive: 4 to 48 mg/day PO divided one to four times per day. 2.5 to 60 mg IM daily (Kenalog). Intra-articular: Small joints 2.5 to 5 mg (Kenalog), 2 to 6 mg (Aristospan); large joints 5 to 15 mg (Kenalog); 10 to 20 mg (Aristospan).
PEDS — Dosing guidelines not established.
UNAPPROVED PEDS — Anti-inflammatory/immuno-suppressive: 0.117 to 1.66 mg/kg/day PO divided four times per day.
FORMS — Trade only: Injection 10 mg/mL, 40 mg/mL, 5 mg/mL, 20 mg/mL (Aristospan).

NOTES — Parenteral form not for IV use. Kenalog and Aristospan contain benzyl alcohol; do not use in neonates.
MOA — Intermediate-acting glucocorticoid.
ADVERSE EFFECTS — Serious: Hypertension, diabetes, osteoporosis, immunosuppression, impaired wound healing, adrenal suppression, peptic ulcer disease, cataracts, postinjection flare, anaphylaxis, angioedema. Frequent: Cushingoid state, N/V, wt gain, myopathy, leukocytosis, skin atrophy, injection site hyper/hypopigmentation, edema.

ENDOCRINE AND METABOLIC: Diabetes-Related—Alpha-Glucosidase Inhibitors

NOTE: Alpha-glucosidase inhibitor administered alone should not cause hypoglycemia. If hypoglycemia occurs, treat with oral glucose rather than sucrose (table sugar). Adverse GI effects (ie, flatulence, diarrhea, abdominal pain) may occur with initial therapy.

ACARBOSE (*Precose, ✳Glucobay*) ▶Gut/K ♀B ▶– $$$
ADULT — DM, Type 2: Initiate therapy with 25 mg PO three times per day with the first bite of each meal. May start with 25 mg PO daily to minimize GI adverse effects. May increase to 50 mg PO three times per day after 4 to 8 weeks. Usual range is 50 to 100 mg PO three times per day. Max dose for patients wt 60 kg or less is 50 mg three times per day, wt greater than 60 kg max is 100 mg three times per day.
PEDS — Not approved in children.
UNAPPROVED ADULT — DM prevention, Type 2: 100 mg PO three times per day or to max tolerated dose.
FORMS — Generic/Trade: Tabs 25, 50, 100 mg.
MOA — Inhibits intestinal alpha-glucoside hydrolase and pancreatic alpha-amylase and delays glucose absorption.
ADVERSE EFFECTS — Serious: Elevated serum transaminases, hypersensitivity, ileus, thrombocytopenia,

pneumatosis cystoidis intestinalis, fulminant hepatitis. Frequent: Flatulence, diarrhea, abdominal pain.
MIGLITOL (*Glyset*) ▶K ♀B ▶– $$$$$
ADULT — DM, Type 2: Initiate therapy with 25 mg PO three times per day with the first bite of each meal. Use 25 mg PO daily to start if GI adverse effects. May increase dose to 50 mg PO three times per day after 4 to 8 weeks, max 300 mg/day.
PEDS — Not approved in children.
FORMS — Trade only: Tabs 25, 50, 100 mg.
NOTES — Consider reducing dose of insulin or sulfonylurea if used in combination.
MOA — Inhibits intestinal alpha-glucoside hydrolase and delays glucose absorption.
ADVERSE EFFECTS — Serious: ileus, pneumatosis cystoides intestinalis. Frequent: Flatulence, diarrhea, abdominal pain, rash, transient decrease in serum iron.

ENDOCRINE AND METABOLIC: Diabetes-Related—Combinations

NOTE: Metformin-containing products may cause life-threatening lactic acidosis, usually in setting of decreased tissue perfusion, hypoxia, hepatic dysfunction, or impaired renal clearance. Avoid if ethanol abuse, heart failure (requiring treatment), hepatic impairment, or hypoxic states (cardiogenic shock, septicemia, acute MI). Assess eGFR prior to treatment and at least annually. Avoid in patients with an eGFR <30 mL/min/1.73 m2; initiation in patients with eGFR 30 to 45 mL/min/1.73 m2 is not recommended. In those already taking metformin if eGFR falls below 45 mL/min/1.73 m2 reassess benefits and risks. Discontinue metformin at the time of or prior to an iodinated contrast imaging procedure and for 48 hours after the procedure in those with eGFR <60 mL/min/1.73 m2; in those with liver disease, alcoholism, or heart failure; or in those administered intra-arterial contrast. Reassess the eGFR post-procedure and reinitiate if renal function stable. Initial GI upset may be minimized by starting with lower dose of metformin component. Glitazone-containing products may cause edema, wt gain, new heart failure, or exacerbate existing heart failure (avoid in NYHA Class III or IV). Monitor for signs of heart failure (rapid wt gain, dyspnea, edema) following initiation or dose increase. If occurs, manage fluid retention and consider discontinuation or dosage decrease. Avoid if liver disease or ALT >2.5 times normal. Monitor LFTs before therapy and periodically thereafter. Discontinue if ALT >3 times upper normal limit. Full effect may not be apparent for up to 12 weeks. May cause resumption of ovulation in premenopausal anovulatory women; recommend contraception use. Sulfonylureascan lead to hemolytic anemia in patients with G6PD deficiency; use caution or consider alternate agents. DPP-IV inhibitors: Report pancreatitis and discontinue drug if occurs. Severe/disabling joint pain reported, consider as possible cause of arthralgia and discontinue if occurs. SGLT2 Inhibitors: Check renal function prior to initiation and periodically. Do not use in DM Type 1 or DKA. DKA and euglycemic DKA reported; if signs/symptoms of acidosis then assess for ketoacidosis regardless of glucose level. May cause hypotension, check volume status prior to use. Consider reducing dose of insulin or insulin secretagogue prior to initiation to avoid hypoglycemia. Monitor for and treat genital fungal or urinary tract infections if occur. May increase LDL.

ACTOPLUS METACTOPLUS MET XR (pioglitazone + metformin) ▶KL ♀C ▶? $$$$$
ADULT — DM, Type 2: 1 tab PO daily to two times per day. If inadequate control with metformin monotherapy, start 15/500 or 15/850 mg PO one to two times per day. If inadequate control with pioglitazone monotherapy, start 15/500 mg two times per day or 15/850 mg daily. Max 45/2550 mg/day. Extended release, start 1 tab (15/1000 mg or 30/1000 mg) daily with evening meal. Max: 45/2000 mg/day.
PEDS — Not approved nor recommended in children.
FORMS — Generic/Trade: Tabs 15/500, 15/850 mg. Trade only: Extended-release (Actoplus Met XR) tabs: 15/1000, 30/1000 mg.
NOTES — Urinary bladder tumors reported; advise patients to report macroscopic hematuria or dysuria.
MOA — Combination product that increases insulin sensitivity, decreases hepatic gluconeogenesis.
ADVERSE EFFECTS — Serious: Potential hepatotoxicity, heart failure exacerbation, resumption of ovulation, macular edema, lactic acidosis, decreased vitamin B12, fracture, bladder tumor. Frequent: Asthenia, anemia, edema, wt gain, headache, dyslipidemia, diarrhea, increased LFTs, N/V, flatulence, abdominal discomfort, diarrhea, headache, taste disturbance.

AVANDAMET (rosiglitazone + metformin) ▶KL ♀C ▶? $$$$
ADULT — DM, Type 2, initial therapy (drug-naive): Start 2/500 mg PO one or two times per day. If inadequate control with metformin alone, select tab strength based on adding 4 mg/day rosiglitazone to existing metformin dose. If inadequate control with rosiglitazone alone, select tab strength based on adding 1000 mg/day metformin to existing rosiglitazone dose. Max 8/2000 mg/day.
PEDS — Not approved in children.
FORMS — Trade only: Tabs 2/500, 2/1000 mg.
MOA — Combination product that increases insulin sensitivity, decreases hepatic gluconeogenesis.
ADVERSE EFFECTS — Serious: Potential hepatotoxicity, heart failure, resumption of ovulation, lactic acidosis, decreased vitamin B12, macular edema, fracture in women, myocardial infarction. Frequent: Asthenia, anemia, edema, weight gain or loss, headache, dyslipidemia, diarrhea, increased LFTs, N/V, flatulence, abdominal discomfort, headache, taste disturbance.

DUETACT (pioglitazone + glimepiride) ▶LK ♀C ▶– $$$$$
ADULT — DM, Type 2: Start 30/2 mg PO daily. Start up to 30/4 mg PO daily if prior glimepiride therapy, or 30/2 mg PO daily if prior pioglitazone therapy; max 30/4 mg/day. Give with breakfast or the first main meal of the day. In the elderly, the malnourished, or those with renal/hepatic impairment, precede therapy with trial of glimepiride 1 mg/day and then titrate Duetact more slowly.
PEDS — Not approved nor recommended in children.
FORMS — Generic/Trade: Tabs 30/2, 30/4 mg pioglitazone/glimepiride.

NOTES — Urinary bladder tumors reported; advise patients to report macroscopic hematuria or dysuria.
MOA — Combination product that stimulates pancreatic beta-cell insulin release and increases insulin sensitivity in adipose tissue, skeletal muscle, and liver.
ADVERSE EFFECTS — Serious: Potential hepatotoxicity, heart failure exacerbation, resumption of ovulation, hypoglycemia, hypersensitivity, anaphylaxis, angioedema, Stevens-Johnsons Syndrome, SIADH, disulfiram-like reaction, cholestatic jaundice, marrow suppression, hemolytic anemia, thrombocytopenia, eosinophilia, hepatic porphyria, increased LFTs, macular edema, fracture, bladder tumor. Frequent: Edema, wt gain, upper respiratory tract infection, headache, fatigue, N/V/D, dyspepsia, rash, pruritus, blurred vision.

GLUCOVANCE (glyburide + metformin) ▶KL ♀B ▶? $$$
ADULT — DM, Type 2, initial therapy (drug-naive): Start 1.25/250 mg PO daily or two times per day with meals; max 10/2000 mg daily. Inadequate control with a sulfonylurea or metformin alone: Start 2.5/500 or 5/500 mg PO two times per day with meals; max 20/2000 mg daily.
PEDS — Not approved in children.
FORMS — Generic/Trade: Tabs 1.25/250, 2.5/500, 5/500 mg.
MOA — Combination product that stimulates pancreatic beta-cell insulin release, decreases hepatic gluconeogenesis, and increases insulin sensitivity.
ADVERSE EFFECTS — Serious: Hypoglycemia, hypersensitivity, SIADH, disulfiram-like reaction, cholestatic jaundice, aplastic anemia, hemolytic anemia, leukopenia, thrombocytopenia, agranulocytosis, pancytopenia, eosinophilia, hepatic porphyria, increased LFTs, hepatitis, liver failure, lactic acidosis, decreased serum vitamin B12. Frequent: Diarrhea, N/V, flatulence, abdominal discomfort, headache, fatigue, rash, weight gain or loss, taste disturbance.

GLYXAMBI (empagliflozin + linagliptin) ▶LK ♀C ▶? $$$$$
ADULT — DM, Type 2: 1 tab (10 mg empagliflozin/ 5 mg linagliptin) PO daily in morning, with or without food. May increase to 25 mg empagliflozin/5 mg linagliptin PO daily.
PEDS — Not approved in children.
FORMS — Trade only: 10/5, 25/5 mg empagliflozin/linagliptin tabs.
NOTES — Do not use if CrCl <45 mL/min. Monitor for and discontinue if hypersensitivity reaction; reaction can occur early or late in therapy.
MOA — Combination of inhibitor of sodium-glucose cotransporter 2 (SGLT2) which blocks reabsorption of glucose from the kidney and increases glucose loss in the urine and a dipeptidyl peptidase IV (DPP-IV) inhibitor that slows inactivation of incretin hormones, resulting in increased glucose-stimulated insulin secretion and decreased glucagon secretion

(cont.)

GLYXAMBI (*cont.*)

ADVERSE EFFECTS — Serious: hypotension, renal dysfunction, hypoglycemia, pancreatitis, hypersensitivity, urticaria, angioedema, bronchial hyperreactivity. Frequent: genital fungal infections, urinary tract infections, increased urination, increased LDL, nasopharyngitis, arthralgia, back pain, headache.

INVOKAMET (canagliflozin + metformin) ▶KL ♀– ?/X/X ▶? $$$$$

ADULT — DM, Type 2: 1 tab PO twice daily. In patients not taking metformin, start with low dose of 500 mg metformin with gradual dose titration for GI tolerance. In patients not taking canagliflozin, start 50 mg canagliflozin. If eGFR 45 to less than 60 mL/min, max canagliflozin dose is 100 mg/day.

PEDS — Not approved in children.

FORMS — Trade only: 50/500, 50/1000, 150/500, 150/1000 canagliflozin/metformin tabs.

NOTES — Do not use if eGFR <45 mL/min. Acute kidney injury and renal impairment reported, monitor renal function during therapy and consider holding during reduced oral intake or fluid losses. May cause hyperkalemia, check K+ levels.

MOA — Combination product of sodium-glucose cotransporter 2 (SGLT2) inhibitor which blocks reabsorption of glucose from the kidney and increases glucose loss in the urine and biguanide that decreases hepatic gluconeogenesis and increases insulin sensitivity.

ADVERSE EFFECTS — Serious: hypotension, hyperkalemia, renal dysfunction, hypoglycemia, hypersensitivity, lactic acidosis, decreased serum vitamin B12, bone fracture, decreased bone mineral density, falls. Frequent: genital fungal infections, urinary tract infections, increased urination, increased LDL, diarrhea, N/V, flatulence, abdominal discomfort, headache, weakness, taste disturbance.

JANUMET (sitagliptin + metformin, *Janumet XR*) ▶K ♀B ▶? $$$$$

ADULT — DM, Type 2: Individualize based on patient's current therapy. Immediate-release: Start 1 tab PO two times per day. Extended-release: 1 tab PO daily. If inadequate control with metformin monotherapy, start 50/500 or 50/1000 two times per day based on current metformin dose. Extended-release: Start 100 mg sitagliptin daily plus current daily metformin. If inadequate control on sitagliptin monotherapy: Immediate-release: Start 50/500 two times per day. Extended-release: Start 100/1000 mg daily. Max 100/2000 mg daily. Give with meals.

PEDS — Not approved in children.

FORMS — Trade only: Immediate-release tabs 50/500, 50/1000 mg, extended-release tabs 100/1000, 50/500, 50/1000 mg sitagliptin/metformin.

NOTES — Not for use in Type 1 DM or DKA. Assess renal function and hematologic parameters prior to initiating and at least annually thereafter. Assess renal function more often if risk factors for dysfunction and discontinue if renal dysfunction. Do not split, crush, or chew extended-release formulation. Discontinue if signs of hypersensitivity, including

anaphylaxis, angioedema, and severe dermatologic reactions.

MOA — Combination product that decreases hepatic gluconeogenesis, increases insulin sensitivity and slows inactivation of incretin hormones.

ADVERSE EFFECTS — Serious: Lactic acidosis, hypersensitivity, decreased serum vitamin B12, pancreatitis. Frequent: Diarrhea, N/V, flatulence, abdominal discomfort, headache, wt loss, taste disturbance, URI, nasopharyngitis, athralgia, myalgia, pain in extremity, back pain, pruritis.

JENTADUETO (linagliptin + metformin, *Jentadueto XR*) ▶KL ♀– ?/?/? ▶? $$$$$

ADULT — DM, Type 2: Immediate release: If prior metformin, start 2.5 mg linagliptin and current metformin dose PO two times per day. If no prior metformin, start 2.5/500 mg linagliptin/metformin PO two times per day. If current linagliptin/metformin, start at current doses. Extended-release: If prior metformin, start 5 mg linagliptin and current metformin dose PO daily. If no prior metformin, start 5/1000 mg linagliptin/metformin extended-release PO daily. If prior linagliptin/metformin, switch to 5 mg linagliptin and current metformin dose PO daily. Max 5/2000 mg daily.

PEDS — Not approved in peds.

FORMS — Trade only: Immediate release tabs 2.5/500, 2.5/850, 2.5/1000 mg linagliptin/metformin. Extended release tabs 2.5/1000, 5/1000 linagliptin/extended-release metformin

NOTES — Not for use in Type 1 DM or DKA. May cause hypoglycemia when added to sulfonylurea or insulin therapy; consider reducing dose of sulfonylurea or insulin to decrease risk of hypoglycemia. Metformin may lower B12 levels, monitor hematologic parameters annually. Monitor for pancreatitis at initiation of therapy and dosage increases; discontinue drug if occurs. Monitor for and discontinue if hypersensitivity reaction; reaction can occur early or late in therapy.

MOA — Combination product that decreases hepatic gluconeogenesis, increases insulin sensitivity and slows inactivation of incretin hormones.

ADVERSE EFFECTS — Serious: Hypoglycemia, pancreatitis, hypersensitivity, lactic acidosis, B12 deficiency, mouth ulcerations.. Frequent: nasopharyngitis, diarrhea, N/V, flatulence, myalgia.

KAZANO (alogliptin + metformin) ▶K – ♀B ▶? $$$$$

ADULT — DM, Type 2: Individualize based on patient's current therapy. 1 tab PO two times per day. Max 25/2000 mg/day. Give with meals.

PEDS — Not approved in children.

FORMS — Trade only: 12.5/500, 12.5/1000 mg alogliptin/metformin.

NOTES — Not for use in Type 1 DM or DKA. Assess renal function and hematologic parameters prior to initiating and at least annually thereafter. Assess renal function more often if risk factors for dysfunction and discontinue if renal dysfunction. Discontinue if signs of hypersensitivity, including anaphylaxis, angioedema, and severe dermatologic

(cont.)

KAZANO (*cont.*)

reactions. Consider risk/benefit in those with or at risk for heart failure. Postmarketing reports of hepatic failure, discontinue if liver injury detected and do not restart if no identified etiology for liver injury.

MOA — Combination product that decreases hepatic gluconeogenesis, increases insulin sensitivity and slows inactivation of incretin hormones.

ADVERSE EFFECTS — Serious: Lactic acidosis, hypersensitivity, decreased serum vitamin B12, hepatic failure, pancreatitis. Frequent: Diarrhea, N/V, flatulence, abdominal discomfort, headache, taste disturbance, URI, nasopharyngitis, UTI, back pain, HTN.

KOMBIGLYZE XR (saxagliptin + metformin, ✱ *Komboglyze*) ▸♀B ▶? $$$$$

ADULT — DM, Type 2: If inadequately controlled on metformin alone, start 2.5 to 5 mg of saxagliptin plus current dose of metformin; give once daily with evening meal. If inadequately controlled on saxagliptin, start 5/500 mg once daily with evening meal. Max: 5/2000 mg/day.

PEDS — Not approved in children.

FORMS — Trade only: Tabs 5/500, 2.5/1000, 5/1000 mg.

NOTES — Reduce saxagliptin dose to 2.5 mg when administered with strong CYP3A4/5 inhibitors such as ketoconazole; use individual products instead of combination product if needed to achieve appropriate dose. Not for use in Type 1 DM or DKA. Assess renal function periodically. To minimize risk of hypoglycemia if used with insulin or a sulfonylurea, consider lower dose of insulin or sulfonylurea. Do not split, crush, or chew. Hypersensitivity, including angioedema, reported; caution if history of angioedema to other DPP4 inhibitors.

MOA — Combination product with dipeptidyl peptidase IV (DPP-IV) inhibitor that slows inactivation of incretin hormones, resulting in increased glucose-stimulated insulin secretion and decreased glucagon secretion and a biguanide that decreases hepatic gluconeogenesis and increases insulin sensitivity.

ADVERSE EFFECTS — Serious: Lactic acidosis, decreased serum vitamin B12, hypersensitivity, angioedema, hypoglycemia, lymphopenia, pancreatitis. Frequent: Diarrhea, N/V, flatulence, abdominal discomfort, headache, wt loss, taste disturbance, URI, UTI, nasopharyngitis, peripheral edema.

METAGLIP (glipizide + metformin) ▸KL ♀C ▶? $$$

ADULT — DM, Type 2, initial therapy (drug-naive): Start 2.5/250 mg PO daily to 2.5/500 mg PO twice per day with meals; max 10/2000 mg daily. Inadequate control with a sulfonylurea or metformin alone: Start 2.5/500 or 5/500 mg PO twice per day with meals; max 20/2000 mg daily.

PEDS — Not approved in children.

FORMS — Generic only: Tabs 2.5/250, 2.5/500, 5/500 mg.

MOA — Combination product that stimulates pancreatic beta-cell insulin release, decreases hepatic gluconeogenesis, and increases insulin sensitivity.

ADVERSE EFFECTS — Serious: Hypoglycemia, hypersensitivity, SIADH, disulfiram-like reaction, cholestatic jaundice, hepatocellular jaundice, aplastic anemia, hemolytic anemia, leukopenia, thrombocytopenia, agranulocytosis, pancytopenia, eosinophilia, hepatic porphyria, increased LFTs, lactic acidosis, decreased serum vitamin B12. Frequent: Weight gain or loss, fatigue, diarrhea, nausea, dyspepsia, rash, vomiting, flatulence, asthenia, abdominal discomfort, headache, taste disturbance.

OSENI (alogliptin + pioglitazone) ▸KL – ♀C ▶? $$$$$

ADULT — DM, Type 2: Individualize based on patient's current therapy. 1 tab PO daily. Max 25/45 mg/day. If CrCl 30 to 59 mL/min, reduce dose of alogliptin to 12.5 mg daily.

PEDS — Not approved in children.

FORMS — Trade only: Tabs 12.5/15, 12.5/30, 12.5/45, 25/15, 25/30, 25/45 mg alogliptin/pioglitazone.

NOTES — Do not use in Type 1 DM or DKA. Not recommended for patients with severe renal impairment or ESRD. Discontinue if signs of hypersensitivity, including anaphylaxis, angioedema, and severe dermatologic reactions. Consider risk/benefit in those with or at risk for heart failure. Postmarketing reports of hepatic failure, discontinue if liver injury detected and do not restart if no identified etiology for liver injury. Urinary bladder tumors reported with pioglitazone; advise patients to report macroscopic hematuria or dysuria. Reports of fracture risk with pioglitazone.

MOA — Combination of dipeptidyl peptidase IV (DPP-IV) inhibitor that slows inactivation of incretin hormones, resulting in increased glucose-stimulated insulin secretion and decreased glucagon secretion and thiazolidinedione that increases insulin sensitivity in adipose tissue, skeletal muscle, and liver.

ADVERSE EFFECTS — Serious: Hepatotoxicity, liver failure, heart failure exacerbation, resumption of ovulation, macular edema, fracture, bladder tumor, hypersensitivity, anaphylaxis, angioedema, pancreatitis. Frequent: Edema, wt gain, nasopharyngitis, HA, URI, myalgia.

PRANDIMET (repaglinide + metformin) ▸KL ♀C ▶? $$$$$

ADULT — DM, Type 2, initial therapy (drug-naive): Start 1/500 mg PO daily before meals; max 10/2500 mg daily or 4/1000 mg/meal. Inadequate control with metformin alone: Start 1/500 mg PO two times per day before meals. Inadequate control with repaglinide alone: Start 500 mg metformin component PO two times per day before meals. In patients taking repaglinide and metformin concomitantly: Start at current dose and titrate to achieve adequate response.

PEDS — Not approved in children.

FORMS — Trade: Tabs 1/500, 2/500 mg.

(cont.)

PRANDIMET (*cont.*)

NOTES — May take dose immediately preceding meal to as long as 30 min before the meal. Patients should be advised to skip dose if skipping meal. Do not use with NPH insulin.

MOA — Combination product that stimulates pancreatic beta-cell insulin release, decreases hepatic gluconeogenesis, and increases insulin sensitivity.

ADVERSE EFFECTS — Serious: Hypoglycemia, hypersensitivity, thrombocytopenia, leukopenia, increased serum transaminases, lactic acidosis, decreased serum vitamin B12. Frequent: Headache, diarrhea, arthralgia, N/V, flatulence, abdominal discomfort, weight loss, taste disturbance.

SYNJARDY (**empagliflozin + metformin**) ▶KL ♀C ▶?
$$$$$
ADULT — DM, Type 2: 1 tab PO twice daily. In patients not taking metformin, start with low dose of 500 mg metformin with gradual dose titration for GI tolerance. In patients not taking empagliflozin, start 5 mg empagliflozin. Titrate as tolerated for glycemic control. Max: 25/2000 mg empagliflozin/metformin per day.

PEDS — Not approved for use in children.

FORMS — Trade only: 5/500, 5/1000, 12.5/500, 12.5/1000 mg empagliflozin/metformin tabs.

NOTES — Do not use if eGFR <45 mL/min.

MOA — Combination product of sodium-glucose cotransporter 2 (SGLT2) inhibitor which blocks reabsorption of glucose from the kidney and increases glucose loss in the urine and biguanide that decreases hepatic gluconeogenesis and increases insulin sensitivity.

ADVERSE EFFECTS — Serious: hypotension, renal dysfunction, hypoglycemia, lactic acidosis, euglycemic ketoacidosis, renal dysfunction. Frequent: genital fungal infections, urinary tract infections, increased urination, increased LDL, diarrhea, N/V, flatulence, abdominal discomfort, headache, weakness, taste disturbance.

XIGDUO XR (**dapagliflozin + metformin**) ▶KL ♀C ▶?
$$$$$
ADULT — DM, Type 2: 1 tab PO once daily in the morning with food. Individualize starting dose based on current treatment.

PEDS — Not approved in children.

UNAPPROVED ADULT — DM, Type 2: 1 tab PO once daily in the morning with food. Individualize starting dose based on current treatment.

FORMS — Trade only: 5/500, 5/1000, 10/500, 10/1000 mg dapagliflozin/metformin extended-release tabs.

NOTES — Do not use if eGFR <60 mL/min. Acute kidney injury and renal impairment reported, monitor renal function during therapy and consider holding during reduced oral intake or fluid losses. Possible increase in bladder cancer observed, use with caution in those with history of bladder cancer and do not use if active bladder cancer.

MOA — Combination product of sodium-glucose cotransporter 2 (SGLT2) inhibitor which blocks reabsorption of glucose from the kidney and increases glucose loss in the urine and biguanide that decreases hepatic gluconeogenesis and increases insulin sensitivity.

ADVERSE EFFECTS — Serious: hypotension, hyperkalemia, renal dysfunction, hypoglycemia, hypersensitivity, lactic acidosis, decreased serum vitamin B12. Frequent: genital fungal infections, urinary tract infections, increased urination, increased LDL, nasopharyngitis, diarrhea, N/V, flatulence, abdominal discomfort, headache, weight loss, taste disturbance.

ENDOCRINE AND METABOLIC: Diabetes-Related—DPP-4 inhibitors

NOTE: Not for use in Type 1 DM or DKA. When adding to sulfonylurea or insulin therapy, consider reducing dose of sulfonylurea or insulin to decrease risk of hypoglycemia. Monitor for pancreatitis at initiation of therapy and dosage increases; discontinue drug if occurs. Risk of pancreatitis increased if prior pancreatitis. Discontinue if signs of hypersensitivity, including anaphylaxis, angioedema, and severe dermatologic reactions. Severe/disabling joint pain reported, consider as possible cause of arthralgia and discontinue if occurs.

ALOGLIPTIN (*Nesina*) ▶K − ♀?/?/? ▶? $$$$$
WARNING — Consider risk/benefit in those with or at risk for heart failure. Postmarketing reports of hepatic failure, discontinue if liver injury detected and do not restart if no identified etiology for liver injury.

ADULT — DM, Type 2: 25 mg PO daily. If CrCl 30 to 59 mL/min, reduce dose to 12.5 mg daily; if CrCl <30 mL/min, then give 6.25 mg daily.

PEDS — Not approved in children.

FORMS — Trade only: Tabs 6.25, 12.5, 25 mg.

MOA — Dipeptidyl peptidase IV (DPP-IV) inhibitor that slows inactivation of incretin hormones, resulting in increased glucose-stimulated insulin secretion and decreased glucagon secretion.

ADVERSE EFFECTS — Serious: Hypersensitivity, anaphylaxis, angioedema, hepatic failure, pancreatitis. Frequent: nasopharyngitis, HA, URI.

LINAGLIPTIN (*Tradjenta*, *✷Trajenta*) ▶L − ♀B ▶? $$$$$
ADULT — DM, Type 2: 5 mg PO once daily.

PEDS — Not approved in children.

FORMS — Trade only: Tab 5 mg.

NOTES — Monitor for and discontinue if hypersensitivity reaction; reaction can occur early or late in therapy.

MOA — Dipeptidyl peptidase IV (DPP-IV) inhibitor that slows inactivation of incretin hormones, resulting in increased glucose-stimulated insulin secretion and decreased glucagon secretion.

ADVERSE EFFECTS — Serious: hypoglycemia, pancreatitis, hypersensitivity, urticaria, angioedema, bronchial hyperreactivity, mouth ulcerations. Frequent: nasopharyngitis, arthralgia, back pain, headache.

SAXAGLIPTIN (*Onglyza*) ▶LK ♀B ▶? $$$$$
WARNING — None
ADULT — DM, Type 2: 2.5 or 5 mg PO daily. If CrCl is ≤50 mL/min, reduce dose to 2.5 mg daily.
PEDS — Not approved in children.
FORMS — Trade only: Tabs 2.5, 5 mg.
NOTES — Assess renal function periodically. Reduce dose when administered with strong CYP3A4/5 inhibitors such as ketoconazole. Consider risk/benefit in those with or at risk for heart failure.
MOA — Dipeptidyl peptidase IV (DPP-IV) inhibitor that slows inactivation of incretin hormones, resulting in increased glucose-stimulated insulin secretion and decreased glucagon secretion.
ADVERSE EFFECTS — Serious: hypersensitivity, angioedema, hypoglycemia, lymphopenia,

pancreatitis. Frequent: URI, UTI, headache, GI, nasopharyngitis, peripheral edema.

SITAGLIPTIN (*Januvia*) ▶K ♀B ▶? $$$$$
ADULT — DM, Type 2: 100 mg PO daily. If CrCl 30 to 49 mL/min, reduce dose to 50 mg daily; if CrCl less than 30 mL/min, then give 25 mg daily.
PEDS — Not approved in children.
FORMS — Trade only: Tabs 25, 50, 100 mg.
MOA — Dipeptidyl peptidase IV (DPP-IV) inhibitor that slows inactivation of incretin hormones, resulting in increased glucose-stimulated insulin secretion and decreased glucagon secretion.
ADVERSE EFFECTS — Serious: Hypersensitivity, anaphylaxis, angioedema, pancreatitis. Frequent: URI, nasopharyngitis, HA, increased serum transaminases, constipation, vomiting, arthralgia, myalgia, pain in extremity, back pain, pruritis.

ENDOCRINE AND METABOLIC: Diabetes-Related—GLP-1 agonists

NOTE: Start with low dose to increase GI tolerance. Not recommended in severe GI disease, including gastroparesis. Take medications that require rapid GI absorption at least 1 h prior to exenatide immediate-release or liraglutide. May give SC in upper arm, abdomen, or thigh. May promote slight wt loss. Risk of hypoglycemia is higher when used with insulin or insulin secretagogue (sulfonylurea, meglitinides); therefore, consider reduction in sulfonylurea or insulin dose. Pancreatitis reported, monitor for signs and symptoms including abdominal pain and vomiting upon initiation and dose increases. Discontinue if pancreatitis occurs. Has not been studied in those with history of pancreatitis. Not recommended as 1st-line therapy or for use in DM, Type 1 or DKA. Abiglutide, dulaglutide, liraglutide and extended-release exenatide: Thyroid C-cell tumors reported in animal studies with GLP-1 agonists. Contraindicated if history or family history of medullary thyroid cancer or in patients with multiple endocrine neoplasia syndrome type 2. Counsel patients on risk of thyroid tumors.

ALBIGLUTIDE (*Tanzeum*) ▶proteolysis ♀C ▶? $$$$$
ADULT — DM, Type 2, adjunctive therapy: 30 mg SC once weekly. May increase to 50 mg SC once weekly.
PEDS — Not approved in children.
FORMS — Trade only: 30, 50 mg single-dose pen.
NOTES — May be given any time of day without regard to meals. In those with renal impairment, check renal function if reporting severe GI reactions. Concurrent use with mealtime insulin has not been studied.
MOA — Incretin analog that reduces fasting and postprandial glucose by increasing glucose-stimulated insulin secretion, decreasing glucagon secretion, slowing gastric emptying and reducing appetite
ADVERSE EFFECTS — Serious: pancreatitis, hypersensitivity, hypoglycemia. Frequent: Nausea, diarrhea, upper respiratory tract infection, injection site reaction, cough, back pain, arthralgia, sinusitis, influenza.

DULAGLUTIDE (*Trulicity*) ▶proteolysis ♀C ▶? $$$$$
ADULT — DM, Type 2: Start 0.75 mg SC once weekly. May increase to 1.5 mg SC once weekly.
PEDS — Not approved in children.
FORMS — Trade only: 0.75, 1.5 mg single-dose pen; 0.75, 1.5 mg single-dose prefilled syringe.
NOTES — May be given any time of day without regard to meals. Monitor renal function in patients with renal impairment reporting severe GI reactions. Concurrent use with basal insulin has not been studied.
MOA — Incretin analog that reduces fasting and postprandial glucose by increasing glucose-stimulated

insulin secretion, decreasing glucagon secretion, slowing gastric emptying and reducing appetite.
ADVERSE EFFECTS — Serious: pancreatitis, hypoglycemia, hypersensitivity. Common: nausea, diarrhea, vomiting, abdominal pain, decreased appetite.

EXENATIDE (*Byetta, Bydureon*) ▶ K/proteolysis ♀C ▶? $$$$$
ADULT — DM, Type 2, adjunctive therapy: Immediate-release: 5 mcg SC two times per day (within 1 h before the morning and evening meals, or 1 h before the two main meals of the day at least 6 h apart). May increase to 10 mcg SC two times per day after 1 month. Extended-release: 2 mg SC once weekly anytime of day without regard to meals.
PEDS — Not approved in children.
FORMS — Trade only: Byetta, prefilled pen (60 doses each) 5 mcg/dose, 1.2 mL; 10 mcg/dose, 2.4 mL. Bydureon (extended-release): 2 mg/vial; 2 mg/prefilled pen (single-use).
NOTES — Protect from light. Prior to initial use, keep refrigerated. After initial use, store at temperature below 78°F; do not freeze. Discard pen 30 days after 1st use. Multidose prefilled pens for use by one individual only; risk for bloodborne pathogen transmission. Avoid use if renal insufficiency (CrCl <30 mL/min). Caution recommended if increasing dose from 5 to 10 mcg in patients with CrCl 30 to 50 mL/min (immediate release). Monitor for kidney dysfunction. Do not substitute for insulin in the insulin-dependent; concurrent use with any insulin (Bydureon) or mealtime insulin (Byetta) has not been studied.

(cont.)

EXENATIDE (*cont.*)

Use with short- or rapid-acting insulins not recommended. May potentiate warfarin. Serious injection-site reactions (abcess, cellulitis, necrosis) may occur with extended-release; advise patients to seek attention if pain, swelling, blisters, or open wounds.

MOA — Incretin analog that reduces fasting and postprandial glucose by increasing glucose-stimulated insulin secretion, decreasing glucagon secretion, slowing gastric emptying and reducing appetite.

ADVERSE EFFECTS — Serious: angioedema, hypersensitivity, anaphylaxis, pancreatitis, renal dysfunction, serious injection-site reactions (abcess, cellulitis, necrosis). Frequent: hypoglycemia, N/V, diarrhea, constipation, flatulence, dizziness, headache.

LIRAGLUTIDE (*Victoza, Saxenda*) ▶proteolysis ♀ C (Victoza), X (Saxenda) ▶? $$$$$

ADULT — DM, Type 2 (Victoza): Start 0.6 mg SC daily for 1 week, then increase to 1.2 mg SC daily. May increase to 1.8 mg SC daily. Chronic weight management for BMI 30 kg/m² or 27 kg/m² with comorbid condition (Saxenda): Start 0.6 mg SC daily for 1 week, then increase at weekly intervals to effective dose of 3 mg SC daily.

PEDS — Not approved in children.

FORMS — Trade only (Victoza): Multidose pen (18 mg/3 mL) delivers doses of 0.6, 1.2, or 1.8 mg. Trade only (Saxenda): Multidose pen (18 mg/3 mL) delivers doses of 0.6, 1.2, 1.8, 2.4, or 3 mg.

NOTES — May be given any time of day without regard to meals. Use caution in patients with renal or hepatic impairment. Concurrent use with mealtime insulin has not been studied. Monitor patients on Saxenda for depression or suicidal behavior. Multidose prefilled pens for use by one individual only; risk for bloodborne pathogen transmission.

MOA — Incretin analog that reduces fasting and postprandial glucose by increasing glucose-stimulated insulin secretion, decreasing glucagon secretion, slowing gastric emptying and reducing appetite.

ADVERSE EFFECTS — Serious: pancreatitis, hypersensitivity, cholelithiasis, hypoglycemia, tachycardia (Saxenda), depression (Saxenda), suicidal thoughts (Saxenda), increased lipase (Saxenda), renal impairment. Frequent: Headache, nausea, diarrhea, constipation, vomiting, dyspepsia, fatigue, dizziness, abdominal pain, anti-liraglutide antibody formation, rash, pruritis.

ENDOCRINE AND METABOLIC: Diabetes-Related—Insulins

INJECTABLE INSULINS*

		Onset (h)	Peak (h)	Duration (h)
Rapid/short-acting	Insulin aspart (NovoLog)	< 0.2	1–3	3–5
	Insulin glulisine (Apidra)	0.30–0.4	1	4–5
	Insulin lispro (Humalog)	0.25–0.5	0.5–2.5	3–5
	Regular (Novolin R, Humulin R)	0.5–1	2–3	5–8
Intermediate/long-acting	NPH (Novolin N, Humulin N)	2–4	4–10	10–16
	Insulin detemir (Levemir)	1–2	6–8	up to 24†
	Insulin glargine (Lantus, Toujeo, Basaglar)	2–4	peakless	24
	Insulin degludec (Tresiba)	1	peakless	>42
Mixtures	Insulin aspart protamine susp/aspart (NovoLog Mix 70/30)	0.25	1–4 (biphasic)	10–16
	Insulin lispro protamine susp/insulin lispro (Humalog Mix 75/25, Humalog Mix 50/50)	< 0.25	1–3 (biphasic)	10–16
	NPH/Reg (Humulin 70/30, Novolin 70/30)	0.5–1	2–10 (biphasic)	10–16
	Insulin degludec/aspart (Ryzodeg 70/30)	0.25	2–3	>24

*These are general guidelines, as onset, peak, and duration of activity are affected by the site of injection, physical activity, body temperature, and blood supply.

†Dose-dependent duration of action, range from 6 to 23 h.

NOTE: Adjust insulin dosing to achieve glycemic control. See table "diabetes numbers" for goals. Administer Humalog, NovoLog, Apidra within 15 min before or immediately after a meal. Administer Ryzodeg with a meal. Administer regular insulin 30 min before meals. Administer inhaled insulin (Afrezza) at the beginning of a meal. May mix NPH with aspart, lispro, glulisine, or regular. Draw up rapid-/short-acting insulin first. Do not mix long-acting insulins with other insulins. Multidose prefilled pens for use by one individual only; risk for bloodborne pathogen transmission.

INSULIN—INHALED SHORT-ACTING (*Afrezza*) ▶K ♀C ▶? $$$$$
WARNING — Contraindicated in patients with asthma, COPD, or other chronic lung diseases; acute bronchospasm reported. Assess for potential lung disease with history, physical exam, and spirometry prior to starting.
ADULT — Diabetes: Insulin naïve: Start 4 units inhaled at each meal. Switching from prandial insulin: 4 to 24 units inhaled per meal depending on prior insulin dose; round up to the nearest 4 units. Switching from premixed insulin: Estimate the mealtime dose by dividing half of the total daily injected premixed dose equally among three meals. Administer 4 to 24 units inhaled per meal depending on prior mealtime insulin dose; round up to the nearest 4 units.
PEDS — Not approved in pediatrics.
FORMS — Trade only: 4, 8, 12 unit cartridges.
NOTES — Not recommended in smokers. Assess pulmonary function with spirometry at baseline, at 6 months, then annually thereafter. Monitor blood glucose.
MOA — Stimulates peripheral glucose uptake, and inhibits hepatic gluconeogenesis.
ADVERSE EFFECTS — Serious: hypoglycemia, acute bronchospasm, decline in pulmonary function, diabetic ketoacidosis, hypokalemia. Common: cough, throat pain/irritation.

INSULIN—INJECTABLE COMBINATIONS (*Humalog Mix 75/25, Humalog Mix 50/50, Humulin 70/30, Novolin 70/30, NovoLog Mix 70/30), ReliOn Novolin 70/30, Ryzodeg 70/30)* ▶LK ♀B/C ▶+ $$$$$
ADULT — Doses vary, but typically total insulin 0.3 to 1 unit/kg/day SC in divided doses (Type 1), and 0.5 to 1.5 unit/kg/day SC in divided doses (Type 2).
PEDS — Not approved in children.
UNAPPROVED PEDS — Diabetes: Maintenance: Total insulin 0.5 to 1 unit/kg/day SC, but doses vary.
FORMS — Trade only: Insulin lispro protamine susp/insulin lispro (Humalog Mix 75/25, Humalog Mix 50/50). Insulin aspart protamine/insulin aspart (NovoLog Mix 70/30). NPH and regular mixtures (Humulin 70/30, Novolin 70/30, ReliOn Novolin 70/30). Insulin degludec/insulin aspart mixture (Ryzodeg 70/30). Insulin available in pen form: NovoLog Mix 70/30 FlexPen, Humulin 70/30, Humalog Mix 75/25 KwikPen, Humalog Mix 50/50 KwikPen, Ryzodeg 70/30 FlexTouch.
MOA — Stimulates peripheral glucose uptake, and inhibits hepatic gluconeogenesis.
ADVERSE EFFECTS — Serious: Hypoglycemia, allergic reaction, hypokalemia. Frequent: Weight gain, lipoatrophy, lipohypertrophy, injection site reaction.

INSULIN—INJECTABLE, SHORT-/RAPID-ACTING (*Apidra, Novolin R, NovoLog, Humulin R, Humalog, ✱NovoRapid*) ▶LK ♀B/C ▶+ $$$$
ADULT — Doses vary, but typically total insulin 0.3 to 0.5 unit/kg/day SC in divided doses (Type 1), and 1 to 1.5 unit/kg/day SC in divided doses (Type 2). Generally, 50 to 70% of insulin requirements are provided by rapid- or short-acting insulin and the remainder from intermediate- or long-acting insulin.
PEDS — Diabetes, age older than 4 yo (Apidra), older than 3 yo (Humalog) or older than 2 yo (NovoLog): Doses vary, but typically total insulin maintenance dose 0.5 to 1 unit/kg/day SC in divided doses. Generally, 50 to 70% of insulin requirements are provided by rapid-acting insulin and the remainder from intermediate- or long-acting insulin.
UNAPPROVED ADULT — DM, Type 2 (ADA): When adding mealtime insulin to basal insulin for uncontrolled DM, start 4 units, 0.1 units/kg or 10% of basal dose with largest meal. Titrate up by 10 to 15% or 1 to 2 units once or twice per week to reach target SMBG. Decrease dose by 10 to 20% or 2 to 4 units for hypoglycemia. Follow same procedure when adding mealtime insulin to a 2nd or 3rd meal in a basal-bolus regimen in uncontrolled DM. Severe hyperkalemia: 5 to 10 units regular insulin plus concurrent dextrose IV. Profound hyperglycemia (eg, DKA): 0.1 unit/kg regular insulin IV bolus, then begin IV infusion 100 units in 100 mL NS (1 unit/mL) at 0.1 units/kg/h. 70 kg: 7 units/h (7 mL/h). Titrate to clinical effect.
UNAPPROVED PEDS — Profound hyperglycemia (eg, DKA): 0.1 unit/kg regular insulin IV bolus, then IV infusion 100 units in 100 mL NS (1 unit/mL) at 0.1 units/kg/h. Titrate to clinical effect. Severe hyperkalemia: 0.1 units/kg regular insulin IV with glucose over 30 min. May repeat in 30 to 60 min or start 0.1 units/kg/h.
FORMS — Trade only: Injection regular 100 units/mL (Novolin R, Humulin R). Injection regular 500 units/mL (Humulin U-500, concentrated). Insulin glulisine (Apidra). Insulin lispro 100 units/mL (Humalog). Insulin aspart (NovoLog). Insulin available in pen form (100 units/mL): Novolin R InnoLet, Humulin R, Apidra SoloSTAR, Humalog KwikPen, NovoLog FlexPen. Insulin lispro 200 units/mL (Humalog U-200 KwikPen). Insulin regular 500 units/mL, concentrated (Humulin R U-500 KwikPen).
NOTES — Apidra, Humalog, and NovoLog approved for use by continuous SC infusion in insulin pump. Do not mix insulins in pump. Consult manufacturer instructions for frequency of reservoir change when used in pump. Caution: Med errors have occurred

(cont.)

INSULIN—INJECTABLE, SHORT-/RAPID-ACTING (*cont.*)

when using concentrated Humulin R U-500, note strength 500 units/mL.

MOA — Stimulates peripheral glucose uptake, and inhibits hepatic gluconeogenesis.

ADVERSE EFFECTS — Serious: Hypoglycemia, allergic reaction, hypokalemia. Frequent: Weight gain, lipoatrophy, lipohypertrophy, injection site reaction.

INSULIN—INJECTABLE, INTERMEDIATE (*Novolin N, Humulin N, ReliOn Novolin N*) ▶LK ♀B/C ▶+ $$$$

ADULT — Diabetes: Doses vary, but typically total insulin 0.3 to 0.5 unit/kg/day SC in divided doses (Type 1), and 1 to 1.5 unit/kg/day SC in divided doses (Type 2). Generally, 50 to 70% of insulin requirements are provided by rapid- or short-acting insulin and the remainder from intermediate- or long-acting insulin.

PEDS — Diabetes: Maintenance: Total insulin 0.5 to 1 unit/kg/day SC, but doses vary. Generally, 50 to 70% of insulin requirements are provided by rapid-acting insulin and the remainder from intermediate- or long-acting insulin.

FORMS — Trade only: Injection NPH (Novolin N, Humulin N, ReliOn Novolin N). Insulin available in pen form: Humulin N KwikPen. Premixed preparations of NPH and regular insulin also available.

MOA — Stimulates peripheral glucose uptake, and inhibits hepatic gluconeogenesis.

ADVERSE EFFECTS — Serious: Hypoglycemia, allergic reaction, hypokalemia. Frequent: Weight gain, lipoatrophy, lipohypertrophy, injection site reaction.

INSULIN—INJECTABLE, LONG-ACTING (*Lantus, Levemir, Toujeo, Tresiba, Basaglar*) ▶LK ♀B/C ▶+ $$$$$

ADULT — Diabetes: Doses vary, but typically total insulin 0.3 to 0.5 units/kg/day SC in divided doses (Type 1), and 1 to 1.5 units/kg/day SC in divided doses (Type 2). Generally, 50 to 70% of insulin requirements are provided by rapid- or short-acting insulin and the remainder from intermediate- or long-acting insulin. Lantus, Type 2 DM: Start 10 units or 0.2 units/kg SC daily (same time everyday) in insulin-naive patients. When transferring from twice-daily NPH, the initial Lantus dose should be reduced by about 20% from the previous total daily NPH dose, then adjust dose based on patient response. Levemir, Type 2 DM: Start 10 units or 0.1 to 0.2 units/kg SC daily in the evening or divided twice daily in insulin-naive patients. When transferring from basal insulin (Lantus, NPH) in Type 1 or 2 DM, change on a unit-to-unit basis; more Levemir may be required than NPH insulin in DM, Type 2. DM, Type 1 (Lantus/Levemir): Start with one-third of total daily insulin dose; remainder of requirements from rapid- or short-acting insulin.

PEDS — DM, Type 1: Lantus (age 6 to 15 yo): See adult dose. Levemir (age 2 to 17 yo): See adult dose.

UNAPPROVED ADULT — DM, Type 2 (ADA): Start 10 units or 0.1 to 0.2 units/kg/day then titrate up by 10 to 15% or 2 to 4 units once or twice per week to reach target fasting blood glucose. Decrease dose by 10 to 20% or 4 units for hypoglycemia.

FORMS — Trade only: Lantus (insulin glargine), Levemir (insulin detemir) 100 units/mL (U-100), 10 mL vial. Insulin available in pen form: Lantus SoloSTAR (glargine, U-100, 3 mL), Toujeo SoloSTAR (glargine, U-300, 1.5 mL), Levemir FlexTouch (detemir, U-100, 3 mL), Tresiba FlexTouch (degludec, U-100, U-200, 3 mL), Basaglar KwikPen (glargine, U-100, 3 mL, avail Dec 16).

MOA — Stimulates peripheral glucose uptake, and inhibits hepatic gluconeogenesis.

ADVERSE EFFECTS — Serious: Hypoglycemia, allergic reaction, hypokalemia. Frequent: Weight gain, lipoatrophy, lipohypertrophy, injection site reaction.

ENDOCRINE AND METABOLIC: Diabetes-Related—Meglitinides

NATEGLINIDE (*Starlix*) ▶L ♀C ▶? $$$$

ADULT — DM, Type 2, monotherapy or in combination with metformin or thiazolidinedione: 120 mg PO three times per day within 30 min before meals; use 60 mg PO three times per day in patients who are near goal A1C.

PEDS — Not approved in children.

FORMS — Generic/Trade: Tabs 60, 120 mg.

NOTES — Not to be used as monotherapy in patients inadequately controlled with glyburide or other antidiabetic agents previously. Patients with severe renal impairment are at risk for hypoglycemic episodes.

MOA — Stimulates pancreatic beta-cell insulin release.

ADVERSE EFFECTS — Serious: Hypoglycemia, jaundice, cholestatic hepatitis, increased LFTs. Frequent: Arthralgia, upper respiratory tract infection, hypersensitivity.

REPAGLINIDE (*Prandin, ✱GlucoNorm*) ▶L ♀C ▶? $$$

ADULT — DM, Type 2: 0.5 to 2 mg PO three times per day within 30 min before a meal. Allow 1 week between dosage adjustments. Usual range is 0.5 to 4 mg PO three to four times per day, max 16 mg/day.

PEDS — Not approved in children.

FORMS — Generic/Trade: Tabs 0.5, 1, 2 mg.

NOTES — May take dose immediately preceding meal to as long as 30 min before the meal. Gemfibrozil and itraconazole increase blood repaglinide levels and may result in an increased risk of hypoglycemia. Do not use with NPH insulin.

MOA — Stimulates pancreatic beta-cell insulin release.

ADVERSE EFFECTS — Serious: Hypoglycemia, hypersensitivity, thrombocytopenia, leukopenia, increased serum transaminases. Frequent: Diarrhea, arthralgia, upper respiratory tract infection.

ENDOCRINE AND METABOLIC: Diabetes-Related—SGLT2 Inhibitors

NOTE: DKA and euglycemic DKA reported; if signs/symptoms of acidosis then assess for ketoacidosis regardless of glucose level. Do not use in DM Type 1 or DKA. May cause hypotension, check volume status prior to use. Consider reducing dose of insulin or insulin secretagogue prior to initiation to avoid hypoglycemia. Monitor for and treat genital fungal or urinary tract infections if occur. May increase LDL. Do not monitor glycemic control with urine glucose tests due to potential for false positive.

CANAGLIFLOZIN (*Invokana*) ▶LK – ♀– ?/X/X ▶? $$$$$
ADULT — DM, Type 2: 100 mg PO daily before first meal of the day. If tolerated and needed for glycemic control, may increase to 300 mg PO daily if eGFR greater than 60 mL/min.
PEDS — Not approved in children.
FORMS — Trade only: Tabs 100, 300 mg.
NOTES — Do not use if eGFR <45 mL/min. May cause hyperkalemia, monitor K+ levels. Acute kidney injury and renal impairment reported, monitor renal function during therapy and consider holding during reduced oral intake or fluid losses. May increase risk of genital fungal infections; treat as indicated. Bone fracture reported; consider risk factors for fracture prior to initiation. May increase LDL, monitor and treat if indicated.
MOA — Inhibitor of sodium-glucose cotransporter 2 (SGLT2) which blocks reabsorption of glucose from the kidney and increases glucose loss in the urine.
ADVERSE EFFECTS — Serious: hypotension, hyperkalemia, renal dysfunction, hypoglycemia, hypersensitivity, bone fracture, euglycemic diabetic ketoacidosis. Frequent: genital fungal infections, urinary tract infections, increased urination, increased LDL.

DAPAGLIFLOZIN (*Farxiga*, ✽*Forxiga*) ▶LK ♀C ▶– $$$$$
ADULT — DM, Type 2: 5 mg PO daily in the morning, with or without food. If tolerated and needed for glycemic control, may increase to 10 mg PO daily.

FORMS — Trade only: Tabs 5, 10 mg
NOTES — Do not use if eGFR <60 mL/min. Acute kidney injury and renal impairment reported, monitor renal function during therapy and consider holding during reduced oral intake or fluid losses. Possible increase in bladder cancer observed, use with caution in those with history of bladder cancer and do not use if active bladder cancer.
MOA — Inhibitor of sodium-glucose cotransporter 2 (SGLT2) which blocks reabsorption of glucose from the kidney and increases glucose loss in the urine.
ADVERSE EFFECTS — Serious: hypotension, hyperkalemia, renal dysfunction, hypoglycemia, hypersensitivity. Frequent: genital fungal infections, urinary tract infections, increased urination, increased LDL.

EMPAGLIFLOZIN (*Jardiance*) ▶LK ♀C ▶? $$$$$
ADULT — DM, Type 2: Start 10 mg PO daily in morning, with or without food. May increase up to 25 mg PO daily in morning, with or without food.
PEDS — Not approved in children.
FORMS — Trade only: 10, 25 mg.
NOTES — Do not use if eGFR <45 mL/min.
MOA — Inhibitor of sodium-glucose cotransporter 2 (SGLT2) which blocks reabsorption of glucose from the kidney and increases glucose loss in the urine.
ADVERSE EFFECTS — Serious: hypotension, renal dysfunction, hypoglycemia. Frequent: genital fungal infections, urinary tract infections, increased urination, increased LDL.

ENDOCRINE AND METABOLIC: Diabetes-Related—Sulfonylureas—1st Generation

NOTE: Sulfonylureas can lead to hemolytic anemia in patients with G6PD deficiency; use caution or consider alternate agents.

CHLORPROPAMIDE ▶LK ♀C ▶– $$$
ADULT — DM, Type 2: Initiate therapy with 100 to 250 mg PO daily. Titrate after 5 to 7 days by increments of 50 to 125 mg at intervals of 3 to 5 days to obtain optimal control. Max 750 mg/day.
PEDS — Not approved in children.
FORMS — Generic only: Tabs 100, 250 mg.
NOTES — Clinical use in the elderly has not been properly evaluated. Elderly are more prone to hypoglycemia and/or hyponatremia possibly from renal impairment or drug interactions. May cause disulfiram-like reaction with alcohol.
MOA — Stimulates pancreatic beta-cell insulin release.
ADVERSE EFFECTS — Serious: Hypoglycemia, hypersensitivity, SIADH, disulfiram-like reaction, cholestatic jaundice, hepatitis, hepatic porphyria, increased serum transaminases, aplastic anemia,

hemolytic anemia, leukopenia, thrombocytopenia, agranulocytosis, pancytopenia, eosinophilia. Frequent: Weight gain, fatigue, diarrhea, nausea, dyspepsia, rash.

TOLAZAMIDE ▶LK ♀C ▶? $$$$
ADULT — DM, Type 2: Initiate therapy with 100 mg PO daily in patients with fasting blood glucose less than 200 mg/dL, and in patients who are malnourished, underweight, or elderly. Initiate therapy with 250 mg PO daily in patients with fasting blood glucose more than 200 mg/dL. Give with breakfast or the first main meal of the day. If daily doses exceed 500 mg, divide the dose two times per day. Max 1000 mg/day.
PEDS — Not approved in children.
FORMS — Generic only: Tabs 250, 500 mg.
MOA — Stimulates pancreatic beta-cell insulin release.

(cont.)

TOLAZAMIDE (*cont.*)

ADVERSE EFFECTS — Serious: Hypoglycemia, hypersensitivity, SIADH, disulfiram-like reaction, cholestatic jaundice, aplastic anemia, hemolytic anemia, leukopenia, thrombocytopenia, agranulocytosis, pancytopenia, eosinophilia, hepatic porphyria, increased serum transaminases. Frequent: Weight gain, fatigue, diarrhea, nausea, dyspepsia, rash.

TOLBUTAMIDE ▶LK ♀C ▶+ $$$

ADULT — DM, Type 2: Start 1 g PO daily. Maintenance dose is usually 250 mg to 2 g PO daily. Total daily dose may be taken in the morning, divide doses if GI intolerance occurs. Max 3 g/day.

PEDS — Not approved in children.

FORMS — Generic only: Tabs 500 mg.

MOA — Stimulates pancreatic beta-cell insulin release.

ADVERSE EFFECTS — Serious: Hypoglycemia, hypersensitivity, SIADH, disulfiram-like reaction, cholestatic jaundice, aplastic anemia, hemolytic anemia, leukopenia, thrombocytopenia, agranulocytosis, pancytopenia, eosinophilia, hepatic porphyria, increased serum transaminases. Frequent: Weight gain, fatigue, diarrhea, nausea, dyspepsia, rash.

ENDOCRINE AND METABOLIC: Diabetes-Related—Sulfonylureas—2nd Generation

NOTE: Sulfonylureas can lead to hemolytic anemia in patients with G6PD deficiency; use caution or consider alternate agents.

GLICLAZIDE (✤*Diamicron, Diamicron MR*) ▶KL ♀C ▶? $

ADULT — Canada only, DM, Type 2: Immediate-release: Start 80 to 160 mg PO daily, max 320 mg PO daily (160 mg or more per day should be in divided doses). Modified-release: Start 30 mg PO daily, max 120 mg PO daily.

PEDS — Not approved in children.

FORMS — Generic/Trade: Tabs 80 mg (Diamicron). Trade only: Tabs, modified-release 30 mg (Diamicron MR).

NOTES — Immediate- and modified-release not equipotent; 80 mg of immediate-release can be changed to 30 mg of modified-release.

MOA — Stimulates pancreatic beta-cell insulin release.

ADVERSE EFFECTS — Serious: Hypoglycemia, hypersensitivity, disulfiram-like reaction, cholestatic jaundice, aplastic anemia, hemolytic anemia, leukopenia, thrombocytopenia, agranulocytosis, pancytopenia, eosinophilia, hepatic porphyria, increased LFTs. Frequent: Weight gain, fatigue, diarrhea, nausea, dyspepsia, rash.

GLIMEPIRIDE (*Amaryl*) ▶LK ♀C ▶– $$

ADULT — DM, Type 2: Initiate therapy with 1 to 2 mg PO daily. Start with 1 mg PO daily in elderly, malnourished patients or those with renal or hepatic insufficiency. Give with breakfast or the first main meal of the day. Titrate in increments of 1 to 2 mg at 1- to 2-week intervals based on response. Usual maintenance dose is 1 to 4 mg PO daily, max 8 mg/day.

PEDS — Not approved in children.

FORMS — Generic/Trade: Tabs 1, 2, 4 mg.

NOTES — Allergy may develop if allergic to other sulfonamide derivatives.

MOA — Stimulates pancreatic beta-cell insulin release.

ADVERSE EFFECTS — Serious: Hypoglycemia, hypersensitivity, SIADH, disulfiram-like reaction, cholestatic jaundice, aplastic anemia, hemolytic anemia, leukopenia, thrombocytopenia, agranulocytosis, pancytopenia, eosinophilia, hepatic porphyria, increased serum transaminases. Frequent: Weight gain, fatigue, diarrhea, nausea, dyspepsia, rash.

GLIPIZIDE (*Glucotrol, Glucotrol XL*) ▶LK ♀C ▶? $

ADULT — DM, Type 2: Initiate therapy with 5 mg PO daily. Give 2.5 mg PO daily to geriatric patients or those with liver disease. Adjust dose in increments of 2.5 to 5 mg to a usual maintenance dose of 10 to 20 mg/day, max 40 mg/day. Doses more than 15 mg should be divided two times per day. Extended-release (Glucotrol XL): Initiate therapy with 5 mg PO daily. Usual dose is 5 to 10 mg PO daily, max 20 mg/day.

PEDS — Not approved in children.

FORMS — Generic/Trade: Tabs 5, 10 mg. Extended-release tabs 2.5, 5, 10 mg.

NOTES — Maximum effective dose is generally 20 mg/day.

MOA — Stimulates pancreatic beta-cell insulin release.

ADVERSE EFFECTS — Serious: Hypoglycemia, hypersensitivity, SIADH, disulfiram-like reaction, cholestatic jaundice, hepatocellular injury, aplastic anemia, hemolytic anemia, leukopenia, thrombocytopenia, agranulocytosis, pancytopenia, eosinophilia, hepatic porphyria, increased serum transaminases. Frequent: Weight gain, fatigue, diarrhea, nausea, dyspepsia, rash.

GLYBURIDE (*DiaBeta, Glynase PresTab,* ✤*Euglucon*) ▶LK ♀B ▶? $

WARNING — Contraindicated with bosentan.

ADULT — DM, Type 2: Initiate therapy with 2.5 to 5 mg PO daily. Start with 1.25 mg PO daily in elderly or malnourished patients or those with renal or hepatic insufficiency. Give with breakfast or the first main meal of the day. Titrate in increments of no more than 2.5 mg at weekly intervals based on response. Usual maintenance dose is 1.25 to 20 mg PO daily or divided two times per day, max 20 mg/day. Micronized tabs: Initiate therapy with 1.5 to 3 mg PO daily. Start with 0.75 mg PO daily in elderly, malnourished patients or those with renal or hepatic insufficiency. Give with breakfast or the first main meal of the day. Titrate in increments of no more than 1.5 mg at weekly intervals based on response. Usual maintenance dose is 0.75 to 12 mg PO daily, max 12 mg/day. May divide dose two times per day if more than 6 mg/day.

(cont.)

GLYBURIDE (cont.)

PEDS — Not approved in children.

FORMS — Generic/Trade: Tabs (scored) 1.25, 2.5, 5 mg. Micronized tabs (scored) 1.5, 3, 6 mg.

NOTES — Maximum effective dose is generally 10 mg/day.

MOA — Stimulates pancreatic beta-cell insulin release.

ADVERSE EFFECTS — Serious: Hypoglycemia, hypersensitivity, SIADH, disulfiram-like reaction, cholestatic jaundice, hepatitis, liver failure, increased serum transaminases, aplastic anemia, hemolytic anemia, leukopenia, thrombocytopenia, agranulocytosis, pancytopenia, eosinophilia, hepatic porphyria. Frequent: Weight gain, fatigue, diarrhea, nausea, dyspepsia, rash.

ENDOCRINE AND METABOLIC: Diabetes-Related—Thiazolidinediones

NOTE: May cause edema, wt gain, new heart failure, or exacerbate existing heart failure (contraindicated in NYHA Class III or IV), especially in combination with insulin. Monitor for signs of heart failure (rapid wt gain, dyspnea, edema) following initiation or dose increase. If occurs, manage fluid retention and consider discontinuation or dosage decrease. Avoid if liver disease or ALT greater than 2.5 times normal. Monitor LFTs before therapy and periodically thereafter. Discontinue if ALT greater than 3 times upper normal limit. Full effect may not be apparent for up to 12 weeks. May cause resumption of ovulation in premenopausal anovulatory women; recommend contraception use. Reports of fracture risk.

PIOGLITAZONE (*Actos*) ▶L ♀C ▶− $$$$$

ADULT — DM, Type 2: Start 15 to 30 mg PO daily, may adjust dose after 3 months to max 45 mg/day.

PEDS — Not approved nor recommended in children.

FORMS — Generic/Trade: Tabs 15, 30, 45 mg.

NOTES — Do not use in Type 1 DM or DKA. Urinary bladder tumors reported; advise patients to report macroscopic hematuria or dysuria.

MOA — Increases insulin sensitivity in adipose tissue, skeletal muscle, and liver.

ADVERSE EFFECTS — Serious: Hepatotoxicity, liver failure, heart failure exacerbation, resumption of ovulation, macular edema, fracture, bladder tumor. Frequent: Edema, wt gain, upper respiratory tract infection, headache, myalgia.

ROSIGLITAZONE (*Avandia*) ▶L ♀C ▶− $$$$

ADULT — DM, Type 2 monotherapy or in combination with metformin or sulfonylurea: Start 4 mg PO daily or divided two times per day, may increase after 8 to 12 weeks to max 8 mg/day.

PEDS — Not approved in children younger than 18 yo.

FORMS — Trade only: Tabs 2 and 4 mg.

MOA — Increases insulin sensitivity in adipose tissue, skeletal muscle, and liver.

ADVERSE EFFECTS — Serious: Potential hepatotoxicity, heart failure, resumption of ovulation, macular edema, fracture, myocardial infarction, hypersensitivity. Frequent: Edema, weight gain, upper respiratory tract infection, headache, back pain, dyslipidemia.

ENDOCRINE AND METABOLIC: Diabetes-Related—Other

DEXTROSE (*Glutose, B-D Glucose, Insta-Glucose, Dex-4*) ▶L ♀C ▶? $

ADULT — Hypoglycemia: 0.5 to 1 g/kg (1 to 2 mL/kg) up to 25 g (50 mL) of 50% soln by slow IV injection. Hypoglycemia in conscious diabetics: 10 to 20 g PO q 10 to 20 min prn.

PEDS — Hypoglycemia in neonates: 0.25 to 0.5 g/kg/dose (5 to 10 mL of 25% dextrose in a 5 kg infant). Severe hypoglycemia or older infants may require larger doses up to 3 g (12 mL of 25% dextrose) followed by a continuous IV infusion of 10% dextrose. Non-neonates may require 0.5 to 1 g/kg.

UNAPPROVED ADULT — Hypoglycemia: 15 to 20 g PO once, repeat in 15 minutes if continued hypoglycemia per self-monitoring.

FORMS — OTC Generic/Trade: Chewable tabs 4 g (Dex-4), 5 g (Glutose). Trade only: Oral gel 40%.

NOTES — Do not exceed an infusion rate of 0.5 g/kg/h.

MOA — Elevates blood glucose.

ADVERSE EFFECTS — Serious: None. Frequent: Nausea.

GLUCAGON (*GlucaGen*) ▶LK ♀B ▶? $$$$$

ADULT — Hypoglycemia: 1 mg IV/IM/SC. If no response within 15 min, may repeat dose 1 to 2 times (preferred via IV for repeat). Diagnostic aid for GI tract radiography: 1 mg IV/IM/SC.

PEDS — Hypoglycemia in children wt greater than 20 kg (Glucagon) or wt greater than 25 kg (GlucaGen) or age 6 or older when weight unknown (GlucaGen): Same as adults. Hypoglycemia in children wt less than 20 kg (Glucagon): 0.5 mg IV/IM/SC or 20 to 30 mcg/kg. Hypoglycemia in children wt less than 25 kg or younger than age 6 when weight unknown (GlucaGen): 0.5 mg IV/IM/SC. If no response in 5 to 20 min, may repeat dose 1 to 2 times.

UNAPPROVED ADULT — The following indications are based upon limited data. Esophageal obstruction caused by food: 1 mg IV over 1 to 3 min. Symptomatic bradycardia/hypotension, especially with beta-blocker therapy: 3 to 10 mg IV bolus (0.05 mg/kg general recommendation) may repeat in 10 min; may be followed by continuous infusion of 1 to 5 mg/h or 0.07 mg/kg/h. Infusion rate should be titrated to the desired response.

(cont.)

GLUCAGON (*cont.*)

FORMS — Trade/generic: Injection 1 mg. Trade only: GlucaGen Diagnostic Kit, 1 mg; GlucaGen HypoKit 1 mg, Glucagon Emergency Kit 1 mg.

NOTES — Reconstitute prior to use; yields 1 mg/mL solution. Should be reserved for refractory/severe cases or when IV dextrose cannot be administered. Advise patients to educate family members and coworkers how to administer a dose. Give supplemental carbohydrates when patient responds.

MOA — Inhibits glycogen synthesis, enhances glucose formation, and increases hepatic glycogenolysis; has relaxant effect on the GI tract; temporarily inhibits GI tract movement for diagnostic procedures.

ADVERSE EFFECTS — Serious: Generalized allergic reaction, hypotension. Frequent: N/V.

METFORMIN (*Glucophage, Glucophage XR, Glumetza, Fortamet, Riomet*) ▶K ♀B ▶? $$$

ADULT — DM, Type 2: Immediate-release: Start 500 mg PO one to two times per day or 850 mg PO daily with meals. Increase by 500 mg q week or 850 mg q 2 weeks to a maximum of 2550 mg/day. Higher doses may be divided three times per day with meals. Extended-release: Glucophage XR: 500 mg PO daily with evening meal; increase by 500 mg q week to max 2000 mg/day (may divide two times per day). Glumetza: 1000 mg PO daily with evening meal; increase by 500 mg q week to max 2000 mg/day (may divide two times per day). Fortamet: 500 to 1000 mg daily with evening meal; increase by 500 mg q week to max 2500 mg/day. All products started at low doses to improve GI tolerability, gradually increase as tolerated.

PEDS — DM, Type 2, 10 yo or older: Start 500 mg PO one to two times per day (Glucophage) with meals, increase by 500 mg q week to max 2000 mg/day in divided doses (10 to 16 yo). Glucophage XR and Fortamet are indicated for age 17 yo or older.

UNAPPROVED ADULT — Polycystic ovary syndrome: 500 mg PO three times per day or 850 mg PO two times per day. Prevention/delay DM Type 2 (with lifestyle modifications): 850 mg PO daily for 1 month, then increase to 850 mg PO two times per day.

FORMS — Generic/Trade: Tabs 500, 850, 1000 mg, extended-release 500, 750 mg. Trade only, extended-release (Fortamet, Glumetza): 500, 1000 mg. Trade only (Riomet): Oral soln 500 mg/5 mL.

NOTES — May reduce the risk of progression to Type 2 DM in those with impaired glucose tolerance, but less effectively than intensive lifestyle modification. Metformin-containing products may cause life-threatening lactic acidosis, usually in setting of decreased tissue perfusion, hypoxia, hepatic dysfunction, unstable congestive heart failure, or impaired renal clearance. Avoid if ethanol abuse, hepatic insufficiency, or hypoxic states (cardiogenic shock, septicemia, acute MI). Assess eGFR prior to treatment and at least annually. Avoid in patients with an eGFR <30 mL/min/1.73 m²; initiation in patients with eGFR 30 to 45 mL/min/1.73 m² is not recommended. In those already taking metformin, if eGFR falls below 45 mL/min/1.73 m²,reassess benefits and risks. Discontinue metformin at the time of or prior to an iodinated contrast imaging procedure and for 48 h after the procedure in those with eGFR <60 mL/min/1.73 m²; in those with liver disease, alcoholism, or heart failure; or in those administered intra-arterial contrast. Reassess the eGFR post-procedure and reinitiate if renal function stable.

MOA — Decreases hepatic gluconeogenesis and increases insulin sensitivity.

ADVERSE EFFECTS — Serious: Lactic acidosis, decreased serum vitamin B12. Frequent: Diarrhea, N/V, flatulence, abdominal discomfort, headache, weight loss, taste disturbance.

PRAMLINTIDE (*Symlin, SymlinPen*) ▶K ♀C ▶? $$$$$

WARNING — May cause severe insulin-induced hypoglycemia, especially in Type 1 DM, usually within 3 h. Avoid if hypoglycemic unawareness, gastroparesis, GI motility medications, alpha-glucosidase inhibitors, A1C more than 9%, poor compliance, or hypersensitivity to the metacresol preservative. Appropriate patient selection, careful patient instruction, and insulin dose adjustments (reduction in premeal short-acting insulin of 50%) are critical for reducing the hypoglycemia risk.

ADULT — DM, Type 1 with mealtime insulin therapy: Initiate 15 mcg SC immediately before major meals and titrate by 15 mcg increments (if significant nausea has not occurred for at least 3 days) to maintenance 30 to 60 mcg as tolerated. If significant nausea, decrease to 30 mcg. DM, Type 2 with mealtime insulin therapy: Initiate 60 mcg SC immediately before major meals and increase to 120 mcg as tolerated (if significant nausea has not occurred for 3 to 7 days). If significant nausea, decrease dose to 60 mcg.

PEDS — Not approved in children.

FORMS — Trade only: 1000 mcg/mL pen injector (SymlinPen) 1.5, 2.7 mL.

NOTES — Keep unopened vials refrigerated. Opened vials can be kept at room temperature or refrigerated up to 28 days. Multidose prefilled pens for use by one individual only; risk for bloodborne pathogen transmission. May give SC in abdomen or thigh. Take medications that require rapid onset 1 h prior or 2 h after. Careful patient selection and skilled healthcare supervision are critical for safe and effective use. Monitor pre-/postmeal and bedtime glucose. Decrease initial premeal short-acting insulin doses by 50% including fixed-mix insulin (ie, 70/30). Do not mix with insulin. Use new needle and syringe for each dose.

MOA — Amylin analog that reduces postprandial hyperglycemia by slowing gastric emptying and decreasing postprandial glucagon secretion. It also decreases caloric intake by decreasing appetite.

ADVERSE EFFECTS — Serious: Severe hypoglycemia, systemic allergic reaction, pancreatitis. Frequent: N/V, headache, abdominal pain, hypoglycemia, injection site reactions.

ENDOCRINE AND METABOLIC: Diagnostic Agents

CORTICOTROPIN (*H.P. Acthar Gel*) ▶K ♀C ▶– $$$$$
ADULT — Diagnostic testing of adrenocortical function: 80 units IM or SC. Acute exacerbation of multiple sclerosis: 80 to 120 units IM daily for 2 to 3 weeks.
PEDS — Infantile spasms: 75 units/m^2 IM twice daily. After 2 weeks taper dose over a 2-week period until discontinuation.
NOTES — Limited therapeutic value in conditions responsive to corticosteroid therapy; corticosteroids should be the treatment of choice if responsive. Prolonged use in children may inhibit skeletal growth. May decrease bone density in adults. Cosyntropin preferred for diagnostic testing as it is less allergenic and more potent. Increased susceptibility to infections. Do not give live or live attenuated vaccines during therapy. Monitor for adrenal insufficiency after prolonged therapy. Cushing's syndrome, elevations in BP, salt and water retention, and hypokalemia may occur. Increased risk of GI perforation and bleeding. May cause behavioral and mood disorders. May worsen DM or myasthenia gravis.
MOA — Stimulates the adrenal cortex to secrete cortisol, corticosterone, aldosterone and weakly androgenic substances.
ADVERSE EFFECTS — Serious: Hypersensitivity, convulsions, infections, cardiac hypertrophy, hyperglycemia, BP elevations. Frequent: Electrolyte imbalances, menstrual irregularities, increased appetite, weight gain, mood changes, fluid retention.
COSYNTROPIN (*Cortrosyn*, *✱Synacthen*) ▶L ♀C ▶? $$$
ADULT — Rapid screen for adrenocortical insufficiency: 0.25 mg IM/IV over 2 min; measure serum cortisol before and 30 to 60 min after.

PEDS — Rapid screen for adrenocortical insufficiency: 0.25 mg (0.125 mg if age younger than 2 yo) IM/IV over 2 min; measure serum cortisol before and 30 to 60 min after.
MOA — Stimulates the adrenal cortex to produce and secrete hormones.
ADVERSE EFFECTS — Serious: Hypersensitivity. Frequent: None (since used diagnostically).
METYRAPONE (*Metopirone*) ▶KL ♀C ▶? $$$
WARNING — May cause acute adrenal insufficiency.
ADULT — Diagnostic aid for testing hypothalamic-pituitary adrenocorticotropic hormone (ACTH) function: Specialized single- and multiple-test dose available.
PEDS — ACTH function: Specialized single- and multiple-test dose available.
UNAPPROVED ADULT — Cushing's syndrome: Dosing varies.
FORMS — Trade only: Caps 250 mg. Only available from manufacturer: 1-855-674-7663.
NOTES — Ability of adrenals to respond to exogenous ACTH should be demonstrated before metyrapone is employed as a test. In the presence of hypo- or hyperthyroidism, response to the test may be subnormal. May suppress aldosterone synthesis. May cause dizziness and sedation.
MOA — Inhibits endogenous adrenal corticosteroid synthesis.
ADVERSE EFFECTS — Serious: Acute adrenal insufficiency, bone marrow suppression, neutropenia, hypotension. Frequent: Sedation, dizziness, headache, rash, abdominal discomfort, vomiting.

ENDOCRINE AND METABOLIC: Minerals

CALCIUM ACETATE (*PhosLo, Eliphos, Phoslyra*) ▶K ♀C ▶? $
ADULT — Phosphate binder to reduce serum phosphorus in end-stage renal disease: Initially 2 tabs/caps or 10 mL of soln PO three times per day with each meal. Titrate dose gradually based on serum phosphorus. Usual dose 3 to 4 tabs/caps or 15 to 20 mL per meal.
PEDS — Not approved in children.
UNAPPROVED PEDS — Titrate to response.
FORMS — Generic/Trade: Gelcaps 667 mg (169 mg elem Ca). Tabs 667 mg (169 mg elem Ca). Trade only: Soln (Phoslyra): 667 mg (169 mg elemental calcium)/5 mL.
NOTES — Avoid calcium supplements and antacids with calcium. Monitor serum calcium twice weekly initially and during dosage adjustment. Monitor for signs of hypercalcemia and discontinue if occurs. Consider decreasing or discontinuing vitamin D supplementation if mild hypercalcemia occurs. Maintain serum calcium-phosphorous product (Ca × P) less than 55. Hypercalcemia may aggravate digoxin toxicity.

MOA — Binds with dietary phosphate to form a nonabsorbable complex.
ADVERSE EFFECTS — Serious: Severe hypercalcemia (with confusion, delirium, stupor, coma), renal calculi. Frequent: Mild hypercalcemia, constipation, anorexia, N/V.
CALCIUM CARBONATE (*Caltrate, Mylanta Children's, Os-Cal, Oyst-Cal, Tums, Viactiv, ✱Calsan*) ▶K ♀+ (? 1st trimester) ▶? $
ADULT — Supplement: 1 to 2 g elem Ca/day or more PO with meals divided two to four times per day. Prevention of osteoporosis: 1000 to 1500 mg elem Ca/day PO divided two to three times per day with meals. The adequate intake in most adults is 1000 to 1200 mg elem Ca/day. Antacid: 1000 to 3000 mg (2 to 4 tab) PO q 2 h prn or 1 to 2 pieces gum chewed prn, max 7000 mg/day.
PEDS — Hypocalcemia: Neonates: 50 to 150 mg elem Ca/kg/day PO in 4 to 6 divided doses. Children: 45 to 65 mg elem Ca/kg/day PO divided four times per day. Adequate intake for children (in elem calcium): Age younger than 6 mo: 210 mg/day when fed human milk and 315 mg/day when fed cow's

(cont.)

CALCIUM CARBONATE (*cont.*)

milk; 6 to 12 mo: 270 mg/day when fed human milk + solid food and 335 mg/day when fed cow's milk + solid food; 1 to 3 yo: 500 mg/day; 4 to 8 yo: 800 mg/day; 9 to 18 yo 1300 mg/day.

FORMS — OTC Generic/Trade: Tabs 500, 650, 750, 1000, 1250, 1500 mg. Chewable tabs 400, 500, 750, 850, 1000, 1177, 1250 mg. Caps 1250 mg. Gum 300, 450 mg. Susp 1250 mg/5 mL. Calcium carbonate is 40% elem Ca and contains 20 mEq of elem Ca/g calcium carbonate. Not more than 500 to 600 mg elem Ca/dose. Available in combination with sodium fluoride, vitamin D, and/or vitamin K. Trade examples: Caltrate 600 + vitamin D = 600 mg elemental Ca/200 units vitamin D, Os-Cal 500 + D = 500 mg elemental Ca/200 units vitamin D, Os-Cal Extra D = 500 mg elemental Ca/400 units vitamin D, Tums (regular strength) = 200 mg elemental Ca, Tums (ultra) = 400 mg elemental Ca, Viactiv (chewable) 500 mg elemental Ca + 100 units vitamin D + 40 mcg vitamin K.

NOTES — Decreases absorption of levothyroxine, tetracycline, and fluoroquinolones.

MOA — Antacid, mineral supplement.

ADVERSE EFFECTS — Serious: Severe hypercalcemia (with confusion, delirium, stupor, coma), renal calculi. Frequent: Mild hypercalcemia, constipation, anorexia, N/V.

CALCIUM CHLORIDE ▶K ♀+ ▶+ $

ADULT — Hypocalcemia: 500 to 1000 mg slow IV q 1 to 3 days. Magnesium intoxication: 500 mg IV. Hyperkalemic ECG changes: Dose based on ECG.

PEDS — Hypocalcemia: 0.2 mL/kg IV up to 10 mL/day. Cardiac resuscitation: 0.2 mL/kg IV.

UNAPPROVED ADULT — Has been used in calcium channel blocker toxicity and to treat or prevent calcium channel blocker–induced hypotension.

UNAPPROVED PEDS — Has been used in calcium channel blocker toxicity.

FORMS — Generic only: Injectable 10% (1000 mg/10 mL) 10 mL ampules, vials, syringes.

NOTES — Calcium chloride contains 14.4 mEq Ca/g versus calcium gluconate 4.7 mEq Ca/g. For IV use only; do not administer IM or SC. Avoid extravasation. Administer no faster than 0.5 to 1 mL/min, preferably via central line or deep vein. Use cautiously in patients receiving digoxin; inotropic and toxic effects are synergistic and may cause arrhythmias. Usually not recommended for hypocalcemia associated with renal insufficiency because calcium chloride is an acidifying salt.

MOA — Antagonizes the cardiotoxic effects of hyperkalemia.

ADVERSE EFFECTS — Serious: Vasodilation, hypotension. Frequent: Irritation at infusion site.

CALCIUM CITRATE (*Citracal*) ▶K ♀+ ▶+ $

ADULT — 1 to 2 g elem Ca/day or more PO with meals divided two to four times per day. Prevention of osteoporosis: 1000 to 1500 mg elem Ca/day PO divided two to three times per day with meals. The adequate intake in most adults is 1000 to 1200 mg elem Ca/day.

PEDS — Not approved in children.

FORMS — OTC Trade/generic (mg elem Ca/units vitamin D): 200/250, 250/200, 315/250, 600/500 (slow release); some products available with magnesium and/or phosphorus. Chewable gummies: 250 mg with 250 units vitamin D.

NOTES — Calcium citrate is 21% elem Ca. Not more than 500 to 600 mg elem Ca/dose. Decreases absorption of levothyroxine, tetracycline, and fluoroquinolones. Acidic environment not needed for absorption; preferred calcium salt in patients on PPI or H2RA.

MOA — Essential mineral that maintains the nervous, muscular, and skeletal systems and cell membrane and capillary permeability.

ADVERSE EFFECTS — Serious: Severe hypercalcemia (with confusion, delirium, stupor, coma), renal calculi. Frequent: Mild hypercalcemia, constipation, anorexia, N/V.

CALCIUM GLUCONATE ▶K ♀+ ▶+ $

ADULT — Emergency correction of hypocalcemia: 7 to 14 mEq slow IV prn. Hypocalcemic tetany: 4.5 to 16 mEq IM prn. Hyperkalemia with cardiac toxicity: 2.25 to 14 mEq IV while monitoring ECG. May repeat after 1 to 2 min. Magnesium intoxication: 4.5 to 9 mEq IV, adjust dose based on patient response. If IV not possible, give 2 to 5 mEq IM. Exchange transfusions: 1.35 mEq calcium gluconate IV concurrent with each 100 mL of citrated blood. Oral calcium gluconate: 1 to 2 g elem Ca/day or more PO with meals divided two to four times per day. Prevention of osteoporosis: 1000 to 1500 mg elem Ca/day PO with meals in divided doses.

PEDS — Emergency correction of hypocalcemia: Children: 1 to 7 mEq IV prn. Infants: 1 mEq IV prn. Hypocalcemic tetany: Children: 0.5 to 0.7 mEq/kg IV three to four times per day. Neonates: 2.4 mEq/kg/day IV in divided doses. Exchange transfusions: Neonates: 0.45 mEq IV/100 mL of exchange transfusions. Oral calcium gluconate: Hypocalcemia: Neonates: 50 to 150 mg elem Ca/kg/day PO in 4 to 6 divided doses; children: 45 to 65 mg elem Ca/kg/day PO divided four times per day.

UNAPPROVED ADULT — Has been used in calcium channel blocker toxicity and to treat or prevent calcium channel blocker–induced hypotension.

UNAPPROVED PEDS — Has been used in calcium channel blocker toxicity.

FORMS — Generic only: Injectable 10% (1000 mg/10 mL, 4.65 mEq/10 mL) 1, 10, 50, 100 mL. OTC Generic only: Tabs 500, 650, 700 mg. Chewable tabs 650 mg.

NOTES — Calcium gluconate is 9.3% elem Ca and contains 4.6 mEq elem Ca/g calcium gluconate. Administer IV calcium gluconate not faster than 0.5 to 2 mL/min. Use cautiously in patients receiving digoxin; inotropic and toxic effects are synergistic and may cause arrhythmias.

(cont.)

CALCIUM GLUCONATE (*cont.*)

MOA — Essential mineral that maintains the nervous, muscular, and skeletal systems and cell membrane and capillary permeability; antagonizes the cardiotoxic effects of hyperkalemia.

ADVERSE EFFECTS — Serious: Severe hypercalcemia (with confusion, delirium, stupor, coma), renal calculi; with IV: vasodilation, hypotension, arrhythmia, syncope and cardiac arrest. Frequent: Mild hypercalcemia, constipation, anorexia, N/V, irritation at infusion site (for IV).

COPPER GLUCONATE ▶L – ♀A ▶? $

ADULT — Supplementation: 2 to 5 mg PO daily. RDA: Adults: 900 mcg PO daily; pregnancy: 1000 mcg PO daily. Breastfeeding: 1300 mcg PO daily.

PEDS — RDA: 14 to 18 yo: 890 mcg PO daily; 9 to 13 yo: 700 mcg PO daily; 4 to 8 yo: 440 mcg PO daily; 1 to 3 yo: 340 mcg PO daily; 7 to 12 mo: 220 mcg PO daily; 0 to 6 mo: 200 mcg PO daily.

FORMS — OTC Generic: 2, 5 mg.

MOA — Essential element required for iron metabolism, CNS function and immune system activity.

ADVERSE EFFECTS — Serious: cirrhosis, hemoglobinuria. Common: arthralgias, myalgias, hypertension, dermatitis, N/V, diarrhea, abdominal pain, headache.

FERRIC CARBOXYMALTOSE (*Injectafer*) ▶NA ♀C ▶? $$$$$

ADULT — Iron deficiency anemia (unsatisfactory response to oral iron, nondialysis dependent): If less than 50 kg: 15 mg/kg elemental iron IV for 2 doses, separated by at least 7 days. If 50 kg or greater: 750 mg elemental iron IV for 2 doses, separated by at least 7 days. Max: 1500 mg per course.

FORMS — Trade only: 750 mg iron/15 mL vial.

NOTES — Hypersensitivity reported, monitor during and at least 30 min following administration. Monitor for hypertension.

MOA — Essential mineral needed for hemoglobin, myoglobin, and enzymatic function.

ADVERSE EFFECTS — Serious: Hypersensitivity reactions, severe hypertension. Frequent: Nausea, hypertension, flushing, hypophosphatemia, dizziness.

FERRIC GLUCONATE COMPLEX (*Ferrlecit*) ▶KL ♀B ▶? $$$$$

WARNING — Potentially fatal hypersensitivity reactions rarely reported with sodium ferric gluconate complex. Facilities for CPR must be available during dosing.

ADULT — Iron deficiency in chronic hemodialysis patients: 125 mg elem iron IV over 10 min or diluted in 100 mL NS IV over 1 h. Most hemodialysis patients require 1 g of elem iron over 8 consecutive hemodialysis session.

PEDS — Iron deficiency in chronic hemodialysis, age 6 yo or older: 1.5 mg/kg elem iron diluted in 25 mL NS and administered IV over 1 h at 8 sequential dialysis sessions. Max 125 mg/dose.

UNAPPROVED ADULT — Iron deficiency in cancer- and chemotherapy-induced anemia: 125 mg elem iron IV over 60 min, repeat weekly for 8 doses, or 200 mg IV over 3 to 4 h repeated q 3 weeks for 5 doses.

NOTES — Potentially fatal hypersensitivity reactions, including serious hypotension, reported with sodium ferric gluconate complex. Facilities for CPR must be available during dosing.

MOA — Essential mineral needed for hemoglobin, myoglobin, and enzymatic function.

ADVERSE EFFECTS — Serious: Anaphylactic reaction, chest pain, hypotension, shock, cardiac arrest, iron overdose. Frequent: Arthralgia, backache, chills, dizziness, fever, flushing, headache, infusion site reaction, malaise, myalgia, N/V.

FERRIC PYROPHOSPHATE CITRATE (*Triferic*) ▶NA ♀C ▶? $$$$$

ADULT — Iron replacement to maintain hemoglobin in CKD on hemodialysis: Add one ampule to 2.5 gallons of bicarbonate concentrate hemodialysate at each dialysis session. Final concentration 2 micromolar or 110 mcg/L of triferic iron.

PEDS — Safety and efficacy in pediatrics not established.

NOTES — Hypersensitivity reactions; observe during dialysis and until stable clinically.

MOA — Essential mineral needed for hemoglobin, myoglobin, and enzymatic function.

ADVERSE EFFECTS — Serious: AV fistula thrombosis/hemorrhage, hypotension, dyspnea. Common: headache, peripheral edema, fever, fatigue, muscle spasm, back pain.

SIDE EFFECTS —

FERROUS GLUCONATE (*Fergon*) ▶K ♀+ ▶+ $

WARNING — Severe iron toxicity possible in overdose, especially in children. Store out of reach of children and in child-resistant containers. Iron overdose is a leading cause of poisoning in children younger than 6 yo.

ADULT — Iron deficiency: 800 to 1600 mg ferrous gluconate (100 to 200 mg elem iron) PO divided three times per day. RDA (elem iron): 8 mg for adult males age 19 yo or older, 18 mg for adult premenopausal females age 19 to 50 yo, 8 mg for females age 51 yo or older, 27 mg during pregnancy, 10 mg during lactation if age 14 to 18 yo and 9 mg if age 19 to 50 yo. Upper limit: 45 mg/day.

PEDS — Mild to moderate iron deficiency: 3 mg/kg/day of elem iron PO in 1 to 2 divided doses. Severe iron deficiency: 4 to 6 mg/kg/day PO in 3 divided doses. RDA (elem iron): 0.27 mg for age younger than 6 mo, 11 mg for age 7 to 12 mo, 7 mg for age 1 to 3 yo, 10 mg for age 4 to 8 yo, 8 mg for age 9 to 13 yo, 11 mg for males age 14 to 18 yo, 15 mg for females age 14 to 18 yo.

UNAPPROVED ADULT — Adjunct to epoetin to maximize hematologic response: 200 mg elem iron/day PO.

UNAPPROVED PEDS — Adjunct to epoetin to maximize hematologic response: 2 to 3 mg/kg elem iron/day PO.

FORMS — OTC Generic/Trade: Tabs (ferrous gluconate) 240 mg (27 mg elemental iron). Generic only: Tabs 324, 325 mg.

NOTES — Ferrous gluconate is 12% elem iron. For iron deficiency, 4 to 6 months of therapy generally

(cont.)

FERROUS GLUCONATE *(cont.)*

necessary to replete stores even after hemoglobin has returned to normal. Do not take within 2 h of antacids, tetracyclines, levothyroxine, or fluoroquinolones. May cause black stools, constipation, or diarrhea.

MOA — Essential mineral needed for hemoglobin, myoglobin, and enzymatic function.

ADVERSE EFFECTS — Serious: Hypersensitivity, iron overdose. Frequent: Constipation, N/V, diarrhea, black stools.

FERROUS SULFATE *(Fer-in-Sol, Feosol, Slow FE, ✦Ferodan, Slow-Fe)* ▶K ♀+ ▶+ $

WARNING — Severe iron toxicity possible in overdose, especially in children. Store out of reach of children and in child-resistant containers. Iron overdose is a leading cause of poisoning in children younger than 6 yo.

ADULT — Iron deficiency: 500 to 1000 mg ferrous sulfate (100 to 200 mg elem iron) PO divided three times per day. For iron supplementation RDA, see ferrous gluconate.

PEDS — Mild to moderate iron deficiency: 3 mg/kg/day of elem iron PO in 1 to 2 divided doses; Severe Iron deficiency: 4 to 6 mg/kg/day PO in 3 divided doses. For Iron supplementation RDA see ferrous gluconate.

UNAPPROVED ADULT — Adjunct to epoetin to maximize hematologic response: 200 mg elem iron/day PO.

FORMS — OTC Generic/Trade (mg ferrous sulfate): Tabs, extended-release 160 mg. Tabs 200, 324, 325 mg. OTC Generic only (mg ferrous sulfate): Soln 75 mg/0.6 mL. Elixir 220 mg/5 mL.

NOTES — Iron sulfate is 20% elem iron. For iron deficiency, 4 to 6 months of therapy generally necessary. Do not take within 2 h of antacids, tetracyclines, levothyroxine, or fluoroquinolones. May cause black stools, constipation, or diarrhea.

MOA — Essential mineral needed for hemoglobin, myoglobin, and enzymatic function.

ADVERSE EFFECTS — Serious: Hypersensitivity, iron overdose. Frequent: Constipation, N/V, diarrhea, black stools, tooth staining (liquid preparations).

FERUMOXYTOL *(Feraheme)* ▶KL ♀C ▶? $$$$$

WARNING — Observe for hypersensitivity for at least 30 min following infusion, life-threatening hypersensitivity reported.

ADULT — Iron deficiency in chronic kidney disease: Give 510 mg IV infusion, followed by 510 mg IV infusion for 1 dose given 3 to 8 days after initial injection. May re-administer if persistent/recurrent iron deficiency anemia.

PEDS — Not studied in pediatrics.

NOTES — Monitor hemoglobin and iron studies at least 1 month following 2nd dose. May alter MRI imaging studies. Contraindicated in anemias not due to iron deficiency.

MOA — Superparamagnetic iron oxide to provide essential mineral needed for hemoglobin, myoglobin, and enzymatic function.

ADVERSE EFFECTS — Serious: Anaphylactic reaction, hypersensitivity, hypotension, iron overdose, syncope, cardiac arrest, arrhythmia, ischemic event, heart failure. Frequent: Diarrhea, nausea, dizziness, constipation, peripheral edema.

FLUORIDE *(Fluori-tab, ✦Fluor-A-Day)* ▶K ♀? ▶? $

ADULT — Prevention of dental cavities: 10 mL of topical rinse swish and spit daily.

PEDS — Prevention of dental caries: Dose based on age and fluoride concentrations in water. See table.

FORMS — Generic only: Chewable tabs 0.25, 0.5, 1 mg. Gtts 0.125, 0.25, 0.5 mg/dropperful. Soln 0.2 mg/mL. Gel 0.1, 0.5, 1.23%. Rinse (sodium fluoride) 0.05, 0.1, 0.2%.

NOTES — In communities without fluoridated water, fluoride supplementation should be used until 13 to 16 yo. Chronic overdosage of fluorides may result in dental fluorosis (mottling of tooth enamel) and osseous changes. Use rinses and gels after brushing and flossing and before bedtime.

MOA — Trace element that promotes tooth remineralization and inhibits cariogenesis.

ADVERSE EFFECTS — Serious: Increased bone fracture, allergic rash. Frequent: Rash, eczema, gastric distress, headache, tooth staining (liquid preparations).

FLUORIDE SUPPLEMENTATION

Age	<0.3 ppm in drinking water	0.3–0.6 ppm in drinking water	>0.6 ppm in drinking water
0–6 mo	none	none	none
6 mo–3 yo	0.25 mg PO daily	none	none
3–6 yo	0.5 mg PO daily	0.25 mg PO daily	none
6–16 yo	1 mg PO daily	0.5 mg PO daily	none

JADA 2010;141:1480–1489.

IRON DEXTRAN (*InFeD, DexFerrum, ✦Dexiron, Infufer*) ▸KL ♀C ▶? $$$$$

WARNING — Administer a test dose prior to 1st dose. Parenteral iron therapy has resulted in anaphylactic reactions, even with test dose and after uneventful test doses. Potentially fatal hypersensitivity reactions have been reported with iron dextran injection. Facilities for CPR must be available during dosing. Use only when clearly warranted.

ADULT — Iron deficiency: Dose based on patient wt and hemoglobin. Total dose (mL) = 0.0442 × (desired Hb − observed Hb) × wt (kg) + [0.26 × wt (kg)]. For wt, use lesser of lean body wt or actual body wt. Iron replacement for blood loss: Replacement iron (mg) = blood loss (mL) × hematocrit. Max daily IM dose 100 mg.

PEDS — Not recommended for infants younger than 4 mo. Iron deficiency in children greater than 5 kg: Dose based on patient wt and hemoglobin. Dose (mL) = 0.0442 × (desired Hb − observed Hb) × wt (kg) + [0.26 × wt (kg)]. For wt, use lesser of lean body wt or actual body wt. Iron replacement for blood loss: Replacement iron (mg) = blood loss (mL) × hematocrit. Max daily IM dose: Infant wt less than 5 kg, give 25 mg; children 5 to 10 kg give 50 mg; children wt greater than 10 kg give 100 mg.

UNAPPROVED ADULT — Adjunct to epoetin to maximize hematologic response. Total dose (325 to 1500 mg) as a single, slow (6 mg/min) IV infusion has been used.

UNAPPROVED PEDS — Adjunct to epoetin to maximize hematologic response.

NOTES — A 0.5 mL IV test dose (0.25 mL in infants) over 30 sec or longer should be given at least 1 h before therapy. Infuse no faster than 50 mg/min. For IM administration, use Z-track technique.

MOA — Essential mineral needed for hemoglobin, myoglobin, and enzymatic function.

ADVERSE EFFECTS — Serious: Anaphylactic reaction, chest pain, hypotension, shock, cardiac arrest, iron overdose. Frequent: Arthralgia, backache, chills, dizziness, fever, flushing, headache, infusion site reaction, malaise, myalgia, N/V.

IRON POLYSACCHARIDE (*Niferex, Niferex-150, Nu-Iron 150, Ferrex 150*) ▸K ♀+ ▶+ $$

WARNING — Severe iron toxicity possible in overdose, especially in children. Store out of reach of children and in child-resistant containers. Iron overdose is a leading cause of poisoning in children younger than 6 yo.

ADULT — Iron deficiency: 50 to 200 mg PO divided one to three times per day. For iron supplementation RDA see ferrous gluconate.

PEDS — Mild to moderate iron deficiency: 3 mg/kg/day of elem iron PO in 1 to 2 divided doses. Severe iron deficiency: 4 to 6 mg/kg/day PO in 3 divided doses. For iron supplementation RDA see ferrous gluconate.

UNAPPROVED ADULT — Adjunct to epoetin to maximize hematologic response: 200 mg elem iron/day PO.

UNAPPROVED PEDS — Adjunct to epoetin to maximize hematologic response: 2 to 3 mg/kg elem iron/day PO.

FORMS — OTC Trade only: Caps 60 mg (Niferex). OTC Generic/Trade: Caps 150 mg (Niferex-150, Nu-Iron 150, Ferrex 150), Elixir 100 mg/5 mL (Niferex). 1 mg iron polysaccharide = 1 mg elemental iron.

NOTES — For iron deficiency, 4 to 6 months of therapy generally necessary. Do not take within 2 h of antacids, tetracyclines, levothyroxine, or fluoroquinolones. May cause black stools, constipation, or diarrhea.

MOA — Essential mineral needed for hemoglobin, myoglobin, and enzymatic function.

ADVERSE EFFECTS — Serious: Hypersensitivity, iron overdose. Frequent: Constipation, N/V, diarrhea, black stools.

IRON SUCROSE (*Venofer*) ▸KL ♀B ▶? $$$$$

WARNING — Potentially fatal hypersensitivity reactions have been rarely reported with iron sucrose injection. Facilities for CPR must be available during dosing.

ADULT — Iron deficiency in chronic hemodialysis patients: 5 mL (100 mg elem iron) IV over 5 min or diluted in 100 mL NS IV over 15 min or longer. Iron deficiency in non-dialysis-dependent chronic kidney disease patients: 10 mL (200 mg elem iron) IV over 5 min or 500 mg diluted in 250 mL NS IV over 4 h.

PEDS — Iron deficiency in chronic hemodialysis, dependent or non-dialysis-dependent chronic kidney disease (2 yo or older): 0.5 mg/kg slow IV injection or infusion. Max: 100 mg elemental iron. Give injection over 5 min or dilute in in 25 mL of NS and administer IV over 5 to 60 min.

UNAPPROVED ADULT — Iron deficiency: 5 mL (100 mg elem iron) IV over 5 min or diluted in 100 mL NS IV over 15 min or longer.

NOTES — Most hemodialysis patients require 1 g of elem iron over 10 consecutive hemodialysis sessions. Non-dialysis patients require 1 g of elemental iron divided and given over 14 days. Observe patients for at least 30 minutes following administration; anaphylaxis reported.

MOA — Essential mineral needed for hemoglobin, myoglobin, and enzymatic function.

ADVERSE EFFECTS — Serious: Anaphylaxis, chest pain, hypotension, shock, cardiac arrest, iron overdose. Frequent: Arthralgia, backache, chills, dizziness, fever, flushing, headache, infusion site reaction, malaise, myalgia, N/V.

MAGNESIUM CHLORIDE (*Slow-Mag*) ▸K ♀A ▶+ $

ADULT — Dietary supplement: 2 tabs PO daily. RDA (elem Mg): Adult males: 400 mg if 19 to 30 yo, 420 mg if older than 30 yo. Adult females: 310 mg if 19 to 30 yo, 320 mg if older than 30 yo.

PEDS — Not approved in children.

UNAPPROVED ADULT — Hypomagnesemia: 300 mg elem magnesium PO divided four times per day.

FORMS — OTC Trade only: Enteric-coated tab 64 mg. 64 mg tab Slow-Mag = 64 mg elemental magnesium.

(cont.)

MAGNESIUM CHLORIDE (*cont.*)

NOTES — May cause diarrhea. May accumulate in renal insufficiency.

MOA — Essential mineral needed for muscle function, organ function, potassium and calcium absorption.

ADVERSE EFFECTS — Serious: Potential magnesium intoxication. Frequent: Diarrhea, weakness, N/V.

MAGNESIUM GLUCONATE (*Magtrate, Mangonate, Mag-G, ✽Maglucate*) ▶K ♀A ▶+ $

ADULT — Dietary supplement: 500 to 1000 mg/day PO divided three times per day. RDA (elem Mg): Adult males: 19 to 30 yo: 400 mg; older than 30 yo: 420 mg. Adult females: 19 to 30 yo: 310 mg; older than 30 yo: 320 mg.

PEDS — Not approved in children.

UNAPPROVED ADULT — Hypomagnesemia: 300 mg elem magnesium PO divided four times per day. Unproven efficacy for oral tocolysis following IV magnesium sulfate.

UNAPPROVED PEDS — Hypomagnesemia: 10 to 20 mg elem magnesium/kg/dose PO four times per day. RDA (elem Mg): Age 0 to 6 mo: 30 mg/day; age 7 to 12 mo: 75 mg/day; age 1 to 3 yo: 80 mg; age 4 to 8 yo: 130 mg; age 9 to 13 yo: 240 mg; age 14 to 18 yo (males): 410 mg; age 14 to 18 yo (females): 360 mg.

FORMS — OTC Generic only: Tabs 500 mg (27 mg elemental Mg).

NOTES — May cause diarrhea. Use caution in renal failure; may accumulate.

MOA — Essential mineral needed for muscle function, organ function, potassium and calcium absorption.

ADVERSE EFFECTS — Serious: Potential magnesium intoxication. Frequent: Diarrhea, weakness, N/V.

MAGNESIUM OXIDE (*Mag-200, Mag-Ox 400, Mag-Caps, Uro-Mag*) ▶K ♀A ▶+ $

ADULT — Dietary supplement: 400 to 800 mg PO daily. RDA (elem Mg): Adult males: 19 to 30 yo: 400 mg; older than 30 yo 420 mg. Adult females: 19 to 30 yo: 310 mg; older than 30 yo: 320 mg.

PEDS — Not approved in children.

UNAPPROVED ADULT — Hypomagnesemia: 300 mg elem magnesium PO four times per day. Has also been used as oral tocolysis following IV magnesium sulfate (unproven efficacy) and in the prevention of calcium-oxalate kidney stones.

FORMS — OTC Generic/Trade: Caps/Tabs: 140 (84.5 mg elemental Mg); Tabs only: 200 (elemental), 250 (elemental), 400 (241 mg elemental Mg), 420 (253 mg elemental Mg), 500 mg (elemental).

NOTES — Take with food. Magnesium oxide is approximately 60% elemental magnesium. May accumulate in renal insufficiency.

MOA — Essential mineral needed for muscle function, organ function, potassium and calcium absorption.

ADVERSE EFFECTS — Serious: Potential magnesium intoxication. Frequent: Diarrhea, weakness, N/V.

MAGNESIUM SULFATE ▶K ♀D C/D ▶+ $

ADULT — Hypomagnesemia: Mild deficiency: 1 g IM q 6 h for 4 doses; severe deficiency: 2 g IV over 1 h (monitor for hypotension). Hyperalimentation: Maintenance requirements not precisely known; adults generally require 8 to 24 mEq/day. Seizure prevention in severe preeclampsia or eclampsia: ACOG recommendations: 4 to 6 g IV loading dose, then 1 to 2 g/h IV continuous infusion for at least 24 h. Or per product information: Total initial dose of 10 to 14 g administered via IV infusion and IM doses (4 g IV infusion with 5 g IM injections in each buttock). Initial dose is followed by 4 to 5 g IM into alternate buttocks q 4 h prn or initial dose is followed by 1 to 2 g/h constant IV infusion. Max: 30 to 40 g/24 h.

PEDS — Not approved in children.

UNAPPROVED ADULT — Preterm labor: 6 g IV over 20 min, then 1 to 3 g/h titrated to decrease contractions. Has been used as an adjunctive bronchodilator in very severe acute asthma (2 g IV over 10 to 20 min), and in chronic fatigue syndrome. Torsades de pointes: 1 to 2 g IV in D5W over 5 to 60 min.

UNAPPROVED PEDS — Hypomagnesemia: 25 to 50 mg/kg IV/IM q 4 to 6 h for 3 to 4 doses, max single dose 2 g. Hyperalimentation: Maintenance requirements not precisely known; infants require 2 to 10 mEq/day. Acute nephritis: 20 to 40 mg/kg (in 20% soln) IM prn. Adjunctive bronchodilator in very severe acute asthma: 25 to 100 mg/kg IV over 10 to 20 min.

NOTES — 1000 mg magnesium sulfate contains 8 mEq elem magnesium. Do not give faster than 1.5 mL/min (of 10% soln) except in eclampsia or seizures. Use caution in renal insufficiency; may accumulate. Monitor urine output, patellar reflex, respiratory rate, and serum magnesium level. Concomitant use with terbutaline may lead to fatal pulmonary edema. IM administration must be diluted to a 20% soln. If needed, may reverse toxicity with calcium gluconate 1 g IV. Continuous use in pregnancy beyond 5 to 7 days may cause fetal harm.

MOA — Essential mineral needed for muscle function, organ function, potassium and calcium absorption; blocks neuromuscular transmission to prevent or control convulsions.

ADVERSE EFFECTS — Serious: Magnesium intoxication (in recipient of drug or in newborn of pregnant woman receiving Mg), cardiac depression, CNS depression, respiratory paralysis, hypotension, stupor, hypothermia, circulatory collapse. Frequent: Flushing, sweating, depressed reflexes.

PHOSPHORUS (*Neutra-Phos, K-Phos*) ▶K ♀C ▶? $

ADULT — Dietary supplement: 1 cap/packet (Neutra-Phos) PO four times per day or 1 to 2 tabs (K-Phos) PO four times per day after meals and at bedtime. Severe hypophosphatemia (less than 1 mg/dL): 0.08 to 0.16 mmol/kg IV over 6 h. In TPN, 310 to 465 mg/day (10 to 15 mM) IV is usually adequate, although higher amounts may be necessary in hypermetabolic states. RDA for adults is 800 mg.

(cont.)

PHOSPHORUS (cont.)

PEDS — RDA (elem phosphorus): 0 to 6 mo: 100 mg; 6 to 12 mo: 275 mg; 1 to 3 yo: 460 mg; 4 to 8 yo: 500 mg; 9 to 18: 1250 mg. Severe hypophosphatemia (less than 1 mg/dL): 0.25 to 0.5 mmol/kg IV over 4 to 6 h. Infant TPN: 1.5 to 2 mmol/kg/day in TPN.

FORMS — OTC Trade only: (Neutra-Phos, Neutra-Phos K) tab/cap/packet 250 mg (8 mmol) phosphorus. Rx: Trade only: (K-Phos) tab 250 mg (8 mmol) phosphorus.

NOTES — Dissolve caps/tabs/powder in 75 mL water prior to ingestion.

MOA — Essential mineral needed for bone metabolism and enzymatic functions.

ADVERSE EFFECTS — Serious: Phosphate intoxication with reciprocal hypocalcemic tetany (with IV). Frequent: Laxative-like effect, nausea, abdominal pain, vomiting.

POTASSIUM ▶K ♀C ▶? $

ADULT — Hypokalemia: 20 to 40 mEq/day or more IV or immediate-release PO. Intermittent infusion: 10 to 20 mEq/dose IV over 1 to 2 h prn. Consider monitoring for infusions greater than 10 mEq/h. Prevention of hypokalemia: 20 to 40 mEq/day PO one to two times per day.

PEDS — Not approved in children.

UNAPPROVED ADULT — Diuretic-induced hypokalemia: 20 to 60 mEq/day PO.

UNAPPROVED PEDS — Hypokalemia: 2.5 mEq/kg/day given IV/PO one to two times per day. Intermittent infusion: 0.5 to 1 mEq/kg/dose IV at 0.3 to 0.5 mEq/kg/h prn. Infusions faster than 0.5 mEq/kg/h require continuous monitoring.

FORMS — Injectable, many different products in a variety of salt forms (ie, chloride, bicarbonate,

POTASSIUM (ORAL FORMS)*

Effervescent Granules	
20 mEq	Klorvess Effervescent, K-vescent
Effervescent Tabs	
10 mEq	Effer-K
20 mEq	Effer-K
25 mEq	Effer-K, K+Care ET, K-Lyte, K-Lyte/Cl, Klor-Con/EF
50 mEq	K-Lyte DS, K-Lyte/Cl 50
Liquids	
20 mEq/15 mL	Cena-K, Kaochlor S-F, K-G Elixir, Kaochlor 10%, Kay Ciel, Kaon, Kaylixir, Kolyum, Potasalan, Twin-K
30 mEq/15 mL	Rum-K
40 mEq/15 mL	Cena-K, Kaon-Cl 20%
45 mEq/15 mL	Tri-K
Powders	
15 mEq/pack	K+Care
20 mEq/pack	Gen-K, K+Care, Kay Ciel, K-Lor, Klor-Con
25 mEq/pack	K+Care, Klor-Con 25
Tabs/Caps	
8 mEq	K+8, Klor-Con 8, Slow-K, Micro-K
10 mEq	K+10, K-Norm, Kaon-Cl 10, Klor-Con M10, Klotrix, K-Tab, K-Dur 10, Micro-K 10
20 mEq	Klor-Con M20, K-Dur 20

* Table provides examples and is not intended to be all inclusive.

(cont.)

POTASSIUM (*cont.*)

citrate, acetate, gluconate), available in tabs, caps, liquids, effervescent tabs, packets. Potassium gluconate is available OTC. See table.

NOTES — Use potassium chloride for hypokalemia associated with alkalosis; use potassium bicarbonate, citrate, acetate, or gluconate when associated with acidosis.

MOA — Intracellular cation that participates in numerous essential physiological processes.

ADVERSE EFFECTS — Serious: Hyperkalemia, gastrointestinal toxicity (obstruction, bleed, ulcer, perforation, esophagitis). Frequent: N/V, diarrhea, abdominal pain, infusion site irritation (IV).

ZINC ACETATE (*Galzin*) ▶Minimal absorption ♀A ▶— $$$

ADULT — RDA (elemental Zn): Adult males: 11 mg daily. Adult females: 8 to 12 mg daily. Zinc deficiency: 25 to 50 mg (elemental) daily. Wilson's disease, previously treated with chelating agent: 25 to 50 mg (elemental) PO three times per day.

PEDS — RDA (elem Zn): Age 7 mo to 3 yo: 3 mg; 4 to 8 yo: 5 mg; 9 to 13 yo: 8 mg; 14 to 18 yo (males): 8 mg; 14 to 18 yo (females): 9 to 14 mg. Zinc deficiency: 0.5 to 1 mg elemental zinc mg/kg/day divided two to three times per day. Wilson's disease (age 10 yo or older): 25 to 50 mg (elemental) three times per day.

FORMS — Trade only: Caps 25, 50 mg elemental zinc.

NOTES — Poorly absorbed; take 1 h before or 2 to 3 h after meals. Decreases absorption of tetracycline and fluoroquinolones.

MOA — Nutritional supplement. Blocks intestinal absorption of copper.

ADVERSE EFFECTS — Serious: Sideroblastic anemia, pancreatitis. Frequent: N/V.

ZINC SULFATE (*Orazinc*) ▶Minimal absorption ♀A ▶— $

ADULT — RDA (elemental Zn): Adult males: 11 mg daily. Adult females: 8 to 12 mg daily. Zinc deficiency: 25 to 50 mg (elemental) PO daily.

PEDS — RDA (elemental Zn): Age 7 mo to 3 yo: 3 mg; 4 to 8 yo: 5 mg; 9 to 13 yo: 8 mg; 14 to 18 yo (males): 8 mg; 14 to 18 yo (females): 9 to 14 mg. Zinc deficiency: 0.5 to 1 mg elemental zinc mg/kg/day PO divided two to three times per day.

UNAPPROVED ADULT — Wound healing in zinc deficiency: 200 mg PO three times per day.

FORMS — OTC Generic/Trade: Tabs 66, 110, 220 mg.

NOTES — Zinc sulfate is 23% elemental Zn. Decreases absorption of tetracycline and fluoroquinolones. Poorly absorbed; increased absorption on empty stomach; however, administration with food decreases GI upset.

MOA — Nutritional supplement.

ADVERSE EFFECTS — Serious: Sideroblastic anemia, pancreatitis. Frequent: N/V.

ENDOCRINE AND METABOLIC: Nutritionals

BANANA BAG ▶KL ♀+ ▶+ $

UNAPPROVED ADULT — Alcoholic malnutrition (example formula): Add thiamine 100 mg + folic acid 1 mg + IV multivitamins to 1 liter NS and infuse over 4 h. Magnesium sulfate 2 g may be added. "Banana bag" is jargon and not a valid drug order; also known as "rally pack"; specify individual components.

MOA — Mixture of vitamin supplements that mediates glucose utilization to prevent Wernicke-Korsakoff syndrome in alcoholism.

ADVERSE EFFECTS — Serious: Hypersensitivity, anaphylaxis, cyanosis, pulmonary edema, GI hemorrhage, cardiovascular shock. Frequent: Injection-site reaction, feeling of warmth, pruritus, sweating, N/V, restlessness, angioedema.

LEVOCARNITINE (*Carnitor*) ▶KL ♀B ▶? $$$$$

ADULT — Prevention of levocarnitine deficiency in dialysis patients: 10 to 20 mg/kg IV at each dialysis session. Titrate dose based on serum concentration.

PEDS — Prevention of deficiency in dialysis patients: 10 to 20 mg/kg IV at each dialysis session. Titrate dose based on serum concentration.

FORMS — Generic/Trade: Caps, 250, 300, 400 mg. Tabs 330, 500 mg. Oral soln 1 g/10 mL.

NOTES — Adverse neurophysiologic effects may occur with long-term, high doses of oral levocarnitine in patients with renal dysfunction. Only the IV formulation is indicated in patients receiving hemodialysis.

MOA — Facilitates long-chain fatty acid utilization.

ADVERSE EFFECTS — Serious: Seizures. Frequent: N/V, body odor, mild myasthenia.

RALLY PACK ▶KL ♀C ▶— $

UNAPPROVED ADULT — See "Banana Bag." "Rally pack" is jargon and not a valid drug order; specify individual components.

MOA — Mixture of vitamin supplements that mediates glucose utilization to prevent Wernicke-Korsakoff syndrome in alcoholism.

ADVERSE EFFECTS — Serious: Hypersensitivity, anaphylaxis, cyanosis, pulmonary edema, GI hemorrhage, cardiovascular shock. Frequent: Injection-site reaction, feeling of warmth, pruritus, sweating, N/V, restlessness, angioedema.

ENDOCRINE AND METABOLIC: Phosphate Binders

FERRIC CITRATE (*Auryxia*) ▶KL ♀B ▶? $$$$$

ADULT — Treatment of hyperphosphatemia in end-stage renal disease on dialysis: Start 2 tabs PO three times daily with meals. Titrate by 1 to 2 tabs q

week to achieve target serum phosphorous levels. Max 12 tabs/day.

PEDS — Not approved for use in children.

FORMS — Trade only (Tabs): 210 mg ferric iron (equivalent to 1 g ferric citrate).

(cont.)

FERRIC CITRATE (*cont.*)

NOTES — Do not use in iron overload. Monitor ferritin and TSAT. Adjust IV iron as needed if on concomitant therapy. Keep out of reach of children, iron products are a leading cause of poisoning children younger than 6 yo.

MOA — Binds dietary phosphate in GI tract creating ferric phosphate precipitate which is insoluble and excreted in the stool, thereby lowering the phosphate concentration in the serum.

ADVERSE EFFECTS — Serious: iron overload. Common: diarrhea, discolored feces, constipation, N/V.

LANTHANUM CARBONATE (*Fosrenol*) ▶Not absorbed ♀C ▶? $$$$$

ADULT — Treatment of hyperphosphatemia in end-stage renal disease: Start 1500 mg/day PO in divided doses with meals. Titrate dose q 2 to 3 weeks in increments of 750 mg/day until acceptable serum phosphate is reached. Most will require 1500 to 3000 mg/day to reduce serum phosphate less than 6.0 mg/dL. Chew or crush tabs completely before swallowing; not to be swallowed whole.

PEDS — Not approved in children.

FORMS — Trade only: Chewable tabs 500, 750, 1000 mg. Oral powder 750, 1000 mg.

NOTES — Divided doses up to 3750 mg/day have been used. Caution if acute peptic ulcer, ulcerative colitis, or Crohn's disease. Serious GI obstructions and perforations reported; contraindicated if pre-existing bowel obstruction, ileus, and fecal impaction. Avoid medications known to interact with antacids within 2 h. May be radio-opaque enough to appear on abdominal x-ray.

MOA — Binds dietary phosphate forming highly insoluble complexes that are eliminated through the GI tract.

ADVERSE EFFECTS — Serious: Dialysis graft occlusion, GI perforation. Frequent: N/V, abdominal pain, diarrhea.

SEVELAMER (*Renagel, Renvela*) ▶Not absorbed ♀C ▶? $$$$$

ADULT — Hyperphosphatemia in kidney disease on dialysis: Start 800 to 1600 mg PO three times per day with meals, adjust according to serum phosphorus concentration.

PEDS — Not approved in children.

FORMS — Trade only (Renagel—sevelamer hydrochloride): Tabs 400, 800 mg. (Renvela—sevelamer carbonate): Tabs 800 mg. Powder: 800, 2400 mg packets.

NOTES — Titrate by 800 mg/meal at 2-week intervals to keep phosphorus less than 5.5 mg/dL; highest daily dose in studies: Renagel, 13 g; Renvela, 14 g. If significant interaction expected, separate timing of administration and/or monitor clinical response or blood levels of concomitant medication. Caution in GI motility disorders, including severe constipation. Contraindicated if bowel obstruction. Dysphagia and esophageal tablet retention reported; consider susp form if history of swallowing difficulties.

MOA — Binds intestinal phosphate preventing absorption.

ADVERSE EFFECTS — Serious: Hypophosphatemia, intestinal obstruction, dysphagia, bowel perforation. Frequent: N/V, dyspepsia, diarrhea, flatulence, constipation.

SUCROFERRIC OXYHYDROXIDE (*Velphoro*) ▶not absorbed ♀B ▶+ $$$$$

ADULT — Hyperphosphatemia in kidney disease on dialysis: Start 1 tab (500 mg) PO three times daily with meals, adjust weekly according to serum phosphorus concentrations. Tablets must be chewed.

FORMS — Trade only: Tabs 500 mg.

NOTES — Titrate at weekly intervals to achieve serum phosphorous 5.5 mg/dL or less. Not studied in GI or hepatic disorders.

MOA — Binds intestinal phosphate preventing absorption.

ADVERSE EFFECTS — Common: discolored feces, diarrhea, nausea, altered taste.

ENDOCRINE AND METABOLIC: Thyroid Agents

LEVOTHYROXINE (*Synthroid, Tirosint, Unithroid, T4, ✱Eltroxin, Euthyrox*) ▶L ♀A ▶+ $

WARNING — Do not use for obesity/wt loss; possible serious or life-threatening toxic effects when used in euthyroid patients.

ADULT — Hypothyroidism: Start 100 to 200 mcg PO daily (healthy adults) or 12.5 to 50 mcg PO daily (elderly or CV disease), increase by 12.5 to 25 mcg/day at 3- to 8-week intervals. Usual maintenance dose 100 to 200 mcg PO daily, max 300 mcg/day. Myxedema coma: 300 to 500 mcg IV once, then 50 to 100 mcg daily until able to tolerate PO therapy.

PEDS — Hypothyroidism: 0 to 6 mo: 8 to 10 mcg/kg/day PO; 6 to 12 mo: 6 to 8 mcg/kg/day PO; 1 to 5 yo: 5 to 6 mcg/kg/day PO; 6 to 12 yo: 4 to 5 mcg/kg/day PO; older than 12 yo: 2 to 3 mcg/kg/day PO, max 300 mcg/day.

UNAPPROVED ADULT — Hypothyroidism: 1.6 mcg/kg/day PO; start with lower doses (25 mcg PO daily) in elderly and patients with cardiac disease. Myxedema coma: 200 to 400 mcg IV once, then 1.2 mcg/kg/day IV until able to tolerate PO therapy.

FORMS — Generic/Trade: Tabs 25, 50, 75, 88, 100, 112, 125, 137, 150, 175, 200, 300 mcg. Trade only: Caps (Tirosint) 13, 25, 50, 75, 88, 100, 112, 125, 137, 150 mcg.

NOTES — May crush tabs for infants and children. Give IV at ¾ oral dose then adjust based on tolerance and therapeutic response. Consistent use of same preparation (brand or same generic) preferred as products may not be therapeutically interchangable; reevaluate thyroid function when switching.

MOA — Synthetic thyroid derivative that increases metabolic rate of body tissues.

(cont.)

LEVOTHYROXINE (*cont.*)

ADVERSE EFFECTS — Serious: Hyperthyroidism (arrhythmia, heart failure, angina, cardiac arrest), pseudotumor cerebri. Frequent: Palpitations, tachycardia, tremor, headache, nervousness, insomnia, diarrhea, vomiting, weight loss, menstrual irregularity, sweating, heat intolerance.

LIOTHYRONINE (*T3, Cytomel, Triostat*) ▶L ♀A ▶? $$

WARNING — Do not use for obesity/weight loss; possible serious or life-threatening toxic effects when used in euthyroid patients.

ADULT — Mild hypothyroidism: 25 mcg PO daily, increase by 12.5 to 25 mcg/day at 1- to 2-week intervals to desired response. Usual maintenance dose 25 to 75 mcg PO daily. Goiter: 5 mcg PO daily, increase by 5 to 10 mcg/day at 1- to 2-week intervals. Usual maintenance dose 75 mcg PO daily. Myxedema: 5 mcg PO daily, increase by 5 to 10 mcg/day at 1- to 2-week intervals. Usual maintenance dose 50 to 100 mcg/day.

PEDS — Congenital hypothyroidism: 5 mcg PO daily, increase by 5 mcg/day at 3- to 4-day intervals to desired response.

FORMS — Generic/Trade: Tabs 5, 25, 50 mcg.

NOTES — Levothyroxine is preferred maintenance treatment for hypothyroidism. Start therapy at 5 mcg/day in children and elderly and increase by 5 mcg increments only. Rapidly absorbed from the GI tract. Monitor T3 and TSH. Elderly may need lower doses due to potential decreased renal function.

MOA — Synthetic thyroid derivative that increases metabolic rate of body tissues.

ADVERSE EFFECTS — Serious: Hyperthyroidism (arrhythmia, heart failure, angina, cardiac arrest), pseudotumor cerebri. Frequent: Palpitations, tachycardia, tremor, headache, nervousness, insomnia, diarrhea, vomiting, weight loss, menstrual irregularity, sweating, heat intolerance.

METHIMAZOLE (*Tapazole*) ▶L ♀D ▶+ $$$

ADULT — Hyperthyroidism. Mild: 5 mg PO three times per day. Moderate: 10 mg PO three times per day. Severe: 20 mg PO three times per day (q 8 h intervals). Maintenance dose is 5 to 30 mg/day.

PEDS — Hyperthyroidism: 0.4 mg/kg/day PO divided q 8 h. Maintenance dose is half of the initial dose, max 30 mg/day.

UNAPPROVED ADULT — Start 10 to 30 mg PO daily, then adjust.

FORMS — Generic/Trade: Tabs 5, 10 mg.

NOTES — Check CBC for evidence of marrow suppression if fever, sore throat, or other signs of infection. Propylthiouracil preferred over methimazole in 1st trimester of pregnancy.

MOA — Inhibits synthesis of thyroid hormones.

ADVERSE EFFECTS — Serious: Agranulocytosis, granulocytopenia, thrombocytopenia, aplastic anemia, leukopenia, interstitial pneumonitis, dermatitis, hepatotoxicity, periarteritis, nephritis, hypoprothrombinemia. Frequent: N/V, rash, pruritus, headache, dizziness, vertigo, drowsiness, alopecia, constipation, paresthesia, neuritis, hyperpigmentation.

POTASSIUM IODIDE (*Iosat, SSKI, Thyrosafe, ThyroShield*) ▶L ♀D ▶– $

WARNING — Do not use for obesity.

ADULT — Thyroidectomy preparation: 50 to 250 mg PO three times per day for 10 to 14 days prior to surgery. Thyroid storm: 1 mL (Lugol's) PO three times per day at least 1 h after initial propylthiouracil or methimazole dose. Thyroid blocking in radiation emergency: 130 mg PO daily for 10 days or as directed by state health officials.

PEDS — Thyroid blocking in radiation emergency: Birth to 1 mo: 16 mg (⅛ of a 130 mg tab) PO daily. 1 mo to 3 yo: 32 mg (¼ of a 130 mg tab) PO daily. Age 3 to 18 yo: 65 mg (½ of a 130 mg tab) PO daily, or 130 mg PO daily in adolescents greater than 70 kg. Duration is until risk of exposure to radioiodines no longer exists.

FORMS — OTC Trade only: Tabs 130 mg (Iosat). Trade only Rx: Soln 1 g/mL (30, 240 mL, SSKI). OTC Generic only: Tabs 65 mg (Thyrosafe), Soln 65 mg/mL (30 mL, ThyroShield).

MOA — Elemental substance used therapeutically to block thyroid uptake or suppress thyroid hormone synthesis and release.

ADVERSE EFFECTS — Serious: Agranulocytosis, granulocytopenia, thrombocytopenia, aplastic anemia, leukopenia, interstitial pneumonitis, exfoliative dermatitis, vasculitis, hepatotoxicity. Frequent: N/V, rash, pruritus, headache, dizziness, drowsiness, alopecia, constipation, paresthesia, neuritis, hyperpigmentation.

PROPYLTHIOURACIL (*PTU, ✱Propyl Thyracil*) ▶L ♀D (but preferred over methimazole in 1st trimester) ▶+ $$$$

WARNING — Acute liver failure and severe liver injury reported, including fatal injury and need for liver transplantation. Use only if patient cannot tolerate methimazole or if not a candidate for radioactive iodine therapy or surgery.

ADULT — Hyperthyroidism: 100 to 150 mg PO three times per day. Severe hyperthyroidism and/or large goiters: 200 to 400 mg PO three times per day. Continue initial dose for approximately 2 months. Adjust dose to desired response. Usual maintenance dose 100 to 150 mg/day. Thyroid storm: 200 mg PO q 4 to 6 h once daily, decrease dose gradually to usual maintenance dose.

PEDS — Hyperthyroidism in children age 6 to 10 yo: 50 mg PO daily to three times per day. Children or older than 10 yo: 50 to 100 mg PO three times per day. Continue initial dose for 2 months, then maintenance dose is ⅓ to ⅔ the initial dose.

UNAPPROVED PEDS — Hyperthyroidism in neonates: 5 to 10 mg/kg/day PO divided q 8 h. Children: 5 to 7 mg/kg/day PO divided q 8 h.

FORMS — Generic only: Tabs 50 mg.

NOTES — Monitor CBC for marrow suppression if fever, sore throat, or other signs of infection. Vasculitic syndrome with positive antineutrophilic cytoplasmic antibodies (ANCAs) reported requiring discontinuation. Propylthiouracil preferred over methimazole in 1st trimester of pregnancy.

(cont.)

PROPYLTHIOURACIL (*cont.*)

MOA — Inhibits synthesis of thyroid hormones.

ADVERSE EFFECTS — Serious: Agranulocytosis, granulocytopenia, thrombocytopenia, aplastic anemia, leukopenia, interstitial pneumonitis, exfoliative dermatitis, vasculitis, hepatotoxicity. Frequent: N/V, rash, pruritus, headache, dizziness, drowsiness, alopecia, constipation, paresthesia, neuritis, hyperpigmentation.

SODIUM IODIDE I-131 (*Hicon*) ▶K ♀X ▶– $$$$$

ADULT — Specialized dosing for hyperthyroidism and thyroid carcinoma.

PEDS — Not approved in children.

FORMS — Generic/Trade: Caps, oral soln: Radioactivity range varies at the time of calibration. Hicon is a kit containing caps and a concentrated oral soln for dilution and cap preparation.

NOTES — Hazardous substance, handle with necessary precautions and use proper disposal. Avoid if preexisting vomiting or diarrhea. Discontinue antithyroid therapy at least 3 days before starting. Low serum chloride or nephrosis may increase uptake; renal insufficiency may decrease excretion and thus increase radiation exposure. Ensure adequate hydration before and after administration. Follow low-iodine diet for 1 to 2 weeks before treatment. Women should have negative pregnancy test prior to treatment and be advised not to conceive for at least 6 months.

MOA — Radioactive iodide that is trapped by thyroid tissue; radiation exposure results in cell destruction.

ADVERSE EFFECTS — Serious: Hypersensitivity, bone marrow suppression (high doses), acute thyroid crises, chromosomal abnormalities, death, sialadenitis, hypoparathyroidism, solid cancers. Frequent: Hypothyroidism.

THYROID—DESICCATED (*Nature-Throid, Westhroid, Thyroid USP, Armour Thyroid*) ▶L ♀A ▶? $

WARNING — Do not use for wt loss; possible serious or life-threatening toxic effects when used in euthyroid patients.

ADULT — Hypothyroidism: Start 30 mg PO daily, increase by 15 mg/day at 2- to 3-week intervals to a max dose of 180 mg/day.

PEDS — Congenital hypothyroidism: 15 mg PO daily. Increase at 2-week intervals.

FORMS — Generic/Trade: Tabs 15, 30, 60, 90, 120, 180, 240, 300 mg. Trade only: Tabs (Westhroid) 16.25, 32.5, 65, 130 mg. Tabs (Nature-Throid) 16.25, 32.5, 48.75, 65, 81.25, 97.5, 113.75, 130, 146.25, 162.5, 195, 260, 325 mg.

NOTES — Combination of levothyroxine (T4) and liothyronine (T3) with ratio of 4.2:1. Each grain (65 mg) of desiccated thryoid contains 38 mcg T4 and 9 mcg T3. Levothyroxine is recommended as the preferred supplement for primary hypothyroidism per American Thyroid Association.

MOA — Thyroid hormones from animal thyroid gland that increases metabolic rate of body tissues.

ADVERSE EFFECTS — Serious: Hyperthyroidism (arrhythmia, heart failure, angina, cardiac arrest), pseudotumor cerebri, hypersensitivity. Frequent: Palpitations, tachycardia, tremor, headache, nervousness, insomnia, diarrhea, vomiting, weight loss, menstrual irregularity, sweating, heat intolerance.

THYROLAR LIOTRIX (**levothyroxine + liothyronine**) ▶L ♀A ▶? $

WARNING — Do not use for wt loss; possible serious or life-threatening toxic effects when used in euthyroid patients.

ADULT — Hypothyroidism: 1 tab PO daily, starting with small doses initially (¼ to ½ strength), then increase at 2-week intervals.

PEDS — Not approved in children.

FORMS — Trade only: Tabs T4/T3 12.5 mcg/3.1 mcg (¼ strength), 25 mcg/6.25 mcg (half-strength), 50 mcg/12.5 mcg (#1), 100 mcg/25 mcg (#2), 150 mcg/37.5 mcg (#3).

NOTES — Combination of levothyroxine (T4) and liothyronine (T3).

MOA — Synthetic thyroid derivative that increases metabolic rate of body tissues.

ADVERSE EFFECTS — Serious: Hyperthyroidism (arrhythmia, heart failure, angina, cardiac arrest), pseudotumor cerebri. Frequent: Palpitations, tachycardia, tremor, headache, nervousness, insomnia, diarrhea, vomiting, weight loss, menstrual irregularity, sweating, heat intolerance.

ENDOCRINE AND METABOLIC: Vitamins

ASCORBIC ACID (*vitamin C, ✣Redoxon*) ▶K ♀C ▶? $

ADULT — Prevention of scurvy: 70 to 150 mg/day PO. Treatment of scurvy: 300 to 1000 mg/day PO. RDA females: 75 mg/day; males: 90 mg/day. Smokers: Add 35 mg/day more than nonsmokers.

PEDS — Prevention of scurvy: Infants: 30 mg/day PO. Treatment of scurvy: Infants: 100 to 300 mg/day PO. Adequate daily intake for infants 0 to 6 mo: 40 mg; 7 to 12 mo: 50 mg. RDA for children: 1 to 3 yo: 15 mg; 4 to 8 yo: 25 mg; 9 to 13 yo: 45 mg; 14 to 18 yo: 75 mg (males), 65 mg (females).

UNAPPROVED ADULT — Urinary acidification with methenamine: More than 2 g/day PO. Idiopathic

methemoglobinemia: 150 mg/day or more PO. Wound healing: 300 to 500 mg/day or more PO for 7 to 10 days. Severe burns: 1 to 2 g/day PO.

FORMS — OTC Generic only: Tabs 25, 50, 100, 250, 500, 1000 mg. Chewable tabs 100, 250, 500 mg. Timed-release tabs 500, 1000, 1500 mg. Timed-release caps 500 mg. Lozenges 60 mg. Liquid 35 mg/0.6 mL. Oral soln 100 mg/mL. Syrup 500 mg/5 mL.

NOTES — Use IV/IM/SC ascorbic acid for acute deficiency or when oral absorption is uncertain. Avoid excessive doses in diabetics, patients prone to renal calculi, those undergoing stool occult blood

(cont.)

ASCORBIC ACID (cont.)

tests (may cause false-negative), those on sodium-restricted diets, and those taking anticoagulants (may decrease INR). Doses in adults more than 2 g/day may cause osmotic diarrhea.

MOA — Water-soluble vitamin with antioxidant properties.

ADVERSE EFFECTS — Serious: Renal calculi, hypersensitivity. Frequent: Injection-site irritation (if IV).

CALCITRIOL (Rocaltrol) ▶L ♀C ▶? $$

ADULT — Hypocalcemia in chronic renal dialysis: Oral: 0.25 mcg PO daily, increase by 0.25 mcg q 4 to 8 weeks until normocalcemia achieved. Most hemodialysis patients require 0.5 to 1 mcg/day PO. Hypocalcemia and/or secondary hyperparathyroidism in chronic renal dialysis IV: 1 to 2 mcg, 3 times a week; increase dose by 0.5 to 1 mcg q 2 to 4 weeks. If PTH decreased less than 30%, then increase dose; if PTH decreased 30 to 60%, then maintain current dose; if PTH decreased more than 60%, then decrease dose; if PTH 1.5 to 3 times the upper normal limit, then maintain current dose. Hypoparathyroidism: 0.25 mcg PO q am; increase dose q 2 to 4 weeks if inadequate response. Most adults respond to 0.5 to 2 mcg/day PO. Secondary hyperparathyroidism in predialysis patients: 0.25 mcg PO q am; may increase dose to 0.5 mcg q am.

PEDS — Hypoparathyroidism 1 to 5 yo: 0.25 to 0.75 mcg PO q am. Age 6 yo or older: Give 0.25 mcg PO q am; increase dose in 2 to 4 weeks; usually respond to 0.5 to 2 mcg/day PO. Secondary hyperparathyroidism in predialysis patients, younger than 3 yo: 0.01 to 0.015 mcg/kg/day PO. Age 3 yo or older: 0.25 mcg q am; may increase dose to 0.5 mcg q am.

UNAPPROVED ADULT — Psoriasis vulgaris: 0.5 mcg/day PO or 0.5 mcg/g petrolatum topically daily.

FORMS — Generic/Trade: Caps 0.25, 0.5 mcg. Oral soln 1 mcg/mL. Injection 1 mcg/mL.

NOTES — Calcitriol is the activated form of vitamin D. During titration period, monitor serum calcium at least twice a week. Successful therapy requires an adequate daily calcium intake. Topical preparation must be compounded (not commercially available).

MOA — Vitamin D analogue that suppresses PTH secretion, bone resorption and increases gastrointestinal calcium absorption thus affecting bone homeostasis.

ADVERSE EFFECTS — Serious: Vitamin D toxicity/overdose, anaphylaxis, hypersensitivity, mild acidosis, renal toxicity, pancreatitis, arrhythmia, overt psychosis, elevated serum transaminases. Frequent: Weakness, headache, N/V, dry mouth, constipation, muscle pain, bone pain, metallic taste, irritability, weight loss, conjunctivitis, dyslipidemia, hypertension.

CYANOCOBALAMIN (vitamin B12, Nascobal, B-12 Compliance Injection, Physicians EZ Use B-12) ▶K ♀C ▶+ $

ADULT — See also "unapproved adult" dosing. Maintenance of nutritional deficiency following IM correction: 500 mcg (1 spray 1 nostril) intranasal weekly (Nascobal). Pernicious anemia: 100 mcg IM/SC daily, for 6 to 7 days, then every other day for 7 doses, then q 3 to 4 days for 2 to 3 weeks, then q month. Other patients with vitamin B12 deficiency: 30 mcg IM daily for 5 to 10 days, then 100 to 200 mcg IM q month. RDA for adults is 2.4 mcg.

PEDS — Nutritional deficiency: 100 mcg/24 h deep IM/SC for 10 to 15 days then at least 60 mcg/month IM/deep SC. Pernicious anemia: 30 to 50 mcg/24 h for 14 days or more to total dose of 1000 to 5000 mcg deep IM/SC then 100 mcg/month deep IM/SC. Adequate daily intake for infants: 0 to 6 mo: 0.4 mcg; 7 to 11 mo: 0.5 mcg. RDA for children: 1 to 3 yo: 0.9 mcg; 4 to 8 yo: 1.2 mcg; 9 to 13 yo: 1.8 mcg; 14 to 18 yo: 2.4 mcg.

UNAPPROVED ADULT — Pernicious anemia and nutritional deficiency states: 1000 to 2000 mcg PO daily for 1 to 2 weeks, then 1000 mcg PO daily. Prevention and treatment of cyanide toxicity associated with nitroprusside.

UNAPPROVED PEDS — Prevention/treatment of nitroprusside-associated cyanide toxicity.

FORMS — OTC Generic only: Tabs 100, 250, 500, 1000, 5000 mcg. Extended-release Tabs 1000 mcg. SL Tabs 2500 mcg. Lozenges 50, 100, 250, 500 mcg. Rx Trade only: Nasal spray 500 mcg/spray (Nascobal 2.3 mL). Rx Trade/Generic: Injection 1000 mcg/mL.

NOTES — Prime nasal pump before use per package insert directions. Although official dose for deficiency states is 100 to 200 mcg IM q month, some give 1000 mcg IM periodically. Oral supplementation is safe and effective for B12 deficiency even when intrinsic factor is not present. Monitor B12, folate, iron, and CBC.

MOA — Water-soluble vitamin required for purine nucleotides synthesis and amino acid metabolism.

ADVERSE EFFECTS — Serious: Anaphylaxis (IM), angioedema (IM). Frequent: Asthenia, dizziness, headache, infection, glossitis, nausea, paresthesia, rash, rhinitis (nasal), nasopharyngitis (nasal), nasal discomfort (nasal).

DOXERCALCIFEROL (Hectorol) ▶L ♀B ▶? $$$$$

ADULT — Secondary hyperparathyroidism on dialysis: Oral: If PTH greater than 400 pg/mL, start 10 mcg PO 3 times a week; if PTH greater than 300 pg/mL, increase by 2.5 mcg/dose q 8 weeks prn; if PTH 150 to 300 pg/mL, maintain current dose; if PTH less than 100 pg/mL, stop for 1 week, then resume at a dose at least 2.5 mcg lower. Max 60 mcg/week. IV: If PTH greater than 400 pg/mL, 4 mcg IV 3 times a week at the end of dialysis; if PTH decreased by less than 50% and greater than 300 pg/mL, increase by 1 to 2 mcg q 8 weeks as necessary; if PTH decreased by greater than 50% and greater than 300 pg/mL, maintain current dose; if PTH 150 to 300 pg/mL, maintain current dose; if PTH less than 100 pg/mL, stop for 1 week, then resume at a dose that is at least 1 mcg lower. Max 18 mcg/week. Secondary hyperparathyroidism not on dialysis: If PTH greater

(cont.)

DOXERCALCIFEROL (*cont.*)

than 70 pg/mL (Stage 3) or greater than 110 pg/mL (Stage 4), start 1 mcg PO daily; if PTH greater than 70 pg/mL (Stage 3) or greater than 110 pg/mL (Stage 4), increase by 0.5 mcg/dose q 2 weeks; if PTH 35 to 70 pg/mL (Stage 3) or 70 to 110 pg/mL (Stage 4), maintain current dose; if less than 35 pg/mL (Stage 3) or less than 70 pg/mL (Stage 4), stop for 1 week, then resume at a dose that is at least 0.5 mcg lower. Max 3.5 mcg/day.

PEDS — Not approved in children.

FORMS — Generic/Trade: Caps 0.5, 1, 2.5 mcg.

NOTES — Monitor PTH, serum calcium, and phosphorus weekly during dose titration; may need to monitor patients with hepatic insufficiency more closely. Serious hypersensitivity including anaphylaxis reported; monitor for reactions.

MOA — Vitamin D analogue that suppresses PTH secretion and bone resorption thus affecting bone homeostasis.

ADVERSE EFFECTS — Serious: Vitamin D toxicity/overdose, hypersensitivity/anaphylaxis, mild acidosis, renal toxicity, pancreatitis, arrhythmia, overt psychosis, elevated serum transaminases. Frequent: Weakness, headache, N/V, dry mouth, constipation, muscle pain, bone pain, metallic taste, irritability, weight loss, conjunctivitis, dyslipidemia, hypertension.

ERGOCALCIFEROL (*vitamin D2, Calciferol, Drisdol,* ✚*OsteoForte*) ▶L ♀A (C if exceed RDA) ▶+ $

ADULT — Familial hypophosphatemia (vitamin D–resistant rickets): 12,000 to 500,000 units PO daily. Hypoparathyroidism: 50,000 to 200,000 units PO daily. Adequate daily intake: 18 to 70 yo: 600 units (15 mcg); older than 70 yo: 800 units (20 mcg).

PEDS — Adequate daily intake: 1 to 18 yo 600 units (15 mcg). Hypoparathyroidism: 1.25 to 5 mg PO daily.

UNAPPROVED ADULT — Osteoporosis prevention and treatment (age 50 or older): 800 to 1000 units PO daily with calcium supplements. Fanconi syndrome: 50,000 to 200,000 units PO daily. Osteomalacia: 1000 to 5000 units PO daily. Anticonvulsant-induced osteomalacia: 2000 to 50,000 units PO daily. Vitamin D deficiency: 50,000 units PO weekly or biweekly for 8 to 12 weeks.

UNAPPROVED PEDS — Familial hypophosphatemia: 400,000 to 800,000 units PO daily, increased by 10,000 to 20,000 units/day q 3 to 4 months as needed. Hypoparathyroidism: 50,000 to 200,000 units PO daily. Fanconi syndrome: 250 to 50,000 units PO daily.

FORMS — OTC Generic only: Caps 400, 1000, 5000 units. Soln 8000 units/mL (Calciferol). Rx Generic/Trade: Caps 50,000 units. Rx Generic only: Caps 25,000 units.

NOTES — 1 mcg ergocalciferol = 40 units vitamin D. Sufficient level of 25(OH) vitamin D is greater than 20 ng/mL; optimal is greater than 30 ng/mL. Vitamin D2 (ergocalciferol) is less effective than vitamin D3 (cholecalciferol) in maintaining 25-OH

vitamin D levels; higher doses may be needed. IM or high-dose oral therapy may be necessary if malabsorption exists. Familial hypophosphatemia also requires phosphate supplementation; hypoparathyroidism also requires calcium supplementation.

MOA — Fat-soluble vitamin needed for calcium homeostasis (GI absorption, renal resorption, mobilization from bone).

ADVERSE EFFECTS — Serious: Vitamin D toxicity/overdose, hypersensitivity, mild acidosis, renal toxicity, pancreatitis, arrhythmia, overt psychosis, elevated serum transaminases. Frequent: Weakness, headache, N/V, dry mouth, constipation, muscle pain, bone pain, metallic taste, irritability, weight loss, conjunctivitis, dyslipidemia, hypertension.

FOLGARD (**folic acid + cyanocobalamin + pyridoxine**) ▶K ♀? ▶? $

ADULT — Nutritional supplement: 1 tab PO daily.

PEDS — Not approved in children.

FORMS — OTC Trade only: Folic acid 0.8 mg + cyanocobalamin 0.115 mg + pyridoxine 10 mg tab.

NOTES — Folic acid doses greater than 0.1 mg may obscure pernicious anemia, preventable with the concurrent cyanocobalamin.

MOA — Combination product containing 3 water-soluble vitamins that lowers plasma homocysteine.

ADVERSE EFFECTS — Serious: Masking pernicious anemia, sensory neuropathic syndromes. Frequent: Unstable gait, numb feet, awkwardness of the hands, perioral numbness, decreased sensations (touch, temperature, vibrations), paresthesia, photosensitivity, ataxia, asthenia, headache, infection, glossitis, nausea, rhinitis.

FOLGARD RX (**folic acid + cyanocobalamin + pyridoxine**) ▶K – ♀ ▶? $

ADULT — Nutritional supplement: 1 tab PO daily.

PEDS — Not approved in children.

FORMS — Trade only: Folic acid 2.2 mg + cyanocobalamin 1000 mcg + pyridoxine 25 mg tab.

NOTES — Folic acid doses greater than 0.1 mg may obscure pernicious anemia, preventable with the concurrent cyanocobalamin.

MOA — Combination product containing 3 water-soluble vitamins that lowers plasma homocysteine.

ADVERSE EFFECTS — Serious: Masking pernicious anemia, sensory neuropathic syndromes. Frequent: Unstable gait, numb feet, awkwardness of the hands, perioral numbness, decreased sensations (touch, temperature, vibrations), paresthesia, photosensitivity, ataxia, asthenia, headache, infection, glossitis, nausea, rhinitis.

FOLIC ACID (*folate*) ▶K ♀A ▶+ $

ADULT — Megaloblastic anemia: 1 mg PO/IM/IV/SC daily. When symptoms subside and CBC normalizes, give maintenance dose of 0.4 mg PO daily and 0.8 mg PO daily in pregnant and lactating females. RDA for adults: 0.4 mg, 0.6 mg for pregnant females, and 0.5 mg for lactating women. Max recommended daily dose 1 mg.

PEDS — Megaloblastic anemia: Infants: 0.05 mg PO daily, maintenance of 0.04 mg PO daily; Children:

(cont.)

FOLIC ACID (*cont.*)

0.5 to 1 mg PO daily, maintenance of 0.4 mg PO daily. Adequate daily intake for infants: 0 to 6 mo: 65 mcg; 7 to 12 mo: 80 mcg. RDA for children: 1 to 3 yo: 150 mcg; 4 to 8 yo: 200 mcg; 9 to 13 yo: 300 mcg, 14 to 18 yo: 400 mcg.
UNAPPROVED ADULT — Hyperhomocysteinemia: 0.5 to 1 mg PO daily.
FORMS — OTC Brand/Generic: Tabs 0.4, 0.8 mg. Rx Generic: Tabs 1 mg.
NOTES — Folic acid doses greater than 0.1 mg/day may obscure pernicious anemia. Prior to conception all women should receive 0.4 mg/day to reduce the risk of neural tube defects in infants. Consider high dose (up to 4 mg) in women with prior history of infant with neural tube defect. Use oral route except in cases of severe intestinal absorption.
MOA — Water-soluble vitamin that stimulates red blood cell, white blood cell, and platelet production, and is a cofactor for transformylation reactions.
ADVERSE EFFECTS — Serious: Masking pernicious anemia. Frequent: None.

FOLTX (folic acid + cyanocobalamin + pyridoxine) ▶K ♀A ▶+ $$

ADULT — Nutritional supplement for end-stage renal failure, dialysis, hyperhomocysteinemia, homocystinuria, nutrient malabsorption, or inadequate dietary intake: 1 tab PO daily.
PEDS — Not approved in children.
FORMS — Trade only: Folic acid 2.5 mg/cyanocobalamin 2 mg/pyridoxine 25 mg tab.
NOTES — Folic acid doses greater than 0.1 mg may obscure pernicious anemia, preventable with the concurrent cyanocobalamin.
MOA — Combination product containing 3 water-soluble vitamins that lowers plasma homocysteine.
ADVERSE EFFECTS — Serious: Masking pernicious anemia, sensory neuropathic syndromes. Frequent: Unstable gait, numb feet, awkwardness of the hands, perioral numbness, decreased sensations (touch, temperature, vibrations), paresthesia, photosensitivity, ataxia, asthenia, headache, infection, glossitis, nausea, rhinitis.

MULTIVITAMINS (MVI) ▶LK ♀+ ▶+ $

WARNING — Severe iron toxicity possible in overdose, especially in children. Store out of reach of children and in child-resistant containers. Iron overdose is a leading cause of poisoning in children younger than 6 yo.
ADULT — Dietary supplement: Dose varies by product.
PEDS — Dietary supplement: Dose varies by product.
FORMS — OTC and Rx: Many different brands and forms available with and without iron (tabs, caps, chewable tabs, gtts, liquid).
NOTES — Do not take within 2 h of antacids, tetracyclines, levothyroxine, or fluoroquinolones.
MOA — Combination vitamin that usually contains vitamins A, D, E, B1, B2, B3, B5, B6, B12, and C, biotin and folic acid.
ADVERSE EFFECTS — Usually no adverse effects in recommended doses (see individual vitamins).

NEPHRO-VITE RX (ascorbic acid + folic acid + niacin + thiamine + riboflavin + pyridoxine + pantothenic acid + biotin + cyanocobalamin) ▶K ♀? ▶? $

ADULT — Nutritional supplement for chronic renal failure, dialysis, hyperhomocysteinemia, or inadequate dietary vitamin intake: 1 tab PO daily. If on dialysis, take after treatment.
PEDS — Not approved in children.
FORMS — Generic/Trade: Vitamin C 60 mg/folic acid 1 mg/niacin 20 mg/thiamine 1.5 mg/riboflavin 1.7 mg/pyridoxine 10 mg/pantothenic acid 10 mg/biotin 300 mcg/cyanocobalamin 6 mcg.
NOTES — Folic acid doses greater than 0.1 mg/day may obscure pernicious anemia (preventable with the concurrent cyanocobalamin).
MOA — Combination product containing water-soluble vitamins.
ADVERSE EFFECTS — Serious: Masking pernicious anemia. Frequent: Mild transient diarrhea.

NEPHROCAP (ascorbic acid + folic acid + niacin + thiamine + riboflavin + pyridoxine + pantothenic acid + biotin + cyanocobalamin) ▶K ♀? ▶? $$$$

ADULT — Nutritional supplement for chronic renal failure, uremia, impaired metabolic functions of the kidney, and to maintain levels when the dietary intake of vitamins is inadequate or excretion and loss are excessive: 1 cap PO daily. If on dialysis, take after treatment.
PEDS — Not approved in children.
FORMS — Generic/Trade: Vitamin C 100 mg/folic acid 1 mg/niacin 20 mg/thiamine 1.5 mg/riboflavin 1.7 mg/pyridoxine 10 mg/pantothenic acid 5 mg/biotin 150 mcg/cyanocobalamin 6 mcg.
NOTES — Folic acid doses greater than 0.1 mg/day may obscure pernicious anemia (preventable with the concurrent cyanocobalamin).
MOA — Combination product containing water-soluble vitamins.
ADVERSE EFFECTS — Serious: Masking pernicious anemia. Frequent: Mild transient diarrhea.

NIACIN (*vitamin B3, nicotinic acid, Niacor, Slo-Niacin, Niaspan*) ▶K ♀C ▶? $

ADULT — Niacin deficiency: 100 mg PO daily. RDA: 16 mg for males, 14 mg for females. Hyperlipidemia: Start 50 to 100 mg PO two to three times per day with meals, increase slowly, usual maintenance range 1.5 to 3 g/day, max 6 g/day. Extended-release (Niaspan): Start 500 mg at bedtime with a low-fat snack for 4 weeks, increase prn q 4 weeks to max 2000 mg.
PEDS — Safety and efficacy not established for doses that exceed nutritional requirements. Adequate daily intake for infants: 0 to 6 mo: 2 mg; 7 to 12 mo: 3 mg. RDA for children: 1 to 3 yo: 6 mg; 4 to 8 yo: 8 mg; 9 to 13 yo: 12 mg; 14 to 18 yo: 16 mg (males) and 14 mg (females).
UNAPPROVED ADULT — Pellagra: 50 to 100 mg three to four times per day, up to 500 mg PO daily.
FORMS — OTC Generic only: Tabs 50, 100, 250, 500 mg. Timed-release caps 250, 500 mg. Timed-release tabs 250, 500 mg. Liquid 50 mg/5 mL. Trade only:

(cont.)

NIACIN (cont.)

250, 500, 750 mg (Slo-Niacin). Rx: Generic/Trade: Timed-release tabs 500, 750, 1000 mg (Niaspan, $$$$). Trade only: Tabs 500 mg (Niacor).

NOTES — Start with low doses and increase slowly to minimize flushing; 325 mg aspirin (non-EC) 30 to 60 min prior to niacin ingestion will minimize flushing. Use caution in diabetics, patients with gout, peptic ulcer, liver, or gallbladder disease. Extended-release formulations may have greater hepatotoxicity. Niacin has not been shown to reduce CV morbidity/mortality in patients on statins.

MOA — Water-soluble vitamin that serves as a coenzyme for oxidation-reduction reactions. Decreases lipoproteins associated with high LDL-cholesterol and triglycerides and increases lipoproteins associated with low HDL-cholesterol.

ADVERSE EFFECTS — Serious: Hepatotoxicity, diabetes, peptic ulcer disease, gout, hypotension, myopathy, creatine kinase increase, hepatitis. Frequent: Flushing, dyspepsia, vomiting, abdominal pain, rash, burning paresthesias.

PARICALCITOL (Zemplar) ▶L ♀C ▶? $$$$$

ADULT — Prevention/treatment of secondary hyperparathyroidism with renal insufficiency: If PTH less than 500 pg/mL, start 1 mcg PO daily or 2 mcg PO three times per week. If PTH greater than 500 pg/mL, start 2 mcg PO daily or 4 mcg PO three times per week. Can increase PO dose by 1 mcg daily or 2 mcg three times per week based on PTH in 2- to 4-week intervals. Prevention/treatment of secondary hyperparathyroidism with renal failure (CrCl <15 mL/min): PO: To calculate initial dose, divide baseline iPTH by 80 then administer this dose in mcg three times per week. To titrate dose based on response, divide recent iPTH by 80 then administer this dose in mcg three times per week. IV: Initially 0.04 to 0.1 mcg/kg (2.8 to 7 mcg) IV three times per week during dialysis. Can increase IV dose 2 to 4 mcg based on PTH in 2- to 4-week intervals. PO/IV: If PTH level decreased less than 30%, increase dose; if PTH level decreased 30 to 60%, maintain current dose; if PTH level decreased greater than 60%, decrease dose.

PEDS — Prevention/treatment of secondary hyperparathyroidism with renal failure (CrCl <15 mL/min): 0.04 to 0.1 mcg/kg (2.8 to 7 mcg) IV three times per week at dialysis; increase dose by 2 to 4 mcg or 0.04 mcg/kg q 2 to 4 weeks until desired PTH level is achieved. Max dose 0.24 mcg/kg (16.8 mcg).

FORMS — Generic/Trade: Caps 1, 2, 4 mcg.

NOTES — Monitor serum PTH, calcium, and phosphorus. IV doses up to 0.24 mcg/kg (16.8 mcg) have been administered. Do not initiate PO therapy in renal failure until calcium is 9.6 mg/dL or lower. Avoid prescription-based doses of vitamin D and derivatives to minimize the risk of hypercalcemia. Monitor closely (eg, twice weekly) during dosage adjustment for acute hypercalcemia. Chronic hypercalcemia may lead to vascular and soft tissue calcification. Do not administer with aluminum-containing medications; risk of aluminum toxicity. Risk of digoxin toxicity if hypercalcemia.

MOA — Vitamin D analogue that suppresses PTH secretion and bone resorption thus affecting bone homeostasis.

ADVERSE EFFECTS — Serious: Vitamin D toxicity/overdose, hypersensitivity, mild acidosis, renal toxicity, pancreatitis, arrhythmia, overt psychosis, elevated serum transaminases, angioedema, serum creatinine increase, hypercalcemia. Frequent: Weakness, headache, N/V, dry mouth, constipation, muscle pain, bone pain, metallic taste, irritability, weight loss, conjunctivitis, dyslipidemia, hypertension.

PHYTONADIONE (vitamin K, Mephyton, AquaMephyton) ▶L ♀C ▶+ $$$

WARNING — Severe reactions, including fatalities, have occurred during and immediately after IV injection, even with diluted injection and slow administration. Restrict IV use to situations where other routes of administration are not feasible.

ADULT — Excessive oral anticoagulation: Dose varies based on INR. INR 4.5 to 10: 2012 CHEST guidelines recommend against routine vitamin K administration; INR greater than 10 with no bleeding: 2012 CHEST guidelines recommend giving vitamin K, but do not specify a dose, 2008 guidelines previously recommended 5 to 10 mg PO; serious bleeding and elevated INR: 5 to 10 mg slow IV infusion. Hypoprothrombinemia due to other causes: 2.5 to 25 mg PO/IM/SC. Adequate daily intake: 120 mcg (males) and 90 mcg (females).

PEDS — Hemorrhagic disease of the newborn: Prophylaxis: 0.5 to 1 mg IM 1 h after birth; Treatment: 1 mg SC/IM.

UNAPPROVED PEDS — Nutritional deficiency: Children: 2.5 to 5 mg PO daily or 1 to 2 mg IM/SC/IV. Excessive oral anticoagulation: Infants: 1 to 2 mg IM/SC/IV q 4 to 8 h. Children: 2.5 to 10 mg PO/IM/SC/IV, may be repeated 12 to 48 h after PO dose or 6 to 8 h after IM/SC/IV dose.

FORMS — Trade only: Tabs 5 mg.

NOTES — Excessive doses of vitamin K in a patient receiving warfarin may cause warfarin resistance for up to a week. Avoid IM administration in patients with a high INR.

MOA — Fat-soluble vitamin that promotes formation of clotting factors.

ADVERSE EFFECTS — Serious: Anaphylactic reaction. Frequent: Injection-site reaction, flushing sensation, "peculiar" taste sensation.

PYRIDOXINE (vitamin B6) ▶K ♀A ▶+ $

ADULT — Dietary deficiency: 10 to 20 mg PO daily for 3 weeks. Prevention of deficiency due to isoniazid in high-risk patients: 10 to 25 mg PO daily. Treatment of neuropathies due to isoniazid: 50 to 200 mg PO daily. Isoniazid overdose (greater than 10 g): 4 g IV followed by 1 g IM over 30 min, repeat until total dose of 1 g for each g of isoniazid ingested. RDA for adults: 19 to 50 yo: 1.3 mg; older than 50 yo: 1.7

(cont.)

PYRIDOXINE (*cont.*)

mg (males), 1.5 mg (females). Max recommended: 100 mg/day.

PEDS — Adequate daily intake for infants: 0 to 6 mo: 0.1 mg; 7 to 12 mo: 0.3 mg. RDA for children: 1 to 3 yo: 0.5 mg; 4 to 8 yo: 0.6 mg; 9 to 13 yo: 1 mg; 14 to 18 yo: 1.3 (boys) and 1.2 mg (girls).

UNAPPROVED ADULT — Premenstrual syndrome: 50 to 500 mg/day PO. Hyperoxaluria type I and oxalate kidney stones: 25 to 300 mg/day PO. Prevention of oral contraceptive–induced deficiency: 25 to 40 mg PO daily. Hyperemesis of pregnancy: 10 to 50 mg PO q 8 h. Has been used in hydrazine poisoning.

UNAPPROVED PEDS — Dietary deficiency: 5 to 10 mg PO daily for 3 weeks. Prevention of deficiency due to isoniazid: 1 to 2 mg/kg/day PO daily. Treatment of neuropathies due to isoniazid: 10 to 50 mg PO daily. Pyridoxine-dependent epilepsy: Neonatal: 25 to 50 mg/dose IV; older infants and children: 100 mg/dose IV for 1 dose then 100 mg PO daily.

FORMS — OTC Generic only: Tabs 25, 50, 100, 250, 500 mg. Timed-release tab 100, 200 mg; Oral soln 200 mg/5 mL.

MOA — Water-soluble vitamin that is a coenzyme involved in numerous metabolic transformations of proteins and amino acids.

ADVERSE EFFECTS — Serious: Sensory neuropathic syndromes. Frequent: Unstable gait, numb feet, awkwardness of the hands, perioral numbness, decreased sensations (touch, temperature, vibrations), paresthesia, photosensitivity, ataxia.

RIBOFLAVIN (*vitamin B2*) ▶K ♀A ▶+ $

ADULT — Deficiency: 5 to 25 mg/day PO. RDA for adults: 1.3 mg (males) and 1.1 mg (females), 1.4 mg for pregnant women, 1.6 mg for lactating women.

PEDS — Deficiency: 5 to 10 mg/day PO. Adequate daily intake for infants: 0 to 6 mo: 0.3 mg; 7 to 12 mo: 0.4 mg. RDA for children: 1 to 3 yo: 0.5 mg; 4 to 8 yo: 0.6 mg; 9 to 13 yo: 0.9 mg; 14 to 18 yo: 1.3 mg (males) and 1 mg (females).

UNAPPROVED ADULT — Prevention of migraine headaches: 400 mg PO daily.

FORMS — OTC Generic only: Tabs 25, 50, 100 mg.

NOTES — May cause yellow/orange discoloration of urine.

MOA — Water-soluble vitamin that catalyzes oxidative-reduction reactions.

ADVERSE EFFECTS — Serious: None. Frequent: Yellow discoloration of urine.

THIAMINE (*vitamin B1*) ▶K ♀A ▶+ $

ADULT — Beriberi: 10 to 20 mg IM three times per week for 2 weeks. Wet beriberi with MI: 10 to 30 mg IV three times per day. Wernicke encephalopathy: 50 to 100 mg IV and 50 to 100 mg IM for 1 dose, then 50 to 100 mg IM daily until patient resumes normal diet. Give before starting glucose. RDA for adults: 1.2 mg (males) and 1.1 mg (females).

PEDS — Beriberi: 10 to 25 mg IM daily or 10 to 50 mg PO daily for 2 weeks then 5 to 10 mg PO daily for 1 month. Adequate daily intake infants: 0 to 6 mo: 0.2

mg; 7 to 12 mo: 0.3 mg. RDA for children: 1 to 3 yo: 0.5 mg; 4 to 8 yo: 0.6 mg; 9 to 13 yo: 0.9 mg; 14 to 18 yo: 1.2 mg (males), 1.0 mg (females).

FORMS — OTC Generic only: Tabs 50, 100, 250, 500 mg. Enteric-coated tabs 20 mg.

MOA — Water-soluble vitamin needed for carbohydrate metabolism, normal growth maintenance, nerve impulse transmission, and acetylcholine synthesis.

ADVERSE EFFECTS — Serious: Hypersensitivity, anaphylaxis, cyanosis, pulmonary edema, GI hemorrhage, cardiovascular shock. Frequent: Injection site reaction, feeling of warmth, pruritus, sweating, N/V, restlessness, angioedema.

VITAMIN A ▶L ♀A (C if exceed RDA, X in high doses) ▶+ $

ADULT — Treatment of deficiency states: 100,000 units IM daily for 3 days, then 50,000 units IM daily for 2 weeks. RDA: 1000 mcg RE (males), 800 mcg RE (females). Max recommended daily dose in nondeficiency 3000 mcg (see notes).

PEDS — Treatment of deficiency states: Infants: 7500 to 15,000 units IM daily for 10 days; children 1 to 8 yo: 17,500 to 35,000 units IM daily for 10 days. Kwashiorkor: 30 mg IM of water-soluble palmitate followed by 5000 to 10,000 units PO daily for 2 months. Xerophthalmia: Older than 1 yo: 110 mg retinyl palmitate PO or 55 mg IM plus 110 mg PO next day. Administer another 110 mg PO prior to discharge. Vitamin E (40 units) should be coadministered to increase efficacy of retinol. RDA for children: 0 to 6 mo: 400 mcg (adequate intake); 7 to 12 mo: 500 mcg; 1 to 3 yo: 300 mcg; 4 to 8 yo: 400 mcg; 9 to 13 yo: 600 mcg; 14 to 18 yo: 900 mcg (males), 700 mcg (females).

UNAPPROVED ADULT — Test for fat absorption: 7000 units/kg (2100 RE/kg) PO for 1 dose. Measure serum vitamin A concentrations at baseline and 4 h after ingestion. Dermatologic disorders such as follicularis keratosis: 50,000 to 500,000 units PO daily for several weeks.

UNAPPROVED PEDS — Has been tried in reduction of malaria episodes in children older than 12 mo and to reduce the mortality in HIV-infected children.

FORMS — OTC Generic only: Caps 8,000, 10,000, 15,000, 25,000 units; Tabs 10,000 units. Rx: Generic: Trade only: Soln 50,000 units/mL.

NOTES — 1 RE (retinol equivalent) = 1 mcg retinol or 6 mcg beta-carotene. Continued vitamin A/retinol intake of 2000 mcg/day or more may increase risk of hip fracture in postmenopausal women.

MOA — Fat-soluble vitamin needed for vision, dental development, growth, steroid synthesis, epithelial differentiation, embryonic development and reproduction.

ADVERSE EFFECTS — Serious: Vitamin A toxicity/overdose, hypersensitivity. Frequent: None.

VITAMIN D3 (*cholecalciferol*) ▶L – ♀ ▶+ $

ADULT — Familial hypophosphatemia (vitamin D–resistant rickets): 12,000 to 500,000 units PO daily. Hypoparathyroidism: 50,000 to 200,000 units PO daily. Adequate daily intake adults: 1 to 70 yo:

(cont.)

VITAMIN D3 (*cont.*)

600 units; older than 70 yo: 800 units. Max recommended daily dose in nondeficiency: 4000 units.

PEDS — Adequate daily intake: 1 to 18 yo 600 units. Hypoparathyroidism: 1.25 to 5 mg PO daily.

UNAPPROVED ADULT — Osteoporosis prevention and treatment (age 50 or older): 800 to 1000 units PO daily with calcium supplements.

UNAPPROVED PEDS — Familial hypophosphatemia: 400,000 to 800,000 units PO daily, increased by 10,000 to 20,000 units/day q 3 to 4 months as needed. Hypoparathyroidism: 50,000 to 200,000 units PO daily. Fanconi syndrome: 250 to 50,000 units PO daily.

FORMS — OTC Generic: 200, 400, 800, 1000, 2000, 4000, 5000 units (caps/tabs). Trade only: Soln 400, 1000, 2000, 4000 units/drop.

NOTES — Sufficient level of 25(OH) Vitamin D is greater than 20 ng/mL; optimal is greater than 30 ng/mL.

MOA — Fat-soluble vitamin needed for calcium homeostasis (GI absorption, renal resorption, mobilization from bone).

ADVERSE EFFECTS — Serious: Vitamin D toxicity/overdose, hypersensitivity, mild acidosis, renal toxicity, pancreatitis, arrhythmia, overt psychosis, elevated serum transaminases. Frequent: Weakness, headache, N/V, dry mouth, constipation, muscle pain, bone pain, metallic taste, irritability, weight loss, conjunctivitis, dyslipidemia, hypertension.

VITAMIN E (*tocopherol, ✤Aquasol E*) ▶L ♀A ▶? $

ADULT — RDA: 22 units (natural, d-alpha-tocopherol) or 33 units (synthetic, d,l-alpha-tocopherol) or 15 mg (alpha-tocopherol). Max recommended 1000 mg (alpha-tocopherol).

PEDS — Adequate daily intake (alpha-tocopherol): Infants 0 to 6 mo: 4 mg; 7 to 12 mo: 6 mg. RDA for children (alpha-tocopherol): 1 to 3 yo: 6 mg; 4 to 8 yo: 7 mg; 9 to 13 yo: 11 mg; 14 to 18 yo: 15 mg.

UNAPPROVED PEDS — Nutritional deficiency: Neonates: 25 to 50 units PO daily. Children: 1 unit/kg PO daily. Cystic fibrosis: 5 to 10 units/kg PO daily (use water-soluble form), max 400 units/day.

FORMS — OTC Generic only: Tabs 200, 400 units. Caps 73.5, 100, 147, 165, 200, 330, 400, 500, 600, 1000 units. Gtts 50 mg/mL.

NOTES — 1 mg alpha-tocopherol equivalents equals ~1.5 units. Natural vitamin E (d-alpha-tocopherol) recommended over synthetic (d,l-alpha-tocopherol). Higher doses may increase risk of bleeding. Large randomized trials have failed to demonstrate cardioprotective effects.

MOA — Fat-soluble vitamin that protects cellular constituents from oxidation.

ADVERSE EFFECTS — Serious: Vitamin E toxicity/overdose. Frequent: None.

ENDOCRINE AND METABOLIC: Other

AMMONUL (*sodium phenylacetate + sodium benzoate*) ▶KL ♀C ▶? $$$$$

ADULT — Acute hyperammonemia with encephalopathy in urea cycle enzyme deficiency: 55 mL/m² IV over 90 to 120 min, followed by maintenance 55 mL/m² over 24 h. Stop when hyperammonemia resolved or oral nutrition and medications are tolerated.

PEDS — Acute hyperammonemia with encephalopathy in urea cycle enzyme deficiency: If wt 20 kg or less, then 2.5 mL/kg IV over 90 to 120 min, followed by maintenance 2.5 mL/kg over 24 h. If greater than 20 kg, then 55 mL/m² IV over 90 to 120 min, followed by maintenance 55 mL/m² over 24 h. Consider coadministration of arginine in hyperammonemic infants. Stop when hyperammonemia resolved or oral nutrition and medications are tolerated.

FORMS — Single-use vial 50 mL (10% sodium phenylacetate/10% sodium benzoate).

NOTES — Administer through a central line. Closely monitor if renal insufficiency. Monitor plasma ammonia level, neurologic status, electrolytes, blood pH, blood pCO2 and clinical response. May cause hypokalemia. Consider coadministration of antiemetic. Penicillin and probenecid may affect renal secretion.

MOA — Serves an alternative to urea which effectively reduces waste nitrogen levels via hepatic conjugation and renal secretion.

ADVERSE EFFECTS — Serious: Neurotoxicity, brain edema, convulsions, pancytopenia, cardiac arrest, metabolic acidosis. Frequent: N/V, pyrexia, hyperglycemia, hypokalemia, hypotension, mental impairment.

BROMOCRIPTINE (*Cycloset, Parlodel*) ▶L ♀B ▶— $$$$$

ADULT — Type 2 DM: Start 0.8 mg PO q am, may increase by 0.8 weekly to max 4.8 mg. Hyperprolactinemia: Start 1.25 to 2.5 mg PO at bedtime, then increase q 3 to 7 days to usual effective dose of 2.5 to 15 mg/day, max 40 mg/day. Acromegaly: Usual effective dose is 20 to 30 mg/day, max 100 mg/day. Doses greater than 20 mg/day can be divided two times per day. Also approved for Parkinson's disease, but rarely used. Take with food to minimize dizziness and nausea.

PEDS — Not approved in children.

UNAPPROVED ADULT — Neuroleptic malignant syndrome: 2.5 to 5 mg PO 2 to 6 times per day. Hyperprolactinemia: 2.5 to 7.5 mg/day vaginally if GI intolerance occurs with PO dosing.

FORMS — Generic: Tabs 2.5 mg. Generic/Trade: Caps 5 mg. Trade only: Tabs 0.8 mg (Cycloset).

NOTES — Take with food to minimize dizziness and nausea. Ergots have been associated with potentially life-threatening fibrotic complications. Seizures, CVA, HTN, arrhythmias, and MI have been reported. Should not be used for postpartum

(cont.)

BROMOCRIPTINE (*cont.*)

lactation suppression. Contraindicated in Raynaud's syndrome. Avoid concomitant use of other ergot medications.

MOA — Dopamine agonist (ergot).

ADVERSE EFFECTS — Serious: Orthostatic hypotension, syncope, sleep attacks, shock, MI, stroke, arrhythmias, seizures, psychosis; retroperitoneal, pleural, pericardial, or cardiac valvular fibrosis, erythromelalgia, neutropenia and other blood dyscrasias, hemolytic anemia, adrenal insufficiency, hepatotoxicity, melanoma. Frequent: N/V, anorexia, diarrhea, constipation, abdominal pain, headache, dizziness, drowsiness, fatigue, confusion, orthostatic hypotension, edema, hallucinations, hypothyroidism, Parkinson's disease only: abnormal involuntary movements, urge to gamble, melanoma.

CABERGOLINE ▶L ♀B ▶– $$$$$

ADULT — Hyperprolactinemia: Initiate therapy with 0.25 mg PO twice a week. Increase by 0.25 mg twice a week at 4-week intervals up to a maximum of 1 mg twice a week.

PEDS — Not approved in children.

UNAPPROVED ADULT — Acromegaly: 0.5 mg PO twice a week. Increase prn up to 3.5 mg/week based on plasma IGF-1 levels.

FORMS — Generic: Tabs 0.5 mg.

NOTES — Monitor serum prolactin levels. Hepatically metabolized; use with caution in hepatic insufficiency. Contraindicated if cardiac vascular disease; perform pre-treatment cardiovascular evaluation for valvular disease. Associated with valvular disease, especially during use for Parkinson's with higher doses and longer durations of use, but also reported with lower doses in hyperprolactinemia. Monitor for valvular disease via echocardiogram q 6 to 12 months or as clinically indicated. Discontinue if signs of valvular thickening, regurgitation, or restriction. Postmarketing reports of pathological gambling, increased libido, and hypersexuality. Reports of fibrosis. Monitor for signs of pleural fibrosis (dyspnea, shortness of breath, cough), retroperitoneal fibrosis (renal insufficiency, flank pain, abdominal mass), and cardiac fibrosis (cardiac failure).

MOA — Dopamine agonist that decreases prolactin secretion.

ADVERSE EFFECTS — Serious: Hypotension, pulmonary fibrosis, pleural fibrosis, retroperitoneal fibrosis, pericardial fibrosis, increased ESR, valvulopathy. Frequent: Nausea, headache, dizziness, fatigue, lightheadedness, vomiting, abdominal cramps, rhinorrhea.

CALCITONIN (*Miacalcin, Fortical, ✦Calcimar*) ▶Plasma ♀C ▶? $$$

ADULT — Osteoporosis: 100 units SC/IM every other day or 200 units (1 spray) intranasal daily (alternate nostrils). Paget's disease: 50 to 100 units SC/IM daily or 3 times per week. Hypercalcemia: 4 units/kg SC/IM q 12 h. May increase after 2 days to maximum of 8 units/kg q 6 h.

PEDS — Not approved in children.

UNAPPROVED ADULT — Acute osteoporotic vertebral fracture pain: 100 units SC/IM daily or 200 units intranasal daily (alternate nostrils).

UNAPPROVED PEDS — Osteogenesis imperfecta, age 6 mo to 15 yo: 2 units/kg SC/IM 3 times per week with oral calcium supplements.

FORMS — Generic/Trade: Nasal spray 200 units/activation in 3.7 mL bottle (minimum of 30 doses/bottle).

NOTES — Skin test before using injectable product: 1 unit intradermally and observe for local reaction. Hypocalcemic effect diminishes in 2 to 7 days, therefore, only useful during acute short-term management of hypercalcemia.

MOA — Polypeptide hormone that decreases the rate of bone resorption.

ADVERSE EFFECTS — Serious: Antibody formation, hypersensitivity, anaphylaxis, bronchospasm, malignancy. Frequent: Nasal irritation, rhinitis, back pain, arthralgia, epistaxis, headache, sinusitis, dizziness, N/V, flushing, rash, abdominal pain, diarrhea, injection site irritation/urticaria (for SC/IM), tremor.

CINACALCET (*Sensipar*) ▶LK ♀C ▶? $$$$$

ADULT — Treatment of secondary hyperparathyroidism in dialysis patients: 30 mg PO daily. May titrate q 2 to 4 weeks through sequential doses of 60, 90, 120, and 180 mg daily to target intact parathyroid hormone level of 150 to 300 pg/mL. Treatment of hypercalcemia in parathyroid carcinoma or primary hyperparathyroidism unable to undergo parathyroidectomy: 30 mg PO two times per day. May titrate q 2 to 4 weeks through sequential does of 60 mg two times per day, 90 mg two times per day, and 90 mg three to four times per day as necessary to normalize serum calcium levels.

PEDS — Not approved in children.

FORMS — Trade only: Tabs 30, 60, 90 mg.

NOTES — Monitor serum calcium and phosphorus 1 week after initiation or dose adjustment, then monthly after a maintenance dose has been established. Intact parathyroid hormone should be checked 1 to 4 weeks after initiation or dose adjustment, and then 1 to 3 months after a maintenance dose has been established. For parathyroid carcinoma, monitor serum calcium within 1 week after initiation or dose adjustment, then q 2 months after a maintenance dose has been established. Withhold if serum calcium falls below less than 7.5 mg/dL or if signs and symptoms of hypocalcemia. May restart when calcium level reaches 8.0 mg/dL or when signs and symptoms of hypocalcemia resolve. Re-initiate using the next lowest dose. Use calcium-containing phosphate binder and/or vitamin D to raise calcium if it falls between 7.5 and 8.4 mg/dL. Seizure threshold reduced; QT may be prolonged; and arrhythmia, worsening heart failure, or hypotension may occur if hypocalcemia. Reduce dose or discontinue if intact parathyroid hormone level is less than 150 to 300 pg/mL to prevent adynamic bone disease. Do not check parathyroid

(cont.)

CINACALCET *(cont.)*

hormone levels within 12 h after administration of a dose. Inhibits metabolism by CYP2D6; may increase levels of flecainide, vinblastine, thioridazine, TCAs. Dose adjustment may be needed when initiating/ discontinuing a strong CYP3A4 inhibitor (eg, keto-conazole, erythromycin, and itraconazole). Closely monitor parathyroid hormone and serum calcium if moderate to severe hepatic impairment.

MOA — Lowers parathyroid hormone levels and decreases serum calcium by increasing sensitivity of the calcium-sensing receptor to extracellular calcium.

ADVERSE EFFECTS — Serious: Seizures, adynamic bone disease, hypocalcemia, hypotension, worsening heart failure, arrhythmia, hypersensitivity. Frequent: N/V, diarrhea, myalgia, dizziness, rash.

CONIVAPTAN *(Vaprisol)* ▶LK ♀C ▶? $$$$$

ADULT — Euvolemic or hypervolemic hyponatremia: Loading dose of 20 mg IV over 30 min, then continuous infusion 20 mg over 24 h for 2 to 4 days. Titrate to desired serum sodium. Max dose 40 mg daily as continuous infusion.

PEDS — Not approved in children.

NOTES — No benefit expected in anuric patients. Avoid concurrent use of CYP3A4 inhibitors (ketoconazole, itraconazole, clarithromycin, ritonavir, indinavir). May increase digoxin levels. Discontinue if hypovolemia, hypotension, or rapid rise in serum sodium (greater than 12 mEq/L/24 h) occurs. Rapid correction of serum sodium may cause osmotic demyelination syndrome. Requires frequent monitoring of serum sodium, volume, and neurologic status. Administer through large veins and change infusion site daily to minimize irritation. Not approved for hyponatremia in heart failure. Increased exposure to conivaptan in renal or hepatic impairment. Not recommended if CrCl <30 mL/min.

MOA — Selective vasopressin V2-receptor antagonist that promotes free water excretion to raise sodium levels.

ADVERSE EFFECTS — Serious: hypotension, hypovolemia. Frequent: Infusion site reactions, constipation, nausea, diarrhea, vomiting, infection, electrolyte changes, polyuria, erythema, hypotension, hypertension.

DENOSUMAB *(Prolia)* ▶? ♀X ▶? $$$$

ADULT — Postmenopausal osteoporosis: 60 mg SC q 6 months. Osteoporosis in men: 60 mg SC q 6 months. Increase bone mass in men receiving androgen deprivation therapy for nonmetastatic prostate cancer: 60 mg SC q 6 months. Increase bone mass in women receiving adjuvant aromatase inhibitor therapy for breast cancer at high risk of fracture: 60 mg SC q 6 months.

PEDS — Not approved in children.

FORMS — Trade only: 60 mg/1 mL vial (Prolia), prefilled syringe.

NOTES — Must correct hypocalcemia before administration; monitor serum calcium in all patients. In those predisposed to hypocalcemia and disturbances of mineral metabolism (eg, severe renal impairment or dialysis, hypoparathyroidism, thyroid/parathyroid surgery, malabsorption syndromes, excision of small intestine) monitor serum calcium, phosphorous, and magnesium within 14 days of administration. Elevations in PTH also noted in renal insufficiency. Prior to treatment, consider dental exam and appropriate preventive dentistry, particularly with risk factors (eg, cancer, chemotherapy, angiogenesis inhibitors, corticosteroids, poor oral hygiene). While on therapy, avoid invasive dental procedures when possible. Administered by a healthcare professional SC in upper arm, upper thigh, or abdomen. Give calcium 1000 mg and at least 400 international units vitamin D daily. Prolia contains same active ingredient (denosumab) as Xgeva; see Oncology section for Xgeva indications. Potential for hypercalcemia following treatment discontinuation in patients with growing skeletons.

MOA — RANK ligand (RANKL) inhibitor that decreases bone resorption.

ADVERSE EFFECTS — Serious: Hypocalcemia, serious infections, serious dermatologic reactions, cellulitis, osteonecrosis of the jaw, pancreatitis, hypersensitivity, anaphylaxis. Frequent: Dermatitis, rash, eczema, back pain, pain in extremity, hypercholesterlemia, musculoskeletal pain, cystitis, constipation.

DESMOPRESSIN *(DDAVP, Stimate, ✽Minirin, Octostim)* ▶LK ♀B ▶? $$$$$

WARNING — Adjust fluid intake downward to decrease potential water intoxication and hyponatremia; use cautiously in those at risk.

ADULT — Diabetes insipidus: 10 to 40 mcg (0.1 to 0.4 mL) intranasally daily or divided two to three times per day or 0.05 to 1.2 mg PO daily or divided two to three times per day or 0.5 to 1 mL (2 to 4 mcg) SC/IV daily in 2 divided doses. Hemophilia A, von Willebrand's disease: 0.3 mcg/kg IV over 15 to 30 min; 300 mcg intranasally if wt 50 kg or more (1 spray in each nostril), 150 mcg intranasally if wt less than 50 kg (single spray in 1 nostril). Primary nocturnal enuresis: 0.2 to 0.6 mg PO at bedtime.

PEDS — Diabetes insipidus 3 mo to 12 yo: 5 to 30 mcg (0.05 to 0.3 mL) intranasally once or twice daily or 0.05 mg PO daily. Hemophilia A, von Willebrand's disease (age 3 mo or older for IV, age 11 mo 12 yo for nasal spray): 0.3 mcg/kg IV over 15 to 30 min; 300 mcg intranasally if wt 50 kg or greater (1 spray in each nostril), 150 mcg intranasally if wt less than 50 kg (single spray in 1 nostril). Primary nocturnal enuresis, age 6 yo or older: 0.2 to 0.6 mg PO at bedtime.

UNAPPROVED ADULT — Uremic bleeding: 0.3 mcg/kg IV single dose or q 12 h (onset 1 to 2 h; duration 6 to 8 h after single dose). Intranasal is 20 mcg/day (onset 24 to 72 h; duration 14 days during 14-day course).

UNAPPROVED PEDS — Hemophilia A and type 1 von Willebrand's disease: 2 to 4 mcg/kg intranasally or 0.2 to 0.4 mcg/kg IV over 15 to 30 min.

(cont.)

DESMOPRESSIN (*cont.*)

FORMS — Trade only: Stimate nasal spray 150 mcg/0.1 mL (1 spray), 2.5 mL bottle (25 sprays). Generic/Trade (DDAVP nasal spray): 10 mcg/0.1 mL (1 spray), 5 mL bottle (50 sprays). Note difference in concentration of nasal soln. Rhinal tube: 2.5 mL bottle with 2 flexible plastic tube applicators with graduation marks for dosing. Tabs 0.1, 0.2 mg.

NOTES — Monitor serum sodium and for signs/symptoms of hyponatremia including headache, wt gain, altered mental status, muscle weakness/cramps, seizure, coma, or respiratory arrest. Restrict fluid intake 1 h before to 8 h after PO administration. Hold PO treatment for enuresis during acute illnesses that may cause fluid/electrolyte imbalances. Start at lowest dose with diabetes insipidus. IV/SC doses are approximately 1/10 the intranasal dose. Anaphylaxis reported with both IV and intranasal forms. Do not give if type IIB von Willebrand's disease. Changes in nasal mucosa may impair absorption of nasal spray. Refrigerate nasal spray; stable for 3 weeks at room temperature. 10 mcg = 40 units desmopressin.

MOA — Synthetic vasopressin analogue with a rapid onset that promotes water resorption (anti-diuretic effect). Increases Factor VIII and von Willebrand's factor activity.

ADVERSE EFFECTS — Serious: Anaphylaxis, seizures (hyponatremia-associated), hyponatremia, fluid overload, chest pain, thrombotic events (rare). Frequent: Abdominal pain, flushing, headache, nasal congestion, nausea, rhinitis, agitation, balanitis, chills, increased blood pressure, sore throat, local irritation, epistaxis.

DIAZOXIDE (*Proglycem*) ▶L ♀C ▶– $$$$$

ADULT — Hypoglycemia from hyperinsulinism: Initially 3 mg/kg/day PO divided equally q 8 h, usual maintenance dose 3 to 8 mg/kg/day divided equally q 8 to 12 h, max 10 to 15 mg/kg/day.

PEDS — Hypoglycemia from hyperinsulinism: Neonates and infants, initially 10 mg/kg/day divided equally q 8 h, usual maintenance dose 8 to 15 mg/kg/day divided equally q 8 to 12 h; children, same as adult.

FORMS — Trade only: Susp 50 mg/mL (30 mL).

NOTES — Close monitoring of blood glucose required. Consider reduced dose in renal impairment. Used for hyperinsulinism associated with islet cell adenoma, carcinoma, or hyperplasia; extrapancreatic malignancy, leucine sensitivity in children, nesidioblastosis. Avoid if hypersensitivity to thiazides or sulfonamide derivatives. Caution in gout; may increase uric acid. Monitor for edema and heart failure exacerbation during administration; diuretic therapy may be needed. Monitor for signs/symptoms of pulmonary hypertension when used in newborns and infants.

MOA — Inhibits insulin release from the pancreas

ADVERSE EFFECTS — Serious: heart failure, diabetic ketoacidosis, hyperosmolar nonketotic coma, tachycardia, thrombocytopenia, hypotension, pulmonary hypertension (newborns/infants). Common: hirsutism, hyperglycemia, glycosuria, N/V, anorexia, diarrhea, loss of taste, sodium/water retention, increased uric acid.

MIFEPRISTONE (*Korlym*) ▶L ♀X ▶– $$$$$

ADULT — Hyperglycemia in Cushing's syndrome (failed surgery or not surgical candidate): 300 mg PO once daily with meal. Titrate to max of 1200 mg daily as tolerated. Max 20 mg/kg/day. In renal impairment or mild to moderate hepatic impairment, max 600 mg/day.

PEDS — Not approved in peds.

FORMS — Trade only: Tabs 300 mg.

NOTES — Contraindicated in pregnancy; antiprogestational effects result in termination. Confirm no pregnancy prior to initiation and if treatment is interrupted for more than 14 days in women of reproductive age. Do not use in women with endometrial hyperplasia or carcinoma or unexplained vaginal bleeding. Not for use in Type 2 DM unrelated to Cushing's syndrome. Monitor for signs and symptoms of adrenal insufficiency.

MOA — Cortisol receptor blockade

ADVERSE EFFECTS — Serious: pregnancy termination, adrenal insufficiency, hypokelemia, vaginal bleeding, endometrial changes, QT interval prolongation. Frequent: N/V, fatigue, HA, arthralgia, edema, decreased appetite, dizziness, HTN.

PARATHYROID HORMONE (*Natpara*) ▶LK ♀C ▶? $$$$$

WARNING — Osteosarcoma in animal studies; avoid in those at risk (eg, Paget's disease, prior skeletal radiation). Available through a restricted access program.

ADULT — Hypocalcemia in hypoparathyroidism: Start 50 mcg SC once daily in thigh (alternate thigh every other day). Adjust dose by 25 mcg q 4 weeks to max of 100 mcg to achieve serum calcium 8 to 9 mg/dL.

PEDS — Not approved for use in children.

FORMS — Trade only: 25, 50, 75, 100 mcg dose strength cartridges. Available through restricted-access program (NATPARA REMS).

NOTES — Before initiation, confirm 25(OH) vitamin D stores sufficient and serum calcium above 7.5 mg/dL. Decrease dose of active vitamin D by 50% upon initiation. Monitor serum calcium within 3 to 7 days. See product information for detailed instructions of how to adjust drug, active vitamin D, and calcium supplement doses.

MOA — Parathyroid hormone that increases renal tubular calcium reabsorption, bone turnover, and intestinal calcium absorption (through conversion of 25 OH vitamin D to 1,25 OH2 vitamin D).

ADVERSE EFFECTS — Serious: hypercalcemia, hypocalcemia. Common: Paresthesia, headache, nausea, loss of sensitivity to touch, diarrhea, vomiting, arthralgia, hypercalciuria, pain in extremity.

PATIROMER (*Veltassa*) ▶not absorbed ♀– 0/0/0 ▶+ $$$$$

WARNING — Binds to PO medications; give other PO meds 6 h before or 6 h after patiromer.

ADULT — Hyperkalemia: 8.4 g PO daily with food. Adjust by 8.4 g daily on weekly basis as needed to achieve desired serum K+.

(cont.)

PATIROMER (*cont.*)

PEDS — Not approved for use in children.

FORMS — Trade only: 8.4, 16.8, 22.2 g packets.

MOA — Binds potassium in GI tract to increase fecal excretion of potassium and reduce serum potassium levels.

ADVERSE EFFECTS — Serious: hypomagnesemia, hypersensitivity. Common: constipation, diarrhea, nausea, abdominal discomfort, flatulence.

SODIUM POLYSTYRENE SULFONATE (*Kayexalate*)
▶Fecal excretion ♀C ▶? $

ADULT — Hyperkalemia: 15 g PO one to four times per day or 30 to 50 g retention enema (in sorbitol) q 6 h prn. Retain for 30 min to several h. Irrigate with tap water after enema to prevent necrosis.

PEDS — Hyperkalemia: 1 g/kg PO q 6 h.

UNAPPROVED PEDS — Hyperkalemia: 1 g/kg PR q 2 to 6 h.

FORMS — Generic only: Susp 15 g/60 mL. Powdered resin.

NOTES — 1 g binds approximately 1 mEq of potassium. Avoid in bowel obstruction, constipation, or abnormal bowel function, including patients without a bowel movement post-surgery. Avoid administration with sorbitol as intestinal necrosis has been reported. Discontinue use if constipation develops. Follow aspiration cautions during oral administration.

MOA — Cation exchange resin that reduces potassium in exchange for sodium.

ADVERSE EFFECTS — Serious: Hypokalemia, hypocalcemia, hypomagnesemia, intestinal obstruction, intestinal necrosis, serious GI events (bleeding, perforation). Frequent: Sodium and water retention, gastric irritation, anorexia, N/V, constipation.

SOMATROPIN (*human growth hormone, Genotropin, Gentropin MiniQuick, Humatrope, Norditropin FlexPro, Nutropin AQ NuSpin, Nutropin AQ Pen, Omnitrope, Saizen, Serostim, Valtropin, Zomacton, Zorbitive*) ▶LK ♀B/C ▶? $$$$$

WARNING — Avoid in patients with Prader-Willi syndrome who are severely obese, have severe respiratory impairment or sleep apnea, or unidentified respiratory infection; fatalities have been reported.

ADULT — Growth hormone deficiency (Genotropin, Humatrope, Norditropin FlexPro, Nutropin AQ NuSpin, Omnitrope, Saizen): Doses vary according to product. AIDS wasting or cachexia (Serostim): 0.1 mg/kg SC daily, max 6 mg daily. Short bowel syndrome (Zorbtive): 0.1 mg/kg SC daily, max 8 mg daily.

PEDS — Growth hormone deficiency (Genotropin, Humatrope, Norditropin FlexPro, Nutropin AQ NuSpin, Omnitrope, Saizen, Zomacton): Doses vary according to product used. Turner syndrome (Genotropin, Humatrope, Norditropin FlexPro, Nutropin AQ NuSpin): Doses vary according to product used. Growth failure in Prader-Willi syndrome (Genotropin, Omnitrope): Individualized dosing. Idiopathic short stature (Genotropin, Humatrope): Individualized dosing. SHOX deficiency (Humatrope): Individualized dosing. Short stature in Noonan syndrome (Norditropin FlexPro): Individualized dosing. Growth failure in chronic renal insufficiency (Nutropin AQ NuSpin): Individualized dosing. Short stature in small for gestational age children (Humatrope, Norditropin FlexPro, Omnitrope): Individualized dosing.

FORMS — Single-dose vials (powder for injection with diluent): Omnitrope: 5.8 mg vial. Saizen 5, 8.8 mg vial. Zomacton: 5, 10 mg vial. Zorbtive: 8.8 mg vial. Cartridges: Genotropin MiniQuick: 0.2, 0.4, 0.6, 0.8, 1, 1.2, 1.4, 1.6, 1.8, 2 single-use injection; 5.8, 13.8 mg cartridges. Humatrope: 6, 12, 24 mg pen cartridges; 5 mg vial (powder for injection with diluent). Pens: Norditropin FlexPro: 5, 10, 15, 30 mg. Nutropin AQ NuSpin: 5, 10, 20 mg. Omnitrope: 5, 10 mg. Saizen Click.Easy 8.8 mg. Serostim: 4, 5, 6 mg single-dose vials.

NOTES — Do not use in children with closed epiphyses. Contraindicated in active malignancy or critical illness. Increased risk of developing a second neoplasm in childhood cancer survivors who received radiation to the brain/head. Monitor glucose for insulin resistance; use with caution if DM or risk for DM. Transient and dose-dependent fluid retention may occur in adults. May cause hypothyroidism. Monitor thyroid function periodically. Evaluate patients with Prader-Willi syndrome for upper airway obstruction and sleep apnea prior to treatment; control wt and monitor for signs and symptoms of respiratory infection. Avoid if pre-proliferative or proliferative diabetic retinopathy. Perform funduscopic exam initially and then periodically. Monitor other hormonal replacement treatments closely in patients with hypopituitarism. Risk of pancreatitis may be greater in children, especially girls with Turner syndrome; consider pancreatitis if persistent abdominal pain.

MOA — Recombinantly derived human growth hormone that stimulates production of IGF-1.

ADVERSE EFFECTS — Serious: Diabetes, impaired glucose tolerance, antibody production, leukemia, pancreatitis, intracranial hypertension, dyspnea, malignancy. Frequent: Edema, increased nevi size, gynecomastia, headache, localized pain, weakness, hyperglycemia, injection-site pain, hypothyroidism, hypertension, sleep apnea.

TERIPARATIDE (*Forteo*) ▶LK ♀C ▶– $$$$$

WARNING — Osteosarcoma in animal studies; avoid in those at risk (eg, Paget's disease, prior skeletal radiation).

ADULT — Treatment of postmenopausal osteoporosis, treatment of men and women with glucocorticoid-induced osteoporosis, or to increase bone mass in men with primary or hypogonadal osteoporosis and high risk for fracture: 20 mcg SC daily in thigh or abdomen for no longer than 2 years.

PEDS — Not approved in children.

FORMS — Trade only: 28-dose pen injector (20 mcg/dose).

(cont.)

TERIPARATIDE (*cont.*)

NOTES — Take with calcium and vitamin D. Pen-like delivery device requires education, and should be discarded 28 days after 1st injection even if not empty.

MOA — Parathyroid hormone analogue that stimulates trabecular and cortical bone formation.

ADVERSE EFFECTS — Serious: Orthostatic hypotension, HTN, angina, hypercalcemia, hyperuricemia. Frequent: Dizziness, leg cramps/spasms, back spasm, asthenia, arthralgia, depression, insomnia, dyspepsia.

TOLVAPTAN (*Samsca*) ▶K ♀C ▶? $$$$$

WARNING — Start and restart therapy in the hospital setting to closely monitor serum sodium. Avoid rapid correction of serum sodium (greater than 12 mEq/L/24 h); rapid correction may cause osmotic demyelination causing death or symptoms including dysarthria, dysphagia, lethargy, seizures, or coma. Slower correction advised in higher risk patients including malnutrition, alcoholism, or advanced liver disease.

ADULT — Euvolemic or hypervolemic hyponatremia (sodium less than 125 mEq/L): Start 15 mg PO daily. Titrate to desired serum sodium. If needed, increase q 24 h or more slowly to 30 mg PO daily; max dose 60 mg daily.

PEDS — Not approved in children.

FORMS — Trade only: Tabs 15, 30 mg.

NOTES — Avoid fluid restriction for first 24 h. May use for hyponatremia secondary to heart failure or SIADH. May use in hyponatremia with sodium greater than 125 mEq/L if resistant to fluid restriction and symptomatic. Do not use if urgent rise in serum sodium needed or serious neurologic symptoms. Requires frequent monitoring of serum sodium, volume, and neurologic status; monitor potassium if baseline K+ greater than 5 mEq/L. Avoid concurrent use of strong or moderate CYP3A4 inhibitors or inducers. Reports of liver injury, including fatal hepatotoxicity; do not use if underlying liver disease and limit use to 30 days.

MOA — Selective vasopressin V2-receptor antagonist that promotes free water excretion to raise sodium levels.

ADVERSE EFFECTS — Serious: Hypotension, hypovolemia, GI bleed (in cirrhosis), osmotic demyelination syndrome, hypernatremia, hepatotoxicity, hypersensitivity (anaphylactic shock). Frequent: Thirst, dry mouth, asthenia, constipation, polyuria, hyperglycemia.

ENT

ENT COMBINATIONS (selected). Formulations and names change frequently.

	Decongestant	Antihistamine	Antitussive	Typical Adult Doses
OTC				
Benadryl-D Allergy/ Sinus Tablets	phenylephrine	diphenhydramine	–	1 tab q 4 h
Claritin-D 12-h, Alavert D-12	pseudoephedrine	loratadine	–	1 tab q 12 h
Claritin-D 24-h	pseudoephedrine	loratadine	–	1 tab daily
Dimetapp Cold & Allergy Elixir	phenylephrine	brompheniramine	–	20 mL q 4 h
Dimetapp DM Cold & Cough	phenylephrine	brompheniramine	dextromethorphan	20 mL q 4 h
Drixoral Cold & Allergy	pseudoephedrine	dexbrompheniramine	–	1 tab q 12 h
Mucinex-DM Extended- Release	–	–	guaifenesin, dextromethorphan	1–2 tabs q 12 h
Robitussin CF	phenylephrine	–	guaifenesin, dextromethorphan	10 mL q 4 h*
Robitussin DM, Mytussin DM	–	–	guaifenesin, dextromethorphan	10 mL q 4 h*
Robitussin PE, Guiatuss PE	phenylephrine	–	guaifenesin	10 mL q 4 h*B
Triaminic Cold & Allergy	phenylephrine	chlorpheniramine	–	10 mL q 4 h*
Rx Only				
Allegra-D 12-h	pseudoephedrine	fexofenadine	–	1 tab q 12 h
Allegra-D 24-h	pseudoephedrine	fexofenadine	–	1 tab daily
Bromfenex	pseudoephedrine	brompheniramine	–	1 cap q 12 h
Clarinex-D 24-h	pseudoephedrine desloratadine	desloratadine	–	1 tab daily
Deconamine	pseudoephedrine	chlorpheniramine	–	1 tab or 10 mL tid–qid
Deconamine SR, Chlordrine SR	pseudoephedrine hlorpheniramine	chlorpheniramine	–	1 tab q 12 h

(cont.)

ENT COMBINATIONS (selected). Formulations and names change frequently. (*continued*)

	Decongestant	Antihistamine	Antitussive	Typical Adult Doses
Rx Only				
Deconsal I	phenylephrine	–	guaifenesin	1–2 tabs q 12 h
Dimetane-DX	pseudoephedrine	brompheniramine	dextromethorphan	10 mL PO q 4 h
Duratuss	phenylephrine	–	guaifenesin	1 tab q 12 h
Duratuss HD©II	phenylephrine	–	guaifenesin, hydrocodone	5-10 mL q 4–6 h
Entex PSE, Guaifenex PSE 120	pseudoephedrine	–	guaifenesin	1 tab q 12 h
Histussin D ©II	pseudoephedrine	–	hydrocodone	5 mL qid
Histussin HC ©II	phenylephrine	chlorpheniramine	hydrocodone	10 mL q 4 h
Humibid DM	–	–	guaifenesin, dextromethorphan	1 tab q 12 h
Hycotuss ©II	–	–	guaifenesin, hydrocodone	5 mL after meals & at bedtime
Phenergan/ Dextromethorphan	promethazine	promethazine	dextromethorphan	5 mL q 4–6 h
Phenergan VC	phenylephrine	promethazine	–	5 mL q 4–6 h
Phenergan VC w/codeine ©V	phenylephrine	promethazine	codeine	5 mL q 4–6 h
Robitussin AC ©V (generic only)	–	–	guaifenesin, codeine	10 mL q 4 h*
Robitussin DAC ©V (generic only)	pseudoephedrine	–	guaifenesin, codeine	10 mL q 4 h*
Rondec Syrup	phenylephrine	chlorpheniramine	–	5 mL qid†
Rondec DM Syrup	phenylephrine	chlorpheniramine	dextromethorphan	5 mL qid†
Rondec Oral Drops	phenylephrine	chlorpheniramine	–	0.75 to 1 mL qid

(cont.)

ENT COMBINATIONS (selected). Formulations and names change frequently. (*continued*)

	Decongestant	Antihistamine	Antitussive	Typical Adult Doses
Rx Only				
Rondec DM Oral Drops	phenylephrine	chlorpheniramine	dextromethorphan	0.75 to 1 mL qid
Rynatan	phenylephrine	chlorpheniramine	–	1–2 tabs q 12 h
Rynatan-P Pediatric	phenylephrine	chlorpheniramine	–	2.5–5 mL q 12 h*
Semprex-D	pseudoephedrine	acrivastine	–	1 cap q 4–6 h
Tanafed (generic only)	pseudoephedrine	chlorpheniramine	–	10–20 mL q 12 h*
Tussionex ©II	–	chlorpheniramine	hydrocodone	5 mL q 12 h

tid = three times per day; qid = four times per day
*5 mL/dose if 6–11 yo. 2.5 mL if 2–5 yo.
†2.5 mL/dose if 6–11 yo. 1.25 mL if 2–5 yo.
‡Also contains acetaminophen.

ENT: Antihistamines—Non-Sedating

NOTE: Antihistamines ineffective when treating the common cold.

DESLORATADINE (*Clarinex*, ✱*Aerius*) ▶LK ♀C ▶+ $
WARNING — Some products contain phenylalanine.
ADULT — Allergic rhinitis/urticaria: 5 mg PO daily.
PEDS — Allergic rhinitis/urticaria: 2 mL (1 mg) PO daily for age 6 to 11 mo, ½ teaspoonful (1.25 mg) PO daily for age 12 mo to 5 yo, 1 teaspoonful (2.5 mg) or 2.5 mg ODT PO daily for age 6 to 11 yo, 5 mg PO daily for age older than 12 yo.
FORMS — Generic/Trade: Tabs 5 mg. Orally disintegrating tabs 2.5, 5 mg. Trade only: Syrup 0.5 mg/mL.
NOTES — Increase dosing interval in liver or renal insufficiency to every other day. Use a measured dropper for syrup.
MOA — Antihistamine.
ADVERSE EFFECTS — Serious: None. Frequent: None.
FEXOFENADINE (*Allegra*) ▶LK ♀C ▶+ $
WARNING — Some products contain phenylalanine.
ADULT — Allergic rhinitis, urticaria: 60 mg PO two times per day or 180 mg PO daily. 60 mg PO daily if decreased renal function.
PEDS — Allergic rhinitis, urticaria: 30 mg PO two times per day or orally disintegrating tab two times per day for age 2 to 11 yo. Use adult dose for age 12 yo or older. 30 mg PO daily if decreased renal function. Urticaria: 15 mg (2.5 mL) twice daily for age 6 mo to younger than 2 yo. 15 mg PO daily if decreased renal function.
FORMS — OTC Generic/Trade: Tabs 30, 60, 180 mg. Susp 30 mg/5 mL. Trade only: Orally disintegrating tab 30 mg.
NOTES — Avoid taking with fruit juice due to a large decrease in bioavailability. Do not remove orally disintegrating tab from its blister package until time of administration.
MOA — Antihistamine.
ADVERSE EFFECTS — Serious: None. Frequent: None.
LORATADINE (*Claritin, Claritin Hives Relief, Claritin RediTabs, Alavert, Tavist ND*) ▶LK ♀B ▶+ $
WARNING — Some products contain phenylalanine.
ADULT — Allergic rhinitis/urticaria: 10 mg PO daily.
PEDS — Allergic rhinitis/urticaria: 5 mg PO daily (syrup) for age 2 to 5 yo, 10 mg PO daily for age older than 6 yo.
FORMS — OTC Generic/Trade: Tabs 10 mg. Fast-dissolve tabs (Alavert, Claritin RediTabs) 5, 10 mg. Syrup 1 mg/mL. Rx Trade only (Claritin): Chewable tabs 5 mg; Liqui-gel caps 10 mg.

(cont.)

LORATADINE (*cont.*)

NOTES — Decrease dose in liver failure or renal insufficiency. Fast-dissolve tabs dissolve on tongue without water. ND indicates nondrowsy (Tavist).

MOA — Antihistamine.
ADVERSE EFFECTS — Serious: None. Frequent: None.

ENT: Antihistamines—Other

NOTE: Antihistamines ineffective when treating the common cold. Contraindicated in narrow-angle glaucoma, BPH, stenosing peptic ulcer disease, and bladder obstruction. Use half the normal dose in the elderly. May cause drowsiness and/or sedation, which may be enhanced with alcohol, sedatives, and other CNS depressants. Deaths have occurred in children younger than 2 yo attributed to toxicity from cough and cold medications; the FDA does not recommend their use in this age group.

CARBINOXAMINE (*Palgic, Karbinal ER*) ▶L ♀C ▶– $$$
ADULT — Allergic/vasomotor rhinitis/urticaria: 4 to 8 mg PO three to four times per day.
PEDS — Allergic/vasomotor rhinitis/urticaria: Give 2 mg PO three to four times per day for age 2 to 3 yo, give 2 to 4 mg PO three to four times per day for age 3 to 6 yo, give 4 to 6 mg PO three to four times per day for age 6 yo or older.
FORMS — Generic/Trade: Oral soln 4 mg/5 mL. Tabs 4 mg. Trade only: Extended-release suspension 4 mg/5 mL (Karbinal ER).
NOTES — Decrease dose in hepatic impairment.
MOA — Antihistamine.
ADVERSE EFFECTS — Serious: None. Frequent: Sedation, dizziness.

CETIRIZINE (*Zyrtec, ✦Reactine, Aller-Relief*) ▶LK ♀B ▶– $
ADULT — Allergic rhinitis/urticaria: 5 to 10 mg PO daily.
PEDS — Allergic rhinitis/urticaria: Age 6 yo and older: 5 to 10 mg PO daily. Age 2 to 5 yo: initial dose 2.5 mg PO daily, max dose 2.5 mg twice a day or 5 mg once a day. Age 12 mo to < 2 yo: 2.5 mg daily with max dose of 2.5 mg twice a day. Age 6 mos to < 12 mos: 2.5 mg daily.
FORMS — OTC Generic/Trade: Tabs 5, 10 mg. Syrup 5 mg/5 mL. Chewable tabs, grape flavored 5, 10 mg. Trade only: oral disintegrating tab 10 mg, caps 10 mg.
NOTES — Decrease dose in renal or hepatic impairment.
MOA — Antihistamine.
ADVERSE EFFECTS — Serious: None. Frequent: Sedation in 14%.

CHLORPHENIRAMINE (*Chlor-Trimeton, Aller-Chlor*) ▶LK ♀B ▶– $
ADULT — Allergic rhinitis: 4 mg PO q 4 to 6 h. 8 mg PO q 8 to 12 h (timed-release) or 12 mg PO q 12 h (timed-release). Max 24 mg/day.
PEDS — Allergic rhinitis: 2 mg PO q 4 to 6 h (up to 12 mg/day) for age 6 to 11 yo, give adult dose for age 12 yo or older.
UNAPPROVED PEDS — Allergic rhinitis, age 2 to 5 yo: 1 mg PO q 4 to 6 h (up to 6 mg/day). Timed-release, age 6 to 11 yo: 8 mg PO q 12 h prn.
FORMS — Generic/Trade: Tabs 4 mg. Syrup 2 mg/5 mL. Tabs, extended-release 12 mg.
MOA — Antihistamine.

ADVERSE EFFECTS — Serious: None. Frequent: Sedation.

CLEMASTINE (*Tavist-1*) ▶LK ♀B ▶– $
ADULT — Allergic rhinitis: 1.34 mg PO two times per day. Max 8.04 mg/day. Urticaria/angioedema: 2.68 mg PO one to three times per day. Max 8.04 mg/day.
PEDS — Allergic rhinitis: Give 0.67 mg PO two times per day. Max 4.02 mg/day for age 6 to 12 yo, give adult dose for age 12 yo or older. Urticaria/angio-edema: Give 1.34 mg PO two times per day (up to 4.02 mg/day) for age 6 to 12 yo, give adult dose for age 6 to 12 yo.
UNAPPROVED PEDS — Allergic rhinitis for age younger than 6 yo: 0.05 mg/kg/day (as clemastine base) PO divided two to three times per day. Max dose 1 mg/day.
FORMS — OTC Generic/Trade: Tabs 1.34 mg. Rx: Generic only: Tabs 2.68 mg. Syrup 0.5 mg/5 mL.
NOTES — 1.34 mg is equivalent to 1 mg clemastine base.
MOA — Antihistamine.
ADVERSE EFFECTS — Serious: None. Frequent: Sedation, dry mouth.

CYPROHEPTADINE (*Periactin*) ▶LK ♀B ▶– $$
ADULT — Allergic rhinitis/urticaria: Start 4 mg PO three times per day, usual effective dose is 12 to 16 mg/day. Max 32 mg/day.
PEDS — Allergic rhinitis/urticaria: Start 2 mg PO two to three times per day (up to 12 mg/day) for age 2 to 6 yo. Start 4 mg PO two to three times per day (up to 16 mg/day) for age 7 to 14 yo.
UNAPPROVED ADULT — Appetite stimulant: 2 to 4 mg PO three times per day 1 h before meals. Prevention of migraine headaches: 2 mg PO two times per day. Treatment of acute serotonin syndrome: 12 mg PO/NG followed by 2 mg q 2 h until symptoms clear, then 8 mg q 6 h maintenance while syndrome remains active.
UNAPPROVED PEDS — Migraine prophylaxis: 0.2 to 0.4 mg/kg/day given in two divided doses, max dose 0.5 mg/kg/day.
FORMS — Generic only: Tabs 4 mg. Syrup 2 mg/5 mL.
NOTES — Also used for vasomotor rhinitis, reactions to blood, adjunct for anaphylaxis treatment, and dermatographism
MOA — Antihistamine/serotonin antagonist.
ADVERSE EFFECTS — Serious: None. Frequent: Sedation.

DIPHENHYDRAMINE (*Benadryl, Banophen, Aller-Max, Diphen, Diphenhist, Dytan, Siladryl, Sominex, *Allerdryl, Nytol*) ▶LK ♀B ▶– $

ADULT — Allergic rhinitis, urticaria, hypersensitivity reactions: 25 to 50 mg PO/IM/IV q 4 to 6 h. Max 300 to 400 mg/day. Motion sickness: 25 to 50 mg PO pre-exposure and q 4 to 6 h prn. Drug-induced parkinsonism: 10 to 50 mg IV/IM. Antitussive: 25 mg PO q 4 h. Max 100 mg/day. EPS: 25 to 50 mg PO three to four times per day or 10 to 50 mg IV/IM three to four times per day. Insomnia: 25 to 50 mg PO at bedtime.

PEDS — Hypersensitivity reactions: Give 12.5 to 25 mg PO q 4 to 6 h or 5 mg/kg/day PO/IV/IM divided four times per day for age 6 to 11 yo, give adult dose for age 12 yo or older. Max 150 mg/day. Antitussive (syrup): Give 6.25 mg PO q 4 h (up to 25 mg/day) for age 2 to 5 yo, give 12.5 mg PO q 4 h (up to 50 mg/day) for age 6 to 12 yo. EPS: 12.5 to 25 mg PO three to four times per day or 5 mg/kg/day IV/IM divided four times per day, max 300 mg/day. Insomnia, age 12 yo or older: 25 to 50 mg PO at bedtime.

FORMS — OTC Trade only: Tabs 25, 50 mg. Chewable tabs 12.5 mg. OTC and Rx: Generic only: Caps 25, 50 mg. Softgel cap 25 mg. OTC Generic/Trade: Soln 6.25 or 12.5 mg per 5 mL. Rx: Trade only: (Dytan) Susp 25 mg/mL. Chewable tabs 25 mg.

NOTES — Anticholinergic side effects are enhanced in the elderly and may worsen dementia or delirium. Avoid use with donepezil, rivastigmine, or galantamine.

MOA — Antihistamine.

ADVERSE EFFECTS — Serious: None. Frequent: Sedation, dry mouth.

HYDROXYZINE (*Atarax, Vistaril*) ▶L ♀C ▶– $

WARNING — Can prolong QT interval.

ADULT — Pruritus: 25 to 100 mg IM/PO three to four times per day or prn. Anxiety: 50-100 mg four times per day.

PEDS — Pruritus: Give 50 mg/day PO divided four times per day for age younger than 6 yo, give 50 to 100 mg/day PO divided four times per day for age 6 or older.

FORMS — Generic only: Tabs 10, 25, 50 mg. Caps 100 mg. Generic/Trade: Caps 25, 50 mg. Susp 25 mg/5 mL (Vistaril). Caps = Vistaril; Tabs = Atarax.

NOTES — Atarax (hydrochloride salt), Vistaril (pamoate salt).

MOA — Antihistamine.

ADVERSE EFFECTS — Serious: None. Frequent: Sedation.

LEVOCETIRIZINE (*Xyzal*) ▶K ♀B ▶– $$$

ADULT — Allergic rhinitis/urticaria: 2.5-5 mg PO daily.

PEDS — Allergic rhinitis/urticaria: Give 1.25 mg daily for age 6 mo to 5 yo. Give 2.5 mg PO daily for age 6 to 11 yo, give 5 mg PO daily for age 12 or older.

FORMS — Generic/Trade: Tabs, scored 5 mg. Oral soln 2.5 mg/5 mL (148 mL).

NOTES — Decrease dose in renal impairment.

MOA — Antihistamine.

ADVERSE EFFECTS — Serious: None. Frequent: Sedation.

MECLIZINE (*Antivert, Bonine, Medivert, Meclicot, Meni-D*) ▶L ♀B ▶? $

ADULT — Motion sickness: 25 to 50 mg PO 1 h prior to travel, then 25 to 50 mg PO daily.

PEDS — Not approved in children.

UNAPPROVED ADULT — Vertigo: 25 mg PO one to four times per day prn.

FORMS — Rx/OTC/Generic/Trade: Tabs 12.5, 25 mg. Chewable tabs 25 mg. Rx/Trade only: Tabs 50 mg.

NOTES — FDA classifies meclizine as "possibly effective" for vertigo. May cause dizziness and drowsiness.

MOA — Antihistamine.

ADVERSE EFFECTS — Serious: Tachycardia, confusion. Frequent: Dry mouth, constipation, drowsiness, dizziness, blurred vision, urinary retention, rash.

ENT: Antitussives / Expectorants

BENZONATATE (*Tessalon, Tessalon Perles, Zonatuss*) ▶L ♀C ▶? $$

ADULT — Cough: 100 to 200 mg PO three times per day. Max 600 mg/day.

PEDS — Cough: Give adult dose for age older than 10 yo.

FORMS — Generic/Trade: Softgel caps 100, 200 mg. Trade only: Caps 150 mg (Zonatuss).

NOTES — Swallow whole. Do not chew. Numbs mouth; possible choking hazard.

MOA — Local anesthetic.

ADVERSE EFFECTS — Serious: None. Frequent: None.

DEXTROMETHORPHAN (*Benylin, Delsym, DexAlone, Robitussin Cough, Vick's 44 Cough*) ▶L ♀+ ▶+ $

ADULT — Cough: 10 to 20 mg PO every 4 hours or 30 mg PO every 6 to 8 hours. 60 mg PO ever 12 hours (Delsym).

PEDS — Cough: age 4 to 6 yo: 2.5 to 7.5 mg every 4 to 8 hours. Age 6 to 12 yo: 5 to 10 mg every 4 hours. Not for use in children under 4 yo.

FORMS — OTC Trade only: Caps 15 mg. Susp, extended-release 30 mg/5 mL (Delsym). Generic/Trade: Syrup 5, 7.5, 10, 15 mg/5 mL. Generic only: Lozenges 5, 7.5 mg.

NOTES — Contraindicated with MAOIs due to potential for serotonin syndrome. Use caution with other serotonergic drugs such as SSRIs and tramadol.

MOA — Cough suppressant by depressing medullary cough center.

ADVERSE EFFECTS — Serious: None. Frequent: None.

GUAIFENESIN (*Robitussin, Hytuss, Guiatuss, Mucinex*) ▶L ♀C ▶+ $
ADULT — Expectorant: 100 to 400 mg PO q 4 h. 600 to 1200 mg PO q 12 h (extended-release). Max 2.4 g/day.
PEDS — Expectorant: 50 to 100 mg/dose for age 2 to 5 yo, give 100 to 200 mg/dose for age 6 to 11 yo, give adult dose for age 12 yo or older.
UNAPPROVED PEDS — Expectorant: Give 25 mg PO q 4 h (up to 150 mg/day) for age 6 to 11 mo, give 50 mg PO q 4 h (up to 300 mg/day) for age 12 to 23 mo.

FORMS — OTC Generic/Trade: Extended-release tabs 600, 1200 mg. Liquid, Syrup 100 mg/5 mL, 200 mg/5 mL. OTC Trade only: Oral disintegrating tabs 50, 100 mg (Mucinex). OTC Generic only: Tabs 200, 400 mg.
NOTES — Lack of convincing studies to document efficacy.
MOA — Expectorant.
ADVERSE EFFECTS — Serious: None. Frequent: None.

ENT: Combination Products—OTC

NOTE: Decongestants in some ENT combination products can increase BP, aggravate anxiety, or cause insomnia (use caution). Some contain sedating antihistamines. Sedation can be enhanced by alcohol and other CNS depressants. Some states have restricted or ended OTC sale of pseudoephedrine and pseudoephedrine combination products or reclassified it as a scheduled drug due to the potential for diversion to methamphetamine labs. Deaths have occurred in children younger than 2 yo attributed to toxicity from cough and cold medications; the FDA does not recommend their use in this age group.

ACTIFED COLD AND ALLERGY (**phenylephrine + chlorpheniramine**) ▶L ♀C ▶+ $
ADULT — Allergic rhinitis/nasal congestion: 1 tab PO q 4 to 6 h. Max 4 tabs/day.
PEDS — Allergic rhinitis/nasal congestion: Give ½ tab PO q 4 to 6 h (up to 2 tabs/day) for age 6 to 12 yo, give adult dose for age older than 12 yo.
FORMS — OTC Generic/Trade: Tabs 10 mg phenylephrine/4 mg chlorpheniramine.
MOA — Decongestant/antihistamine combination.
ADVERSE EFFECTS — Serious: None. Frequent: Insomnia, palpitations, sedation.

ACTIFED COLD AND SINUS (**pseudoephedrine + chlorpheniramine + acetaminophen**) ▶L ♀C ▶+ $$
ADULT — Allergic rhinitis/nasal congestion/headache: 2 caps PO q 6 h. Max 8 caps/day.
PEDS — Allergic rhinitis/nasal congestion/headache: Age older than 12 yo: Use adult dose.
FORMS — OTC Generic only: Tabs 30 mg pseudoephedrine/2 mg chlorpheniramine/500 mg acetaminophen.
MOA — Decongestant/antihistamine/analgesic combination.
ADVERSE EFFECTS — Serious: None. Frequent: Insomnia, palpitations, sedation.

ALAVERT D-12 (**pseudoephedrine + loratadine**) ▶LK ♀B ▶– $
ADULT — Allergic rhinitis/nasal congestion: 1 tab PO two times per day.
PEDS — Not approved in children.
FORMS — OTC Generic/Trade: Tabs, 12 h extended-release, 120 mg pseudoephedrine/5 mg loratadine.
NOTES — Decrease dose to 1 tab PO daily with CrCl <30 mL/min. Avoid in hepatic insufficiency.
MOA — Decongestant/antihistamine combination.
ADVERSE EFFECTS — Serious: None. Frequent: Insomnia, palpitations, sedation.

ALEVE COLD AND SINUS (**naproxen + pseudoephedrine**) ▶L ♀C (D in 3rd trimester) ▶+ $
ADULT — Nasal/sinus congestion, fever, and pain: 1 cap PO q 12 h.

PEDS — Nasal/sinus congestion, fever, and pain: Age older than 12 yo: Use adult dose.
FORMS — OTC Trade only: Extended-release caps: 220 mg naproxen sodium/120 mg pseudoephedrine.
MOA — Decongestant/analgesic/antipyretic.
ADVERSE EFFECTS — Serious: Hypersensitivity, GI bleeding, nephrotoxicity. Frequent: Insomnia, palpitations.

ALLERFRIM (**pseudoephedrine + triprolidine**) ▶L ♀C ▶+ $
ADULT — Allergic rhinitis/nasal congestion: 1 tab or 10 mL PO q 4 to 6 h. Max 4 tabs/day or 40 mL/day.
PEDS — Allergic rhinitis/nasal congestion: Give ½ tab or 5 mL PO q 4 to 6 h (up to 2 tabs/day or 20 mL/day) for age 6 to 12 yo, give adult dose for age older than 12 yo.
FORMS — OTC Trade only: Tabs 60 mg pseudoephedrine/2.5 mg triprolidine. Syrup 30 mg pseudoephedrine/1.25 mg triprolidine/5 mL.
MOA — Decongestant/antihistamine combination.
ADVERSE EFFECTS — Serious: None. Frequent: Insomnia, palpitations, sedation.

APRODINE (**pseudoephedrine + triprolidine**) ▶L ♀C ▶+ $
ADULT — Allergic rhinitis/nasal congestion: 1 tab or 10 mL PO q 4 to 6 h. Max 4 tabs/day or 40 mL/day.
PEDS — Allergic rhinitis/nasal congestion: Age older than 12 yo: Use adult dose. 6 to 12 yo: ½ tab or 5 mL PO q 4 to 6 h. Max 2 tabs/day or 20 mL/day.
FORMS — OTC Generic/Trade: Tabs 60 mg pseudoephedrine/2.5 mg triprolidine. Syrup 30 mg pseudoephedrine/1.25 mg triprolidine/5 mL.
MOA — Decongestant/antihistamine combination.
ADVERSE EFFECTS — Serious: None. Frequent: Insomnia, palpitations, sedation.

BENADRYL-D ALLERGY AND SINUS (**phenylephrine + diphenhydramine**) ▶L ♀C ▶– $
ADULT — Allergic rhinitis/nasal congestion: 1 tab PO q 4 h. Max 6 tabs/day.
PEDS — Allergic rhinitis/nasal congestion: Age older than 12 yo: Use adult dose.

(cont.)

BENADRYL-D ALLERGY AND SINUS (*cont.*)
FORMS — OTC Trade only: Tabs 10/25 mg phenylephrine/diphenhydramine.
MOA — Decongestant/antihistamine combination.
ADVERSE EFFECTS — Serious: None. Frequent: Insomnia, palpitations, sedation.

Cheracol D Cough (**guaifenesin + dextromethorphan**) ▶L ♀C ▶? $
ADULT — Cough: 10 mL PO q 4 h.
PEDS — Cough: Give 2.5 mL PO q 4 h (up to 15 mL/day) for age 2 to 5 yo, give 5 mL PO q 4 h for age 6 to 11 yo, give adult dose for age 12 yo or older.
FORMS — OTC Generic/Trade: Syrup 100 mg guaifenesin/10 mg dextromethorphan/5 mL.
MOA — Expectorant/cough suppressant combination.
ADVERSE EFFECTS — Serious: None. Frequent: None.

CHILDREN'S ADVIL COLD (**ibuprofen + pseudoephedrine**) ▶L ♀C (D in 3rd trimester) ▶+ $
ADULT — Not approved for use in adults.
PEDS — Nasal congestion/sore throat/fever: Give 5 mL PO q 6 h for age 2 to 5 yo, give 10 mL PO q 6 h for age 6 to 11 yo.
FORMS — OTC Generic only: Susp: 100 mg ibuprofen/15 mg pseudoephedrine/5 mL. Grape flavor, alcohol-free.
NOTES — Shake well before using. Do not use for more than 7 days for cold, sinus, and flu symptoms.
MOA — Decongestant/anti-inflammatory/antipyretic combination.
ADVERSE EFFECTS — Serious: Allergic reactions. Frequent: Insomnia, palpitations.

CLARITIN-D 12 HR (**pseudoephedrine + loratadine**) ▶LK ♀B ▶+ $
ADULT — Allergic rhinitis/nasal congestion: 1 tab PO two times per day.
PEDS — Not approved in children.
FORMS — OTC Generic/Trade: Tabs, 12 h extended-release 120 mg pseudoephedrine/5 mg loratadine.
NOTES — Decrease dose to 1 tab PO daily with CrCl <30 mL/min. Avoid in hepatic insufficiency.
MOA — Decongestant/antihistamine combination.
ADVERSE EFFECTS — Serious: None. Frequent: Insomnia, palpitations, sedation.

CLARITIN-D 24 HR (**pseudoephedrine + loratadine**) ▶LK ♀B ▶+ $
ADULT — Allergic rhinitis/nasal congestion: 1 tab PO daily.
PEDS — Not approved in children.
FORMS — OTC Generic/Trade: Tabs, 24 h extended-release 240 mg pseudoephedrine/10 mg loratadine.
NOTES — Decrease dose to 1 tab PO every other day with CrCl <30 mL/min. Avoid in hepatic insufficiency.
MOA — Decongestant/antihistamine combination.
ADVERSE EFFECTS — Serious: None. Frequent: Insomnia, palpitations, sedation.

CORICIDIN HBP CONGESTION AND COUGH (**guaifenesin + dextromethorphan**) ▶LK ♀B ▶+ $$
ADULT — Productive cough: 1 to 2 softgels PO q 4 h. Max 12 softgels/day.

PEDS — Productive cough: Give adult dose for age 12 yo or older.
FORMS — OTC Trade only: Softgels 200 mg guaifenesin/10 mg dextromethorphan.
MOA — Expectorant/cough suppressant combination.
ADVERSE EFFECTS — Serious: None. Frequent: None.

CORICIDIN HBP COUGH AND COLD (**chlorpheniramine + dextromethorphan**) ▶LK ♀B ▶+ $
ADULT — Rhinitis/cough: 1 tab q 6 h. Max 4 doses/day.
PEDS — Rhinitis/cough: Give adult dose for age 12 yo or older.
FORMS — OTC Trade only: Tabs 4 mg chlorpheniramine/30 mg dextromethorphan.
MOA — Antihistamine/cough suppressant combination.
ADVERSE EFFECTS — Serious: None. Frequent: Sedation.

DIMETAPP COLD AND ALLERGY (**phenylephrine + brompheniramine**) ▶LK ♀C ▶– $
ADULT — Allergic rhinitis/nasal congestion: 20 mL PO q 4 h. Max 4 doses/day.
PEDS — Allergic rhinitis/nasal congestion: 10 mL PO q 4 h for age 6 to 11 yo, give adult dose for 12 yo or older.
FORMS — OTC Trade only: Liquid, Tabs 2.5 mg phenylephrine/1 mg brompheniramine per tab or 5 mL.
NOTES — Grape flavor, alcohol-free.
MOA — Decongestant/antihistamine combination.
ADVERSE EFFECTS — Serious: None. Frequent: Insomnia, palpitations, sedation.

DIMETAPP COLD AND COUGH (**phenylephrine + brompheniramine + dextromethorphan**) ▶LK ♀C ▶– $
ADULT — Nasal congestion/cough: 20 mL PO q 4 h. Max 6 doses/day.
PEDS — Nasal congestion/cough: Give 10 mL PO q 4 h (up to 6 doses/day) for age 6 to 11 yo, give adult dose for 12 yo or older.
FORMS — OTC Trade only: Liquid 2.5 mg phenylephrine/1 mg brompheniramine/5 mg dextromethorphan/5 mL.
NOTES — Red grape flavor, alcohol-free.
MOA — Decongestant/antihistamine/cough suppressant combination.
ADVERSE EFFECTS — Serious: None. Frequent: Insomnia, palpitations, sedation.

DIMETAPP NIGHTTIME COLD AND CONGESTION (**phenylephrine + diphenhydramine**) ▶LK ♀C ▶– $
ADULT — Nasal congestion/runny nose/fever/cough/sore throat: 20 mL PO q 4 h. Max 5 doses/day.
PEDS — Nasal congestion/runny nose/fever/cough/sore throat: Give 10 mL PO q 4 h (up to 5 doses/day) for age 6 to 11 yo, give adult dose for 12 yo or older.
FORMS — OTC Trade only: Syrup 2.5 mg phenylephrine and 6.25 mg diphenhydramine.
NOTES — Bubble gum flavor, alcohol-free.
MOA — Decongestant/antihistamine/cough suppressant/analgesic combination.
ADVERSE EFFECTS — Serious: Hepatotoxicity. Frequent: Insomnia, palpitations, sedation.

MUCINEX D (guaifenesin + pseudoephedrine) ▶L ♀C ▶? $
WARNING — Multiple strengths; write specific product on Rx.
ADULT — Cough/congestion: 2 tabs (600/60) PO q 12 h; max 4 tabs/24 h. 1 tab (1200/120) PO q 12 h; max 2 tabs/24 h.
PEDS — Cough: Give adult dose for age 12 yo or older.
FORMS — OTC Trade only: Tabs, extended-release 600/60, 1200/120 mg guaifenesin/pseudoephedrine.
NOTES — Do not crush, chew, or break the tab. Take with a full glass of water.
MOA — Decongestant/expectorant combination.
ADVERSE EFFECTS — Serious: None. Frequent: Insomnia, palpitations.

MUCINEX DM (guaifenesin + dextromethorphan) ▶L ♀C ▶? $
WARNING — Multiple strengths; write specific product on Rx.
ADULT — Cough: 1 to 2 tabs (600/30) PO q 12 h; max 4 tabs/24 h. 1 tab (1200/60) PO q 12 h; max 2 tabs/24 h.
PEDS — Cough: Give adult dose for age 12 yo or older.
FORMS — OTC Trade only: Tabs, extended-release 600/30, 1200/60 mg guaifenesin/dextromethorphan.
NOTES — DM indicates dextromethorphan. Do not crush, chew, or break the tab. Take with a full glass of water.
MOA — Expectorant/cough suppressant combination.
ADVERSE EFFECTS — Serious: None. Frequent: None.

ROBITUSSIN DM (guaifenesin + dextromethorphan) ▶L ♀C ▶+ $
ADULT — Cough: 10 mL PO q 4 h. Max 60 mL/day.
PEDS — Cough: Give 2.5 mL PO q 4 h (up to 15 mL/day) for age 2 to 5 yo, give 5 mL PO q 4 h (up to 30 mL/day) for age 6 to 11 yo, give adult dose for 12 yo or older.
FORMS — OTC Generic/Trade: Syrup 100 mg guaifenesin/10 mg dextromethorphan/5 mL.
NOTES — Alcohol-free. DM indicates dextromethorphan.
MOA — Expectorant/cough suppressant combination.
ADVERSE EFFECTS — Serious: None. Frequent: None.

ROBITUSSIN PEAK COLD CF (phenylephrine + guaifenesin + dextromethorphan) ▶L ♀C ▶– $
ADULT — Nasal congestion/cough: 10 mL PO q 4 h.
PEDS — Nasal congestion/cough: Give 2.5 mL PO q 4 h for age 2 to 5 yo, give 5 mL PO q 4 h for age 6 to 11 yo, give adult dose for 12 yo or older.
FORMS — OTC Generic/Trade: Syrup 5 mg phenylephrine/100 mg guaifenesin/10 mg dextromethorphan/5 mL.
NOTES — CF indicates cough formula.
MOA — Decongestant/expectorant/cough suppressant combination.
ADVERSE EFFECTS — Serious: None. Frequent: Insomnia, palpitations.

TRIAMINIC CHEST AND NASAL CONGESTION (phenylephrine + guaifenesin) ▶LK ♀C ▶– $
ADULT — Child-only preparation.
PEDS — Chest/nasal congestion: Give 5 mL PO q 4 h (up to 6 doses/day) for age 2 to 6 yo, give 10 mL PO q 4 h (up to 6 doses/day) for age 6 to 12 yo.
FORMS — OTC Trade only, yellow label: Syrup 2.5 mg phenylephrine/50 mg guaifenesin/5 mL, tropical flavor.
MOA — Decongestant/expectorant combination.
ADVERSE EFFECTS — Serious: None. Frequent: Insomnia, palpitations.

TRIAMINIC COLD AND ALLERGY (phenylephrine + chlorpheniramine) ▶LK ♀C ▶– $
ADULT — Child-only preparation.
PEDS — Allergic rhinitis/nasal congestion: 10 mL PO q 4 h to max 6 doses/day for age 6 to 12 yo.
FORMS — OTC Trade only, orange label: Syrup 2.5 mg phenylephrine/1 mg chlorpheniramine/5 mL, orange flavor.
MOA — Decongestant/antihistamine combination.
ADVERSE EFFECTS — Serious: None. Frequent: Insomnia, palpitations, sedation.

TRIAMINIC COUGH AND SORE THROAT (dextromethorphan + acetaminophen) ▶LK ♀C ▶– $
ADULT — Child-only preparation.
PEDS — Cough/sore throat: Give PO q 4 h to max 5 doses/day: 5 mL or 1 softchew tab per dose for age 2 to 6 yo, give 10 mL or 2 softchew tabs per dose for age 7 to 12 yo.
FORMS — OTC Trade only, purple label: Syrup, Softchew tabs 5 mg dextromethorphan/160 mg acetaminophen/5 mL or tab, grape flavor.
MOA — Cough suppressant/analgesic combination.
ADVERSE EFFECTS — Serious: Hepatotoxicity. Frequent: Insomnia, palpitations.

TRIAMINIC DAY TIME COLD AND COUGH (phenylephrine + dextromethorphan) ▶LK ♀C ▶– $
ADULT — Child-only preparation.
PEDS — Nasal congestion/cough: Give PO q 4 h to max 6 doses/day: 5 mL or 1 strip per dose for age 2 to 6 yo, give 10 mL or 2 strips per dose for age 7 to 12 yo.
FORMS — OTC Trade only, red label: Syrup, thin strips 2.5 mg phenylephrine/5 mg dextromethorphan/5 mL, cherry flavor.
NOTES — Allow strips to dissolve on the tongue.
MOA — Decongestant/cough suppressant combination.
ADVERSE EFFECTS — Serious: None. Frequent: Insomnia, palpitations, sedation.

TRIAMINIC FLU COUGH AND FEVER (acetaminophen + chlorpheniramine + dextromethorphan) ▶LK ♀C ▶– $
ADULT — Child-only preparation.
PEDS — Fever/cough: 10 mL PO q 6 h to max 4 doses/day for age 6 to 12 yo.
FORMS — OTC Trade only, pink label: Syrup 160 mg acetaminophen/1 mg chlorpheniramine/7.5 mg dextromethorphan/5 mL, bubble gum flavor.

(cont.)

TRIAMINIC FLU COUGH AND FEVER (cont.)

MOA — Analgesic/antihistamine/cough suppressant combination.
ADVERSE EFFECTS — Serious: None. Frequent: Insomnia, palpitations.

***TRIAMINIC NIGHT TIME COLD AND COUGH* (phenyleph-rine + diphenhydramine)** ▶LK ♀C ▶– $
ADULT — Child-only preparation.

PEDS — Nasal congestion/cough: 10 mL PO q 4 h to max 6 doses/day for age 6 to 12 yo.
FORMS — OTC Trade only, blue label: Syrup 2.5 mg phenylephrine/6.25 mg diphenhydramine/5 mL, grape flavor.
MOA — Decongestant/antihistamine combination.
ADVERSE EFFECTS — Serious: None. Frequent: Insomnia, palpitations, sedation.

ENT: Combination Products—Rx Only

NOTE: Decongestants in some ENT combination products can increase BP, aggravate anxiety, or cause insomnia (use caution). Some contain sedating antihistamines. Sedation can be enhanced by alcohol and other CNS depressants. Deaths have occurred in children younger than 2 yo attributed to toxicity from cough and cold medications; the FDA does not recommend their use in this age group.

***ALLEGRA-D 12-HOUR* (fexofenadine + pseudoephed-rine)** ▶LK ♀C ▶+ $$
ADULT — Allergic rhinitis/nasal congestion: 1 tab PO q 12 h.
PEDS — Not approved in children.
FORMS — OTC Generic/Trade: Tabs, extended-release 60/120 mg fexofenadine/pseudoephedrine.
NOTES — Decrease dose to 1 tab PO daily with decreased renal function. Take on an empty stomach. Avoid taking with fruit juice due to a large decrease in bioavailability.
MOA — Decongestant/antihistamine combination.
ADVERSE EFFECTS — Serious: None. Frequent: Insomnia, palpitations.

***ALLEGRA-D 24-HOUR* (fexofenadine + pseudoephed-rine)** ▶LK ♀C ▶+ $$
ADULT — Allergic rhinitis/nasal congestion: 1 tab PO daily.
PEDS — Not approved in children.
FORMS — OTC: Generic/Trade: Tabs, extended-release 180/240 mg fexofenadine/pseudoephedrine.
NOTES — Decrease dose to 1 tab PO every other day with decreased renal function. Take on an empty stomach. Avoid taking with fruit juice due to a large decrease in bioavailability.
MOA — Decongestant/antihistamine combination.
ADVERSE EFFECTS — Serious: None. Frequent: Insomnia, palpitations.

***CHERATUSSIN AC* (guaifenesin + codeine)** ▶L ♀C ▶? ©V $
ADULT — Cough: 10 mL PO q 4 h. Max 60 mL/day.
PEDS — Cough: Give 1.25 to 2.5 mL PO q 4 h (up to 15 mL/day) for age 6 to 23 mo, give 2.5 to 5 mL PO q 4 h (up to 30 mL/day) for age 2 to 5 yo, give 5 mL PO q 4 h (up to 30 mL/day) for age 6 to 11 yo, give adult dose for age 12 or older.
FORMS — Generic/Trade: Syrup 100 mg guaifenesin/10 mg codeine/5 mL. Sugar-free.
MOA — Expectorant/cough suppressant combination.
ADVERSE EFFECTS — Serious: Respiratory depression/arrest. Frequent: N/V, constipation, sedation.

***CHERATUSSIN DAC* (pseudoephedrine + guaifenesin + codeine)** ▶L ♀C ▶? ©V $
ADULT — Nasal congestion/cough: 10 mL PO q 4 h. Max 40 mL/day.

PEDS — Nasal congestion/cough: Give 5 mL PO q 4 h (up to 20 mL/day) for age 6 to 11 yo, give adult dose for 12 yo or older.
FORMS — Generic/Trade: Syrup 30 mg pseudoephedrine/100 mg guaifenesin/10 mg codeine/ 5 mL. Sugar-free.
NOTES — DAC indicates decongestant and codeine.
MOA — Decongestant/expectorant/cough suppressant combination.
ADVERSE EFFECTS — Serious: Respiratory depression/arrest. Frequent: N/V, constipation, sedation, insomnia, palpitations.

***CHLORDRINE SR* (pseudoephedrine + chlorphenira-mine)** ▶LK ♀C ▶– $
ADULT — Allergic rhinitis/nasal congestion: 1 cap PO q 12 h. Max 2 caps/day.
PEDS — Allergic rhinitis/nasal congestion: 1 cap PO daily for age 6 to 11 yo, use adult dose for age 12 yo or older.
FORMS — Generic only: Caps, sustained-release 120 mg pseudoephedrine/8 mg chlorpheniramine.
MOA — Decongestant/antihistamine combination.
ADVERSE EFFECTS — Serious: None. Frequent: Insomnia, palpitations, sedation.

***CLARINEX-D 12 HOUR* (pseudoephedrine + deslorata-dine)** ▶LK ♀C ▶+ $$$$$
ADULT — Allergic rhinitis: 1 tab PO q 12 h.
PEDS — Allergic rhinitis, age 12 yo or older: Use adult dose.
FORMS — Trade only: Tabs, extended-release 120 mg pseudoephedrine/2.5 mg desloratadine.
NOTES — Swallow tabs whole. Avoid with hepatic or renal insufficiency.
MOA — Decongestant/antihistamine combination.
ADVERSE EFFECTS — Serious: None. Frequent: Insomnia, palpitations.

***ENTEX LIQUID* (phenylephrine + guaifenesin)** ▶L ♀C ▶– $$$
ADULT — Nasal congestion/cough: 5 mL PO every 4 hours, max 6 doses/day.
PEDS — Nasal congestion/cough: Age 12 and over: use adult dose. Age 6 to 11 yo: give 2.5 mL PO every 4 hours. Age 2 to 5 yo: give 1.25 mL every 4 hours. Max 6 doses/day for all age groups. Not recommended in children under 1 yo.

(cont.)

ENTEX LIQUID (*cont.*)

FORMS — Generic/Trade: Liquid 10 mg phenyl-ephrine/100 mg guaifenesin/5 mL. Punch flavor, alcohol-free.

MOA — Decongestant/expectorant combination.

ADVERSE EFFECTS — Serious: None. Frequent: Insomnia, palpitations.

GUIATUSS AC (**guaifenesin + codeine**) ▶L ♀C ▶? ©V $

ADULT — Cough: 10 mL PO q 4 h. Max 60 mL/day.

PEDS — Cough: Give 5 mL PO q 4 h (up to 30 mL/day) for age 6 to 11 yo, give adult dose for 12 yo or older.

FORMS — Generic only: Syrup 100 mg guaifenesin/10 mg codeine/5 mL. Sugar-free.

NOTES — AC indicates before meals and codeine.

MOA — Expectorant/cough suppressant combination.

ADVERSE EFFECTS — Serious: Respiratory depression/arrest. Frequent: N/V, constipation, sedation.

GUIATUSSIN DAC (**pseudoephedrine + guaifenesin + codeine**) ▶L ♀C ▶– ©V $$$

ADULT — Nasal congestion/cough: 10 mL PO q 4 h. Max 40 mL/day.

PEDS — Nasal congestion/cough: Give 5 mL PO q 4 h (up to 20 mL/day) for age 6 to 11 yo, give adult dose for 12 yo or older.

FORMS — Generic only: Syrup 30 mg pseudoephedrine/100 mg guaifenesin/10 mg codeine/5 mL. Sugar-free.

NOTES — DAC indicates decongestant and codeine.

MOA — Decongestant/expectorant/cough suppressant combination.

ADVERSE EFFECTS — Serious: Respiratory depression/arrest. Frequent: N/V, constipation, sedation, insomnia, palpitations.

HALOTUSSIN AC (**guaifenesin + codeine**) ▶L ♀C ▶? ©V $

ADULT — Cough: 10 mL PO q 4 h. Max 60 mL/day.

PEDS — Cough: Give 5 mL PO q 4 h (up to 30 mL/day) for age 6 to 11 yo, give adult dose for age 12 yo or older.

FORMS — Generic only: Syrup 100 mg guaifenesin/10 mg codeine/5 mL. Sugar-free.

NOTES — AC indicates before meals and codeine.

MOA — Expectorant/cough suppressant combination.

ADVERSE EFFECTS — Serious: Respiratory depression/arrest. Frequent: N/V, constipation, sedation.

HALOTUSSIN DAC (**pseudoephedrine + guaifenesin + codeine**) ▶L ♀C ▶– ©V $$$

ADULT — Nasal congestion/cough: 10 mL PO q 4 h. Max 40 mL/day.

PEDS — Nasal congestion/cough: Give 5 mL PO q 4 h (up to 20 mL/day) for age 6 to 11 yo, give adult dose for 12 yo or older.

FORMS — Generic only: Syrup 30 mg pseudoephedrine/100 mg guaifenesin/10 mg codeine/5 mL. Sugar-free.

NOTES — DAC indicates decongestant and codeine.

MOA — Decongestant/expectorant/cough suppressant combination.

ADVERSE EFFECTS — Serious: Respiratory depression/arrest. Frequent: N/V, constipation, sedation, insomnia, palpitations.

HYCODAN (**hydrocodone + homatropine**) ▶L ♀C ▶– ©II $$

ADULT — Cough: 1 tab or 5 mL PO q 4 to 6 h. Max 6 doses/day.

PEDS — Cough: Give 2.5 mg (based on hydrocodone) PO q 4 to 6 h prn (up to 15 mg/day) for age 6 to 12 yo, give adult dose for age older than 12 yo.

FORMS — Generic only: Syrup 5 mg hydrocodone/1.5 mg homatropine methylbromide/5 mL. Generic/trade: Tabs 5/1.5 mg.

NOTES — May cause drowsiness/sedation. Dosing based on hydrocodone content.

MOA — Cough suppressant.

ADVERSE EFFECTS — Serious: Respiratory depression/arrest. Frequent: N/V, constipation, sedation.

NOVAFED A (**pseudoephedrine + chlorpheniramine**) ▶LK ♀C ▶– $

ADULT — Allergic rhinitis/nasal congestion: 1 cap PO q 12 h. Max 2 caps/day.

PEDS — Allergic rhinitis/nasal congestion: 1 cap PO daily for age 6 to 12 yo, use adult dose for age older than 12 yo.

FORMS — Generic only: Caps, sustained-release 120 mg pseudoephedrine/8 mg chlorpheniramine.

MOA — Decongestant/antihistamine combination.

ADVERSE EFFECTS — Serious: None. Frequent: Insomnia, palpitations, sedation.

PALGIC DS (**pseudoephedrine + carbinoxamine**) ▶L ♀C ▶– $$

ADULT — Allergic rhinitis/nasal congestion: 10 mL PO four times per day.

PEDS — Allergic rhinitis/nasal congestion: Give up to the following PO four times per day: 1.25 mL for age 1 to 3 mo, 2.5 mL for age 3 to 6 mo, 3.75 mL for age 6 to 9 mo, 3.75 to 5 mL for age 9 to 18 mo, 5 mL for age 18 mo to 6 yo, use adult dose for age older than 6 yo.

FORMS — Generic/Trade: Syrup 25 mg pseudoephedrine/2 mg carbinoxamine/5 mL. Alcohol- and sugar-free.

NOTES — Carbinoxamine has potential for sedation similar to diphenhydramine.

MOA — Decongestant/antihistamine combination.

ADVERSE EFFECTS — Serious: None. Frequent: Insomnia, palpitations, sedation.

PHENERGAN VC (**phenylephrine + promethazine**) ▶LK ♀C ▶? $

WARNING — Promethazine contraindicated if age younger than 2 yo due to risk of fatal respiratory depression; caution in older children.

ADULT — Allergic rhinitis/congestion: 5 mL PO q 4 to 6 h. Max 30 mL/day.

PEDS — Allergic rhinitis/congestion: Give 1.25 to 2.5 mL PO q 4 to 6 h (up to 15 mL/day) for age 2 to 5 yo, give 2.5 to 5 mL PO q 4 to 6 h for age 6 to 12 yo (up to 20 mL/day), give adult dose for age 12 yo or older.

FORMS — Trade unavailable. Generic only: Syrup 6.25 mg promethazine/5 mg phenylephrine/ 5 mL.

NOTES — VC indicates vasoconstrictor.

MOA — Decongestant/antihistamine combination.

ADVERSE EFFECTS — Serious: None. Frequent: Insomnia, palpitations, sedation.

PHENERGAN VC W/CODEINE (phenylephrine + promethazine + codeine) ▶LK ♀C ▶? ©V $$$$
WARNING — Promethazine contraindicated if younger than 2 yo due to risk of fatal respiratory depression; caution in older children.
ADULT — Allergic rhinitis/congestion/cough: 5 mL PO q 4 to 6 h. Max 30 mL/day.
PEDS — Allergic rhinitis/congestion/cough: Give 1.25 to 2.5 mL PO q 4 to 6 h (up to 10 mL/day) for age 2 to 5 yo, give 2.5 to 5 mL PO q 4 to 6 h for age 6 to 12 yo (up to 20 mL/day), give adult dose for age 12 yo or older.
FORMS — Trade unavailable. Generic only: Syrup 5 mg phenylephrine/6.25 mg promethazine/10 mg codeine/5 mL.
MOA — Decongestant/antihistamine/cough suppressant combination.
ADVERSE EFFECTS — Serious: Respiratory depression/arrest. Frequent: N/V, constipation, sedation, insomnia, palpitations.

PHENERGAN WITH CODEINE (promethazine + codeine) ▶LK ♀C ▶? ©V $
WARNING — Promethazine contraindicated if younger than 6 yo due to risk of fatal respiratory depression; caution in older children.
ADULT — Allergic rhinitis/cough: 5 mL PO q 4 to 6 h. Max 30 mL/day.
PEDS — Allergic rhinitis/cough: 2.5 to 5 mL for age 6 to 11 yo. Adult dosing for age 12 yo and older.
FORMS — Trade unavailable. Generic only: Syrup 6.25 mg promethazine/10 mg codeine/5 mL.
MOA — Antihistamine/cough suppressant combination.
ADVERSE EFFECTS — Serious: Respiratory depression/arrest. Frequent: N/V, constipation, sedation.

PHENERGAN/DEXTROMETHORPHAN (promethazine + dextromethorphan) ▶LK ♀C ▶? $
WARNING — Promethazine contraindicated if younger than 2 yo due to risk of fatal respiratory depression; caution in older children.
ADULT — Allergic rhinitis/cough: 5 mL PO q 4 to 6 h. Max 30 mL/day.
PEDS — Allergic rhinitis/cough: Give 1.25 to 2.5 mL PO q 4 to 6 h (up to 10 mL/day) for age 2 to 5 yo, give 2.5 to 5 mL PO q 4 to 6 h (up to 20 mL/day) for age 6 to 12 yo, give adult dose for age 12 yo or older.
FORMS — Trade unavailable. Generic only: Syrup 6.25 mg promethazine/15 mg dextromethorphan/5 mL.
MOA — Decongestant/cough suppressant combination.
ADVERSE EFFECTS — Serious: None. Frequent: Sedation.

PSEUDO-CHLOR (pseudoephedrine + chlorpheniramine) ▶LK ♀C ▶– $
ADULT — Allergic rhinitis/nasal congestion: 1 cap PO q 12 h. Max 2 caps/day.
PEDS — Allergic rhinitis/nasal congestion: Age older than 12 yo: Use adult dose.
FORMS — Generic only: Caps, sustained-release 120 mg pseudoephedrine/8 mg chlorpheniramine.

MOA — Decongestant/antihistamine combination.
ADVERSE EFFECTS — Serious: None. Frequent: Insomnia, palpitations, sedation.

REZIRA (hydrocodone + pseudoephedrine) ▶LK – ♀C ▶– ©II $$$$
ADULT — Nasal congestion/cough: 5 mL q 4 to 6 h. Max 20 mL/day.
PEDS — Not approved in children.
FORMS — Trade: Syrup 5 mg hydrocodone/60 mg pseudoephedrine/5 mL.
MOA — Decongestant/cough suppressant combination.
ADVERSE EFFECTS — Serious: respiratory depression. Common: sedation, insomnia, palpitations.

ROBITUSSIN AC (guaifenesin + codeine) ▶L ♀C ▶? ©V $
ADULT — The "Robitussin AC" brand is no longer produced; corresponding generics include Cheratussin AC, Guiatuss AC, and Guaifenesin AC.
MOA — Expectorant/cough suppressant combination.
ADVERSE EFFECTS — Serious: Respiratory depression/arrest. Frequent: N/V, constipation, sedation.

ROBITUSSIN DAC (pseudoephedrine + guaifenesin + codeine) ▶L ♀C ▶– ©V $$$
ADULT — The "Robitussin DAC" brand is no longer produced; corresponding generics include Cheratussin DAC and Guaifenesin DAC.
MOA — Decongestant/expectorant/cough suppressant combination.
ADVERSE EFFECTS — Serious: Respiratory depression/arrest. Frequent: N/V, constipation, sedation, insomnia, palpitations.

RONDEC INFANT DROPS (phenylephrine + chlorpheniramine) ▶L ♀C ▶– $
PEDS — Allergic rhinitis/nasal congestion: Give the following dose PO four times per day: 0.75 mL for age 6 to 12 mo, 1 mL for age 13 to 24 mo.
FORMS — Generic only: Gtts 3.5 mg phenylephrine/1 mg chlorpheniramine/mL, grape flavor, 30 mL. Alcohol- and sugar-free.
MOA — Decongestant/antihistamine combination.
ADVERSE EFFECTS — Serious: None. Frequent: Insomnia, palpitations, sedation.

SEMPREX-D (pseudoephedrine + acrivastine) ▶LK ♀C ▶– $$$$
ADULT — Allergic rhinitis/nasal congestion: 1 cap PO q 4 to 6 h. Max 4 caps/day.
PEDS — Not approved in children.
FORMS — Trade only: Caps 60 mg pseudoephedrine/8 mg acrivastine.
MOA — Decongestant/antihistamine combination.
ADVERSE EFFECTS — Serious: None. Frequent: Insomnia, palpitations, sedation.

TUSSICAPS (chlorpheniramine + hydrocodone) ▶L ♀C ▶– ©II $$$$$
ADULT — Allergic rhinitis/cough: 1 full-strength cap PO q 12 h. Max 2 caps/day.
PEDS — Allergic rhinitis/congestion/cough: Give half-strength cap PO q 12 h (up to 2 caps/day) for age 6 to 12 yo, give adult dose for age older than 12 yo.

(cont.)

TUSSICAPS (*cont.*)

FORMS — Trade only: Caps, extended-release 4/5 mg (half-strength), 8/10 mg (full-strength) chlorpheniramine/hydrocodone.

MOA — Antihistamine/cough suppressant combination.

ADVERSE EFFECTS — Serious: Respiratory depression/arrest. Frequent: N/V, constipation, sedation.

TUSSIONEX (chlorpheniramine + hydrocodone) ▶L ♀C ▶– ©II $$$

ADULT — Allergic rhinitis/cough: 5 mL PO q 12 h. Max 10 mL/day.

PEDS — Allergic rhinitis/cough: 2.5 mL PO q 12 h (up to 5 mL/day) for age 6 to 12 yo, give adult dose for age older than 12 yo.

FORMS — Generic/Trade: Extended-release susp 8 mg chlorpheniramine/10 mg hydrocodone/5 mL.

MOA — Antihistamine/cough suppressant combination.

ADVERSE EFFECTS — Serious: Respiratory depression/arrest. Frequent: N/V, constipation, sedation.

ZUTRIPRO (hydrocodone + chlorpheniramine + pseudoephedrine) ▶LK – ♀C ▶– ©II $$$$$

ADULT — Cough/nasal congestion/allergic rhinitis: 5 mL PO q 4 to 6 h. Max 20 mL/day.

PEDS — Not approved in children.

FORMS — Trade: Syrup 5 mg hydrocodone/4 mg chlorpheniramine/60 mg pseudoephedrine/5 mL.

MOA — Decongestant/antihistamine/cough suppressant combination.

ADVERSE EFFECTS — Serious: respiratory depression/arrest. Common: sedation, palpitations, insomnia.

ZYRTEC-D (cetirizine + pseudoephedrine) ▶LK ♀C ▶– $

ADULT — Allergic rhinitis/nasal congestion: 1 tab PO q 12 h.

PEDS — Not approved in children.

FORMS — OTC Generic/Trade: Tabs, extended-release 5 mg cetirizine/120 mg pseudoephedrine.

NOTES — Decrease dose to 1 tab PO daily with decreased renal or hepatic function. Take on an empty stomach.

MOA — Decongestant/antihistamine combination.

ADVERSE EFFECTS — Serious: None. Frequent: Insomnia, palpitations, sedation.

ENT: Decongestants

NOTE: See ENT: Nasal Preparations for nasal spray decongestants (oxymetazoline, phenylephrine). Systemic decongestants are sympathomimetic and may aggravate HTN, anxiety, BPH, and insomnia. Use cautiously in such patients. Some states have restricted or ended OTC sale of pseudoephedrine or reclassified it as schedule III or V drug due to the potential for diversion to methamphetamine labs. Deaths have occurred in children younger than 2 yo attributed to toxicity from cough and cold medications; the FDA does not recommend their use in this age group.

PHENYLEPHRINE (*Sudafed PE*) ▶L ♀C ▶+ $

ADULT — Nasal congestion: 10 mg PO q 4 h prn. Max 6 doses/day.

PEDS — Nasal congestion, age older than 12 yo: Use adult dose.

FORMS — OTC Trade only: Tabs 10 mg.

NOTES — Avoid with MAOIs.

MOA — Decongestant.

ADVERSE EFFECTS — Serious: None. Frequent: Dizziness, anxiety, insomnia.

PSEUDOEPHEDRINE (*Sudafed, Sudafed 12 Hour, Efidac/24, Dimetapp Decongestant Infant Drops, PediaCare Infants' Decongestant Drops, Triaminic Oral Infant Drops*) ▶L ♀C ▶+ $

ADULT — Nasal congestion: 60 mg PO q 4 to 6 h. 120 mg PO q 12 h (extended-release). 240 mg PO daily (extended-release). Max 240 mg/day.

PEDS — Nasal congestion: Give 15 mg PO q 4 to 6 h for age 2 to 5 yo, give 30 mg PO q 4 to 6 h for age 6 to 12 yo, use adult dose for age older than 12 yo.

FORMS — OTC Generic/Trade: Tabs 30, 60 mg. Tabs, extended-release 120 mg (12 h). Soln 15, 30 mg/5 mL. Trade only: Tabs, extended-release 240 mg (24 h). Rx only in some states.

NOTES — 12 to 24 h extended-release dosage forms may cause insomnia; use a shorter-acting form if this occurs.

MOA — Decongestant.

ADVERSE EFFECTS — Serious: None. Frequent: Insomnia, palpitations.

ENT: Ear Preparations

AURALGAN (benzocaine—otic + antipyrine) ▶Not absorbed ♀C ▶? $

ADULT — Otitis media, adjunct: Instill 2 to 4 gtts (or enough to fill the ear canal) three to four times per day or q 1 to 2 h prn. Cerumen removal: Instill 2 to 4 gtts (or enough to fill the ear canal) three times per day for 2 to 3 days to detach cerumen, then prn for discomfort. Insert cotton plug moistened with soln after instillation.

PEDS — Otitis media, adjunct: Use adult dose. Cerumen removal: Use adult dose.

FORMS — Generic only: Otic soln 10, 15 mL.

MOA — Local anesthetic/analgesic.

ADVERSE EFFECTS — Serious: None. Frequent: None.

CARBAMIDE PEROXIDE (*Debrox, Murine Ear*) ▶Not absorbed ♀? ▶? $

ADULT — Cerumen impaction: Instill 5 to 10 gtts into ear two times per day for up to 4 days.

PEDS — Not approved in children.

(cont.)

CARBAMIDE PEROXIDE (*cont.*)

FORMS — OTC Generic/Trade: Otic soln 6.5%, 15 mL.

NOTES — Drops should remain in ear for several minutes. Do not use for more than 4 days. Remove excess wax by flushing with warm water using a rubber bulb ear syringe.

MOA — Cerumenolytic that emulsifies/disperses ear wax.

ADVERSE EFFECTS — Serious: None. Frequent: None.

CIPRO HC OTIC (ciprofloxacin—otic + hydrocorti-sone—otic) ▶Not absorbed ♀C ▶– $$$$$

ADULT — Otitis externa: Instill 3 gtts into affected ear(s) two times per day for 7 days.

PEDS — Otitis externa, age 1 yo or older: Use adult dose.

FORMS — Trade only: Otic susp 10 mL.

NOTES — Shake well. Contains benzyl alcohol.

MOA — Fluoroquinolone antibiotic/anti-inflammatory combination.

ADVERSE EFFECTS — Serious: None. Frequent: None.

CIPRODEX OTIC (ciprofloxacin—otic + dexametha-sone—otic) ▶Not absorbed ♀C ▶– $$$$$

ADULT — Otitis externa: Instill 4 gtts into affected ear(s) two times per day for 7 days.

PEDS — Otitis externa and otitis media with tympa-nostomy tubes, age 6 mo or older: Instill 4 gtts into affected ear(s) two times per day for 7 days.

FORMS — Trade only: Otic susp 7.5 mL.

NOTES — Shake well. Warm susp by holding bottle in hands for 1 to 2 min before instilling.

MOA — Fluoroquinolone antibiotic/anti-inflammatory combination.

ADVERSE EFFECTS — Serious: None. Frequent: None.

CIPROFLOXACIN—OTIC (*Cetraxal*) ▶Not absorbed ♀C ▶– $$$$

ADULT — Otitis externa: Instill 1 single-use container into affected ear(s) twice per day for 7 days.

PEDS — Otitis externa, age 1 yo or older: Use adult dose. Bilateral otitis with effusion undergoing tym-panostomy tube placement: Single dose intratym-panic injection of 0.1 mL into each ear following suctioning of the middle ear effusion.

FORMS — Trade only: 0.25 mL single-use containers with 0.2% ciprofloxacin soln, #14. Otic Suspension 1 mL vial of 60 mg/mL.

NOTES — Protect from light.

MOA — Fluoroquinolone antibiotic.

ADVERSE EFFECTS — Serious: None. Frequent: None.

CORTISPORIN OTIC (hydrocortisone—otic + poly-myxin—otic + neomycin—otic) ▶Not absorbed ♀? ▶? $$

ADULT — Otitis externa: Instill 4 gtts in affected ear(s) three to four times per day up to 10 days.

PEDS — Otitis externa: Instill 3 gtts in affected ear(s) three to four times per day up to 10 days.

FORMS — Generic/Trade: Otic soln 10 mL. Generic only: Otic susp 10 mL.

NOTES — Caveats with perforated TMs or tympanos-tomy tubes: (1) Risk of neomycin ototoxicity, espe-cially if use prolonged or repeated; (2) Use susp rather than acidic soln.

MOA — Antibiotic/anti-inflammatory combination.

ADVERSE EFFECTS — Serious: Ototoxicity. Frequent: None.

CORTISPORIN TC OTIC (hydrocortisone—otic + neomycin—otic + thonzonium + colistin) ▶Not absorbed ♀? ▶? $$$

ADULT — Otitis externa: Instill 5 gtts in affected ear(s) three to four times per day up to 10 days.

PEDS — Otitis externa: Instill 4 gtts in affected ear(s) three to four times per day up to 10 days.

FORMS — Generic only: Otic susp, 5 mL. Trade only: Otic susp, 10 mL.

MOA — Antibiotic/anti-inflammatory combination.

ADVERSE EFFECTS — Serious: None. Frequent: None.

DOMEBORO OTIC (acetic acid + aluminum acetate) ▶Not absorbed ♀? ▶? $$$

ADULT — Otitis externa: Instill 4 to 6 gtts in affected ear(s) q 2 to 3 h.

PEDS — Otitis externa: Instill 2 to 3 gtts in affected ear(s) q 3 to 4 h.

FORMS — Generic only: Otic soln 60 mL.

NOTES — Insert a saturated wick. Keep moist for 24 h.

MOA — Antibacterial.

ADVERSE EFFECTS — Serious: None. Frequent: None.

FLUOCINOLONE—OTIC (*DermOtic*) ▶L ♀C ▶? $$$$$

ADULT — Chronic eczematous external otitis: Instill 5 gtts in affected ear(s) two times per day for 7 to 14 days.

PEDS — Chronic eczematous external otitis: Age 2 yo or older: Use adult dose.

FORMS — Generic/Trade: Otic oil 0.01% 20 mL.

NOTES — Contains peanut oil.

MOA — Anti-inflammatory.

ADVERSE EFFECTS — Serious: None. Frequent: Burning, itching, irritation.

OFLOXACIN—OTIC (*Floxin Otic*) ▶Not absorbed ♀C ▶– $$$

ADULT — Otitis externa: Instill 10 gtts in affected ear(s) daily for 7 days. Chronic suppurative otitis media: Instill 10 gtts in affected ear(s) two times per day for 14 days.

PEDS — Otitis externa: Instill 5 gtts in affected ear(s) daily for 7 days for age 1 to 12 yo, use adult dose for age 12 yo or older. Chronic suppurative oti-tis media for age older than 12 yo: Use adult dose. Acute otitis media with tympanostomy tubes, age 1 to 12 yo: Instill 5 gtts in affected ear(s) two times per day for 10 days.

FORMS — Generic/Trade: Otic soln 0.3% 5, 10 mL. Trade only: "Singles": Single-dispensing containers 0.25 mL (5 gtts), 2 per foil pouch.

MOA — Fluoroquinolone antibiotic.

ADVERSE EFFECTS — Serious: None. Frequent: None.

SWIM-EAR (isopropyl alcohol + anhydrous glycerins) ▶Not absorbed ♀? ▶? $

ADULT — Otitis externa, prophylaxis: Instill 4 to 5 gtts in ears after swimming, showering, or bathing.

PEDS — Otitis externa, prophylaxis: Use adult dose.

FORMS — OTC Trade only: Otic soln 30 mL.

MOA — Drying agent.

ADVERSE EFFECTS — Serious: None. Frequent: None.

ENT: Mouth and Lip Preparations

CEVIMELINE (*Evoxac*) ▶L ♀C ▶– $$$$$
WARNING — May alter cardiac conduction/heart rate; caution in heart disease. May worsen bronchospasm in asthma/COPD.
ADULT — Dry mouth due to Sjögren's syndrome: 30 mg PO three times per day.
PEDS — Not approved in children.
FORMS — Generic/Trade: Caps 30 mg.
NOTES — Contraindicated in narrow-angle glaucoma, acute iritis, and severe asthma. May potentiate beta-blockers.
MOA — Cholinergic agonist.
ADVERSE EFFECTS — Serious: AV block, arrhythmias, brady/tachycardia, pulmonary edema, bronchospasm, blurred vision, cholecystitis. Frequent: Sweating, nausea, rhinitis, flushing.

CHLORHEXIDINE GLUCONATE (*Peridex, Periogard*) ▶Fecal excretion ♀B ▶? $
ADULT — Gingivitis: Twice per day as an oral rinse, morning and evening after brushing teeth. Rinse with 15 mL of undiluted soln for 30 sec. Do not swallow. Spit after rinsing.
PEDS — Not approved in children.
FORMS — Generic/Trade: Oral rinse 0.12% 15 mL, 118 mL, and 473 mL bottles.
MOA — Antibacterial.
ADVERSE EFFECTS — Serious: Hypersensitivity. Frequent: Staining of teeth, calculus formation, and altered taste.

DEBACTEROL (**sulfuric acid + sulfonated phenolics**) ▶Not absorbed ♀C ▶+ $$
ADULT — Aphthous stomatitis, mucositis: Apply to dry ulcer. Rinse with water.
PEDS — Not approved in children younger than 12 yo.
FORMS — Trade only: 1 mL prefilled, single-use applicator.
NOTES — 1 application per ulcer treatment. Dry ulcer area with cotton swab. Apply to ulcer and ring of normal mucosa around it for 5 to 10 sec. Rinse and spit. Return of ulcer pain right after rinsing indicates incomplete application; can be reapplied immediately once. Avoid eye contact. If excess irritation, rinse with dilute bicarbonate soln.
MOA — Topical analgesic + cauterizing agent.
ADVERSE EFFECTS — Serious: None. Frequent: Brief stinging during application.

GELCLAIR (**maltodextrin + propylene glycol**) ▶Not absorbed ♀+ ▶+ $$$$$
ADULT — Aphthous ulcers, mucositis, stomatitis: Rinse mouth with 1 packet three times per day or prn.
PEDS — Not approved in children.
FORMS — Trade only: 15, 90 packets/box.
NOTES — Mix packet with 3 tablespoons of water. Swish for 1 min, then spit. Do not eat or drink for 1 h after treatment.
MOA — Protective barrier.
ADVERSE EFFECTS — Serious: None. Frequent: None.

LIDOCAINE—VISCOUS (*Xylocaine*) ▶LK ♀B ▶+ $
WARNING — Avoid swallowing during oral or labial use due to GI absorption and toxicity. Measure dose exactly. May apply to small areas in mouth with a cotton-tipped applicator.
ADULT — Mouth or lip pain: 15 to 20 mL topically or swish and spit q 3 h. Max 8 doses/day.
PEDS — Use with extreme caution, as therapeutic doses approach potentially toxic levels. Use the lowest effective dose. Mouth or lip pain, age older than 3 yo: 3.75 to 5 mL topically or swish and spit up to q 3 h.
FORMS — Generic/Trade: Soln 2%, 15 mL unit dose, 100 mL bottle. Soln 4%, 50 mL.
NOTES — High risk of adverse effects and overdose in children. Consider benzocaine as a safer alternative. Clearly communicate the amount, frequency, max daily dose, and mode of administration (eg, cotton pledget to individual lesions, ½ dropper to each cheek q 4 h, or 20 min before meals). Do not prescribe on a "prn" basis without specified dosing intervals.
MOA — Local anesthetic.
ADVERSE EFFECTS — Serious: Hypersensitivity. Frequent: Burning, stinging.

MAGIC MOUTHWASH (**diphenhydramine + Mylanta + sucralfate**) ▶LK ♀ ▶– $$$
ADULT — See components.
PEDS — Not approved in children.
UNAPPROVED ADULT — Stomatitis: 5 mL PO swish and spit or swish and swallow three times per day before meals and prn.
UNAPPROVED PEDS — Stomatitis: Apply small amounts to lesions prn.
FORMS — Compounded susp. A standard mixture is 30 mL diphenhydramine liquid (12.5 mg/5 mL)/60 mL Mylanta or Maalox/4 g Carafate.
NOTES — Variations of this formulation are available. The dose and decision to swish and spit or swallow may vary with the indication and/or ingredient. Some preparations may contain Kaopectate, nystatin, tetracycline, hydrocortisone, 2% lidocaine, cherry syrup (for children). Check local pharmacies for customized formulations. Avoid diphenhydramine formulations that contain alcohol: May cause stinging of mouth sores.
MOA — Antihistamine/antacid/antiulcer combination.
ADVERSE EFFECTS — Serious: None. Frequent: Sedation, constipation, diarrhea.

PILOCARPINE (*Salagen*) ▶L ♀C ▶– $$$$
ADULT — Dry mouth due to radiation of head and neck: 5 mg PO three times per day. May increase to 10 mg PO three times per day. Dry mouth due to Sjögren's syndrome: 5 mg PO four times per day.
PEDS — Not approved in children.
UNAPPROVED ADULT — Dry mouth due to Sjögren's syndrome: 2% pilocarpine eye gtts: Swish and swallow 4 gtts diluted in water three times per day ($).

(cont.)

PILOCARPINE (cont.)
FORMS — Generic/Trade: Tabs 5, 7.5 mg.
NOTES — Contraindicated in narrow-angle glaucoma, acute iritis, and severe asthma. May potentiate beta-blockers. Reduce dose to 5 mg PO twice daily in moderate hepatic impairment.

MOA — Cholinergic agonist.
ADVERSE EFFECTS — Serious: AV block, arrhythmias, brady/tachycardia, pulmonary edema, bronchospasm, blurred vision. Frequent: Sweating, urinary frequency, nausea, diarrhea, flushing, dizziness.

ENT: Nasal Preparations—Corticosteroids

NOTE: Decrease to the lowest effective dose for maintenance therapy. Tell patients to prime pump before first use and shake well before each subsequent use.

BECLOMETHASONE—NASAL (Beconase AQ, Qnasl) ▶L ♀C ▶? $$$$
ADULT — Allergic rhinitis/nasal polyp prophylaxis: Beconase AQ: 1 to 2 spray(s) in each nostril two times per day. Allergic rhinitis: Qnasl 80 mcg/spray 2 sprays in each nostril daily, max of 4 sprays/day.
PEDS — Allergic rhinitis/nasal polyp prophylaxis: 1 spray in each nostril three times per day for age 6 to 12 yo, give adult dose for age older than 12 yo. Beconase AQ: 1 to 2 spray(s) in each nostril two times per day for age older than 6 yo. Allergic rhinitis: age 4-11 yo: Qnasl 40 mcg/spray 1 spray in each nostril once daily, max of 2 sprays/day. Age 12 and older: use adult dose.
FORMS — Trade only: Beconase AQ 42 mcg/spray, 200 sprays/bottle. Qnasl: 40 mcg/spray, 60 or 120 sprays/bottle. Qnasl: 80 mcg/spray, 120 sprays/bottle.
NOTES — AQ (aqueous) formulation may cause less stinging.
MOA — Steroidal anti-inflammatory.
ADVERSE EFFECTS — Serious: Hypersensitivity, anaphylactoid reactions, urticaria, angioedema, bronchospasm, rash. Frequent: Nasal irritation.
BUDESONIDE—NASAL (Rhinocort Allergy Spray, Rhinocort Aqua) ▶L ♀B ▶? $$$$
ADULT — Allergic rhinitis: 1 to 4 sprays per nostril daily.
PEDS — Allergic rhinitis age 6 yo or older: 1 to 2 sprays per nostril daily.
FORMS — Generic/Trade: Nasal inhaler 120 sprays/bottle. Trade only: Rhinocort Allergy Spray available OTC ($).
NOTES — CYP3A4 inhibitors such as ketoconazole, erythromycin, ritonavir, etc significantly increase systemic concentrations, possibly causing adrenal suppression.
MOA — Steroidal anti-inflammatory.
ADVERSE EFFECTS — Serious: Hypersensitivity. Frequent: Nasal irritation.
CICLESONIDE—NASAL (Omnaris, Zetonna) ▶L ♀C ▶? $$$$$
ADULT — Allergic rhinitis: Omnaris: 2 sprays per nostril daily, max dose 200 mcg/day (4 sprays/day). Zetonna: 1 actuation per nostril daily, max dose 74 mcg/day (2 sprays/day).
PEDS — Allergic rhinitis, seasonal: Omnaris: Give adult dose for age 6 yo or older. Zetonna: Give adult dose for age 12 yo or older. Allergic rhinitis,

perennial: Omnaris and Zetonna: Give adult dose for age 12 yo or older.
FORMS — Trade only: Nasal spray, 50 mcg/spray, 120 sprays/bottle (Omnaris). Nasal aerosol, 37 mcg/actuation, 60 actuations/canister (Zetonna).
MOA — Steroidal anti-inflammatory.
ADVERSE EFFECTS — Serious: None. Frequent: Epistaxis, headache.
FLUNISOLIDE—NASAL (Nasalide, ✦Rhinalar) ▶L ♀C ▶? $$$
ADULT — Allergic rhinitis: 2 sprays per nostril two times per day, may increase to three times per day. Max 8 sprays/nostril/day.
PEDS — Allergic rhinitis, age 6 to 14 yo: 1 spray per nostril three times per day or 2 sprays per nostril two times per day. Max 4 sprays/nostril/day.
FORMS — Generic only: Nasal soln 0.025%
MOA — Steroidal anti-inflammatory.
ADVERSE EFFECTS — Serious: Hypersensitivity. Frequent: Nasal irritation.
FLUTICASONE—NASAL (Flonase, Veramyst) ▶L ♀C ▶? $
ADULT — Allergic rhinitis, perennial nonallergic rhinitis: 2 sprays per nostril daily or 1 spray per nostril two times per day, decrease to 1 spray per nostril daily when appropriate.
PEDS — Allergic rhinitis, age 4-11 yo: 1 spray in each nostril daily. Age 12-17 yo: 2 sprays in each nostril daily, with a 1 spray daily maintenance dose as appropriate. Perennial nonallergic rhinitis, age 4-17 yo: 1 spray each nostril daily with a maximal dose of 2 sprays each nostril, and maintenance dose of 1 spray each nostril daily as appropriate.
FORMS — Generic: fluticasone Rx nasal spray 0.05% 15.8 mL 120 sprays/bottle. Brand: Flonase OTC nasal spray 0.05% 9.9 mL 60 sprays/bottle and 15.8 mL 120 sprays/bottle
NOTES — CYP3A4 inhibitors such as ketoconazole, erythromycin, ritonavir, etc significantly increase systemic concentrations, possibly causing adrenal suppression.
MOA — Steroidal anti-inflammatory.
ADVERSE EFFECTS — Serious: Hypersensitivity. Frequent: Nasal irritation.
MOMETASONE—NASAL (Nasonex) ▶L ♀C ▶? $$$$$
ADULT — Prevention or treatment of symptoms of allergic rhinitis: 2 sprays per nostril daily. Treatment of nasal polyps: 2 sprays per nostril two times per day (once daily may also be effective).

(cont.)

MOMETASONE—NASAL (*cont.*)

PEDS — Prevention or treatment of symptoms of allergic rhinitis, age 12 yo or older: Use adult dose. 2 to 11 yo: 1 spray per nostril daily.

FORMS — Generic/Trade: Nasal spray, 120 sprays/bottle.

MOA — Steroidal anti-inflammatory.

ADVERSE EFFECTS — Serious: Hypersensitivity. Frequent: Nasal irritation.

TRIAMCINOLONE—NASAL (*Nasacort AQ, Nasacort HFA, Tri-Nasal, AllerNaze*) ▶L ♀C ▶– $

ADULT — Allergic rhinitis: 2 sprays per nostril daily. May reduce to 1 spray per nostril daily once controlled.

PEDS — Allergic rhinitis: 1 spray each nostril daily for age 2 to < 6 yo, 1 spray each nostril and may increase to 2 sprays each nostril for 6 to < 12 yo.

FORMS — Trade only: OTC: Nasal spray, 55 mcg/spray, 120 sprays/bottle (Nasacort Allergy 24HR) . Generic only: Rx: Nasal spray, 55 mcg/spray, 120 sprays/bottle.

NOTES — AQ (aqueous) formulation may cause less stinging. Decrease to lowest effective dose after allergy symptom improvement.

MOA — Steroidal anti-inflammatory.

ADVERSE EFFECTS — Serious: Hypersensitivity. Frequent: Nasal irritation.

ENT: Nasal Preparations—Other

NOTE: For nasal sprays except saline, oxymetazoline, and phenylephrine, tell patients to prime pump before first use and shake well before each subsequent use.

AZELASTINE—NASAL (*Astelin, Astepro*) ▶L ♀C ▶? $$$$

ADULT — Allergic/vasomotor rhinitis: 1 to 2 sprays/nostril two times per day.

PEDS — Allergic rhinitis: 1 spray/nostril two times per day for age 5 to 11 yo, give adult dose for 12 yo or older. Vasomotor rhinitis: Give adult dose for 12 yo or older.

FORMS — Generic/Trade: Astepro 0.15% nasal spray 200 sprays/bottle. Generic only: 0.1% nasal spray 200 sprays/bottle.

MOA — Antihistamine.

ADVERSE EFFECTS — Serious: Atrial fibrillation. Frequent: Bitter taste, sedation.

CETACAINE (benzocaine + tetracaine + butamben) ▶LK ♀C ▶? $$

WARNING — Do not use on the eyes. Hypersensitivity (rare). Methemoglobinemia (rare).

ADULT — Topical anesthesia of mucous membranes: Spray: Apply for 1 sec or less. Liquid or gel: Apply with cotton applicator directly to site.

PEDS — Use adult dose.

FORMS — Trade only: (14%/2%/2%) Spray 56 mL. Topical liquid 56 mL. Topical gel 5, 29 g.

NOTES — Do not hold cotton applicator in position for extended time due to increased risk of local reactions. Do not use multiple applications. Maximum anesthesia occurs 1 min after application; duration 30 min. May result in potentially dangerous methemoglobinemia; use minimum amount needed.

MOA — Local anesthetic combination.

ADVERSE EFFECTS — Serious: Hypersensitivity, methemoglobinemia. Frequent: Erythema, pruritus.

CROMOLYN—NASAL (*NasalCrom*) ▶LK ♀B ▶+ $

ADULT — Allergic rhinitis: 1 spray per nostril three to four times per day up to 6 times per day.

PEDS — Allergic rhinitis, for age 2 yo or older: Use adult dose.

FORMS — OTC Generic/Trade: Nasal inhaler 200 sprays/bottle 13, 26 mL.

NOTES — Therapeutic effects may not be seen for 1 to 2 weeks.

MOA — Anti-inflammatory mast-cell stabilizer.

ADVERSE EFFECTS — Serious: None. Frequent: None.

DYMISTA (azelastine—nasal + fluticasone—nasal) ▶L – ♀C ▶? $$$$$

ADULT — Seasonal allergic rhinitis: 1 spray per nostril 2 times per day.

PEDS — Seasonal allergic rhinitis: Give adult dose for age 12 yo or older.

FORMS — Trade only: Nasal spray: 137 mcg azelastine/50 mcg fluticasone/spray, 120 sprays/bottle.

NOTES — CYP3A4 inhibitors such as ketoconazole, erythromycin, ritonavir, etc significantly increase systemic concentrations of fluticasone, possibly causing adrenal suppression.

MOA — Intranasal antihistamine/anti-inflammatory steroid combination.

ADVERSE EFFECTS — Serious: Atrial fibrillation, hypersensitivity. Frequent: Bitter taste, sedation, nasal irritation.

IPRATROPIUM—NASAL (*Atrovent Nasal Spray*) ▶L ♀B ▶? $$

ADULT — Rhinorrhea due to allergic/nonallergic rhinitis: 2 sprays (0.03%) per nostril two to three times per day or 2 sprays (0.06%) per nostril four times per day. Rhinorrhea due to common cold: 2 sprays (0.06%) per nostril three to four times per day.

PEDS — Rhinorrhea due to allergic/nonallergic rhinitis: Give adult dose (0.03% strength) for age 6 yo or older, give adult dose (0.06% strength) for age 5 yo or older. Rhinorrhea due to common cold: 2 sprays (0.06% strength) per nostril three times per day for age 5 yo or older.

UNAPPROVED ADULT — Vasomotor rhinitis: 2 sprays (0.06%) in each nostril three to four times per day.

FORMS — Generic/Trade: Nasal spray 0.03%, 30 mL (345 sprays)/bottle, 0.06%, 15 mL (165 sprays)/bottle.

MOA — Anticholinergic.

ADVERSE EFFECTS — Serious: Hypersensitivity. Frequent: Nasal irritation, epistaxis.

LEVOCABASTINE—NASAL (✱*Livostin*) ▶L (but minimal absorption) ♀C ▶– $$

ADULT — Canada only. Allergic rhinitis: 2 sprays per nostril two times per day; increase prn to 2 sprays per nostril three to four times per day.

PEDS — Not approved in children younger than 12 yo.

FORMS — Trade only: Nasal spray 0.5 mg/mL, plastic bottles of 15 mL. 50 mcg/spray.

NOTES — Nasal spray is devoid of CNS effects. Safety and efficacy in patients older than 65 yo have not been established.

MOA — Antihistamine.

ADVERSE EFFECTS — Frequent: Nasal irritation.

OLOPATADINE—NASAL (*Patanase*) ▶L ♀C ▶? $$$$$

ADULT — Allergic rhinitis: 2 sprays/nostril two times per day.

PEDS — Allergic rhinitis, age 12 yo or older: Use adult dose. For age 6 to 11 yo: 1 spray/nostril two times per day.

FORMS — Generic/Trade: Nasal spray 0.6% soln, 240 sprays/bottle.

MOA — Antihistamine.

ADVERSE EFFECTS — Serious: None. Frequent: Epistaxis, nasal irritation, bitter taste, sedation.

OXYMETAZOLINE (*Afrin, Dristan 12 Hr Nasal, Nostrilla, Vicks Sinex 12 Hr*) ▶L ♀C ▶? $

WARNING — Use with caution in patients with BPH, CAD or HTN.

ADULT — Nasal congestion: 2 to 3 sprays or gtts (0.05%) per nostril two times per day for no more than 3 days.

PEDS — Nasal congestion: 2 to 6 yo: no FDA-approved dose. Not recommended in children under 2 yo.

FORMS — OTC Generic/Trade: Nasal spray 0.05% 15, 30 mL; Nose gtts 0.05% 20 mL with dropper.

NOTES — Overuse (more than 3 to 5 days) may lead to rebound congestion. If this occurs, taper to use in 1 nostril only, alternating sides, then discontinue. Substituting an oral decongestant or nasal steroid may also be useful.

MOA — Alpha-1 agonist decongestant.

ADVERSE EFFECTS — Serious: None. Frequent: Stinging, rebound congestion.

PHENYLEPHRINE—NASAL (*Neo-Synephrine*) ▶L ♀C ▶? $

WARNING — Use caution in patients with BPH or taking MAO inhibitors.

ADULT — Nasal congestion: 2 to 3 sprays or gtts (0.25 or 0.5%) per nostril q 4 h prn for no more than 3 days. Use 1% soln for severe congestion.

PEDS — Nasal congestion, age 6-11 yo: Give 2 to 3 gtts or sprays (0.25%) per nostril no more than q 4 h prn for no more than 3 days. For 12 yo or older: use adult dose.

FORMS — OTC Generic/Trade: Nasal gtts/spray 0.25, 0.5, 1% (15 mL).

NOTES — Overuse (more 3 to 5 days) may lead to rebound congestion. If this occurs, taper to use in 1 nostril only, alternating sides, then discontinue. Rebound may persist for several weeks. Substituting oral decongestants, oral antihistamines, nasal saline, or nasal steroids may help.

MOA — Alpha agonist decongestant.

ADVERSE EFFECTS — Serious: None. Frequent: Stinging, rebound congestion.

SALINE NASAL SPRAY (*SeaMist, Entsol, Pretz, NaSal, Ocean,* ✱*hydraSense*) ▶Not metabolized ♀A ▶+ $

WARNING — If water source possibly impure, boil water or use distilled water.

ADULT — Nasal dryness: 1 to 3 sprays per nostril prn.

PEDS — Nasal dryness: 1 to 3 gtts per nostril prn.

UNAPPROVED ADULT — Chronic sinusitis, allergic rhinitis and nasal congestion: 1 to 3 gtts per nostril prn.

UNAPPROVED PEDS — Chronic sinusitis, allergic rhinitis and nasal congestion: 1 to 3 gtts per nostril prn.

FORMS — Generic/Trade (OTC): Nasal spray 0.4, 0.5, 0.65, 0.75%. Nasal gtts 0.4, 0.65%. Trade only: Preservative-free nasal spray 3% (Entsol).

NOTES — May be prepared at home by combining: ¼ teaspoon salt with 8 ounces (1 cup) warm water. Add ¼ teaspoon baking soda (optional) and put in spray bottle, ear syringe, neti pot, or any container with a small spout. Discard after 1 week.

MOA — Moisturizer and irrigant.

ADVERSE EFFECTS — Serious: None. Frequent: None.

GASTROENTEROLOGY

HELICOBACTER PYLORI THERAPY

- Triple therapy PO for 10 to 14 days: clarithromycin 500 mg two times per day plus amoxicillin 1 g two times per day (or metronidazole 500 mg two times per day) plus PPI*
- Quadruple therapy PO for 14 days: bismuth subsalicylate 525 mg (or 30 mL) four times per day plus metronidazole four times per day plus tetracycline 500 mg four times per day plus a PPI* or an H2 blocker[†]
- PPI or H2 blocker may need to be continued past 14 days to heal the ulcer.

*PPIs include esomeprazole 40 mg daily, lansoprazole 30 mg two times per day, omeprazole 20 mg two times per day, pantoprazole 40 mg two times per day, rabeprazole 20 mg two times per day, pantoprazole 40 mg two times per day, rabeprazole 20 mg two times per day.
[†]H2 blockers include cimetidine 400 mg two times per day, famotidine 20 mg two times per day, nizatidine 150 mg two times per day, ranitidine 150 mg two times per day. Adapted from *Treat Guidel Med Lett* 2008:55.

GASTROENTEROLOGY: Antidiarrheals

BISMUTH SUBSALICYLATE (*Pepto-Bismol, Kaopectate*) ▶K ♀D ▶? $

WARNING — Avoid in children and teenagers with chickenpox or flu due to possible association with Reye's syndrome.

ADULT — Diarrhea: 2 tabs or 30 mL (262 mg/15 mL) PO q 30 to 60 min up to 8 doses/day for up to 2 days.

PEDS — Diarrhea: 100 mg/kg/day divided into 5 doses or ⅓ tab, chew tab, or 5 mL (262 mg/15 mL) q 30 to 60 min prn up to 8 doses/day for age 3 to 6 yo; ⅔ tab, chew tab, or 10 mL (262 mg/15 mL) q 30 to 60 min prn up to 8 doses/day for age 7 to 9 yo; 1 tab or chew tab or 15 mL (262 mg/15 mL) q 30 to 60 min prn up to 8 doses/day for age 10 to 12 yo. Do not take for more than 2 days.

UNAPPROVED ADULT — Prevention of traveler's diarrhea: 2.1 g/day or 2 tabs four times per day before meals and at bedtime. Has been used as part of a multidrug regimen for Helicobacter pylori.

UNAPPROVED PEDS — Chronic infantile diarrhea: 2.5 mL (262 mg/15 mL) PO q 4 h for age 2 to 24 mo, 5 mL (262 mg/15 mL) PO q 4 h for age 25 to 48 mo, 10 mL (262 mg/15 mL) PO q 4 h for age 49 to 70 mo.

FORMS — OTC Generic/Trade: Chewable tabs 262 mg. Susp 262, 525, 750 mg/15 mL. Caplets 262 mg (Pepto-Bismol). OTC Trade only: Susp 87 mg/5 mL (Kaopectate Children's Liquid).

NOTES — Use with caution in patients already taking salicylates or warfarin, children recovering from chickenpox or flu. Decreases absorption of tetracycline. May darken stools or tongue. Children's Pepto-Bismol contains calcium carbonate.

MOA — Antidiarrheal.

ADVERSE EFFECTS — Frequent: None.

IMODIUM MULTI-SYMPTOM RELIEF (loperamide + simethicone) ▶L ♀C ▶+ $

ADULT — Diarrhea: 2 tabs/caps PO initially, then 1 tab/cap PO after each unformed stool to a max of 4 tabs/caps/day.

PEDS — Diarrhea: 1 cap PO initially, then ½ tab/cap PO after each unformed stool (up to 2 tabs/caps/day for age 6 to 8 yo or wt 48 to 59 lbs, up to 3 tabs/caps/day for age 9 to 11 yo or wt 60 to 95 lbs).

FORMS — OTC Generic/Trade: Caplets, Chewable tabs 2 mg loperamide/125 mg simethicone.

NOTES — Not for C. difficile–associated diarrhea, toxigenic bacterial diarrhea, or most childhood diarrhea (difficult to exclude toxigenic).

MOA — Antidiarrheal, inhibits peristalsis of intestinal muscles.

ADVERSE EFFECTS — Frequent: Sedation in children.

LOMOTIL (diphenoxylate + atropine) ▶L ♀C ▶– ©V $

ADULT — Diarrhea: 2 tabs or 10 mL PO four times per day.

PEDS — Diarrhea: 0.3 to 0.4 mg diphenoxylate/kg/24 h in 4 divided doses. Max daily dose 20 mg. Not recommended for younger than 2 yo; give 1.5 to 3 mL PO four times per day for age 2 yo or wt 11 to 14 kg; 2 to 3 mL PO four times per day for age 3 yo or wt 12 to 16 kg; 2 to 4 mL PO four times per day for age 4 yo or wt 14 to 20 kg; 2.5 to 4.5 mL PO four times per day for age 5 yo or wt 16 to 23 kg; 2.5 to 5 mL PO four times per day for age 6 to 8 yo or wt 17 to 32 kg; 3.5 to 5 mL PO four times per day for 9 to 12 yo or wt 23 to 55 kg.

FORMS — Generic/Trade: Oral soln or tab 2.5 mg/0.025 mg diphenoxylate/atropine per 5 mL or tab.

NOTES — Give with food to decrease GI upset. May cause atropinism in children, especially with Down syndrome, even at recommended doses. Can cause delayed toxicity. Has been reported to cause severe respiratory depression, coma, brain damage, death after overdose in children. Naloxone reverses toxicity. Do not use for C. difficile–associated diarrhea, toxigenic bacterial diarrhea, or most childhood diarrhea (difficult to exclude toxigenic).

MOA — Antidiarrheal, inhibits peristalsis of intestinal muscles.

ADVERSE EFFECTS — Frequent: Nervousness, dizziness, headache, depression, restlessness.

LOPERAMIDE (*Imodium, Imodium AD, *Loperacap, Diarr-Eze*) ▶L ♀C ▶+ $

WARNING — Discontinue if abdominal distention or ileus. Caution in children due to variable response.

ADULT — Diarrhea: 4 mg PO initially, then 2 mg after each unformed stool to max 16 mg/day.

(cont.)

LOPERAMIDE (*cont.*)

PEDS — Diarrhea: First day: 1 mg PO three times per day for age 2 to 5 yo or wt 13 to 20 kg, 2 mg PO two times per day for age 6 to 8 yo or wt 21 to 30 kg, 2 mg PO three times per day for age 9 to 12 yo or wt greater than 30 kg. After 1st day: Give 0.1 mg/kg PO after each loose stool; daily dose not to exceed daily dose of first day.

UNAPPROVED ADULT — Chronic diarrhea or ileostomy drainage: 4 mg initially then 2 mg after each stool until symptoms are controlled, then reduce dose for maintenance treatment, average adult maintenance dose 4 to 8 mg daily as a single dose or in divided doses.

UNAPPROVED PEDS — Chronic diarrhea: Limited information. Average doses of 0.08 to 0.24 mg/kg/day PO in 2 to 3 divided doses. Max 2 mg/dose. Max 16 mg/day.

FORMS — OTC Generic/Trade: Tabs 2 mg. Oral soln 1 mg/5 mL. Oral soln 1 mg/7.5 mL.

NOTES — Not for C. difficile–associated diarrhea, toxigenic bacterial diarrhea, or most childhood diarrhea (difficult to exclude toxigenic). Doses greater than 16 mg/day have been used.

MOA — Antidiarrheal, inhibits peristalsis of intestinal muscles.

ADVERSE EFFECTS — Frequent: Sedation in children.

MOTOFEN (**difenoxin + atropine**) ▶L ♀C ▶– ©IV $$$$$

ADULT — Diarrhea: 2 tabs PO initially, then 1 tab after each loose stool q 3 to 4 h prn (up to 8 tabs/day).

PEDS — Not approved in children. Contraindicated younger than 2 yo.

FORMS — Trade only: Tabs difenoxin 1 mg + atropine 0.025 mg.

NOTES — Do not use for C. difficile–associated diarrhea, toxigenic bacterial diarrhea, or most childhood diarrhea (difficult to exclude toxigenic). May cause atropinism in children, especially with Down syndrome, even at recommended doses. Can cause delayed toxicity. Has been reported to cause severe respiratory depression, coma, brain damage, death after overdose in children. Difenoxin is the primary metabolite of diphenoxylate.

MOA — Antidiarrheal, inhibits peristalsis of intestinal muscles.

ADVERSE EFFECTS — Frequent: Anticholinergic effects, nervousness, dizziness, headache, depression, restlessness.

OPIUM (***opium tincture, paregoric***) ▶L ♀C ▶? ©II $$$

ADULT — Diarrhea: Paregoric: 5 to 10 mL PO daily (up to four times). Opium tincture: 0.6 mL (range 0.3 to 1 mL) PO q 2 to 6 h prn up to four times a day

PEDS — Diarrhea: 0.25 to 0.5 mL/kg paregoric PO daily (up to four times per day).

FORMS — Trade only: Opium tincture 10% (deodorized opium tincture, 10 mg morphine equivalent/mL). Generic only: Paregoric (camphorated opium tincture, 2 mg morphine equivalent/5 mL).

NOTES — Opium tincture contains 25 times more morphine than paregoric. Do not use for C. difficile–associated diarrhea, toxigenic bacterial diarrhea, or most childhood diarrhea.

MOA — Antidiarrheal, inhibits peristalsis of intestinal muscles.

ADVERSE EFFECTS — Frequent: Palpitations, hypotension, bradycardia, dizziness, drowsiness, weakness, urinary retention. Severe: Possible biliary tract spasm.

GASTROENTEROLOGY: Antiemetics—5-HT3 Receptor Antagonists

AKYNZEO (**palonosetron + netupitant**) ▶L ♀C ▶ $$$$$

WARNING — Hypersensitivity reactions, including anaphylaxis, have been reported.

ADULT — Prevention of N/V with chemo: 1 capsule PO prior to chemo.

PEDS — Not approved in children younger than 18 yo.

FORMS — Trade only: Capsule (0.5 mg palonosetron + 300 mg netupitant).

MOA — 5-HT3 receptor antagoist + substance P/neurokinin 1 receptor antagonist

ADVERSE EFFECTS — Frequent: headache, asthenia, fatigue, constipation, erythemia.

DOLASETRON (**Anzemet**) ▶LK ♀B ▶? $$$$

ADULT — Prevention of N/V with chemo: 100 mg PO single dose 60 min before chemo. Prevention/treatment of post-op N/V: 12.5 mg IV 15 min before end of anesthesia (prevention) or at onset of N/V (treatment).

PEDS — Prevention of N/V with chemo: 1.8 mg/kg up to 100 mg PO single dose 60 min before chemo for age 2 to 16 yo. Prevention/Treatment of Post-op N/V: 2 to 16 yo: 0.35 mg/kg IV (max 12.5 mg) IV 15 min before end of anesthesia (prevention) or at onset of N/V (treatment). Or 1.2 mg/kg (max 100 mg) PO within 2 hr before surgery (prevention).

UNAPPROVED ADULT — N/V due to radiotherapy: 0.3 mg/kg IV as a single dose.

FORMS — Trade only: Tabs 50, 100 mg. Injectable no longer available in Canada.

NOTES — Use caution in patients of any age who have or may develop prolongation of QT interval (ie, hypokalemia, hypomagnesemia, concomitant antiarrhythmic therapy, cumulative high-dose anthracycline therapy). Cimetidine may increase serum concentrations, rifampin may reduce serum concentrations. May increase the risk of serotonin syndrome.

MOA — Antiemetic, serotonin antagonist blocking chemoreceptor trigger zone.

ADVERSE EFFECTS — Frequent: headache. Severe: Prolongation of cardiac conduction intervals, particularly QTc, ventricular tachycardia, ventricular fibrillation.

GASTROENTEROLOGY: Antiemetics 259

GRANISETRON (*Sustol, Sancuso*) ▶L ♀B ▶? $$$$

ADULT — Prevention of N/V with chemo: Transdermal (Sancuso): 1 patch to upper outer arm at least 24 h (but up to 48 h) before chemotherapy. Remove 24 h after completion of chemotherapy. Can be worn up to 7 days depending on the duration of chemo. 10 mcg/kg IV within 30 min of chemo. 2 mg once daily PO or 1 mg twice daily PO to start up to 1 h before chemotherapy. 10 mg SC (Sustol) 30 min prior to chemo. Prevention of N/V with radiation: 2 mg PO within 1 h prior of radiation.

PEDS — Prevention of N/V with chemo: 2 to 16 years: 10 mcg/kg IV within 30 min of chemo.

FORMS — Trade only: Transdermal patch (Sancuso) 34.3 mg of granisetron delivering 3.1 mg/24 h. Generic only: Tablet 1 mg.

NOTES — May increase the risk of serotonin syndrome. Do not expose patch to sunlight or heat (e.g., heating pad).

MOA — Antiemetic, serotonin antagonist blocking chemoreceptor trigger zone.

ADVERSE EFFECTS — Frequent: Headache. Severe: Arrhythmias, QT prolongation.

ONDANSETRON (*Zofran, Zuplenz*) ▶L ♀B ▶? $$$$$

WARNING — Avoid in patients with congenital long QT syndrome. ECG monitoring is recommended in patients with electrolyte abnormalities, CHF, brady-arrhythmias, or patients taking other medications that can prolong QT interval. May increase the risk of serotonin syndrome.

ADULT — Prevention of N/V with chemo: 0.15 mg/kg IV (max 16 mg) 30 min prior to chemo and repeated at 4 and 8 h after 1st dose. Alternatively, 8 mg PO 30 min before moderately emetogenic chemo and 8 h later. Can be given q 12 h for 1 to 2 days after completion of chemo. For single-day highly emetogenic chemo, 24 mg PO 30 min before chemo. Prevention of post-op nausea: 4 mg IV over 2 to 5 min or 4 mg IM IV or IM doses s 30 minutes before end of anesthesia or 16 mg PO 1 h before anesthesia. Prevention of N/V associated with radiotherapy: 8 mg PO three times per day.

PEDS — Prevention of N/V with chemo: IV: 0.15 mg/kg (max 16 mg) 30 min prior to chemo and repeated at 4 and 8 h after 1st dose for age older than 6 mo. PO: Give 4 mg 30 minutes prior to chemo and repeat at 4 and 8 h after 1st dose for age 4 to 11 yo. Can be given q 8 h PO for 1 to 2 days after completion of chemo. Give 8 mg PO 30 min before chemo and 8 h later for age 12 yo or older. Prevention of post-op

N/V: 0.1 mg/kg IV over 2 to 5 min for age 1 mo to 12 yo if wt 40 kg or less; give 4 mg IV over 2 to 5 min if wt greater than 40 kg. IV doses should be given 30 min before end of surgery

UNAPPROVED ADULT — Has been used in hyperemesis associated with pregnancy.

UNAPPROVED PEDS — Use with caution if younger than 4 yo. Dosing based on BSA: Give 1 mg PO three times per day for BSA less than 0.3 m^2, give 2 mg PO three times per day for BSA 0.3 to 0.6 m^2, give 3 mg PO three times per day for BSA 0.6 to 1 m^2, give 4 mg PO three times per day for BSA greater than 1 m^2. Use caution in infants younger than 6 mo.

FORMS — Generic/Trade: Tabs 4, 8, 24 mg. Orally disintegrating tabs 4, 8 mg. Oral soln 4 mg/5 mL. Trade only: Oral film (Zuplenz) 4, 8 mg.

NOTES — Can prolong QT interval. Max oral dose if severe liver disease is 8 mg/day. Max IV dose is 16 mg. Use following abdominal surgery or in those receiving chemotherapy may mask a progressive ileus or gastric distension. Contraindicated with apomorphine; concomitant use can lead to hypotension and loss of consciousness. May increase risk of serotonin syndrome.

MOA — Antiemetic, serotonin antagonist blocking chemoreceptor trigger zone.

ADVERSE EFFECTS — Frequent: Headache, fever, diarrhea, constipation, transient increases in LFTs. Severe: Transient blindness, especially with IV, arrhythmia, QT prolongation, Stevens-Johnson syndrome and toxic epidermal necrolysis.

PALONOSETRON (*Aloxi*) ▶L ♀B ▶? $$$$$

ADULT — Prevention of N/V with chemo: 0.25 mg IV over 30 sec, 30 min prior to chemo. Prevention of postop N/V: 0.075 mg IV over 10 sec just prior to anesthesia.

PEDS — Prevention of N/V with chemo (1 mo to 17 yo): 20 mcg/kg (max 1.5 mg) over 15 min, 30 min prior to chemo.

UNAPPROVED PEDS — Limited information suggests 3 mcg/kg (max 0.25 mg) IV is effective and safe in children older than 2 yo.

FORMS — Trade only: Injectable.

NOTES — May increase the risk of serotonin syndrome.

MOA — Antiemetic, serotonin antagonist blocking chemoreceptor trigger zone.

ADVERSE EFFECTS — Frequent: Headache, constipation. Severe: Arrhythmia, QT prolongation, serotonin syndrome.

GASTROENTEROLOGY: Antiemetics—Other

APREPITANT (*Emend, fosaprepitant*) ▶L ♀B ▶? $$$$$

ADULT — Prevention of N/V with moderately to highly emetogenic chemo, in combination with a corticosteroid and a 5-HT3 antagonist: 125 mg PO on day 1 (1 h prior to chemo), then 80 mg PO q am on days 2 and 3. Prevention of postop N/V: 40 mg PO within 3 h prior to anesthesia.

PEDS — Prevention of N/V with moderately to highly emetogenic chemo, in combination with a corticosteroid and a 5-HT3 antagonist in children 6 months and older: 3 mg/kg (max 125 mg) PO on day 1, then 2 mg/kg (max 80mg) PO on days 2 and 3.

FORMS — Trade only (aprepitant): Caps 40, 80, 125 mg. Susp 125 mg. IV form is fosaprepitant.

(cont.)

APREPITANT (cont.)

NOTES — Use caution with other medications metabolized by CYP3A4 hepatic enzyme system and an inducer of the CYP2C9 hepatic enzyme system. Contraindicated with pimozide. May decrease efficacy of oral contraceptives; women should use alternate/back-up method. Monitor INR in patients receiving warfarin. Fosaprepitant is a prodrug of aprepitant.

MOA — Antiemetic, substance P/neurokinin-1 receptor antagonist.

ADVERSE EFFECTS — Frequent: Fatigue, diarrhea, constipation, muscular weakness, hiccups. Severe: Hypersensitivity and anaphylactic reactions.

DICLEGIS (doxylamine + pyridoxine, ✸ Diclectin) ▶LK ♀A ▶– $$$$$

WARNING — Avoid taking with MAO inhibitors.

ADULT — N/V due to pregnancy: 2 tabs PO at bedtime. If not controlled, can increase to a max of 4 tabs daily (1 tab PO q am, 1 tab PO mid-afternoon, 2 tabs PO at bedtime).

PEDS — Not indicated for children.

FORMS — Trade: Tabs doxylamine 10 mg and pyridoxine 10 mg.

MOA — Unknown.

ADVERSE EFFECTS — Frequent: drowsiness, somnolence.

DIMENHYDRINATE (Dramamine, ✸Gravol) ▶LK ♀B ▶– $

ADULT — Nausea: 50 to 100 mg/dose PO/IM/IV q 4 to 6 h prn. Max PO dose 400 mg/24 h, max IV/IM dose 600 mg/24 h. Canada only: 50 to 100 mg/dose PR q 6 to 8 h prn.

PEDS — Nausea: Not recommended for age younger than 2 yo. Give 12.5 to 25 mg PO q 6 to 8 h or 5 mg/kg/day (up to 75 mg/day) PO divided q 6 h for age 2 to 5 yo, give 25 to 50 mg (up to 150 mg/day) PO q 6 to 8 h or for age 6 to 12 yo.

FORMS — OTC Generic/Trade: Tabs 50 mg. Trade only: Chewable tabs 25, 50 mg. Canada only: Supps 25, 50, 100 mg.

NOTES — May cause drowsiness. Use with caution in conditions that may be aggravated by anticholinergic effects (ie, prostatic hypertrophy, asthma, narrow-angle glaucoma). Available as suppositories in Canada.

MOA — Antihistamine.

ADVERSE EFFECTS — Frequent: Blurred vision, dry mouth, dizziness. Severe: Hallucinations, psychosis.

DOMPERIDONE ▶L ♀? ▶ $$

ADULT — Canada only. Postprandial dyspepsia: 10 to 20 mg PO three to four times per day, 30 min before a meal. N/V: 20 mg PO three to four times per day.

PEDS — Not approved in children.

UNAPPROVED ADULT — Has been used for diabetic gastroparesis, chemotherapy/radiation-induced N/V. Has also been used to increase milk production in lactating mothers although this is not currently recommended due to safety concerns.

UNAPPROVED PEDS — Use in children generally not recommended except for chemotherapy- or radiation-induced N/V: 200 to 400 mcg/kg PO q 4 to 8 h.

FORMS — Canada only. Trade/Generic: Tabs 10, 20 mg.

NOTES — Similar in efficacy to metoclopramide but less likely to cause EPS.

MOA — Dopamine antagonist at GI muscle receptors and chemoreceptor trigger zone, resulting in improved gastric emptying.

ADVERSE EFFECTS — Serious: Cardiac dysrhythmia. Frequent: galactorrhea, gynecomastia.

DOXYLAMINE (Unisom Nighttime Sleep Aid SleepTabs, others) ▶L ♀A ▶? $

PEDS — Not approved in children younger than 12 yo.

UNAPPROVED ADULT — N/V due to pregnancy: 12.5 mg PO two to four times per day; often used in combination with pyridoxine.

FORMS — OTC, Generic/Trade: Tabs 25 mg. Chewable tab 5 mg (Aldex-N).

NOTES — Some Unisom products contain diphenhydramine instead of doxylamine.

MOA — Anticholinergic and sedative.

ADVERSE EFFECTS — Frequent: None.

DRONABINOL (Syndros, Marinol) ▶L ♀C ▶– ©III $$$$$

ADULT — Nausea with chemo: 5 mg/m² PO 1 to 3 h before chemo then 5 mg/m²/dose q 2 to 4 h after chemo for 4 to 6 doses/day. Dose can be increased to max 15 mg/m². Syndros: 4.2 mg/m² PO 1 to 3 hours before chemo, on an empty stomach, then eery 2 to 4 hours after chemotherapy for up to 4 to 6 doses daily. Anorexia associated with AIDS: Initially 2.5 mg PO two times per day before lunch and dinner. If indicated and tolerated, increase to 20 mg/day. Syndros: 2.1 mg PO twice daily, 1 hour before luch and dinner.

PEDS — Nausea with chemo: 5 mg/m² PO 1 to 3 h before chemo then 5 mg/m²/dose PO q 2 to 4 h after chemo (up to 4 to 6 doses/day). Dose can be increased to max 15 mg/m². Not approved for anorexia associated with AIDS in children. Syndros is not approved for any indications in children.

UNAPPROVED ADULT — Appetite stimulant: 2.5 mg PO twice daily (for dronabinol, not Syndros).

UNAPPROVED PEDS — Nausea with chemo: 5 mg/m² PO 1 to 3 h before chemo then 5 mg/m²/dose PO q 2 to 4 h after chemo (up to 4 to 6 doses/day). Dose can be increased to max 15 mg/m² (for dronabinol, not Syndros).

FORMS — Generic/Trade: Caps 2.5, 5, 10 mg. Oral soln (Syndros) 5 mg/mL.

NOTES — Patient response varies; individualize dosing (start with low doses in elderly). Additive CNS effects with alcohol, sedatives, hypnotics, psychotomimetics. Caution if history of seizures.

MOA — Unknown.

ADVERSE EFFECTS — Frequent: Drowsiness, dizziness, anxiety, detachment, mood changes, anorexia. Severe: Syncope.

DROPERIDOL (Inapsine) ▶L ♀C ▶? $

WARNING — Cases of fatal QT prolongation and/or torsade des pointes have occurred in patients receiving droperidol at or below recommended doses (some without risk factors for QT prolongation).

(cont.)

DROPERIDOL (*cont.*)

Reserve for nonresponse to other treatments, and perform 12-lead ECG prior to administration and continue ECG monitoring 2 to 3 h after treatment. Avoid if prolonged baseline QT.

ADULT — Antiemetic premedication: 0.625 to 2.5 mg IV or 2.5 mg IM then 1.25 mg prn.

PEDS — Pre-op: 0.088 to 0.165 mg/kg IV for age 2 to 12 yo. Children older than 12 yo: 2.5 mg IM/IV, additional doses of 1.25 mg can be given with caution. Post-op antiemetic: 0.01 to 0.03 mg/kg/dose IV q 6 to 8 h prn. Usual dose 0.05 to 0.06 mg/kg/dose (up to 0.1 mg/kg/dose).

UNAPPROVED ADULT — Chemo-induced nausea: 2.5 to 5 mg IV/IM q 3 to 4 h prn.

UNAPPROVED PEDS — Chemo-induced nausea: 0.05 to 0.06 mg/kg/dose IV/IM q 4 to 6 h prn.

NOTES — Has no analgesic or amnestic effects. Consider lower doses in geriatric, debilitated, or high-risk patients such as those receiving other CNS depressants. May cause hypotension or tachycardia, extrapyramidal reactions, drowsiness.

MOA — Alters action of dopamine to sedate and reduce emesis.

ADVERSE EFFECTS — Frequent: QTc prolongatioon, restlessness, anxiety, dystonic reactions. Severe: Cardiac arrest, sedation, hypotension, seizures, extrapyramidal reactions.

METOCLOPRAMIDE (*Reglan, Metozolv ODT, ✦Maxeran*) ▶K ♀B ▶? $

WARNING — Irreversible tardive dyskinesia with high dose or long-term (greater than 3 months) use.

ADULT — GERD: 10 to 15 mg PO four times per day 30 min before meals and at bedtime. Diabetic gastroparesis: 10 mg PO/IV/IM 30 min before meals and at bedtime. Prevention of chemo-induced emesis: 1 to 2 mg/kg PO/IV/IM 30 min before chemo then q 2 h for 2 doses then q 3 h for 3 doses prn. Prevention of post-op nausea: 10 to 20 mg IM/IV near end of surgical procedure, may repeat q 3 to 4 h prn. Intubation of small intestine: 10 mg IV. Radiographic exam of upper GI tract: 10 mg IV.

PEDS — Intubation of small intestine: 0.1 mg/kg IV for age younger than 6 yo; 2.5 to 5 mg IV for age 6 to 14 yo. Radiographic exam of upper GI tract: 0.1 mg/kg IV for age younger than 6 yo; 2.5 to 5 mg IV for age 6 to 14 yo.

UNAPPROVED ADULT — Prevention/treatment of chemo-induced emesis: 3 mg/kg IV over 1 h followed by continuous IV infusion of 0.5 mg/kg/h for 12 h. Migraine treatment: 10 mg IV. Migraine adjunct: 10 mg PO 5 to 10 min before ergotamine/analgesic/sedative.

UNAPPROVED PEDS — Gastroesophageal reflux: 0.4 to 0.8 mg/kg/day in 4 divided doses. Prevention of chemo-induced emesis: 1 to 2 mg/kg 30 min before chemo and then q 3 h prn (up to 5 doses/day or 5 to 10 mg/kg/day).

FORMS — Generic/Trade: Tabs 5, 10 mg. Trade: Orally disintegrating tabs 5, 10 mg (Metozolv). Generic only: Oral soln 5 mg/5 mL.

NOTES — To reduce incidence and severity of akathisia, consider giving IV doses over 15 min. If extrapyramidal reactions occur (especially with high IV doses) give diphenhydramine IM/IV. Adjust dose in renal dysfunction. Irreversible tardive dyskinesia with high dose or long-term (greater than 12 weeks) use. Avoid use greater than 12 weeks except in rare cases where benefit outweighs risk of tardive dyskinesia. May cause drowsiness, agitation, seizures, hallucinations, galactorrhea, hyperprolactinemia, constipation, diarrhea. Increases cyclosporine and ethanol absorption. Do not use if bowel perforation or mechanical obstruction present. Levodopa decreases metoclopramide effects.

MOA — Dopamine blockade; inhibits chemoreceptor trigger zone.

ADVERSE EFFECTS — Frequent: Restlessness, drowsiness, diarrhea, asthenia.

NABILONE (*Cesamet*) ▶L ♀C ▶– ©II $$$$$

ADULT — N/V in cancer chemotherapy patients with poor response to other agents: 1 to 2 mg PO two times per day, 1 to 3 h before chemotherapy. Max dose 6 mg/day in 3 divided doses.

PEDS — Not approved in children.

UNAPPROVED PEDS — Children 4 yo or older: wt less than 18 kg: 0.5 mg PO two times per day, wt 18 to 30 kg: 1 mg PO two times per day, wt 30 kg or greater: 1 mg PO three times per day.

FORMS — Trade only: Caps 1 mg.

NOTES — Contraindicated in known sensitivity to marijuana or other cannabinoids. Use with caution with current or past psychiatric reactions. Additive CNS effects with alcohol, sedatives, hypnotics, psychotomimetics. Additive cardiac effects with amphetamines, antihistamines, anticholinergic medications.

MOA — Synthetic cannabinoid with antiemetic properties.

ADVERSE EFFECTS — Frequent: Drowsiness, vertigo, dry mouth, euphoria, ataxia, headache, impaired concentration. Serious: Psychotic reactions, seizures, hallucinations.

PHOSPHORATED CARBOHYDRATES (*Emetrol*) ▶L ♀A ▶+ $

ADULT — Nausea: 15 to 30 mL PO q 15 min until nausea subsides or up to 5 doses.

PEDS — Nausea: 2 to 12 yo: 5 to 10 mL q 15 min until nausea subsides or up to 5 doses.

UNAPPROVED ADULT — Morning sickness: 15 to 30 mL PO upon rising, repeat q 3 h prn. Motion sickness or nausea due to drug therapy or anesthesia: 15 mL/dose.

UNAPPROVED PEDS — Regurgitation in infants: 5 to 10 mL PO 10 to 15 min prior to each feeding. Motion sickness or nausea due to drug therapy or anesthesia: 5 mL/dose.

FORMS — OTC Generic/Trade: Soln containing dextrose, fructose, and phosphoric acid.

NOTES — Do not dilute. Do not ingest fluids before or for 15 min after dose. Monitor blood glucose in diabetic patients.

(cont.)

PHOSPHORATED CARBOHYDRATES (*cont.*)

MOA — Hyperosmolar effect on GI wall to reduce contraction.

ADVERSE EFFECTS — Frequent: Abdominal pain, diarrhea (in high doses).

PROCHLORPERAZINE (*Compazine, ✻Stemetil*) ▶LK ♀C ▶? $

ADULT — N/V: 5 to 10 mg PO/IM three to four times per day (up to 40 mg/day). Sustained release: 10 mg PO q 12 h or 15 mg PO q am. Suppository: 25 mg PR q 12 h. IV/IM: 5 to 10 mg IV over at least 2 min q 3 to 4 h prn (up to 40 mg/day); 5 to 10 mg IM q 3 to 4 h prn (up to 40 mg/day).

PEDS — N/V: Not recommended in age younger than 2 yo or wt less than 10 kg, 0.4 mg/kg/day PO/PR in 3 to 4 divided doses for age older than 2 yo; 0.1 to 0.15 mg/kg/dose IM; IV not recommended in children.

UNAPPROVED ADULT — Migraine: 10 mg IV/IM or 25 mg PR single dose for acute headache.

UNAPPROVED PEDS — N/V during surgery: 5 to 10 mg IM 1 to 2 h before anesthesia induction, may repeat in 30 min; 5 to 10 mg IV 15 to 30 min before anesthesia induction, may repeat once.

FORMS — Generic only: Tabs 5, 10, 25 mg. Generic/Trade: Supp 25 mg.

NOTES — May cause extrapyramidal reactions (especially in elderly), hypotension (with IV), arrhythmias, sedation, seizures, hyperprolactinemia, gynecomastia, dry mouth, constipation, urinary retention, leukopenia, thrombocytopenia. Elderly more prone to adverse effects. Brand name Compazine no longer available.

MOA — Blocks post-synaptic dopaminergic receptors.

ADVERSE EFFECTS — Frequent: None. Severe: Cardiac arrest, hypotension, extrapyramidal signs.

PROMETHAZINE (*Phenergan*) ▶LK ♀C ▶– $

WARNING — Contraindicated if age younger than 2 yo due to risk of fatal respiratory depression; caution in older children. Risks of severe tissue injury associated with IV administration including gangrene. Preferred route of administration is deep IM injection, SC injection is contraindicated.

ADULT — N/V: 12.5 to 25 mg q 4 to 6 h PO/IM/PR prn. Motion sickness: 25 mg PO/PR 30 to 60 min prior to departure and q 12 h prn. Hypersensitivity reactions: 25 mg IM/IV, may repeat in 2 h. Allergic conditions: 12.5 mg PO/PR/IM/IV four times per day or 25 mg PO/PR at bedtime.

PEDS — N/V: 0.25 to 1 mg/kg/dose PO/IM/PR (up to 25 mg/dose) q 4 to 6 h prn for age 2 yo or older.

Motion sickness: 0.5 mg/kg (up to 25 mg/dose) PO 30 to 60 min prior to departure and q 12 h prn. Hypersensitivity reactions: 6.25 to 12.5 mg PO/PR/IM/IV q 6 h prn for age older than 2 yo.

UNAPPROVED ADULT — N/V: 12.5 to 25 mg IV q 4 h prn.

UNAPPROVED PEDS — N/V: 0.25 mg/kg/dose IV q 4 h prn for age 2 yo or older.

FORMS — Generic only: Tabs 12.5, 25, 50 mg. Syrup 6.25 mg/5 mL. Generic/Trade: Supp 12.5, 25, 50 mg.

NOTES — May cause sedation, extrapyramidal reactions (especially with high IV doses), hypotension with rapid IV administration, anticholinergic side effects, eg, dry mouth, blurred vision. Brand name Phenergan no longer available.

MOA — Antihistamine; blocks post-synaptic dopaminergic receptors.

ADVERSE EFFECTS — Frequent: Sedation, dry mouth. Severe: Cardiac arrest, hypotension, extrapyramidal signs, cholestatic jaundice.

SCOPOLAMINE (*Transderm-Scop, ✻Transderm-V*) ▶L ♀C ▶+ $$$

ADULT — Motion sickness: 1 disc behind ear at least 4 h before travel and q 3 days prn. Prevention of postop N/V: Apply patch behind ear 4 h before surgery, remove 24 h after surgery.

PEDS — Not approved for age younger than 12 yo.

UNAPPROVED PEDS — Preop and antiemetic: 6 mcg/kg/dose IM/IV/SC (max dose 0.3 mg/dose). May repeat q 6 to 8 h. Has also been used in severe drooling.

FORMS — Trade only: Topical disc 1.5 mg/72 h, box of 4. Injectable soln.

NOTES — Dry mouth common. Also causes drowsiness, blurred vision.

MOA — Acetylcholine blockage at parasympathetic sites.

ADVERSE EFFECTS — Frequent: Blurred vision, photophobia.

TRIMETHOBENZAMIDE (*Tigan*) ▶LK ♀C ▶? $$

ADULT — N/V: 300 mg PO q 6 to 8 h, 200 mg IM q 6 to 8 h.

PEDS — Not approved for use in children.

UNAPPROVED PEDS — 100 to 200 mg PO q 6 to 8 h if wt 13.6 to 40.9 kg.

FORMS — Generic/Trade: Caps 300 mg.

NOTES — Not for IV use. May cause sedation. Reduce starting dose in the elderly or if reduced renal function to minimize risk of adverse effects.

MOA — Inhibits chemoreceptor trigger zone.

ADVERSE EFFECTS — Frequent: Drowsiness. Severe: EPS.

GASTROENTEROLOGY: Antiulcer—Antacids

***ALKA-SELTZER* (acetylsalicylic acid + citrate + bicarbonate)** ▶LK ♀? (− 3rd trimester) ▶? $

ADULT — Relief of upset stomach: 2 regular-strength tabs in 4 oz water q 4 h PO prn (up to 8 tabs daily for age younger than 60 yo, up to 4 tabs daily for age 60 yo or older) or 2 extra-strength tabs in 4 oz water q 6

h PO prn (up to 7 tabs daily for age younger than 60 yo, up to 3 tabs daily for age 60 yo or older).

PEDS — Not approved in children.

FORMS — OTC Generic/Trade: Regular-strength, original: Aspirin 325 mg + citric acid 1000 mg + sodium bicarbonate 1916 mg. Regular-strength

(cont.)

ALKA-SELTZER (cont.)

lemon-lime and cherry: 325 mg + 1000 mg + 1700 mg. Extra-strength: 500 mg + 1000 mg + 1985 mg. Not all forms of Alka-Seltzer contain aspirin (eg, Alka-Seltzer Heartburn Relief).

NOTES — Avoid aspirin-containing forms in children and teenagers due to risk of Reye's syndrome.

MOA — Antacid.

ADVERSE EFFECTS — Frequent: None. Serious: Sodium content may worsen BP or heart failure; peptic ulcer.

ALUMINUM HYDROXIDE (*Alternagel, Amphojel, Alu-Tab, Alu-Cap, ✻Basaljel, Mucaine*) ▶K ♀C ▶? $

ADULT — Hyperphosphatemia in chronic renal failure (short-term treatment only to avoid aluminum accumulation): 300 to 600 mg PO with meals. Titrate prn. Upset stomach, indigestion: 5 to 10 mL or 300 to 600 mg PO 6 times per day, between meals and at bedtime and prn.

PEDS — Not approved in children.

UNAPPROVED ADULT — Symptomatic reflux: 15 to 30 mL PO q 30 to 60 min. Long-term management of reflux disease: 15 to 30 mL PO 1 and 3 h after meals and at bedtime prn. Peptic ulcer disease: 15 to 45 mL or 1 to 3 tabs PO 1 and 3 h after meals and at bedtime. Prophylaxis against GI bleeding (titrate dose to maintain gastric pH greater than 3.5): 30 to 60 mL or 2 to 4 tab PO q 1 to 2 h.

UNAPPROVED PEDS — Peptic ulcer disease: 5 to 15 mL PO 1 and 3 h after meals and at bedtime. Prophylaxis against GI bleeding (titrate dose to maintain gastric pH greater than 3.5): Neonates 0.5 to 1 mL/kg/dose PO q 4 h. Infants 2 to 5 mL PO q 1 to 2 h. Child: 5 to 15 mL PO q 1 to 2 h.

FORMS — OTC Generic/Trade: Susp 320, 600 mg/ 5 mL.

NOTES — For concentrated suspensions, use ½ the recommended dose. May cause constipation. Avoid administration with tetracyclines, digoxin, iron, isoniazid, buffered/enteric aspirin, diazepam, fluoroquinolones.

MOA — Antacid.

ADVERSE EFFECTS — Frequent: Constipation, chalky taste, stomach cramps, fecal impaction.

GAVISCON (aluminum hydroxide + magnesium carbonate) ▶K ♀? ▶? $

ADULT — 15 to 30 mL (regular-strength) or 10 mL (extra-strength) PO four times per day prn.

PEDS — Not approved in children.

UNAPPROVED PEDS — Peptic ulcer disease: 5 to 15 mL PO after meals and at bedtime.

FORMS — OTC Trade only: Tabs: Extra-strength (Al hydroxide 160 mg + Mg carbonate 105 mg). Liquid: Regular-strength (Al hydroxide 95 mg + Mg carbonate 358 mg per 15 mL), extra-strength (Al hydroxide 254 mg + Mg carbonate 237.5 mg per 5 mL).

NOTES — Contains alginic acid or sodium alginate, which is considered an "inactive" ingredient. Alginic acid forms foam barrier which floats in stomach to minimize esophageal contact with acid. Chronic use may cause metabolic alkalosis. Contains sodium.

MOA — Antacid, "foam barrier" in stomach to minimize esophageal contact with acid (alginic acid).

ADVERSE EFFECTS — Frequent: Diarrhea, constipation. Serious: Sodium content may worsen BP or heart failure.

MAALOX (aluminum hydroxide + magnesium hydroxide) ▶K ♀C ▶? $

ADULT — Heartburn/indigestion: 10 mL to 20 mL PO four times per day, after meals and at bedtime and prn.

PEDS — Not approved in children.

UNAPPROVED ADULT — Peptic ulcer disease: 15 mL to 45 mL PO 1 h and 3 h after meals and at bedtime. Symptomatic reflux: 15 mL to 30 mL PO q 30 min to 60 min prn. Long-term management of reflux disease: 15 mL to 30 mL PO 1 h and 3 h after meals and at bedtime prn. Prophylaxis against GI bleeding (titrate dose to maintain gastric pH greater than 3.5): 30 mL to 60 mL PO q 1 h to 2 h.

UNAPPROVED PEDS — Peptic ulcer disease: 5 mL to 15 mL PO 1 h and 3 h after meals and at bedtime. Prophylaxis against GI bleeding (titrate dose to maintain gastric pH greater than 3.5): Neonates 1 mL/kg/dose PO q 4 h. Infants 2 mL to 5 mL PO q 1 h to 2 h. Child: 5 mL to 15 mL PO q 1 h to 2 h.

FORMS — OTC Generic/Trade: Susp (225/200 mg per 5 mL). Other strengths available.

NOTES — Maalox Extra Strength and Maalox TC are more concentrated than Maalox. Maalox Plus has added simethicone. May cause constipation or diarrhea. Avoid concomitant administration with tetracyclines, digoxin, iron, isoniazid, buffered/enteric aspirin, diazepam, fluoroquinolones. Avoid chronic use in patients with renal dysfunction due to potential for magnesium accumulation.

MOA — Antacid.

ADVERSE EFFECTS — Frequent: None.

MYLANTA (aluminum hydroxide + magnesium hydroxide + simethicone) ▶K ♀C ▶? $

ADULT — Heartburn/indigestion: 10 to 20 mL between meals and at bedtime.

PEDS — Safe dosing has not been established.

UNAPPROVED ADULT — Peptic ulcer disease: 15 to 45 mL PO 1 and 3 h after meals and at bedtime. Symptomatic reflux: 15 to 30 mL PO q 30 to 60 min. Long-term management of reflux: 15 to 30 mL PO 1 and 3 h postprandially and at bedtime prn.

UNAPPROVED PEDS — Peptic ulcer disease: 5 to 15 mL PO or 0.5 to 2 mL/kg/dose (max 15 mL/dose) after meals and and at bedtime.

FORMS — OTC Generic/Trade: Liquid (various concentrations, eg, regular-strength, maximum-strength, supreme).

NOTES — May cause constipation or diarrhea. Avoid concomitant administration with tetracyclines, fluoroquinolones, digoxin, iron, isoniazid, buffered/enteric aspirin, diazepam. Avoid chronic use in renal dysfunction.

MOA — Antacid.

ADVERSE EFFECTS — Frequent: None.

ROLAIDS (calcium carbonate + magnesium hydroxide) ▶K ♀? ▶? $
ADULT — 2 to 4 tabs PO q 1 h prn, max 12 tabs/day (regular-strength) or 10 tabs/day (extra-strength).
PEDS — Not approved in children.
FORMS — OTC Trade only: Tabs, regular-strength (Ca carbonate 550 mg, Mg hydroxide 110 mg), extra-strength (Ca carbonate 675 mg, Mg hydroxide 135 mg).
NOTES — Chronic use may cause metabolic alkalosis.
MOA — Antacid.
ADVERSE EFFECTS — Frequent: None. Serious: None.

GASTROENTEROLOGY: Antiulcer—H2 Antagonists

CIMETIDINE (*Tagamet, Tagamet HB*) ▶LK ♀B ▶+ $
ADULT — Treatment of duodenal or gastric ulcer: 800 mg PO at bedtime or 300 mg PO four times per day with meals and at bedtime or 400 mg PO two times per day. Prevention of duodenal ulcer: 400 mg PO at bedtime. Erosive esophagitis: 800 mg PO two times per day or 400 mg PO four times per day. Prevention or treatment of heartburn (OTC product only approved for this indication): 200 mg PO prn, max 400 mg/day for up to 14 days. Hypersecretory conditions: 300 mg PO four times per day with meals and at bedtime. Patients unable to take oral medications: 300 mg IV/IM q 6 to 8 h or 37.5 mg/h continuous IV infusion. Prevention of upper GI bleeding in critically ill patients: 50 mg/h continuous infusion.
PEDS — 16 yo and older: Duodenal ulcer/benign gastric ulcer: 300 mg IV/IM q 6 to 8 h. GI bleed: 50 mg/h IV. Pathological hypersecretory: 300 mg IV/IM q 6 to 8 h.
UNAPPROVED ADULT — Prevention of aspiration pneumonitis during surgery: 300 to 600 mg PO or 200 to 400 mg IV 60 to 90 min prior to anesthesia. Has been used as adjunctive therapy with H1 antagonist for severe allergic reactions.
UNAPPROVED PEDS — Treatment of duodenal or gastric ulcers, erosive esophagitis, hypersecretory conditions: Neonates: 5 to 10 mg/kg/day PO/IV/IM divided q 8 to 12 h. Infants: 10 to 20 mg/kg/day PO/IV/IM divided q 6 h. Children: 20 to 40 mg/kg/day PO/IV/IM divided q 6 h. Chronic viral warts in children: 25 to 40 mg/kg/day PO in divided doses.
FORMS — Tabs 200, 300, 400, 800 mg. Rx Generic only: Oral soln 300 mg/5 mL. OTC Generic/Trade: Tabs 200 mg.
NOTES — May cause dizziness, drowsiness, headache, diarrhea, nausea. Decreased absorption of ketoconazole, itraconazole. Increased levels of carbamazepine, cyclosporine, diazepam, labetalol, lidocaine, theophylline, phenytoin, procainamide, quinidine, propranolol, TCAs, valproic acid, warfarin. Stagger doses of cimetidine and antacids. Decrease dose with CrCl less than 30 mL/min.
MOA — Histamine-2 receptor blocker.
ADVERSE EFFECTS — Frequent: Drowsiness, dizziness, agitation, diarrhea, N/V.

FAMOTIDINE (*Pepcid, Pepcid AC, Maximum Strength Pepcid AC*) ▶LK ♀B ▶? $
ADULT — Treatment of duodenal ulcer: 40 mg PO at bedtime or 20 mg PO two times per day. Maintenance of duodenal ulcer: 20 mg PO at bedtime. Treatment of gastric ulcer: 40 mg PO at bedtime. GERD: 20 mg PO two times per day. Treatment or prevention of heartburn: (OTC product only approved for this indication) 10 to 20 mg PO prn, up to 2 tabs per day. Hypersecretory conditions: 20 mg PO q 6 h. Patients unable to take oral medications: 20 mg IV q 12 h.
PEDS — GERD: 0.5 mg/kg/day PO daily for up to 8 weeks for age younger than 3 mo; 0.5 mg/kg PO two times per day for age 3 to 12 mo; 1 mg/kg/day PO divided two times per day or 2 mg/kg/day PO daily, max 40 mg PO two times per day for age 1 to 16 yo. Peptic ulcer: 0.5 mg/kg/day PO at bedtime or divided two times per day up to 40 mg/day.
UNAPPROVED ADULT — Prevention of aspiration pneumonitis during surgery: 40 mg PO prior to anesthesia. Upper GI bleeding: 20 mg IV q 12 h. Has been used as adjunctive therapy with H1 antagonist for severe allergic reactions.
UNAPPROVED PEDS — Treatment of hypersecretory conditions: 0.25 mg/kg IV q 12 h (max 40 mg daily) or 1 to 1.2 mg/kg/day PO in 2 to 3 divided doses, max 40 mg/day.
FORMS — Generic/Trade: Tabs 10 mg (OTC, Pepcid AC Acid Controller), 20 mg (Rx and OTC, Maximum Strength Pepcid AC), 40 mg. Rx Generic/Trade: Susp 40 mg/5 mL.
NOTES — May cause dizziness, headache, constipation, diarrhea. Decreased absorption of ketoconazole, itraconazole. Adjust dose in patients with CrCl <50 mL/min.
MOA — Histamine-2 receptor blocker.
ADVERSE EFFECTS — Frequent: Dizziness, headache, nausea. Severe: Convulsion in renal impairment, interstitial pneumonia, Stevens-Johnson syndrome, rhabdomyolysis.

NIZATIDINE (*Axid*) ▶K ♀B ▶? $$$$
ADULT — Treatment of duodenal or gastric ulcer: 300 mg PO at bedtime or 150 mg PO two times per day. Maintenance of duodenal ulcer: 150 mg PO at bedtime. GERD: 150 mg PO two times per day. Treatment or prevention of heartburn: (OTC product only approved for this indication) 75 mg PO prn, max 150 mg/day.
PEDS — Esophagitis, GERD: 150 mg PO two times per day for age 12 yo or older.
UNAPPROVED ADULT — Has been used as adjunctive therapy with H1 antagonist for severe allergic reactions.
UNAPPROVED PEDS — 6 mo to 11 yo (limited data): 5 to 10 mg/kg/day PO in 2 divided doses.

(cont.)

NIZATIDINE *(cont.)*

FORMS — Generic only: Caps 150, 300 mg. Oral soln 15 mg/mL (120, 480 mL).

NOTES — May cause dizziness, headache, constipation, diarrhea. Decrease absorption of ketoconazole, itraconazole. Adjust dose if CrCl <50 mL/min.

MOA — Histamine-2 receptor blocker.

ADVERSE EFFECTS — Frequent: Dizziness, headache, nausea, constipation.

PEPCID COMPLETE (famotidine + calcium carbonate + magnesium hydroxide) ▶LK ♀B ▶? $

ADULT — Treatment of heartburn: 1 tab PO prn. Max 2 tabs/day.

PEDS — Not approved in children younger than 12 yo. In children 12 yo or older, use adult dosing for OTC product.

FORMS — OTC trade/generic: Chewable tabs, famotidine 10 mg with Ca carbonate 800 mg and Mg hydroxide 165 mg.

MOA — Histamine-2 receptor blocker, antacid.

ADVERSE EFFECTS — Frequent: Dizziness, headache, nausea.

RANITIDINE (Zantac, Zantac EFFERdose, Zantac 75, Zantac 150, Peptic Relief) ▶K ♀B ▶? $

ADULT — Treatment of duodenal ulcer: 150 mg PO two times per day or 300 mg at bedtime. Treatment of gastric ulcer or GERD: 150 mg PO two times per day. Maintenance of duodenal or gastric ulcer: 150 mg PO at bedtime. Treatment of erosive esophagitis: 150 mg PO four times per day. Maintenance of erosive esophagitis: 150 mg PO two times per day. Prevention/treatment of heartburn: (OTC product only approved for this indication) 75 to 150 mg PO prn, max 300 mg/day. Hypersecretory conditions: 150 mg PO two times per day. Patients unable to take oral meds: 50 mg IV/IM q 6 to 8 h or 6.25 mg/h continuous IV infusion.

PEDS — Treatment of duodenal or gastric ulcers: 2 to 4 mg/kg PO two times per day (max 300 mg) or 2 to 4 mg/kg/day IV q 6 to 8 h for ages 1 mo to 16 yo. GERD, erosive esophagitis: 2.5 to 5 mg/kg PO two times per day (max 200 mg/day) or 2 to 4 mg/kg/day IV divided q 6 to 8 h (max 200 mg/day). Maintenance of duodenal or gastric ulcers: 2 to 4 mg/kg/day PO daily (max 150 mg).

UNAPPROVED ADULT — Prevention of upper GI bleeding in critically ill patients: 6.25 mg/h continuous IV infusion (150 mg/day). Has been used as adjunctive therapy with H1 antagonist for severe allergic reactions.

UNAPPROVED PEDS — Treatment of duodenal or gastric ulcers, GERD, hypersecretory conditions: Premature and term infants younger than 2 weeks of age: 1 mg/kg/day PO two times per day or 1.5 mg/kg IV for one dose, then 12 h later 0.75 to 1 mg/kg IV q 12 h. Continuous infusion 1.5 mg/kg for 1 dose then 0.04 to 0.08 mg/kg/h infusion. Neonates: 1 to 2 mg/kg PO two times per day or 2 mg/kg/24 h IV divided q 12 h. Infants and children: 2 to 4 mg/kg/24 h IV/IM divided q 6 to 12 h or 1 mg/kg IV loading dose followed by 0.08 to 0.17 mg/kg/h continuous IV infusion.

FORMS — Generic/Trade: Tabs 75 mg (OTC: Zantac 75), 150 mg (OTC and Rx: Zantac 150), 300 mg. Syrup 75 mg/5 mL. Rx Generic only: Caps 150, 300 mg.

NOTES — May cause dizziness, sedation, headache, drowsiness, rash, nausea, constipation, diarrhea. Elevations in SGPT have been observed when H2-antagonists have been administered IV in greater-than-recommended dosages for 5 days or longer. Bradycardia can occur if the IV form is injected too rapidly. Variable effects on warfarin, decreased absorption of ketoconazole, itraconazole. Dissolve effervescent tabs in water. Stagger doses of ranitidine and antacids. Adjust dose in patients with CrCl less than 50 mL/min.

MOA — Histamine-2 receptor blocker.

ADVERSE EFFECTS — Frequent: Dizziness, headache, nausea, constipation, taste changes, stool or tongue darkening.

GASTROENTEROLOGY: Antiulcer—Helicobacter pylori Treatment

PREVPAC (lansoprazole + amoxicillin + clarithromycin, ✲ HP-Pac) ▶LK ♀C ▶? $$$$$

ADULT — Active duodenal ulcer associated with H. pylori: 1 dose PO two times per day for 10 to 14 days.

PEDS — Not approved in children.

FORMS — Generic/Trade: Each dose consists of lansoprazole 30 mg cap + amoxicillin 1 g (two 500 mg caps), + clarithromycin 500 mg tab.

NOTES — See components.

MOA — Antimicrobial treatment for Helicobacter pylori.

ADVERSE EFFECTS — See components. Frequent: Diarrhea, headache, altered taste. Severe: Colitis, hypersensitivity reactions such as serum-sickness-like reactions, erythema multiforme, Stevens-Johnson syndrome, and exfoliative dermatitis, hepatic dysfunction, hemolytic anemia.

PYLERA (bismuth subcitrate potassium + metronidazole + tetracycline) ▶LK ♀D ▶– $$$$$

ADULT — Duodenal ulcer associated with H. pylori: 3 caps PO four times per day (after meals and at bedtime) for 10 days. To be given with omeprazole 20 mg PO two times per day.

PEDS — Not approved in children.

FORMS — Trade only: Each cap contains bismuth subcitrate potassium 140 mg + metronidazole 125 mg + tetracycline 125 mg.

NOTES — See components.

MOA — Antimicrobial treatment for Helicobacter pylori.

ADVERSE EFFECTS — Frequent: Diarrhea, headache, altered taste. Severe: Colitis, hypersensitivity reactions such as serum-sickness, erythema multiforme, Stevens-Johnson syndrome, and exfoliative dermatitis; hepatic dysfunction, hemolytic anemia.

GASTROENTEROLOGY: Antiulcer—Proton Pump Inhibitors

NOTE: Due to the effects on gastric acid secretion, all proton pump inhibitors can reduce the absorption of drugs such as ampicillin, ketoconazole, atazanavir, nelfinavir, iron salts, erlotinib, and mycophenolate or increase the absorption of drugs such as digoxin .

DEXLANSOPRAZOLE (*Dexilant, Dexilant SoluTab*) ▶L ♀B ▶ – $$$$$
- ADULT — Healing of erosive esophagitis: 60 mg PO once daily for up to 8 weeks. Maintenance of erosive esophagitis: 30 mg PO once daily for up to 6 months. Symptomatic nonerosive GERD: 30 mg PO once daily for 4 weeks.
- PEDS — 12 year and older: use adult dosing. Not approved in children younger than 12 years.
- FORMS — Trade only: Cap 30, 60 mg. Orally-disintegrating tablet 30 mg (Dexilant SoluTab).
- NOTES — Take without regard to meals. Many drug interactions. Capsule can be opened and mixed with applesauce or water. Long-term use may result in a reduction of vitamin B12 levels.
- MOA — Na-K-ATPase inhibitor
- ADVERSE EFFECTS — Frequent: diarrhea, abdominal pain, nausea, upper respiratory tract infection, vomiting, and flatulence.. Severe: Pancreatitis, severe skin reactions, hypersensitivity.

ESOMEPRAZOLE (*Nexium*) ▶L ♀B ▶? $
- ADULT — Erosive esophagitis: 20 to 40 mg PO daily for 4 to 8 weeks. Maintenance of erosive esophagitis: 20 mg PO daily. Zollinger-Ellison: 40 mg PO two times per day. GERD: 20 mg PO daily for 4 weeks. Prevention of NSAID–associated gastric ulcer: 20 to 40 mg PO daily for up to 6 months. H. pylori eradication: 40 mg PO daily with amoxicillin 1000 mg PO two times per day and clarithromycin 500 mg PO two times per day for 10 days.
- PEDS — GERD: wt less than 20 kg: 10 mg PO daily; wt 20 kg or more: 10 to 20 mg daily. Alternatively, 2.5 mg (for 3 kg to 5 kg), 5 mg (for 5.1 kg to 7.5 kg), or 10 mg (for 7.6 kg to 12 kg) PO once daily for up to 6 weeks for age 1 mo to younger than 1 yo, 10 to 20 mg PO daily for up to 8 weeks for age 1 to 11 yo, 20 to 40 mg PO daily for up to 8 weeks for age 12 to 17 yo.
- FORMS — Rx Generic/Trade: Caps, delayed-release 20, 40 mg. Trade only: Delayed-release granules for oral susp 2.5, 5, 10, 20, 40 mg per packet. OTC/Trade: Caps, delayed-release 20 mg.
- NOTES — Concomitant administration with voriconazole, an inhibitor of CYP2C19 and CYP3A4, may lead to a more than doubling of esomeprazole exposure. Esomeprazole may reduce the efficacy of clopidogrel. Use caution with high-dose methotrexate. May increase serum chromogranin A levels, which may cause false-positive results in diagnostic investigations for neuroendocrine tumors. Long-term use may cause reduction in vitamin B12 levels.
- MOA — H-K ATPase proton pump inhibitor.
- ADVERSE EFFECTS — Frequent: Headache, dizziness, rash, diarrhea, N/V, taste perversion. Severe: Anaphylaxis, toxic epidermal necrolysis, Stevens-Johnson syndrome, erythema multiforme, pancreatitis, hepatitis.

LANSOPRAZOLE (*Prevacid*) ▶L ♀B ▶? $$$
- ADULT — Heartburn: 15 mg PO daily. Erosive esophagitis: 30 mg PO daily for 4 weeks or 30 mg IV daily for 7 days or until taking PO. Maintenance therapy following healing of erosive esophagitis: 15 mg PO daily. NSAID–induced gastric ulcer: 30 mg PO daily for 8 weeks (treatment), 15 mg PO daily for up to 12 weeks (prevention). GERD: 15 mg PO daily for up to 8 weeks. Duodenal ulcer treatment and maintenance: 15 mg PO daily. Gastric ulcer: 30 mg PO daily for up to 8 weeks. Part of a multidrug regimen for H. pylori eradication: 30 mg PO two times per day with amoxicillin 1000 mg PO two times per day and clarithromycin 500 mg PO two times per day for 10 to 14 days (see table) or 30 mg PO three times per day with amoxicillin 1000 mg PO three times per day for 14 days. Hypersecretory conditions: 60 mg PO daily.
- PEDS — Not effective in patients with symptomatic GERD age 1 mo to younger than 1 yo. Esophagitis and GERD: 1 to 11 yo, less than 30 kg: 15 kg PO daily up to 12 weeks; 12 to 17 yo, 30 kg or greater: 30 mg PO daily up to 12 weeks.
- FORMS — OTC Generic/Trade: Caps 15 mg. Rx Generic/Trade: 15, 30 mg. Orally disintegrating tabs 15, 30 mg.
- NOTES — Take before meals. May reduce absorption of vitamin B12. Potential for PPIs to reduce the response to clopidogrel. Evaluate the need for a PPI in clopidogrel-treated patients and consider H2-blocker/antacid. Orally disintegrating tabs can be dissolved in water (15 mg tab in 4 mL, 30 mg tab in 10 mL) and administered via an oral syringe or nasogastric tube at least 8 French within 15 min. Delayed-release orally disintegrating tabs should not be broken or cut.
- MOA — H-K ATPase proton pump inhibitor.
- ADVERSE EFFECTS — Frequent: fatigue, dizziness, headache, abdominal pain, diarrhea, nausea, increased appetite. Severe: Pancreatitis, severe skin reactions, myositis, interstitial nephritis.

OMEPRAZOLE (*Prilosec, ✦Losec*) ▶L ♀C ▶? $
- WARNING — Serum chromogranin A levels increase and may cause false-positive results in diagnostic investigations for neuroendocrine tumors. Long-term use may cause reduction in vitamin B12 levels.
- ADULT — GERD, duodenal ulcer, erosive esophagitis: 20 mg PO daily. Heartburn (OTC): 20 mg PO daily for 14 days. Gastric ulcer: 40 mg PO daily. Hypersecretory conditions: 60 mg PO daily. Part of a multidrug regimen for H. pylori eradication: 20 mg PO two times per day with amoxicillin 1000 mg PO two times per day and clarithromycin 500 mg PO

(cont.)

OMEPRAZOLE (*cont.*)

two times per day for 10 days, with additional 18 days of omeprazole 20 mg PO daily if ulcer present (see table). Or 40 mg PO daily with clarithromycin 500 mg PO three times per day for 14 days, with additional 14 days of omeprazole 20 mg PO daily if ulcer present.

PEDS — GERD, acid-related disorders, maintenance of healing erosive esophagitis in children 1 to 16 yo: 5 mg PO daily for wt 5 to 9 kg, 10 mg PO daily for wt 10 to 19 kg, give 20 mg PO daily for wt 20 kg or greater.

UNAPPROVED PEDS — Gastric or duodenal ulcers, hypersecretory states: 0.2 to 3.5 mg/kg/dose PO daily. GERD: 1 mg/kg/day PO one or two times per day.

FORMS — Rx Generic/Trade: Caps 10, 20, 40 mg. Trade only: Granules for oral susp 2.5 mg, 10 mg. OTC Trade only: Cap 20 mg.

NOTES — Take before meals. Caps contain enteric-coated granules; do not chew. Caps may be opened and administered in acidic liquid (eg, apple juice) or 1 tablespoon of applesauce. May increase levels of diazepam, warfarin, and phenytoin. May decrease absorption of ketoconazole, itraconazole, iron, ampicillin, and digoxin. Reduces plasma levels of atazanavir. Concomitant administration with voriconazole, an inhibitor of CYP2C19 and CYP3A4, may lead to a more than doubling of omeprazole exposure. Avoid administration with sucralfate. Use caution with high-dose methotrexate. Omeprazole may reduce the efficacy of clopidogrel.

MOA — H-K ATPase proton pump inhibitor.

ADVERSE EFFECTS — Frequent: Headache, dizziness, rash, diarrhea, N/V, taste perversion. Severe: Stevens-Johnson syndrome, erythema multiforme, stomatitis, agitation, pancytopenia, agranulocytosis, other blood dyscrasias, pancreatitis, psychiatric disturbances.

PANTOPRAZOLE (*Protonix, ✦Pantoloc, Tecta*) ▶L ♀B ▶? $

ADULT — Treatment of erosive esophagitis associated with GERD: 40 mg PO daily for 8 to 16 weeks. Maintenance of erosive esophagitis: 40 mg PO once daily. Zollinger-Ellison syndrome and other hypersecretory conditions: 40 mg PO twice daily or 80 mg IV q 8 to 12 h for 7 days until taking PO.

PEDS — Erosive esophagitis associated with GERD, 5 yo or older: 15 kg to less than 40 kg: 20 mg PO daily for up to 8 weeks. 40 kg or greater: 40 mg PO daily for up to 8 weeks.

UNAPPROVED ADULT — Has been studied as part of various multidrug regimens for H. pylori eradication. Reduce peptic ulcer re-bleeding after hemostasis: 80 mg IV bolus, then 8 mg/h continuous IV infusion for 3 days, followed by oral therapy (or 40 mg IV q 12 h for 4 to 7 days if unable to tolerate PO).

UNAPPROVED PEDS — GERD associated with a history of erosive esophagitis: 0.5 to 1 mg/kg/day (max 40 mg/day).

FORMS — Generic/Trade: Tabs 20, 40 mg. Trade only: Granules for susp 40 mg/packet.

NOTES — Use caution with high-dose methotrexate. Do not coadminister with atazanavir or nelfinavir. Concomitant warfarin use may require monitoring. May interfere with the absorption of drugs where gastric pH is important for bioavailability. May reduce absorption of vitamin B12 with long-term use.

MOA — H-K ATPase proton pump inhibitor.

ADVERSE EFFECTS — Frequent: Headache. Serious: rhabdomyolysis, anaphylaxis, angioedema, severe dermatologic reactions, hepatocellular damage, interstitial nephritis, pancreatitis, pancytopenia, agranulocytosis.

RABEPRAZOLE (*AcipHex, ✦Pariet*) ▶L ♀C ▶? $$$$$

ADULT — GERD: 20 mg PO daily for 4 to 16 weeks. Duodenal ulcers: 20 mg PO daily for 4 weeks. Zollinger-Ellison syndrome: 60 mg PO daily, may increase up to 100 mg daily or 60 mg two times per day. Part of a multidrug regimen for H. pylori eradication: 20 mg PO two times per day, with amoxicillin 1000 mg PO two times per day and clarithromycin 500 mg PO two times per day for 7 days.

PEDS — GERD: Children 1 yo to 11 yo: less than 15 kg: 5 mg PO once daily, may increase to 10 mg; 15 kg or greater: 10 mg PO once daily. Children 12 yo or older: 20 mg PO daily up to 8 weeks.

FORMS — Generic/Trade: Tabs 20 mg. Trade only: Sprinkle caps (open and sprinkle on soft food or liquid) 5, 10 mg.

NOTES — Does not appear to interact with clopidogrel. May reduce absorption of vitamin B12 with long-term use. Contraindicated in atients receiving rilpivirine-containing products. Long-term use may cause a reduction in vitamin B12 levels.

MOA — H-K ATPase proton pump inhibitor.

ADVERSE EFFECTS — Frequent: Headache. Serious: rhabdomyolysis, anaphylaxis, angioedema, severe dermatologic reactions, hepatocellular damage, interstitial nephritis, pancreatitis, pancytopenia.

ZEGERID (omeprazole + bicarbonate) ▶L ♀C ▶? $

ADULT — Duodenal ulcer, GERD, erosive esophagitis: 20 mg PO daily for 4 to 8 weeks. Gastric ulcer: 40 mg PO once daily for 4 to 8 weeks. Reduction of risk of upper GI bleed in critically ill (susp only): 40 mg PO, then 40 mg 6 to 8 h later, then 40 mg once daily thereafter for up to 14 days.

PEDS — Not approved in children.

FORMS — OTC Trade only ($): Omeprazole/sodium bicarbonate caps 20 mg/1.1 g. Rx Generic/Trade ($$$$$): Caps 20 mg/1.1 g and 40 mg/1.1 g. Trade only: Powder packets for susp 20 mg/1.68 g and 40 mg/1.68 g.

NOTES — Omeprazole may reduce the efficacy of clopidogrel. Serum chromogranin A levels increase and may cause false-positive results in diagnostic investigations for neuroendocrine tumors. Long-term use may cause a reduction in vitamin B12 levels. Increased risk of adverse effects when taken with methotrexate.

(cont.)

ZEGERID (*cont.*)

MOA — H-K ATPase proton pump inhibitor plus antacid combination.

ADVERSE EFFECTS — Frequent: Headache, dizziness, rash, diarrhea, N/V, taste perversion. Severe: Stevens-Johnson syndrome, erythema multiforme, stomatitis, agitation, pancytopenia, agranulocytosis, other blood dyscrasias, pancreatitis, psychiatric disturbances.

GASTROENTEROLOGY: Antiulcer—Other

DICYCLOMINE (*Bentyl, ✲Bentylol*) ▶LK ♀B ▶– $

WARNING — May cause psychosis or delirium, especially in elderly or those with preexisting psychiatric disease.

ADULT — Treatment of functional bowel/irritable bowel syndrome (irritable colon, spastic colon, mucous colon): Initiate with 20 mg PO four times per day and increase to 40 mg PO four times per day, if tolerated. Patients who are unable to take oral medications: 20 mg IM q 6 h.

PEDS — Not approved in children.

UNAPPROVED PEDS — Treatment of functional/irritable bowel syndrome: Infants 6 mo or older: 5 mg PO three to four times per day. Children: 10 mg PO three to four times per day.

FORMS — Generic/Trade: Tabs 20 mg. Caps 10 mg.

NOTES — Although some use lower doses (ie, 10 to 20 mg PO four times per day), the only adult oral dose proven to be effective is 160 mg/day.

MOA — Inhibits effect of acetylcholine at parasympathetic receptors.

ADVERSE EFFECTS — Frequent: None specific but generally similar to other anticholinergic drugs.

DONNATAL (**phenobarbital + hyoscyamine + atropine + scopolamine**) ▶LK ♀C ▶– $$$

ADULT — Adjunctive therapy of irritable bowel syndrome or adjunctive treatment of duodenal ulcers: 1 to 2 tabs/caps or 5 to 10 mL PO three to four times per day or 1 extended-release tab PO q 8 to 12 h.

PEDS — Adjunctive therapy of irritable bowel syndrome, adjunctive treatment of duodenal ulcers: 0.1 mL/kg/dose q 4 h, max 5 mL. Alternative dosing regimen: Give 0.5 mL PO q 4 h or 0.75 mL PO q 6 h for wt 4.5 kg, give 1 mL PO q 4 h or 1.5 mL PO q 6 h for wt 9.1 kg, give 1.5 mL PO q 4 h or 2 mL PO q 6 h for wt 13.6 kg, give 2.5 mL PO q 4 h or 3.75 mL PO q 6 h for wt 22.7 kg, give 3.75 mL PO q 4 h or 5 mL PO q 6 h for wt 34 kg, give 5 mL PO q 4 h or 7.5 mL PO q 6 h for wt 45 kg or greater.

FORMS — Generic/trade: Phenobarbital 16.2 mg + hyoscyamine 0.1 mg + atropine 0.02 mg + scopolamine 6.5 mcg in each tab or 5 mL. Trade only: Extended-release tabs, 48.6 + 0.3111 + 0.0582 + 0.0195 mg.

NOTES — The FDA has classified Donnatal as "possibly effective" for treatment of irritable bowel syndrome and duodenal ulcer. Heat stroke may occur in hot weather. Can cause anticholinergic side effects; use caution in narrow-angle glaucoma, BPH, etc.

MOA — Anticonvulsant, inhibits effect of acetylcholine at parasympathetic receptors.

ADVERSE EFFECTS — Frequent: xerostomia, blurred vision, urinary retention and hesitancy, N/V, dizziness.

HYOSCINE (*✲Buscopan*) ▶LK ♀C ▶? $$

ADULT — Canada: GI or bladder spasm: 10 to 20 mg PO/IV up to 60 mg daily (PO) or 100 mg daily (IV).

PEDS — Not approved in children.

FORMS — Canada Trade only: Tabs 10 mg.

NOTES — May cause dizziness, drowsiness, blurred vision, dry mouth, N/V, urinary retention. Contraindicated in narrow-angle glaucoma, obstructive conditions (eg, pyloric, duodenal or other intestinal obstructive lesions, ileus, and obstructive uropathies), and myasthenia gravis.

MOA — Anticholinergic that counteracts urinary and GI smooth muscle contraction.

ADVERSE EFFECTS — Serious: Heat stroke, paralytic ileus, increased ocular pressure, psychosis, anaphylaxis. Frequent: Dry mouth, urinary retention, constipation, headache, dizziness, drowsiness, fever, weakness, impotence, suppressed lactation, confusion, blurred vision, tachycardia, palpitations, anhidrosis, mydriasis, cycloplegia, loss of taste.

HYOSCYAMINE (*Anaspaz, A-spaz, Cystospaz, ED Spaz, Hyosol, Hyospaz, Levbid, Levsin, Medispaz, NuLev, Spacol, Spasdel, Symax*) ▶LK ♀C ▶– $

ADULT — Bladder spasm, control gastric secretion, GI hypermotility, irritable bowel syndrome: 0.125 to 0.25 mg PO/SL q 4 h or prn. Extended-release 0.375 to 0.75 mg PO q 12 h. Max 1.5 mg/day.

PEDS — Bladder spasm: Use adult dosing in age older than 12 yo. To control gastric secretion, GI hypermotility, irritable bowel syndrome, and others: Initial oral dose by wt for age younger than 2 yo: Give 12.5 mcg for 2.3 kg, give 16.7 mcg for 3.4 kg, give 20.8 mcg for 5 kg, give 25 mcg for 7 kg, give 31.3 to 33.3 mcg for 10 kg, give 45.8 mcg for 15 kg. Alternatively, if age younger than 2 yo: 3 gtts for wt 2.3 kg, give 4 gtts for 3.4 kg, give 5 gtts for 5 kg, give 6 gtts for 7 kg, give 8 gtts for 10 kg, give 11 gtts for 15 kg. Doses can be repeated q 4 h prn, but max daily dose is six times initial dose. Initial oral dose by wt for age 2 to 12 yo: Give 31.3 to 33.3 mcg for 10 kg, give 62.5 mcg for 20 kg, give 93.8 mcg for 40 kg, and give 125 mcg for 50 kg. Doses may be repeated q 4 h, but max daily dose should not exceed 750 mcg.

FORMS — Generic/Trade: Tabs 0.125. SL tabs 0.125 mg. Chewable tabs 0.125 mg. Extended-release tabs 0.375 mg. Elixir 0.125 mg/5 mL. Gtts 0.125 mg/1 mL.

NOTES — May cause dizziness, drowsiness, blurred vision, dry mouth, N/V, urinary retention.

(cont.)

HYOSCYAMINE (*cont.*)

Contraindicated in narrow-angle glaucoma, obstructive conditions (eg, pyloric, duodenal, or other intestinal obstructive lesions; ileus; achalasia; GI hemorrhage; and obstructive uropathies), unstable cardiovascular status, and myasthenia gravis.

MOA — Anticholinergic that counteracts urinary and GI smooth muscle contraction.

ADVERSE EFFECTS — Serious: Heat stroke, paralytic ileus, increased ocular pressure, psychosis. Frequent: Dry mouth, urinary retention, constipation, headache, dizziness, drowsiness, fever, weakness, impotence, suppressed lactation, confusion, blurred vision, tachycardia, palpitations, anhidrosis, mydriasis, cycloplegia, loss of taste.

MEPENZOLATE (*Cantil*) ▶K + gut ♀B ▶? $$$$$

ADULT — Adjunctive therapy in peptic ulcer disease: 25 to 50 mg PO four times per day, with meals and at bedtime.

PEDS — Not approved in children.

FORMS — Trade only: Tabs 25 mg.

NOTES — Contraindicated in narrow-angle glaucoma, obstructive uropathy, paralytic ileus, toxic megacolon, obstructive diseases of GI tract, intestinal atony in elderly/debilitated, myasthenia gravis, unstable CV status, acute GI bleed.

MOA — Post-ganglionic parasympathetic inhibitor.

ADVERSE EFFECTS — Frequent: Drowsiness, blurred vision, constipation, headache, dry mouth, urinary retention, tachycardia.

MISOPROSTOL (*PGE1, Cytotec*) ▶LK ♀X ▶– $$$$

WARNING — Contraindicated in desired early or preterm pregnancy due to its abortifacient property. Pregnant women should avoid contact/exposure to the tabs. Uterine rupture reported with use for labor induction and medical abortion.

ADULT — Prevention of NSAID–induced gastric ulcers: 200 mcg PO four times per day. If not tolerated, use 100 mcg PO four times per day.

PEDS — Not approved in children.

UNAPPROVED ADULT — Cervical ripening and labor induction: 25 mcg intravaginally q 3 h to 6 h (or 50 mcg q 6 h). First-trimester pregnancy failure: 800 mcg intravaginally, repeat on day 3 if expulsion incomplete. Medical abortion 63 days gestation or less: With mifepristone, see mifepristone; with methotrexate: 800 mcg intravaginally 5 to 7 days after 50 mg/m² IM methotrexate. Pre-op cervical ripening: 400 mcg intravaginally 3 h to 4 h before mechanical cervical dilation. Postpartum hemorrhage: 400 mcg to 600 mcg PO or PR single dose. Treatment of duodenal ulcers: 100 mcg to 200 mcg PO four times per day. Alternatively, 400 mcg PO twice daily has been tried.

UNAPPROVED PEDS — Improvement in fat absorption in cystic fibrosis in children 8 yo to 16 yo: 100 mcg PO four times per day.

FORMS — Generic/Trade: Oral tabs 100, 200 mcg.

NOTES — Contraindicated with prior C-section. Oral tabs can be inserted into the vagina for labor induction/cervical ripening. Monitor for uterine hyperstimulation and abnormal fetal heart rate. Risk factors for uterine rupture: Prior uterine surgery and 5 previous pregnancies or more.

MOA — Prostaglandin E1 analog, uterine stimulant.

ADVERSE EFFECTS — Serious: Uterine hyperstimulation, uterine rupture. Frequent: Diarrhea, abdominal pain.

PROPANTHELINE (*Pro-Banthine*) ▶LK ♀C ▶– $$$$

ADULT — Adjunctive therapy in peptic ulcer disease: 7.5 to 15 mg PO 30 min before meals and 30 mg at bedtime.

PEDS — Not approved in children.

UNAPPROVED ADULT — Irritable bowel, pancreatitis, urinary bladder spasms: 7.5 to 15 mg PO three times per day and 30 mg at bedtime.

UNAPPROVED PEDS — Antisecretory effects: 1 to 2 mg/kg/day PO in 3 to 4 divided doses. Antispasmodic effects: 2 to 3 mg/kg/day PO divided q 4 to 6 h and at bedtime.

FORMS — Generic only: Tabs 15 mg.

NOTES — For elderly adults and those with small stature use 7.5 mg dose. May cause constipation, dry mucous membranes.

MOA — Antispasmodic.

ADVERSE EFFECTS — Frequent: anticholinergic effects

SIMETHICONE (*Mylicon, Gas-X, Phazyme, ✱Ovol*) ▶not absorbed ♀C but + ▶? $

ADULT — Excessive gas in GI tract: 40 to 360 mg PO after meals and at bedtime prn, max 500 mg/day.

PEDS — Excessive gas in GI tract: 20 mg PO four times per day prn, max 240 mg/day for age younger than 2 yo, 40 mg PO four times per day prn for age 2 to 12 yo (max 500 mg/day).

UNAPPROVED PEDS — Although used to treat infant colic (in approved dose for gas), several studies suggest no benefit.

FORMS — OTC Generic/Trade: Chewable tabs 80, 125 mg. Gtts 40 mg/0.6 mL. Trade only: Softgels 166 mg (Gas-X), 180 mg (Phazyme). Strips, oral (Gas-X) 62.5 mg (adults), 40 mg (children).

NOTES — For administration to infants, may mix dose in 30 mL of liquid. Chewable tabs should be chewed thoroughly.

MOA — Theoretically, relieves gas pressure and bloating.

ADVERSE EFFECTS — Frequent: None.

SUCRALFATE (*Carafate, ✱Sulcrate*) ▶not absorbed ♀B ▶? $$

ADULT — Duodenal ulcer: 1 g PO four times per day, 1 h before meals and at bedtime. Maintenance therapy of duodenal ulcer: 1 g PO two times per day.

PEDS — Not approved in children.

UNAPPROVED ADULT — Gastric ulcer, reflux esophagitis, NSAID–induced GI symptoms, stress ulcer prophylaxis: 1 g PO four times per day 1 h before meals and at bedtime. Oral and esophageal ulcers due to radiation/chemo/sclerotherapy: (susp only) 5 to 10 mL swish and spit/swallow four times per day.

(cont.)

SUCRALFATE (*cont.*)

UNAPPROVED PEDS — Reflux esophagitis, gastric or duodenal ulcer, stress ulcer prophylaxis: 40 to 80 mg/kg/day PO divided q 6 h. Alternative dosing: 500 mg PO four times per day for age younger than 6 yo, give 1 g PO four times per day for age 6 yo or older.

FORMS — Generic/Trade: Tabs 1 g. Susp 1 g/10 mL.

NOTES — May cause constipation. May reduce the absorption of cimetidine, ciprofloxacin, digoxin, ketoconazole, levothyroxine, itraconazole, phenytoin, ranitidine, tetracycline, theophylline and warfarin; separate doses by at least 2 h. Antacids should be separated by at least 30 min. Hyperglycemia has been reported in patients with diabetes.

MOA — Forms synthetic barrier against peptic acid.

ADVERSE EFFECTS — Frequent: Constipation. Severe: hypersensitivity reactions.

GASTROENTEROLOGY: Laxatives—Bulk-Forming

METHYLCELLULOSE (*Citrucel*) ▶not absorbed ♀+ ▶? $

ADULT — Laxative: 1 heaping tablespoon in 8 oz cold water PO daily or 2 caplets PO daily (up to six doses per day).

PEDS — Laxative: Age 6 to 12 yo: 1½ heaping teaspoons in 4 oz cold water daily (up to 6 doses per day) PO prn.

FORMS — OTC Trade only: Regular and sugar-free packets and multiple-use canisters, Clear-mix soln, Caplets 500 mg.

NOTES — Must be taken with water to avoid esophageal obstruction or choking.

MOA — Osmotic effect in intestinal lumen.

ADVERSE EFFECTS — Frequent: None.

POLYCARBOPHIL (*FiberCon, Konsyl Fiber, Equalactin*) ▶not absorbed ♀+ ▶? $

ADULT — Laxative: 2 tabs (1250 mg) PO four times per day prn.

PEDS — Laxative: 6 to 12 yo: 625 mg PO up to four times per day prn; 12 yo or older: 2 tabs (1250 mg) PO four times per day prn.

UNAPPROVED ADULT — Diarrhea: 2 tabs (1250 mg) PO q 30 min prn. Max daily dose 6 g.

UNAPPROVED PEDS — Diarrhea: 500 mg PO q 30 min prn (up to 1 g polycarbophil/day for age 3 to 5 yo, and 2 g/day for age older than 6 yo).

FORMS — OTC Generic/Trade: Tabs/Caps 625 mg. OTC Trade only: Chewable tabs 625 mg (Equalactin).

NOTES — When used as a laxative, take dose with at least 8 oz of fluid. Do not administer concomitantly with tetracycline; separate by at least 2 h.

MOA — Bulk-forming laxatives.

ADVERSE EFFECTS — Frequent: None. Severe: Esophageal obstruction, hypersensitivity.

PSYLLIUM (*Metamucil, Fiberall, Konsyl, Hydrocil*) ▶not absorbed ♀+ ▶? $

ADULT — Laxative: 1 rounded tsp in liquid, 1 packet in liquid or 1 wafer with liquid PO daily (up to three times per day).

PEDS — Laxative (children 6 to 11 yo): ½ to 1 rounded tsp in liquid, ½ to 1 packet in liquid or 1 wafer with liquid PO daily (up to three times per day).

UNAPPROVED ADULT — Reduction in cholesterol: 1 rounded tsp in liquid, 1 packet in liquid or 1 to 2 wafers with liquid PO three times per day. Prevention of GI side effects with orlistat: 6 g in liquid with each orlistat dose or 12 g in liquid at bedtime.

FORMS — OTC Generic/Trade: Regular and sugar-free powder, granules, caps, wafers, including various flavors and various amounts of psyllium.

NOTES — Powders and granules must be mixed with 8 oz water/liquid prior to ingestion. Start with 1 dose/day and gradually increase to minimize gas and bloating. Can bind with warfarin, digoxin, potassium-sparing diuretics, salicylates, tetracycline, and nitrofurantoin; space at least 3 h apart.

MOA — Adsorbs water to bulk stool.

ADVERSE EFFECTS — Frequent: None. Severe: Bronchospasm, anaphylaxis.

GASTROENTEROLOGY: Laxatives—Osmotic

GLYCERIN (*Fleet-glycerin*) ▶not absorbed ♀C ▶? $

ADULT — Constipation: 1 adult suppository or 5 mL to 15 mL as an enema PR prn.

PEDS — Constipation: 0.5 mL/kg/dose as an enema PR prn in neonates, 1 infant suppository or 2 to 5 mL rectal soln as an enema PR prn for age younger than 6 yo, 1 adult suppository or 5 to 15 mL of rectal soln as enema PR prn for age 6 yo or older.

FORMS — OTC Generic/Trade: Supp, infant and adult. Soln (Fleet Babylax) 4 mL/applicator.

MOA — Softens and lubricates stool.

ADVERSE EFFECTS — Frequent: None.

LACTULOSE (*Enulose, Kristalose*) ▶not absorbed ♀B ▶? $$

ADULT — Constipation: 15 mL to 30 mL (syrup) or 10 g to 20 g (powder for oral soln) PO daily. Evacuation of barium following barium procedures: 15 mL to 30 mL (syrup) PO daily, may increase to 60 mL. Acute hepatic encephalopathy: 30 mL to 45 mL syrup/dose PO q 1 h until laxative effect observed or 300 mL in 700 mL water or saline PR as a retention enema q 4 h to 6 h. Prevention of encephalopathy: 30 mL to 45 mL syrup PO three to four times per day.

PEDS — Prevention or treatment of encephalopathy: Infants: 2.5 to 10 mL/day (syrup) PO in 3 to 4 divided doses. Children/adolescents: 40 to 90 mL/day (syrup) PO in 3 to 4 divided doses.

UNAPPROVED ADULT — Restoration of bowel movements in hemorrhoidectomy patients: 15 mL syrup PO two times per day on days before surgery and for 5 days following surgery.

(cont.)

LACTULOSE (*cont.*)

UNAPPROVED PEDS — Constipation: 7.5 mL syrup PO daily, after breakfast.

FORMS — Generic/Trade: Syrup 10 g/15 mL. Trade only (Kristalose): 10, 20 g packets for oral soln.

NOTES — May be mixed in water, juice, or milk to improve palatability. Packets for oral soln should be mixed in 4 oz of water or juice. Titrate dose to produce 2 to 3 soft stools/day.

MOA — Converts NH3 to NH4+ to prevent rediffusion into plasma.

ADVERSE EFFECTS — Frequent: Flatulence, diarrhea.

MAGNESIUM CITRATE ▶K ♀B ▶? $

ADULT — Evacuate bowel prior to procedure: 150 to 300 mL PO once or in divided doses.

PEDS — Evacuate bowel prior to procedure: 2 to 4 mL/kg PO once or in divided doses for age younger than 6 yo. 100 to 150 mL PO once or in divided doses for age 6 to 12 yo.

FORMS — OTC Generic only: Soln 300 mL/bottle. Low-sodium and sugar-free available.

NOTES — Use caution with impaired renal function. May decrease absorption of phenytoin, ciprofloxacin, benzodiazepines, and glyburide. May cause additive CNS depression with CNS depressants. Chill to improve palatability.

MOA — Osmotic effect in intestinal lumen.

ADVERSE EFFECTS — Frequent: None. Severe: Electrolyte disturbances, CNS depression.

MAGNESIUM HYDROXIDE (*Milk of Magnesia*) ▶K ♀+ ▶? $

ADULT — Laxative: 30 to 60 mL regular strength (400 mg per 5 mL), 15 to 30 mL (800 mg per 5 mL strength) or 10 to 20 mL (1200 mg per 5 mL) PO as a single dose or divided doses. Antacid: 5 to 15 mL/dose PO four times per day prn or 622 to 1244 mg PO four times per day prn.

PEDS — Laxative: 0.5 mL/kg regular strength (400 mg per 5 mL) PO as a single dose or in divided doses for age younger than 2 yo, 5 to 15 mL/day PO as a single dose or in divided doses for age 2 to 5 yo, 15 to 30 mL PO in a single dose or in divided doses for age 6 to 11 yo. Antacid: 5 to 15 mL/dose regular strength (400 mg per 5 mL) PO four times per day prn for age older than 12 yo.

FORMS — OTC Generic/Trade: Susp 400 mg/5 mL. Trade only: Chewable tabs 311, 400 mg. Generic only: Susp 800 mg/5 mL, (concentrated) 1200 mg/5 mL, sugar-free 400 mg/5 mL.

NOTES — Use caution with impaired renal function.

MOA — Osmotic effect in intestinal lumen.

ADVERSE EFFECTS — Frequent: Diarrhea.

POLYETHYLENE GLYCOL (*MiraLax, GlycoLax*, ✽*Lax-A-Day, Restoralax*) ▶not absorbed ♀C ▶? $

ADULT — Constipation: 17 g (1 heaping tablespoon) in 4 to 8 oz water, juice, soda, coffee, or tea PO daily.

PEDS — Not approved in children.

UNAPPROVED PEDS — Children older than 6 mo: 0.5 to 1.5 g/kg/day PO, max 17 g/day.

FORMS — OTC Generic/Trade: Powder for oral soln 17 g/scoop, 17 g packets. Rx Generic/Trade: Powder for oral soln 17 g/scoop.

NOTES — Takes 1 to 3 days to produce bowel movement. Indicated for up to 14 days.

MOA — Osmotic laxative.

ADVERSE EFFECTS — Frequent: Nausea, fullness, bloating. Serious: Risk of aspiration in children.

POLYETHYLENE GLYCOL WITH ELECTROLYTES (*GoLYTELY, Colyte, Suclear, Suprep, TriLyte, NuLYTELY, MoviPrep, HalfLytely, ✽Klean-Prep, Electropeg, Peg-Lyte*) ▶not absorbed ♀C ▶? $

ADULT — Bowel cleansing prior to GI examination: 240 mL PO q 10 min or 20 to 30 mL/min NG until 4 L are consumed or rectal effluent is clear. MoviPrep: 240 mL q 15 min for 4 doses (over 1 h) the night before plus additional clear liquid and 240 mL q 15 min for 4 doses (over 1 h) plus additional clear liquid on the morning of the colonoscopy. Alternatively, 240 mL q 15 min for 4 doses (over 1 h) at 6 pm on the evening before the colonoscopy and then 1.5 h later, 240 mL q 15 min for 4 doses (over 1 h) plus additional clear liquid on the evening before the colonoscopy (MoviPrep only). Suclear: Dose 1 PO evening before and dose 2 PO morning of colonoscopy with additional liquid after each dose. Alternatively, dose 1 PO early evening before and dose 2 PO 2 h after starting dose 1 on evening before colonoscopy with additional liquid with each dose. Suprep: 1 diluted bottle PO evening before and morning of (at least 2 h before procedure) colonoscopy. Additional water after each dose.

PEDS — Bowel prep: (NuLYTELY, TriLyte): 25 mL/kg/h PO/NG, until rectal effluent is clear, max 4 L for age older than 6 mo.

UNAPPROVED ADULT — Chronic constipation: 125 to 500 mL/day PO daily (up to two times per day). Whole bowel irrigation in iron overdose: 1500 to 2000 mL/h.

UNAPPROVED PEDS — Bowel cleansing prior to GI examination: 25 to 40 mL/kg/h PO/NG for 4 to 10 h or until rectal effluent is clear or 20 to 30 mL/min NG until 4 L are consumed or rectal effluent is clear. Whole bowel irrigation in iron overdose: 9 mo to 6 yo: 500 mL/h; 6 yo to 12 yo 1000 mL/h; older than 12 yo, use adult dose.

FORMS — Generic/Trade: Powder for oral soln in disposable jug 4 L or 2 L (MoviPrep). Trade only: GoLYTELY Packet for oral soln to make 3.785 L. Suclear: Dose 1 (16 oz) and dose 2 (2 L bottle) for reconstitution. Suprep: Two 6 oz bottles.

NOTES — Solid food should not be given within 2 h of soln. Effects should occur within 1 to 2 h. Chilling improves palatability.

MOA — Osmotic and cathartic effect in intestinal lumen.

ADVERSE EFFECTS — Frequent: Nausea, fullness, bloating. Severe: Hypersensitivity reactions, ischemic colitis, electrolyte and fluid imbalances, anaphylaxis, fever, chills, dehydration.

PREPOPIK (sodium picosulfate) ▶minimal absorption ♀B ▶? $

ADULT — Bowel cleansing prior to colonoscopy: Preferred method: 1 packet (diluted in 5 oz water) evening before the colonoscopy and second packet (diluted in 5 oz water) morning prior to colonoscopy. Alternatively, first dose during afternoon or early evening before the colonoscopy and second dose 6 h later in evening before colonoscopy. Additional clear liquids should be consumed.

PEDS — Not approved for use in children.

FORMS — Trade: 2 packets of 16 g powder for reconstitution.

NOTES — Use caution in patients with renal dysfunction and in patients at risk for aspiration.

MOA — Osmotic and cathartic effect in intestinal lumen.

ADVERSE EFFECTS — Frequent: nausea, headache, vomiting, abdominal bloating, pain and cramping, watery diarrhea hypermagnesemia, acute reduction in GFR.

SODIUM PHOSPHATE (Fleet-sodium phosphate, Fleet EZ-Prep, Accu-Prep, OsmoPrep, Visicol, ✸Enemol, Phoslax) ▶not absorbed ♀C ▶? $

WARNING — Phosphate-containing bowel cleansing regimens have been reported to cause acute phosphate nephropathy. Risk factors include advanced age, kidney disease or decreased intravascular volume, bowel obstruction or active colitis, and medications that affect renal perfusion or function such as diuretics, ACE inhibitors, ARBs, and maybe NSAIDs. Use extreme caution in bowel cleansing. Also associated with ischemic colitis and electrolyte and fluid imbalances.

ADULT — Constipation: 1 adult or pediatric enema PR or 20 to 30 mL of oral soln PO prn (max 45 mL/24 h). Prep prior to colonoscopy: Visicol: Evening before colonoscopy: 3 tabs with 8 oz clear liquid q 15 min until 20 tabs are consumed. Day of colonoscopy: Starting 3 to 5 h before procedure, 3 tabs with 8 oz clear liquid q 15 min until 20 tabs are consumed. OsmoPrep: 32 tabs PO with total of 2 quarts clear liquids as follows: evening before procedure: 4 tabs PO with 8 oz of clear liquids q 15 min for a total of 20 tabs; day of procedure: 3 to 5 h before procedure, 4 tabs with 8 oz of clear liquids q 15 min for a total of 12 tabs.

PEDS — Laxative: 2 to 11 yo: 1 pediatric enema (67.5 mL) PR prn. 5 to 9 yo: 5 mL of oral soln PO prn. 10 to 12 yo: 10 mL of oral soln PO prn.

UNAPPROVED ADULT — Visicol: Evening before colonoscopy: 3 tabs with 8 oz clear liquid q 15 min until 20 tabs are consumed. Day of colonoscopy: Starting 3 to 5 h before procedure, 3 tabs with 8 oz clear liquid q 15 min until 8 to 12 tabs are consumed.

FORMS — OTC Generic/Trade: Adult enema, oral soln. OTC Trade only: Pediatric enema, bowel prep. Rx Trade only: Visicol, OsmoPrep tabs ($$$$) 1.5 g.

NOTES — Taking the last 2 doses of Visicol with ginger ale appears to minimize residue. Excessive doses (more than 45 mL/24 h) of oral products may lead to serious electrolyte disturbances. Use with caution in severe renal impairment.

MOA — Osmotic and cathartic effect in intestinal lumen.

ADVERSE EFFECTS — Frequent: Bloating, nausea, abdominal pain, and vomiting. Severe: Electrolyte and fluid imbalances, ischemic colitis, arrhythmias, seizures, aspiration.

SORBITOL ▶not absorbed ♀C ▶? $

ADULT — Laxative: 30 to 150 mL (of 70% soln) PO or 120 mL (of 25 to 30% soln) PR. Cathartic: 4.3 mL/kg PO.

PEDS — Laxative: Children 2 to 11 yo: 2 mL/kg (of 70% soln) PO or 30 to 60 mL (of 25 to 30% soln) PR.

UNAPPROVED PEDS — Cathartic: 4.3 mL/kg of 35% soln (diluted from 70% soln) PO single dose.

FORMS — Generic only: Soln 70%.

NOTES — When used as a cathartic, can be given with activated charcoal to improve taste and decrease gastric transit time of charcoal. May precipitate electrolyte changes.

MOA — Osmotic and cathartic effect in intestinal lumen.

ADVERSE EFFECTS — Serious: Pulmonary congestion, angina-like pain, acidosis, electrolyte loss, convulsions. Frequent: Hyperglycemia, diarrhea, tachycardia, diuresis, urinary retention, blurred vision, dry mouth, thirst, dehydration, edema, N/V, rhinitis, chills, vertigo, headache, urticaria.

SUPREP (sodium sulfate + potassium sulfate + magnesium sulfate) ▶not absorbed ♀C ▶? $$$

ADULT — Evening before colonoscopy: Dilute 1 bottle to 16 oz with water and drink, then drink 32 oz water over next hour. Next morning, repeat both steps. Compete 1 h before colonoscopy.

PEDS — Not approved in children.

FORMS — Trade: Two 6 oz bottles for dilution.

MOA — osmotic

ADVERSE EFFECTS — Frequent: discomfort, abdominal fullness, nausea, cramping, vomiting.

GASTROENTEROLOGY: Laxatives—Stimulant

BISACODYL (Correctol, Dulcolax, Feen-a-Mint, Fleet-bisacodyl) ▶L ♀C ▶? $

ADULT — Constipation/colonic evacuation prior to a procedure: 5 to 15 mg PO once daily prn, 10 mg PR once daily prn.

PEDS — Constipation/colonic evacuation prior to a procedure: 0.3 mg/kg/day PO once daily prn.

Children younger than 2 yo: 5 mg PR once daily prn; 2 to 11 yo: 5 to 10 mg PO or PR once daily prn; 12 yo or older: 10 mg PO or PR once daily prn.

FORMS — OTC Generic/Trade: Tabs 5 mg; Supp 10 mg. OTC Trade only: Enema, 10 mg/30 mL.

NOTES — Oral tab has onset of 6 to 10 h. Onset of action of supp is approximately 15 to 60 min. Do not

(cont.)

BISACODYL (*cont.*)

chew tabs; swallow whole. Do not give within 1 h of antacids or dairy products. Chronic use of stimulant laxatives may be habit forming.
MOA — Direct colonic stimulant.
ADVERSE EFFECTS — Frequent: None.

CASCARA ▶L ♀C ▶+ $

ADULT — Constipation: 5 mL/day of aromatic fluid extract PO at bedtime prn.
PEDS — Constipation: Infants: 1.25 mL/day of aromatic fluid extract PO daily prn. Children 2 to 11 yo: 2.5 mL/day of aromatic fluid extract PO daily prn.
FORMS — Rx Generic only: Liquid aromatic fluid extract.
NOTES — Cascara sagrada fluid extract is 5 times more potent than cascara sagrada aromatic fluid extract. Chronic use of stimulant laxatives may be habit forming.
MOA — Direct irritation of intestinal mucosa.
ADVERSE EFFECTS — Frequent: Lightheadedness, fluid/electrolyte imbalance, abdominal cramps, nausea, diarrhea, discoloration of urine.

CASTOR OIL ▶not absorbed ♀X ▶? $

ADULT — Constipation: 15 to 60 mL PO daily prn. Colonic evacuation prior to procedure: 15 to 60 mL of castor oil or 30 to 60 mL emulsified castor oil PO as a single dose 16 h prior to procedure.
PEDS — Colonic evacuation prior to procedure: 1 to 5 mL of castor oil or 2.5 to 7.5 mL emulsified castor oil PO as a single dose 16 h prior to procedure for age younger than 2 yo. 5 to 15 mL of castor oil or 7.5 to 30 mL of emulsified castor oil PO as a single dose 16 h prior to procedure for age 2 to 11 yo.

FORMS — OTC Generic only: Oil 60, 120, 180, 480 mL.
NOTES — Emulsions somewhat mask the bad taste. Onset of action approximately 2 to 6 h. Do not give at bedtime. Chill or administer with juice to improve taste.
MOA — Softens and lubricates stool.
ADVERSE EFFECTS — Frequent: None.

SENNA (*Senokot, SenokotXTRA, Ex-Lax, Fletcher's Castoria*) ▶L ♀C ▶+ $

ADULT — Laxative or evacuation of the colon for bowel or rectal examinations: 10 to 15 mL or 2 tabs PO at bedtime. Max daily dose 30 mL of syrup or 8 tabs.
PEDS — Laxative: 10 to 20 mg/kg/dose PO at bedtime. Alternative regimen: 1 mo to 2 yo: 1.25 to 2.5 mL syrup PO at bedtime, max 5 mL/day; 2 to 5 yo: 2.5 to 3.75 mL syrup PO at bedtime, max 7.5 mL/day; 6 to 12 yo: 5 to 7.5 mL syrup PO at bedtime, max 15 mL/day.
FORMS — OTC Generic/Trade (all dosing is based on sennosides content; 1 mg sennosides is equivalent to 21.7 mg standardized senna concentrate): Syrup 8.8 mg/5 mL. Liquid 33.3 mg senna concentrate/mL (Fletcher's Castoria). Tabs 8.6, 15, 17, 25 mg. Chewable tabs 10, 15 mg.
NOTES — Effects occur 6 to 24 h after oral administration. Use caution in renal dysfunction. Chronic use of stimulant laxatives may be habit forming.
MOA — Enhances GI motility.
ADVERSE EFFECTS — Frequent: Potential for severe diaper rash in children wearing diapers.

GASTROENTEROLOGY: Laxatives—Stool Softener

DOCUSATE (*Colace, Docu-Soft, DOK, Dulcolax, Docu-Liquid, Enemeez, Fleet Sof-Lax, Octycine, Silace*) ▶L ♀A ▶? $

ADULT — Constipation: Docusate calcium: 240 mg PO daily. Docusate sodium: 50 to 500 mg/day PO in 1 to 4 divided doses.
PEDS — Constipation: Docusate sodium: 10 to 40 mg/day for age younger than 3 yo, 20 to 60 mg/day for age 3 to 6 yo, 40 to 150 mg/day for age 6 to 12 yo. In all cases, doses are divided up to four times per day.
UNAPPROVED ADULT — Docusate sodium, Constipation: Can be given as a retention enema: Mix 50 to 100 mg docusate liquid with saline or water retention enema for rectal use. Cerumen

removal: Instill 1 mL liquid (not syrup) in affected ear; allow to remain for 10 to 15 min, then irrigate with 50 mL lukewarm NS if necessary.
UNAPPROVED PEDS — Docusate sodium: Cerumen removal: Instill 1 mL liquid (not syrup) in affected ear; allow to remain for 10 to 15 min, then irrigate with 50 mL lukewarm NS if necessary.
FORMS — Docusate calcium OTC Generic/Trade: Caps 240 mg. Docusate sodium OTC Generic/Trade: Caps 50, 100, 250 mg. Liquid 50 mg/5 mL. Syrup 20 mg/5 mL. Docusate sodium OTC Trade only (Enemeez): Enema, rectal 283 mg/5 mL.
NOTES — Takes 1 to 3 days to notably soften stools.
MOA — Softens stool, cerumen.
ADVERSE EFFECTS — Frequent: Abdominal cramping.

GASTROENTEROLOGY: Laxatives—Other or Combinations

LUBIPROSTONE (*Amitiza*) ▶gut ♀C ▶? $$$$$

WARNING — Avoid if symptoms or history of mechanical GI obstruction.
ADULT — Chronic idiopathic constipation: 24 mcg PO two times per day with food and water. Irritable bowel syndrome with constipation in age 18 yo or older: 8 mcg PO two times per day. Opioid-induced

constipation in adults with chronic, non-cancer pain: 24 mcg PO two times per day with food and water.
PEDS — Not approved in children.
FORMS — Trade only: Caps 8, 24 mcg.
NOTES — Reduce dose with moderate to severe hepatic dysfunction. Has not been studied with

(cont.)

LUBIPROSTONE (*cont.*)

diphenylheptane opioids such as methadone-induced constipation. Swallow capsules whole.

MOA — Chloride channel activator which enhances intestinal fluid secretion, thereby increasing intestinal motility.

ADVERSE EFFECTS — Frequent: Nausea, diarrhea, headache, abdominal pain/distension, flatulence.

MINERAL OIL (*Kondremul, Fleet Mineral Oil Enema, Liqui-Doss, ♣Lansoÿl*) ▶not absorbed ♀C ▶? $

ADULT — Laxative: 15 to 45 mL PO in a single dose or in divided doses, 60 to 150 mL PR.

PEDS — Laxative: Children 6 to 11 yo: 5 to 15 mL PO in a single dose or in divided doses. Children 2 to 11 yo: 30 to 60 mL PR.

FORMS — OTC Generic/Trade: Oil (30, 480 mL), Enema (Fleet). OTC Trade only: Oral liquid (Liqui-Doss) 13.5 mg/15 mL. Oral microemulsion (Kondremul) 2.5 mg/5 mL.

NOTES — Use with caution in children younger than 4 yo and elderly or debilitated patients due to concerns for aspiration pneumonitis. Although usual directions for plain mineral oil are to administer at bedtime, this increases risk of lipid pneumonitis. Mineral oil emulsions may be administered with meals.

MOA — Softens and lubricates stool.

ADVERSE EFFECTS — Frequent: None.

PERI-COLACE (**docusate + sennosides**) ▶L ♀C ▶? $

ADULT — Constipation: 2 to 4 tabs PO once daily or in divided doses prn.

PEDS — Constipation, 2 to 6 yo: Up to 1 tab PO daily prn. 6 to 12 yo: 1 to 2 tabs PO daily prn.

FORMS — OTC Generic/Trade: Tabs 50 mg docusate + 8.6 mg sennosides.

NOTES — Chronic use of stimulant laxatives (casanthranol) may be habit forming.

MOA — Softens stool.

ADVERSE EFFECTS — Frequent: Abdominal cramping.

SENOKOT-S (**senna + docusate**) ▶L ♀C ▶+ $

ADULT — 2 tabs PO daily, max 4 tabs two times per day.

PEDS — 2 to 6 yo: ½ tab PO daily, max 1 tab two times per day. 6 to 12 yo: 1 tab PO daily, max 2 tabs two times per day.

FORMS — OTC Generic/Trade: Tabs 8.6 mg senna concentrate + 50 mg docusate.

NOTES — Effects occur 6 to 12 h after oral administration. Use caution in renal dysfunction. Chronic use of stimulant laxatives may be habit forming.

MOA — Natural product; enhances GI motility and softens stool.

ADVERSE EFFECTS — Frequent: None.

GASTROENTEROLOGY: Ulcerative Colitis

BALSALAZIDE (*Colazal, Giazo*) ▶minimal absorption ♀B ▶? $$$$$

ADULT — Ulcerative colitis: 2.25 g PO three times per day (Colazal) for 8 to 12 weeks or 3 x 1.1 g (3.3 g) PO twice per day for 8 weeks (Giazo). Giazo is for males only, not approved for use in females.

PEDS — 5 to 17 yo (Colazal): Mild to moderately active ulcerative colitis: 2.25 g PO three times per day for 8 weeks. Alternatively, 750 mg PO three times per day for 8 weeks.

FORMS — Generic/Trade (Colazal): Caps 750 mg. Trade (Giazo): Tabs 1.1 g.

NOTES — Contraindicated in salicylate allergy. Caution with renal insufficiency.

MOA — Mesalamine prodrug, inhibits cyclooxygenase pathways.

ADVERSE EFFECTS — Frequent: Headache, abdominal pain, nausea, diarrhea, vomiting, respiratory infection, arthralgias. Severe: Cholestatic jaundice, cirrhosis, liver failure, hypersensitivity, pericarditis.

MESALAMINE (*5-aminosalicylic acid, Apriso, 5-Aspirin, Lialda, Pentasa, Canasa, Rowasa, Delzicol, Asacol HD♣Mesasal, Salofalk*) ▶gut ♀C ▶? $$$$$

ADULT — Ulcerative colitis: Delzicol: 800 mg PO three times a day (treatment) or 800 mg PO twice a day (maintenance). Pentasa: 1 g PO four times per day. Lialda: 2.4 to 4.8 g PO daily with a meal for 8 weeks. Asacol HD: 1.6 g PO three times a day for 6 weeks. Rectal susp: 4 g (60 mL) PR retained for 8 h at bedtime. Maintenance of remission of ulcerative colitis: Apriso: 1.5 g (4 caps) PO q am. Lialda: 2.4 g PO daily.

Ulcerative proctitis: Canasa suppository: 500 mg PR two to three times per day or 1000 mg PR at bedtime.

PEDS — Active ulcerative colitis 5 yo and older: 17 kg to 32 kg: 36 to 71 mg/kg/day (max 1.2 g/day); 33 kg to 53 kg: 37 to 61 mg/kg/day (max 2.0 g/day); 54 kg to 90 kg: 27 to 44 mg/kg/day (max 2.4 g/day).

UNAPPROVED ADULT — Active Crohn's: 0.4 to 4.8 g/day PO in divided doses. Maintenance of remission of Crohn's: 2.4 g/day in divided doses.

FORMS — Trade only: Delayed-release caps (Delzicol) 400 mg. Controlled-release caps 250, 500 mg (Pentasa). Delayed-release tabs 800 mg (Asacol HD), 1200 mg (Lialda). Rectal supp 1000 mg (Canasa). Controlled-release caps 0.375 g (Apriso). Generic/Trade: Rectal susp 4 g/60 mL (Rowasa).

NOTES — Avoid in salicylate sensitivity or hepatic dysfunction. Reports of hepatic failure in patients with pre-existing liver disease. Pentasa can be opened and mixed with water or applesauce in patients who cannot swallow a capsule. May decrease digoxin levels. May discolor urine yellow-brown. Most common adverse effects include headache, abdominal pain, fever, rash. Two Delzicol are not bioequivalent to Asacol HD. The coating of Asacol and Asacol HD contain the inactive chemical, dibutyl phthalate (DBP). In animal studies at doses more than 190 times the human dose, maternal DBP was associated with external and skeletal malformations and adverse effects on the male reproductive system. Use may cause false elevations of urinary normetanephrine concentrations.

(cont.)

MESALAMINE (*cont.*)

MOA — Unknown.

ADVERSE EFFECTS — Frequent: Headache, malaise, abdominal pain, cramps, flatulence, gas, hair loss. Severe: Cytopenias, myo- and pericarditis, hepatitis, pneumonitis, nephritis, anaphylactic reaction, angioedema, Steven-Johnson syndrome, drug reaction with eosinophilia and systematic symptoms (DRESS).

OLSALAZINE (*Dipentum*) ▶L ♀C ▶– $$$$$

ADULT — Maintenance of remission of ulcerative colitis in patients intolerant to sulfasalazine: 500 mg PO two times per day with food.

PEDS — Not approved in children.

UNAPPROVED ADULT — Crohn's disease: 1.5 to 3 g/ day PO in divided doses with food.

FORMS — Trade only: Caps 250 mg.

NOTES — Diarrhea in up to 17%. Avoid in salicylate sensitivity.

MOA — Unknown.

ADVERSE EFFECTS — Frequent: Diarrhea, cramps, abdominal pain.

SULFASALAZINE—GASTROENTEROLOGY (*Azulfidine, Azulfidine EN-tabs,* ✱*Salazopyrin En-tabs*) ▶L ♀B ▶? $$

WARNING — Beware of hypersensitivity, marrow suppression, renal and liver damage, central nervous system effects, irreversible neuromuscular and CNS changes, fibrosing alveolitis.

ADULT — Induction of remission, ulcerative colitis: Initial dose of 500 to 1000 mg PO four times per day. Maintenance of remission: 500 mg PO four times per day.

PEDS —Induction of remission, ulcerative colitis, age 6 yo or older: Initially 40 to 60 mg/kg/day PO divided into 3 to 6 doses. Max 75 mg/kg/day. Maintenance of remission: 30 mg/kg/day PO divided into 4 doses.

FORMS — Generic/Trade: Tabs 500 mg, scored. Enteric-coated, delayed-release (EN-tabs) 500 mg.

NOTES — Contraindicated in children younger than 2 yo. Avoid with hepatic or renal dysfunction, intestinal or urinary obstruction, porphyria, or sulfonamide or salicylate sensitivity. Monitor CBC q 2 to 4 weeks for 3 months then q 3 months. Monitor LFTs, CBC, and renal function. Oligospermia and infertility, and photosensitivity may occur. May decrease folic acid, digoxin, cyclosporine, and iron levels. May turn body fluids, contact lenses, or skin orange-yellow. Enteric-coated (Azulfidine EN, Salazopyrin EN) tabs may cause fewer GI adverse effects. Supplement with folic acid during pregnancy. Reports of bloody stools or diarrhea in breastfed infants of mothers taking sulfasalazine.

MOA — Colonic antiinflammatoru, immunosuppressant.

ADVERSE EFFECTS — Serious: Agranulocytosis, hemolytic anemia, nephro/hepatotoxicity, hepatic failure, drug rash and other severe skin reactions, hypersensitivity, anaphylaxis, angioedema, neural tube defect, reversible male infertility, infections associated with myelosuppression and severe hypersensitivity reactions. Frequent: Nausea, dyspepsia, rash.

VEDOLIZUMAB (*Entyvio*) ▶? ♀B ▶? $$$$$

ADULT — Active ulcerative colitis or Crohn's disease, moderate to severe: 300 mg IV infused over 30 minutes at weeks 0, 2, 6, and then q 8 weeks. Discontinue if no benefit by week 14. Indicated for patients intolerant or unresponsive to TNF-blockers, or corticosteroid-dependent or -intolerant.

NOTES — Avoid live vaccines unless potential benefit exceeds risk; bring immunizations up to date before using vedolizumab. May cause infusion and hypersensitivity reactions. Increased risk of infection; do not start during serious infection and consider holding if one occurs. Do not coadminister with natalizumab, another integrin antagonist that can cause progressive multifocal leukoencephalopathy. Do not coadminister with TNF-blockers.

MOA — Humanized IgG1 antibody that is an integrin receptor antagonist; reduces inflammation by inhibiting T-lymphocyte migration into gut lymph tissue.

ADVERSE EFFECTS — Serious: Hypersensitivity and infusion-related reactions including anaphylaxis; increased risk of infection; possible risk of progressive multifocal leukoencephalopathy. Frequent: headache, nausea, fever, fatigue, cough, rash, pruritus, infection (bronchitis, nasopharyngitis, influenza, sinusitis, upper respiratory tract infection), pain (arthralgia; oropharyngeal, extremity, and back pain). Increased LFTs.

GASTROENTEROLOGY: Other GI Agents

ALOSETRON (*Lotronex*) ▶L ♀B ▶? $$$$$

WARNING — Can cause severe constipation and ischemic colitis. Concomitant use with fluvoxamine, a potent CYP1A2 inhibitor, is contraindicated. Use caution with moderate CYP1A2 inhibitors such as quinolone antibiotics and cimetidine. Use caution with strong inhibitors of CYP3A4 such as ketoconazole, clarithromycin, protease inhibitors, voriconazole, and itraconazole.

ADULT — Diarrhea-predominant irritable bowel syndrome in women who have failed conventional therapy: 0.5 mg PO twice a day for 4 weeks; discontinue in patients who become constipated. If well tolerated and symptoms not controlled after 4 weeks, may increase to 1 mg PO two times per day. Discontinue if symptoms not controlled in 4 weeks on 1 mg PO two times per day.

PEDS — Not approved in children.

FORMS — Generic/Trade: Tabs 0.5, 1 mg.

NOTES — Prescribers should complete REMs program prior to prescribing.

MOA — Selective 5-HT3 receptor antagonist.

(cont.)

ALOSETRON (cont.)

ADVERSE EFFECTS — Frequent: Constipation, nausea, abdominal pain. Severe: Severe constipation, ischemic colitis.

ALPHA-GALACTOSIDASE (*Beano*) ▶minimal absorption ♀? ▶? $

ADULT — 1 tab per ½ cup gassy food, 2 to 3 tabs PO (chew, swallow, or crumble) or 1 melt-away tab per typical meal.

PEDS — Not approved in age younger than 12 yo.

FORMS — OTC Trade only: Tabs, melt-away tabs.

NOTES — Beano produces 2 to 6 g of carbohydrates for every 100 g of food treated by Beano; may increase glucose levels.

MOA — Enzyme that breaks down complex sugars in gassy foods making them more digestible.

ADVERSE EFFECTS — Frequent: None. Severe: None.

ALVIMOPAN (*Entereg*) ▶intestinal flora ♀B ▶? $$$$$

WARNING — Increased risk of myocardial infarction in a clinical trial of patients taking alvimopan long-term. Only available through a restricted program for short-term use (15 doses).

ADULT — To accelerate time to upper and lower gastrointestinal recovery following partial bowel resection with primary anastomosis, short-term (up to 15 doses) only: 12 mg PO 30 min to 5 h prior to surgery, then 12 mg PO two times per day starting the day after surgery for up to 7 days.

PEDS — Not approved in children.

FORMS — Trade only: Caps 12 mg.

NOTES — Only available to hospitals that are authorized to use the medication (requires hospital DEA number to be dispensed). Contraindicated in patients who have taken therapeutic doses of opioids for more than 7 consecutive days. Not for use in those with severe hepatic or renal disease, or for gastric primary pancreatic anastomosis. Serum concentrations in patients of Japanese descent may be up to 2-fold greater than Caucasian subjects with same dose. Monitor Japanese patients for adverse events.

MOA — Peripherally acting mu-opioid receptor antagonist used for post operative ileus.

ADVERSE EFFECTS — Frequent: Anemia, dyspepsia, hypokalemia, back pain, urinary retention. Severe: Myocardial infarction.

BUDESONIDE (*Entocort EC, Uceris*) ▶L ♀C ▶? $$$$$

ADULT — Mild to moderate Crohn's, induction of remission: 9 mg PO daily for up to 8 weeks. May repeat 8-week course for recurring episodes. 1 metered dose applied to rectal area twice daily for 2 weeks followed by 1 metered dose once daily for 4 weeks (Uceris foam). Maintenance: 6 mg PO daily for 3 months (Entocort only). Mild to moderate ulcerative colitis, induction of remission: 9 mg PO q am for up to 8 weeks.

PEDS — Mild to moderate Crohn's disease in children 8 to 17 years: 9 mg PO q am for up to 8 weeks, then 6 mg PO q am for 2 weeks.

UNAPPROVED PEDS — Mild to moderate Crohn's in children younger than 8 years: 0.45 mg/kg up to 9 mg PO daily for 8 to 12 weeks for age 9 yo or older.

FORMS — Generic/Trade: Caps 3 mg. Trade only: Extended-release tabs (Uceris) 9 mg. (Uceris for ulcerative colitis, only).Rectal foam (Uceris) 2 mg/metered dose, 14 actuactions/canister.

NOTES — May taper dose to 6 mg for 2 weeks prior to discontinuation (Entocort).

MOA — Affects cell motility and protein synthesis; anti-inflammatory.

ADVERSE EFFECTS — Frequent: Palpitations, nervousness, dizziness, headache, pruritus, rash, GI irritation, nausea, bitter taste, hyperglycemia, increased infection rate. Severe: Anaphylaxis.

CHENODIOL (*Chenodal*) ▶bile L ♀X ▶? varies by therapy

ADULT — Gallstone dissolution: 13 to 16 mg/kg/day in two divided doses, morning and night, starting with 250 mg two times per day the first 2 weeks and increasing by 250 mg/day each week thereafter until the recommended or max tolerated dose is reached.

PEDS — Not approved for use in children.

FORMS — Generic: Tabs 250 mg.

NOTES — Monitor LFTs.

MOA — Bile acid

ADVERSE EFFECTS — Frequent: increases in LFTs, diarrhea.

CHLORDIAZEPOXIDE—CLIDINIUM ▶K ♀D ▶– $$$$

ADULT — Irritable bowel syndrome: 1 to 2 caps PO three to four times per day.

PEDS — Not approved in children.

FORMS — Generic: Caps, chlordiazepoxide 5 mg + clidinium 2.5 mg.

NOTES — May cause drowsiness. After prolonged use, gradually taper to avoid withdrawal symptoms. Contains ingredients formerly contained in Librax.

MOA — Anticholinergic/benzodiazepine.

ADVERSE EFFECTS — Frequent: Dry mouth, drowsiness, ataxia, memory impairment, rash, decreased libido, xerostomia, changes in appetite, micturation difficulties. Severe: CNS, respiratory depression.

CHOLIC ACID (*Cholbam*) ▶bile L ♀? ▶? $$$$$

ADULT — Bile synthesis disorders: 10 to 15 mg/kg PO once daily or in two divided doses. Familial triglyceridemia: 11 to 17 mg/kg PO once daily or in two divided doses.

PEDS — Use adult dosing.

FORMS — Trade: Capsules 50, 250 mg.

NOTES — Monitor LFTs during therapy. Discontinue if no improvement in 3 months. Separate dosing from bile acid sequestrants and aluminum-containing antacids.

MOA — Primary bile acid

ADVERSE EFFECTS — Frequent: diarrhea, reflux esophagitis, malaise, jaundice, skin lesion, nausea, abdominal pain, intestinal poly, UTI.

CONTRAVE (naltrexone + bupropion) ▶LK ♀X ▶? $$$$$

WARNING — Antidepressants (bupropion) increase the risk of suicidal thoughts in children, adolescents, and young adults. Neuropsychiatric reactions

(cont.)

CONTRAVE (*cont.*)

have occurred in patients taking bupropion for smoking cessation.

ADULT — Obese or overweight with comorbidities: 1 tab PO daily for 1 week, then 1 tab PO twice daily for 1 week, then 2 tabs PO q am and 1 tab PO q pm for 1 week, then 2 tabs PO twice daily.

PEDS — Not approved in children younger than 18 yo.

FORMS — Trade only: Tabs (naltrexone 8 mg + bupropion 90 mg).

MOA — opioid antagonist + aminoketone antidepressant

ADVERSE EFFECTS — See components

CROFELEMER (*Fulyzaq*) ▶minimal absorption ♀C ▶? $$$$$

ADULT — Noninfectious AIDS diarrhea: 125 mg PO twice daily.

PEDS — Not approved in children younger than 18 yo.

FORMS — Trade: Delayed-release tab 125 mg.

NOTES — Rule out infectious causes of diarrhea before initiating.

MOA — Inhibits cAMP-stimulated cystic fibrosis transmembrane conductance regulator chloride ion channel, and calcium-activated Cl channels at the luminal membrane of enterocytes

ADVERSE EFFECTS — Common: flatulence, bronchitis, cough.

ELUXADOLINE (*Viberzi*) ▶glucuronidation ♀? ?/?/?/? ▶©IV $$$$$

WARNING — Monitor patients who do not have a gallbladder for new or worsening abdominal pain with or without vomiting, and biliary pain, pancreatic enzyme elevation due to risk of Sphincter of Oddi spasm and pancreatitis.

ADULT — Diarrhea-predominant IBS: 100 mg PO twice daily. Reduce dose to 75 mg PO twice daily in patients who cannot tolerate the higher dose, those do not have a gallbladder, those with mild to moderate heaptic impairmen, and patients who are receiving OATP1B1 inhibitors such as cycliosporine, alfentanil, ergotamine, fentanyl, sirolimus, tacrolimus, others.

PEDS — Not approved for use in children.

FORMS — Rx, Trade: tabs 75 mg, 100 mg.

NOTES — Discontinue therapy in patients who develop severe constipation for more than 4 days.

MOA — Mu-opioid receptor agonist, delta opioid receptor antagonist, kappa opioid receptor agonist.

ADVERSE EFFECTS — Frequent: constipation, nausea, abdominal pain. Severe: Sphincter of Oddi spasm, pancreatitis

GLYCOPYRROLATE (*Robinul, Robinul Forte, Cuvposa*) ▶K ♀B ▶? $$$$

ADULT — Peptic ulcer disease: 1 to 2 mg PO two to three times per day. Preop/intraoperative respiratory antisecretory effect: 4 mcg/kg IV 30-60 minutes before anesthesia or at the time the preanesthetic narcotic or sedative is administered..

PEDS — Chronic drooling in children 3 to 16 yo (Cuvposa): 0.02 mg/kg three times per day, 1 h before or 2 h after meals. Increase by 0.02 mg/kg q

5 to 7 days to a max of 0.1 mg/kg three times a day, not to exceed 1.5 to 3 mg based on weight.

UNAPPROVED ADULT — Drooling: 0.1 mg/kg PO two to three times per day or 1 mg PO twice daily, max 6 mg/day.

FORMS — Trade: Soln 1 mg/5 mL (480 mL, Cuvposa). Generic/Trade: Tabs 1, 2 mg.

NOTES — Contraindicated in narrow-angle glaucoma, obstructive uropathy, paralytic ileus or GI obstruction, myasthenia gravis, severe ulcerative colitis, toxic megacolon, and unstable cardiovascular status in acute hemorrhage.

MOA — Inhibits effects of acetylcholine.

ADVERSE EFFECTS — Frequent: Dry skin, dry mouth/throat, constipation, vomiting, flushing, nasal congestion, urinary retention, dry nose, local irritation.

LACTASE (*Lactaid*) ▶not absorbed ♀+ ▶+ $

ADULT — Swallow or chew 3 caps (original-strength), 2 caps (extra-strength), 1 cap (Ultra) with 1st bite of dairy foods. Adjust dose based on response.

PEDS — Titrate dose based on response.

FORMS — OTC Generic/Trade: Caps, Chewable tabs.

MOA — Replenish lactase enzymes.

ADVERSE EFFECTS — Frequent: None.

LINACLOTIDE (*Linzess, ✦Constella*) ▶gut – ♀C ▶? $$$$$

WARNING — Contraindicated in pediatric patients younger than 6 yo. Avoid use in children 6 through 17 yo.

ADULT — Irritable bowel syndrome: 290 mcg PO daily. Chronic idiopathic constipation: 145 mcg PO once daily.

PEDS — Not approved in children younger than 18 years old.

FORMS — Trade: Caps 145, 290 mcg.

NOTES — Take on empty stomach, 30 minutes before food. For patients trouble swallowing a capsule or with an NG tube, open capsule and mix with water or applesauce prior to administration. Do not use in patients with mechanical GI obstruction.

MOA — guanylate cyclase-C (GC-C) agonist.

ADVERSE EFFECTS — Frequent: diarrhea, abdominal pain, flatulence, abdominal distension.

LORCASERIN (*Belviq*) ▶L ♀X ▶ $$$$$

WARNING — Contraindicated in pregnancy.

ADULT — Obesity or overweight with comorbidities: 10 mg PO twice a day. Discontinue if 5% wt loss not achieved by 12 weeks.

PEDS — Not approved for use in children.

FORMS — Trade: Tabs 10 mg.

NOTES — Can cause serotonin syndrome when given with other serotonergic or antidopaminergic agent. Monitor for signs or symptoms of valvular heart disease. Can cause cognitive impairment. May be associated with psychiatric diseases. May cause priapism.

MOA — Selective serotonin 2C receptor agonist

ADVERSE EFFECTS — Frequent: headache, dizziness, fatigue, nausea, dry mouth, constipation, hypoglycemia in diabetic patients. Severe: serotonin syndrome, valvular heart disease.

METHYLNALTREXONE (*Relistor*) ▶unchanged ♀B ▶?
$$$$$

ADULT — Opioid-induced constipation with chronic non-cancer pain:12 mcg SC once daily or 450 mg PO once daily in the morning. Opioid-induced constipation in patients with advanced illness who are receiving palliative care, when response to laxative therapy has not been sufficient: Less than 38 kg: 0.15 mg/kg SC every other day; 38 kg to 61 kg: 8 mg SC every other day; 62 kg to 114 kg: 12 mg SC every other day; 115 kg or greater: 0.15 mg/kg SC every other day.

PEDS — Not approved in children.

FORMS — Rx, Trade: Single-use vial 12 mg/0.6 mL soln for SC injection; single-use prefilled syringe 8 mg/0.4 mL and 12 mg/0.6 mL soln for SC injection. Tabs 150 mg.

NOTES — Discontinue all maintenance laxative upon initiation, and resume only if needed. Do not use with GI obstruction or lesions of GI tract. If severe or persistent diarrhea develops, stop medication and consult physician. Usual dose every other day, but no more frequently than once daily. For CrCl less than 30 mL/min, reduce dose by half. When using the oral form, take with water, on an empty stomach, 30 minutes before the first meal of the day.

MOA — Peripherally acting opioid antagonist

ADVERSE EFFECTS — Frequent: Abdominal pain, flatulence, nausea, dizziness, diarrhea, hyperhidrosis. Severe: GI perforation

NALOXEGOL (*Movantik*) ▶L ♀C ▶– $$$$$

WARNING — Monitor for opioid withdrawal reactions. Contraindicated in bowel obstruction and in patients taking strong CYP3A4 inhibitors (eg, clarithromycin, ketoconazole).

ADULT — Opioid-induced constipation: 25 mg PO once daily, if not tolerated reduce dose to 12.5 mg.

PEDS — Not approved in children younger than 18 yo.

FORMS — Trade only: Tabs 12.5, 25 mg.

NOTES — Many drug interactions. Reduce dose in CrCl <60 mL/min.

MOA — Opioid antagonist

ADVERSE EFFECTS — Frequent: abdominal pain, diarrhea, nausea, vomiting, flatulence, headache.

NEOMYCIN—ORAL (*Neo-Fradin*) ▶minimal absorption ♀D ▶? $$$

ADULT — Suppression of intestinal bacteria (given with erythromycin): 1 g PO at 19 h, 18 h, and 9 h prior to procedure (eg, 1 pm, 2 pm, 11 pm on prior day). Alternative regimen 1 g PO q 1 h for 4 doses then 1 g PO q 4 h for 5 doses. Hepatic encephalopathy: 4 to 12 g/day PO divided q 4 to 6 h for 5 to 6 days. Diarrhea caused by enteropathogenicE. coli: 3 g/day PO divided q 6 h.

PEDS — Suppression of intestinal bacteria (given with erythromycin): 25 mg/kg PO at 19 h, 18 h and 9 h prior to procedure (eg, 1 pm, 2 pm, 11 pm on prior day). Alternative regimen 90 mg/kg/day PO divided q 4 h for 2 days. Hepatic encephalopathy: 50 to 100 mg/kg/day PO divided q 6 to 8 h for 5 to 6

days. Diarrhea caused by enteropathogenic E. coli: 50 mg/kg/day PO divided q 6 h for 2 to 3 days.

FORMS — Generic only: Tabs 500 mg. Trade only: Soln 125 mg/5 mL.

NOTES — Increased INR with warfarin, decreased levels of digoxin, methotrexate.

MOA — Inhibits bacterial protein synthesis.

ADVERSE EFFECTS — Frequent: None. Severe: nephrotoxicity, neurotoxicity.

OBETICHOLIC ACID (*Ocaliva*) ▶L bile ♀? ?/?/? ▶? $$$$$

WARNING — Adjust the dosage for patients with moderate or severe hepatic impairment. Monitor for increased LFTs. Discontinue in patients who develop complete biliary obstruction. Monitor for reductions in HDL. Can cause severe pruritis.

ADULT — Primary biliary cholangit s, with ursodiol if no response to ursodiol for at least year or without ursodiol in those intolerant to ursodiol: 5 mg PO daily . Can be increased to 10 mg once daily in 3 months if inadequate response.

PEDS — Not approved for use in children.

FORMS — Trade only: Tabs 5, 10 mg.

MOA — Agonist for FXR, a receptor which regulates bile acid, inflammatory, fibrotic, and metabolic pathways.

ADVERSE EFFECTS — Frequent: pruritis, fatigue, abdominal discomfort, arthralgia. Severe: liver failure.

OCTREOTIDE (*Sandostatin, Sandostatin LAR*) ▶LK ♀B ▶? $$$$$

ADULT — Diarrhea associated with carcinoid tumors: 100 to 600 mcg/day SC/IV in 2 to 4 divided doses for 2 weeks or 20 mg IM (Sandostatin LAR) q 4 weeks for 2 months. Adjust dose based on response. Diarrhea associated with vasoactive intestinal peptide-secreting tumors: 200 to 300 mcg/day SC/IV in 2 to 4 divided doses for 2 weeks or 20 mg IM (Sandostatin LAR) q 4 weeks for 2 months. Adjust dose based on response.

PEDS — Not approved in children.

UNAPPROVED ADULT — Variceal bleeding: Bolus 25 to 50 mcg IV followed by 25 to 50 mcg/h continuous IV infusion. AIDS diarrhea: 25 to 250 mcg SC three times per day, max 500 mcg SC q 8 h. Irritable bowel syndrome: 100 mcg as a single dose to 125 mcg SC two times per day. GI and pancreatic fistulas: 50 to 200 mcg SC/IV q 8 h.

UNAPPROVED PEDS — Diarrhea: Initially 1 to 10 mcg/kg SC/IV q 12 h. Congenital hyperinsulinism: 1 to 40 mcg/kg SC daily. Hypothalamic obesity in children 6 to 17 yo: 40 mg IM q 4 weeks (Sandostatin LAR) or 5 to 15 mcg/kg SC daily.

FORMS — Generic/Trade: Injection vials 0.05, 0.1, 0.2, 0.5, 1 mg. Trade only: Long-acting injectable susp (Sandostatin LAR) 10, 20, 30 mg.

NOTES — For the treatment of variceal bleeding, most studies treat for 3 to 5 days. Individualize dose based on response. Dosage reduction often necessary in elderly. May cause hypoglycemia, hyperglycemia; caution especially in diabetes. May cause hypothyroidism, cardiac arrhythmias. Increases

(cont.)

OCTREOTIDE (*cont.*)

bioavailability of bromocriptine. Sandostatin LAR only indicated for patients who are stabilized on Sandostatin.

MOA — Mimics natural somatostatin.

ADVERSE EFFECTS — Frequent: Sinus bradycardia, chest pain, fatigue, headache, malaise, fever, dizziness, pruritis, hyperglycemia, abdominal pain, nausea, diarrhea. Severe: Hepatitis, progressive abdominal distension, severe epigastric pain.

ORLISTAT (*Alli, Xenical*) ▸gut ♀X ▶? $$$

ADULT — Weight loss and wt management: 60 mg to 120 mg PO three times per day with meals or up to 1 h after meals.

PEDS — Children 12 to 16 yo: 60 mg to 120 mg PO three times per day with meals. Not approved in age younger than 12 yo.

FORMS — OTC Trade only (Alli): Caps 60 mg. Rx Trade only (Xenical): Caps 120 mg.

NOTES — All patients should take a vitamin containing fat-soluble vitamins (A, E, D, K, beta carotene). May cause fatty stools, fecal urgency, flatus with discharge, and oily spotting in more than 20% of patients. GI adverse effects greater when taken with high-fat diet. Has been associated with liver damage. Can reduce the effect of levothyroxine, amiodarone and antiepileptic drugs or increase the effects of warfarin. Administer orlistat and levothyroxine at least 4 h apart. Administer cyclosporine 3 h after orlistat. Monitor INR and antiepileptic serum concentrations.

MOA — Inhibits gastric and pancreatic lipases.

ADVERSE EFFECTS — Frequent: CNS effects, oily stool, fecal incontinence, flatus with discharge Severe: Cholelithiasis, nephrolithiasis, nephropathy, pancreatitis, severe liver injury with hepatocellular necrosis or acute hepatic failure.

PANCREATIN (*Creon, Ku-Zyme, ✣Entozyme*) ▸gut ♀C ▶? $$$

ADULT — Enzyme replacement (initial dose): 8000 to 24,000 units lipase (1 to 2 caps/tabs) PO with meals and snacks.

PEDS — Enzyme replacement (initial dose): 2000 units lipase PO with meals for age younger than 1 yo, 4000 to 8000 units lipase PO with meals or 4000 units lipase with snacks for age 1 to 6 yo, 4000 to 12,000 units lipase PO with meals and snacks for age 7 to 12 yo.

FORMS — Tabs, Caps with varying amounts of lipase, amylase, and protease.

NOTES — Titrate dose to stool fat content. Products are not interchangeable. Avoid concomitant calcium carbonate and magnesium hydroxide because these may affect the enteric coating. Do not crush/chew microspheres or tabs. Possible association of colonic strictures and high doses of lipase (greater than 16,000 units/kg/meal) in pediatric patients.

MOA — Replaces endogenous enzymes.

ADVERSE EFFECTS — Frequent: None.

PANCRELIPASE (*Creon, Pancreaze, Pancrecarb, Cotazym, Ku-Zyme HP, Ultresa, Viokace, Zenpep*) ▸gut ♀C ▶? $$$

ADULT — Enzyme replacement (initial dose): 500 lipase units/kg per meal, max 2500 lipase units/kg per meal.

PEDS — Enzyme replacement (initial dose, varies by wt): Infants (up to 12 mo): 2000 to 4000 lipase units per 120 mL of formula or per breastfeeding. 12 mo or older to younger than 4 yo: 1000 lipase units/kg, max 2500 lipase units/kg per meal. 4 yo or older: 500 lipase units/kg per meal, max 2500. lipase units/kg per meal.

FORMS — Tabs, Caps, Powder with varying amounts of lipase, amylase, and protease.

NOTES — Titrate dose to stool fat content. Products are not interchangeable. Avoid concomitant calcium carbonate and magnesium hydroxide because these may affect the enteric coating. Do not crush/chew. Possible association of colonic strictures and high doses of lipase (greater than 16,000 units/kg/meal) in pediatric patients.

MOA — Replaces endogenous enzymes.

ADVERSE EFFECTS — Frequent: None.

PINAVERIUM (*Dicetel*) ▶? ♀C ▶– $$$

ADULT — Canada only. Irritable bowel syndrome: 50 mg PO three times per day, may increase to max of 100 mg three times per day.

PEDS — Not for children.

FORMS — Trade only: Tabs 50, 100 mg.

NOTES — Take with a full glass of water during meal or snack.

MOA — Calcium antagonist; blocks voltage-dependent calcium channels at the smooth muscle cell level; highly selective for intestinal smooth muscle.

ADVERSE EFFECTS — Frequent: Epigastric pain, nausea, constipation.

QSYMIA (**phentermine + topiramate**) ▸KL ♀X ▶– ©IV $$$$$

WARNING — Contraindicated in pregnancy, glaucoma, hyperthyroidism, and during 14 days after MAO inhibitor.

ADULT — Obesity or overweight with comorbidities: 3.75 mg/23 mg PO once daily for 14 days, then increase to 7.5 mg/46 mg PO once daily. Can increase dose if 3% wt loss not achieved after 12 weeks. Max dose 15 mg/92 mg PO daily. Discontinue if 5% wt loss not achieved on max dose for 12 weeks. Taper gradually by taking a dose every other day for at least 1 week before discontinuing to avoid potential seizures.

PEDS — Not approved for use in children.

FORMS — Trade: Tabs 3.75/23, 7.5/46, 11.25/69, 15/92 mg (phentermine/topiramate).

NOTES — Do not exceed 7.5 mg/46 mg in moderate to severe renal impairment or moderate hepatic impairment. May increase heart rate. Monitor for suicidal thoughts or depression. Measure creatinine and electrolytes before and during treatment. Monitor for hypoglycemia in patients with diabetes.

MOA — See components.

ADVERSE EFFECTS — See components.

RECTIV (*nitroglycerin—rectal*) ►L ♀C ►? $$$$$

ADULT — Chronic anal fissures: Apply 1 inch intra-anally q 12 h for up to 3 weeks.

PEDS — Not approved in children younger than 18 yo.

FORMS — Trade only: Oint 0.4% 30 g.

NOTES — Use within 8 weeks of opening. Do not use with PDE5 inhibitors.

MOA — Relaxation of the internal anal sphincter muscle

ADVERSE EFFECTS — Frequent: headache, dizziness.

SECRETIN (*SecreFlo, ChiRhoStim*) ►serum ♀C ►? $$$$$

ADULT — Stimulation of pancreatic secretions, to aid in diagnosis of exocrine pancreas dysfunction: Test dose 0.2 mcg IV. If tolerated, 0.2 mcg/kg IV over 1 min. Stimulation of gastrin to aid in diagnosis of gastrinoma: Test dose 0.2 mcg IV. If tolerated, 0.4 mcg/kg IV over 1 min. Identification of ampulla of Vater and accessory papilla during ERCP: 0.2 mcg/kg IV over 1 min.

PEDS — Not approved in children.

UNAPPROVED PEDS — Has been tried in autism, but does not appear to be effective.

NOTES — Previously known as SecreFlo. Contraindicated in acute pancreatitis.

MOA — Increases volume and bicarbonate content of secreted pancreatic juices.

ADVERSE EFFECTS — Frequent: Abdominal discomfort, hypotension, diaphoresis, flushing, nausea.

TEDUGLUTIDE (*Gattex*) ► ♀B ►? $$$$$

WARNING — May accelerate neoplastic growth, may cause intestinal obstruction or fluid overload or pancreatic and biliary disease.

ADULT — Short bowel syndrome patients receiving IV TPN: 0.05 mg/kg (max 3.8 mg) SC daily.

PEDS — Not approved in children.

FORMS — Trade only: 5 mg/vial, powder for reconstitution.

MOA — glucagon-like peptide-2

ADVERSE EFFECTS — Frequent: abdominal pain, injection site reactions, nausea, headache, abdominal distension, vomiting. Severe: neoplastic growth, intestinal obstruction, biliary and pancreatic disease, fluid overload.

URSODIOL (*Actigall, URSO, URSO Forte*) ►bile ♀B ►? $$$

ADULT — Radiolucent gallstone dissolution (Actigall): 8 to 10 mg/kg/day PO divided in 2 to 3 doses. Prevention of gallstones associated with rapid wt loss (Actigall): 300 mg PO two times per day. Primary biliary cirrhosis (URSO): 13 to 15 mg/kg/day PO divided in 2 to 4 doses.

PEDS — Not approved in children.

UNAPPROVED ADULT — Cholestasis of pregnancy: 300 to 600 mg PO two times per day.

UNAPPROVED PEDS — Biliary atresia: 10 to 15 mg/kg/day PO once daily. Cystic fibrosis with liver disease: 15 to 30 mg/kg/day PO divided two times per day. TPN-induced cholestasis: 30 mg/kg/day PO divided three times per day.

FORMS — Generic/Trade: Caps 300 mg, Tabs 250, 500 mg.

NOTES — Do not use in patients with complete biliary obstruction. Gallstone dissolution requires months of therapy. Complete dissolution does not occur in all patients and 5-year recurrence up to 50%. Does not dissolve calcified cholesterol stones, radiopaque stones, or radiolucent bile pigment stones. Monitor LFTs and bilirubin. Avoid concomitant antacids, cholestyramine, colestipol, estrogen, oral contraceptives.

MOA — Decreases cholesterol content of bile and bile stones.

ADVERSE EFFECTS — Frequent: Diarrhea, constipation, nausea, vomiting, dizziness. Serious: Thrombocytopenia, hypersensitivity reactions.

HEMATOLOGY/ANTICOAGULANTS

HEMATOLOGY/ANTICOAGULANTS: Anticoagulants - Direct Thrombin Inhibitors

ARGATROBAN ▸L ♀B ▶– $$$$$

ADULT — Prevention/treatment of thrombosis in HIT: Start 2 mcg/kg/min IV infusion. Get PTT at baseline and 2 h after starting infusion. Adjust dose (up to 10 mcg/kg/min) until PTT is 1.5 to 3 times baseline (but not more than 100 sec). Percutaneous coronary intervention in those with or at risk for HIT: Bolus 350 mcg/kg IV over 3 to 5 min then 25 mcg/kg/min infusion. Target activated clotting time (ACT): 300 to 450 sec. If ACT less than 300 sec, give 150 mcg/kg bolus and increase infusion rate to 30 mcg/kg/min. If ACT more than 450 sec, reduce infusion rate to 15 mcg/kg/min. Maintain ACT 300 to 450 sec for the duration of the procedure.

PEDS — Not approved in children.

NOTES — ACCP recommends starting max of 2 mcg/kg/min with lower doses of 0.5 to 1.2 mcg/kg/min in patients with heart failure, multiorgan failure, anasarca, or postcardiac surgery. Argatroban prolongs INR with warfarin; discontinue when INR greater than 4 on combined therapy, recheck INR in 4 to 6 h and restart argatroban if INR subtherapeutic.

MOA — Direct thrombin inhibitor, synthetic derivative of L-arginine.

ADVERSE EFFECTS — Serious: Major bleeding, hypotension. Frequent: Fever, diarrhea.

BIVALIRUDIN (*Angiomax*) ▸proteolysis/K ♀B ▶? $$$$$

ADULT — Anticoagulation in patients without HIT or without HIT and thrombosis syndrome, undergoing PCI/PTCA: 0.75 mg/kg IV bolus, then 1.75 mg/kg/h IV infusion for duration of procedure (with provisional Gp IIb/IIIa inhibition for patients with conditions listed in REPLACE-2 clinical trial; see prescribing information for details). Check activated clotting time 5 minutes after bolus dose given; give additional bolus of 0.3 mg/kg needed. May continue infusion up to 4 h post-procedure (should be considered post-STEMI to reduce risk of stent thrombosis), then may additionally infuse 0.2 mg/kg/h for up to 20 h more. Anticoagulation in patients with HIT or with HIT and thrombosis syndrome undergoing PCI: 0.75 mg/kg IV bolus, then 1.75 mg/kg/h IV infusion for duration of procedure and optionally up to 4 h post-procedure. May additionally infuse 0.2 mg/kg/h for up to 20 h more. For CrCl <30 mL/min, reduce infusion dose to 1 mg/kg/h after bolus. For patients on dialysis, reduce infusion dose to 0.25 mg/kg/h after bolus. Use with aspirin 300 to 325 mg PO daily.

PEDS — Not approved in children.

UNAPPROVED ADULT — NSTEMI, with early invasive strategy: (with or without Gp IIb/IIIa inhibition): 0.1 mg/kg bolus, then 0.25 mg/kg/h continued until diagnostic procedure or PCI. Use with dual antiplatelet therapy.

NOTES — Interferes with INR; INR may not be useful for determining dose of warfarin while on bivalirudin. Monitor activated clotting time. Former trade name Hirulog.

MOA — Direct thrombin inhibitor (reversible).

ADVERSE EFFECTS — Serious: Major bleeding, acute stent thrombosis in STEMI patients undergoing PCI. Frequent: Back pain, nausea.

DABIGATRAN (*Pradaxa*) ▸K ♀C ▶? $$$$$

WARNING — Increased risk of thrombotic event, including stroke, when discontinued. Consider coverage with alternative anticoagulant unless discontinuing due to life-threatening bleeding. Risk of spinal/epidural hematoma if spinal puncture or neuraxial anesthesia during treatment; monitor for neurologic impairment.

ADULT — Stroke prevention in atrial fibrillation: CrCl greater than 30 mL/min with no interacting medications: 150 mg PO two times per day; CrCL between 30 and 50 mL/min with p-glycoprotein inhibitors (dronedarone and ketoconazole) or CrCL between 15 and 30 mL/min without interacting medications: 75 mg PO two times per day; CrCl less than 15 mL/min or CrCl between 15 and 30 mL/min with p-glycoprotein inhibitor: contraindicated. Per ACCP CHEST guidelines, not recommended if CrCl is less than 30 mL/min. Treatment of DVT/PE: CrCl greater than 30 mL/min: 150 mg PO two times per day after 5 to 10 days of parenteral anticoagulation. Reduction in risk of DVT/PE: CrCl greater than 30 mL/min:150 mg PO two times per day after previous treatment. VTE prevention in hip replacement surgery: CrCl greater than 30 mL/min: 110 mg orally one dose given 1 to 4 h after surgery or start 220 mg once if started on postop day 1, then 220 mg daily for 28 to 35 days. CrCl <50 mL/min with p-glycoprotein inhibitor: contraindicated.

PEDS — Not approved in children.

UNAPPROVED ADULT — VTE prevention in knee replacement: Start 110 mg for one dose given 1 to 4 h after surgery or start 220 mg once if started on postop day 1, then 220 mg daily for 10 days.

FORMS — Trade only: Caps 75, 110, 150 mg.

NOTES — Do not break, open, or chew capsules; administer with a full glass of water. Must be stored in original container and used within 4 months or discarded; protect from moisture. Check renal function at baseline and periodically to dose adjust appropriately. May cause gastritis. Avoid use with P-glycoprotein inducers, including rifampin. Potent P-glycoprotein inhibitors may increase exposure and risk of bleeding, particularly if renal dysfunction; see dose adjustment in adult FDA dosing for concomitant use with dronedarone and ketoconazole. Discontinue 1 to 2 days (if CrCl is ≥50 mL/min) or 3 to 5 days (if CrCl <50 mL/min) before invasive

(cont.)

DABIGATRAN (*cont.*)

procedures. When transitioning from warfarin, stop warfarin and start dabigatran when INR is less than 2. When transitioning from heparin/LMWH, timing of initiation depends on renal function; see prescribing information. Serious, sometimes fatal, bleeding has been reported. Contraindicated for use in prosthetic heart valves. Removed by hemodialysis, but experience limited for use during bleeding. Idarucizumab available for reversal in emergency surgery or life-threatning/uncontrolled bleeding.

MOA — Direct thrombin inhibitor

ADVERSE EFFECTS — Serious: bleeding, hypersensitivity (anaphylaxis, angioedema), thrombotic event (stroke), thrombocytopenia, esophageal ulcers. Frequent: dyspepsia, gastritis, hypersensitivity (urticaria, rash, and pruritus).

DESIRUDIN (*Iprivask*) ▶K ♀C ▶? $$$$$

WARNING — High risk of spinal/epidural hematoma if spinal puncture or neuraxial anesthesia before/during treatment. Risk increased by drugs that affect hemostasis including NSAIDs, antiplatelets, and other anticoagulants. Risk also increased by use of indwelling catheters, history of trauma or repeated epidural punctures, spinal deformity, or spinal surgery.

ADULT — DVT prophylaxis (hip replacement surgery): 15 mg SC q 12 h. (If CrCl is 31 to 60 mL/min, give 5 mg SC q 12 h; if CrCl <31 mL/min, give 1.7 mg SC q 12 h.)

PEDS — Not approved in children.

NOTES — ACCP guidelines recommend against use if CrCl <30 mL/min and against repeated use due to risk of anaphylaxis. Severe anaphylactic reactions resulting in death have been reported upon initial or re-exposure.

MOA — Direct thrombin inhibitor.

ADVERSE EFFECTS — Serious: Anaphylaxis, major hemorrhage (including fatal, intracranial, intraspinal, intraocular), hypotension. Frequent: Injection site reactions, hematoma, minor bleeding, nausea.

HEMATOLOGY/ANTICOAGULANTS: Anticoagulants—Factor Xa Inhibitors

NOTE: See Cardiovascular section for antiplatelet drugs and thrombolytics. Contraindicated in active major bleeding. High risk of spinal/epidural hematoma if spinal puncture or neuraxial anesthesia before/during treatment (see 2010;35:64-101.); optimal timing between administration and neuraxial procedures unknown. Risk of bleeding increased by oral anticoagulants, aspirin, dipyridamole, dextran, glycoprotein IIb/IIIA inhibitors, NSAIDs (including ketorolac), clopidogrel, and thrombolytics. Monitor platelets, Hb, stool for occult blood.

APIXABAN (*Eliquis*) ▶LK ♀B ▶? $$$$$

WARNING — Discontinuation increases risk of thrombotic events, including stroke. If discontinued for a reason other than bleeding, strongly consider coverage with alternative anticoagulant during periods of interruption.

ADULT — Nonvalvular atrial fibrillation: 5 mg PO two times per day. If at least two of the following characteristics: Age 80 yo or older, wt 60 kg or less, serum creatinine 1.5 mg/dL or greater, then decrease dose to 2.5 mg PO two times daily. In ESRD on hemodialysis: 5 mg PO two times per day; if at least one of the following characteristics: Age 80 yo or older, wt 60 kg or less, then decrease dose to 2.5 mg PO two times daily. DVT prophylaxis in hip or knee replacement: 2.5 mg PO two times per day. Treatment of DVT/PE: 10 mg PO two times daily for 7 days, then 5 mg PO two times daily. Reduction in risk of recurrence of DVT/PE: 2.5 mg PO two times daily after initial therapy for treatment (minimum 6 months).

PEDS — Not approved in children.

FORMS — Trade only: Tabs 2.5, 5 mg.

NOTES — For atrial fibrillation, when transitioning from warfarin, start apixaban when INR below 2.0. When transitioning from apixaban to warfarin, note that apixaban impacts INR and the effect is highly variable; labeling recommends discontinuing apixaban and starting a parenteral anticoagulant with warfarin at the time the next apixaban dose is due. When transitioning from apixaban to anticoagulants other than warfarin, labeling recommends discontinuing apixaban and starting the new anticoagulant at the time the next apixaban dose is due. Avoid concomitant use with strong inducers of CYP3A4 and P-glycoprotein or strong dual inhibitors of CYP3A4 and P-glycoprotein.

MOA — Direct Factor Xa inhibitor

ADVERSE EFFECTS — Serious: Major bleeding (GI, intracranial, intraocular, fatal). Common: minor bleeding (bruising, nosebleeds), nausea, anemia.

EDOXABAN (*Savaysa*) ▶K ♀C ▶? $$$$$

WARNING — Do not use if CrCl greater than 95 mL/min; reduced efficacy. Discontinuation increases risk of thrombotic events, including stroke. If discontinued for a reason other than bleeding, strongly consider coverage with alternative anticoagulant during periods of interruption.

ADULT — Nonvalvular atrial fibrillation: CrCl greater than 50 up to and including 95 mL/min: 60 mg PO daily. CrCl 15 to 50 mL/min: 30 mg PO daily. Treatment of DVT/PE: 60 mg PO daily after 5 to 10 days of parenteral anticoagulation. CrCl 15 to 50 mL/min or body weight less than or equal to 60 kg or certain P-glycoprotein inhibitors: 30 mg PO daily after 5 to 10 days of parenteral anticoagulation.

PEDS — Not approved in children.

FORMS — Trade only: 15, 30, 60 mg tabs.

NOTES — Check renal function at baseline and periodically to dose adjust appropriately.

(cont.)

EDOXABAN (*cont.*)

Discontinue at least 24 h before invasive procedures. When transitioning from warfarin, stop warfarin and start edoxaban when INR is less than 2.5. When transitioning from oral anticoagulants other than warfarin or LMWH, start edoxaban when next dose of this anticoagulant is due. When transitioning from heparin, start 4 h after stopping heparin. Serious, sometimes fatal, bleeding has been reported. Not recommended for use in mechanical heart valves or moderate to severe mitral stenosis.

MOA — Direct Factor Xa inhibitor

ADVERSE EFFECTS — Serious: Major bleeding (GI, intracranial, intraocular, fatal), anemia, abnormal LFTs. Common: minor bleeding (bruising, nosebleeds), nausea, rash.

FONDAPARINUX (*Arixtra*) ▶K ♀B ▶? $$$$$

ADULT — DVT prophylaxis, hip/knee replacement or hip fracture surgery, abdominal surgery: 2.5 mg SC daily starting 6 to 8 h postop (giving earlier increases risk of bleeding). Usual duration is 5 to 9 days; extend prophylaxis up to 24 additional days (max 32 days) in hip fracture surgery. DVT/PE treatment based on wt: Wt less than 50 kg: 5 mg SC daily; wt between 50 and 100 kg: 7.5 mg SC daily; wt greater than 100 kg: 10 mg SC daily for at least 5 days and therapeutic oral anticoagulation.

PEDS — Not approved in children. Because risk for bleeding is increased if wt less than 50 kg, bleeding may be a particular concern in pediatrics.

UNAPPROVED ADULT — Unstable angina or non-ST-elevation MI: 2.5 mg SC daily until hospital discharge or for up to 8 days. ST-elevation MI and creatinine less than 3 mg/dL: 2.5 mg IV loading dose, then 2.5 mg SC daily until hospital discharge or for up to 8 days. Heparin-induced thrombocytopenia with thrombosis: 5 mg SC daily if less than 50 kg; 7.5 mg SC daily if 50 to 100 kg; 10 mg SC daily if greater than 100 kg.

FORMS — Generic/Trade: Prefilled syringes 2.5 mg/0.5 mL, 5 mg/0.4 mL, 7.5 mg/0.6 mL, 10 mg/0.8 mL.

NOTES — May cause thrombocytopenia; however, lacks in vitro cross-reactivity with heparin-induced thrombocytopenia antibodies. Risk of major bleeding increased in elderly. Contraindicated if CrCl <30 mL/min due to increased bleeding risk. Caution advised if CrCl 30 to 50 mL/min. Monitor renal function in all patients; discontinue if severely impaired or labile. In DVT prophylaxis, contraindicated if body wt less than 50 kg. Protamine ineffective for reversing anticoagulant effect. Factor VIIa partially reverses anticoagulant effect in small studies. Risk of catheter thrombosis in PCI; use in conjunction with anticoagulant with anti-IIa activity. Store at room temperature.

MOA — Synthetic pentasaccharide sequence of heparin that binds with antithrombin III to inactivate factor Xa.

ADVERSE EFFECTS — Serious: Major bleeding (especially in elderly, low body weight, or renal dysfunction), thrombocytopenia (rare), spinal/epidural hematomas associated with neuraxial anesthesia/spinal punctures before/during treatment, anaphylaxis. Frequent: None.

RIVAROXABAN (*Xarelto*) ▶K – ♀C ▶? $$$$$

WARNING — Premature discontinuation without alternative anticoagulation increases risk of thrombotic events. If discontinued for a reason other than bleeding, strongly consider coverage with alternative anticoagulant during periods of interruption. Not studied for anticoagulation for prosthetic heart valves. Do not use for acute PE if hemodynamically unstable or planned thrombolysis or pulmonary embolectomy. Spinal or epidural hematomas reported; consider risk/benefit if neuraxial intervention required. Avoid use with combined P-glycoprotein and strong CYP3A4 inhibitors/inducers.

ADULT — DVT prophylaxis in knee or hip replacement: 10 mg PO daily, if CrCl <30 mL/min, avoid use. Start at least 6 to 10 h post-surgery after hemostasis. Continue for 35 days in hip replacement and 12 days in knee replacement. Nonvalvular atrial fibrillation: 20 mg PO daily with the evening meal if CrCl >50 mL/min; reduce dose to 15 mg PO daily with the evening meal if CrCl 15 to 50 mL/min, avoid use if CrCl <15 mL/min. DVT/PE treatment and to reduce risk of DVT/PE recurrence: 15 mg PO two times daily with food for 21 days, then 20 mg PO daily with food. If CrCl 30 to 49 mL/min: 15 mg PO twice daily with food for 3 weeks, then 15 mg PO daily with food.

FORMS — Trade only: Tabs 10, 15, 20 mg.

NOTES — Periodically assess renal function as clinically necessary and modify therapy accordingly. For DVT prophylaxis, DVT/PE treatment, and to reduce the risk of recurrence of DVT/PE, avoid if CrCl <30 mL/min. For DVT prophylaxis, caution if CrCl 30 to 50 mL/min due to increased rivaroxaban exposure. For atrial fibrillation, when transitioning from warfarin, start rivaroxaban when INR below 3.0. Rivaroxaban affects INR, so initial measurements of INR during transition may be unreliable. When transitioning from LMWH or other oral anticoagulant, start rivaroxaban 0 to 2 h before next scheduled evening administration of the anticoagulant. When transitioning from heparin, start rivaroxaban when heparin drip infusion is discontinued.

MOA — Direct Factor Xa inhibitor

ADVERSE EFFECTS — Serious: major bleeding, thrombocytopenia, agranulocytosis, jaundice, cholestasis, hepatitis, hypersensitivity, anaphylactic shock, Stevens-Johnson syndrome, syncope. Frequent: wound secretion, pain in extremity, muscle spasm, pruritis, blister, transaminase elevations.

HEMATOLOGY/ANTICOAGULANTS: Anticoagulants—Low Molecular Weight Heparins (LWMH)

NOTE: Contraindicated in active major bleeding. High risk of spinal/epidural hematoma if spinal puncture or neuraxial anesthesia before/during treatment; optimal timing between LMWH administration and neuraxial procedures is unknown, see product information for guidance. Risk of bleeding increased by indwelling epidural catheters, traumatic or repeated epidural/spinal punctures, spinal deformity/surgery, and drugs affecting hemostasis including anticoagulants, platelet inhibitors, and NSAIDs. Monitor platelets, Hb, stool for occult blood. Use caution and consider monitoring anti-Xa levels if CrCl less than 30 mL/min, pregnancy, morbidly obese, underweight, or abnormal coagulation/bleeding. Contraindicated in patients with heparin or pork allergy, history of heparin-induced thrombocytopenia. Drug effect can be partially reversed with protamine. For DVT/PE prevention post-orthopedic surgery: Longer prophylaxis may be warranted based on individual thromboembolic risk. ACCP recommendations suggest that patients with total hip or knee replacement or hip fracture surgery receive prophylaxis for at least 10 days; consider extended prophylaxis (28 to 35 days) in hip replacement or hip fracture surgery.

DALTEPARIN (*Fragmin*) ▶KL ♀B ▶+ $$$$$
ADULT — DVT prophylaxis, acute medical illness with restricted mobility: 5000 units SC daily for 12 to 14 days. DVT prophylaxis, abdominal surgery: 2500 units SC 1 to 2 h preop and daily postop for 5 to 10 days. DVT prophylaxis, abdominal surgery in patients with malignancy: 5000 units SC evening before surgery and daily postop for 5 to 10 days. Alternatively, 2500 units SC 1 to 2 h preop and 12 h later, then 5000 units SC daily for 5 to 10 days. DVT prophylaxis, hip replacement: Give SC for up to 14 days. Preop start (day of surgery): 2500 units 2 h preop and 4 to 8 h postop, then 5000 units daily starting at least 6 h after 2nd dose. Preop start (evening before surgery): 5000 units SC given evening before surgery then 5000 units daily starting at least 4 to 8 h postop (approximately 24 h between doses). Postop start regimen: 2500 units 4 to 8 h postop, then 5000 units daily starting at least 6 h after 1st dose. Treatment of DVT/PE in cancer: 200 units/kg SC daily for 1 month, then 150 units/kg SC daily for 5 months. Max 18,000 units/day, round to nearest commercially available syringe dose (if CrCl <30 mL/min then target therapeutic anti-Xa level of 0.5 to 1.5 units/mL; recheck 4 to 6 h after dose following at least 3 to 4 doses). Unstable angina or non-Q-wave MI: 120 units/kg up to 10,000 units SC q 12 h with aspirin (75 to 165 mg/day PO) until clinically stable.
PEDS — Not approved in children.
UNAPPROVED ADULT — Therapeutic anticoagulation: 200 units/kg SC daily or 100 to 120 units/kg SC two times per day. Venous thromboembolism in pregnancy. Prevention: 5000 units SC daily. Treatment: 100 units/kg SC q 12 h or 200 units/kg SC daily. To avoid unwanted anticoagulation during delivery, stop LMWH 24 h before elective induction of labor.
FORMS — Trade only: Single-dose syringes 2500, 5000 units/0.2 mL, 7500 units/0.3 mL, 10,000 units/1 mL, 12,500 units/0.5 mL, 15,000 units/0.6 mL, 18,000 units/0.72 mL; Multidose vial 10,000 units/mL, 9.5 mL and 25,000 units/mL, 3.8 mL.
MOA — Low molecular weight heparin, antithrombin activator that preferentially inhibits factor Xa and inhibits factor IIa.
ADVERSE EFFECTS — Serious: Major bleeding, HIT (rare), spinal/epidural hematomas associated with neuraxial anesthesia/spinal punctures before/

during treatment. Frequent: Asymptomatic increase in hepatic transaminases, injection site pain.

ENOXAPARIN (*Lovenox*) ▶KL ♀B ▶+ $$$$$
ADULT — See table.
PEDS — Not approved in children.
UNAPPROVED ADULT — DVT prophylaxis after major trauma: 30 mg SC q 12 h starting 12 to 36 h postinjury if hemostasis achieved. DVT prophylaxis in acute spinal cord injury: 30 mg SC q 12 h. Venous thromboembolism in pregnancy: Prevention: 40 mg SC daily. Treatment: 1 mg/kg SC q 12 h. To avoid unwanted anticoagulation during delivery, stop LMWH 24 h before elective induction of labor.
UNAPPROVED PEDS — Therapeutic anticoagulation: Age younger than 2 mo: 1.5 mg/kg/dose SC q 12 h titrated to anti-Xa level of 0.5 to 1 units/mL. Age 2 mo or older: 1 mg/kg/dose SC q 12 h titrated to anti-Xa level of 0.5 to 1 units/mL. DVT prophylaxis: Age younger than 2 mo: 0.75 mg/kg/dose q 12 h. Age 2 mo or older: 0.5 mg/kg/dose q 12 h.
FORMS — Generic/Trade: Syringes 30, 40 mg; graduated syringes 60, 80, 100, 120, 150 mg. Concentration is 100 mg/mL except for 120, 150 mg, which are 150 mg/mL. All syringes also available preservative free. Available as Multidose vial 300 mg.
NOTES — In PCI, if last enoxaparin administration was more than 8 h before balloon inflation, give 0.3 mg/kg IV bolus. Use caution in mechanical heart valves, especially in pregnancy; reports of valve thrombosis (maternal and fetal deaths reported). Congenital anomalies linked to enoxaparin use during pregnancy; causality unclear. Multidose formulation contains benzyl alcohol, which can cause hypersensitivity and cross placenta in pregnancy.
MOA — Low molecular weight heparin, antithrombin activator that preferentially inhibits factor Xa and inhibits factor IIa.
ADVERSE EFFECTS — Serious: Major bleeding, thrombocytopenia (rare), hemorrhagic anemia, eosinophilia, hepatocellular/cholestatic liver injury, osteoporosis with long-term therapy, spinal/epidural hematomas associated with neuraxial anesthesia/spinal punctures before/during treatment. Reports of valve thrombosis when used for thromboprophylaxis in patients with prosthetic heart valves, especially pregnant women (maternal and fetal deaths reported). Frequent: Asymptomatic increase in hepatic transaminases, injection site reactions, peripheral edema.

ENOXAPARIN ADULT DOSING

Indication	Dose	Dosing in Renal Impairment (CrCl <30 mL/min)*
DVT prophylaxis		
Abdominal surgery	40 mg SC once daily	30 mg SC once daily
Knee replacement	30 mg SC q 12 h	30 mg SC once daily
Hip replacement	30 mg SC q 12 h or 40 mg SC once daily	30 mg SC once daily
Medical patients	40 mg SC once daily	30 mg SC once daily
Acute DVT		
Inpatient treatment with or without PE	1 mg/kg SC q 12 h or 1.5 mg/kg SC once daily	1 mg/kg SC once daily
Outpatient treatment without PE	1 mg/kg SC q 12 h	1 mg/kg SC once daily
Acute coronary syndrome		
Unstable angina and non-Q-wave MI with aspirin	1 mg/kg SC q 12 h with aspirin	1 mg/kg SC once daily
Acute STEMI in patients younger than 75 yo with aspirin†	30 mg IV bolus with 1 mg/kg SC dose, then 1 mg/kg SC q 12 h (max 100 mg/dose for the 1st two doses)	30 mg IV bolus with 1 mg/kg SC dose, then 1 mg/kg SC once daily
Acute STEMI in patients 75 yo or older with aspirin†	No IV bolus, 0.75 mg/kg SC q 12 h (max 75 mg/dose for the 1st two doses)	No IV bolus, 1 mg/kg SC once daily

DVT = Deep vein thrombosis, PE = pulmonary embolism.

*Not FDA-approved in dialysis.

†If used with thrombolytics, SC dose should be started between 15 min before and 30 min after thrombolytic dose.

HEMATOLOGY/ANTICOAGULANTS: Anticoagulants—Other

HEPARIN ▸Reticuloendothelial system ♀C but + ▶+ $$
ADULT — Venous thrombosis/pulmonary embolus treatment: Load 80 units/kg IV, then initiate infusion at 18 units/kg/h. Adjust based on coagulation testing (PTT)—see Table. DVT prophylaxis: 5000 units SC q 8 to 12 h. Prevention of thromboembolism in pregnancy: 5000 to 10,000 units SC q 12 h. Treatment of thromboembolism in pregnancy: 80 units/kg IV load, then infuse 18 units/kg/h with dose titrated to achieve full anticoagulation for at least 5 days. Then continue via SC route with at least 10,000 units SC q 8 to 12 h adjusted to achieve PTT of 1.5 to 2.5 times control. To avoid unwanted anticoagulation during delivery, stop SC heparin 24 h before elective induction of labor.
PEDS — Venous thrombosis/pulmonary embolus treatment: Load 50 units/kg IV, then 25 units/kg/h infusion.
UNAPPROVED ADULT — Venous thrombosis/pulmonary embolus treatment (unmonitored): Load 333 units/kg SC, then 250 units/kg SC q 12 h based on max 100 kg wt. Venous thrombosis/pulmonary embolus treatment (monitored): Initial dose 17,500 units or 250 units/kg SC twice daily with dose adjustment to achieve and maintain an APTT prolongation that corresponds to plasma heparin levels of 0.3 to 0.7 units/mL anti-Xa activity when measured 6 h after injection. Acute coronary syndromes with or without PCI: 60 units/kg IV, then 12 units/kg/h infusion, adjust according to aPTT or antiXa. See Table.
UNAPPROVED PEDS — Venous thrombosis/pulmonary embolus treatment: Load 75 units/kg IV over 10 min, then 28 units/kg/h if age younger than 1 yo, 20 units/kg/h if age 1 yo or older.
FORMS — Generic only: 1000, 5000, 10,000, 20,000 units/mL in various vial and syringe sizes.
NOTES — Beware of HIT, which may present as a serious thrombotic event. When HIT suspected/diagnosed, discontinue all heparin sources and use alternative

(cont.)

HEPARIN (cont.)

anticoagulant. HIT can occur up to several weeks after heparin discontinued. Monitor for elevated LFTs, hyperkalemia/hypoaldosteronism. Osteoporosis with long-term use. Bleeding risk increased by high dose; concomitant thrombolytic or platelet GPIIb/IIIa receptor inhibitor; recent surgery, trauma, or invasive procedure; concomitant hemostatic defect. Monitor platelets, Hb, stool for occult blood. Anti-Xa is an alternative to PTT for monitoring. Drug effect can be reversed with protamine. Do not administer heparin preserved with benzyl alcohol to neonates, infants, or pregnant or lactating women. Do not use heparin sodium injection product as a "catheter lock flush"; fatal medication errors have occurred.

MOA — Antithrombin activator that inhibits factors Xa and IIa.

ADVERSE EFFECTS — Serious: Major bleeding, HIT, elevated LFTs, hyperkalemia/hypoaldosteronism, osteoporosis (with long-term use). Frequent: None.

WARFARIN (**Coumadin, Jantoven**) ▶L ♀X, (D for mechanical heart valve replacement) ▶+ $

HEPARIN DOSING FOR ACUTE CORONARY SYNDROME (ACS)

ST elevation myocardial infarction (STEMI)	Adjunct to thrombolytics: For use with alteplase, reteplase, or tenecteplase: Bolus 60 units/kg IV load (max 4000 units), then initial infusion 12 units/kg/h (max 1000 units/h) adjusted to achieve target PTT 1.5 to 2 times control.
Unstable angina/non-ST elevation myocardial infarction (UA/NSTEMI)	Initial treatment: Bolus 60 units/kg IV load (max 4000 units), then initiate infusion at 12 to 15 units/kg/h (max 1000 units) and adjusted to achieve target PTT 1.5 to 2.5 times control.
Percutaneous coronary intervention (PCI)	With prior anticoagulant therapy but *without* concurrent GPIIb/IIIa inhibitor planned: Additional heparin as needed (2000 to 5000 units) to achieve target ACT 250–300 seconds for HemoTec or 300–350 seconds for Hemochron.
	With prior anticoagulant therapy but *with* planned concurrent GPIIb/IIIa inhibitor: Additional heparin as needed (2000 to 5000 units) to achieve target 200–250 seconds.
	Without prior anticoagulant therapy but *without* concurrent GPIIb/IIIa inhibitor planned: Bolus 70–100 units/kg with target ACT 250–300 seconds for HemoTec or 300–350 seconds for Hemochron.
	Without prior anticoagulant therapy but *with* planned concurrent GPIIb/IIIa inhibitor: Bolus 50–70 units/kg with target ACT 200–250 seconds.

References: *J Am Coll Cardiol* 2011;57:1946. *Circulation* 2011;124:e608. *Circulation* 2004;110:e82–292. *J Am Coll Cardiol* 2009;54:2235.

WEIGHT-BASED HEPARIN DOSING FOR DVT/PE*

Initial dose	80 units/kg IV bolus, then 18 units/kg/h; check PTT in 6 h
PTT less than 35 sec (less than 1.2 × control)	80 units/kg IV bolus, then increase infusion rate by 4 units/kg/h
PTT 35–45 sec (1.2–1.5 × control)	40 units/kg IV bolus, then increase infusion by 2 units/kg/h
PTT 46–70 sec (1.5–2.3 × control)	No change
PTT 71–90 sec (2.3–3 × control)	Decrease infusion rate by 2 units/kg/h
PTT greater than 90 sec (greater than 3 × control)	Hold infusion for 1 h, then decrease infusion rate by 3 units/kg/h

*PTT = Activated partial thromboplastin time. Reagent-specific target PTT may differ; use institutional nomogram when available. Consider establishing a max bolus dose/max initial infusion rate or use an adjusted body wt in obesity. Monitor PTT 6 h after heparin initiation and 6 h after each dosage adjustment. When PTT is stable within therapeutic range, monitor every morning. Therapeutic PTT range corresponds to anti-factor Xa activity of 0.3–0.7 units/mL. Check platelets between days 3 and 5. Can begin warfarin on 1 day of heparin; continue heparin for at least 4 to 5 days of combined therapy.
Adapted from *Ann Intern Med* 1993;119;874. *Chest* 2012:141:e28S, e154S. *Circulation* 2001;103:2994.

(cont.)

WARFARIN—SELECTED DRUG INTERACTIONS

Assume possible interactions with any medication. When starting/stopping a chronic medication, the INR should be checked at least weekly for 2 to 3 weeks and dose adjusted accordingly. When starting an interacting anti-infective agent, the National Quality Forum recommends checking the INR within 3 to 7 days. Similarly, monitor if significant change in diet (including supplements) or illness resulting in decreased oral intake. For further information regarding mechanism or management, refer to the *Tarascon Pocket Pharmacopoeia* drug interactions database (mobile or Web edition).

Increased anticoagulant effect of warfarin / Increased risk of bleeding

Monitor INR when agents below started, stopped, or dosage changed. Consider alternative agent. Acetaminophen ≥ 2 g/day for ≥ 3 to 4 days, allopurinol, amiodarone*, anabolic steroids, ASA[¶], cefixime, cefoperazone, cefotetan, celecoxib, chloramphenicol, cimetidine[†], corticosteroids, danazol, danshen, disulfiram, dong quai, erlotinib, etravirine, fibrates, fish oil, fluconazole, fluoroquinolones, fluorouracil, fluvoxamine, fosphenytoin (acute), garlic supplements, gemcitabine, gemfibrozil, glucosamine-chondroitin, ginkgo, ifosfamide, imatinib, isoniazid, itraconazole, ketoconazole, leflunomide, levothyroxine[#], macrolides[‡], metronidazole, miconazole (intravaginal), neomycin (PO for >1 to 2 days), NSAIDs[¶], olsalazine, omeprazole, paroxetine, penicillin (high-dose IV), pentoxifylline, phenytoin (acute), propafenone, quinidine, quinine, statins[§], sulfonamides, tamoxifen, testosterones tetracyclines, tramadol, tigecycline, tipranavir, TCAs, valproate, voriconazole, vorinostat, vitamin A (high-dose), vitamin E, zafirlukast, zileuton

Decreased anticoagulant effect of warfarin / Increased risk of thrombosis

Monitor INR when agents below started, stopped, or dosage changed. Consider alternative agent. Aprepitant, cefotetan, azathioprine, barbiturates, bosentan, carbamazepine, coenzyme Q-10, dicloxacillin, fosphenytoin (chronic), ginseng (American), griseofulvin, mercaptopurine, mesalamine, methimazole[#], mitotane, nafcillin, oral contraceptives**, phenytoin (chronic), primidone, propylthiouracil[#], raloxifene, ribavirin, rifabutin, rifampin, rifapentine, ritonavir, St. John's wort, vitamin C (high-dose). *Use alternative to agents below. Or give at different times of day and monitor INR when agent started, stopped, or dose/dosing schedule changed.* Cholestyramine, colestipol[††], sucralfate

*Interaction may be delayed; monitor INR for several weeks after starting and several months after stopping amiodarone. May need to decrease warfarin dose by 33 to 50%.
[†]Famotidine, nizatidine or ranitidine, are alternatives.
[‡]Azithromycin appears to have lower risk of interaction than clarithromycin or erythromycin.
[§]Pravastatin appears to have lower risk of interaction.
[#]Hyperthyroidism/thyroid replacement increases metabolism of clotting factors, increasing response to warfarin therapy and increased bleed risk (typically requires lowering warfarin dose). Reversal of hyperthyroidism (as with methimazole, propylthiouracil) will decrease metabolism of clotting factors and decrease response to warfarin (typically requires increasing warfarin dose).
[¶]Does not necessarily increase INR, but increases bleeding risk. Check INR frequently and monitor for GI bleeding.
**Does not necessarily decrease INR, but may induce hypercoagulability.
[††]Likely lower risk than cholestyramine
Adapted from: Coumadin product information; *Am Fam Phys* 1999; 59:635; *Chest* 2004;126:204S;
Hansten and Horn's Drug Interactions Analysis and Management; Ann Intern Med 2004;141:23; *Arch Intern Med* 2005;165:1095. *Tarascon Pocket Pharmacopoeia* drug interactions database (Mobile or Web edition). National Quality Forum http://www.qualityforum.org.

THERAPEUTIC GOALS FOR ANTICOAGULATION WITH WARFARIN

INR Range*	Indication
2.0–3.0	Atrial fibrillation, deep venous thrombosis, pulmonary embolism, bioprosthetic heart valve (mitral position), mechanical prosthetic heart valve (aortic position)
2.5–3.5	Mechanical prosthetic heart valve (mitral position)

*Aim for an INR in the middle of the INR range (eg, 2.5 for range of 2 to 3 and 3.0 for range of 2.5 to 3.5).
Adapted from: *Chest* 2012;141:e422S, e425S, e533S, e578S; see these guidelines for additional
information and other indications.

(cont.)

WARFARIN (*cont.*)

WARNING — Major or fatal bleeding possible. Higher risk during initiation and when INR elevated. Additional risk factors include: High intensity of anticoagulation (INR greater than 4.0), age 65 yo or older, highly variable INRs, history of GI bleed, hypertension, cerebrovascular disease, heart disease, anemia, malignancy, trauma, renal insufficiency, and long duration of therapy. Regular monitoring of INR needed; monitor those at higher risk more frequently. Educate patients about signs and symptoms of bleeding, measures to reduce risk, and how to manage/seek treatment if bleeding occurs. Many important drug interactions that increase/decrease INR, see table.

ADULT — Oral anticoagulation for prophylaxis/treatment of DVT/PE, thromboembolic complications associated with A-fib, mechanical and bioprosthetic heart valves: Individualize dosing. Start 2 to 5 mg PO daily for 1 to 2 days, then adjust dose to maintain therapeutic PT/INR. Consider using an initial dose of less than 5 mg/day if elderly, malnourished, liver disease, or high bleeding risk. For healthy outpatients, 2012 ACCP CHEST guidelines recommend starting at 10 mg PO daily for 2 days, then adjust dose to maintain therapeutic

INR. See product information if CYP2C9 or VKOR1C genotypes are known. Target INR of 2 to 3 for most indications, 2.5 to 3.5 for mechanical mitral heart valve. See table for specific target INR.

PEDS — Not approved in children.

FORMS — Generic/Trade: Tabs 1, 2, 2.5, 3, 4, 5, 6, 7.5, 10 mg.

NOTES — Clinical factors that may affect maintenance dose needed to achieve target PT/INR include age, race, wt, sex, medications, and comorbidities. Many important drug interactions that increase/decrease INR, see table for significant drug interactions. Warfarin onset of action is within 24 h, peak effect delayed by 3 to 4 days. Most patients can begin warfarin at the same time as injectable (heparin/LMWH/fondaparinux) therapy. Continue injectable therapy until the INR has been in the therapeutic range for 24 h. Tissue necrosis in protein C or S deficiency. See phytonadione (vitamin K) entry for management of abnormally high INR.

MOA — Inhibits vitamin K-dependent coagulation factors II, VII, IX, X. Also inhibits biologic anticoagulant proteins C&S.

ADVERSE EFFECTS — Serious: Major bleeding, tissue necrosis in protein C or S deficiency (rare), systemic cholesterol microembolization, purple toe syndrome. Frequent: Bruising.

HEMATOLOGY/ANTICOAGULANTS: Antihemophilic Agents

ANTI-INHIBITOR COAGULANT COMPLEX (*Feiba NF,* *✷Feiba NF*) ▶L ♀C ▶? $$$$$

ADULT — Hemophilia A or B with factor VIII inhibitors, XI and XII (if surgery or active bleeding): 50 to 100 units/kg IV; specific dose and frequency based on site of bleeding, max 200 units/kg/day.

PEDS — Not approved in children.

FORMS — Trade only: Single-dose vials 500, 1000, 2500 units/vial.

NOTES — Contraindicated if normal coagulation. Human plasma product, thus risk of infectious agent transmission. Avoid in active or impending disseminated intravascular coagulation (DIC).

MOA — Coagulation factors II, IX, X and activated factor VII with factor VIII inhibitor bypassing activity that shortens the APTT of plasma containing factor VIII inhibitor.

ADVERSE EFFECTS — Serious: DIC, thromboembolic events, myocardial infarction, anaphylaxis, infectious agent transmission. Frequent: Hypersensitivity (rash, urticaria), anamnestic response (increase in factor VIII inhibitor titer).

FACTOR 1_VIIA (*NovoSeven RT, ✷NiaStase*) ▶L ♀C ▶? $$$$$

WARNING — Serious thrombotic events reported when used outside of labeled indications, including fatal arterial and venous events. Thrombotic events also reported when used for labeled uses. Monitor all patients for thrombosis. Patients with DIC, advanced atherosclerotic disease, crush

injury, or septicemia may be at increased risk for thrombosis. Use with caution in those with thromboembolic risk factors. If DIC or thrombosis confirmed, reduce dose or stop treatment depending on symptoms.

ADULT — Hemophilia A or B: Individualize factor VIIa dose.

PEDS — Hemophilia A or B: Individualize factor VIIa dose.

UNAPPROVED ADULT — Serious bleeding with INR elevation or life-threatening bleeding (ACCP guidelines): Varying doses have been shown effective (10 mcg/kg to max cumulative dose 400 mcg/kg). Factor VIIa has a short half-life; monitor for desired effect. Intracerebral hemorrhage (within 4 h of symptom onset): 40 to 160 mcg/kg IV over 1 to 2 min. Perioperative blood loss in retropubic prostatectomy: 20 or 40 mcg/kg IV bolus.

FORMS — Trade only: NovoSeven RT: 1, 2, 5, 8 mg/vial.

NOTES — Caution if hypersensitivity to mouse, hamster, or bovine proteins.

MOA — Coagulation factor that acts as a cofactor in extrinsic pathway of coagulation by conversion of Factor IX to IXa and X to Xa.

ADVERSE EFFECTS — Serious: DIC, hemorrhage, hemarthrosis, arterial and venous thromboembolic events. Frequent: Fever, plasma fibrinogen decrease, hyper/hypotension, allergic reactions, infusion site reactions.

FACTOR 2_VIII (*Advate, Alphanate, Helixate FS, Hemofil M, Humate P, Koate, Kogenate FS, Kovaltry, Monoclate P, Novoeight, Nuwiq, Recombinate, Xyntha*) ▶L ♀C ▶? $$$$$
ADULT — Hemophilia A: Individualize factor VIII dose. Surgical procedures in patients with von Willebrand disease (Alphanate, Humate P): Individualized dosing. Bleeding in patients with von Willebrand disease (Humate P): Individualized dosing.
PEDS — Hemophilia A: Individualize factor VIII dose.
FORMS — Specific formulation usually chosen by specialist in hemophilia treatment center. Recombinant formulations: Advate, Helixate, Kogenate, Kovaltry, Novoeight, Nuwig, Recombinate, Xyntha. Human plasma–derived formulations: Alphanate, Hemofil M, Humate P, Koate, Monoclate P.
NOTES — Risk of HIV/hepatitis transmission varies by product; no such risk with recombinant product. Reduced response with development of factor VIII inhibitors. Hemolysis with large/repeated doses in patients with A, B, AB blood type.
MOA — Coagulation factor in the intrinsic coagulation pathway, activated factor VIII acts as a cofactor for conversion of Factor X to Xa.
ADVERSE EFFECTS — Serious: HIV/hepatitis transmission (risk varies by product; no such risk if recombinant). Reduced response with development of factor VIII inhibitors (antibodies). Hemolysis with large/repeated doses in patients with A, B, AB blood type. Frequent: Allergic reactions, infusion site reactions.

FACTOR 3_IX (*AlphaNine SD, Aprolix, Benefix, Ixinity, Mononine, Rixubis, ✱Immunine VH*) ▶L ♀C ▶? $$$$$
ADULT — Hemophilia B: Individualize factor IX dose.
PEDS — Hemophilia B: Individualize factor IX dose.
FORMS — Specific formulation usually chosen by specialist in hemophilia treatment center.
NOTES — Risk of HIV/hepatitis transmission varies by product. AlphaNine SD and Mononine are human derived; Alprolix, Benefix, Ixinity and Rixubis are recombinant products. Products that contain factors II, VII, and X may cause thrombosis in at-risk patients. Stop infusion if signs of DIC.
MOA — Coagulation factor in the intrinsic coagulation pathway. Activated factor IXa in combination with Factor VIII:C activates Factor X to Xa.
ADVERSE EFFECTS — Serious: HIV/hepatitis transmission (risk varies by product). Products that contain factors II, VII, & X may cause thrombosis in at-risk patients. Frequent: Infusion-related fever, chills, flushing, nausea, IV-site discomfort.

HEMATOLOGY/ANTICOAGULANTS: Colony-Stimulating Factors

FILGRASTIM(FILGRASTIM-SNDZ)TBO-FILGRASTIM, G-CSF (*Neupogen, Granix, Zarxio*) ▶L ♀C ▶? $$$$$
ADULT — Neutropenia from myelosuppressive chemotherapy in nonmyeloid malignancies or AML with induction or consolidation chemotherapy (Neupogen, Zarxio): 5 mcg/kg/day SC/IV until postnadir ANC is at least 10,000/mm³ for no more than 2 weeks. Can increase by 5 mcg/kg/day with each cycle prn. Neutropenia from myelosuppressive chemotherapy (Granix):5 mcg/kg/day SC until nadir passed and neutrophil count recovered. Bone marrow transplant (Neupogen, Zarxio): 10 mcg/kg/day IV infusion over 4 to 24 h or 24-h SC infusion. Administer 1st dose at least 24 h after cytotoxic chemotherapy and at least 24 h after bone marrow. Adjust to neutrophil response (see prescribing information). Peripheral blood progenitor cell collection (Neupogen, Zarxio): 10 mcg/kg/day in donors for at least 4 days (usually 6 to 7 days) before the 1st leukapheresis and continued until the final leukapheresis. Consider decreased dose if WBC greater than 100,000/mm³. Severe chronic congenital neutropenia (Neupogen, Zarxio):Start 6 mcg/kg SC two times per day. Severe ideopathic or cyclic chronic neutropenia(Neupogen, Zarxio): Start 5 mcg/kg SC daily. Acute exposure to myelosuppressive doses of radiation (Neupogen):10 mcg/kg SC daily.
PEDS — Neutropenia from myelosuppressive chemotherapy (Neupogen, Zarxio): 5 mcg/kg/day SC/IV for no more than 2 weeks until postnadir ANC is at least 10,000/mm³. 10,000/mm³ for no more than 2 weeks. Can increase by 5 mcg/kg/day with each cycle prn. Bone marrow transplant (Neupogen, Zarxio): 10 mcg/ kg/day IV infusion over 4 to 24 h or 24 h SC infusion. Administer 1st dose at least 24 h after cytotoxic chemotherapy and at least 24 h after bone marrow. Adjust to neutrophil response (see product information). Peripheral blood progenitor cell collection (Neupogen, Zarxio): 10 mcg/kg/day in donors for at least 4 days (usually 6 to 7 days) before the 1st leukapheresis and continued until the final leukapheresis. Consider decreased dose if WBC greater than 100,000/mm³. Severe chronic congenital neutropenia (Neupogen, Zarxio): Start 6 mcg/kg SC two times per day. Severe chronic ideopathic or cyclic neutropenia: Start 5 mcg/ kg SC daily. Acute exposure to myelosuppressive doses of radiation (Neupogen):10 mcg/kg SC daily.
UNAPPROVED ADULT — AIDS: 0.3 to 3.6 mcg/kg/day.
FORMS — Trade: Single-dose vials (Neupogen): 300 mcg/1 mL, 480 mcg/1.6 mL. Biosimilars, Single-dose syringes: Granix, tbo-filgrastim: 300 mcg/0.5 mL, 480 mcg/0.8 mL; Zarxio, filgrastim-sndz: 300 mcg/0.5 mL, 480 mcg/0.8 mL.
NOTES — Allergic-type reactions, bone pain, cutaneous vasculitis. Do not give within 24 h before/after cytotoxic chemotherapy. Store in refrigerator; use within 24 h when kept at room temperature.
MOA — Granulocyte colony-stimulating factor, a colony-stimulating factor that stimulates neutrophil production.
ADVERSE EFFECTS — Serious: Allergic-type reactions, cutaneous vasculitis, osteoporosis, thrombocytopenia, splenomegaly, glomerulonephritis. Frequent: Bone pain, increased levels of LDH and alkaline phosphatase.

PEGFILGRASTIM (*Neulasta, Neulasta Onpro*) ▶Plasma ♀C ▶? $$$$$
ADULT — To reduce febrile neutropenia after chemo for nonmyeloid malignancies: 6 mg SC once each chemo cycle. To increase survival after acute exposure to myleosuppressive radiation: 6 mg SC for two doses administered one week apart
PEDS — Myelosuppressive chemo: weight-based dosing given SC once; less than 10 kg give 0.1 mg/kg; 10 to 20 kg give 1.5 mg; 21 to 30 kg give 2.5 mg; 31 to 44 kg give 5 mg, 45 kg or above see adult dosing. Myelosuppresive radiation: give weight-based dosing above SC for two doses administered one week apart.
FORMS — Trade only: Single-dose syringe (Neulasta, Neulasta Onpro) or syringe kit (Neulasta Onpro) 6 mg/0.6 mL
NOTES — Bone pain common. Do not give in the time period between 14 days prior to and 24 h after cytotoxic chemo. Store in refrigerator. Stable at room temperature for no more than 48 h. Protect from light. Syringe not marked for dosing pediatric patients; direct administration to those requiring dosing of less than 6 mg not recommended .
MOA — Long-acting form of filgrastim that is conjugated to polyethylene glycol (pegylated).
ADVERSE EFFECTS — Serious: cutaneous vasculitis, leukocytosis, splenomegaly, capillary leak syndrome, glomerulonephritis. Frequent: Bone pain, reversible increases in LDH, alkaline phosphatase, uric acid.

SARGRAMOSTIM (*GM-CSF, Leukine*) ▶L ♀C ▶? $$$$$
ADULT — Specialized dosing for leukemia, bone marrow transplantation.
PEDS — Not approved in children.
MOA — Granulocyte-macrophage colony-stimulating factor, a colony-stimulating factor that stimulates the production of neutrophils, monocytes, and eosinophils.
ADVERSE EFFECTS — Serious: Capillary leak syndrome, dyspnea due to sequestration of WBCs in lungs (rare). Frequent: Fluid retention, fever, asthenia, headache, bone pain, chills, myalgia.

HEMATOLOGY/ANTICOAGULANTS: Erythropoiesis Stimulating Agents

NOTE: May exacerbate HTN; contraindicated if uncontrolled HTN. Not for immediate correction of anemia. Evaluate iron stores before and during treatment; most patients eventually require iron supplements. Consider other causes of anemia if no response. Chronic kidney disease: Increased risk of death and serious cardiovascular events, including myocardial infarction, stroke, venous thromboembolism, and vascular access thrombosis; in controlled trials, these events were demonstrated when Hb of greater than 11 g/dL was targeted. Cancer: May shorten time to tumor progression in cancer patients. To minimize risks, use lowest effective dose.

DARBEPOETIN (*Aranesp*) ▶cellular sialidases, L ♀C ▶? $$$$$
WARNING — Not approved for use in cancer patients unless anemia is caused by concurrent myelosuppressive chemotherapy; discontinue when chemotherapy completed. Not for patients receiving myelosuppressive chemotherapy in whom anticipated outcome is cure.
ADULT — Anemia of chronic renal failure: 0.45 mcg/kg IV/SC q week, or 0.75 mcg/kg SC q 2 weeks for some nondialysis patients. Maintenance dose may be lower in predialysis patients than dialysis patients. Initiate when Hb less than 10 g/dL; decrease dose or discontinue when Hb approaches or exceeds 11 g/dL if on dialysis or 10 g/dL if not on dialysis. Anemia in cancer chemo patients: Initially 2.25 mcg/kg SC q week, or 500 mcg SC q 3 weeks. For weekly administration, max 4.5 mcg/kg/dose. Adjust dose based on Hb to maintain lowest level to avoid transfusion. Weekly dose conversion to darbepoetin (D) from erythropoietin (E): 6.25 mcg D for less than 2500 units E; 12.5 mcg D for 2500 to 4999 units E; 25 mcg D for 5000 to 10,999 units E; 40 mcg D for 11,000 to 17,999 units E; 60 mcg D for 18,000 to 33,999 units E; 100 mcg D for 34,000 to 89,999 units E; 200 mcg D for 90,000 units E or greater. Give D once a week for patients taking E 2 to 3 times per week; give D once q 2 weeks for patients taking E once a week. Monitor Hb weekly until stable, then at least monthly.
PEDS — Anemia of chronic renal failure: 0.45 mcg/kg IV/SC q week, or 0.75 mcg/kg SC q 2 weeks for some nondialysis patients. Maintenance dose may be lower in predialysis patients than dialysis patients. Initiate when Hb less than 10 g/dL; decrease dose or discontinue when Hb approaches or exceeds 12 g/dL.
UNAPPROVED ADULT — Chemotherapy-induced anemia: 3 mcg/kg or 200 mcg SC q 2 weeks.
FORMS — Trade only: Single-dose vials: 25, 40, 60, 100, 200, 300, 500 mcg/1 mL, and 150 mcg/0.75 mL. Single-dose prefilled syringes or autoinjectors: 10 mcg/0.4mL, 25 mcg/0.42 mL, 40 mcg/0.4 mL, 60 mcg/0.3 mL, 100 mcg/0.5 mL, 150 mcg/0.3 mL, 200 mcg/0.4 mL, 300 mcg/0.6 mL, 500 mcg/1 mL.
NOTES — Use only 1 dose per vial/syringe; discard any unused portion. Do not shake. Protect from light.
MOA — Long-acting form of erythropoietin that gains its increased serum half-life and biologic activity from increased sialic acid content; stimulates erythroid progenitor cells to increase RBC production.
ADVERSE EFFECTS — Serious: Hypertension, seizures, pure red cell aplasia, thrombotic events, severe anemia secondary to antibodies. Frequent: Iatrogenic iron deficiency, myalgia/arthralgia, headache, edema, GI complaints.

EPOETIN ALFA (*Epogen, Procrit, erythropoietin alpha,* ✱*Eprex*) ▶L ♀C ▶? $$$$$
WARNING — Consider antithrombotic DVT prophylaxis, especially in the perioperative period. Not approved for use in cancer patients unless anemia is caused by concurrent myelosuppressive chemotherapy; discontinue when chemotherapy completed. Not for patients receiving myelosuppressive chemotherapy in whom anticipated outcome is cure.
ADULT — Anemia of chronic renal failure: Initial dose 50 to 100 units/kg IV/SC 3 times per week. Initiate when Hb less than 10 g/dL; decrease dose or discontinue when Hb approaches or exceeds 11 g/dL if on dialysis or 10 g/dL if not on dialysis. Maintain lowest level to avoid transfusion. Zidovudine-induced anemia in HIV-infected patients: 100 to 300 units/kg IV/SC 3 times per week. Anemia in cancer chemo patients: 150 to 300 units/kg SC 3 times per week or 40,000 units SC once a week. Start only if Hb less than 10 g/dL and 2 additional months of myelosuppression therapy planned. Adjust dose based on Hb to maintain lowest level to avoid transfusion. Reduction of allogeneic blood transfusion in surgical patients: 300 units/kg/day SC for 10 days preop, on the day of surgery, and 4 days postop. Or 600 units/kg SC once a week starting 21 days preop and ending on day of surgery (4 doses).
PEDS — Anemia in cancer chemo (5 yo or older): 600 units/kg IV q week until completion of chemo. Anemia of chronic renal failure on dialysis (1 mo to 16 yo): Initial dose 50 units/kg IV/SC 3 times per week. Initiate when Hb less than 10 g/dL; decrease dose or discontinue when Hb approaches or exceeds 11 g/dL if on dialysis or 10 g/dL. Maintain lowest level to avoid transfusion.
UNAPPROVED PEDS — Anemia of chronic renal failure: Initial dose 50 to 100 units/kg IV/SC 3 times per week. Zidovudine-induced anemia in HIV-infected patients: 100 units/kg SC 3 times per week; max 300 units/kg/dose.
FORMS — Trade only: Single-dose 1-mL vials 2000, 3000, 4000, 10,000, 40,000 units/mL. Multidose vials 10,000 units/mL, 2 mL; 20,000 units/mL, 1 mL.
NOTES — Single-dose vials contain no preservatives. Use 1 dose per vial; do not re-enter vial. Discard unused portion.
MOA — Stimulates erythroid progenitor cells to increase red blood cell production.
ADVERSE EFFECTS — Serious: Hypertension in patients with chronic renal failure, seizures, pure red cell aplasia, thrombotic events, severe anemia secondary to antibodies. Frequent: Iatrogenic iron deficiency, headache, arthralgia, fever.

METHOXY POLYETHYLENE GLYCOL-EPOETIN BETA (*Mircera*) ▶L ♀C ▶? $$$$
WARNING — Not approved for use in cancer patients.
ADULT — Anemia of chronic renal failure: Initial dose 0.6 mcg/kg IV/SC q2weeks. Initiate when Hb less than 10 g/dL; decrease dose or discontinue when Hb approaches or exceeds 11 g/dL if on dialysis or 10 g/dL if not on dialysis. Maintain lowest dose to maintain Hb sufficient to avoid transfusion.
PEDS — Not approved for use in pediatrics.
FORMS — Trade only: Single-dose pre-filled syringe 30, 50, 75, 100, 120, 150, 200, 250, 360 mcg.
MOA — Stimulates erythroid progenitor cells to increase red blood cell production.
ADVERSE EFFECTS — Serious: Hypertension in patients with chronic renal failure, seizures, pure red cell aplasia, thrombotic events, anaphylaxis, Stevens-Johnson syndrome. Frequent: diarrhea, nasopharyngitis.

HEMATOLOGY/ANTICOAGULANTS: Other Hematological Agents

AMINOCAPROIC ACID (*Amicar*) ▶K ♀D ▶? $ IV $$$$$
Oral
ADULT — To improve hemostasis when fibrinolysis contributes to bleeding: 4 to 5 g IV/PO over 1 h, then 1 g/h for 8 h or until bleeding controlled.
PEDS — Not approved in children.
UNAPPROVED ADULT — Prevention of recurrent subarachnoid hemorrhage: 6 g IV/PO q 4 h (6 doses/day). Reduction of postop bleeding after cardiopulmonary bypass: 5 g IV, then 1 g/h for 6 to 8 h.
UNAPPROVED PEDS — To improve hemostasis when fibrinolysis contributes to bleeding: 100 mg/kg or 3 g/m² IV infusion during 1st h, then continuous infusion of 33.3 mg/kg/h or 1 g/m²/h. Max dose of 18 g/m²/day. IV prep contains benzyl alcohol; do not use in newborns.
FORMS — Trade only: Tabs 500, 1000 mg. Syrup 250 mg/mL
NOTES — Contraindicated in active intravascular clotting. Do not use in DIC without heparin. Can cause intrarenal thrombosis, hyperkalemia. Skeletal muscle weakness, necrosis with prolonged use; monitor CPK. Use with estrogen/oral contraceptives can cause hypercoagulability. Rapid IV administration can cause hypotension, bradycardia, arrhythmia.
MOA — Inhibits fibrinolysis.
ADVERSE EFFECTS — Serious: Skeletal muscle weakness and necrosis with prolonged use. Rapid IV administration can cause hypotension, bradycardia, arrhythmia. Frequent: None.

ANAGRELIDE (*Agrylin*) ▶LK ♀C ▶? $$$$$
ADULT — Thrombocythemia due to myeloproliferative disorders (including essential thrombocythemia): Start 0.5 mg PO four times per day or 1 mg PO two times per day, then after 1 week adjust to lowest effective dose that maintains platelet count less than 600,000/mcL. Max 10 mg/day or 2.5 mg as a single dose. Usual dose 1.5 to 3 mg/day.
PEDS — Limited data. Thrombocythemia due to myeloproliferative disorders (including essential thrombocythemia): Start 0.5 mg PO daily, then after

(cont.)

ANAGRELIDE (*cont.*)

1 week adjust to lowest effective dose that maintains platelet count less than 600,000/mcL. Max 10 mg/day or 2.5 mg as a single dose. Usual dose 1.5 to 3 mg/day.

FORMS — Generic/Trade: Caps 0.5 mg. Generic only: Caps 1 mg.

NOTES — Caution with heart disease, may cause hypotension, vasodilation, tachycardia, palpitations, heart failure, QTc prolongation, torsades; obtain baseline ECG and consider periodic monitoring. Contraindicated in severe hepatic impairment, use with caution in mild to moderate hepatic impairment. Monitor LFTs baseline and during therapy. Caution in lung disease and renal insufficiency. Dosage should be increased by not more than 0.5 mg/day in any 1 week.

MOA — Unknown; a decrease in megakaryocyte hypermaturation may decrease platelet production.

ADVERSE EFFECTS — Serious: May cause cardiovascular events including hypotension, vasodilation, supraventricular tachycardia, palpitations, heart failure, QTc prolongation and torsades, renal failure, tubulointerstitial nephritis, pulmonary disorders, hepatotoxicity. Frequent: Headache, diarrhea, edema, palpitation, abdominal pain.

DEFERASIROX (*Exjade, Jadenu*) ▶L ♀– ?/?/? ▶? $$$$$

WARNING — Monitor renal and hepatic function closely. Renal impairment, including failure and death, has been reported; assess serum creatinine and creatinine clearance twice before therapy and monthly thereafter. Fatal hepatic failure has been reported; monitor LFTs and bilirubin baseline, q 2 weeks for 1 month, then monthly. GI bleeding reported, especially if thrombocytopenia or advanced hematologic malignancies; risk increased with concurrent ulcerogenic drugs. Severe skin reactions reported; monitor for and discontinue if Stevens-Johnson syndrome or erythema multiforme suspected.

ADULT — Chronic iron overload due to blood transfusions: Exjade: 20 mg/kg PO daily; adjust dose q 3 to 6 months based on ferritin trends. Max 40 mg/kg/day. Jadenu: 14 mg/kg PO daily; adjust dose monthly based on ferritin trends. Max 28 mg/kg/day. Chronic iron overload in non-transfusion-dependent thalassemia syndromes: Exjade: 10 mg/kg PO daily; adjust dose based on ferritin and liver iron concentration. Max 20 mg/kg/day. Jadenu: 7 mg/kg PO daily; adjust dose based on ferritin and liver iron concentration. Max 14 mg/kg/day.

PEDS — Chronic iron overload due to blood transfusions: Exjade: 20 mg/kg PO daily; adjust dose q 3 to 6 months based on ferritin trends. Max 40 mg/kg/day. Jadenu: 14 mg/kg PO daily; adjust dose monthly based on ferritin trends. Max 28 mg/kg/day. Chronic iron overload in non-transfusion-dependent thalassemia syndromes: Exjade: 10 mg/kg PO daily; adjust dose based on ferritin and liver iron concentration. Max 20 mg/kg/day. Jadenu: 7 mg/kg PO daily; adjust dose based on ferritin and liver iron concentration. Max 14 mg/kg/day.

FORMS — Trade only: Exjade: 125, 250, 500 mg tabs for dissolving into oral susp; Jadenu: 90, 180, 360 mg tabs.

NOTES — Calculate dose to the nearest whole tablet. Conversion from Exjade to Jadenu: dose for Jadenu should be 30% lower (round to nearest whole tablet). Do not use if CrCl <40 mL/min, serum creatinine greater than twice upper limit of normal. Do not use if severe (Child-Pugh C) hepatic impairment. Reduce starting dose by 50% in moderate (Child-Pugh B) hepatic impairment or in renal impairment (CrCl 40 to 60 mL/min). Closely monitor patients with mild hepatic impairment. Contraindicated if high-risk for myelodysplastic syndrome, advanced malignancy, poor performance status or platelet count less than 50 per 10^9/L. Give Exjade on an empty stomach 30 min or more before food. Give Jadenu on an empty stomach or light meal (<7% fat; < 250 cal). Reports of fatal cytopenias; monitor CBC regularly. Perform auditory and ophthalmic testing before initiation of therapy and yearly thereafter. Do not take with aluminum-containing antacids. May decrease serum ferritin and liver iron concentrations. See product information for detailed information regarding criteria of iron overload.

MOA — Chelates free serum iron.

ADVERSE EFFECTS — Serious: Renal failure, tubulointerstitial nephritis, hepatic failure, hearing disturbance/loss, ocular disturbances, optic neuritis, neutropenia, thrombocytopenia, GI hemorrhage/ulcer, erythema multiforme, Stevens-Johnson Syndrome. Frequent: Fever, headache, abdominal pain, cough, diarrhea, creatinine increase, N/V, rash, arthralgia, fatigue, skin rashes.

ECULIZUMAB (*Soliris*) ▶Serum ♀C ▶? $$$$$

WARNING — Increased risk of meningococcal infections. Administer meningococcal vaccine at least 2 weeks prior to therapy and revaccinate according to current guidelines. Monitor patients for early signs of meningococcal infections, evaluate, and treat with antibiotics as necessary.

ADULT — Reduction of hemolysis in paroxysmal nocturnal hemoglobinuria: 600 mg IV infusion q 7 days for 4 weeks, then 900 mg for 5th dose 7 days later, then 900 mg q 14 days. Atypical hemolytic uremic syndrome: 900 mg IV infusion weekly for 4 weeks, then 1200 mg for 5th dose 1 week later, then 1200 mg q 14 days. Administer infusion over 35 minutes.

PEDS — Not approved in children.

NOTES — Contraindicated if active meningococcal infection or without current meningococcal vaccination. Increases risk of infection with encapsulated bacteria, including Streptococcus pneumoniae and Haemophilus influenzae type B (Hib). Consider appropriate immunization. Caution if systemic infection. Dose may be given within 2 days of scheduled dosing date. Give supplemental dose after plasmapheresis, plasma exchange or fresh frozen plasma infusion; see product

(cont.)

ECULIZUMAB (*cont.*)

information for dosing. Monitor LDH (if used for paroxysmal nocturnal hemoglobinuria) or LDH, platelets, and serum creatinine (if used for atypical hemolytic uremic syndrome) during therapy. Monitor following discontinuation for hemolysis for 8 weeks (if used for paroxysmal nocturnal hemoglobinuria) or thrombotic microangiopathy for 12 weeks (if used for atypical hemolytic uremic syndrome).

MOA — Recombinant humanized monoclonal antibody that inhibits complement mediated intravascular hemolysis.

ADVERSE EFFECTS — Serious: meningococcal infections, serious infection. Frequent: Hypersensitivity, infusion reaction, headache, nasopharyngitis, back pain, nausea.

ELTROMBOPAG (*Promacta*, *✱Revolade*) ▶LK ♀C ▶? $$$$$

WARNING — Hepatotoxicity; may increase risk of hepatic decompensation in patients with chronic hepatitis C in combination with interferon and ribavirin. Obtain serum transaminases and bilirubin at baseline and q 2 weeks during dose adjustment, then monthly. If abnormal, repeat LFTs within 3 to 5 days. If LFTs remain abnormal, monitor weekly until LFTs return to baseline, stabilize, or resolve. Discontinue if ALT is 3 or more times upper limit of normal and increasing, persistent for at least 4 weeks, hepatotoxicity symptoms, or with increased direct bilirubin.

ADULT — Thrombocytopenia in ITP (unresponsive to steroids, immunoglobulins, or splenectomy): Start 50 mg PO daily. In hepatic insufficiency or East Asian ancestry, start 25 mg daily. Adjust to achieve platelet count of 50,000; max 75 mg daily. Thrombocytopenia in patients with chronic hepatitis C (to allow the initiation and maintenance of interferon-based therapy): 25 mg PO daily. Adjust q 2 weeks to achieve a platelet count that allows antiviral therapy, max 100 mg daily. Severe aplastic anemia: Start 50 mg PO daily. In hepatic insufficiency or East Asian ancestry, start 25 mg daily. Adjust to achieve platelet count of 50,000; max 150 mg daily.

PEDS — Thrombocytopenia in ITP, 6 yo or older (unresponsive to steroids, immunoglobulins, or splenectomy): Start 50 mg PO daily. In hepatic insufficiency or East Asian ancestry, start 25 mg daily. Adjust to achieve platelet count of 50,000, max 75 mg daily.

FORMS — Trade only: Tabs 12.5, 25, 50, 75 mg.

NOTES — Give on empty stomach (1 h before or 2 h after meal); separate from medications and food containing iron, Ca, magnesium, selenium, and zinc with an interval of at least 4 h. Monitor CBC weekly until platelet counts stabilize, then monthly. In ITP, discontinue if no response after 4 weeks on 75 mg daily. Not for use to normalize platelet count; goal is increase platelet count to a level that reduces bleeding or allows antiviral therapy. Discontinuation may worsen thrombocytopenia; monitor CBC weekly for 4 weeks after discontinuation. Monitor peripheral blood for signs of marrow fibrosis. Portal vein thrombosis reported in patients with chronic liver disease.

MOA — thrombopoietin receptor agonist

ADVERSE EFFECTS — Serious: hepatotoxicity, marrow fibrosis, thromboembolism, thrombotic microangiopathy. Frequent: nausea, vomiting, menorrhagia, myalgia, paresthesia, cataract, dyspepsia, ecchymosis, increased serum transaminases, conjunctival hemorrhage.

HYDROXYUREA (*Hydrea, Droxia*) ▶LK ♀X/X/X ▶– $$$

WARNING — Mutagenic and clastogenic; may cause secondary leukemia. Instruct patients to report promptly fever, sore throat, signs of local infection, bleeding from any site, or symptoms suggestive of anemia. Cutaneous vasculitic toxicities, including vasculitic ulcerations and gangrene, have been reported most often in patients on interferon therapy.

ADULT — Sickle cell anemia (Droxia): Start 15 mg/kg PO daily while monitoring CBC q 2 weeks. If WBC is 2500/mm³ or greater, platelet count is 95,000/mm³ or greater, and Hb is above 5.3 g/dL, then increase dose q 12 weeks by 5 mg/kg/day (max 35 mg/kg/day). Head and neck cancer with radiation (Hydrea): 15 mg/kg PO daily. Resistant chronic myeloid leukemia: 15 mg/kg PO daily. Give concomitant folic acid.

PEDS — Not approved in children.

UNAPPROVED ADULT — Essential thrombocythemia at high risk for thrombosis: 0.5 to 1 g PO daily adjusted to keep platelets less than 400/mm³. Also has been used for HIV, psoriasis, polycythemia vera.

UNAPPROVED PEDS — Sickle cell anemia.

FORMS — Generic/Trade: Caps 500 mg. Trade only: (Droxia) Caps 200, 300, 400 mg.

NOTES — Reliable contraception is recommended. Monitor CBC and renal function. Reduce dose for CrCl <60 ml/min. Elderly may need lower doses. Minimize exposure to the drug by wearing gloves during handling. Avoid live vaccines.

MOA — Antimetabolite.

ADVERSE EFFECTS — Serious: Bone marrow suppression, nephrotoxicity. Frequent: Bone marrow suppression, erythropoiesis, mucositis, rash.

IDARUCIZUMAB (*Praxbind*) ▶? Biodegradation ♀?/?/? ▶? $$$$$

ADULT — Reversal of dabigatran anticoagulation for emergency surgery/procedures or life-threatening/uncontrolled bleeding: 5 g IV.

PEDS — Not approved in pediatrics.

FORMS — Trade only: 2.5 g/50 mL vial.

NOTES — Given as two consecutive 2.5g IV infusion or IV bolus doses. May increase thromboembolic risk when anticoagulation is reversed. Monitor coagulation parameters. Limited data supporting additional 5 g IV. Discontinue if hypersensitivity reaction. Patients with history of hereditary fructose intolerance may experience serious adverse reactions due to sorbitol excipient.

MOA — Humanized monocloonal antibody fragment the provides specific reversal for dabigatran by

(cont.)

IDARUCIZUMAB *(cont.)*

binding to dabigatran and its metabolites thereby neutralizing their anticoagulant effect

ADVERSE EFFECTS — Serious: hypersensitivity, thromboembolic risk, hyperkalemia. Common: headache, delirum, constipation, fever.

PLERIXAFOR (*Mozobil*) ▸K ♀D ▶? $$$$$

ADULT — Hematopoietic stem cell mobilization with G-CSF for autologous transplantation in non-Hodgkin's lymphoma and multiple myeloma: Patients less than or equal to 83 kg give 20 mg dose or 0.24 mg/kg (actual body wt) SC once daily for up to 4 days. Patients greater than 83 kg give 0.24 mg/kg (actual body wt) SC once daily for up to 4 days, max 40 mg/day.

PEDS — Not approved in children.

FORMS — Trade only: Single-dose vials 20 mg/mL, 1.2 mL vial.

NOTES — Use with G-CSF; initiate after patient has received G-CSF daily for 4 days. Administer 11 h prior to apheresis. If CrCl <50 mL/min, decrease dose to 0.16 mg/kg. Do not use in leukemia. Monitor CBC, may increase WBC and decrease platelets. May mobilize tumor cells from marrow. Evaluate for splenic rupture if left upper abdominal, scapular, or shoulder pain. Risk of anaphylaxis; administer in healthcare setting and monitor for at least 30 minutes.

MOA — CXCR4 chemokine antagonist.

ADVERSE EFFECTS — Serious: Leukocytosis, thrombocytopenia, splenic rupture, anaphylactic shock, nightmares. Frequent: Diarrhea, nausea, fatigue, injection site reactions, headache, arthralgia, dizziness, vomiting.

PROTAMINE ▸Plasma ♀C ▶? $

WARNING — Hypotension, cardiovascular collapse, pulmonary edema/vasoconstriction/hypertension may occur. May be more common with higher doses, overdose, or repeated doses, including previous exposure to protamine or protamine-containing drugs (including insulin). Other risk factors include fish allergy, vasectomy, LV dysfunction, and pulmonary hemodynamic instability.

ADULT — Heparin overdose: Within 30 minutes of IV heparin: 1 mg antagonizes about 100 units heparin. If greater than 30 minutes since heparin: 0.5 mg antagonizes about 100 units heparin. Due to short half-life of heparin (60 to 90 min), use IV heparin doses only from last several hours to calculate dose of protamine. SC heparin may require prolonged administration of protamine. Give IV over 10 min in doses of no greater than 50 mg.

PEDS — Not approved in children.

UNAPPROVED ADULT — Reversal of low-molecular-weight heparin: If within 8 h of LMWH dose: Give 1 mg protamine per 100 anti-Xa units of dalteparin or 1 mg protamine per 1 mg enoxaparin. Smaller doses advised if greater than 8 h since LMWH administration. Give additional 0.5 mg protamine per 100 anti-Xa units of dalteparin or 0.5 mg protamine per 1 mg enoxaparin if aPTT remains prolonged 2 to 4 h after 1st infusion of protamine.

UNAPPROVED PEDS — Heparin overdose: Within 30 min of last heparin dose, give 1 mg protamine per 100 units of heparin received; between 30 and 60 min since last heparin dose, give 0.5 to 0.75 mg protamine per 100 units of heparin received; between 60 and 120 min since last heparin dose, give 0.375 to 0.5 mg protamine per 100 units of heparin; more than 120 min since last heparin dose, give 0.25 to 0.375 mg protamine per 100 units of heparin.

NOTES — Severe hypotension/anaphylactoid reaction possible with too rapid administration. Additional doses of protamine may be required in some situations (neutralization of SC heparin, heparin rebound after cardiac surgery). Monitor aPTT to confirm. Incomplete neutralization of LMWHs.

MOA — Binds with and neutralizes heparin and partially reverses LMWHs.

ADVERSE EFFECTS — Serious: Severe hypotension/anaphylactoid reaction with too rapid administration, allergic reactions in patients with fish allergy, previous exposure to protamine (including insulin), pulmonary edema, circulatory collapse. Frequent: Back pain, transient flushing.

PROTEIN C CONCENTRATE (*Ceprotin*) ▸Serum ♀C ▶? $$$$$

ADULT — Severe congenital protein C deficiency (prevention and treatment of venous thrombosis and purpura fulminans): Individualized dosing.

PEDS — Severe congenital protein C deficiency (prevention and treatment of venous thrombosis and purpura fulminans): Individualized dosing.

NOTES — Product contains heparin; do not use if history of heparin-induced thrombocytopenia. Check platelets and discontinue if heparin-induced thrombocytopenia suspected. Product contains sodium. Made from pooled human plasma, may transmit infectious agents.

MOA — Concentrated protein C from human blood donors that controls the coagulation system to prevent excessive procoagulant responses to activating stimuli.

ADVERSE EFFECTS — Serious: Hypersensitivity, hemothorax, hypotension, thrombocytopenia. Frequent: Rash, itching, lightheadedness.

PROTHROMBIN COMPLEX CONCENTRATE (*Kcentra*) ▸N/A ♀C ▶? $$$$$

WARNING — Weigh risk/benefit of reversing vitamin K antagonist, especially if history of thromboembolic event. Not studied if thromboembolic event within the last 3 months. Fatal bleeding and thromboembolic complications reported.

ADULT — Vitamin K antagonist reversal for acute major bleed or urgent surgery/invasive procedure: Individualized dosing based on pre-treatment INR and body weight. INR 2 to less than 4: 25 units of Factor IX/kg body weight (max: 2500 units); INR 4 to 6: 35 units of Factor IX/kg body weight (max: 3500 units); INR greater than 6: 50 units of Factor IX/kg body weight (max 5000 units).

PEDS — Not approved in pediatrics.

(cont.)

PROTHROMBIN COMPLEX CONCENTRATE (cont.)

FORMS — Brand: 500, 1000 unit vial.

NOTES — Give vitamin K to maintain reversal. Repeat dosing has not been studied therefore is not recommended. Do not administer if anaphylactic reactions to human albumin. Contains heparin; do not administer in HIT.

MOA — Contains clotting factors (Factors II, VII, IX, X, Protein C, Protein S) to replace depleted clotting factors.

ADVERSE EFFECTS — Serious: thromboembolism (stroke, pulmonary embolism, deep vein thrombosis), hypersensitivity, hypotension, anemia. Common: headache, N/V.

ROMIPLOSTIM (Nplate) ▶L ♀C ▶? $$$$$

ADULT — Chronic immune idiopathic thrombocytopenic purpura: 1 mcg/kg SC weekly. Adjust by 1 mcg/kg weekly to achieve and maintain platelet count at least 50,000 cells/mcL; max 10 mcg/kg weekly. Hold dose if platelet count is 400,000 cells/mcL or greater.

PEDS — Not approved in children.

NOTES — Use only for chronic ITP; do not use if low platelets from other causes. Use only if increased risk of bleeding and insufficient response to corticosteroids, immunoglobulins, or splenectomy. Do not use to normalize platelet counts; excessive therapy may increase risk of thrombosis. May increase risk for fibrous deposits in bone marrow. Monitor CBC (platelets and peripheral blood smears) weekly until stable dose; then monthly. Platelet counts may drop below baseline following discontinuation; monitor CBC for 2 weeks following cessation of therapy. May increase risk of hematologic malignancies, especially if myelodysplastic syndrome. Available only through restricted distribution program. To minimize errors, follow specific administration instructions in product information.

MOA — Throbopoietin receptor agonist.

ADVERSE EFFECTS — Serious: Thrombosis, bone marrow fibrosis, hypersensitivity, angioedema. Frequent: Headache, arthralgia, dizziness, insomnia, myalgia, pain in extremity, shoulder pain, dyspepsia, paresthesia.

THROMBIN—TOPICAL   (Evithrom,   Recothrom, Thrombin-JMI) ▶? ♀C ▶? $$$

WARNING — The bovine form (Thrombin-JMI) has been associated with rare but potentially fatal abnormalities in hemostasis ranging from asymptomatic alterations in PT and/or aPTT to severe bleeding or thrombosis. Hemostatic abnormalities are likely due to antibody formation, may cause factor V deficiency, and are more likely with repeated applications. Consult hematologist if abnormal coagulation, bleeding, or thrombosis after topical thrombin use.

ADULT — Hemostatic aid for minor bleeding: Apply topically to site of bleeding; dose depends on area to be treated.

PEDS — Hemostatic aid for minor bleeding (Evithrom): Apply topically to site of bleeding; dose depends on area to be treated. Recothrom/Thrombin-JMI not approved in children.

NOTES — Do not inject; for topical use only. Do not use for severe or brisk arterial bleeding. Thaw Evithrom prior to use. Reconstitute Recothrom and Thrombin-JMI prior to use. Evithrom is human-derived and carries risk of viral transmission. Recothrom is a recombinant product; risk of allergic reaction in known hypersensitivity to snake proteins; contraindicated in hypersensitivity to hamster proteins. Thrombin-JMI is a bovine origin product; contraindicated in hypersensitivity to products of bovine origin.

MOA — Promotes clot formation by activating platelets and catalyzing the conversion of fibrinogen to fibrin.

ADVERSE EFFECTS — Serious: Anaphylaxis, antibody development, hemostatic abnormalities, thrombosis, severe bleeding. Frequent: Pruritus, incision/procedure site complications.

TRANEXAMIC ACID (Cyklokapron, Lysteda) ▶K ♀B ▶– $$$$

WARNING — Do not use with combined hormonal contraceptives; risk of thromboembolism.

ADULT — Prophylaxis/reduction of bleeding during tooth extraction in hemophilia patients: 10 mg/kg IV immediately before surgery, then 10 mg/kg PO 3 to 4 times per day for 2 to 8 days following surgery. Heavy menstrual bleeding (Lysteda): 1300 mg PO three times per day for up to 5 days during menstruation.

PEDS — Not approved in children.

FORMS — Generic/Trade (Lysteda, PO): Tabs 650 mg. Generic/Trade (Cyklokapron, IV): 100 mg/mL, 10 mL vial.

NOTES — Dose adjust in renal impairment.

MOA — Competitively inhibits plasminogen activator and noncompetitively plasmin (at higher doses).

ADVERSE EFFECTS — Severe: Hypotension (infusion rate limiting), DVT, PE, vision abnormalities, convulsions. Frequent: N/V, diarrhea, giddiness, menstrual discomfort.

HERBAL AND ALTERNATIVE THERAPIES

NOTE: In the United States, herbal and alternative therapies are regulated as dietary supplements, not drugs. Premarketing evaluation and FDA approval are not required unless specific therapeutic claims are made. Because these products are not required to demonstrate safety and efficacy, it is unclear whether many of them have any health benefit and some can cause harm. In addition, the actual ingredients may vary considerably from the ingredients on the label, and may be adulterated.

CHAMOMILE (*Matricaria recutita—German chamomile, Anthemis nobilis—Roman chamomile*) ▶? ♀–▶? $

UNAPPROVED ADULT — Oral extract: Modest benefit in study for generalized anxiety disorder, but little to no benefit in study for primary chronic insomnia. Topical: Efficacy unclear for skin infections or inflammation. Does not appear to reduce mucositis caused by 5-fluorouracil or radiation.

UNAPPROVED PEDS — Supplements not for use in children. Efficacy and safety unclear for treatment of infant colic with multi-ingredient teas/extracts of chamomile, fennel, and lemon balm.

FORMS — Not by prescription.

NOTES — Theoretical concern (no clinical evidence) for drug interactions due to increased sedation, increased risk of bleeding (contains coumarin derivatives), delayed GI absorption of other drugs (due to antispasmodic effect). Increased INR with warfarin attributed to chamomile in a single case.

MOA — Contains compounds with antispasmodic, antiinflammatory, antimicrobial, and mild sedative effects in animal and in vitro studies.

ADVERSE EFFECTS — Rare allergic reactions including anaphylaxis, contact dermatitis. Cross-hypersensitivity with other plants in Compositae family, including arnica, chrysanthemum, echinacea, feverfew, ragweed, Artemisia. Topical application to the eye can cause conjunctivitis.

MILK THISTLE (*Silybum marianum, Legalon, silymarin, Thisilyn*) ▶LK ♀–▶–$

UNAPPROVED ADULT — Hepatic cirrhosis (efficacy unclear): 100 to 200 mg PO three times per day of standardized extract (70 to 80% silymarin). Alcoholic liver disease guidelines recommend against use. Appears ineffective for chronic hepatitis C; the American Gastroenterological Association recommends against use. Amatoxin-containing mushroom poisoning (possibly effective): IV silibinin (Legalon SIL) available from NIH study by calling 1-866-520-4412; oral milk thistle has been used when IV silibinin is not available.

UNAPPROVED PEDS — Not for use in children.

FORMS — Not by prescription.

NOTES — May inhibit CYP2C9 (conflicting study results); monitor for reduced response to losartan.

MOA — Hepatoprotectant with antioxidant, membrane-stabilizing, liver cell regeneration properties. Silibinin inhibits OATP 1B3 and NTCP transport of amatoxin into hepatocytes.

ADVERSE EFFECTS — Serious: Anaphylaxis. Other: GI distress, abdominal distension, diarrhea, headache, skin reactions, arthralgias.

ALOE VERA (*acemannan, burn plant*) ▶LK ♀ oral – topical + ? ▶ oral – topical + ? $

UNAPPROVED ADULT — Topical: Efficacy unclear for seborrheic dermatitis, psoriasis, genital herpes, partial-thickness skin burns. Does not prevent radiation-induced skin injury. Do not apply to surgical incisions; impaired healing reported. Oral: Efficacy unclear for active ulcerative colitis or type 2 diabetes.

UNAPPROVED PEDS — Not for use in children.

FORMS — Not by prescription.

NOTES — OTC laxatives containing aloe latex were removed from the US market due to concerns about increased risk of colon cancer. Cases of Henoch-Schonlein purpura and hepatotoxicity reported with oral administration.

MOA — Topical: Constituents of gel from within leaves have skin-moisturizing, immunomodulatory, anti-inflammatory, and antiviral activity in vitro. Oral: Aloe latex contains anthraquinone glycosides (stimulant laxative). Pancreatic beta cell stimulation in vitro.

ADVERSE EFFECTS — Topical: Contact dermatitis, pruritus. Oral: Abdominal cramping, diarrhea. Potassium depletion or electrolyte imbalance possible with chronic administration. Hepatotoxicity (hypersensitivity probable mechanism). Henoch-Schonlein purpura (several case reports).

ALPHA LIPOIC ACID (*lipoic acid, thioctic acid, ALA*) ▶intracellular ♀C ▶? $

UNAPPROVED ADULT — Diabetic peripheral neuropathy (possibly effective): 600 mg PO daily. American Academy of Neurology found evidence insufficient to support or refute use. May lower blood sugar (little or no effect on A1C) and is used as adjunct in patients with diabetes at doses of 600 to 1200 mg daily. Does not appear effective for burning mouth syndrome.

UNAPPROVED PEDS — Not for use in children.

FORMS — Not by prescription

NOTES — Considered an important nutrient, but has not been studied as a supplement in pregnancy, lactation, and children.

MOA — Antioxidant.

ADVERSE EFFECTS — Rash, N/V (dose-related), vertigo (dose-related), low blood sugar, urine odor. Hypoglycemic episodes in patients with insulin autoimmune syndrome. Case report of acute cholestatic hepatitis.

ANDROSTENEDIONE (*andro*) ▶L, peripheral conversion to estrogens and androgens ♀–▶–$

UNAPPROVED ADULT — Was marketed as anabolic steroid to enhance athletic performance. Tell

(cont.)

ANDROSTENEDIONE (*cont.*)

patients to avoid; may cause androgenic (primarily in women) and estrogenic (primarily in men) side effects.

UNAPPROVED PEDS — Not for use in children.

FORMS — Not by prescription.

NOTES — Banned as dietary supplement by FDA. Also banned by many athletic organizations. In theory, chronic use may increase risk of hormone-related cancers (prostate, breast, endometrial, ovarian). Increase in androgen levels could exacerbate hyperlipidemia.

MOA — Anabolic steroid precursor; converted to estrogen and testosterone.

ADVERSE EFFECTS — Potential long-term effects include: Testicular atrophy, impotence, and gynecomastia in men; acne, male pattern baldness, deep voice, hirsutism, clitoral enlargement, abnormal menstrual cycles, and thromboembolism in women; premature puberty and short stature in children/adolescents. May exacerbate hyperlipidemia. Case report of priapism.

ARISTOLOCHIC ACID (*Aristolochia, Mu Tong, Fangchi*) ▶? ♀– ▶– $

UNAPPROVED ADULT — Do not use due to well-documented risk of nephrotoxicity. Was promoted for wt loss.

UNAPPROVED PEDS — Do not use.

FORMS — Not by prescription.

NOTES — Banned by FDA due to risk of nephrotoxicity and cancer. Possible adulterant in other Chinese herbal products like Akebia, Clematis, Stephania, and others. Rule out aristolochic acid nephrotoxicity in cases of unexplained renal failure.

MOA — Nephrotoxic (causes interstitial renal fibrosis). Also caused lymphoma and kidney, bladder, stomach, and lung cancer in animal studies.

ADVERSE EFFECTS — Serious: End-stage renal disease and urothelial carcinoma reported in humans.

ARNICA (*Arnica montana*) ▶? ♀– ▶– $

UNAPPROVED ADULT — Toxic if taken by mouth. Topical preparations promoted for treatment of bruises, aches, and sprains, but insufficient data to assess efficacy. Do not use on open wounds.

UNAPPROVED PEDS — Not for use in children.

FORMS — Not by prescription.

NOTES — Repeated topical application can cause skin reactions.

MOA — Contains derivatives of thymol. Thymol is a subcutanuos vasodilator, may have anti-inflammatory and analgesic effects. Helenalin in the product is a GI toxin.

ADVERSE EFFECTS — Repeated topical application can cause skin reactions. Contact dermatitis; cross-hypersensitivity possible with other plants in Compositae family, including chamomile, chrysanthemum, echinacea, feverfew, ragweed, Artemisia. If ingested, may cause gastroenteritis and GI bleeding.

ARTICHOKE LEAF EXTRACT (*Cynara scolymus*) ▶? ♀? ▶? $

UNAPPROVED ADULT — May reduce total cholesterol, but clinical significance is unclear. Possibly effective for functional dyspepsia. Does not appear to prevent alcohol-induced hangover.

UNAPPROVED PEDS — Not for use in children.

FORMS — Not by prescription.

NOTES — Advise against use by patients with bile duct obstruction or gallstones.

MOA — Contains cynarine, a choleretic that increases bile secretion.

ADVERSE EFFECTS — Contact dermatitis (rare).

ASTRAGALUS (*Astragalus membranaceus, huang qi, Jin Fu Kang*) ▶? ♀? ▶? $

UNAPPROVED ADULT — Used with other herbs in traditional Chinese medicine for CHD, CHF, chronic kidney disease, viral infections, upper respiratory tract infections. Early studies suggested that astragalus might improve efficacy of platinum-based chemotherapy for non-small-cell lung cancer. But an astragalus-based herbal formula (Jin Fu Kang) did not affect survival in phase II study of non-small-cell lung cancer.

UNAPPROVED PEDS — Not for use in children.

FORMS — Not by prescription.

NOTES — Not used for more than 3 weeks without close follow-up in traditional Chinese medicine. In theory, may enhance activity of drugs for diabetes, HTN, and anticoagulation.

MOA — Has immunostimulant properties. Contains saponins, astragalosides, high-weight polysaccharides, amino acids, and trace minerals.

ADVERSE EFFECTS — GI discomfort, facial flushing, low blood pressure reported with IV administration.

BILBERRY (*Vaccinium myrtillus, huckleberry, Tegens*) ▶Bile, K ♀– ▶– $

UNAPPROVED ADULT — Insufficient data to evaluate efficacy for macular degeneration or cataracts. Does not appear to improve night vision.

UNAPPROVED PEDS — Supplements not for use in children.

FORMS — Not by prescription.

NOTES — High doses may impair platelet aggregation, affect clotting time, and cause GI distress.

MOA — Contains bioflavonoids (antioxidants) and anthocyanosides (stabilize collagen).

ADVERSE EFFECTS — GI distress, rash. High doses may impair platelet aggregation and affect clotting time.

BITTER MELON (*Momordica charantia, ampalaya, karela*) ▶? ♀– ▶– $$

UNAPPROVED ADULT — Efficacy unclear for type 2 diabetes.

UNAPPROVED PEDS — Not for use in children. Two cases of hypoglycemic coma in children ingesting bitter melon tea.

FORMS — Not by prescription.

MOA — Mechanism of hypoglycemic action unknown but contains insulin-like peptide. MAP30 protein

(cont.)

BITTER MELON (*cont.*)

in seeds has in vitro antiviral and antineoplastic activity.

ADVERSE EFFECTS — Two cases of hypoglycemic coma in children ingesting bitter melon tea. Seeds can cause hemolytic anemia in G6PD deficiency. Can cause diarrhea and abdominal pain.

BITTER ORANGE (*Citrus aurantium, Seville orange*) ▶K ♀–▶– $

UNAPPROVED ADULT — Marketed as substitute for ephedra in weight-loss dietary supplements; safety and efficacy not established.

UNAPPROVED PEDS — Not for use in children.

FORMS — Not by prescription.

NOTES — Contains sympathomimetics including synephrine and octopamine. Synephrine banned by some sports organizations. Do not use within 14 days of an MAOI. Juice may inhibit intestinal CYP3A4.

MOA — Contains sympathomimetics, including synephrine (similar to phenylephrine) and octopamine. May increase blood pressure and heart rate. Juice contains furocoumarin which inhibits CYP3A4.

ADVERSE EFFECTS — Treatment-resistant hypertension. Supplements containing synephrine linked to reports of rhabdomyolysis, MI, stroke, ischemic colitis, and ventricular tachycardia. Ephedra, a related compound, was banned from US market due to similar adverse effects. Bitter orange peel oil may be phototoxic.

BLACK COHOSH (*Cimicifuga racemosa, Remifemin, Menofem*) ▶Bile, feces ♀–▶– $

UNAPPROVED ADULT — Ineffective for relief of menopausal symptoms.

UNAPPROVED PEDS — Not for use in children.

FORMS — Not by prescription.

NOTES — US Pharmacopoeia concluded black cohosh is possible cause of hepatotoxicity in 30 case reports. Does not alter vaginal epithelium, endometrium, or estradiol levels in postmenopausal women.

MOA — Contains triterpene glycosides. Mechanism of action unknown, but does not appear to interact directly with estrogen receptors.

ADVERSE EFFECTS — GI distress, rash. United States Pharmacopoeia determined black cohosh to be possible cause of hepatotoxicity in 30 case reports.

BUTTERBUR (*Petasites hybridus, Petadolex*) ▶? ♀–▶– $$

UNAPPROVED ADULT — Migraine prophylaxis (effective): Petadolex 50 to 75 mg PO two times per day. American Academy of Neurology and American Headache Society recommend for migraine prophylaxis. Allergic rhinitis prophylaxis (possibly effective): Petadolex 50 mg PO two times per day. Efficacy unclear for asthma.

UNAPPROVED PEDS — Not for use in children.

FORMS — Not by prescription. Standardized pyrrolizidine-free extracts: Petadolex tabs 50, 75 mg.

NOTES — Do not use raw butterbur; it may contain hepatotoxic pyrrolizidine alkaloids which processing

removes. Butterbur is related to Asteraceae and Compositae; consider the potential for cross-allergenicity between plants in these families.

MOA — Cerebrovascular smooth muscle relaxant and inhibitor of leukotriene synthesis.

ADVERSE EFFECTS — Serious: None reported. Frequent: Nausea, burping, stomach pain. No long-term safety data.

CESIUM CHLORIDE ▶K ♀–▶– $$$

UNAPPROVED ADULT — Promoted for end-stage cancer, but no evidence of benefit and can cause life-threatening torsades.

FORMS — Not by prescription.

NOTES — Prolonged toxicity (QT interval prolongation, life-threatening torsades, hypokalemia) due to extremely long half-life (200 days to steady-state). Prussian blue speeds elimination.

MOA — Non-radioactive alkali metal (not to be confused with radioactive cesium-137). Claims that cesium kills tumor cells by increasing intracellular pH are unproven. Cesium prolongs QT interval by blocking potassium channels.

ADVERSE EFFECTS — Syncope, QT interval prolongation, torsades de pointes, hypokalemia, diarrhea, paresthesias.

CHASTEBERRY (*Vitex agnus castus fruit extract, Femaprin*) ▶? ♀–▶– $

UNAPPROVED ADULT — Premenstrual syndrome (possibly effective): 20 mg PO daily of extract ZE 440 (Femaprin).

UNAPPROVED PEDS — Not for use in children.

FORMS — Not by prescription.

NOTES — Liquid formulations may contain alcohol. Avoid concomitant dopamine antagonists such as haloperidol or metoclopramide.

MOA — Higher doses may reduce prolactin levels by binding to dopamine D2 receptors in the pituitary. Low doses may increase serum prolactin levels.

ADVERSE EFFECTS — Rash, acne, GI upset, intermenstrual bleeding.

CHONDROITIN ▶K ♀? ▶? $

UNAPPROVED ADULT — Does not appear effective for relief of OA pain overall. Chondroitin 400 mg PO three times per day + glucosamine may improve pain in subgroup of patients with moderate to severe knee OA.

UNAPPROVED PEDS — Not for use in children.

FORMS — Not by prescription.

NOTES — Chondroitin content not standardized and known to vary. Cosamin DS contains 3 mg manganese/cap; tolerable upper limit of manganese is 11 mg/day. Some products made from bovine cartilage. Case reports of increased INR/bleeding with warfarin in patients taking chondroitin + glucosamine.

MOA — Glycosaminoglycan that may stimulate production of cartilage matrix.

ADVERSE EFFECTS — GI distress, allergic reactions. Adverse effects appear minor and infrequent. Rare case reports of increased serum transaminases and hepatotoxicity with glucosamine + chondroitin.

CINNAMON (*Cinnamomum cassia, Cinnamomum aromaticum*) ▶? ♀+ in food, – in supplements ▶+ in food, – in supplements $
UNAPPROVED ADULT — Doses of 1 to 6 g/day do not appear to substantially reduce A1C, fasting glucose, or lipids in type 2 diabetes.
UNAPPROVED PEDS — Does not appear to improve glycemic control in adolescents with type 1 diabetes.
FORMS — Not by prescription.
NOTES — A ½ teaspoon of powdered cinnamon is approximately 1 g. Warn that ingesting cinnamon powder in "cinnamon challenge" can cause choking, aspiration, and collapsed lung.
MOA — Increases insulin sensitivity via stimulation of insulin receptor.
ADVERSE EFFECTS — Hypersensitivity reactions including allergic contact stomatitis; nausea; abdominal pain. Collapsed lung reported from ingestion of cinnamon powder in "cinnamon challenge".

COENZYME Q10 (*CoQ-10, ubiquinone*) ▶Bile ♀– ▶– $$
UNAPPROVED ADULT — Heart failure: 100 to 300 mg/day PO divided two to three times per day (conflicting clinical trials; may reduce hospitalization, dyspnea, edema, but AHA/ACC does not recommend). Statin-induced myalgia: 100 to 200 mg PO daily (efficacy unclear; conflicting clinical trials). Prevention of migraine (possibly effective): 100 mg PO three times per day. May be considered for migraine prevention per American Academy of Neurology and American Headache Society. Efficacy unclear for hypertension, improving athletic performance, and preventing progression of Huntington's disease. Appears ineffective for diabetes, amyotrophic lateral sclerosis. Did not improve cancer-related fatigue or quality of life in RCT of women with breast cancer. Does not slow functional decline in early Parkinson's disease.
UNAPPROVED PEDS — Not for use in children.
FORMS — Not by prescription.
NOTES — Case reports of increased INR with warfarin; but a crossover study did not find an interaction.
MOA — Coenzyme in mitochondrial metabolism; also an antioxidant.
ADVERSE EFFECTS — Mild insomnia, increased LFTs, rash, GI distress. Coenzyme q10 in anti-aging cosmetics linked to cases of vitiligo.

CRANBERRY (*CranActin, Vaccinium macrocarpon*) ▶? ♀+ in food, – in supplements ▶+ in food, – in supplements $
UNAPPROVED ADULT — Prevention of UTI (possibly ineffective): 300 mL/day PO cranberry juice cocktail. Usual dose of cranberry juice extract caps/tabs is 300 to 400 mg PO two times per day. Insufficient data to assess efficacy for treatment of UTI. Does not appear to prevent UTI in spinal cord injury; IDSA advises against routine use to reduce bacteriuria/UTI in neurogenic bladder managed with intermittent/indwelling catheter.
UNAPPROVED PEDS — Insufficient data to assess efficacy for prevention/treatment of UTI in children.

Does not appear to prevent UTI in spinal cord injury; IDSA advises against routine use to reduce bacteriuria/UTI in neurogenic bladder managed with intermittent/indwelling catheter.
FORMS — Not by prescription.
NOTES — Numerous case reports of increased INRs and bleeding with warfarin. However, most clinical trials did not find an increase in the INR with cranberry. Approximately 100 calories/6 oz of cranberry juice cocktail. Advise diabetics that some products have high sugar content. Increases urinary oxalate excretion; may increase risk of oxalate kidney stones.
MOA — Proanthocyanidin or fructose appears to block adhesion of bacteria to uroepithelial cells. Although cranberry juice is acidic, it does not appear to significantly change urine pH.
ADVERSE EFFECTS — GI distress and diarrhea with more than 3 L/day.

CREATINE ▶LK ♀– ▶– $
UNAPPROVED ADULT — Promoted to enhance athletic performance. No benefit for endurance exercise, but modest benefit for intense anaerobic tasks lasting less than 30 sec. Usually taken as loading dose of 10 to 20 g/day PO for 4 to 7 days, then 2 to 5 g/day divided 2 times per day. Possibly effective for increasing muscle strength in Duchenne muscular dystrophy, polymyositis/ dermatomyositis. Does not appear effective for myotonic dystrophy Type 1, amyotrophic lateral sclerosis, or to slow progression of Parkinson's disease. Research ongoing in Huntington's disease.
UNAPPROVED PEDS — Not usually for use in children. The AAP strongly discourages performance-enhancing substances by athletes. Possibly effective for increasing muscle strength in Duchenne muscular dystrophy.
FORMS — Not by prescription.
NOTES — Caffeine may antagonize the ergogenic effects of creatine. Creatine is metabolized to creatinine. In young, healthy adults, large doses can increase serum creatinine slightly without affecting CrCl. The effect in elderly is unknown.
MOA — Endogenous product converted in muscle to creatine phosphate which may increase ATP levels and increase the force of muscle contraction. Improved mitochondrial function and antioxidant activity are proposed mechanism in Parkinson's disease.
ADVERSE EFFECTS — Single case of lone atrial fibrillation (causality unclear). Manic switch reported in two patients in pilot study of bipolar depression. Anecdotal reports of GI distress and myalgia. Diarrhea with doses at least 10 g. Creatine is metabolized to creatinine. Supplements slightly increase serum creatinine in young healthy adults; effect in elderly is unknown. Infrequent reports of renal impairment are unconfirmed. Creatine, especially when taken with protein supplements, has led to misdiagnosis of chronic kidney disease.

CURCUMIN (*Meriva, turmeric*) ▶L ♀+ in food, – in supplements ▶+ in food, – in supplements $
UNAPPROVED ADULT — Efficacy unclear for osteo-arthritis, depression, psoriasis, prevention of dementia.
FORMS — Not by prescription.
NOTES — Turmeric is generally regarded as safe as food by FDA. May increase sulfasalazine exposure.
MOA — Curcumin is a yellow pigment in turmeric. May stimulate gall-bladder contraction. Possible anti-infammatory, antimicrobial, hepatoprotective effects.
ADVERSE EFFECTS — Abdominal discomfort and bloating.

DANSHEN (*Salvia miltiorrhiza*) ▶? ♀? ▶? $
UNAPPROVED ADULT — Used for cardiovascular dis-eases in traditional Chinese medicine.
UNAPPROVED PEDS — Not for use in children.
FORMS — Not by prescription.
NOTES — Cases of increased INR with warfarin.
MOA — Tanoshionones may cause coronary artery vasodilation. Fatty acids in danshen may inhibit thromboxane formation and platelet aggregation/adhesion.
ADVERSE EFFECTS — May increase INR with warfarin.

DEHYDROEPIANDROSTERONE (*DHEA, Aslera, Fidelin, prasterone*) ▶Peripheral conversion to estrogens and androgens ♀– ▶– $
UNAPPROVED ADULT — To improve wellbeing in women with adrenal insufficiency: 50 mg PO daily (possibly effective; conflicting clinical trials). Efficacy unclear for treating poor responders to in vitro fertilization. Does not improve cognition, quality of life, or sexual function in elderly. Not recommended as androgen replacement in late-onset male hypogonadism. Used by athletes as a substitute for anabolic steroids, but no convinc-ing evidence of enhanced athletic performance or increased muscle mass. Banned by many sports organizations.
UNAPPROVED PEDS — Not for use in children.
FORMS — Not by prescription.
NOTES — In theory, chronic use may increase risk of hormone-related cancers (prostate, breast, ovarian). But epidemiologic studies found no link between sex hormone serum levels and prostate cancer.
MOA — Adrenal steroid precursor for estrogen and testosterone. Physiologic doses increase androgen and estrogen levels in women, and estrogen levels in men. May increase insulin sensitivity.
ADVERSE EFFECTS — Acne, hirsutism, and decreased HDL with 100-200 mg/day in women. Case reports of mania induction.

DEVIL'S CLAW (*Harpagophytum procumbens, Doloteffin, Harpadol*) ▶? ♀– ▶– $
UNAPPROVED ADULT — OA, acute exacerbation of chronic low-back pain (possibly effective): 2400 mg extract/day (50 to 100 mg harpagoside/day) PO divided two to three times per day.

UNAPPROVED PEDS — Not for use in children.
FORMS — Not by prescription. Extracts standardized to harpagoside content.
MOA — Contains harpagoside and other iridoid glycosides with antiinflammatory and analgesic effects. Appears to inhibit COX-2 (but not COX-1), and nitric oxide synthetase. May increase gas-tric acid secretion. May decrease heart rate and contractility.
ADVERSE EFFECTS — Serious: Bradycardia. Frequent: Dyspepsia, diarrhea. No long-term safety data.

DONG QUAI (*Angelica sinensis*) ▶? ♀ generally consid-ered unsafe ▶? $
UNAPPROVED ADULT — Appears ineffective for post-menopausal symptoms; North American Menopause Society recommends against use. Used for dys-menorrhea, TIA, CVA, PAD, and cardiovascular con-ditions in traditional Chinese medicine.
UNAPPROVED PEDS — Not for use in children.
FORMS — Not by prescription.
NOTES — Increased risk of bleeding with warfarin with/without increase in INR; avoid concurrent use.
MOA — Unknown. In vitro evidence of platelet antag-onism; contains natural coumarins.
ADVERSE EFFECTS — Photosensitivity possible. A case of subarachnoid hemorrhage attributed to supplement containing Siberian ginseng, dong quai, red clover.

ECHINACEA (*E. purpurea, E. angustifolia, E. pallida, EchinaGuard, Echinacin Madaus*) ▶L ♀– ▶– $
UNAPPROVED ADULT — Promoted as immune stimu-lant. Conflicting clinical trials for prevention or treatment of upper respiratory infections. Appears ineffective to treat common cold.
UNAPPROVED PEDS — Not for use in children younger than 12 yo; risk of rash and allergic reac-tions outweighs any benefit. Appears ineffective for treatment of upper respiratory tract infections in children.
FORMS — Not by prescription.
NOTES — Causality unclear for cases of hepato-toxicity, eosinophilia, precipitation of thrombotic thrombocytopenic purpura, and exacerbation of pemphigus vulgaris. Rare allergic reactions including anaphylaxis. Cross-hypersensitivity possible with other plants in Compositae fam-ily. Photosensitivity possible. Could interact with immunosuppressants due to immunomodulating effects. Some experts limit use to 8 weeks and rec-ommend against use in autoimmune disorders.
MOA — May have immunomodulating and/or anti-viral effects.
ADVERSE EFFECTS — Serious: Rare allergic reac-tions including anaphylaxis (may be more common in atopic individuals), photosensitivity possible. Case reports of hepatotoxicity, eosinophilia, pre-cipitation of thrombotic thrombocytopenic purpura and exacerbation of pemphigus vulgaris; causal-ity unclear. Other: GI complaints. Frequent: Rash in children.

ELDERBERRY (*Sambucus nigra, Sambucol*) ▶LK ♀– ▶– $

UNAPPROVED ADULT — Efficacy unclear for influenza, sinusitis, and bronchitis.

UNAPPROVED PEDS — Not for use in children.

FORMS — Not by prescription.

NOTES — Sinupret and Sambucol also contain other ingredients. Eating uncooked elderberries may cause nausea or cyanide toxicity.

MOA — Stimulates cytokine production and inhibits influenza virus replication in vitro. Flowers and berries contain flavonoids and antioxidant with immunomodulating activity. Also reported to have diuretic and hypoglycemic effects.

ADVERSE EFFECTS — Eating uncooked elderberries may cause nausea or cyanide toxicity.

EPHEDRA (*Ephedra sinica, ma huang*) ▶K ♀– ▶– $

UNAPPROVED ADULT — Little evidence of efficacy for obesity, other than modest short-term wt loss. Traditional use as a bronchodilator.

UNAPPROVED PEDS — Not for use in children.

FORMS — Not by prescription.

NOTES — FDA banned ephedra in 2004 because of link to CVA, MI, sudden death, HTN, palpitations, tachycardia, seizures. Risk of harm may increase with dose, strenuous exercise, or use of other stimulants like caffeine. Country mallow (Sida cordifolia) contains ephedrine.

MOA — Contains sympathomimetics, ephedrine and pseudoephedrine, which cause CNS stimulation, bronchodilation, hypertension, and chronotropic and inotropic effects.

ADVERSE EFFECTS — Serious: Linked to stroke, myocardial infarction, sudden death, HTN, tachycardia, seizures, psychiatric symptoms. Case reports of ephedra kidney stones. Frequent: N/V, palpitations, tremor, insomnia.

EVENING PRIMROSE OIL (*Oenothera biennis*) ▶? ♀? ▶? $

UNAPPROVED ADULT — Appears ineffective for premenstrual syndrome, postmenopausal symptoms, atopic dermatitis. Inadequate data to evaluate efficacy for cervical ripening.

UNAPPROVED PEDS — Not for use in children.

FORMS — Not by prescription.

MOA — Contains gamma linolenic acid and linoleic acid, precursors of arachidonic acid and other eicosanoids. Promoted to have anti-inflammatory properties.

ADVERSE EFFECTS — No significant health hazards identified other than mild nausea, diarrhea, headache.

FENUGREEK (*Trigonella foenum-graecum*) ▶? ♀– ▶? $$

UNAPPROVED ADULT — Efficacy unclear for diabetes or hyperlipidemia. Insufficient data to evaluate efficacy as galactagogue.

UNAPPROVED PEDS — Not for use in children.

FORMS — Not by prescription.

NOTES — Case report of increased INR with warfarin possibly related to fenugreek. Can cause maple syrup–like body odor. Fiber content could decrease GI absorption of some drugs.

MOA — A legume that is a good source of fiber. Hydroxyisoleucine may increase glucose-mediated insulin release. Sapogenins may increase biliary cholesterol excretion.

ADVERSE EFFECTS — Abdominal pain, flatulence, diarrhea. Generally regarded as safe as food by FDA.

FEVERFEW (*Chrysanthemum parthenium, MigreLief, Tanacetum parthenium L.*) ▶? ♀– ▶– $

UNAPPROVED ADULT — Prevention of migraine (probably effective): 50 to 100 mg extract PO daily; 2 to 3 fresh leaves PO daily; 50 to 125 mg freeze-dried leaf PO daily. Take either leaf form with or after meals. Benefit of alcoholic extract questioned. Response may take 1 to 2 months. Should be considered for migraine prevention per American Academy of Neurology and American Headache Society. Inadequate data to evaluate efficacy for acute migraine.

UNAPPROVED PEDS — Not for use in children.

FORMS — Not by prescription.

NOTES — May cause uterine contractions; avoid in pregnancy. MigreLief contains feverfew, riboflavin, and magnesium. MigraSpray and Gelstat are homeopathic products that are unlikely to be beneficial.

MOA — Parthenolide may inhibit prostaglandin synthesis or act as serotonin antagonist. Inhibition of platelet aggregation in vitro, but not in humans. Leaves contain tiny amount of melatonin.

ADVERSE EFFECTS — Mouth and lip irritation after chewing fresh leaves. Mild GI complaints. Rebound headache reported after chronic use. Cross-hypersensitivity possible with other composite flowers (arnica, chamomile, echinacea, ragweed, marigolds, chrysanthemums, daisies).

FLAVOCOXID (*Limbrel*) ▶L ♀– ▶– $$$

UNAPPROVED ADULT — OA (efficacy unclear): 250 to 500 mg PO two times per day. Max 2000 mg/day short-term. Taking 1 h before or after meals may increase absorption.

UNAPPROVED PEDS — Not for use in children.

FORMS — Caps 250, 500 mg. Marketed as prescription-only medical food.

NOTES — Hepatotoxicity reported. Be alert for confusion between the brand names, Limbrel and Enbrel, as well as misidentification of flavocoxid as a COX-2 inhibitor. Baicalin, a component of Limbrel, may reduce exposure to rosuvastatin in some patients. Each cap contains 10 mg elemental zinc.

MOA — Contains flavonoids (baicalin, catechin) from Scutellaria baicalensis and Acacia catechu that may inhibit the production of inflammatory prostaglandins and leukotrienes in the arachidonic acid pathway. Flavonoids may also act as antioxidants. Flavocoxid is not a COX-2 inhibitor.

ADVERSE EFFECTS — Rash, synovitis, hypersensitivity, hypersensitivity pneumonitis, increased LFTs, hepatotoxicity. Frequent: Nausea, diarrhea, flatulence.

GARCINIA CAMBOGIA (*Citri Lean*) ▶? ♀– ▶– $
UNAPPROVED ADULT — Appears ineffective for wt loss.
UNAPPROVED PEDS — Not for use in children.
FORMS — Not by prescription.
MOA — Contains hydroxycitric acid which may inhibit lipogenesis.
ADVERSE EFFECTS — Hepatotoxicity and rhabdomyolysis reported mostly with multi-ingredient garcinia wt loss supplements. Case reports with garcinia of hepatotoxicity, acute necrotizing eosinophilic myocarditis, and serotonin syndrome (in combo with SSRI).

GARLIC SUPPLEMENTS (*Allium sativum, Kwai, Kyolic*) ▶LK ♀– ▶– $
UNAPPROVED ADULT — Ineffective for hyperlipidemia; American College of Cardiology does not recommend for this indication. Small reduction in BP, but efficacy for HTN unclear. Does not appear effective for diabetes. Efficacy unclear for prevention of common cold.
UNAPPROVED PEDS — Not for use in children.
FORMS — Not by prescription.
NOTES — Topical application of garlic can cause burn/rash. Significantly decreases saquinavir levels; may also interact with other protease inhibitors. May increase bleeding risk with warfarin with/without increase in INR. However, Kyolic (aged garlic extract) and enteric-coated garlic did not affect the INR in clinical studies.
MOA — May inhibit HMG-CoA reductase; may inhibit platelet aggregation and enhances fibrinolytic activity; may have antioxidant activity; may cause vasodilation.
ADVERSE EFFECTS — GI irritation, bad breath, rash. Topical application can cause burns. Case reports of anaphylaxis to raw garlic, and garlic-induced eosinophilic esophagitis.

GINGER (*Zingiber officinale*) ▶bile ♀? ▶? $
UNAPPROVED ADULT — American Congress of Obstetricians and Gynecologists considers ginger 250 mg PO four times per day a nonpharmacologic option for N/V in pregnancy. Some experts advise pregnant women to limit dose to usual dietary amount (no more than 1 g/day). Acute chemotherapy-induced nausea (efficacy unclear as adjunct to standard antiemetics): 250 to 500 mg PO two times per day for 6 days, starting 3 days before chemo. May have benefit for acute nausea, but not acute vomiting or delayed N/V. Possibly ineffective for prevention of motion sickness. Does not appear effective for postoperative N/V. Benefit appears modest for OA pain, minimal for dysmenorrhea.
UNAPPROVED PEDS — Not for use in children.
FORMS — Not by prescription.
NOTES — Increased INR attributed to ginger in a phenprocoumon-treated patient, but study in healthy volunteers found no effect of ginger on INR or pharmacokinetics of warfarin. Some European countries advise pregnant women to avoid ginger in supplements because it is cytotoxic in vitro. A ½ teaspoon of ground ginger is about 1 g of ginger.

MOA — Gingerols and shogaols may increase rate of gastric emptying. Ginger is cytotoxic in vitro, raising concern about use by pregnant women.
ADVERSE EFFECTS — Heartburn; bruising/flushing; rash. GI irritation possible at high doses.

GINKGO BILOBA (*EGb 761, Ginkgold, Ginkoba*) ▶K ♀– ▶– $
UNAPPROVED ADULT — Dementia (efficacy unclear): 40 mg PO three times per day of standardized extract (24% ginkgo flavone glycosides, 6% terpene lactones). American Psychiatric Association and others find evidence too weak to recommend for Alzheimer's or other dementias. Does not prevent dementia in elderly with normal or mildly impaired cognitive function. Does not improve cognition in healthy younger people or patients with multiple sclerosis. Does not appear to prevent acute altitude sickness. Ineffective for intermittent claudication, tinnitus.
UNAPPROVED PEDS — Not for use in children.
FORMS — Not by prescription.
NOTES — Possible increased risk of stroke. Cases of intracerebral, subdural, and ocular bleeding, but no increase in major bleeding in large clinical trial. Does not appear to increase INR with warfarin, but monitoring for bleeding is advised. May reduce efficacy of efavirenz. A few reports attribute new or worsening seizures to ginkgo supplements, possibly due to contamination with a neurotoxin from ginkgo seeds. Some experts advise caution or avoidance of ginkgo by those with seizures or taking drugs that lower the seizure threshold.
MOA — May decrease capillary fragility or blood viscosity, cause vasodilation, increase peripheral blood flow, affect neurotransmitters, and act as antioxidant.
ADVERSE EFFECTS — Serious: Seizures possible (rare), intracerebral, subdural, ocular bleeding (rare). Higher risk of stroke in clinical trial of ginkgo for prevention of cognitive decline in elderly. Other: GI complaints, headache, allergy, anxiety/restlessness, sleep disturbances.

GINSENG—AMERICAN (*Panax quinquefolius L., Cold-FX, Cold-FX Extra*) ▶K ♀– ▶– $
UNAPPROVED ADULT — Prevention of colds/flu (possible modest efficacy): 1 to 2 caps Cold-FX PO two times per day or 1 cap Cold-FX Extra PO two times per day during flu season. Ineffective for cold treatment. Approved natural product for cold prevention in Canada. Postprandial hyperglycemia in type 2 diabetes (possibly effective): 3 g PO taken with or up to 2 h before meal. Cancer-related fatigue (possibly effective; conflicting data): 1000 mg PO two times per day in am and midafternoon.
UNAPPROVED PEDS — Usually not for use in children. Prevention of colds/flu, age 12 yo and older (possible modest efficacy): 1 to 2 caps Cold-FX PO two times per day or 1 cap Cold-FX Extra PO two times per day during flu season. Ineffective for cold treatment. Approved natural product for cold prevention in Canada.

(cont.)

GINSENG—AMERICAN (*cont.*)

FORMS — Not by prescription.

NOTES — Ginseng content varies widely and some products are mislabeled or adulterated with caffeine. American, Asian, and Siberian ginseng are often misidentified. Decreased INR with warfarin.

MOA — Ginsenosides may increase insulin sensitivity or secretion. Polysaccharides in Cold-FX may have immunomodulating effect; it does not contain ginsenosides.

ADVERSE EFFECTS — None found.

GINSENG—ASIAN (*Panax ginseng, Ginsana, Korean red ginseng*) ▶? ♀– ▶– $

UNAPPROVED ADULT — Promoted to improve vitality and wellbeing: 200 mg PO daily. Ginsana: 2 caps PO daily or 1 cap PO two times per day. Preliminary evidence of efficacy for erectile dysfunction. Efficacy unclear for improving physical or psychomotor performance, diabetes, herpes simplex infections, cognitive or immune function. American Congress of Obstetricians and Gynecologists and North American Menopause Society recommend against use for postmenopausal hot flashes.

UNAPPROVED PEDS — Not for use in children.

FORMS — Not by prescription.

NOTES — Some formulations may contain up to 34% alcohol. Reports of an interaction with the MAOI phenelzine. Ginseng content varies widely and some products are mislabeled or adulterated with caffeine. American, Asian, and Siberian ginseng are often misidentified. May interfere with some digoxin assays.

MOA — Unknown. Considered an adaptogen.

ADVERSE EFFECTS — Hypertension, headache, restlessness, estrogenic effects (swollen breasts, menstrual bleeding). Case reports of mania;QT interval prolongation; hypertensive crisis and TIA;pulmonary thromboembolism; gynecomastia in adolescent boy; DRESS with coadministration of ginseng-lamotrigine.

GINSENG—SIBERIAN (*Eleutherococcus senticosus, Ci-wu-jia*) ▶? ♀– ▶– $

UNAPPROVED ADULT — Does not appear to improve athletic endurance. Did not appear effective in single clinical trial for chronic fatigue syndrome.

UNAPPROVED PEDS — Not for use in children.

FORMS — Not by prescription.

NOTES — May interfere with some digoxin assays. A case report of thalamic CVA attributed to Siberian ginseng plus caffeine.

MOA — Considered an adaptogen. Vasodilatory and antiviral activity reported. Not related to Asian or American ginseng (Panax ginseng or quinquefolius).

ADVERSE EFFECTS — A case of thalamic stroke attributed to Siberian ginseng plus caffeine. A case of subarachnoid hemorrhage attributed to supplement containing Siberian ginseng, dong quai, red clover. Hypertension and dysrhythmia also reported.

GLUCOSAMINE (*Cosamin DS, Dona*) ▶L ♀– ▶– $

UNAPPROVED ADULT — OA: Glucosamine HCl 500 mg PO three times per day or glucosamine sulfate (Dona $$) 1500 mg PO once daily. Appears ineffective overall for OA pain, but glucosamine plus chondroitin may reduce pain in moderate to severe knee OA.

UNAPPROVED PEDS — Not for use in children.

FORMS — Not by prescription.

NOTES — Use cautiously or avoid if shellfish allergy. Cases of increased INR/bleeding with warfarin in patient taking chondroitin with glucosamine.

MOA — May stimulate production of cartilage matrix.

ADVERSE EFFECTS — GI complaints, allergic skin reactions (rare). Well-tolerated in the GAIT study. Rare case reports of increased serum transaminases and hepatotoxicity with glucosamine + chondroitin. Increased intraocular pressure reported with glucosamine.

GOLDENSEAL (*Hydrastis canadensis*) ▶L ♀– ▶– $

UNAPPROVED ADULT — Used in attempt to achieve false-negative urine drug test (efficacy unclear). Often combined with echinacea in cold remedies, but insufficient data to assess efficacy of goldenseal for the common cold or URIs.

UNAPPROVED PEDS — Not for use in children.

FORMS — Not by prescription.

NOTES — Alkaloids in goldenseal with antibacterial activity not well absorbed orally. Oral use contraindicated in pregnancy (may cause uterine contractions), newborns (may cause kernicterus), and HTN (high doses may cause peripheral vasoconstriction). Adding goldenseal directly to urine turns it brown. May inhibit CYP2D6 and 3A4. Berberine, a component of goldenseal, may increase cyclosporine levels.

MOA — Contains isoquinoline alkaloids (berberine and others) with antimicrobial activity.

ADVERSE EFFECTS — Oral use contraindicated in pregnancy (may cause uterine contractions), newborns (may cause kernicterus), and hypertension (high doses may cause peripheral vasoconstriction). Berberine doses more than 500 mg may be toxic; may cause ventricular arrhythmias in patients with heart failure. Possible exacerbation of severe hypernatremia reported in child with type I diabetes.

GRAPE SEED EXTRACT (*Vitis vinifera L.*) ▶? ♀? ▶? $

UNAPPROVED ADULT — Small clinical trials suggest benefit in chronic venous insufficiency. No benefit in study of seasonal allergic rhinitis. Insufficient evidence for treatment of HTN.

UNAPPROVED PEDS — Not for use in children.

FORMS — Not by prescription.

NOTES — Pine bark (Pycnogenol) and grape seed extract are often confused; they both contain oligomeric proanthocyanidins.

MOA — Contains oligomeric proanthocyanidins (OPC/PCO) with antioxidant properties. May inhibit platelet aggregation or reactivity.

ADVERSE EFFECTS — None.

GREEN TEA (*Camellia sinensis, Polyphenon E*) ▶LK ♀+ in moderate amount in food, – in supplements ▶+ in moderate amount in food, – in supplements $

UNAPPROVED ADULT — Minimal efficacy for short-term weight loss, hyperlipidemia. Green tea

(cont.)

GREEN TEA (*cont.*)

catechins (Polyphenon E) did not prevent prostate cancer in men with high-grade prostate intraepithelial neoplasia.

UNAPPROVED PEDS — Not for children.

FORMS — Not by prescription. Green tea extract available in caps standardized to polyphenol content.

NOTES — Case of decreased INR with warfarin attributed to vitamin K in large amount of green tea. Can decrease nadolol exposure; avoid coadministration. May contain caffeine. Cases of hepatotoxicity with supplements (not tea); abnormal LFTs with polyphenon E.

MOA — May contain caffeine (approximately 50 mg/cup of tea), catechins, polyphenols including (−)-epigallocatechin-3-gallate (ECGC; primary catechin in polyphenon E), trace elements, vitamins. Has antioxidant activity.

ADVERSE EFFECTS — Reports of hepatotoxicity with supplements (not tea); abnormal LFTs with Polyphenon E. N/V, insomnia, fatigue, diarrhea, abdominal pain, and confusion reported in clinical trials.

GUARANA (*Paullinia cupana*) ▶? ♀+ in food, − in supplements ▶+ in food, − in supplements $

UNAPPROVED ADULT — Marketed as a source of caffeine in weight-loss dietary supplements; it may provide high doses of caffeine.

UNAPPROVED PEDS — Not for use in children.

FORMS — Not by prescription.

MOA — Stimulant effects. Contains caffeine.

ADVERSE EFFECTS — Sympathomimetic effect may increase the risk of serious cardiovascular adverse effects. Case reports of rhabdomyolysis and seizures possibly related to caffeine intoxication from sports drinks containing caffeine, guarana, garcinia, and other ingredients.

GUGGULIPID (*Commiphora mukul extract, guggul*) ▶? ♀− ▶− $$

UNAPPROVED ADULT — Does not appear effective for hyperlipidemia with doses up to 2000 mg PO three times per day, but may cause a small increase in LDL.

UNAPPROVED PEDS — Not for use in children.

FORMS — Not by prescription.

NOTES — May decrease levels of propranolol and diltiazem.

MOA — Resin from the mukul mirth tree traditionally used in Ayurvedic medicine. Contains E and Z guggalsterones which may facilitate cholesterol catabolism via FXR receptor. May reduce C-reactive protein and improve insulin sensitivity at high doses.

ADVERSE EFFECTS — GI distress, headache, and rash. Allergic contact dermatitis reported with guggulipid anticellulite cream.

HAWTHORN (*Crataegus, Crataegutt, HeartCare*) ▶? ♀− ▶− $

UNAPPROVED ADULT — Symptomatic improvement of mild CHF (NYHA I–II; possibly effective): 80 mg PO two times per day to 160 mg PO three times per day (HeartCare 80 mg tabs), but American College of Cardiology does not recommend. The SPICE study (NYHA II-III) found no benefit for reducing cardiac events with 900 mg/day, but possible reduction of sudden cardiac death for LVEF 25 to 35%. Does not appear effective for HTN.

UNAPPROVED PEDS — Not for use in children.

FORMS — Not by prescription.

NOTES — Unclear whether hawthorn and digoxin should be used together; mechanisms of action may be similar.

MOA — Contains oligomeric procyanidins and flavonoids with positive inotropic and vasodilatory properties, and possible antioxidant activity. May have anti-ischemic activity.

ADVERSE EFFECTS — GI distress, dizziness, palpitations (rare). Some inotropic agents increase mortality in heart failure. Initial presentation of SPICE study did not report increased mortality; hawthorn was safe in combo with other heart failure meds.

HONEY (*Medihoney*) ▶? ♀+ ▶+ $ for oral $$$ for Medihoney

ADULT — Topical for burn/wound care (including pressure ulcers, 1st- and 2nd-degree partial-thickness burns, donor sites, surgical/traumatic wounds): Apply Medihoney to wound for 12 to 24 h/day.

PEDS — Topical for burn/wound care (including pressure ulcers, 1st- and 2nd- degree partial-thickness burns, donor sites, surgical/traumatic wounds): Apply Medihoney to wound for 12 to 24 h/day.

UNAPPROVED ADULT — Constipation (efficacy unclear): 1 to 2 tbsp (30 to 60 g) PO in glass of water. Efficacy of topical honey unclear for prevention of dialysis catheter infections.

UNAPPROVED PEDS — Oral honey not for children younger than 1 yo due to risk of infant botulism. Nocturnal cough due to upper RTI in children (effective): Give PO within 30 min before sleep. Give ½ tsp for 2 to 5 yo, 1 tsp for 6 to 11 yo, 2 tsp for 12 to 18 yo. WHO considers honey a cheap, popular, and safe demulcent for children.

FORMS — Mostly not by prescription. Medihoney is FDA approved.

NOTES — Honey may contain trace amounts of antimicrobials used to treat infection in honeybee hives. Medihoney sterile dressings contain Leptospermum (Manuka) honey that is irradiated to inactivate C. botulinum spores.

MOA — Topical: Antimicrobial due to hygroscopic property, low pH, generation of hydrogen peroxide. May also have anti-inflammatory activity. Leptospermum honey may have unique antimicrobial properties. Oral: May act as a demulcent. Laxative effect due to unabsorbed fructose.

ADVERSE EFFECTS — Serious: Botulism from ingestion of honey by infants younger than 1 yo; anaphylaxis reported after honey ingestion in patient with history of Compositae pollen allergy. Topical: Stinging sensation after application in ~5% of patients; local atopic reaction in atopic patients. Oral: Well-tolerated, diarrhea.

HORSE CHESTNUT SEED EXTRACT (*Aesculus hippocastanum, Venastat*) ▶? ♀– ▶– $

UNAPPROVED ADULT — Chronic venous insufficiency (effective): 1 cap Venastat PO two times per day with water before meals. Response within 1 month. American College of Cardiology found evidence insufficient to recommend for peripheral arterial disease.

UNAPPROVED PEDS — Not for use in children.

FORMS — Not by prescription. Venastat (standardized to 16.7% escin) Caps 600 mg.

NOTES — Venastat does not contain aesculin, a toxin in horse chestnuts.

MOA — Escin increases venous pressure; may prevent leukocyte activation or inhibit elastase and hyaluronidase.

ADVERSE EFFECTS — Mild and infrequent GI distress, dizziness, headache.

KAVA (*Piper methysticum*) ▶K ♀– ▶– $

UNAPPROVED ADULT — Promoted as anxiolytic (possibly effective) or sedative; recommend against use due to hepatotoxicity.

UNAPPROVED PEDS — Not for use in children.

FORMS — Not by prescription.

NOTES — Reports of severe hepatotoxicity leading to liver transplantation. May potentiate CNS effects of benzodiazepines and other sedatives, including alcohol. Warn against driving/hazardous tasks after taking kava. Reversible yellow skin discoloration with long-term use.

MOA — Anxiolytic and sedative effects.

ADVERSE EFFECTS — Serious: Reports of severe hepatotoxicity leading to death or liver transplantation. Most cases used kava products prepared by ethanol or acetone extraction methods. Reversible yellow skin discoloration with long-term use. Case report of rhabdomyolysis.

KOMBUCHA TEA ▶? ♀– ▶– $

UNAPPROVED ADULT — Promoted for many indications, but no evidence of benefit for any condition. FDA advises caution due to a case of fatal metabolic acidosis.

UNAPPROVED PEDS — Not for use in children.

FORMS — Not by prescription.

NOTES — Very acidic (pH <2) fermented drink made from addition of bacterial and yeast culture to sweetened black or green tea. It may contain alcohol, ethyl acetate, acetic acid, and lactate. Lead poisoning possible if brewed in lead-glazed ceramic container. Anthrax and aspergillosis contamination possible.

MOA — Culture of bacteria and yeast (Acetobacter, Candida, Saccharomyces, etc) that is very acidic (pH <2) after preparation.

ADVERSE EFFECTS — Serious: Case reports of hepatotoxicity; anti-Jo1 myositis; fatal metabolic acidosis; hyperthermia with lactic acidosis and acute renal failure. Outbreak of cutaneous anthrax from topical application of B anthracis-contaminated kombucha tea. Lead-poisoning from kobucha tea brewed in lead-glazed ceramic pot. Other: Nausea, vomiting, allergy, rash, head/neck pain.

LICORICE (*CankerMelt, Glycyrrhiza*) ▶bile ♀– ▶– $

UNAPPROVED ADULT — Prevention of postoperative sore throat (possibly effective): Licorice 0.5 g in 30 mL water gargled 5 minutes before anesthesia. Aphthous ulcers (efficacy unclear): Apply CankerMelt oral patch to ulcer for 16 h/day until healed. Insufficient data to assess efficacy for postmenopausal vasomotor symptoms.

UNAPPROVED PEDS — Not for use in children.

FORMS — Not by prescription.

NOTES — Chronic high doses can cause pseudo-primary aldosteronism with hypertension, edema, hypokalemia. Cases of myopathy. Diuretics or stimulant laxatives may potentiate licorice-induced hypokalemia. In the US, "licorice" candy often does not contain licorice. Deglycyrrhizinated licorice does not have mineralocorticoid effects.

MOA — Has in vitro antioxidant, antimicrobial, antiviral, and anti-inflammatory activity. Glycyrrhizin has mineralocorticoid activity (not present in deglycyrrhizinated licorice), and antitussive and expectorant properties. Mucilage also sooths cough.

ADVERSE EFFECTS — Pseudo-primary aldosteronism (with hypertension, edema, hypokalemia) possible with chronic high doses. Licorice-induced hypokalemia led to metabolic alkalosis and rhabdomyolysis in case reports. Case reports of myopathy. Transient visual loss.

MELATONIN ▶L ♀– ▶– $

UNAPPROVED ADULT — To reduce jet lag after flights across more than 5 time zones (effective; especially traveling East; may also help for 2 to 4 time zones): 0.5 to 5 mg PO at bedtime (10 pm to midnight) for 3 to 6 nights starting on day of arrival. Faster onset and better sleep quality with 5 mg. No benefit with use before departure or slow-release formulations. Do not take earlier in day; may cause drowsiness and delay adaptation to local time. To promote daytime sleep in night-shift workers: 1.8 to 3 mg PO prior to daytime sleep. Delayed sleep phase disorder: 0.3 to 5 mg PO 1.5 to 6 h before habitual bedtime. Non-24-hour sleep-wake disorder in blind patients with no light perception: 0.3 to 2 mg each night 1 h before bedtime. Possibly effective for difficulty falling asleep, but not staying asleep. American Academy of Sleep Medicine recommends for jet lag, but not chronic insomnia.

UNAPPROVED PEDS — Not usually used in children. Sleep-onset insomnia in ADHD, age 6 yo or older (possibly effective): 3 to 6 mg PO at bedtime. Insomnia in autism (possibly effective for improving sleep latency and duration): Initial dose of 0.5 to 1 mg PO given 30 to 45 minutes before bedtime, increasing the dose in 1 mg increments q 1 to 3 weeks to a max of 10 mg/dose. Non-24-hour sleep-wake disorder in blind patients with no light perception: 0.3 to 2 mg each night 1 h before bedtime.

FORMS — Not by prescription.

(cont.)

MELATONIN (*cont.*)

NOTES — Some experts warn patients with nocturnal asthma to avoid melatonin supplements; high melatonin levels may be linked to nocturnal asthma. Neurologic adverse events reported in children (causality unclear) include anxiety, panic reaction, visual hallucinations, seizures, fatigue, aggression, abnormal dreams, and headache.

MOA — Pineal hormone related to 5-hydroxytryptamine. Synthesis is controlled by environmental factors including light. Melatonin helps to regulate circadian rhythms, induces pigment lightening of skin cells, and suppresses ovarian function at high doses. May reset endogenous circadian pacemaker.

ADVERSE EFFECTS — Adverse effects with short-term use: Nausea, dizziness, restlessness, headache. May cause drowsiness for 4-5 h after the dose; warn against hazardous tasks. May increase withdrawn behavior in elderly patients with dementia. Case reports of hallucinations, psychosis, ulcerative colitis exacerbation, fixed drug eruption, urticarial vasculitis, autoimmune hepatitis. In 2016, Health Canada and WHO reported 173 pediatric adverse events (causality unclear; 71 serious) including anxiety, panic reaction, visual hallucinations, seizures, fatigue, aggression, abnormal dreams, and headache.

METHYLSULFONYLMETHANE (*MSM, dimethyl sulfone, crystalline DMSO2*) ▶? ♀– ▶– $

UNAPPROVED ADULT — Insufficient data to assess efficacy of oral and topical MSM for arthritis pain.

UNAPPROVED PEDS — Not for use in children.

FORMS — Not by prescription.

NOTES — Can cause nausea, diarrhea, headache. DMSO metabolite promoted as a source of sulfur without odor.

MOA — DMSO metabolite promoted as a source of sulfur without odor.

ADVERSE EFFECTS — Nausea, diarrhea, headache.

NETTLE ROOT (*stinging nettle, Urtica dioica radix*) ▶? ♀– ▶– $

UNAPPROVED ADULT — Efficacy unclear for treatment of BPH or OA.

UNAPPROVED PEDS — Not for use in children.

FORMS — Not by prescription.

NOTES — Can cause allergic skin reactions, mild GI upset, sweating. Case reports of gynecomastia in a man and galactorrhea in a woman.

MOA — May have anti-inflammatory effects. Contains phytosterols.

ADVERSE EFFECTS — Allergic skin reactions, mild GI upset, sweating. Case reports of gynecomastia in a man and galactorrhea in a woman.

NONI (*Morinda citrifolia*) ▶? ♀– ▶– $$$

UNAPPROVED ADULT — Promoted for many medical disorders; but insufficient data to assess efficacy.

UNAPPROVED PEDS — Supplements not for use in children.

FORMS — Not by prescription.

NOTES — Potassium content comparable to orange juice. Hyperkalemia reported in a patient with chronic renal failure. Cases of hepatotoxicity.

MOA — Antineoplastic, anthelmintic, and immunostimulant activity in vitro and in animal studies.

ADVERSE EFFECTS — Hyperkalemia reported in a patient with chronic renal failure. Cases of hepatotoxicity.

PEPPERMINT OIL (*Colpermin, IBGard*) ▶LK ♀+ in food, ? in supplements ▶+ in food, ? in supplements $

UNAPPROVED ADULT — Irritable bowel syndrome (possibly effective): 1 to 2 enteric-coated caps (187 mg peppermint oil/0.2 mL) PO three times per day before meals. Do not crush or chew caps. Efficacy of peppermint oil plus caraway seed is unclear for dyspepsia.

UNAPPROVED PEDS — Irritable bowel syndrome (possibly effective), age 15 yo or old: Use adult dose.

FORMS — Not by prescription. Enteric-coated capsules: Colpermin (187 mg peppermint oil/0.2 mL), IBGard (90 mg ultra-purified peppermint oil/cap; marketed as medical food).

NOTES — Generally regarded as safe as food by FDA. May exacerbate GERD. For irritable bowel syndrome, use enteric-coated caps that deliver peppermint oil to lower GI tract. Drugs that increase gastric pH (antacids, H2 blockers, proton pump inhibitors) may dissolve enteric-coated capsules too soon, causing heart burn and reducing benefit. Separate peppermint oil and antacid doses by at least 2 h.

MOA — Menthol, the apparent active ingredient, has antispasmotic activity.

ADVERSE EFFECTS — Perianal burning, nausea.

POLICOSANOL (*CholeRex*) ▶? ♀– ▶– $

UNAPPROVED ADULT — Ineffective for hyperlipidemia. A Cuban formulation (unavailable in the US) reduced LDL cholesterol in studies by one research group. Studies by others, including a study of a US formulation, found no benefit.

UNAPPROVED PEDS — Not for use in children.

FORMS — Not by prescription.

MOA — Mixture of aliphatic alcohols extracted from sugar cane wax (octacosanol). Mechanism of action in hyperlipidemia unknown.

ADVERSE EFFECTS — Serious: None reported.

PROBIOTICS (*Acidophilus, Align, Bacid, Bifantis, Bifidobacteria, BioGaia, Culturelle, Florastor, Gerber Soothe Colic drops, Lactobacillus, Power-Dophilus, Primadophilus, Saccharomyces boulardii, VSL#3*) ▶? ♀+ ▶+ $

ADULT — VSL#3 approved as medical food. Ulcerative colitis (effective): 1 to 2 sachets/day, 0.5 to 1 DS sachet/day, or 4 to 8 caps/day. Active ulcerative colitis, unresponsive to conventional therapy: 4 to 8 sachets/day or 2 to 4 DS sachets/day. Pouchitis (effective; low quality evidence): 2 to 4 sachets/day or 1 to 2 DS sachets/day. Irritable bowel syndrome (may relieve gas and bloating): 0.5 to 1 sachet/day or 2 to 4 caps daily. Mix with cold non-carbonated beverage or cold food before ingesting immediately; caps can be swallowed whole.

UNAPPROVED ADULT — Antibiotic-associated diarrhea (effective): Saccharomyces boulardii 500 mg PO two times per day (Florastor 2 caps PO two times

(cont.)

PROBIOTICS *(cont.)*

per day) during and up to 2 weeks after a course of antibiotics. IDSA recommends against probiotics to prevent C. difficile–associated diarrhea; safety and efficacy are unclear. Probiotics may reduce GI side effects of H. pylori eradication regimens. Bifidobacterium and some combo products improve abdominal pain and bloating in irritable bowel syndrome. (eg, Align 1 cap PO once daily), but Lactobacillus alone did not improve symptoms. Efficacy of probiotics unclear for traveler's diarrhea (conflicting evidence), Crohn's disease, H. pylori, radiation enteritis. Ineffective to prevent of UTI. Lactobacillus GG appears ineffective to prevent post-antibiotic vulvovaginitis.

UNAPPROVED PEDS — Prevention of antibiotic-associated diarrhea (effective): Lactobacillus GG 10 to 20 billion CFU/day PO given 2 h before/after antibiotic or S. boulardii 250 mg PO two times per day (Florastor 1 cap/packet PO two times per day). IDSA recommends against probiotics to prevent C. difficile–associated diarrhea; safety and efficacy are unclear. Acute gastroenteritis, adjunct to rehydration therapy (effective): Lactobacillus GG at least 10 billion (10^{10}) CFU per day for 5 to 7 days or Saccharomyces boulardii 250 to 750 mg per day for 5 to 7 days. Infant colic (efficacy unclear; conflicting study results): 5 drops of L. reuteri DMS 17938 (Gerber Soothe Colic drops) once daily for 21 days. Ulcerative colitis (effective): VSL #3 1 sachet/day for age 4 to 6 yo and wt 17 to 23 kg; 2 sachet/day for age 7 to 9 yo and wt 24 to 33 kg; 3 sachet/day for age 11 to 14 yo and wt 34 to 53 kg; 4 sachet/day for age 15 to 17 yo and wt 54 to 66 kg. Mix with cold non-carbonated beverage or cold food before ingesting. Efficacy of probiotics unclear for radiation enteritis. Lactobacillus GG does not appear effective for Crohn's disease in children. Research ongoing for prevention and treatment of atopic dermatitis.

FORMS — Mostly not by prescription. Culturelle contains Lactobacillus GG 5 billion CFU per powder packet/chewable tab of Culturelle Kids, 10 billion CFU per cap/chewable tab of Culturelle Digestive Health, 15 billion CFU per cap of Culturelle Health & Wellness, 20 billion CFU per cap of Culturelle Extra Strength Digestive Health. Florastor and Florastor Kids contain Saccharomyces boulardii 250 mg per cap/powder packet (contains lactose). VSL#3 (medical food) contains 450 billion CFA/sachet (nonprescription), 900 billion CFU/DS sachet (Rx only), 225 billion cells/2 caps (non-prescription). VSL#3 contains Bifidobacterium breve, B. longum, B. infantis, Lactobacillus acidophilus, L. plantarum, L. casei, L. bulgaricus, Streptococcus thermophilus. Align contains Bifidobacterium infantis 35624, 1 billion cells/cap. Gerber Soothe Colic drops contains Lactobacillus reuteri DSM 17938, 100 million cells per 5 drops. BioGaia ProTectis containsLactobacillus reuteri DSM 17938, 100 million cells per chewable tab/straw.

NOTES — Do not use probiotics in patients with acute pancreatitis; increased mortality and bowel ischemia reported in clinical trial. Acquired infection possible, especially in immunocompromised or critically-ill patients; bacteremia, endocarditis, abscess reported, with possible contamination of central venous access port in some cases. Microbial type and content vary by product. Pick yogurt products labeled "Live and active cultures." Refrigerate packets of VSL#3; can store at room temp for 2 weeks. May contain gluten.

MOA — Lactobacillus bacteria and Saccharomyces boulardii, a nonpathogenic yeast, are part of gut normal flora. They inhibit pathogen attachment in colon, modulate intestinal inflammation, reduce colonic permeability, and may enhance barrier function. Bifidobacterium infantis may reduce gut transit time.

ADVERSE EFFECTS — Serious: Acquired infection possible, especially in immunocompromised or critically ill patients; bacteremia, endocarditis, abscess reported, with possible contamination of central venous access port in some cases. Increased risk of bowel ischemia and death in clinical trial evaluting probiotics for acute pancreatitis.

PYCNOGENOL *(French maritime pine tree bark)* ▶L ♀?
▶? $

UNAPPROVED ADULT — Promoted for many medical disorders, but efficacy unclear for chronic venous insufficiency, sperm dysfunction, melasma, OA, HTN, type 2 diabetes, diabetic retinopathy, and ADHD.

UNAPPROVED PEDS — Not for use in children.

FORMS — Not by prescription.

NOTES — Pine bark (Pycnogenol) and grape seed extract are often confused; they both contain oligomeric proanthocyanidins.

MOA — Antioxidant. Contains oligomeric proanthocyanidins and bioflavonoids.

ADVERSE EFFECTS — GI distress.

PYGEUM AFRICANUM *(African plum tree)* ▶? ♀– ▶– $

UNAPPROVED ADULT — Benign prostatic hypertrophy (may have modest efficacy): 50 to 100 mg PO two times per day or 100 mg PO daily of standardized extract containing 14% triterpenes.

UNAPPROVED PEDS — Not for use in children.

FORMS — Not by prescription.

NOTES — Appears well-tolerated. Self-treatment could delay diagnosis of prostate cancer.

MOA — Unknown, but may inhibit 5-alpha reductase.

ADVERSE EFFECTS — Well-tolerated, GI distress.

RED CLOVER *(red clover isoflavone extract, Trifolium pratense, Promensil, Trinovin)* ▶Gut, L, K ♀– ▶– $$

UNAPPROVED ADULT — Postmenopasual vasomotor symptoms (efficacy unclear; conflicting studies): Promensil 1 tab PO one or two times per day with meals. Appears ineffective overall, but may have modest benefit for severe symptoms. Efficacy unclear to prevent osteoporosis and treat hyperlipidemia in postmenopausal women. Trinovin (1 tab PO daily) marketed to maintain prostate health and

(cont.)

RED CLOVER (*cont.*)

urinary function in men; efficacy unclear for BPH symptoms.

UNAPPROVED PEDS — Not for use in children.

FORMS — Not by prescription. Isoflavone content (genistein, daidzein, biochanin, formononetin) is 40 mg/tab in Promensil and Trinovin.

NOTES — Does not appear to stimulate endometrium. Effect on breast cancer risk is unclear; some experts recommend against use of isoflavone supplements by women with breast cancer (see Soy entry). No effect on breast density in women with Wolfe P2 or DY mammographic breast density patterns. H2 blockers, proton pump inhibitors, and antibiotics may decrease metabolic activation of isoflavones in GI tract. Ingesting lots of red clover can cause bleeding in cattle; bleeding risk in humans is theoretical.

MOA — Contains isoflavone phytoestrogens (biochanin, formononetin, genistein, daidzein), which may act as selective estrogen receptor modulators. Biochanin and formononetin metabolized to genistein and daidzein.

ADVERSE EFFECTS — Appears well tolerated. May increase hepatic transaminases. Safety of isoflavone supplements unclear in women with breast cancer. A case of subarachnoid hemorrhage attributed to supplement containing Siberian ginseng, dong quai, red clover.

RED YEAST RICE (*Monascus purpureus, Xuezhikang, Zhibituo, Hypocol*) ▶L ♀− ▶− $$

UNAPPROVED ADULT — Hyperlipidemia: Usual dose is 1200 mg PO two times per day. Efficacy for hyperlipidemia depends on whether formulation contains lovastatin or other statins. In the US, red yeast rice should only contain trace amounts of statins, but some products contain up to 10 mg lovastatin per cap. Some clinicians consider red yeast rice an alternative for patients with myalgia from prescription statins. In China, it is approved for secondary prevention of CAD.

UNAPPROVED PEDS — Not for use in children.

FORMS — Not by prescription. Xuezhikang marketed in Asia, Norway (HypoCol).

NOTES — Can cause myopathy. Cases of hepatotoxicity. Consider the potential for lovastatin drug interactions.

MOA — Fermentation product of red yeast (Monascus purpureus) grown on rice; it contains some statins (monacolins) and sterols, including lovastatin (Monocolin K).

ADVERSE EFFECTS — Case reports of myopathy, including rhabdomyolysis in a transplant patient treated with cyclosporine. Case reports of hepatotoxicity, peripheral neuropathy. A potential nephrotoxin, citrinin, can be produced with improper fermentation of red yeast rice and has been found in some products in the US. Usual adverse effects of Xuezhikang/Zibituo: Dizziness, stomach ache, abdominal distension, nausea, diarrhea.

S-ADENOSYLMETHIONINE (*SAM-e*) ▶L ♀? ▶? $$$

UNAPPROVED ADULT — Mild to moderate depression (effective): 800 to 1600 mg/day PO in divided doses with meals. Efficacy unclear for OA and alcoholic liver disease.

UNAPPROVED PEDS — Not for use in children.

FORMS — Not by prescription.

NOTES — Serotonin syndrome possible when co-administered with SSRIs. Do not use within 2 weeks of an MAOI or in bipolar disorder.

MOA — Acts as a methyl group donor in methylation reactions. Mechanism of action in depression and osteoarthritis unknown.

ADVERSE EFFECTS — Anxiety, headache, insomnia, nausea, induction of mania in bipolar disorder.

SAW PALMETTO (*Serenoa repens*) ▶? ♀− ▶− $

UNAPPROVED ADULT — Ineffective for BPH symptoms.

UNAPPROVED PEDS — Not for use in children.

FORMS — Not by prescription.

NOTES — Not for use by women of childbearing potential. Does not interfere with PSA test.

MOA — May have anti-androgenic, anti-estrogenic, and estrogenic effects.

ADVERSE EFFECTS — Adverse reactions are mild and infrequent. May cause nausea, diarrhea, abdominal pain. Single case reports of intraoperative hemorrhage and acute pancreatitis.

SHARK CARTILAGE (*Cartilade*) ▶? ♀− ▶− $$$$$

UNAPPROVED ADULT — Appears ineffective for palliative care of advanced cancer. A derivative of shark cartilage was ineffective in a phase 3 clinical trial for non-small-cell lung cancer.

UNAPPROVED PEDS — Not for use in children.

FORMS — Not by prescription.

NOTES — Cases of hypercalcemia linked to calcium content (elemental calcium 130 mg/cap in Cartilade). Salmonella contamination reported in some products.

MOA — Contains proteins, glycoproteins, and glycosaminoglycans (chondroitin). Inhibits tumor angiogenesis in animal models.

ADVERSE EFFECTS — Hypercalcemia due to calcium content, hyperglycemia, GI distress, constipation, hypotension.

SILVER—COLLOIDAL ▶tissues ♀− ▶− $

UNAPPROVED ADULT — The FDA does not recognize OTC colloidal silver products as safe or effective for any use.

UNAPPROVED PEDS — Not for use in children.

FORMS — Not by prescription. May come as silver chloride, cyanide, iodide, oxide, or phosphate.

NOTES — Silver accumulates in skin (leads to permanent grey tint), conjunctiva, and internal organs with chronic use.

MOA — Suspension of silver particles in a colloidal (gelatinous) base. Silver has antimicrobial effects.

ADVERSE EFFECTS — Serious: Silver accumulates in skin (leads to gray tint), conjunctiva, and internal organs with chronic use.

SOUR CHERRY (*Prunus cerasus, Montmorency cherry***)** ▶LK ♀+ for moderate amount in food, – in supplements ▶+ for moderate amount in food, – in supplements $$
UNAPPROVED ADULT — OA (efficacy unclear): 240 mL juice (~45 to 100 Montmorency cherries/dose) PO two times per day. Prevention of gout (efficacy unclear): 15 mL concentrate (~45 to 60 cherries/dose) PO two times per day. Insomnia (possibly effective): 240 mL juice (~50 Montmorency cherries/dose) or 30 mL concentrate (~90 to 100 Montmorency cherries) PO two times per day. Prevention of exercise-induced muscle damage/pain after strenuous exercise (efficacy unclear): 240 mL or 360 mL juice (~50 to 60 Montmorency cherries/dose) or 30 mL concentrate (~90 Montmorency cherries/dose) PO two times per day. Dilute concentrate before drinking.
FORMS — Not by prescription.
MOA — Contains anthocyanins with antioxidant and anti-inflammatory activit (in vitro inhibitor of COX-1 and -2). Some cultivars contain melatonin.
ADVERSE EFFECTS — Serious: Anaphylaxis. Case report of acute reversible renal failure.

SOY (*Genisoy, Healthy Woman, Novasoy, Phyto soya***)** ▶Gut, L, K ♀+ for food, ? for supplements ▶+ for food, ? for supplements $
UNAPPROVED ADULT — Postmenopausal vasomotor symptoms (modest benefit): Per North American Menopause Society, consider 50 mg/day or more of soy isoflavones for at least 12 weeks. Conflicting clinical trials for reducing postmenopausal bone loss. AHA recommends against isoflavone supplements for treatment or prevention of hyperlipidemia, or breast, endometrial, or prostate cancer. Per American Cancer Society and other experts, breast cancer survivors (including tamoxifen-treated women) can consume up to 2 servings/day of soy foods, but should avoid supplements (including soy powder). In epidemiologic studies of breast cancer survivors, higher consumption of soy foods was linked to lower rates of recurrence (including women treated with tamoxifen), but did not appear to affect mortality. No improvement in poorly-controlled asthma with soy isoflavone supplement.
UNAPPROVED PEDS — Soy foods are regarded as safe for children. No improvement in poorly-controlled asthma with soy isoflavone supplement.
FORMS — Not by prescription.
NOTES — Case report of soy milk decreasing INR with warfarin. Report of soy protein decreasing levothyroxine absorption.
MOA — Contains isoflavone phytoestrogens (genistein, daidzein), which may act as estrogen receptor agonists or antagonists. In 30-50% of the population, gut microbes convert daidzein to equol, a nonsteroidal estrogen. Benefit for postmenopausal symptoms may be limited to equol producers. Soy foods are low in saturated fat and high in fiber, vitamins, and minerals.

ADVERSE EFFECTS — Soy is generally regarded as safe as a food. Protein powder may cause GI complaints. High doses (150 mg/day isoflavones) may cause endometrial hyperplasia.

ST. JOHN'S WORT (*Hypericum perforatum***)** ▶L ♀– ▶– $
UNAPPROVED ADULT — Mild to moderate depression (effective): 300 mg PO three times per day of standardized extract (0.3% hypericin).
UNAPPROVED PEDS — Not for use in children. Does not appear effective for ADHD.
FORMS — Not by prescription.
NOTES — Photosensitivity possible with more than 1800 mg/day. Inducer of hepatic CYP3A4, CYP2C9, CYP2C19, and p-glycoprotein. May enhance antiplatelet effect of clopidogrel. May decrease efficacy of drugs with hepatic metabolism including alprazolam, cyclosporine, methadone, non-nucleoside reverse transcriptase inhibitors, omeprazole, oral contraceptives, oxycodone, protease inhibitors, statins, tacrolimus, voriconazole, zolpidem. May need increased dose of digoxin, theophylline, TCAs. Decreased INR with warfarin. Administration with SSRI/SNRI may cause serotonin syndrome. Do not use within 14 days of an MAOI.
MOA — May inhibit uptake of serotonin, dopamine, norepinephrine, GABA, or L-glutamate.
ADVERSE EFFECTS — Serious: Induction of mania/hypomania, serotonin syndrome. Other: Photosensitivity possible with more than 1800 mg/day, dry mouth, dizziness, GI symptoms, fatigue, headache. Better tolerated than paroxetine in short-term trial for depression.

STEVIA (*Stevia rebaudiana***)** ▶L ♀– ▶? $
ADULT — Rebaudioside A (a component of stevia) is FDA approved as a general purpose sweetener.
PEDS — Rebaudioside A (a component of stevia) is FDA approved as a general purpose sweetener.
UNAPPROVED ADULT — Leaves traditionally used as a sweetener but not enough safety data for FDA approval as such. WHO acceptable daily intake of up to 4 mg/kg/day of steviol glycosides. Health Canada advises a max of 280 mg/day of stevia leaf powder in adults.
UNAPPROVED PEDS — Stevia leaves not for use in children.
FORMS — Not by prescription. Rebaudioside A available as Rebiana, Truvia, Pure Via.
NOTES — Unrefined stevia is available as a dietary supplement in the US, but is not FDA approved as a food sweetener. Rebaudioside A (FDA approved as sweetener) lacks bitter aftertaste of unrefined stevia. Canadian labeling advises against use by pregnant women, children, or those with low BP.
MOA — Leaves of stevia plant contain glycosides (stevioside and rebaudioside). Stevioside is 100-fold sweeter than sucrose; rebaudioside A is even sweeter. Stevia may stimulate insulin secretion by pancreatic beta cells at high glucose levels.
ADVERSE EFFECTS — No effect of rebaudioside A on blood pressure or glycemic control in type 2 diabetes.

TEA TREE OIL (*melaleuca oil, Melaleuca alternifolia*) ▶? ♀– ▶– $

UNAPPROVED ADULT — Not for oral use; CNS toxicity reported. Limited evidence for topical treatment of onychomycosis, tinea pedis, acne vulgaris, dandruff, pediculosis.

UNAPPROVED PEDS — Not for use in children.

FORMS — Not by prescription.

NOTES — Can cause allergic contact dermatitis, especially with concentration of 2% or greater.

MOA — Oil distilled from leave of Melaleuca alternifolia; weak antimicrobial, scabicidal, and antifungal activity in vitro.

ADVERSE EFFECTS — Allergic contact dermatitis; products with concentration of 2% or greater linked to skin reactions. Single case reports of immediate hypersensitivity reaction, and gynecomastia in prepubertal boy.

TRIBULUS TERRESTRIS ▶? — ♀? ▶? $$

UNAPPROVED ADULT — Does not appear effective for erectile dysfunction. Does not increase testosterone levels. Studies in athletes do not show an ergogenic effect.

UNAPPROVED PEDS — Not for use in children.

FORMS — Capsules with 625 mg extract standardized to 125 mg of saponins.

MOA — Unknown.

ADVERSE EFFECTS — Toxic to sheep. Case reports of acute renal failure (causality unclear).

VALERIAN (*Valeriana officinalis, Alluna*) ▶? ♀– ▶– $

UNAPPROVED ADULT — Insomnia (possibly modestly effective; conflicting clinical trials): 400 to 900 mg of standardized extract PO 30 min before bedtime. Response reported in 2 to 4 weeks. Alluna (valerian + hops): 2 tabs PO 1 h before bedtime. American Academy of Sleep Medicine does not recommend for chronic insomnia due to inadequate safety and efficacy data.

UNAPPROVED PEDS — Not for use in children.

FORMS — Not by prescription.

NOTES — Do not combine with CNS depressants. Withdrawal symptoms reported after long-term use. Some products have unpleasant smell.

MOA — Valerenic acid inhibits breakdown of GABA in CNS.

ADVERSE EFFECTS — Headache. Some products have unpleasant smell. Withdrawal symptoms reported after long-term use. Serious: Case reports of possible hepatotoxicity.

WILD YAM (*Dioscorea villosa*) ▶L ♀? ▶? $

UNAPPROVED ADULT — Ineffective as topical "natural progestin."

UNAPPROVED PEDS — Not for use in children.

FORMS — Not by prescription.

MOA — Contains diosgenin which is structurally similar to cholesterol. Was used historically to synthesize progestins, cortisone, and androgens; it is not converted to them or DHEA in the body.

ADVERSE EFFECTS — None known.

WILLOW BARK EXTRACT (*Salicis cortex, salicin*) ▶K ♀– ▶– $

UNAPPROVED ADULT — OA, low-back pain (possibly effective): 60 to 240 mg/day salicin PO divided two to three times per day. Onset of pain relief is approximately 2 h. Often included in multi-ingredient wt-loss supplements based on preliminary research suggesting that aspirin increases thermogenesis.

UNAPPROVED PEDS — Not for use in children.

FORMS — Not by prescription. Some products standardized to 15% salicin content.

NOTES — Contraindicated in 3rd trimester of pregnancy and in patients with intolerance or allergy to aspirin or other NSAIDs. Consider contraindications and precautions that apply to other salicylates. Avoid concomitant use of NSAIDs.

MOA — Antipyretic, anti-inflammatory, and analgesic activity. Inhibits prostaglandin synthesis. Salicin, the primary component, is a prodrug that is metabolized to salicylic acid. Salicin does not irreversibly inhibit platelet aggregation like aspirin. The pharmacologic activity of willow is not due solely to salicin.

ADVERSE EFFECTS — Serious: Anaphylactic reactions possible in patients with a history of aspirin hypersensitivity; risk of gastrointestinal bleeding unclear. Frequent: Dose-related tinnitus; GI complaints.

YOHIMBE (*Corynanthe yohimbe, Pausinystalia yohimbe*) ▶L ♀– ▶– $

UNAPPROVED ADULT — Minimal evidence of efficacy for impotence and as aphrodisiac. Risk of adverse events exceeds any potential benefit.

UNAPPROVED PEDS — Not for use in children.

FORMS — Not by prescription.

NOTES — Warn patients to avoid yohimbe dietary supplements; they may contain substantial doses of yohimbine (potent alpha 2-adrenergic blocker which may be an MOAI). Prescription yohimbine no longer available in the US.

MOA — The primary alkaloid in yohimbe bark is yohimbine, a potent alpha 2-adrenergic receptor blocker that may have MAOI activity.

ADVERSE EFFECTS — Hypertension, tachycardia, anxiety/agitation, panic attacks, headache, gastrointestinal distress. Case report of priapism.

IMMUNOLOGY

ADULT IMMUNIZATION SCHEDULE (for more information see CDC website at cdc.gov)

ADULT IMMUNIZATION SCHEDULE*
Tetanus, diphtheria (Td): For all ages, 1 dose booster q 10 years.
Pertussis: Consider single dose of pertussis in adults younger than 65 yo (as part of Tdap), at least 10 years since last tetanus dose. If patient has never received a pertussis booster, use Boostrix if 10 to 18 yo, Adacel if 11 to 64 yo. Administer 1 dose Tdap during each pregnancy.
Influenza: 1 yearly dose (trivalent or quadrivalent) if age 50 yo or older. If younger than 50 yo, then 1 yearly dose if healthcare worker, pregnant, chronic underlying illness, household contact of person with chronic underlying illness or household contact with children younger than 5 yo, or those who request vaccination. Intranasal vaccine indicated for healthy adults younger than 50 yo. Fluzone High-Dose or Fluad vaccine indicated for 65 yo or older.
Pneumococcal (polysccharide, Pneumovax 23): 1 dose if age 65 yo or older. If younger than 65 yo, consider immunizing if chronic underlying illness, nursing home resident. Consider revaccination 5 years later if high risk or if age 65 yo or older and received primary dose before age 65 yo. Pneumococcal (conjugate, Prevnar 13): 1 dose in high-risk adolescents and adults such as those who are immunocpmpromised, those with asplenia, sickle cell/hemoglobinopathies, renal failure, CSF leak, Cochlear implant, as an adjunct to the polysaccharide vaccine.
Hepatitis A: For all ages with clotting factor disorders, chronic liver disease, or exposure risk (travel to endemic areas, illegal drug use, men having sex with men), 2 doses (0, 6 to 12 months). Twinrix (hepatitis A + B) requires 3-dose series.
Hepatitis B: For all ages with medical (hemodialysis, clotting factor recipients, chronic liver disease), occupational (healthcare or public safety workers with blood exposure), behavioral (illegal drug use, multiple sex partners, those seeking evaluation or treatment of sexually transmitted disease, men having sex with men), or other (household/sex contacts of those with chronic HBV or HIV infections, clients/staff of developmentally disabled, more than 6 months of travel to high-risk areas, inmates of correctional facilities) indications, 3 doses (0, 1–2, 4–6 months). Hemodialysis patients require 4 doses and higher dose (40 mcg).
Measles, mumps, rubella (MMR): If born during or after 1957 and immunity in doubt, see www.cdc.gov.
Varicella: For all ages if immunity in doubt, age 13 yo or older, 2 doses separated by 4 to 8 weeks.

CHILDHOOD IMMUNIZATION SCHEDULE*

Age	Birth	Months							Years		
		1	2	4	6	12	15	18	2	4–6	11–12
Hepatitis B	HB	HB				HB					
Rotavirus			Rota	Rota	Rota@						
DTP			DTaP	DTaP	DTaP		DTaP			DTaP	
H. influenzae b			Hib	Hib	Hib^X	Hib^X					
Pneumococcal**			PCV	PCV	PCV	PCV			(PPSV if indicated*)		
Polio			IPV	IPV	IPV					IPV#	
Influenza†					Influenza (yearly)† ≥6 months						
MMR						MMR				MMR	
Varicella						Varicella				Varicella	
Hepatitis A¶						Hep A × 2¶					
Papillomavirus§,¶											HPV × 3§
Meningococcal^											MCV^

*2016 schedule from the CDC, ACIP, AAP, & AAFP, see CDC website (www.cdc.gov).

**Administer 1 dose Prevnar 13 to all healthy children 24 to 59 mo having an incomplete schedule.

***When immunizing adolescents 10 yo or older, consider Tdap if patient has never received a pertussis booster. (Boostrix if 10 yo or older, Adacel if 11 to 64 yo).

@If using Rotarix, give at 2 and 4 mo (no earlier than 6 weeks). Give at 2, 4, and 6 mo if using Rotateq. Max age for final dose is 8 mo.

#Last IPV on or after 4th birthday, and at least 6 months since last dose.

XIf using PedvaxHib or Comvax, dose at 6 mo not necessary, but booster at 12 to 15 mo indicated.

† For healthy patients age 2 yo or older can use intranasal form. If age younger than 9 yo and receiving for first time, administer 2 doses 4 or more weeks apart for injected form and 6 or more weeks apart for intranasal form. FluLaval, Fluarix, and single-dose Fluzone syringe not indicated in younger than 3 years. Fluvirin not indicated in younger than 4 years. Do not use Afluria in younger than 9 years. Do not use Flucelvax, Fluzone ID or Fluzone HD in children.

¶Two doses 6 to 18 months apart. Twinrix (hep A + hep B) requires 3 doses.

§Second and third doses 2 and 6 months after 1st dose. Also approved (Gardasil only) for males 9 to 26 yo to reduce risk of genital warts. Either the quadrivalent or 9-valent or 2-valent (females only) vaccine can be used. Vaccination may begin as early as 9 years of age.

^Vaccinate all children at age 11 to 12 years with a single dose of Menactra or Menveo, with a booster dose at age 16. For high-risk younger children, refer to CDC for recommendations. Consider Trumendat or Bexero in children 10 years or older who are at risk for meningococcal disease.

TETANUS WOUND CARE (www.cdc.gov)

Cell Paragraph	Unknown or less than 3 prior tetanus immunizations	3 or more prior tetanus immunizations
Non-tetanus-prone wound (eg, clean and minor)	DTaP if < 7 yo, Td if 7-10 yo, Tdap if 11 yo or older and no previous Tdap and Td if previously received Tdap.	Td if more than 10 years since last dose
Tetanus-prone wound (eg, dirt, contamination, punctures, crush components)	DTaP if < 7 yo, Td if 7-10 yo, Tdap if 11 yo or older and no previous Tdap and Td if previously received Tdap. Tetanus immune globulin 250 units IM at different site.	Td if more than 5 years since last dose

If patient age 10 yo or older has never received a pertussis booster consider DTaP (Boostrix if 10 yo or older, Adacel if 11–64 yo).

IMMUNOLOGY: Immunizations

NOTE: For vaccine info see CDC website (www.cdc.gov).

BCG VACCINE ▶immune system ♀C ▶? $$$$
WARNING — BCG infections reported in healthcare workers following exposure from accidental needle sticks or skin lacerations. Nosocomial infections reported in patients receiving parenteral drugs that were prepared in areas in which BCG was reconstituted. Serious infections, including fatal infections, have been reported in patients receiving intravesical BCG.
ADULT — 0.2 to 0.3 mL percutaneously (using 1 mL sterile water for reconstitution).
PEDS — Decrease concentration by 50% using 2 mL sterile water for reconstitution, then 0.2 to 0.3 mL percutaneously for age younger than 1 mo. May revaccinate with full dose (adult dose) after 1 yo if necessary. Use adult dose for age older than 1 mo.
MOA — Active immunity, stimulates antibody production.
ADVERSE EFFECTS — Frequent: None.
Comvax **(haemophilus B vaccine + hepatitis B vaccine)** ▶immune system ♀C ▶? $$$
ADULT — Do not use in adults.
PEDS — Infants born of HBsAg (–) mothers: 0.5 mL IM for 3 doses at 2, 4, and 12 to 15 mo.
NOTES — Combination is made of PedvaxHIB (haemophilus B vaccine) + Recombivax HB (hepatitis B vaccine). For infants 8 weeks of age or older.
MOA — Active immunity, stimulates antibody production.
ADVERSE EFFECTS — Frequent: Acute febrile reaction.
DIPHTHERIA, TETANUS, AND ACELLULAR PERTUSSIS VACCINE (***DTaP, Tdap, Infanrix, Daptacel, Boostrix, Adacel***) ▶immune system ♀C ▶– $$
ADULT — 0.5 mL IM in deltoid as a single dose, 2 to 5 years since last tetanus dose one time only. ACIP recommends Tdap in every pregnancy, preferably between 27 and 35 weeks of gestation.

PEDS — Check immunization history: DTaP is preferred for all DTP doses. Give first dose of 0.5 mL IM at approximately 2 mo, second dose at 4 mo, third dose at 6 mo, fourth dose at 15 to 18 mo, and fifth dose (booster) at 4 to 6 yo. Use Boostrix only if 10 yo or older, and at least 2 to 5 years after the last childhood dose of DTaP. Use Adacel only in 11 to 64 yo and at least 2 to 5 years after last childhood dose of DTaP or Td.
NOTES — When feasible, use same brand for first 3 doses. Do not give if prior DTaP vaccination caused anaphylaxis or encephalopathy within 7 days. Do not use Boostrix or Adacel for primary childhood vaccination series, if prior DTaP vaccination caused anaphylaxis or encephalopathy, or if progressive neurologic disorders (eg, encephalopathy) or uncontrolled epilepsy. For adolescents and adults, only 1 dose should be given, at least 2 to 5 years after last tetanus dose. Specify Adacel/Boostrix vaccine for adolescent and adult booster as pediatric formulations have increased pertussis concentrations and may increase local reaction. No information available on repeat doses in adolescents or adults.
MOA — Active immunity, stimulates antibody production.
ADVERSE EFFECTS — Frequent: Agitation, drowsiness, pain, redness and swelling at injection site, headache, fatigue.
DIPHTHERIA-TETANUS TOXOID (***Td, DT, ✱D2T5***) ▶immune system ♀C ▶? $
ADULT — 0.5 mL IM, second dose 4 to 8 weeks later, and third dose 6 to 12 months later. Give 0.5 mL booster dose at 10-year intervals. Use adult formulation (Td) for adults and children at least 7 yo.
PEDS — 0.5 mL IM for age 6 weeks to 6 yo, second dose 4 to 8 weeks later, and third dose 6 to 12 months later using DT for pediatric use. If immunization of infants begins in the first year of life using

(cont.)

DIPHTHERIA-TETANUS TOXOID (*cont.*)

DT rather than DTP (ie, pertussis is contraindicated), give three 0.5 mL doses 4 to 8 weeks apart, followed by a fourth dose 6 to 12 months later.

FORMS — Injection DT (Peds: 6 weeks to 6 yo). Td (adult and children at least 7 yo).

NOTES — DTaP is preferred for most children age less than 7 yo. Td is preferred for adults and children at least 7 yo.

MOA — Active immunity, stimulates antibody production.

ADVERSE EFFECTS — Frequent: Agitation, drowsiness.

HAEMOPHILUS B VACCINE (*ActHIB, Hiberix, PedvaxHIB*)
▶immune system ♀C ▶? $$

PEDS — Doses vary depending on formulation used and age at first dose. ActHIB: Give 0.5 mL IM for 3 doses at 2-month intervals for age 2 to 6 mo, give 0.5 mL IM for 2 doses at 2-month intervals for age 7 to 11 mo, give 0.5 mL IM for 1 dose for age 12 to 14 mo. A single 0.5 mL IM booster dose is given to previously immunized children at least 15 mo, and at least 2 months after the previous injection. For children age 15 mo to 5 yo at age of first dose, give 0.5 mL IM for 1 dose (no booster). PedvaxHIB: 0.5 mL IM for 2 doses at 2-month intervals for age 2 to 14 mo. If the 2 doses are given before 12 mo, a third 0.5 mL IM (booster) dose is given at least 2 months after the second dose. 0.5 mL IM for 1 dose (no booster) for age 15 mo to 5 yo.

UNAPPROVED ADULT — Asplenia, at least 14 days prior to elective splenectomy, or immunodeficiency: 0.5 mL IM for 1 dose of any Hib conjugate vaccine.

UNAPPROVED PEDS — Asplenia, at least 14 days prior to elective splenectomy, or immunodeficiency age 5 yo or older: 0.5 mL IM for 1 dose of any Hib vaccine.

NOTES — Not for IV use. No data on interchangeability between brands; AAP and ACIP recommend use of any product in children age 12 to 15 mo.

MOA — Active immunity, stimulates antibody production.

ADVERSE EFFECTS — Frequent: Acute febrile reaction, soreness and redness at injection site.

HEPATITIS A VACCINE (*Havrix, Vaqta, ✳Avaxim*)
▶immune system ♀C ▶+ $$$

ADULT — Havrix: 1 mL (1440 ELU) IM, then 1 mL (1440 ELU) IM booster dose 6 to 12 months later. Vaqta: 1 mL (50 units) IM, then 1 mL (50 units) IM booster 6 months later for age 18 yo or older.

PEDS — Havrix: 0.5 mL (720 ELU) IM for 1 dose, then 0.5 mL (720 ELU) IM booster 6 to 12 months after first dose for age 1 to 18 yo. Vaqta: 0.5 mL (25 units) IM for 1 dose, then 0.5 mL (25 units) IM booster 6 to 18 months later for age 1 to 18 yo.

FORMS — Single-dose vial (specify pediatric or adult).

NOTES — Do not inject IV, SC, or ID. Brands may be used interchangeably. Need for boosters is unclear. Postexposure prophylaxis with hepatitis A vaccine alone is not recommended. Should be given 4 weeks prior to travel to endemic area. May be given at the same time as immune globulin, but preferably at different site.

MOA — Active immunity, stimulates antibody production.

ADVERSE EFFECTS — Frequent: Headache, pain, tenderness, warmth, soreness and redness at injection site.

HEPATITIS B VACCINE (*Engerix-B, Recombivax HB*)
▶immune system ♀C ▶+ $$$

ADULT — Engerix-B: 1 mL (20 mcg) IM, repeat in 1 and 6 months for age 20 yo or older. Hemodialysis: Give 2 mL (40 mcg) IM, repeat in 1, 2, and 6 months. Give 2 mL (40 mcg) IM booster when antibody levels decline to less than 10 mIU/mL. Recombivax HB: 1 mL (10 mcg) IM, repeat in 1 and 6 months. Hemodialysis: 1 mL (40 mcg) IM, repeat in 1 and 6 months. Give 1 mL (40 mcg) IM booster when antibody levels decline to less than 10 mIU/mL. Patients with diabetes: ACIP recommends hepatitis B vaccine for all previously unvaccinated diabetics age 19 through 59 yo, vaccinate as soon as possible after diabetes diagnosis.

PEDS — Dosing based on age and maternal HBsAg status. Engerix-B 10 mcg (0.5 mL) IM 0, 1, 6 months for infants of hepatitis B–negative and –positive mothers and children age 15 to 20 yo. Recombivax 5 mcg (0.5 mL) IM 0, 1, 6 months for infants of hepatitis B–negative and –positive mothers and children age 15 to 20 yo. A 2-dose schedule can be used (Recombivax HB) 10 mcg (1 mL) IM at 0 and 4 to 6 months for age 11 to 15 yo.

NOTES — Infants born to hepatitis B–positive mothers should also receive hepatitis B immune globulin and hepatitis B vaccine within 12 h of birth. Not for IV or ID use. May interchange products. CDC states acceptable to administer each of 3 doses to diabetics on a schedule matching convenient timing of healthcare visits scheduled for routine follow up, instead of usual 0, 1, and 6 months. Must still observe minimum intervals between doses. Recombivax HB dialysis formulation is intended for adults only. Avoid if yeast allergy.

MOA — Active immunity, stimulates antibody production.

ADVERSE EFFECTS — Frequent: Dizziness, malaise, pain and tenderness at injection site.

HUMAN PAPILLOMAVIRUS RECOMBINANT VACCINE (*Cervarix, Gardasil*) ▶immune system ♀B ▶? $$$$$

ADULT — Prevention of cervical cancer, vulvar and vaginal cancer in females 9 to 26 yo (HPV2, HPV4, HPV9): 0.5 mL IM at time 0, 2, and 6 months. Prevention of anal cancer, genital warts, anal intraepithelial neoplasia in males 9 to 26 yo (Gardasil only, HPV4 or HPV9): 0.5 mL IM at time 0, 2, and 6 months.

PEDS — Prevention of cervical cancer, vulvar and vaginal cancer in females 9 to 26 yo(HPV2, HPV4, HPV9): 0.5 mL IM at time 0, 2, and 6 months. Prevention of anal cancer, genital warts, anal intraepithelial neoplasia in males 9 to 26 yo

(cont.)

HUMAN PAPILLOMAVIRUS RECOMBINANT VACCINE (*cont.*)

(Gardasil only, HPV4 or HPV9): 0.5 mL IM at time 0, 2, and 6 months.

NOTES — Patients must be counseled to continue to use condoms. Immunosuppression may reduce response. Fainting and falling may occur after vaccination; observe patient for 15 min after vaccination. Cervarix (HPV2) not approved for use in males. Gardasil available as HPV4 and HPV9.

MOA — Active immunity, stimulates antibody production.

ADVERSE EFFECTS — Frequent: Pain, tenderness, pruritus and erythema at injection site, fainting.

INFLUENZA VACCINE—INACTIVATED INJECTION (*Fluad, Afluria, Fluarix, FluLaval, Fluzone, Fluvirin, Flucelvax, Flublok, ✱Influvac, Agriflu, Flulaval Tetra, Fluviral, Vaxigrip*) ▸immune system ♀C ▶+ $

ADULT — 0.5 mL IM or ID (Fluzone ID). Fluarix, FluLaval not indicated in children younger than 3 yo. Fluvirin not indicated in children younger than 4 yo. Afluria not indicated in children younger than 9 yo. Flublok for 18 to 49 yo. Flucelvax for 18 yo and older. Fluzone ID for 18 to 64 yo. Fluzone HD and Fluad for 65 yo and older.

PEDS — Give 0.25 mL IM for age 6 to 35 mo (Fluzone only), repeat dose after 4 weeks if previously unvaccinated. Give 0.5 mL IM for age 3 to 8 yo (Fluzone, Fluarix, FluLaval if 3 yo or older, Fluvirin if 4 yo or older) repeat dose after 4 weeks if previously unvaccinated. Give 0.5 mL IM once a year for age 9 to 12 yo.

NOTES — Fluarix, FluLaval not indicated in children younger than 3 yo. Fluvirin not indicated in children younger than 4 yo. Afluria not indicated in children younger than 9 yo. Flucelvax for 18 yo and older. Fluzone ID for 18 to 64 yo; lower amount of antigen, lower immunogenicity, and higher rate of local reactions compared with standard IM injections. Fluzone HD and Fluad for 65 yo; clinically greater flu prevention, but may be associated with increased rate of local reactions. HD formulation only available as trivalent formulation. Many IM formulations are quadrivalent (2 strains of A and B). Thimerosal-free products available. Optimal administration October to November. Flublok is egg-free product for those 18 to 49 yo with egg allergy.

MOA — Active immunity, stimulates antibody production.

ADVERSE EFFECTS — Frequent: Fever, malaise, pain, tenderness and erythema at injection site. Severe: Allergic or anaphylactoid reactions in egg-allergic persons, Guillain-Barré syndrome, angioedema.

INFLUENZA VACCINE—LIVE INTRANASAL (*FluMist*) ▸immune system ♀C ▶+ $

ADULT — The CDC recommends against the use of FluMist for the 2016-17 season. 1 dose (0.2 mL) intranasally once a year for healthy adults age 18 to 49 yo.

PEDS — The CDC recommends against the use of FluMist for the 2016-17 season. 1 dose (0.2 mL) intranasally for healthy children age 2 to 17 yo, repeat dose after 4 weeks if previously unvaccinated and age 2 to 8 yo. If available, live, intranasal vaccine should be preferentially used for healthy children age 2 through 8 yo who have no contraindications or precautions.

NOTES — Avoid in Guillain-Barré syndrome, chicken egg allergy, aspirin therapy in children (Reye's risk), pregnancy, chronic illness that could increase vulnerability to influenza complications (CHF, asthma, diabetes, renal failure), recurrent wheezing, and in children younger than 2 yo. Optimal administration October to November. Because FluMist is a live vaccine, do not use with immune deficiencies (eg, HIV, malignancy) or altered immune status (eg, taking systemic corticosteroids, chemotherapy, radiation).

MOA — Active immunity, stimulates antibody production.

ADVERSE EFFECTS — Frequent: Fever, malaise. Severe: Allergic or anaphylactoid reactions in egg-allergic persons, Guillain-Barré syndrome, angioedema.

JAPANESE ENCEPHALITIS VACCINE (*Ixiaro*) ▸immune system ♀C ▶? $$$$

ADULT — 1 mL SC for 3 doses on days 0, 7, and 30.

PEDS — 0.5 mL SC for 3 doses on days 0, 7, and 30 for age 1 to 3 yo. Give 1 mL SC for 3 doses on days 0, 7, and 30 for age 3 yo or older.

NOTES — Give at least 10 days before travel to endemic areas. An abbreviated schedule on days 0, 7, and 14 can be given if time limits. A booster dose may be given after 2 years. Avoid in thimerosal allergy.

MOA — Active immunity, stimulates antibody production.

ADVERSE EFFECTS — Frequent: Tenderness, redness and swelling at injection site. Severe: Anaphylactic reaction, angioedema, dyspnea, encephalitis, encephalopathy, erythema nodosum, erythema multiforme, peripheral neuropathy, seizures.

MEASLES, MUMPS, AND RUBELLA VACCINE (*M-M-R II, ✱Priorix*) ▸immune system ♀C ▶+ $$$

ADULT — 0.5 mL (1 vial) SC.

PEDS — 0.5 mL (1 vial) SC for age 12 to 15 mo. Revaccinate prior to elementary and/or middle school according to local health guidelines. If measles outbreak, may immunize infants 6 to 12 mo with 0.5 mL SC; then start 2-dose regimen between 12 and 15 mo.

NOTES — Do not inject IV. Contraindicated in pregnancy. Advise women to avoid pregnancy for 4 weeks following vaccination. Live virus, contraindicated in immunocompromised patients. Avoid if allergic to neomycin or gelatin; caution in egg allergy.

MOA — Active immunity, stimulates antibody production.

ADVERSE EFFECTS — Frequent: Fever, burning, induration, rash. Severe: Allergic reactions, encephalitis, convulsions, erythema multiforme, prolonged high fever, Guillain-Barré syndrome, thrombocytopenia.

MENINGOCOCCAL VACCINE (*Bexsero, Menveo, Menomune-A/C/Y/W-135, Menactra, Trumenba,* ✱*Menjugate*) ▶immune system ♀C ▶? $$$$
WARNING — Reports of associated Guillain-Barré syndrome; avoid if prior history of this condition.
ADULT — 0.5 mL SC (Menomune) or IM (Menactra, Menveo) in high-risk individuals (asplenia, etc), repeat in 2 months. Trumenba: Three-dose series (0.5 mL) starting at 0, 2, and 6 months in those 10 to 25 years. Bexsero: 2 doses (0.5 mL) at 0 and 1 month in those 10 to 25 years. Adult MenB series at age 16-23 years (preferred 16-18 years) is discretionary for average-risk individuals. Supplemental dosing of MenACWY, 5 year revaccination for MenACWY and nondiscretionary dosing of MenB is indicated for asplenia, complement deficiency, other high-risk conditions in adults.
PEDS — Menveo: Four-dose series starting at 2 mo at 2, 4, 6, and 12 months. Menactra: Vaccinate all children 11 to 12 yo, and 16 yo. One dose only if between 13 and 18 yo and previously unvaccinated. Children 10 yo or older: Trumenba: Three-dose series starting at 0, 2, and 6 months. Bexsero: 2 doses at 0 and 1 months.
UNAPPROVED PEDS — 0.5 mL SC for 2 doses separated by 3 months for age 3 to 18 mo. Single dose MenACWY at age 11 or 12 with booster dose at age 16; additional administration of MenB series at age 16 to 23 yo (preferred 16 to 18 yo) is discretionary for average risk individuals. Multiple doses of MenACWY age 2 mo to 18 yo and nondiscretionary dosing of MenB in children older than 10 yo is recommended for asplenia, complement deficiency, other high risk conditions in children.
NOTES — Quadrivalent vaccines (MenACWY) include Menomune, Menactra, Menveo. Serogroup B vaccines (MenB) include Trumenba, Bexsero. Give 2 weeks before elective splenectomy or travel to endemic areas. May consider revaccination every 3 to 5 years in high-risk patients. Do not inject IV. Contraindicated in pregnancy. Do not administer Menactra for at least 4 weeks after completion of pneumococcal vaccination, or efficacy of pneumococcal vaccination will be diminished. Minimum age for administration: 9 mo for Menactra, 2 mo for Menveo, 10 years for MenB vaccines. The two MenB vaccines are not interchangeable; the same vaccine product must be used for all doses. Vaccinate all first-year college students living in dormitories who are unvaccinated. Avoid in thimerosal allergy (except Menactra which is thimerosal-free). Although Trumenba and Bexsero are approved for use in ages 10 to 25 yo, ACIP gives no upper age limit.
MOA — Active immunity, stimulates antibody production.
ADVERSE EFFECTS — Frequent: Pain, erythema, induration, tenderness. Severe: Guillain-Barré syndrome.

PEDIARIX (diphtheria tetanus and acellular pertussis vaccine + hepatitis B vaccine + polio vaccine) ▶immune system ♀C ▶? $$$
PEDS — 0.5 mL at 2, 4, 6 mo IM.
NOTES — Do not administer before 6 weeks of age.
MOA — Active immunity, stimulates antibody production.
ADVERSE EFFECTS — Frequent: Local injection site reactions (pain, swelling, redness), fever, fussiness. Severe: Convulsions, encephalopathy.
PLAGUE VACCINE ▶Immune system ♀C ▶+ $
ADULT — 1 mL IM for 1 dose, then 0.2 mL IM 1 to 3 months after the first injection, then 0.2 mL IM 5 to 6 months after the second injection for age 18 to 61 yo.
PEDS — Not approved in children.
NOTES — Up to 3 booster doses (0.2 mL) may be administered at 6-month intervals in high-risk patients. Jet injector gun may be used for IM administration.
MOA — Active immunity, stimulates antibody production.
ADVERSE EFFECTS — Frequent: Malaise, fever, headache, tenderness, nausea.
PNEUMOCOCCAL 13-VALENT CONJUGATE VACCINE (*Prevnar 13*) ▶immune system ♀C ▶? $$$
ADULT — Indicated for some high-risk adolescents and adults (immunocompromised, asplenic state, sickle cell/hemoglobinopathy, renal failure, CSF leak, Cochlear implant) as an adjunct to the 23-valent pneumococcal vaccine. All adults 65 years and older should receive one dose. Delay 13-valent vaccine at least 1 year after 23-valent vaccine or delay 23-valent vaccine 8 weeks after 13-valent vaccine.
PEDS — 0.5 mL IM for 3 doses at 2 mo, 4 mo, and 6 mo, followed by a 4th dose of 0.5 mL IM at 12 to 15 mo. For previously unvaccinated older infants and children age 7 to 11 mo: 0.5 mL for 2 doses 4 weeks apart, followed by a 3rd dose of 0.5 mL at 12 to 15 mo. For previously unvaccinated older infants and children age 12 to 23 mo: Give 0.5 mL for 2 doses 8 weeks apart. For previously unvaccinated children 24 mo to 5 yo, give a single 0.5 mL dose IM before the 6th birthday.
NOTES — Recommended adult administration relative to PPSV23: Delay PCV13 at least 1 year after PPSV23 or delay PPSV23 8 weeks after PCV13. For IM use only; do not inject IV. Shake susp vigorously prior to administration.
MOA — Active immunity, stimulates antibody production.
ADVERSE EFFECTS — Frequent: Erythema, induration, tenderness. Severe: Component hypersensitivity.
PNEUMOCOCCAL 23-VALENT VACCINE, PPSV23 (*Pneumovax,* ✱*Pneumo 23*) ▶immune system ♀C ▶+ $$
ADULT — All adults 65 yo or older: 0.5 mL IM/SC for 1 dose. Vaccination also recommended for high-risk individuals younger than age 65 yo. Routine revaccination in immunocompetent patients is not

(cont.)

PNEUMOCOCCAL 23-VALENT VACCINEPPSV23 (*cont.*)

recommended, but in those 19 years or older with immunocompromising conditions, a second dose of PPSV23 at least 5 years after the first dose of PPSV23 should be considered. Consider revaccination once in patients age 65 yo or older who were vaccinated before the age of 65 years.

PEDS — 0.5 mL IM/SC for age 2 yo or older. Consider revaccination once in patients at high risk of developing serious pneumococcal infection after 3 to 5 years from initial vaccine in patients who would be 10 yo or younger at time of revaccination.

NOTES — Do not give IV or ID. May be given in conjunction with influenza virus vaccine at different site. OK for high-risk children at least 2 yo who received Prevnar series already to provide additional serotype coverage. Consult CDC guidelines for intervals between PCV13 and PPSV23 pneumococcal vaccines.

MOA — Active immunity, stimulates antibody production.

ADVERSE EFFECTS — Frequent: Induration and soreness at the injection site. Severe: Anaphylaxis, Guillain-Barré syndrome,

POLIO VACCINE (*IPOL*) ▶immune system ♀C ▶? $$

ADULT — Previously unvaccinated adults at increased risk of exposure should receive a complete primary immunization series of 3 doses (2 doses at intervals of 4 to 8 weeks; a third dose at 6 to 12 months after the second dose). Accelerated schedules are available. Travelers to endemic areas who have received primary immunization should receive a single booster in adulthood.

PEDS — 0.5 mL IM/SC at age 2 mo, with second dose at 4 mo, third dose at 6 to 18 mo, and fourth dose at 4 to 6 yo.

NOTES — Oral polio vaccine no longer available.

MOA — Active immunity, stimulates antibody production.

ADVERSE EFFECTS — Frequent; Fever, erythema, induration, pain, irritability, sleepiness, fussiness, crying.

***PROQUAD* (measles, mumps, and rubella vaccine + varicella vaccine)** ▶immune system ♀C ▶? $$$$

ADULT — Not indicated in adults.

PEDS — 0.5 mL (1 vial) SC for age 12 mo to 12 yo.

NOTES — Give at least 1 month after a MMR-containing vaccine and at least 3 months after a varicella-containing vaccine. Do not inject IV. Contraindicated in pregnancy. Following vaccination avoid pregnancy for 3 months and aspirin/salicylates for 6 weeks. Live virus, contraindicated in immunocompromise or untreated TB. Avoid if allergic to neomycin; caution with egg allergies.

MOA — Active immunity, stimulates antibody production.

ADVERSE EFFECTS — Frequent: Fever, pain, tenderness, soreness, swelling, rash. Severe: Allergic reactions, encephalitis, convulsions, erythema multiforme, prolonged high fever, Guillain-Barré syndrome, thrombocytopenia.

RABIES VACCINE (*RabAvert, Imovax Rabies, BioRab*) ▶immune system ♀C ▶? $$$$$

ADULT — Postexposure prophylaxis: Give rabies immune globulin (20 international units/kg) immediately after exposure, then give rabies vaccine 1 mL IM in deltoid region on days 0, 3, 7, 14, and 28. If patients have received pre-exposure immunization, give 1 mL IM rabies vaccine on days 0 and 3 only, without rabies immune globulin. Pre-exposure immunization: 1 mL IM rabies vaccine on days 0, 7, and between days 21 and 28. Or 0.1 mL ID on days 0, 7, and between days 21 and 28. (Imovax Rabies ID vaccine formula only). Repeat q 2 to 5 years based on antibody titer.

PEDS — Same as adults.

NOTES — Do not use ID preparation for postexposure prophylaxis.

MOA — Active immunity, stimulates antibody production.

ADVERSE EFFECTS — Frequent: Pain, swelling, erythema, pruritus. Severe: Immune-complex like reactions, Guillain-Barré syndrome.

ROTAVIRUS VACCINE (*RotaTeq, Rotarix*) ▶immune system ♀- ▶? $$$$$

ADULT — Not recommended.

PEDS — RotaTeq: Give the first dose (2 mL PO) between 6 and 12 weeks of age, and then the second and third doses at 4- to 10-week intervals thereafter (last dose no later than 32 weeks). Rotarix: Give first dose (1 mL) at 6 weeks of age, and second dose (1 mL) at least 4 weeks later, and prior to 24 weeks of age.

FORMS — Trade only: Oral susp 2 mL (RotaTeq), 1 mL (Rotarix).

NOTES — Live vaccine so potential for transmission, especially to immunodeficient close contacts. Safety unclear in immunocompromised infants.

MOA — Active immunity, stimulates antibody production.

ADVERSE EFFECTS — Frequent: Diarrhea, vomiting.

SMALLPOX VACCINE (*ACAM 2000, vaccinia vaccine*) ▶immune system ♀C ▶- Not available to civilians.

ADULT — Prevention of smallpox or monkeypox: Specialized administration using bifurcated needle SC for 1 dose.

PEDS — Specialized administration using bifurcated needle SC for 1 dose for children older than 1 yo.

NOTES — Caution in polymyxin, neomycin, tetracycline, or streptomycin allergy. Avoid in those (or household contacts of those) with eczema or a history of eczema, those with a rash due to other causes (eg, burns, zoster, impetigo, psoriasis), immunocompromised, or pregnancy. Persons with known cardiac disease or at least 3 risk factors for cardiac disease should not be vaccinated.

MOA — Active immunity, stimulates antibody production.

ADVERSE EFFECTS — Frequent: Fever, malaise, swelling/tenderness of regional lymph nodes. Severe: Generalized vaccinia, encephalitis, encephalopathy, eczema vaccinatum, myopericarditis, myocardial infarction, angina, death.

TETANUS TOXOID ▶immune system ♀C ▶+ $$

WARNING — Td is preferred in adults and children age 7 yo or older. DTaP is preferred in children younger than 7 yo. Use fluid tetanus toxoid in assessing cell-mediated immunity only.

ADULT — 0.5 mL IM (adsorbed) for 2 doses 4 to 8 weeks apart. Give third dose 6 to 12 months after second injection. Give booster q 10 years. Assess cell-mediated immunity: 0.1 mL of 1:100 diluted skin-test reagent or 0.02 mL of 1:10 diluted skin-test reagent injected intradermally.

PEDS — 0.5 mL IM (adsorbed) for 2 doses 4 to 8 weeks apart. Give third dose 6 to 12 months after second injection. Give booster q 10 years.

NOTES — May use tetanus toxoid fluid for active immunization in patients hypersensitive to the aluminum adjuvant of the adsorbed formulation: 0.5 mL IM or SC for 3 doses at 4- to 8-week intervals. Give fourth dose 6 to 12 months after third injection. Give booster dose q 10 years. Avoid in thimerosal allergy.

MOA — Active immunity, stimulates antibody production.

ADVERSE EFFECTS — Frequent: Local induration at the injection site, chills, fever. Severe: Hypersensitivity reactions, fever (>103 F), neurological disturbances.

TWINRIX (hepatitis A vaccine + hepatitis B vaccine) ▶immune system ♀C ▶? $$$$

ADULT — 1 mL IM in deltoid only for age 18 yo or older, repeat at 1 and 6 months. All 3 doses required for hepatitis A immunity. Accelerated dosing schedule: 0, 7, 21, and 30 days and booster dose at 12 months.

PEDS — Not approved in children.

NOTES — Not for IV or ID use. 1 mL is equivalent to 720 ELU inactivated hepatitis A + 20 mcg hepatitis B surface antigen. Due to lower antigen dose of hepatitis A in Twinrix product compared with standard 2-dose hep A vaccine, all three doses must be given for hepatitis A immunity in adults.

MOA — Active immunity, stimulates antibody production.

ADVERSE EFFECTS — Frequent: Headache, local pain, tenderness, warmth, dizziness, malaise, urticaria, rash, erythema. Severe: Angioedema, anaphylaxis.

TYPHOID VACCINE—INACTIVATED INJECTION (Typhim Vi, ✱Typherix) ▶immune system ♀C ▶? $$

ADULT — 0.5 mL IM for 1 dose given at least 2 weeks prior to potential exposure. May consider revaccination q 2 years in high-risk patients.

PEDS — Same as adult dose for age 2 yo or older.

NOTES — Recommended for travel to endemic areas.

MOA — Active immunity, stimulates antibody production.

ADVERSE EFFECTS — Frequent: Headache, fever, local tenderness at site, erythema, induration, myalgia.

TYPHOID VACCINE—LIVE ORAL (Vivotif Berna) ▶immune system ♀C ▶? $$

ADULT — 1 cap 1 h before a meal with cold or lukewarm drink every other day for 4 doses to be completed at least 1 week prior to potential exposure. May consider revaccination every 5 years in high-risk patients.

PEDS — Give adult dose for age 6 yo or older.

FORMS — Trade only: Caps.

NOTES — Recommended for travel to endemic areas. Oral vaccine may be inactivated by antibiotics, including antimalarials.

MOA — Active immunity, stimulates antibody production.

ADVERSE EFFECTS — Frequent (oral): Rash, abdominal pain, diarrhea, N/V.

VARICELLA VACCINE (Varivax, ✱Varilrix) ▶immune system ♀C ▶+ $$$$

ADULT — 0.5 mL SC. Repeat 4 to 8 weeks later.

PEDS — 0.5 mL SC for 1 dose for age 1 to 12 yo. Repeat at ages 4 yo to 6 yo. Use adult dose for age 13 yo or older. Not recommended for infants younger than 1 yo.

UNAPPROVED PEDS — Postexposure prophylaxis: 0.5 mL SC within 3 to 5 days of exposure.

NOTES — Do not inject IV. Following vaccination avoid pregnancy for 3 months and aspirin/salicylates for 6 weeks. This live vaccine is contraindicated in immunocompromised.

MOA — Active immunity, stimulates antibody production.

ADVERSE EFFECTS — Frequent: Fever, inflammation at the injection site.

YELLOW FEVER VACCINE (YF-Vax) ▶immune system ♀C ▶+ $$$

ADULT — 0.5 mL SC.

PEDS — 0.5 mL SC into thigh (6 mo to 3 yo) or deltoid region for age 3 yo or older.

NOTES — Must be accredited site to administer vaccination. International Certificate of Vaccination obligatory for some travel destinations. Consult CDC traveler's health website for accredited sites or to apply for accreditation. A booster dose (0.5 mL) may be administered every 10 years.

MOA — Active immunity, stimulates antibody production.

ADVERSE EFFECTS — Frequent: Fever, malaise, headache, myalgia.

ZOSTER VACCINE—LIVE (Zostavax) ▶immune system ♀C ▶? $$$$

ADULT — 0.65 mL SC for 1 dose for age 50 yo or older. However, ACIP recommends immunizing those 60 yo and older.

PEDS — Not approved in children.

NOTES — Avoid if history of anaphylactic/anaphylactoid reaction to gelatin or neomycin, if primary or acquired immunodeficiency states, or if taking immunosuppressives. IDSA guidelines state low-level immunosuppression (methotrexate, azathioprine, 6-mercaptopurine, or prednisone less than 20 mg/day is not a contraindication to vaccination. Do not administer if active untreated TB or in possible pregnancy. Theoretically possible to transmit to pregnant household contact who has not had varicella infection or immunocompromised contact. Do not substitute for Varivax in children.

MOA — Active immunity, boosts pre-existing immunity on individuals who have a history of varicella disease.

ADVERSE EFFECTS — Frequent: Pain, tenderness, pruritus and erythema at injection site.

IMMUNOLOGY: Immunoglobulins

NOTE: Adult IM injections should be given in the deltoid region; injection in the gluteal region may result in suboptimal response.

ANTIVENIN—CROTALIDAE IMMUNE FAB OVINE POLYVALENT (*CroFab*) ▶? ♀C ▶? $$$$$
ADULT — Rattlesnake envenomation: Give 4 to 6 vials IV infusion over 60 min, within 6 h of bite if possible. Administer 4 to 6 additional vials if no initial control of envenomation syndrome, then 2 vials q 6 h for up to 18 h (3 doses) after initial control has been established.
PEDS — Same as adults, although specific studies in children have not been conducted.
NOTES — Contraindicated in allergy to papaya or papain. Start IV infusion slowly over the first 10 min at 25 to 50 mL/h and observe for allergic reaction, then increase to full rate of 250 mL/h.
MOA — Antivenom.
ADVERSE EFFECTS — Frequent: None,

ANTIVENIN—CROTALIDAE POLYVALENT ▶L ♀C ▶? $$$$$
ADULT — Pit viper envenomation: 20 to 40 mL (2 to 4 vials) IV infusion for minimal envenomation, 50 to 90 mL (5 to 9 vials) IV infusion for moderate envenomation; give at least 100 to 150 mL (10 to 15 vials) IV infusion for severe envenomation. Administer within 4 h of bite, less effective after 8 h, and of questionable value after 12 h. May give additional 10 to 50 mL (1 to 5 vials) IV infusion based on clinical assessment and response to initial dose.
PEDS — Larger relative doses of antivenin are needed in children and small adults because of small volume of body fluid to dilute the venom. The dose is not based on wt.
NOTES — Test first for sensitivity to horse serum. Serum sickness may occur 5 to 24 days after dose. IV route is preferred. May give IM.
MOA — Antivenom.
ADVERSE EFFECTS — Frequent: None.

ANTIVENIN—LATRODECTUS MACTANS ▶L ♀C ▶? $$
ADULT — Specialized dosing for black widow spider toxicity; consult poison center.
PEDS — Specialized dosing for black widow spider toxicity; consult poison center.
NOTES — Test first for horse serum sensitivity. Serum sickness may occur 5 to 24 days after dose.
MOA — Antivenom.
ADVERSE EFFECTS — Frequent: None.

BOTULISM IMMUNE GLOBULIN (*BabyBIG*) ▶L ♀? ▶? $$$$$
ADULT — Not approved in age 1 yo or older.
PEDS — Infant botulism: 1 mL (50 mg)/kg IV for age younger than 1 yo.
MOA — Passive immunity.
ADVERSE EFFECTS — Frequent: Mild, transient erythematous rash of face or trunk. Severe: Anaphylaxis, angioedema, urticaria, renal dysfunction/failure.

CYTOMEGALOVIRUS IMMUNE GLOBULIN HUMAN (*CytoGam*) ▶L ♀C ▶? $$$$$
ADULT — Specialized dosing based on indication and time since transplant.

PEDS — Specialized dosing based on indication and time since transplant.
MOA — Passive immunity.
ADVERSE EFFECTS — Frequent: Flushing, fever, pain, N/V. Severe: Anaphylaxis.

HEPATITIS B IMMUNE GLOBULIN (*H-BIG, HyperHep B, HepaGam B, NABI-HB*) ▶L ♀C ▶? $$$
ADULT — Postexposure prophylaxis for needlestick, ocular, mucosal exposure: 0.06 mL/kg IM (usual dose 3 to 5 mL) within 24 h of exposure. Initiate hepatitis B vaccine series within 7 days. Consider a second dose of hepatitis B immune globulin (HBIG) 1 month later if patient refuses hepatitis B vaccine series. Postexposure prophylaxis for sexual exposure: 0.06 mL/kg IM within 14 days of sexual contact. Initiate hepatitis B vaccine series. Prevention of hepatitis B recurrence following liver transplantation in HBsAg-positive (HepaGam B): First dose given during transplantation surgery. Subsequent doses daily for 7 days, then biweekly up to 3 months and monthly thereafter. Doses adjusted based on regular monitoring of HBsAg, HBV-DNA, HBeAg, and anti-HBs antibody levels.
PEDS — Prophylaxis of infants born to HBsAg (+) mothers: 0.5 mL IM within 12 h of birth. Initiate hepatitis B vaccine series within 7 days. If hepatitis B vaccine series is refused, repeat HBIG dose at 3 and 6 mo. Household exposure age younger than 12 mo: Give 0.5 mL IM within 14 days of exposure. Initiate hepatitis B vaccine series.
NOTES — HBIG may be administered at the same time or up to 1 month prior to hepatitis B vaccine without impairing the active immune response from hepatitis B vaccine.
MOA — Passive immunity.
ADVERSE EFFECTS — Frequent: Pain at injection site. Severe: Anaphylaxis, angioedema, urticaria.

IMMUNE GLOBULIN—INTRAMUSCULAR (*Baygam, ✦Gamastan*) ▶L ♀C ▶? $$$$
ADULT — Hepatitis A postexposure prophylaxis for household or institutional contacts: 0.02 mL/kg IM within 2 weeks of exposure. Hepatitis A pre-exposure prophylaxis (ie, travel to endemic area): 0.02 mL/kg IM for length of stay less than 3 months, give 0.06 mL/kg IM and repeat q 4 to 6 months for length of stay longer than 3 months. Measles: 0.2 to 0.25 mL/kg IM within 6 days of exposure, max 15 mL. Varicella zoster: 0.6 to 1.2 mL/kg IM. Rubella exposure in pregnant, susceptible women: 0.55 mL/kg IM. Immunoglobulin deficiency: 0.66 mL/kg IM q 3 to 4 weeks.
PEDS — Not approved in children.
UNAPPROVED PEDS — Measles: 0.2 to 0.25 mL/kg IM within 6 days of exposure. In susceptible immunocompromised children use 0.5 mL/kg IM (max 15 mL) immediately after exposure. Varicella zoster: 0.6 to 1.2 mL/kg IM.

(cont.)

IMMUNE GLOBULIN—INTRAMUSCULAR (cont.)

NOTES — Human-derived product, increased infection risk. Hepatitis A vaccine preferred over immune globulin for age 2 yo or older who plan to travel to high-risk areas repeatedly or for long periods of time.

MOA — Passive immunity.

ADVERSE EFFECTS — Frequent: Pain at injection site, tenderness, muscle stiffness, HA. Severe: Anaphylaxis, angioedema, urticaria, nephrotic syndrome.

IMMUNE GLOBULIN—INTRAVENOUS (Carimune, Flebogamma, Gammagard, Gammaplex, Gamunex, Octagam, Privigen) ▶L ♀C ▶? $$$$$

WARNING — Renal dysfunction, acute renal failure, osmotic nephrosis, and death may be associated with IV immune globulins, especially those containing sucrose. Administer at the minimum concentration available and the minimum practical infusion rate.

ADULT — Idiopathic thrombocytopenic purpura (induction): 400 mg/kg IV daily for 5 days (or 1 g/kg IV daily for 1 to 2 days). Bone marrow transplant: 500 mg/kg IV daily, given 7 and 2 days before transplant, and then weekly until 90 days posttransplant for age older than 20 yo. Primary humoral immunodeficiency: 200 to 300 mg/kg IV each month; increase prn to max 400 to 800 mg/kg/month. B-cell chronic lymphocytic leukemia: Specialized dosing. Chronic inflammatory demyelinating polyneuropathy (CIDP): (Gamunex) 2 g/kg IV loading dose followed by 1 g/kg IV every 3 weeks.

PEDS — Pediatric HIV: 400 mg/kg IV every 28 days. Idiopathic thrombocytopenic purpura (induction): 400 mg/kg IV daily for 5 days (or 1 g/kg IV daily for 1 to 2 days). Kawasaki syndrome (acute): 400 mg/kg IV daily for 4 days (or 2 g/kg IV for 1 dose over 10 h). Primary humoral immunodeficiency: 200 to 300 mg/kg IV each month; increase prn to max 400 to 800 mg/kg/month.

UNAPPROVED ADULT — First-line therapy in severe Guillain-Barré syndrome, chronic inflammatory demyelinating polyneuropathy, multifocal motor neuropathy, severe posttransfusion purpura, inclusion body myositis, fetomaternal alloimmune thrombocytopenia; second-line therapy in stiff-person syndrome, dermatomyositis, myasthenia gravis, and Lambert-Eaton myasthenic syndrome. Various dosing regimens have been used; a common one is myasthenia gravis (induction): 400 mg/kg IV daily for 5 days (total 2 g/kg). Has been used in multiple sclerosis and inflammatory myositis (polymyositis and dermatomyositis), renal transplant rejection, systemic lupus erythematosus, toxic epidermal necrolysis and Stevens-Johnson syndrome, Clostridium difficile colitis, Graves' ophthalmopathy, pemphigus, Wegener's granulomatosis, Churg-Strauss syndrome, and Duchenne muscular dystrophy.

UNAPPROVED PEDS — Myasthenia gravis (induction): 400 mg/kg IV daily for 5 days. Other dosing regimens have been used.

NOTES — Indications and doses vary by product. Follow LFTs, renal function, vital signs, and urine output closely. Contraindicated in IgA deficiency. Use caution (and lower infusion rates) if risk factors for thrombosis, heart failure, or renal insufficiency. Use slower infusion rates for initial doses. Consider pretreatment with acetaminophen and/or diphenhydramine to minimize some infusion-related adverse effects. Human-derived product; although donors are carefully screened, there is risk of transmission of infectious agents.

MOA — Immunomodulatory effects through exogenous immunoglobulins.

ADVERSE EFFECTS — Serious: Acute renal failure, noncardiogenic pulmonary edema, hemolysis, heart failure, stroke, MI, DVT, aseptic meningitis, anaphylaxis. Frequent: Infusion reactions, HA, vomiting, fever, chills, hypotension, rash, back pain, reversible neutropenia, pain at injection site.

IMMUNE GLOBULIN—SUBCUTANEOUS (Vivaglobulin, Hizentra) ▶L ♀C ▶? $$$$$

ADULT — Primary immune deficiency: 100 to 200 mg/kg SC weekly. In patients already receiving IV immune globulin: SC dose is equivalent to (previous IV dose × 1.37) divided by frequency of IV regimen in week.

PEDS — Limited information. Dosing appears to be same as in adults.

NOTES — Do not administer IV. Contraindicated in IgA deficiency. Human-derived product, increased infection risk.

MOA — Passive immunity.

ADVERSE EFFECTS — Serious: Acute hypersensitivity reactions, anaphylaxis. Frequent: Injection site reactions, HA, nausea/vomiting, fever, rash, pain, diarrhea, sore throat.

LYMPHOCYTE IMMUNE GLOBULIN (Atgam) ▶L ♀C ▶? $$$$$

ADULT — Renal allograft recipients: 10 to 30 mg/kg IV daily. Delaying onset of allograft rejection: 15 mg/kg IV daily for 14 days, then every other day for 14 days. Treatment of renal transplant rejection: 10 to 15 mg/kg IV for 14 days. Aplastic anemia: 10 to 20 mg/kg IV daily for 8 to 14 days, then every other day, prn, up to 21 total doses.

PEDS — Limited experience. Has been safely administered to a limited number of children with renal transplant and aplastic anemia at doses comparable to adult doses.

NOTES — Equine product. Doses should be administered over at least 4 h.

MOA — Lymphocyte-specific immunosuppressant.

ADVERSE EFFECTS — Frequent: Fever, chills, skin reactions, systemic infections, abnormal renal function, serum-sickness-like reactions, dyspnea, arthralgia, chest, back, flank pain, diarrhea, N/V. Severe: Anaphylaxis, hemolysis, thrombocytopenia, leukopenia.

RABIES IMMUNE GLOBULIN HUMAN (*Imogam Rabies-HT, HyperRAB S/D*) ▶L ♀C ▶? $$$$$
ADULT — Postexposure prophylaxis: 20 units/kg (0.133 mL/kg), with as much as possible infiltrated around the bite and the rest given IM. Give as soon as possible after exposure. Administer with the 1st dose of vaccine, but in a different extremity.
PEDS — Not approved in children.
UNAPPROVED PEDS — Use adult dosing.
NOTES — Do not repeat dose once rabies vaccine series begins. Do not give to patients who have been completely immunized with rabies vaccine. Do not administer IV.
MOA — Passive immunity.
ADVERSE EFFECTS — Frequent: Pain at injection site, sensitization. Severe: Anaphylaxis, angioedema, skin rash, nephrotic syndrome.

RSV IMMUNE GLOBULIN (*RespiGam*) ▶plasma ♀C ▶? $$$$$
PEDS — Respiratory syncytial virus prophylaxis: 1.5 mL/kg/h for 15 min for age younger than 24 mo. Increase rate as clinical condition permits to 3 mL/kg/h for 15 min, then to a max rate of 6 mL/kg/h. Max total dose/month is 750 mg/kg.
NOTES — May cause fluid overload; monitor vital signs frequently during IV infusion. Respiratory syncytial virus season in North America is typically November through April.
MOA — Passive immunity.
ADVERSE EFFECTS — Frequent: Rash, fever, tachycardia, hypotension, hypertension, vomiting, diarrhea, gastroenteritis.

IMMUNOLOGY: Immunosuppression

BASILIXIMAB (*Simulect*) ▶plasma ♀B ▶? $$$$$
WARNING — To be used only by trained physicians. To be given only in facility with adequate laboratory and supportive medical resources.
ADULT — Specialized dosing for organ transplantation.
PEDS — Specialized dosing for organ transplantation.
MOA — Immunosuppressant, prophylaxis of acute organ rejection.
ADVERSE EFFECTS — Frequent: Administration did not increase the incidence or severity of adverse events over placebo in immunosuppressed patients.

BELATACEPT (*Nulojix*) ▶serum ♀C ▶– $$$$$
WARNING — Should only be prescribed by physicians who are knowledgeable about the drug. Serious adverse effects have been reported.
ADULT — Specialized dosing for organ transplantation.
PEDS — Not approved in children.
MOA — T-cell blocker.
ADVERSE EFFECTS — many

CYCLOSPORINE (*Sandimmune, Neoral, Gengraf*) ▶L ♀C ▶– $$$$$
WARNING — Should only be prescribed by physicians who are knowledgeable about the drug. Many drug interactions. Serious adverse effects can occur. Monitor closely in those with renal or hepatic impairment
ADULT — Specialized dosing for organ transplantation, RA, and psoriasis.
PEDS — Not approved in children.
UNAPPROVED ADULT — Specialized dosing for autoimmune eye disorders, vasculitis, inflammatory myopathies, Behcet's disease, psoriatic arthritis, chronic refractory idiopathic thrombocytopenia.
UNAPPROVED PEDS — Specialized dosing for organ transplantation, chronic refractory idiopathic thrombocytopenia.
FORMS — Generic/Trade: Microemulsion Caps 25, 100 mg. Generic/Trade: Caps (Sandimmune)
25, 100 mg. Soln (Sandimmune) 100 mg/mL. Microemulsion soln (Neoral, Gengraf) 100 mg/mL.
NOTES — Monitor cyclosporine blood concentrations closely. Many drug interactions including atorvastatin, azithromycin, lovastatin, oral contraceptives, rosuvastatin, simvastatin, sirolimus, terbinafine, voriconazole, HIV protease inhibitors, grapefruit juice, and others. Use caution when combining with methotrexate or potassium-sparing drugs such as ACE inhibitors. Do not use with bosentan or dabigatran. Reduce dose in renal dysfunction. Monitor BP and renal function closely. Avoid excess UV light exposure. Monitor patients closely when switching from Sandimmune to microemulsion formulations.
MOA — Immunosuppressant, prophylaxis of acute organ rejection.
ADVERSE EFFECTS — Frequent: Hypertension, hirsutism, hypomagnesemia, hypokalemia, gingival hypertrophy, tremor, nephrotoxicity. Severe: Anaphylaxis, infection and increased risk of lymphoma and other malignancies, especially those of the skin, risk, optic disc edema, benign intracranial hypertension, papilledema, visual impairment, thrombotic microangiopathy, hepatotoxicity, polyoma virus infection, neurotoxicty .

EVEROLIMUS—IMMUNOLOGY (*Zortress*) ▶L ♀C ▶– $$$$$
WARNING — Increased risk of infection and malignancies. Increased risk of kidney graft thrombosis. Increased mortality in heart transplant trials so not recommended in heart transplant patients. Reduce dose of cyclosporine to reduce nephrotoxicity.
ADULT — Specialized dosing for organ transplantation.
PEDS — Not approved for use in children.
FORMS — Trade: Tabs 0.25, 0.5, 0.75 mg.
NOTES — Reduce dose in renal dysfunction. Monitor BP and real function closely. Many drug interactions. Increased risk of infections/malignancy.

(cont.)

EVEROLIMUS (cont.)

MOA — Immunosuppressant, prophylaxis of acute organ rejection

ADVERSE EFFECTS — Severe: delayed wound healing, fluid accumulation, interstitial lung disease, pulmonary hypertension, non-infectious pneumonitis, proteinuria, thrombotic microangiopathy, thrombotic thrombocytopenic purpura, hemolytic uremic syndrome, new onset diabetes, male infertility.

MYCOPHENOLATE MOFETIL (CellCept, Myfortic) ▶? ♀D ▶– $$

WARNING — Has been associated with embryofetal toxicity, lymphoma, malignancy, increased risk of infection, and progressive multifocal leukoencephalopathy (PML).

ADULT — Specialized dosing for organ transplantation. Take 1 h before or 2 h after food.

PEDS — Not approved in children.

UNAPPROVED ADULT — Lupus nephritis: 1000 mg PO two times per day. Has been used in pemphigus, bullous pemphigoid, and refractory uveitis.

UNAPPROVED PEDS — Specialized dosing for organ transplantation.

FORMS — Generic/Trade: Caps 250 mg. Tabs 500 mg. Tabs, extended-release (Myfortic): 180, 360 mg. Trade only (CellCept): Susp 200 mg/mL (160 mL).

NOTES — Avoid live vaccine administration. Increased risk of first trimester pregnancy loss and increased risk of congenital malformations, especially external ear and facial abnormalities. Counsel women regarding pregnancy prevention and planning.

MOA — Immunosuppressant, prophylaxis of acute organ rejection.

ADVERSE EFFECTS — Frequent: GI upset, thrombophlebitis, thrombosis (with IV administration). Severe: Infection, GI bleeding, nephrotic syndrome, bone marrow suppression, leukopenia, lymphoma, malignancy, progressive multifocal leukoencephalopathy, pure red cell aplasia.

SIROLIMUS (Rapamune) ▶L ♀C ▶– $$$$$

WARNING — Increased risk of infection and lymphoma. Combination of sirolimus plus cyclosporine or tacrolimus is associated with hepatic artery thrombosis in liver transplant patients. Combination with tacrolimus and corticosteroids in lung transplant patients may cause bronchial anastomotic dehiscence. Possible increased mortality in stable liver transplant patients after conversion from a calcineurin inhibitor (CNI)-based immunosuppressive regimen to sirolimus. Can cause hypersensitivity reactions including anaphylactic and/or anaphylactoid reactions, angioedema, vasculitis. Many drug interactions. Avoid with strong inhibitors of CYP3A4 and/or P-glycoprotein (ketoconazole, voriconazole, itraconazole, erythromycin, clarithromycin) or strong inducers of CYP3A4 and/or P-glycoprotein (rifampin, rifabutin). Monitor level

if cyclosporine is discontinued or dose has markedly changed.

ADULT — Specialized dosing for organ transplantation and lymphangioleiomyomatosis.

PEDS — Not approved in children.

UNAPPROVED PEDS — Specialized dosing for organ transplantation and lymphangioleiomyomatosis.

FORMS — Generic/Trade: Tabs 0.5, 1, 2 mg. Trade only: Soln 1 mg/mL (60 mL).

NOTES — Wear protective clothing and sunscreen when exposed to sunlight to reduce the risk of skin cancer. Be aware of site-specific assay method, as this may affect reported serum concentrations. Adjust dose by ⅓ to ½ in liver dysfunction. Monitor trough levels, particularly in patients likely to have altered drug metabolism, age 13 yo or older with wt less than 40 kg, hepatic impairment, when changing doses, or with interacting medications. Do not adjust dose more frequently than q 1 to 2 weeks. Oral soln and tabs are clinically equivalent from a dosing standpoint at the 2 mg level; however, this is unknown at higher doses. May cause diabetes.

MOA — Immunosuppressant, prophylaxis of acute organ rejection in solid organ transplant.

ADVERSE EFFECTS — Frequent: Hypertension, edema, chest pain, fever, headache, pain, insomnia, rash, abdominal pain, renal dysfunction, nausea, diarrhea, anemia, thrombocytopenia, arthralgia, dyspnea. Hyperlipidemia in up to 90% of patients. May cause diabetes. Severe: Hepatic artery thrombosis in liver transplant patients, hypersensitivity reactions, progressive multifocal leukoencephalopathy, nephrotic syndrome, exfoliative dermatitis, impaired wound healing, angioedema, vasculitis, interstitial lung disease, pulmonary hypertension, hemolytic uremic syndrome/thrombotic thrombocytopenic purpura/thrombotic microangiopathy, increased risk of infections such as tuberculosis, especially when used with calcineurin inhibitor.

TACROLIMUS (Astagraf XL, Hecoria, Prograf, FK 506, Envarsus XR, ✦Advagraf) ▶L ♀C ▶– $$$$$

ADULT — Specialized dosing for organ transplantation.

PEDS — Specialized dosing for organ transplantation.

UNAPPROVED ADULT — RA (approved in Canada), active vasculitis, systemic lupus erythematosus nephritis, and vasculitis.

FORMS — Generic/Trade: Caps 0.5, 1, 5 mg. Trade only: Extended-release caps (Astagraf XL) 0.5, 1, 5 mg. (Envarsus XR) 0.75, 1, 4 mg.

NOTES — Reduce dose in renal dysfunction. Monitor BP and renal function closely. Neurotoxic, especially in high doses. Many drug interactions including some herbal products such as Schisandra. Increased risk of infections, QT prolongation, gastrointestinal perforation.

MOA — Immunosuppressant, prophylaxis of acute organ rejection.

(cont.)

TACROLIMUS (*cont.*)

ADVERSE EFFECTS — Frequent: Hypertension, peripheral edema, headache, insomnia, pain, fever, pruritus, N/V, diarrhea, abdominal pain, tremors, paresthesias. Severe: Anaphylaxis, edema, hypertrophic cardiomyopathy, gastrointestinal perforation, myocardial hypertrophy, ECG abnormalities including QT prolongation and Torsades de Pointes, paralysis, stroke, hemolytic uremic syndrome, nephrotoxicity, secondary malignancy.

IMMUNOLOGY: Other

HYMENOPTERA VENOM ▶Serum ♀C ▶? $$$$

ADULT — Specialized desensitization dosing protocol.

PEDS — Specialized desensitization dosing protocol.

NOTES — Venom products available: Honeybee (Apis mellifera) and yellow jacket (Vespula sp.), yellow hornet (Dolichovespula arenaria), white-faced hornet (D. maculata), and wasp (Polistes sp.). Mixed vespid venom protein (yellow jacket, yellow hornet, and white-faced hornet) is also available.

MOA — Desensitization protein.

ADVERSE EFFECTS — Frequent: Erythema, swelling, pruritus, burning. Severe: Systemic reactions, anaphylaxis, death.

RILONACEPT (*Arcalyst*) ▶? ♀? ▶? $$$$$

ADULT — Familial cold auto-inflammatory syndrome (FCAS) and Muckle-Wells syndrome (MWS): Begin therapy with a loading dose of 320 mg (160 mg SC on the same day at two different sites), then 160 mg SC once weekly.

PEDS — Familial cold auto-inflammatory syndrome (FCAS) and Muckle-Wells syndrome (MWS): Begin therapy with a loading dose of 4.4 mg/kg (max 320 mg) SC in one or two doses, then 2.2 mg/kg (max 160 mg) SC once weekly.

NOTES — Increased risk of infections.

MOA — interleukin 1 blocker

ADVERSE EFFECTS — Frequent: injection site reactions.

TUBERCULIN PPD (*Aplisol, Tubersol, Mantoux, PPD*) ▶L ♀C ▶+ $

ADULT — 5 tuberculin units (0.1 mL) intradermally. Consider two-step testing in those who are going to be retested periodically (e.g., health care workers, nursing home residents).

PEDS — Same as adult dose. AAP recommends screening at 12 mo, 4 to 6 yo, and 14 to 16 yo.

NOTES — Avoid SC injection. Read 48 to 72 h after intradermal injection. Repeat testing in patients with known prior positive PPD; may cause scarring at injection site.

MOA — Skin test for diagnosis of tuberculosis.

ADVERSE EFFECTS — Frequent: Ulceration, necrosis, vesiculation.

NEUROLOGY

Dermatomes

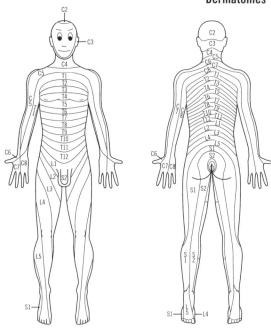

MOTOR FUNCTION BY NERVE ROOTS

Level	Motor Function
C3/C4/C5	Diaphragm
C5/C6	Deltoid/biceps
C7/C8	Triceps
C8/T1	Finger flexion/ intrinsics
T1–T12	Intercostal/ abd muscles
L2/L3	Hip flexion
L2/L3/L4	Hip adductor/quads
L4/L5	Ankle dorsiflexion
S1/S2	Ankle plantarflexion
S2/S3/S4	Rectal tone

LUMBOSACRAL NERVE ROOT COMPRESSIONS	Root	Motor	Sensory	Reflex
	L4	quadriceps	medial foot	knee-jerk
	L5	dorsiflexors	dorsum of foot	medial hamstring
	S1	plantarflexors	lateral foot	ankle-jerk

GLASGOW COMA SCALE

Eye Opening	Verbal Activity	Motor Activity
		6. Obeys commands
4. Spontaneous	5. Oriented	5. Localizes pain
3. To command	4. Confused	4. Withdraws to pain
2. To pain	3. Inappropriate	3. Flexion to pain
1. None	2. Incomprehensible	2. Extension to pain
	1. None	1. None

NEUROLOGY: Alzheimer's Disease—Cholinesterase Inhibitors

NOTE: Avoid concurrent use of anticholinergic agents. Use caution in asthma/COPD. May be coadministered with memantine.

DONEPEZIL (*Aricept*) ▶LK ♀C ▶? $
ADULT — Alzheimer's disease: Start 5 mg PO at bedtime. May increase to 10 mg PO at bedtime in 4 to 6 weeks. Max 10 mg/day for mild to moderate disease. For moderate to severe disease (MMSE 10 or less), may increase after 3 months to 23 mg/day. ODT form should be dissolved on the top of the tongue.

PEDS — Not approved in children.
UNAPPROVED ADULT — Dementia in Parkinson's disease: 5 to 10 mg/day.
FORMS — Generic/Trade: Tabs 5, 10, 23 mg. Orally disintegrating tabs 5, 10 mg.
NOTES — Some clinicians start with 5 mg PO every other day to minimize GI side effects. Avoid

(cont.)

DONEPEZIL (*cont.*)

concurrent use of anticholinergic medications when possible.

MOA — Reversible acetylcholinesterase inhibitor.

ADVERSE EFFECTS — Serious: Cholinergic crisis, seizures, bradycardia, syncope, hypotension, respiratory depression, QTc prolongation, rhabomyolysis. Frequent: N/V, diarrhea, anorexia, weight loss, insomnia, muscle cramps, fatigue, ecchymosis.

GALANTAMINE (*Razadyne, Razadyne ER, ✷Reminyl*) ▶LK ♀C ▶? $$$$

ADULT — Alzheimer's disease (mild to moderate): Immediate-release: Start 4 mg PO two times per day with food; increase to 8 mg two times per day after at least 4 weeks. May increase to 12 mg PO two times per day after another 4 weeks or more. Extended-release: Start 8 mg PO every am with food; increase to 16 mg every am after at least 4 weeks. May increase to 24 mg every am after another 4 weeks or more.

PEDS — Not approved in children.

UNAPPROVED ADULT — Dementia in Parkinson's disease: 4 to 8 mg PO two times per day (immediate-release).

FORMS — Generic/Trade: Tabs 4, 8, 12 mg. Extended-release caps 8, 16, 24 mg. Oral soln 4 mg/mL.

NOTES — Indicated for mild to moderate AD. Do not exceed 16 mg/day in renal or hepatic impairment. Avoid use in severe hepatic or renal impairment. Use caution with CYP3A4 and CYP2D6 inhibitors. Avoid abrupt discontinuation. Restart at the lowest dose if therapy has been interrupted for several days or more. May exaggerate neuromuscular blocking agents used during anesthesia. May increase risk of GI bleeds in predisposed patients, for example those on NSAIDs. Avoid concurrent use of anticholinergics if possible.

MOA — Reversible acetylcholinesterase inhibitor.

ADVERSE EFFECTS — Serious: Cholinergic crisis, seizures, bradycardia, syncope, hypotension, Stevens Johnson syndrome and other serious skin ractions, bronchospasm, hallucinations, hepatotoxicity. Frequent: N/V, diarrhea, anorexia, weight loss, muscle cramps.

RIVASTIGMINE (*Exelon, Exelon Patch*) ▶L cholinesterase-mediated hydrolysis ♀B ▶? $$$$$

ADULT — Alzheimer's disease (mild to moderate): Start 1.5 mg PO two times per day with food. Increase to 3 mg two times per day after at least 2 weeks. May increase to 4.5 mg twice daily and then 6 mg twice daily at two-week intervals. Usual effective dose is 6 to 12 mg/day. Max 12 mg/day. Patch: Start 4.6 mg/24 h once daily; may increase after 1 month or more to recommended dose of 9.5 mg/24 h, max 13.3 mg/24 h. Rotate sites. Dementia in Parkinson's disease (mild to moderate): Start 1.5 mg PO twice daily with food. Increase by 3 mg/day at intervals of 4 weeks or more to max 12 mg/day. May increase to 4.5 mg twice daily then 6 mg twice daily at 4 week intervals. Max 12 mg/day. Patch: Use dosing for Alzheimer's disease.

PEDS — Not approved in children.

FORMS — Generic/Trade: Caps 1.5, 3, 4.5, 6 mg. Trade only: Transdermal patch: 4.6 mg/24 h, 9.5 mg/24 h, 13.3 mg/24 h. Oral solution 2 mg/mL.

NOTES — Restart treatment with the lowest daily dose (ie, 1.5 mg PO two times per day) if discontinued for 3 days or more to reduce the risk of severe vomiting. When changing from PO to patch, patients taking less than 6 mg/day can be placed on 4.6 mg/24 h patch. For those taking 6 to 12 mg/day, may start with 9.5 mg/24 h patch. Have patient start the day after stopping oral dosing. Rotate application sites and do not apply to same spot for 14 days. Patches have been associated with contact dermatitis. Reduce dose and titrate more slowly for moderate to severe renal insufficiency, mild to moderate hepatic insufficiency, and low body mass. Patients with these conditions may only tolerate lower doses. May increase risk of GI bleeding in predisposed patients, for example those taking NSAIDs. May exaggerate response to neuromuscular blocking agents during anesthesia.

MOA — Reversible acetylcholinesterase inhibitor.

ADVERSE EFFECTS — Serious: Cholinergic crisis, seizures, bradycardia, syncope, hypotension, respiratory depression, bronchospasm, hepatitis. Frequent: N/V, diarrhea, dyspepsia, anorexia, weight loss, muscle cramps, headache, dizziness, asthenia.

NEUROLOGY: Alzheimer's Disease—NMDA Receptor Antagonists

MEMANTINE (*Namenda, Namenda XR, ✷Ebixa*) ▶KL ♀B ▶? $$$

ADULT — Alzheimer's disease (moderate to severe): Start 5 mg PO daily. Increase by 5 mg/day at weekly intervals to max 20 mg/day. Doses greater than 5 mg/day should be divided two times per day. Reduce dose to 5 mg twice daily with severe renal impairment. Extended-release: Start 7 mg once daily. Increase at weekly intervals to target dose of 28 mg/day. Reduce to 14 mg/day in severe renal impairment.

PEDS — Not approved in children.

FORMS — Generic/Trade: Tabs 5, 10 mg. Oral soln 2 mg/mL. Trade only: Extended-release caps 7, 14, 21, 28 mg.

NOTES — May be used in combination with acetylcholinesterase inhibitors. Reduce target dose to 5 mg PO twice daily in severe renal impairment (CrCl 5 to 29 mL/min). No dosage adjustment needed for mild to moderate renal impairment. When switching to extended-release caps patients taking 10 mg two times per day can be changed to 28 mg/day of ER after last regular dose. Patients switched from 5 mg two times per day can be changed to 14 mg/day of ER.

(cont.)

MEMANTINE (cont.)

MOA — N-methyl-D-aspartate (NMDA) receptor antagonist.

ADVERSE EFFECTS — Serious: Heart failure, pancreatitis, hepatitis, suicidal ideation, acute renal failure, Stevens Johnson syndrome. Frequent: Hypertension, dizziness, headache, constipation, confusion.

NAMZARIC (memantine extended-release + donepezil) ▶KL ♀C ▶?

ADULT — Moderate to severe Alzheimer's dementia (patients already stabilized on memantine plus donepezil): For patients stabilized on donepezil 10 mg alone start Namzaric 7 mg/10 mg PO once daily in the evening. Increase weekly by 7 mg/day of memantine to recommended dose of 28 mg/10 mg. For patients already stabilized on memantine 10 mg twice daily or 28 mg/day of extended-release, start recommended dose of Namzaric 28 mg/10 mg PO once daily in the evening. Reduce maintenance dose to 14/10 mg for severe renal insufficiency (CrCl 5 to 29 mL/min).

PEDS — Not approved for use in children or adolescents.

FORMS — Trade only: Caps, extended-release memantine + donepezil 7 mg/10 mg, 14/10, 21 mg/10 mg, 28/10 mg.

NOTES — Can be taken with or without food. Contents of capsules can be mixed in applesauce and given. Can cause exaggerated response to muscle relaxants during anesthesia.

MOA — NMDA receptor antagonist and acetylcholinesterase inhibitor.

ADVERSE EFFECTS — Memantine. Serious: none. Frequent: Headache, diarrhea, dizziness. Donepezil. Serious: Cholinergic crisis, seizures, bradycardia, syncope, hypotension, respiratory depression. Frequent: N/V, diarrhea, anorexia, insomnia, muscle cramps, fatigue, ecchymosis.

NEUROLOGY: Anticonvulsants

NOTE: Avoid rapid discontinuation of anticonvulsants, because this can precipitate seizures or other withdrawal symptoms. Increased risk of suicidal ideation or behaviors with antiepileptic drugs. Monitor closely for signs of depression, anxiety, hostility, hypomania/mania, or suicidality. Symptoms may develop within 1 week of initiation, and risk continues for at least 24 weeks.

BIVARACETAM (Briviact) ▶L Primarily hydrolyzed, some by CYP2C19 ♀C Consider enrolling in registry ▶? ©V

ADULT — Partial onset seizures: Start 50 mg PO/IV twice daily. May reduce to 25 mg PO/IV twice daily or increase to 100 mg PO/IV twice daily based on efficacy and tolerability. Reserve IV use for when PO not possible. For all stages of hepatic impairment reduce initial dose to 25 mg twice daily with a max dose of 75 mg twice daily.

PEDS — Not approved for use in children and adolescents under the age of 16 yo. Adolescents 16 yo and above use adult dosing.

FORMS — Trade only: Tabs 10, 25, 50, 75, 100 mg. Oral soln 10 mg/mL.

NOTES — Dosage adjustments are not required for renal impairment. Coadministration with alcohol can lead to excessive sedation.

MOA — High and selective affinity for synaptic vesicle protein 2A in the brain

ADVERSE EFFECTS — Serious: suicidal ideation/behavior, hypesensitvity, bronchospasm, angioedema, leukopenia. Frequent: somnolence, fatigue, dizziness, ataxia, nausea, vomiting.

CARBAMAZEPINE (Tegretol, Tegretol XR, Carbatrol, Epitol, Equetro) ▶LK ♀D ▶+ $$

WARNING — Risk of aplastic anemia, agranulocytosis, and hyponatremia; contraindicated if prior bone marrow depression. Monitor CBC and serum sodium at baseline and periodically.

ADULT — Epilepsy: Start 200 mg PO twice per day. Increase by 200 mg/day at weekly intervals, divided into three or four doses per day (immediate-release), or two times per day (extended-release), or four times per day (susp) to usual max 1000 mg/day. Doses up to 1600 mg/day have been used in rare instances. Trigeminal neuralgia: Start 100 mg PO twice per day or 50 mg PO four times per day (susp); increase by 200 mg/day until pain relief. Usual range 400 to 800 mg/day. Max 1200 mg/day. Bipolar disorder, acute manic/mixed episodes (Equetro): Start 200 mg PO two times per day; increase by 200 mg/day to max 1600 mg/day. See "unapproved adult" section for alternative bipolar dosing.

PEDS — Epilepsy, Age 13 yo and older use adult dosing. Age 6 to 12 yo: Start 100 mg PO twice daily (immediate-release or extended-release) or ½ teaspoon (50 mg) suspension four times daily. Increase by 100 mg/day at weekly intervals divided into three or four daily doses (immediate-release tabs or suspension) or two times per day (extended-release). Max 1000 mg/day. Age younger than 6 yo: Start 10 to 20 mg/kg/day PO divided into two to three doses per day (immediate-release tabs) or four times per day (susp). Increase weekly prn. Max 35 mg/kg/day.

UNAPPROVED ADULT — Neuropathic pain: Start 100 mg PO two times per day; usual effective dose is 200 mg PO two to four times per day. Max 1200 mg/day. Mania (American Psychiatric Association guidelines): Start 200 to 600 mg/day divided into three or four doses per day (standard-release) or two times per day (extended-release), then increase by 200 mg/day q 2 to 4 days. Mean effective dose is 1000 mg/day. Max 1600 mg/day.

UNAPPROVED PEDS — Bipolar disorder (manic or mixed phase): Start 100 to 200 mg PO daily or two times per day; titrate to usual effective dose of 200 to 600 mg/day for children and up to 1200 mg/day for adolescents.

(cont.)

CARBAMAZEPINE (*cont.*)

FORMS — Generic/Trade: Tabs 200 mg, Chewable tabs 100 mg, Susp 100 mg/5 mL. Extended-release tabs (Tegretol XR) 100, 200, 400 mg. Extended-release caps (Carbatrol) 100, 200, 300 mg. Trade only: Extended-release caps (Equetro) 100, 200, 300 mg.

NOTES — Usual therapeutic level is 4 to 12 mcg/mL. Stevens-Johnson syndrome, hepatitis, aplastic anemia, and hyponatremia may occur. Monitor CBC and LFTs. Many drug interactions. Should not be used for absence or atypical absence seizures. Dangerous and possibly fatal skin reactions are more common with the HLA-B*1502 allele (most common in people of Asian and Indian ancestry); screen new patients for this allele prior to starting therapy. The HLA-A*3101 allele may also be associated with increased risk of cutaneous reactions.

MOA — Anticonvulsant, sodium channel blocker.

ADVERSE EFFECTS — Serious: Aplastic anemia and other blood dyscrasias, hepatotoxicity, SIADH/hyponatremia, rash, Stevens-Johnson syndrome, toxic epidermal necrolysis, drug reaction with eosinophilia and systemic symptoms (DRESS), hypersensitivity reactions, suicidality, vanishing bile duct syndrome. Frequent: Drowsiness, ataxia, dizziness, confusion, N/V, blurred vision, nystagmus.

CLOBAZAM (*ONFI, ✽Frisium*) ▶L ♀C ▶– ©IV $$$$$

WARNING — Use caution in the elderly; may accumulate and cause side effects such as psychomotor impairment.

ADULT — Epilepsy (Lennox-Gastaut syndrome), adjunctive: Weight greater than 30 kg: Start 5 mg PO twice per day. Increase to 10 mg PO twice daily after 1 week then to 20 mg PO twice daily after 2 weeks. Weight 30 kg or less: Start 5 mg PO daily. Increase to 5 mg PO twice per day after 1 week, then 10 mg PO twice per day after 2 weeks. Canada, epilepsy (Lennox-Gastaut syndrome), adjunctive: Start 5 to 15 mg PO daily. Gradually increase prn to max 80 mg/day. Geriatric dosing: Start 5 mg PO daily. Titrate according to weight to 10 mg to 20 mg per day as tolerated and required. Max 40 mg/day.

PEDS — US, epilepsy (Lennox-Gastaut syndrome), adjunctive: Children 2 yo and older, weight greater than 30 kg: Start 5 mg PO twice per day. Increase to 10 mg PO twice daily after 1 week then to 20 mg PO twice daily after 2 weeks. Weight 30 kg or less: Start 5 mg PO daily. Increase to 5 mg PO twice per day after 1 week, then 10 mg PO twice per day after 2 weeks. Canada, epilepsy, adjunctive: Start 0.5 to 1 mg/kg PO daily for age younger than 2 yo or 5 mg daily for age 2 to 16 yo: Then may increase prn to max 40 mg/day.

FORMS — Trade only: Tabs 10, 20 mg. Oral susp 2.5 mg/mL.

NOTES — Reduce initial doses and titrate more slowly in CYP2D6 poor-metabolizers.

MOA — Benzodiazepine; potentiates GABA-ergic transmission.

ADVERSE EFFECTS — Serious: Respiratory and CNS depression, tolerance, dependence, suicidality, Stevens-Johnson syndrome, toxic epidermal necrolysis. Frequent: Drowsiness, dizziness, fatigue.

ESLICARBAZEPINE (*Aptiom*) ▶L ♀C ▶? Enters breastmilk $$$$$

ADULT — Partial seizures, adjunct or monotherapy: Start 400 mg PO once daily. May start 800 mg PO once daily if the need for seizure control outweighs risks of side effects. Increase dose weekly by 400 to 600 mg to recommended dose of 800 mg to 1600 mg once daily based on response and tolerability. Reserve the 1600 mg/day dose for those not responding to 1200 mg/day. Do not use with oxcarbazepine.

PEDS — Not approved for children and adolescents.

FORMS — Trade only: Tabs 200, 400, 600, 800 mg.

NOTES — May reduce efficacy of oral contraceptives. Enzyme-inducing or -inhibiting drugs may affect serum concentrations. See package insert for dosing recommendations. Reduce initial and maintenance doses by 50% if CrCl <50 mL/min.

MOA — Inhibition of voltage gated sodium channels.

ADVERSE EFFECTS — Serious: Stevens-Johnson syndrome, toxic epidermal necrolysis, drug reaction with eosinophilia and systemic symptoms (DRESS), hypersensitivity, hyponatremia, cognitive dysfunction, elevated LFTs. Frequent: dizziness, nausea, vomiting, ataxia, diplopia, somnolence, headache, blurred vision, asthenia, fatigue, rash, dysarthria, tremor.

ETHOSUXIMIDE (*Zarontin*) ▶LK ♀?/?/?. Briggs assigned a "C" rating. ▶+ $$$$

ADULT — Absence seizures: Start 500 mg PO given once daily or divided twice per day. Increase by 250 mg/day q 4 to 7 days prn. Max 1.5 g/day.

PEDS — Absence seizures: Start 250 mg PO daily or divided two times per day for age 3 to 6 yo. Use adult dosing for age older than 6 yo. The optimal dose for pediatric patients is approximately 20 mg/kg/day.

UNAPPROVED PEDS — Absence seizures, age younger than 3 yo: Start 15 mg/kg/day PO divided two times per day. Increase q 4 to 7 days prn. Usual effective dose is 15 to 40 mg/kg/day divided two times per day. Max 500 mg/day.

FORMS — Generic/Trade: Caps 250 mg. Syrup 250 mg/5 mL.

NOTES — Usual therapeutic level is 40 to 100 mcg/mL. Monitor CBC for blood dyscrasias. Use caution in hepatic and renal impairment. May increase the risk of tonic-clonic seizures in some patients.

MOA — Reduces 3Hz thalamic oscillations that underlie 3Hz spike-wave discharges of absence epilepsy by inhibition of T-type calcium channels.

ADVERSE EFFECTS — Serious: Blood dyscrasias, hepatotoxicity, Stevens-Johnson syndrome, drug-induced lupus, suicidality, drug reaction with eosinophilia and systemic symptoms (DRESS). Frequent: N/V, anorexia, weight loss, abdominal pain, rash, drowsiness, irritability, headache, fatigue, ataxia, euphoria.

ETHOTOIN (*Peganone*) ▶L ♀D ▶+ $$$$$
ADULT — Generalized tonic–clonic or complex partial seizures: Start 1 g or less per day given in 4 to 6 divided doses after food. Usual effective dose is 2 to 3 g/day.
PEDS — Generalized tonic–clonic or complex partial seizures: Start 750 mg/day or less in 4 to 6 divided doses after food. Usual effective dose is 0.5 to 1 g/day. Max 2 to 3 g/day.
FORMS — Trade only: Tabs 250 mg.
NOTES — Usual therapeutic level is 15 to 50 mcg/mL. Doses less than 2 g/day are usually ineffective in adults. Give after food to reduce GI side effects.
MOA — Increases seizure threshold through modulation of sodium and calcium channels.
ADVERSE EFFECTS — Serious: lymphadenopathy, drug-induced lupus, suicidality. Frequent: ataxia, diplopia, dizziness, fatigue, fever, headache, N/V, nystagmus, rash.

EZOGABINE (*POTIGA*) ▶KL – ♀C ▶? $$$$$
WARNING — Associated with retinal abnormalities with fundoscopic features similar to retinal pigment dystrophies, which can affect visual acuity, and may cause retinal damage and vision loss. Ophthalmic exams should be done q 6 months including visual acuity and dilated fundus photography. Discontinue if pigment abnormalities or visual changes occur unless no other options for seizure control.
ADULT — Partial-onset seizures, adjunctive: Start 100 mg PO three times per day. Increase weekly by no more than 50 mg three times daily to usual maintenance dose of 200 to 400 mg PO three times daily or max of 250 mg three times daily if older than 65 yo.
PEDS — Not approved for use in children or adolescents.
FORMS — Trade: Tabs 50, 200, 300, 400 mg.
NOTES — Taper dose over at least 3 weeks when discontinuing. Reduce dose to max of 200 mg three times daily for CrCl <50 mL/min or severe hepatic impairment, or 250 mg three times daily for moderate hepatic impairment. Reserve for patients who have failed other alternative agents. Consider changing to an alternate agent if skin discoloration occurs.
MOA — Enhances transmembrane potassium currents by opening the potassium channel
ADVERSE EFFECTS — Serious: urinary retention, confusion, psychosis, prolonged QT interval, suicidal ideation, skin discoloration. Frequent: dizziness, ataxia, somnolence, fatigue, tremor, diplopia, memory impairment, disturbance in attention, asthenia, blurred vision.

FELBAMATE (*Felbatol*) ▶KL ♀C ▶– $$$$$
WARNING — Aplastic anemia and fatal hepatic failure have occurred.
ADULT — Severe, refractory epilepsy, partial seizures: Start 1200 mg/day PO divided three to four times per day. Increase by 600 mg/day every 2 weeks to max 3600 mg/day.

PEDS — Lennox-Gastaut syndrome, adjunctive therapy, age 2 to 14 yo: Start 15 mg/kg/day PO in 3 to 4 divided doses. Increase by 15 mg/kg/day at weekly intervals to max 45 mg/kg/day.
FORMS — Generic/Trade: Tabs 400, 600 mg. Oral susp 600 mg/5 mL.
NOTES — Not a 1st-line agent. Use only after discussing the risks and obtaining written informed consent. Many drug interactions. Reduce dose by 50% in renally impaired.
MOA — Increases seizure threshold by blocking glycine binding to NMDA receptors.
ADVERSE EFFECTS — Serious: Aplastic anemia, hepatotoxicity, liver failure, purpura, maculopapular rash, suicidality. Frequent: Insomnia, headache, anxiety, N/V, diarrhea, constipation, rhinitis.

FOSPHENYTOIN (*Cerebyx*) ▶L ♀D ▶+ $
ADULT — Status epilepticus: Load 15 to 20 mg "phenytoin equivalents" (PE) per kg IV no faster than 100 to 150 mg PE/min. Nonemergent loading dose: 10 to 20 mg PE/kg IM/IV at rate no greater than 150 mg PE/min. Maintenance: 4 to 6 mg PE/kg/day in divided doses. Non-emergent use when oral phenytoin not possible: Load 10 to 20 mg PE IV (rate no faster than 150 mg PE/min) or IM. Initial maintenance dose 4 to 6 mg PE/kg/day in divided doses. Use oral phenytoin whenever possible. When substituted for oral phenytoin an equivalent number of phenytoin equivalents may be used.
PEDS — Not approved in children.
UNAPPROVED PEDS — Status epilepticus: 15 to 20 mg PE/kg IV at a rate less than 2 mg PE/kg/min. Nonemergent use age older than 7 yo: 4 to 6 mg PE/kg/24 h IV/IM no faster than 100 to 150 mg PE/min.
NOTES — Fosphenytoin is dosed in "phenytoin equivalents" (PE). The maximal infusion rate is 150 PE per minute because of risk of hypotension and cardiac arrhythias. Use beyond 5 days has not been systematically studied. Monitor ECG and vital signs continuously during and after infusion. Contraindicated in cardiac conduction block. Use cardiac monitoring when giving intravenously. Many drug interactions. Usual therapeutic level is 10 to 20 mcg/mL in normal hepatorenal function. Renal/hepatic disease may change protein binding and levels. Low albumin levels may increase free fraction.
MOA — Prodrug for phenytoin. Increases seizure threshold by modulating sodium and calcium channels.
ADVERSE EFFECTS — Serious: Cardiovascular collapse, CNS depression, hypotension, arrhythmias, hypersensitivity reactions, drug reaction with eosinophilia syndrome and systemic symptoms (DRESS)/multiorgan hypersensitivity syndrome, Stevens-Johnson syndrome, blood dyscrasias, hepatotoxicity, suicidality. Frequent: Nystagmus, dizziness, pruritus, paresthesia, headache, drowsiness, ataxia.

GABAPENTIN (*Neurontin, Horizant, Gralise*) ▶K ♀C ▶? $$$$

ADULT — Partial seizures, adjunctive therapy: Start 300 mg PO three times daily. Gradually increase to recommended dose of 300 to 600 mg PO three times per day. Doses of up to 2400 mg/day have been well tolerated. Max 3600 mg/day divided three times per day. Postherpetic neuralgia, immediate-release tabs: Start 300 mg PO on day 1; increase to 300 mg two times per day on day 2, and to 300 mg three times per day on day 3. Usual maintenance dose 1800 mg/day divided three times per day. Doses as high as 3600 mg/day have been used but are not more effective. Postherpetic neuralgia (Gralise): Start 300 mg PO once daily with evening meal. Increase to 600 mg on day 2, 900 mg on days 3 to 6, 1200 mg on days 7 to 10, 1500 mg on days 11 to 14, and 1800 mg on day 15. Max 1800 mg/day. Postherpetic neuralgia (Horizant): Start 600 mg PO q am for 3 days, then increase to 600 mg PO twice per day. Max 1200 mg/day. Restless legs syndrome (Horizant): 600 mg PO once daily around 5 pm taken with food.

PEDS — Partial seizures, adjunctive therapy: Start 10 to 15 mg/kg/day PO divided three times per day for age 3 to 11 yo. Titrate over 3 days to recommeded dose of 40 mg/kg/day (3 yo to 4 yo) or 25 mg/kg/day to 35 mg/kg/day (5 yo to 11 yo). Give in 3 divided doses. Use adult dosing for age 12 yo and older.

UNAPPROVED ADULT — Neuropathic pain: 300 mg PO three times per day, max 3600 mg/day in 3 to 4 divided doses. Migraine prophylaxis: Start 300 mg PO daily, then gradually increase to 1200 to 2400 mg/day in 3 to 4 divided doses. Restless legs syndrome: Start 300 mg PO at bedtime. Max 3600 mg/day divided three times per day. Hot flashes: 300 mg PO three times per day.

UNAPPROVED PEDS — Neuropathic pain: Start 5 mg/kg PO at bedtime. Increase to 5 mg/kg twice per day on day 2 and 5 mg/kg three times per day on day 3. Titrate to usual effective level of 8 to 35 mg/kg/24 h.

FORMS — Generic only: Tabs 100, 300, 400 mg. Generic/Trade: Caps 100, 300, 400 mg. Tabs 100, 300, 400, 600, 800 mg. Soln 50 mg/mL. Trade only: Tabs, extended-release 300, 600 mg (gabapentin enacarbil, Horizant). Trade only (Gralise): Tabs 300, 600 mg.

NOTES — Reduce dose in renal impairment (CrCl <60 mL/min); table in prescribing information. Discontinue gradually over 1 week or longer. Do not substitute other brands for Gralise because of bio-availability differences.

MOA — Unknown. Does not appear to be a GABA analog.

ADVERSE EFFECTS — Serious: Leukopenia, rhabdomyolysis. Frequent: Fatigue, drowsiness, dizziness, ataxia, nystagmus, tremor, peripheral edema, weight gain, suicidality. Peds only: Emotional lability, hostility, hyperactivity.

LACOSAMIDE (*Vimpat*) ▶KL ♀C ▶? ©V $$$$$

ADULT — Partial onset seizures, adjunctive (17 yo and older): Start 50 mg PO/IV two times per day. Increase weekly by 50 mg two times per day to recommended dose of 100 to 200 mg two times per day. Max recommended 400 mg/day (max 300 mg/day in mild/mod hepatic or severe renal impairment CrCl 30 mL/min or less). Alternative initiation: Load with 200 mg PO/IV followed 12 h later by 100 mg PO two times per day for one week. May then increase weekly as required by 50 mg two times per day to max recommended dose of 400 mg/day. Partial onset seizures, monotherapy: Start 100 mg PO/IV two times per day. May increase weekly by 50 mg two times per day to recommended range of 150 mg to 200 mg two times per day. Alternative initiation: Load with 200 mg PO/IV followed 12 h later by 100 mg twice daily for 1 week. May then increase weekly as required by 50 mg two times per day to recommended range of 150 mg to 200 mg two times per day. Conversion to monotherapy: Initiate and titrate lacosamide to usual dose of 150 mg to 200 mg twice daily and maintain for at least 3 days before tapering off the concomitant drug. Loading and intravenous dosing should be monitored. Doses of 600 mg/day are not more effective than 400 mg/day.

PEDS — Not approved in children or adolescents under the age of 17 yo. For 17 yo and above, use adult dosing.

FORMS — Trade only: Tabs 50, 100, 150, 200 mg. Oral Sol 10 mg/mL.

NOTES — Use caution in patients with cardiac conduction problems or taking drugs that increase the PR interval. Infusion rate for IV should not exceed 15 to 60 minutes with 30 to 60 minutes preferred unless rapid administration is needed. Avoid with severe renal impairment. Use with caution if given with other drugs that increase the PR interval.

MOA — Enhances slow inactivation of voltage-gated sodium channels.

ADVERSE EFFECTS — Severe: Increased PR interval, AV block, suicidality, syncope, agranulocytosis. Frequent: Dizziness, ataxia, nausea/vomiting, diplopia, vertigo, blurred vision, headache.

LAMOTRIGINE—NEUROLOGY (*Lamictal, Lamictal CD, Lamictal ODT, Lamictal XR*) ▶LK ♀C Possible risk of cleft palate or lip. ▶– $$$$

WARNING — Potentially life-threatening rashes (eg, Stevens-Johnson syndrome) have been reported in 0.3% of adults and 0.8% of children, usually within 2 to 8 weeks of initiation; discontinue at first sign of rash. Drug interaction with valproate; see adjusted dosing guidelines. Life-threatening drug reaction with eosinophilia and systemic symptoms (DRESS) has been reported.

ADULT — Partial seizures, Lennox-Gastaut syndrome, or generalized tonic–clonic seizures, adjunctive therapy with other anticonvulsants (not valproate or enzyme inducers); age older than 12 yo: Start

(cont.)

LAMOTRIGINE—NEUROLOGY (*cont.*)

25 mg PO daily for 2 weeks, then 50 mg PO daily for 2 weeks. Increase by 50 mg/day every 1 to 2 weeks to usual maintenance dose of 225 to 375 mg/day divided twice per day. Extended-release (generalized tonic–clonic and partial seizures): Start 25 mg PO daily for weeks 1 to 2, then increase to 50 mg/day for weeks 3 to 4. Increase to 100 mg/day on week 5 then increase weekly by 50 mg/day to target dose of 300 to 400 mg/day. Partial seizures, Lennox-Gastaut syndrome, or generalized tonic–clonic seizures, adjunctive therapy (with an enzyme-inducing anticonvulsant) age older than 12 yo: Immediate-release: Start 50 mg PO daily for 2 weeks, then 50 mg PO twice per day for 2 weeks. Increase by 100 mg/day every 1 to 2 weeks to usual maintenance dose of 300 mg to 500 mg/day divided twice per day. Extended-release (generalized tonic–clonic and partial seizures):Start 50 mg PO daily for weeks 1 to 2, then increase to 100 mg PO daily for weeks 3 to 4. Then increase by 100 mg/day at weekly intervals to target dose of 400 to 600 mg/day. Partial seizures, Lennox-Gastaut syndrome, or generalized tonic–clonic seizures, adjunctive therapy (with valproate) age older than 12 yo: Start 25 mg PO every other day for 2 weeks, then 25 mg PO daily for 2 weeks. Increase by 25 to 50 mg/day every 1 to 2 weeks to usual maintenance dose of 100 to 400 mg/day (when used with valproate + other inducers of glucuronidation) or 100 to 200 mg/day (when used with valproate alone) given once daily or divided twice per day. Extended-release (generalized tonic–clonic and partial seizures): Start 25 mg PO every other day for weeks 1 to 2, then increase to 25 mg/day for weeks 3 to 4. Then increase to 50 mg/day on week 5 and increase weekly by 50 mg/day to target dose of 200 to 250 mg/day. Partial seizures, conversion to monotherapy from adjunctive therapy (with a single enzyme-inducing anticonvulsant), immediate-release: (age 16 yo and older): Use preceding guidelines to gradually increase the dose to 250 mg PO twice per day; then taper the enzyme-inducing anticonvulsant by 20% per week over 4 weeks. Extended-release: Achieve dose of 500 mg/day then begin to reduce the enzyme-inducing AED by 20% decrements weekly over a 4-week period. Two weeks after the enzyme-inducing AED is discontinued Lamictal XR can be decreased no faster than 100 mg/day each week to the target dose of 250 to 300 mg/day. Partial seizures, conversion to monotherapy from adjunctive therapy (with valproate), immediate-release(ages 16 yo and older): Use preceding guidelines to achieve a dose of 200 mg/day and maintain it. Then begin to decrease valproate by decrements of no greater than 500 mg/day per week to a dose of 500 mg/day and maintain this for 1 week. Then increase lamotrigine to 300 mg/day and reduce valproate simultaneously to 250 mg/day and maintain for 1 week. Then stop the valproate and increase lamotrigine by 100 mg/day every week until a maintenance dose of 500 mg/day is

achieved. Extended-release: Achieve a dose of 150 mg/day and maintain it. Then begin to decrease valproate by 500 mg/day per week to 500 mg/day and maintain for 1 week. Then simultaneously increase Lamictal XR to 200 mg/day and decrease valproate to 250 mg/day and maintain for 1 week. Then increase Lamictal XR to 250 mg to 300 mg per day and discontinue valproate. Partial seizures, conversion to monotherapy from other AEDs (not valproate or enzyme inducers) extended-release: Achieve a dose of 250 to 300 mg/day of Lamictal XR then begin to withdraw the other AED by 20% decrements weekly over a 4-week period. No specific guidelines have been developed for conversion from other anticonvulsants (not inducers or valproate) to monotherapy with lamotrigine immediate-release. See psychiatry section for bipolar disorder dosing.

PEDS — Partial seizures, Lennox-Gastaut syndrome or generalized tonic–clonic seizures, adjunctive therapy with an enzyme-inducing anticonvulsant (age 2 to 12 yo): Start 0.6 mg/kg/day PO divided twice per day for 2 weeks, then 1.2 mg/kg/day PO divided twice per day for 2 weeks. Increase every 1 to 2 weeks by 1.2 mg/kg/day (rounded down to the nearest whole tab) to usual maintenance dose of 5 to 15 mg/kg/day divided twice per day. Max 400 mg/day. Partial seizures, Lennox-Gastaut syndrome, or generalized tonic–clonic seizures, adjunctive therapy with valproate (age 2 to 12 yo): Start 0.15 mg/kg/day PO (given daily or divided twice per day) for 2 weeks, then 0.3 mg/kg/day PO (given daily or divided twice per day) for 2 weeks. Increase every 1 to 2 weeks by 0.3 mg/kg/day (rounded down to nearest whole tab) to usual maintenance dose of 1 to 5 mg/kg/day (lamotrigine + valproate and other anticonvulsants) or 1 to 3 mg/kg/day if used with valproate alone. Max 200 mg/day. Partial seizures, Lennox-Gastaut syndrome, or generalized tonic–clonic seizures, adjunctive therapy with other anticonvulsants (not valproate or enzyme inducers) (age 2 to 12 yo): Start 0.3 mg/kg/day (given daily or divided twice per day) for 2 weeks, then 0.6 mg/kg/day divided twice per day for 2 weeks. Increase every 1 to 2 weeks by 0.6 mg/kg/day (rounded down to nearest whole tab) to usual maintenance dose of 4.5 to 7.5 mg/kg/day divided twice per day. Max 300 mg/day. Age older than 12 yo: Use adult dosing for all of the preceding indications including for Lamictal XR. Partial seizures, conversion to monotherapy (ages 16 yo and older): Use adult dosing.

UNAPPROVED ADULT — Initial monotherapy for partial seizures: Start 25 mg PO daily. Usual maintenance dose is 100 to 300 mg/day divided twice per day. Max 500 mg/day.

UNAPPROVED PEDS — Initial monotherapy for partial seizures: Start 0.5 mg/kg/day given daily or divided twice per day. Max 10 mg/kg/day. Newly diagnosed absence seizures: Usual effective dose is 2 to 15 mg/kg/day. Titrate gradually from a low starting dose as for other seizure types.

(cont.)

LAMOTRIGINE—NEUROLOGY (cont.)

FORMS — Generic/Trade: Tabs 25, 100, 150, 200 mg. Chewable dispersible tabs (Lamictal CD) 5, 25 mg. Extended-release tabs (Lamictal XR) 25, 50, 100, 200, 250, 300 mg. Orally disintegrating tabs (Lamictal ODT) 25, 50, 100, 200 mg.

NOTES — Drug interactions with valproate and enzyme-inducing antiepileptic drugs (ie, carbamazepine, phenobarbital, phenytoin, primidone); may need to adjust dose. May increase carbamazepine toxicity. Women taking estrogen-containing oral contraceptives without an enzyme-inducing anticonvulsant will generally require an increase of the lamotrigine maintenance dose by up to 2-fold. Consider increasing the lamotrigine dose when the contraceptive is started. Taper lamotrigine by 25% or less of daily dose every week over a 2-week period if the contraceptive is stopped. Preliminary evidence suggests that exposure during the 1st trimester of pregnancy is associated with a risk of cleft palate and/or cleft lip.

MOA — Blocks sodium channels and inhibits the release of glutamate.

ADVERSE EFFECTS — Serious: Stevens-Johnson syndrome, toxic epidermal necrolysis, hypersensitivity reactions, drug reaction with eosinophilia and systemic symptoms (DRESS), blood dyscrasias, multiorgan failure, suicidality, aseptic meningitis. Frequent: Rash, dizziness, diplopia, ataxia, drowsiness, headache, blurred vision, N/V, somnolence, insomnia.

LEVETIRACETAM (*Spritam, Keppra, Keppra XR*) ▶K ♀C ▶? $$$

ADULT — Partial seizures, juvenile myoclonic epilepsy (JME), or primary generalized tonic–clonic seizures (GTC), adjunctive: Start 500 mg PO/IV twice per day (Keppra or Spritam) or 1000 mg PO once daily (Keppra XR, partial seizures only); increase by 1000 mg/day every 2 weeks prn to max 3000 mg/day (partial seizures) or to recommended dose of 3000 mg/day (JME or GTC, and doses less than 3000 mg/day have not been adequately studied). IV route not approved for GTC or if age younger than 16 yo. Doses above 3000 mg are not more effective.

PEDS — Partial seizures, adjunctive therapy, Keppra, age 16 years and older use adult dosing. Keppra Soln: Age 1 mo to less than 6 mo, start 14 mg/kg/day PO given twice daily (7 mg/kg per dose). Increase every 2 weeks by 14 mg/kg/day given twice daily to recommended dose of 42 mg/kg/day (21 mg/kg twice daily). Age 6 mo to under 4 yo, start 20 mg/kg/day PO given twice daily (10 mg/kg per dose). Increase every 2 weeks by 20 mg/kg/day given twice daily to recommended dose of 50 mg/kg/day given twice daily (25 mg/kg twice daily). Age 4 yo to less than 16 yo, start 20 mg/kg/day PO given twice daily (10 mg/kg twice daily). Increase every 2 weeks by 20 mg/kg/day given twice daily to recommended dose of 60 mg/kg/day given twice daily (30 mg/kg twice daily). May reduce the dose if max not

tolerated. Keppra Tabs: Ages 4 yo to under 16 yo, (20kg-40 kg), start 250 mg PO twice daily. Increase every 2 weeks by 500 mg/day (250 mg twice daily) to max recommended dose of 750 mg twice daily (1500 mg/day). For weight over 40 kg, start 500 mg PO twice daily. Increase every 2 weeks by 1000 mg/day (500 mg twice daily) to max recommended dose of 1500 mg twice daily. Extended-release (Keppra XR), ages 12 yo and older, start 1000 mg PO daily. Increase every 2 weeks by 1000 mg/day to max recommended dose of 3000 mg/day. Spritam, age 4 yo or older and wt over 40 kg, start 500 mg PO twice daily. Increase every 2 weeks by 1000 mg/day to max recommended dose of 1500 mg twice daily (3000 mg/day). Age over 4 yo and wt 20-40 kg, start 250 mg PO twice daily. Increase every 2 weeks by 500 mg/day to max dose of 750 mg twice daily (1500 mg). Juvenile myoclonic epilepsy, adjunctive therapy, Keppra: age 12 yo or older: See adult dosing (IV approved for 16 yo or older only). Spritam, age 12 yo and older: Use adult dosing. Primary generalized tonic–clonic seizures (GTC), adjunctive therapy, Keppra, age 6 to 15 yo: Start 20 mg/kg/day PO (or IV if 16 yo or older) divided twice per day. Increase by 20 mg/kg/day every 2 weeks to recommended dose of 60 mg/kg/day divided twice daily. Age 16 yo and older: Use adult dosing. Patients over 20 kg may take either solution or tablets. Spritam, age 6 yo and older and wt over 40 kg, start 500 mg PO twice daily. Increase every 2 weeks by 1000 mg/day to recommended dose of 3000 mg/day (1500 mg twice daily). Age 6 yo and older and wt 20-40 kg, start 250 mg PO twice daily. Increase every 2 weeks by 500 mg/day to max recommended dose of 1500 mg/day (750 mg twice daily). Do not use in patients under 20 kg.

UNAPPROVED ADULT — Myoclonus: Start 500 to 1000 mg/day in divided doses. May increase to max 1500 to 3000 mg/day or 50 mg/kg/day.

FORMS — Generic/Trade: Tabs 250, 500, 750, 1000 mg. Oral soln 100 mg/mL. Tabs, extended-release 500, 750 mg. Trade: orally disintegrating tablet (Spritam) 250, 500, 750, 1000 mg.

NOTES — Drug interactions unlikely. Decrease dose in renal dysfunction (CrCl <80 mL/min). See package table for details. Emotional lability, hostility, and depression may occur. Use same dose when switching between IV and PO forms. Spritam should be placed on the tongue and followed with a sip of water to dissolve before swallowing. It may also be placed in a small amount of liquid and allowed to dissolve and then swallowed.

MOA — Unknown but may involve opposition of negative modulators of GABA and glycine-gated currents and inhibition of N-type calcium currents.

ADVERSE EFFECTS — Serious: Pancytopenia, pancreatitis, psychosis, depression, panic attacks, suicidality, drug reaction with esosinophilia and systemic symptoms (DRESS). Frequent: Drowsiness, dizziness, fatigue, asthenia, nervousness, emotional lability, hostility, ataxia.

METHSUXIMIDE (*Celontin*) ▶L ♀C ▶? $$$
ADULT — Refractory absence seizures: Start 300 mg PO daily for one week; increase weekly by 300 mg/day. Max 1200 mg/day.
PEDS — Refractory absence seizures: Start 300 mg PO daily for one wek; increase weekly by 300 mg/day. Max 1200 mg/day.
UNAPPROVED PEDS — Refractory absence seizures: Start 10 to 15 mg/kg/day PO in 3 to 4 divided doses; increase weekly prn. Max 30 mg/kg/day.
FORMS — Trade only: Caps 150, 300 mg.
NOTES — Monitor CBC, UA, and LFTs.
MOA — Inhibits low threshold calcium (T) currents.
ADVERSE EFFECTS — Serious: pancytopenia and other blood dyscrasias, drug-induced lupus, Stevens-Johnson syndrome, suicidality. Frequent: N/V, weight loss, anorexia, constipation, drowsiness, ataxia, dizziness.

OXCARBAZEPINE (*Trileptal, Oxtellar XR*) ▶LK ♀C ▶– $$$$$
WARNING — Serious multiorgan hypersensitivity reactions and life-threatening rashes (eg, Stevens-Johnson syndrome, toxic epidermal necrolysis) have occurred, with some fatalities. Consider discontinuation if skin reactions occur.
ADULT — Partial seizures, monotherapy: Start 300 mg PO two times per day. Increase by 300 mg/day every 3 days to usual effective dose of 1200 mg/day. Max 2400 mg/day. Partial seizures, adjunctive and conversion to monotherapy: Immediate-release: Start 300 mg PO two times per day. Increase by no more than 600 mg/day at weekly intervals to recommended dose of 1200 mg/day (adjunctive) or 2400 mg/day (conversion to monotherapy). Extended-release, adjunctive only: Start 600 mg PO daily. Increase by 600 mg/day weekly if needed, max 2400 mg/day.
PEDS — Partial seizures, adjunctive, age 4 to 16 yo: Start 8 to 10 mg/kg/day not to exceed 600 mg/d given twice daily. Increase over two weeks to recommended dose of 900 mg/day (20 to 29 kg), 1200 mg/day (29.1 to 39 kg), or 1800 mg/day (over 39 kg). Age 2 to younger than 4 yo: Start 8 to 10 mg/kg/day not to exceed 600 mg/d given twice daily. Increase over 2 to 4 weeks to max 60 mg/kg/day given twice daily. For patients under 20 kg a starting dose of 16 to 20 mg/kg/day may be considered. Partial seizures, adjunctive, extended-release, ages 6 to 17 yo: Start 8 to 10 mg/kg once daily not to exceed 600 mg in the first week. Increase weekly by 8 to 10 mg/kg once daily not to exceed 600 mg to achieve target doses of 900 mg/d (20-29 kg), 1200 mg/d (29.1-39 kg), or 1800 mg/d (>39 kg). Partial seizures, initial monotherapy, age 4 to 16 yo: Start 8 to 10 mg/kg/day divided two times per day. Increase by 5 mg/kg/day every 3 days to recommended dose (in mg/day based on wt rounded to nearest 5 kg) as follows: 600 to 900 for wt 20 kg, 900 to 1200 for wt 25 and 30 kg, 900 to 1500 for wt 35 and 40 kg, 1200 to 1500 for wt 45 kg, 1200 to 1800 for wt 50 and 55 kg, 1200 to 2100 for wt 60 and 65 kg, 1500 to 2100 for wt 70 kg.

Partial seizures, conversion to monotherapy, age 4 to 16 yo: Start 8 to 10 mg/kg/day divided two times per day. Increase at weekly intervals by no more than 10 mg/kg/day to target dose listed for initial monotherapy.
FORMS — Generic/Trade: Tabs (scored) 150, 300, 600 mg. Oral susp 300 mg/5 mL. Trade only: Extended-release tabs (Oxtellar XR) 150, 300, 600 mg.
NOTES — Monitor serum sodium. Decrease initial dose by ½ in renal dysfunction (CrCl <30 mL/min). Inhibits CYP2C19 and induces CYP3A4/5. Interactions with other antiepileptic drugs, oral contraceptives, and dihydropyridine calcium channel blockers. From 25% to 30% of patients who have had hypersensitivity reactions to carbamazepine will also react to oxcarbazepine. People with the HLA-B*1502 allele are at increased risk for serious dermatoligic reactions including Steven's Johnson syndrome and toxic epidermal necrolysis. Populations from China, Philippines, Malaysia, and Thailand have a higher proportion with this allele. Consider testing for this allele in at-risk populations.
MOA — Unknown. May inhibit sodium channels, increase potassium conductance, and modulate calcium channels.
ADVERSE EFFECTS — Serious: Stevens-Johnson syndrome, toxic epidermal necrolysis, hyponatremia/SIADH, bone marrow depression, leukopenia, agranulocytosis, aplastic anemia, angioedema, suicidality. Frequent: Dizziness, drowsiness, fatigue, headache, ataxia, diplopia, nystagmus, gait disturbance, tremor, N/V, abdominal pain.

PERAMPANEL (*Fycompa*) ▶L ♀C ▶? ©III $$$$$
ADULT — Partial onset seizures: Without other enzyme-inducing drugs: Start 2 mg PO once daily at bedtime. Increase by 2 mg/day weekly to usual range of 8 to 12 mg/day. Max 12 mg/day. With enzyme-inducing drugs: Start 4 mg PO once daily at bedtime. May increase weekly by 2 mg/day to max 12 mg/day. Mild to moderate hepatic impairment: Start 2 mg PO once daily at bedtime. May increase by 2 mg/day every 2 weeks to max 6 mg/day for mild disease and 4 mg/day for moderate. Avoid in severe hepatic impairment. Generalized tonic–clonic seizures, adjunctive: Without other enzyme-inducing drugs: Start 2 mg PO once daily at bedtime. Increase by 2 mg/day weekly to usual range of 8 to 12 mg/day. Max 12 mg/day. With enzyme-inducing drugs: Start 4 mg PO once daily at bedtime. May increase weekly by 2 mg/day to max 12 mg/day. Mild to moderate hepatic impairment: Start 2 mg PO once daily at bedtime. May increase by 2 mg/day every 2 weeks to max 6 mg/day for mild disease and 4 mg/day for moderate. Avoid in severe hepatic impairment.
PEDS — Partial onset seizures and adjunctive therapy for generalized tonic–clonic seizures: Ages 12 to 17 yo: Use adult dosing.
FORMS — Trade only:Tabs 2, 4, 6, 8, 10, 12 mg. Sus 0.5 mg/mL

(cont.)

PERAMPANEL (*cont.*)

NOTES — May reduce efficacy of levonorgestrel-containing oral contraceptives. Avoid with strong CYP3A inducers.

MOA — Non-competitive antagonist of the AMPA glutamate receptor on postsynaptic neurons.

ADVERSE EFFECTS — Severe: Suicidal thoughts and behavior, aggression, hostility, anger, homicidal ideation/threats. Frequent: Dizziness, gait disturbances, falls, somnolence, fatigue, blurred vision, ataxia, weight gain.

PHENOBARBITAL (*Luminal*) ▶L ♀D Some manufacturers rate it as B ▶– ©IV $

ADULT — Epilepsy: 50 mg to 100 mg PO twice to three times daily. Oral daytime sedation: 30 mg to 120 mg PO divided into two or three doses. Max 400 mg/24 hr. Hypnotic: 100 mg to 320 mg PO at bedtime.

PEDS — Epilepsy: 3 to 6 mg/kg/day PO divided two to three times per day. Alternate dosing: 15 mg to 50 mg PO twice or three times daily. Oral daytime sedation: 6 mg/kg/day divided into three doses.

UNAPPROVED ADULT — Status epilepticus: 20 mg/kg IV at 100 mg/min. May repeat with additional 10 mg/kg every hour for refractory sezures until seiures stop.

UNAPPROVED PEDS — Status epilepticus: 30 mg/kg IV at 100 mg/min. May repeat with additional 10 mg/kg every hour for refractory seizures until seizures stop.

FORMS — Generic only: Tabs 15, 16.2, 30, 32.4, 60, 64.8, 97.2, 100 mg. Elixir 20 mg/5 mL.

NOTES — Usual therapeutic level is 15 to 40 mcg/mL. Monitor cardiopulmonary function closely when administering IV. Decrease dose in renal or hepatic dysfunction. Many drug interactions. Trade product Luminal no longer available. High risk of apnea if IV benzodiazepines are given to patients taking phenobarbital.

MOA — Nonselective CNS depressant.

ADVERSE EFFECTS — Serious: Respiratory and CNS depression, blood dyscrasias, anemia, thrombocytopenia, Stevens-Johnson syndrome, angioedema, suicidality. Frequent: Drowsiness, fatigue, N/V, bradycardia, ataxia, nystagmus, dizziness, cognitive symptoms, paradoxical CNS excitation.

PHENYTOIN (*Dilantin, Phenytek*) ▶L ♀D ▶– $$

ADULT — Status epilepticus: 15 to 20 mg/kg IV at rate no faster than 50 mg/min, then 100 mg IV/PO every 6 to 8 h. Epilepsy: Start 100 mg PO three times daily then titrate to a therapeutic serum concentration for maintenance. Once seizures are controlled may consider once-daily dosing for extended-release caps. Usual max 600 mg/day. Alternative oral loading: 400 mg PO initially, then 300 mg again in 2 h and 4 h. Then 24 hour later begin usual maintenance dosing. Limit dose increases to 10% or less due to saturable metabolism.

PEDS — Epilepsy, age older than 6 yo: 5 mg/kg/day PO divided two to three times per day. Titrate to therapeutic serum concentration. Usual max 300 mg/day. Status epilepticus: 15 to 20 mg/kg IV at a rate no faster than 1 to 3 mg/kg/min or 50 mg/min whichever is slower.

FORMS — Generic/Trade: Extended-release caps 100 mg (Dilantin). Susp 125 mg/5 mL. Extended-release caps 200, 300 mg (Phenytek). Chewable tabs 50 mg (Dilantin Infatabs). Trade only: Extended-release caps 30 mg (Dilantin).

NOTES — Usual therapeutic level is 10 to 20 mcg/mL. Limit dose increases to 10% or less due to saturable metabolism. Monitor ECG and vital signs when administering IV. Many drug interactions. Monitor serum levels closely when switching between forms (free acid vs. sodium salt). The free fraction may be increased in patients with low albumin levels. IV loading doses of 15 to 20 mg/kg have also been recommended. May need to reduce loading dose if patient is already on phenytoin. Avoid in patients known to be positive for HLA-B*1502 due to possible increased risk of Stevens-Johnson syndrome.

MOA — Increases seizure threshold through modulation of sodium and calcium channels.

ADVERSE EFFECTS — Serious: Arrhythmias, blood dyscrasias, Stevens-Johnson syndrome, toxic epidermal necrolysis, hypotension, cardiovascular collapse, thrombocytopenia, anemia, hypersensitivity, local skin necrosis (IV only), suicidality. Frequent: Rash, nystagmus, tremor, ataxia, dizziness, vertigo, sedation, lymphadenopathy. Frequent (chronic use): gingival hyperplasia, osteomalacia, coarse facies.

PREGABALIN (*Lyrica*) ▶K ♀?/?/?R Evidence of teratogenicity in animals. Inadequate human data. Enroll in registry; refer to prescribing information ▶? ©V $$$$$

ADULT — Painful diabetic peripheral neuropathy: Start 50 mg PO three times per day; may increase within 1 week to max 100 mg PO three times per day. Postherpetic neuralgia: Start 150 mg/day PO divided two to three times per day. May increase within 1 week to 300 mg/day divided two to three times per day. If needed and tolerated, may increase to 600 mg/day in two to three divided doses. Partial seizures (adjunctive): Start 75 mg PO twice daily or 50 mg PO three times daily. Increase as needed to max 600 mg/day. Fibromyalgia: Start 75 mg PO two times per day; may increase to 150 mg two times per day within 1 week; max 225 mg two times per day. Neuropathic pain associated with spinal cord injury: Start 75 mg PO two times per day; may increase to 150 mg two times per day within 1 week and then to 300 mg two times per day after 2 to 3 weeks if needed and tolerated.

PEDS — Not approved in children.

FORMS — Trade only: Caps 25, 50, 75, 100, 150, 200, 225, 300 mg. Oral soln 20 mg/mL (480 mL).

NOTES — Adjust dose if CrCl less than 60 mL/min; refer to prescribing information. Warn patients to report changes in visual acuity and muscle pain. May increase creatine kinase. Must taper if discontinuing to avoid withdrawal symptoms. Increased risk of peripheral edema when used in conjunction

(cont.)

PREGABALIN (*cont.*)

with thiazolidinedione antidiabetic agents. Taper off when discontinuing.

MOA — Unknown. Binds to alpha-2-delta subunit of voltage-gated calcium channels and reduces neurotransmitter release.

ADVERSE EFFECTS — Serious: Angioedema, visual field changes, reduced visual acuity, thrombocytopenia, suicidality, peripheral edema. Frequent: Dizziness, somnolence, dry mouth, decreased concentration/attention, blurred vision, peripheral edema, weight gain, ataxia, withdrawal reactions.

PRIMIDONE (*Mysoline*) ▶LK ♀D ▶– $$

ADULT — Epilepsy: Start 100 to 125 mg PO at bedtime. Increase over 10 days to usual maintenance dose of 250 mg PO three to four time per day. Max 2 g/day.

PEDS — Epilepsy, age younger than 8 yo: Start 50 mg PO at bedtime. Increase over 10 days to usual maintenance dose of 125 to 250 mg PO three times per day or 10 to 25 mg/kg/day in divided doses. Age 8 yo and older: use adult dosing.

UNAPPROVED ADULT — Essential tremor: Start 12.5 to 25 mg PO at bedtime. May increase weekly prn by 50 mg/day to 250 mg/day given once daily or in divided doses. Max 750 mg/day.

FORMS — Generic/Trade: Tabs 50, 250 mg.

NOTES — Usual therapeutic level is 5 to 12 mcg/mL. Metabolized to phenobarbital.

MOA — Converted to phenobarbital and PEMA. Nonselective CNS depressant.

ADVERSE EFFECTS — Serious: Respiratory and CNS depression, anemia, thrombocytopenia, suicidality. Frequent: Drowsiness, ataxia, vertigo, lethargy, irritability, emotional lability, nystagmus, rash, N/V, paradoxical CNS excitation.

RUFINAMIDE (*Banzel*) ▶K ♀C ▶? $$$$$

ADULT — Epilepsy, Lennox-Gastaut syndrome (adjunctive): Start 400 to 800 mg/day PO divided two times per day. Increase by 400 to 800 mg/day every 2 days to max/target 3200 mg/day divided two times per day. Give with food. Use lower initial doses of 10 mg/kg in children or 400 mg/d for adults if on valproate.

PEDS — Epilepsy, Lennox-Gastaut syndrome (adjunctive) age 1 yo or older: Start 10 mg/kg/day PO given two times per day. Increase by 10 mg/kg every other day max/target of 45 mg/kg/day or 3200 mg/day divided two times per day. Give with food. Use lower initial doses of 10 mg/kg in children who are also on valproate.

FORMS — Trade only: Tabs 200, 400 mg. Susp 40 mg/mL.

NOTES — Give with food. Use caution for patients with mild to moderate hepatic impairment and avoid in severe hepatic impairment and short QT syndrome. Use lower initial doses of less than 10 mg/kg in children or 400 mg per day in adults if on valproate.

MOA — Modulates activity of sodium channels.

ADVERSE EFFECTS — Serious: Suicidality, multiorgan hypersensitivity, drug reaction and esosinophilia with systemic symtpoms (DRESS), Steven's Johnson symdroms. Frequent: Headache, dizziness, fatigue, somnolence, nausea.

TIAGABINE (*Gabitril*) ▶L ♀C ▶? $$$$$

WARNING — New-onset seizures and status epilepticus may occur when used in patients without epilepsy, particularly when combined with other medications that lower the seizure threshold. Avoid off-label use.

ADULT — Partial seizures, adjunctive therapy with an enzyme-inducing anticonvulsant: Start 4 mg PO daily. Increase by 4 to 8 mg/day prn at weekly intervals to max 56 mg/day divided two to four times per day. Use lower inital doses and slower titration for patients on non-inducing anticonvulsants. Give with food.

PEDS — Partial seizures, adjunctive therapy with an enzyme-inducing anticonvulsant (age 12 to 18 yo): Start 4 mg PO daily. Increase by 4 mg/day prn every 1 to 2 weeks to max 32 mg/day divided two to four times per day. Use lower inital doses and slower titration for patients on non-inducing anticonvulsants. Give with food.

FORMS — Generic/Trade: Tabs 2, 4 mg. Trade only: Tabs 12, 16 mg.

NOTES — Take with food. Dosing is for patients on enzyme-inducing anticonvulsants such as carbamazepine, phenobarbital, phenytoin, or primidone. Reduce dosage in patients who are not taking enzyme-inducing medications and in those with liver dysfunction. The use of tiagabine has been associated with new onset seuzures when used by patients without epilepsy.

MOA — Inhibits presynaptic reuptake of GABA.

ADVERSE EFFECTS — Serious: Stevens-Johnson syndrome, generalized weakness, status epilepticus (with overdose); new onset seizures or status epilepticus (with off-label use), suicidality. Frequent: Dizziness, lightheadedness, asthenia, sedation, tremor, confusion, ataxia, nervousness, depression, decreased concentration, N/V, diarrhea.

TOPIRAMATE—NEUROLOGY (*Qudexy XR, Topamax, Trokendi XR*) ▶K ♀D ▶? $$$$$

ADULT — Partial seizures or primary generalized tonic–clonic seizures, monotherapy (immediate-release): Start 25 mg PO two times per day (week 1), 50 mg two times per day (week 2), 75 mg two times per day (week 3), 100 mg two times per day (week 4), 150 mg two times per day (week 5), then 200 mg two times per day as tolerated. Extended release (Trokendi XR and Qudexy XR: Start 50 mg PO daily. Increase weekly by 50 mg/day for 4 weeks then by 100 mg/day for weeks 5 and 6 to recommended dose of 400 mg once daily. Partial seizures, primary generalized tonic–clonic seizures, or Lennox-Gastaut syndrome, adjunctive therapy (immediate-release): Start 25 to 50 mg PO at bedtime. Increase weekly by 25 to 50 mg each day to usual effective dose of 100 to 200 mg PO two times per day (partial

(cont.)

TOPIRAMATE *(cont.)*

seizures and LGS) or 200 mg PO two times per day (generalized tonic–clonic seizures). Doses greater than 400 mg per day not shown to be more effective. Extended-release (Trokendi XR and Qudexy XR): Start 25 to 50 mg PO once daily. Increase weekly by 25 to 50 mg/kg to effective dose. Recommended dose 200 to 400 mg/day for partial seizures or Lennox-Gastaut syndrome or 400 mg/day for generalized tonic–clonic seizures. Migraine prophylaxis: Start 25 mg PO at bedtime (week 1), then 25 mg two times per day (week 2), then 25 mg every am and 50 mg every pm (week 3), then 50 mg two times per day (week 4 and thereafter).

PEDS — Partial seizures or primary generalized tonic–clonic seizures, monotherapy age older than 10 yo: Use adult dosing. Age 2 yo to younger than 10 yo: Start 25 mg PO nightly (week 1), 25 mg two times daily (week 2), then increase by 25 to 50 mg/day weekly as tolerated to maintenance range based on weight of 75 to 125 mg twice daily (weight up to 11 kg), 100 to 150 mg twice daily (12 to 22 kg), 100 to 175 mg twice daily (23 to 31 kg), 125 to 175 mg twice daily (32 to 38 kg), or 125 to 200 mg twice daily (greater than 38 kg). Extended-release (Trokendi XR and Qudexy XR) age 10 yo and older: Use adult dosing. Extended-release (Qudexy XR age 2 yo to younger than 10 yo) or (Trokendi XR age 6 yo to younger than 10 yo): Start 25 mg PO nightly (week 1), then if tolerated 50 mg once daily (week 2), and increase weekly by 25 to 50 mg/day to maintenance range (based on weight) of 150 to 250 mg once daily (up to 11 kg), 200 to 300 mg once daily (12 to 22 kg), 200 to 350 mg once daily (23 to 31 kg), 250 to 350 mg once daily (32 to 38 kg), or 250 to 400 mg once daily (greater than 38 kg). Partial seizures, primary generalized tonic–clonic seizures, or Lennox-Gastaut syndrome, adjunctive therapy age 2 to 16 yo: Start 1 to 3 mg/kg (max 25 mg) PO at bedtime. Increase by 1 to 3 mg/kg/day every 1 to 2 weeks to usual effective dose of 5 to 9 mg/kg/day divided twice a day. Extended-release (Trokendi XR for 6 yo and older) or (Qudexy XR for 2 yo and older): Start 25 mg PO once daily at night for 1 week (or 1 mg/kg to 3 mg/kg once nightly). Increase at 1- to 2-week intervals by increments of 1 mg/kg to 3 mg/ kg daily to recommended dose of 5 mg/kg to 9 mg/ kg given once daily. Migraine prophylaxis (adolescents 12 yo and older): Use adult dosing.

UNAPPROVED ADULT —Essential tremor: Start 25 mg PO daily. Increase by 25 mg/day at weekly intervals to 100 mg/day; max 400 mg/day. Bipolar disorder: Start 25 to 50 mg PO daily. Titrate prn to max 400 mg/day. Alcohol dependence: Start 25 mg PO every day; increase by 25 mg/day at weekly intervals as tolerated to 300 mg/day for up to 14 weeks total.

FORMS — Generic/Trade: Tabs 25, 50, 100, 200 mg. Sprinkle caps 15, 25 mg.Extended-release caps (Qudexy XR) 25, 50, 100, 150, 200 mg. Trade only: Extended-release caps (Trokendi XR) 25, 50, 100, 200 mg.

NOTES — Give ½ usual adult dose in renal impairment (CrCl <70 mL/min). Confusion, nephrolithiasis, glaucoma, and wt loss may occur. Risk of oligohidrosis and hyperthermia, particularly in children; use caution in warm ambient temperatures and/or with vigorous physical activity. Hyperchloremic, nonanion gap metabolic acidosis may occur; monitor serum bicarbonate and either reduce dose or taper off entirely if this occurs. Max dose tested was 1600 mg/day. Use during pregnancy associated with cleft palate/lip. Report fetal exposure to North American Antiepileptic Drug Pregnancy Registry (888-233-2334). May increase the risk of hyperammonemia if used with valproic acid.

MOA — Unknown. May modulate sodium channels and enhance GABA action.

ADVERSE EFFECTS — Serious: Acute angle-closure glaucoma, visual field defects, nephrolithiasis, oligohidrosis, hyperthermia, metabolic acidosis, suicidality, hyperammonemia, bleeding. Frequent: Somnolence, fatigue, ataxia, psychomotor slowing, cognitive symptoms, confusion, diplopia, nystagmus, dizziness, depression, nervousness, weight loss, paresthesia.

VALPROIC ACID —NEUROLOGY (*Depakene, Depakote, Depakote ER, Depacon, Stavzor, divalproex, sodium valproate, ✳Epival, Deproic*) ▶L ♀D Category X when used for migraine prevention ▶+ $$$$

WARNING — Fatal hepatic failure reported, especially in children younger than 2 yo with comorbidities and on multiple anticonvulsants. Monitor LFTs during 1st 6 months of treatment and periodically thereafter. Should not be used in children under 2 yo. Life-threatening pancreatitis reported; evaluate for abdominal pain, N/V, and/or anorexia and discontinue if pancreatitis occurs. May be more teratogenic than other anticonvulsants (eg, carbamazepine, lamotrigine, and phenytoin) and is associated with neural tube defects, lower IQ in offspring, and other effects. Hepatic failure and clotting disorders have also occurred when used during pregnancy. Use during pregnancy when no other options and provide effective contraception.

ADULT — Epilepsy (complex partial seizures): 10 to 15 mg/kg/day PO or IV infusion over 60 min (rate no faster than 20 mg/min) in divided doses (immediate-release, delayed-release, or IV) or given once daily (Depakote ER). Increase by 5 to 10 mg/kg/day at weekly intervals to max 60 mg/kg/day. Simple and complex absence seizures: Start 15 mg/kg/day and increase weekly as needed by 5 to 10 mg/kg/ day to max of 60 mg/kg/day. For both seizure types, give Depkaote ER once daily. Give delayed-release products (Depakote, Depakote Sprinkles) in divided doses for doses above 250 mg/day. Immediate-release products (Depakene, valproic acid) should be divided twice daily for 500 mg/day and above, and three times daily for doses of 750 mg and above. Migraine prophylaxis: Start 250 mg PO two times per day (Depakote or Stavzor) or 500 mg PO

(cont.)

VALPROIC ACID —NEUROLOGY (*cont.*)

daily (Depakote ER) for 1 week, then increase to max 1000 mg/day PO divided two times per day (Depakote or Stavzor) or given once daily (Depakote ER).

PEDS — Epilepsy (complex partial seizures), ages 10 yo and older: 10 to 15 mg/kg/day PO or IV infusion over 60 min (rate no faster than 20 mg/min). Increase by 5 to 10 mg/kg/day at weekly intervals to max 60 mg/kg/day. Simple and complex absence seizures (ages 10 yo and older): Start 15 mg/kg/day and increase weekly as needed by 5 to 10 mg/kg/day to max dose 60 mg/kg/day. For both seizure types, give Depkaote ER once daily. Give delayed-release products (Depakote, Depakote Sprinkles) in divided doses for doses above 250 mg/day. Immediate-release products (Depakene, valproic acid) should be divided twice daily for 500 mg/day and three times daily for doses of 750 mg and above.

UNAPPROVED ADULT — Status epilepticus (not 1st line): Load 20 to 40 mg/kg IV (rate no faster than 6 mg/kg/min), then continue 4 to 8 mg/kg IV three times per day to achieve therapeutic level. May use lower loading dose if already on valproate.

UNAPPROVED PEDS — Status epilepticus, age older than 2 yo (not 1st line): Load 20 to 40 mg/kg IV over 1 to 5 min, then 5 mg/kg/h adjusted to achieve therapeutic level. May use lower loading dose if already on valproate. Epilepsy (ages 2 to under 10 yo): start 10 to 15 mg/kg/day PO or IV infusion over 60 min (rate no faster than 20 mg/min). Increase by 5 to 10 mg/kg/day at weekly intervals to max 60 mg/kg/day. IV administration should be divided every 6 h. Delayed-release products should be given in 2 to 3 daily doses. Immediate-release products (Depakene, valproic acid) should be divided twice daily for 500 mg/day and above, and three times daily for doses of 750 mg and above.

FORMS — Generic/Trade: Immediate-release caps 250 mg (Depakene), syrup (Depakene, valproic acid) 250 mg/5 mL. Delayed-release tabs (Depakote) 125, 250, 500 mg. Extended-release tabs (Depakote ER) 250, 500 mg. Delayed-release sprinkle caps (Depakote) 125 mg. Trade only (Stavzor): Delayed-release caps 125, 250, 500 mg.

NOTES — May be used for other seizure types in association with complex partial or absence seizures. Contraindicated in urea cycle disorders, hepatic dysfunction, in patients with genetic mutations in mitochondrial DNA polymerase gamma, and migraine prophylaxis in pregnant women. Usual therapeutic anticonvulsant trough level is 50 to 100 mcg/mL. Depakote and Depakote ER are not interchangeable. Depakote ER is approximately 10% less bioavailable than Depakote. Divalproex sodium is released over 8 to 12 h with Depakote (1 to 4 doses/day), and 18 to 24 h with Depakote ER (1 dose/day). Many drug interactions. Patients receiving other anticonvulsants may require higher doses of valproic acid. Reduce dose in the elderly. Hyperammonemia (increased by concurrent topiramate), GI irritation, or thrombocytopenia may occur. Use lower initial dose and titrate slower for patients on rufinamide. Carbapenem antibiotics may reduce serum concentration to ineffective levels.

MOA — May increase GABA levels and modulate sodium channels.

ADVERSE EFFECTS — Serious: Hepatotoxicity, anaphylaxis, polycystic ovarian syndrome, bone marrow suppression, thrombocytopenia, bleeding, pancreatitis, SIADH, Stevens-Johnson syndrome, DRESS, hyperammonemia, suicidality. Frequent: N/V, diarrhea, weight gain, CNS depression, drowsiness, tremor, alopecia, rash, nystagmus, asthenia.

VIGABATRIN (*Sabril*) ▶K ♀C ▶– $$$$$

WARNING — Ophthalmologic abnormalities including permanent vision constriction and loss have been reported. It can occur at any time after treatment starts and even after months or years. Visual field testing should be performed prior to treatment and every 3 months thereafter. Continue testing for 3 to 6 months after the drug is discontinued. Once visual loss occurs, it is not reversible. Given the limitations of visual field testing in children younger than 9 yo, vigabatrin should be used in this age group only if clearly indicated. Do not use with other retinotoxic drugs or for patients who have other irreversible vision loss unless the benefits clearly outweigh the risks. The patient's response and need for continued treatment should be reassessed periodically. Vigabatrin should be withdrawn within 3 months of initiation for complex partial seizures and within 2-4 weeks for infantile spasms if there is no clear response or sooner if treatment failure is obvious.

ADULT — Refractory complex partial seizures (adjunctive treatment): Start 500 mg PO twice daily. May increase in 500 mg increments weekly to usual recommended dose of 1500 mg twice daily.

PEDS — Refractory complex partial seizures (adjunctive treatment 10 to 16 yo, 25 to 60 kg): Start 250 mg PO twice daily. May increase weekly by 500 mg/day to maintenance dose of 1000 mg PO twice daily. Patients over 60 kg should be dosed using adult guidelines. Infantile spasms (monotherapy, 1 month to 2 yo): Start 50 mg/kg/day PO divided twice daily. May increase in increments of 25 to 50 mg/kg/day every 3 days to a max of 150 mg/kg/day in 2 divided doses.

FORMS — Trade only: Tabs 500 mg. Oral powder 500 mg/packet.

NOTES — Due to possible vision loss the drug is only available in a restricted distribution program called SHARE, and patients must be enrolled by calling 1-888-457-4273. Reduce the dose if ClCr <80 mL/min. See package insert for dosing with renal insufficiency.

MOA — Irreversible inhibitor of GABA-transaminase; increases CNS levels of GABA.

ADVERSE EFFECTS — Serious: Ophthalmologic abnormalities, retinal atrophy, optic neuritis, optic

(*cont.*)

VIGABATRIN (*cont.*)

atrophy, peripheral neuropathy, MRI abnormalities in the brain, anemia, edema, suicidality. Frequent: Drowsiness, dizziness, headache, weight gain.

ZONISAMIDE (*Zonegran*) ▶LK ♀?/?/?R ▶? $$$$

ADULT — Partial seizures, adjunctive: Start 100 mg PO daily for 2 weeks, then increase to 200 mg PO daily. May increase prn every 2 weeks to 300 mg then 400 mg/day, given once daily or divided two times per day. Max 600 mg/day but doses greater than 400 mg/day are not more effective.

PEDS — Not approved in children or adolescents under the age of 16 yo. For those 16 yo and above, use adult dosing.

FORMS — Generic/Trade: Caps 25, 50, 100 mg.

NOTES — This is a sulfonamide; contraindicated in sulfa allergy. Fatalities and severe reactions including Stevens-Johnson syndrome, toxic epidermal necrolysis, fulminant hepatic necrosis, and blood dyscrasias have occurred with sulfonamides.

Discontinue if rash occurs. Clearance is affected by CYP3A4 inhibitors or inducers such as phenytoin, carbamazepine, phenobarbital, and valproic acid. Nephrolithiasis may occur. Oligohidrosis and hyperthermia may occur and are more common in children. Patients with renal disease may require slower titration.

MOA — Unknown. May involve inhibition of sodium and calcium channels.

ADVERSE EFFECTS — Serious: Toxic epidermal necrolysis, Stevens-Johnson syndrome, drug reaction with eosinophilia and systemic syndrome (DRESS), hepatic necrosis, agranulocytosis, aplastic anemia, hypersensitivity, nephrolithiasis, psychosis, suicidality, oligohidrosis, hyperthermia, metaboic acidosis. Frequent: Abdominal pain, headache, somnolence, fatigue, N/V, anorexia, dizziness, drowsiness, cognitive symptoms, ataxia, diplopia, confusion, depression, irritability, agitation, insomnia, weight loss.

NEUROLOGY: Migraine Therapy—Triptans (5-HT1 Receptor Agonists)

NOTE: May cause vasospasm. Avoid in ischemic or vasospastic heart disease, cerebrovascular syndromes, peripheral arterial disease, uncontrolled HTN, and hemiplegic or basilar migraine. Do not use within 24 h of ergots or other triptans. Risk of serotonin syndrome if used with SSRIs or MAOIs. May be associated with medication overuse headaches if used 10 or more days per month.

ALMOTRIPTAN (*Axert*) ▶LK ♀C ▶? $$

ADULT — Migraine treatment: 6.25 to 12.5 mg PO. May repeat in 2 h prn. Max 25 mg/day.

PEDS — Migraine treatment: For age 12 yo and older use same dose as adult

FORMS — Generic/Trade: Tabs 6.25, 12.5 mg.

NOTES — MAOIs inhibit almotriptan metabolism; use together only with extreme caution. Do not use with ergots. Use lower doses (6.25 mg) in hepatic or severe renal dysfunction with a daily max of 12.5 mg. Use with caution in patients with known hypersensitivity to sulfonamides.

MOA — Serotonin 5-HT1B/D agonist.

ADVERSE EFFECTS — Serious: Chest pain/tightness, coronary vasospasm, acute MI, arrhythmias, peripheral ischemia, stroke serotonin syndrome, medication overuse headache. Frequent: N/V, headache, paresthesias, sedation, dry mouth.

ELETRIPTAN (*Relpax*) ▶LK ♀C ▶? $$$$

ADULT — Migraine treatment: 20 to 40 mg PO at onset. May repeat after 2 h prn. Max 40 mg/dose or 80 mg/day.

PEDS — Not approved in children.

FORMS — Trade only: Tabs 20, 40 mg.

NOTES — Do not use within 72 h of potent CYP3A4 inhibitors such as ketoconazole, itraconazole, nefazodone, clarithromycin, ritonavir, or nelfinavir.

MOA — Serotonin 5-HT1B/D agonist.

ADVERSE EFFECTS — Serious: Chest pain/tightness, coronary vasospasm, acute MI, arrhythmias, peripheral ischemia, stroke, HTN, seizures, medication overuse headache, serotonin syndrome.

Frequent: Dizziness, somnolence, nausea, asthenia, chest tightness.

FROVATRIPTAN (*Frova*) ▶LK ♀C ▶? $$$$

ADULT — Migraine treatment: 2.5 mg PO. May repeat in 2 h prn. Max 7.5 mg/24 h.

PEDS — Not approved in children.

FORMS — Generic/Trade: Tabs 2.5 mg.

NOTES — There is no evidence that a second dose will be effective when the first dose fails to relive the headache. Do not use with ergots.

MOA — Serotonin 5-HT1B/D agonist.

ADVERSE EFFECTS — Serious: Chest pain/tightness, coronary vasospasm, acute MI, arrhythmias, peripheral ischemia, stroke, HTN. Frequent: N/V, headache, paresthesias, sedation, dizziness, fatigue, dry mouth.

NARATRIPTAN (*Amerge*) ▶KL ♀C ▶? $$

ADULT — Migraine treatment: 1 to 2.5 mg PO. May repeat in 4 h prn. Max 5 mg/24 h.

PEDS — Not approved in children.

FORMS — Generic/Trade: Tabs 1, 2.5 mg.

NOTES — Contraindicated in severe renal or hepatic impairment. For mild to moderate renal or hepatic impairment reduce initial dose to 1 mg and do not exceed 2.5 mg/24h. Do not use with ergots.

MOA — Serotonin 5-HT1B/D agonist.

ADVERSE EFFECTS — Serious: Chest pain/tightness, coronary vasospasm, acute MI, arrhythmias, peripheral ischemia, stroke, HTN, medication overuse headache, serotonin syndrome. Frequent: Paresthesia, dizziness, drowsiness, malaise, fatigue.

RIZATRIPTAN (*Maxalt, Maxalt MLT*) ▸LK ♀C ▶? $$$
ADULT — Migraine treatment: 5 to 10 mg PO; may repeat in 2 h prn. Max 30 mg/24 h.
PEDS — Migraine treatment: Children 6 to 17 yo, 5 mg PO if less than 40 kg and 10 mg PO for 40 kg and above. Do not give more than one dose in 24 h.
FORMS — Generic/Trade: Tabs 5, 10 mg. Orally disintegrating tabs 5, 10 mg.
NOTES — Should not be combined with MAOIs. MLT form dissolves on tongue without liquids. Adult patients receiving propranolol should only receive 5 mg dose and not more than 3 doses per 24 h. For pediatric patients taking propranolol and weighing more than 40 kg only a 5 mg dose one time in 24 h should be used. Do not give to children weighing less than 40 kg and taking propranolol.
MOA — Serotonin 5-HT1B/D agonist.
ADVERSE EFFECTS — Serious: Chest pain/tightness, coronary vasospasm, acute MI, arrhythmias, peripheral ischemia, stroke, HTN, medication overuse headache, serotonin syndrome. Frequent: Asthenia, fatigue, drowsiness, pain/pressure sensation, dizziness, paresthesia.
SUMATRIPTAN (*Zembrace SymTouch, Onzetra Xsail, Imitrex, Alsuma, Sumavel, Zecuity*) ▸LK ♀C ▶+ $
ADULT — Migraine treatment: Imitrex: 1 to 6 mg (6 mg usual) SC. May repeat in 1 h prn if there was some response to first dose. Max 12 mg/24 h. If HA returns after initial SC injection, then single tabs may be used every 2 h prn, max 100 mg/24 h. Zembrace SymTouch: 3 mg SC. May repeat after 1 or more hours if needed up to three times or max of 12 mg/24 h. Tabs: 25 to 100 mg PO (50 mg most common). May repeat every 2 h prn with 25 to 100 mg doses. Max 200 mg/24 h. Initial oral dose of 50 mg appears to be more effective than 25 mg. Intranasal spray: 5 to 20 mg every 2 h. Max 40 mg/24 h. Intranasal powder: 22 mg (11 mg in each nostril). May repeat if needed at least 2 h after the first dose. Max 44 mg/24 h. Transdermal (Zecuity): 1 patch topically, max two patches/24 h with no less than 2 h before 2nd application. No evidence of increased benefit with 2nd patch. Cluster headache treatment: 6 mg SC. May repeat after 1 h or longer prn if there was some response to first dose. Max 12 mg/24 h. Avoid MAOIs.
PEDS — Not approved in children.
UNAPPROVED PEDS — Acute migraine, intranasal spray, for age 8 to 17 yo: Give 20 mg for wt 40 kg or greater or 10 mg for wt 20 to 39 kg intranasally at headache onset. May repeat after 2 h prn.
FORMS — Generic/Trade: Tabs 25, 50, 100 mg. Injection (STATdose System) 4, 6 mg prefilled cartridges. Trade only: Nasal spray (Imitrex Nasal) 5, 20 mg (box of #6). Alsuma, Sumavel: Injection 6 mg prefilled cartridge. Injection (Zembrace SymTouch) 3 mg autoinjector. Zecuity Transdermal Patch (temporarily suspended June, 2016): 6.5 mg/4 h. Generic only: Nasal spray 5, 20 mg (box of #6). Intranasal powder: 11 mg/nosepiece.

NOTES — Should not be combined with MAOIs. Do not use with ergots. Avoid IM/IV route. The Zecuity patch is a battery powered iontophoretic system. The FDA reported in 2016 that some patients have reported burns and scarring at application sites with this patch. Patients reporting moderate to severe pain at the site should remove the patch immediately and contact their healthcare professional. Do not bathe, swim, or shower while wearing the patch. The product was temporarily suspended in June, 2016.
MOA — Serotonin 5-HT1B/D agonist.
ADVERSE EFFECTS — Serious: Chest pain/tightness, coronary vasospasm, acute MI, arrhythmias, peripheral ischemia, stroke, seizures, HTN, medication overuse headache, serotonin syndrome. Frequent: Dizziness, lightheadedness, weakness, myalgias, muscle cramps, N/V, fatigue, drowsiness, flushing, pain/pressure sensation.
TREXIMET (**sumatriptan + naproxen**) ▸LK ♀C ▶– $$$$
WARNING — Risk of GI bleeding and perforation. Increased risk of coronary thrombotic events. Do not use after coronary bypass surgery. Do not use ergots within 24 h of Treximet.
ADULT — Migraine treatment: 1 tab (85/500) PO at onset. Max 2 tabs/24 h separated by at least 2 h.
PEDS — Migraine treatment (ages 12 yo and older):1 tab PO of 10/60 mg at onset. Max dose in 24 h is 1 tab of 85/500 mg.
FORMS — Trade only: Tabs 85 mg sumatriptan + 500 mg naproxen sodium and 10 mg sumatriptan + 60 mg of naproxen sodium.
NOTES — Avoid if CrCl less than 30 mL/min, cerebrovascular, cardiovascular, peripheral vascular disease, uncontrolled HTN, or severe hepatic impairment. Max daily dose for mild to moderate hepatic impairment is one 10/60 mg tablet. Contraindicated with MAOIs.
MOA — Combination of serotonin 5-HT1B/D agonist and anti-inflammatory/analgesic.
ADVERSE EFFECTS — Serious: Serotonin syndrome, renal toxicity, anaphylactic reactions, chest pain/tightness, coronary vasospasm, acute MI, arrhythmias, peripheral ischemia, stroke, seizures, HTN, gastrointestinal bleeding/ulceration, medication overuse headache. Frequent: Dizziness, lightheadedness, weakness, myalgias, muscle cramps, N/V, fatigue, drowsiness, flushing, pain/pressure sensation.
ZOLMITRIPTAN (*Zomig, Zomig ZMT*) ▸L ♀C ▶? $$
ADULT — Migraine treatment (acute): Tabs: 1.25 to 2.5 mg PO every 2 h. Max single dose 5 mg. Max 10 mg/24 h. Orally disintegrating tabs (ZMT): 2.5 mg PO. May repeat in 2 h prn. Max 10 mg/24 h. Nasal spray: 5 mg (1 spray) in 1 nostril. May repeat in 2 h prn. Max 10 mg/24 h.
FORMS — Generic/Trade: Tabs 2.5, 5 mg. Orally disintegrating tabs (ZMT) 2.5, 5 mg. Trade only: Nasal spray 5 mg/spray.

(cont.)

ZOLMITRIPTAN (*cont.*)

NOTES — Use lower doses (less than 2.5 mg) in hepatic dysfunction. May break 2.5 mg tabs in half and reduce max to 5 mg/day. Do not use with ergots.

MOA — Serotonin 5-HT1B/D agonist.

ADVERSE EFFECTS — Serious: Chest pain/tightness, coronary vasospasm, acute MI, arrhythmia, peripheral and splenic ischemia, stroke, HTN, medication overuse headache, serotonin syndrome. Frequent: Asthenia, pain/pressure, diaphoresis, dizziness, drowsiness, dyspepsia, flushing, paresthesia, dysgeusia (nasal spray only).

NEUROLOGY: Migraine Therapy—Other

CAFERGOT (ergotamine + caffeine, *Migergot*) ▶L ♀X ▶– $$$

WARNING — Contraindicated with concomitant use of potent CYP3A4 inhibitors (eg, macrolides, protease inhibitors) due to risk of serious/life-threatening peripheral ischemia. Ergots have been associated with potentially life-threatening fibrotic complications.

ADULT — Migraine and cluster headache treatment: 2 tabs PO at onset, then 1 tab every 30 min prn to max 6 tabs/attack or 10 tabs/week. Vascular headaches (migraine, migraine variants): Migergot: Two supps PR is max dose for one headache. Total weekly dose should not exceed 5 supps. Drug interactions. Fibrotic complications.

PEDS — Not approved in children.

UNAPPROVED PEDS — Migraine treatment: 1 tab PO at onset, then 1 tab every 30 min prn to max 3 tabs/attack.

FORMS — Trade/generic: Tabs 1/100 mg ergotamine/caffeine. Trade (Migergot): supp 2 mg/100 mg ergotamine/caffeine

NOTES — Contraindicated in sepsis, CAD, peripheral arterial disease, HTN, impaired hepatic or renal function, malnutrition, or severe pruritus.

MOA — Vasoconstrictor. Partial agonist/antagonist at alpha-adrenergic and serotonin receptors (ergotamine).

ADVERSE EFFECTS — Serious: Coronary vasospasm, coronary or peripheral ischemia, arrhythmias, HTN; retroperitoneal, pleural, pericardial, or cardiac valvular fibrosis. Frequent: N/V, dry mouth, abdominal pain, localized edema and pruritus, myalgias, leg weakness, peripheral ischemia, paresthesias, asthenia

DIHYDROERGOTAMINE (*D.H.E. 45, Migranal*) ▶L ♀X ▶– $$$$$

WARNING — Contraindicated with concomitant use of potent CYP3A4 inhibitors (eg, macrolides, protease inhibitors) due to risk of serious/life-threatening peripheral ischemia. Ergots have been associated with potentially life-threatening fibrotic complications.

ADULT — Migraine treatment: Soln (DHE 45): 1 mg IV/IM/SC; may repeat every 1 h prn to max 2 mg (IV) or 3 mg (IM/SC) per 24 h. Nasal spray (Migranal): 1 spray (0.5 mg) in each nostril; may repeat in 15 min prn to max 6 sprays (3 mg)/24 h or 8 sprays (4 mg)/week.

PEDS — Not approved in children.

FORMS — Generic/Trade: Nasal spray 0.5 mg/spray (Migranal). Self-injecting soln (D.H.E. 45): 1 mg/mL.

NOTES — Contraindicated in basilar or hemiplegic migraine, sepsis, ischemic or vasospastic cardiac disease, peripheral vascular disease, vascular surgery, impaired hepatic or renal function, or uncontrolled HTN. Avoid concurrent ergotamine, methysergide, or triptan use.

MOA — Serotonin 5-HT1D receptor agonist.

ADVERSE EFFECTS — Serious: Coronary vasoconstriction, MI, ventricular arrhythmias, stroke, HTN, peripheral ischemia; retroperitoneal, pleural, pericardial, or cardiac valvular fibrosis. Frequent: N/V, diarrhea, paresthesia, chest pain. Rhinitis and dysgeusia (nasal spray only).

ERGOTAMINE (*Ergomar*) ▶L ♀X ▶– $$

ADULT — Vascular headache: Start 2 mg SL; may repeat every 30 min to max 6 mg/24 h. Drug interactions. Fibrotic complications.

PEDS — Not approved in children.

FORMS — Trade only: SL tabs (ergotamine tartrate) 2 mg.

NOTES — Avoid use with potent CYP3A4 inhibitors (eg, ritonavir, nelfinavir, indinavir, erythromycin, clarithromycin); severe peripheral vasoconstriction may result.

MOA — Vasoconstrictor. Partial agonist/antagonist at alpha-adrenergic and serotonin receptors (ergotamine).

ADVERSE EFFECTS — Serious: coronary vasospasm, coronary or peripheral ischemia, arrhythmias, HTN; retroperitoneal, pleural, pericardial, or cardiac valvular fibrosis. Frequent: N/V, dry mouth, abdominal pain, localized edema and pruritus, myalgias, leg weakness, peripheral ischemia, paresthesia, asthenia, transient chest pain.

FLUNARIZINE ▶L ♀C ▶– $$

ADULT — Canada only. Migraine prophylaxis: 10 mg PO at bedtime; if side effects occur, then reduce dose to 5 mg at bedtime. Safety of long-term use (more than 4 months) has not been established.

PEDS — Not approved in children.

FORMS — Generic/Trade: Caps 5 mg.

NOTES — Gradual onset of benefit, over 6 to 8 weeks. Not for acute therapy. Contraindicated if history of depression or extrapyramidal disorders.

MOA — Selective calcium channel blocker.

(cont.)

FLUNARIZINE (*cont.*)

ADVERSE EFFECTS — Serious: Depression, extrapyramidal symptoms, tardive syndromes. Frequent: Drowsiness, weight gain.

ISOMETHEPTENE + DICHLORALPHENAZONE + ACETAMINOPHEN ▶L ♀? ▶? ©IV $$

ADULT — Tension and vascular headache treatment: 1 to 2 caps PO every 4 h, to max of 8 caps/day. Migraine treatment: 2 caps PO single dose, then 1 cap every 1 h prn to max 5 caps within 12 h.

PEDS — Not approved in children.

FORMS — Generic only: Caps (isometheptene/dichloralphenazone/acetaminophen) 65/100/325 mg.

NOTES — Midrin brand no longer available. FDA has classified as possibly effective for migraine treatment; however, products containing this combination are not FDA approved. Availability of generics may be inconsistent. Contraindicated in glaucoma, severe renal disease, heart disease, hepatic disease, or concurrent MAOI use. Use caution in HTN, peripheral arterial disease, or recent MI.

MOA — Combination sympathomimetic (vasoconstrictor), CNS depressant, and analgesic.

ADVERSE EFFECTS — Serious: Hepatotoxicity, renal tubular necrosis, chronic analgesic nephropathy. Frequent: Rash, dizziness.

NEUROLOGY: Multiple Sclerosis

ALEMTUZUMAB—NEUROLOGY (*Lemtrada*) ▶proteolysis ♀C ▶?

WARNING — Alemtuzumab can cause serious, possibly fatal autoimmune conditions like immune thrombocytopenia and anti-glomerular basement membrane disease. Monitor CBC with differential, serum creatinine, and urinalysis with cell counts periodically for 48 months after the last dose. Alemtuzumab has also caused serious, life-threatening infusion reactions including anaphylaxis. It must be administered under conditions and by personnel where management of these conditions is possible. These reactions can occur after the usual 2-h monitoring period and patients should be warned. There is an increased risk of malignancies with this drug. These include thyroid cancer, melanoma, and lymphoproliferative disorders. Patients should have baseline and yearly skin exams. Alemtuzumab is only available through a restricted distribution program, and may only be prescribed by certified physicians.

ADULT — Relapsing-remitting multiple sclerosis: First course: 12 mg per day by IV infusion over 4 h for 5 consecutive days (total 60 mg). Second course (12 months after 1st course): 12 mg/day by IV infusion over 4 h for 3 consecutive days (total 36 mg). See entry in Oncology for other uses.

PEDS — Not approved for use in children or adolescents.

FORMS — Trade: Injection 12 mg/1.2 mL

NOTES — Patients should be premedicated with 1000 mg of methylprednisolone or the equivalent immediately before the infusion and for the 1st 3 days of each treatment. In addition, patients should be given antiviral prophylaxis for herpetic infections beginning on the 1st day of each treatment for a minimum of 2 months afterward or until the CD4+ lymphocyte count is 200 cells/mL, whichever occurs later. Patients should complete any necessary immunizations at least 6 weeks prior to treatment. Determine if the patient has a history of varicella (VZV) or has been vaccinated against this virus. If not then consider testing for VZV antibodies and if negative consider vaccination. Do not treat until 6 weeks after vaccination. Monitor patients for at least 2 h after each infusion. Obtain CBC with differential, SCr, urinalysis with cell counts at baseline and then at monthly intervals thereafter. Test thyroid function at baseline and every 3 months after treatment. Contraindicated for patients with HIV infection. This drug is available only through a restricted distribution program. For information call 855-676-6326.

MOA — CD52-directed monoclonal antibody causing cytolysis of T and B lymphocytes

ADVERSE EFFECTS — Serious: Autoimmune disorders, potentially fatal infusion reactions, malignancies including melanoma, thyroid cancer and lymphoproliferative disorders, immune thrombocytopenia, glomerular nephropathies, hyper- or hypothyroidism, infections, pneumonitis. Frequent: rash, headache, pyrexia, nasopharyngitis, nausea, urinary tract infection, fatigue, insomnia, upper respiratory tract infection, herpes viral infection, urticaria, pruritis, thyroid abnormalities, fungal infection, arthralgia, pain in extremeties and back, diarrhea, sinusitis, paresthesi, dizziness, abdominal pain, flushing, and vomiting.

DACLIZUMAB (*Zinbryta*) ▶proteolysis ♀?/?/? ▶?

WARNING — May cause severe liver injury including hepatitis and failure. Obtain transaminase and bilirubin prior to therapy and then monthly for up to 6 months after the last dose. Contraindicted with pre-existing liver disease or impairment. Also associated with Immune-mediated skin reactions, lymphadenopathy, non-infectious colitis, and other immune-mediated disorders. These may require systemic corticosteroids.

ADULT — MS - relapsing forms: 150 mg SC monthly.

PEDS — Not approved for use in children or adolescents under 17 years old.

FORMS — Trade only: Inj 150 mg/mL

NOTES — Available on through the Zinbryta REMS Program. Requirements and enrollment is available at 1-800-456-2255. Reserve for use when there is an inadequate response to at least two other drugs use for MS. Obtain liver function tests, biliruibin, and screen for Hepatitis B and

(cont.)

DACLIZUMAB (*cont.*)

C and TB prior to initiation. Check vaccine status and give live vaccines at least 4 months prior to initiation.

MOA — Binds to the CD25 subunit of IL-2 receptor to modulate lymphocyte activation.

ADVERSE EFFECTS — Serious: Infections, liver damage and failure, hypersensitivity, immune-mediated skin reactions and colitism, lymphadenopathy, depression, suicidal thoughts and behaviors. Frequent: nasopharyngitis, upper respiratory tract infections, rash, influenza, dermatitis, oropharyngeal pain, bronchitis, eczema, lymphadenopathy.

DALFAMPRIDINE (*Ampyra*, ✱*Fampyra*) ▶K – ♀C ▶? $$$$$

WARNING — Risk of drug-induced seizures.

ADULT — Multiple sclerosis (improve walking): 10 mg PO two times per day.

PEDS — Not approved for use in children or adolescents

FORMS — Trade: Extended-release tabs 10 mg.

NOTES — Contraindicated with moderate to severe renal impairment (CrCl less than 50 mL/min) and history of seizures. Monitor serum creatinine annually. Obtained from a specialty pharmacy (Ampyra Patient Support Service 888-883-3053). Do not exceed recommended dose. Do not combine with other forms of 4-aminopyridine.

MOA — Broad spectrum potassium channel blocker.

ADVERSE EFFECTS — Serious: Seizures. Frequent: Urinary tract infection, insomnia, dizziness, headache, nausea, asthenia, back pain, balance disorder, multiple sclerosis relapse, paresthesia, nasopharyngitis, constipation, dyspepsia, pharyngolaryngeal pain.

DIMETHYL FUMARATE (*Tecfidera*) ▶esterases – ♀C ▶? $$$$$

ADULT —Multiple sclerosis (relapsing): Start 120 mg PO twice per day. Increase to maintenance dose of 240 mg twice per day after 7 days.

PEDS — Not approved for use in children.

FORMS — Trade only: delayed-release capsules 120, 240 mg.

NOTES — Obtain CBC prior to initiation of treatment. Discontinue at the first sign or symptom of progressive multifocal leukoencephalopathy. Administration with food or 325 mg of non-enteric coated aspirin 30 minutes prior to administration may reduce flushing. Consider reducing the dose to 120 mg daily if the patient cannot tolerate the maintenance dose of 240 mg per day. After 4 weeks increase back to maintenance level. Discontinue if the patient still does not tolerate it.

MOA — Unknown but may activate the Nuclear factor (Nrf2) pathway.

ADVERSE EFFECTS — Serious: Lymphopenia, progressive multifocal leukoencephalopathy, lymphopenia. Frequent: flushing, abdominal pain, diarrhea, nausea.

FINGOLIMOD (*Gilenya*) ▶L – ♀C ▶? $$$$$

ADULT — Relapsing multiple sclerosis: 0.5 mg PO once daily.

PEDS — Not approved for use in children or adolescents.

FORMS — Trade only: Caps 0.5 mg.

NOTES — Do not use within 6 months of MI, stroke/TIA, unstable angina, AV block, decompensated or Class III or IV heart failure. Observe all patients for bradycardia for 6 h after the 1st dose. Repeat this observation if therapy is reinitiated following discontinuation for more than 14 days. Obtain baseline ECG for patients on drugs such as beta blockers and antiarrhythmics that can cause bradycardia. Contraindicated if QTc >500 msec or treatment with antiarrhythmics. Obtain CBC prior to initiation and consider periodic monitoring. Monitor for infection and consider stopping if a serious infection occurs. Obtain baseline ophthalmic exam and after 3 to 4 months of therapy to monitor for macular edema. Obtain baseline LFTs. Use effective contraception during and for 2 months following therapy. Avoid live attenuated vaccines during and for 2 months following therapy. Avoid use with ketoconazole. Women should use effective contraception during treatment and for 2 months after stopping.

MOA — Sphingosine 1-phosphate receptor modulator reducing lymphocyte egress from lymph nodes

ADVERSE EFFECTS — Serious: bradycardia, AV block, leukopenia, infection, macular edema, posterior reversible encephalopathy syndrome, progressive multifocal leukoencephalopathy, dyspnea, teratogenicity. Frequent: headache, influenza, diarrhea, increased liver enzymes, cough, back pain

GLATIRAMER (*Copaxone, Glatopa*) ▶tissues local hydrolysis ♀B ▶? $$$$$

ADULT — Multiple sclerosis (relapsing-remitting): glatiramer acetate 20 mg/mL: 20 mg SC daily. Copaxone 40 mg/mL: 40 mg SC three times weekly with at least 48 h between doses.

PEDS — Not approved in children.

FORMS — Trade and generic: Prefilled syringes 20 mg per mL for injection. Trade only (Copaxone): 40 mg/mL. The 20 mg/mL and 40 mg/mL are not interchangeable.

NOTES — Do not inject IV. Patients may experience immediate post-injection reaction that includes flushing, chest pain, palpitations, anxiety, dyspnea, tightness of the throat, and urticaria. It is usually self-limited and does not require treatment. Patients should be told to report unusual or prolonged chest pain. Glatopa is considered a therapeutically equivalent generic for Copaxone. Rotate injections sites to avoid lipoatrophy and skin necrosis.

MOA — Immunomodulator.

ADVERSE EFFECTS — Serious: Anaphylaxis. Frequent: Injection site reactions, flu-like symptoms, flushing, dyspnea, chest pain, anxiety, palpitations, asthenia, pain, N/V, arthralgia.

INTERFERON BETA-1A (*Avonex, Rebif*) ▸L ♀C ▶? $$$$$
WARNING — Risk of severe hepatic injury and failure, possibly greater when used with other hepatotoxic drugs. Monitor LFTs. Suicidality risk; use caution in depression.
ADULT — Multiple sclerosis (relapsing forms): Avonex 30 mcg (6 million units) IM every week. May start with lower dose of 7.5 mcg and increase by 7.5 mcg each week until 30 mcg dose is achieved. Rebif: For 22 mcg maintenance dose start 4.4 SC mcg three times weekly for 2 weeks, then increase to 11 mcg three times weekly for 2 weeks, then increase to 22 mcg three times weekly. For 44 mcg maintenance dose start 8.8 mcg SC three times weekly for 2 weeks, then increase to 22 mcg three times weekly for 2 weeks, then increase to 44 mcg three times weekly. Give on the same days each week and at least 48 hours apart.
PEDS — Not approved in children.
FORMS — Trade only (Avonex): Injection 30 mcg single-dose vial with or without albumin. Prefilled syringe 30 mcg. Trade only (Rebif): Titration kit 8.8 mcg prefilled syringe. Prefilled syringe 22, 44 mcg. Autoinjector (Rebidose) Titration Kit 8.8, 22, 44 mcg.
NOTES — Use caution in patients with depression, seizure disorders, or cardiac disease. Follow LFTs and CBC. Avonex: Indicated for the first attack of MS. Rebif: Give same dose 3 days each week, with at least 48 h between doses.
MOA — Immunomodulator.
ADVERSE EFFECTS — Serious: Depression, suicidal ideation, psychosis, hepatotoxicity, anaphylaxis, autoimmune disorders (idiopathic thrombocytopenia, hyper- and hypothyroidism, hepatitis), cytopenias, seizures, cardiomyopathy, heart failure, Steven's Johnson Syndrome, thrombotic thrombocytopenic purpura, SLE. Frequent: Injection site reactions, headache, fever, chills, N/V, diarrhea, flu-like symptoms, fatigue, muscle pain.

INTERFERON BETA-1B (*Extavia, Betaseron*) ▸L ♀C ▶? $$$$$
ADULT — Multiple sclerosis (relapsing-remitting): Start 0.0625 mg SC every other day for weeks 1-2, then 0.125 mg weeks 3-4, then 0.1875 mg weeks 5-6, then increase to 0.25 mg (8 million units) SC every other day.
PEDS — Not approved in children.
FORMS — Trade only: Injection 0.3 mg (9.6 million units) single-dose vial.
NOTES — Observe patient for first dose. Suicidality risk; use caution in depression. Check CBC, platelets, blood chemistries, and LFTs after 1, 3, and 6 months and then periodically. Product can be stored at room temp until reconstituted; then refrigerate and use within 3 h. Consider premedication with analgesics and/or antipyretics to reduce flu-like symptons.
MOA — Immunomodulator.
ADVERSE EFFECTS — Serious: Depression, seizures, suicidality, autoimmune hepatitis, hepatic failure,

hypersensitivity, leukopenia, injection site necrosis, hypertension, lupus erythematosis. Frequent: Injection site reactions, headache, fever, chills, N/V, diarrhea, constipation, abdominal pain, edema, flu-like symptoms, myalgia, palpitations, dizziness, somnolence, increased LFTs, abnormal menses.

NATALIZUMAB (*Tysabri*) ▸Serum ♀C ▶? $$$$$
WARNING — May cause progressive multifocal leukoencephalopathy; avoid concomitant use of other immunomodulators. Risk of severe hepatotoxicity; discontinue if jaundice or evidence of liver injury. Risk of anaphylaxis or other hypersensitivity reactions; permanently discontinue if they occur. Risk factors include prior use of immunosuppressants, duration of therapy, and the presence of anti-JCV antibodies.
ADULT — Refractory, relapsing multiple sclerosis (monotherapy) and Crohn's disease: 300 mg IV infusion over 1 h every 4 weeks.
PEDS — Not approved in children.
NOTES — Not 1st line; recommended only when there has been an inadequate response or failure to tolerate other therapies. Available only through the MS-TOUCH or CD-TOUCH prescribing programs at 800-456-2255. Consider testing for anti-JCV antiboides. The presence of these increases the risk of PML. Observe closely for infusion reactions. Avoid other immunosuppressants when using for Crohn's disease; discontinue if no response by 12 weeks. For patients on steroids, taper them as soon as a benefit is noted and discontinue natalizumab if steroids cannot be tapered off within 6 months. Consider stopping natalizumab in patients who require steroids more than 3 months/year.
MOA — Specific mechanism unknown. Monoclonal antibody that blocks interaction of alpha-4-beta 1-integrin expressed inflammatory cells to vascular endothelium and parenchymal cells in the brain.
ADVERSE EFFECTS — Serious: Progressive multifocal leukoencephalopathy, herpes encephalitis and meningitis, cholelithiasis, hepatotoxicity, depression, suicidality, anaphylaxis, hypersensitivity reactions, infection. Frequent: Infusion reactions, headache, fatigue, arthralgia, urinary urgency/frequency, abdominal discomfort, diarrhea, rash, irregular menstruation/dysmenorrhea.

PEGINTERFERON BETA-1A (*Plegridy*) ▸K ♀C Enroll in registry ▶? $$$$$
ADULT — Multiple sclerosis - relapsing forms: start 63 mcg SC on day 1, then 94 mcg on day 15, then 125 mcg on day 29 and every 14 days thereafter.
PEDS — Not approved for use in children or adolescents.
FORMS — Trade only: Inj Starter pack (63 mcg and 94 mcg), pen 125 mcg
NOTES — Pretreat with analgesics and antipyretics prior to injections to reduce flu-like reactions.
MOA — Unknown
ADVERSE EFFECTS — Serious: Hepatitis, autoimmune hepatitis, hepatic failure, depression, suicidal ideation, seizures, anaphylaxis, heart failure,

(cont.)

PEGINTERFERON BETA-1A (*cont.*)
cariomyopathy, thrombotic microangiopathy, decreased peripheral blood counts, autoimmune disorders. Frequent: injection site reactions, flu-like reactions, fever, headache, myalgia, chills, asthenia, arthralgia.

TERIFLUNOMIDE (*Aubagio*) ▶bile ♀X ▶? $$$$$
WARNING — Severe, potentially fatal hepatotoxicity has been seen with a related drug leflunomide, and it may occur with teriflunomide. Obtain baseline liver function tests within 6 months of initiation, and then monitor ALT at least monthly for 6 months. Discontinue at first sign of liver toxicity and employ methods to accelerate drug elimination such as cholestyramine or charcoal. Teriflunomide is a known teratogen. Patients must use reliable contraception during use, and pregnancy should be avoided while using this drug.

ADULT — Multiple sclerosis, relapsing forms: Recommended dose 7 mg or 14 mg PO once daily.
PEDS — Not approved for use by children or adolescents.
FORMS — Trade only: Tabs 7 and 14 mg.
NOTES — Obtain liver function tests including bilirubin and a CBC prior to initiation of therapy. Repeat LFTs at least monthly for 6 months after starting. Monitor CBC based on signs and symptoms of infection. Screen patients for TB prior to initiation.
MOA — Immunomodulator/pyrimidine synthesis inhibitor
ADVERSE EFFECTS — Serious: hepatotoxicity, teratogenicity, bone marrow suppression, peripheral neuropathy, acute renal failure, hyperensitivity, Steven's Johnson syndrome, toxic epidermal necrolysis, hypertension, interstitial lung disease, thrombocytopenia. Frequent: alopecia, diarrhea, influenza, paresthesia, nausea.

NEUROLOGY: Myasthenia Gravis

EDROPHONIUM (*Tensilon, Enlon*) ▶Plasma ♀C ▶? $
ADULT — Evaluation for myasthenia gravis (diagnostic purposes only): 2 mg IV over 15 to 30 sec (test dose) while on cardiac monitor, then 8 mg IV after 45 sec. Reversal of neuromuscular blockade: 10 mg IV over 30 to 45 sec; repeat prn to max 40 mg.
PEDS — Evaluation for myasthenia gravis (diagnostic purposes only): Give 1 mg IV (test dose), then 1 mg IV q 30 to 45 sec to max 5 mg for wt 34 kg or less, give 2 mg IV (test dose), then 2 mg IV q 30 to 45 sec to max 10 mg for wt greater than 34 kg.
UNAPPROVED ADULT — Reversal of nondepolarizing neuromuscular blocking agents: 0.5 to 1 mg/kg IV together with atropine 0.007 to 0.014 mg/kg.
FORMS — 10 mg/mL MDV vial.
NOTES — Not for maintenance therapy of myasthenia gravis because of short duration of action (5 to 10 min). May give IM. Monitor cardiac function. Atropine should be readily available in case of cholinergic reaction. Contraindicated in mechanical urinary or intestinal obstruction.
MOA — Reversible cholinesterase inhibitor.
ADVERSE EFFECTS — Serious: Arrhythmias, bradycardia, respiratory paralysis, cholinergic toxicity, dysphagia, seizures. Frequent: N/V, abdominal cramping, diarrhea, miosis, lacrimation, diplopia, fasciculations.

PYRIDOSTIGMINE (*Mestinon, Mestinon Timespan, Regonol*) ▶Plasma, K ♀C ▶+ $$$$$
ADULT — Myasthenia gravis, immediate-release tabs: Start 60 mg PO three times per day; gradually increase to usual therapeutic dose of 200 mg PO three times per day. Extended-release tabs: Start 180 mg PO daily or divided two times per day. Max 1500 mg/day. May give 2 mg IM or slow IV injection every 2 to 3 h.
PEDS — Not approved in children.
UNAPPROVED PEDS — Myasthenia gravis, neonates: 5 mg PO q 4 to 6 h or 0.05 to 0.15 mg/kg IM/IV q 4 to 6 h. Myasthenia gravis, children: 7 mg/kg/day PO in 5 to 6 divided doses, or 0.05 to 0.15 mg/kg/dose IM/IV q 4 to 6 h. Max 10 mg IM/IV single dose.
FORMS — Generic/Trade: Tabs 60 mg. Extended-release tabs 180 mg. Trade only: Syrup 60 mg/ 5 mL.
NOTES — Give injection at 1/30th of oral dose when oral therapy is not possible.
MOA — Reversible cholinesterase inhibitor.
ADVERSE EFFECTS — Serious: Cholinergic toxicity, bronchospasm, respiratory paralysis, bradycardia, arrhythmias, cardiac arrest. Frequent: N/V, diarrhea, abdominal cramps/pain, muscle cramps/ weakness, fasciculation, miosis, hypersalivation, increased bronchial secretions.

NEUROLOGY: Parkinsonian Agents—Anticholinergics

NOTE: Anticholinergic medications may cause memory loss, delirium, or psychosis, particularly in elderly patients or those with baseline cognitive impairment. Contraindicated in narrow-angle glaucoma, bowel obstruction, and megacolon.

BENZTROPINE MESYLATE (*Cogentin*) ▶LK ♀C ▶? $
ADULT — Parkinsonism: Start 0.5 to 2 mg/day PO/ IM/IV. Increase in 0.5 mg increments at weekly intervals to max 6 mg/day. May divide doses one to four times per day. Drug-induced extrapyramidal

disorders (EPS): 1 to 4 mg PO/IM/IV given once daily or divided two times per day.
PEDS — Not approved in children.
UNAPPROVED PEDS — Parkinsonism in age older than 3 yo: 0.02 to 0.05 mg/kg/dose given once daily

(cont.)

BENZTROPINE MESYLATE (*cont.*)

or divided two times per day. Use caution; potential for undesired anticholinergic effects.

FORMS — Generic only: Tabs 0.5, 1, 2 mg.

NOTES — Contraindicated in narrow-angle glaucoma. Avoid concomitant use of donepezil, rivastigmine, galantamine, or tacrine. Brand name Cogentin discontinued. Provides fairly rapid onset of action when used for EPS. Some patients may be tapered off after 1-2 weeks to see if it is still needed.

MOA — Anticholinergic.

ADVERSE EFFECTS — Serious: Tachycardia, anticholinergic toxicity, psychosis, delirium. Frequent: Dry mouth, constipation, urinary retention, blurred vision, drowsiness, dizziness, headache, rash, N/V, memory problems.

TRIHEXYPHENIDYL (*Artane*) ▸LK ♀C ▸? $

ADULT — Parkinsonism: start 1 mg PO daily. Increase by 2 mg/day at 3- to 5-day intervals to usual therapeutic dose of 6 to 10 mg/day divided three times per day with meals. Max 15 mg/day.

PEDS — Not approved in children.

UNAPPROVED ADULT — Drug-induced parkinsonism (EPS): start 1 mg PO daily. Increase by 2 mg/day to usual range of 5 - 15 mg/day divided twice daily.

FORMS — Generic only: Tabs 2, 5 mg. Elixir 2 mg/5 mL.

NOTES — Brand name Artane has been discontinued.

MOA — Anticholinergic.

ADVERSE EFFECTS — Serious: Tachycardia, anticholinergic toxicity, psychosis, delirium. Frequent: Dry mouth, constipation, urinary retention, blurred vision, drowsiness, dizziness, headache, rash, N/V, memory problems.

NEUROLOGY: Parkinsonian Agents—COMT Inhibitors

ENTACAPONE (*Comtan*) ▸L ♀C ▸? $$$$$

ADULT — Parkinson's disease, adjunctive: Start 200 mg PO with each dose of carbidopa/levodopa. Max 8 tabs (1600 mg)/day.

PEDS — Not approved in children.

FORMS — Generic/Trade: Tabs 200 mg.

NOTES — Adjunct to carbidopa-levodopa in patients who have end-of-dose "wearing off." May need to reduce the dose of levodopa when entacapoine is initiated. Has no antiparkinsonian effect on its own. Avoid concomitant use of nonselective MAOIs. Use caution in hepatobiliary dysfunction. Avoid rapid withdrawal, which may precipitate neuroleptic malignant syndrome. Use caution if using medications metabolized by COMT such as isoproterenol, epinephrine, norepinephrine, dopamine, and dobutamine because an exaggerated response is possible. Use may be associated with abruptly falling asleep from the drug's impact on L-dopa.

MOA — Blocks dopamine breakdown by inhibiting catechol-o-methyltransferase.

ADVERSE EFFECTS — Serious: Orthostatic hypotension, rhabdomyolysis, hallucinations, delirium, severe diarrhea, impulse control disorders, sudden/unexpected somnolence. Frequent: Dyskinesia, hyperkinesia, N/V, abdominal pain, diarrhea, urine discoloration.

TOLCAPONE (*Tasmar*) ▸LK ♀C ▸? $$$$$

WARNING — Fatal hepatic failure has occurred. Use only in patients on carbidopa-levodopa who fail alternative therapies and provide written informed consent. Monitor LFTs at baseline, every 2 to 4 weeks for 6 months, and then periodically. Discontinue if LFT elevation is more than 2 times upper limit of normal or if there is no clinical benefit after 3 weeks of therapy.

ADULT — Parkinson's disease, adjunctive (not 1st line): Start 100 mg PO three times per day. Increase to 200 mg PO three times per day only if expected benefit justifies the risk. Max 600 mg/day. Only effective when used in combination with carbidopa-levodopa.

PEDS — Not approved in children.

FORMS — Trade only: Tabs 100 mg.

NOTES — Adjunct to carbidopa-levodopa in patients who have refractory end-of-dose "wearing off." Has no antiparkinsonian effect on its own. Contraindicated in hepatic dysfunction. Monitor LFTs. Avoid concomitant use of non-selective MAOIs. Avoid rapid withdrawal, which may precipitate neuroleptic malignant syndrome. Informed consent forms are available from the package labeling for Tasmar that can be found at Drugs@FDA.gov.

MOA — Blocks dopamine breakdown by inhibiting catechol-o-methyltransferase

ADVERSE EFFECTS — Serious: fulminant hepatotoxicity, orthostatic hypotension, hallucinations, severe diarrhea, impulse control disorders. Frequent: dyskinesia, dystonia, anorexia, N/V, diarrhea, constipation, confusion, sleep disorders.

NEUROLOGY: Parkinsonian Agents—Dopaminergic Agents and Combinations

NOTE: Dopaminergic medications may cause hallucinations, particularly when used in combination. They have also been associated with sudden-onset episodes of sleep without warning ("sleep attacks"), and with the development of impulse control disorders such as compulsive gambling, hypersexuality, and hyperphagia. This is more common with dopamine agonists than L-dopa. Avoid rapid discontinuation, which may precipitate neuroleptic malignant syndrome.

APOMORPHINE (*Apokyn*) ▶L ♀C ▶? $$$$$

WARNING — Never administer IV due to risk of severe adverse effects including pulmonary embolism.

ADULT — Acute, intermittent treatment of hypomobility ("off episodes") in Parkinson's disease: Start 0.2 mL SC test dose in the presence of medical personnel. May increase dose by 0.1 mL every few days as tolerated. Max 0.6 mL/dose or 2 mL/day. Monitor for orthostatic hypotension after initial dose and with dose escalation. Potent emetic; pretreat with trimethobenzamide 300 mg PO three times per day (or domperidone 20 mg PO three times per day) starting 3 days prior to use, and continue for at least 6 weeks before weaning. Do not use 5-HT3 antagonist antiemetics.

PEDS — Not approved in children.

FORMS — Trade only: Cartridges (for injector pen, 10 mg/mL) 3 mL.

NOTES — Write doses exclusively in mL rather than mg to avoid errors. First dose should be given by a healthcare provider. Most effective when administered at (or just prior to) the onset of an "off" episode. Avoid concomitant use of 5-HT3 antagonists (eg, ondansetron, granisetron, dolasetron, palonosetron, alosetron), which can precipitate severe hypotension and loss of consciousness. Inform patients that the dosing pen is labeled in mL (not mg), and that it is possible to dial in a dose of medication even if the cartridge does not contain sufficient drug. Rotate injection sites. Restart at 0.2 mL/day if treatment is interrupted for 1 week or more. Use cautiously with hepatic impairment. Reduce starting dose to 0.1 mL in patients with mild or moderate renal failure. Contains sulfites.

MOA — Dopamine agonist (non-ergot).

ADVERSE EFFECTS — Serious: Syncope, orthostatic hypotension, QT prolongation, arrhythmias, myocardial infarction, anaphylaxis, sleep attacks, priapism, inappropriate sexual behavior, impulse control disorders. Frequent: N/V, yawning, chest pain, confusion, hallucinations, sedation, drowsiness, dyskinesia, dizziness, rhinorrhea, peripheral edema, injection site reactions.

CARBIDOPA (*Lodosyn*) ▶LK ♀C ▶? $$$$$

ADULT — Parkinson's disease, adjunct to carbidopa-levodopa: Start 25 mg PO daily with 1st daily dose of carbidopa-levodopa. May give an additional 12.5 to 25 mg with each dose of carbidopa-levodopa prn. Max 200 mg/day.

PEDS — Not approved in children.

FORMS — Generic/Trade: Tabs 25 mg.

NOTES — Adjunct to carbidopa-levodopa to reduce peripheral side effects such as nausea. Also increases the CNS availability of levodopa. Monitor for CNS side effects such as dyskinesias and hallucinations when initiating therapy, and reduce the dose of levodopa as necessary.

MOA — Blocks the peripheral conversion of levodopa to dopamine.

ADVERSE EFFECTS — Serious: melanoma. Frequent: None. The adverse effects of carbidopa/levodopa are due to the levodopa component.

CARBIDOPA-LEVODOPA (*Rytary, DUOPA, Sinemet, Sinemet CR, Parcopa*) ▶L ♀C ▶– $$$$

ADULT — Parkinsonism: Standard-release and orally disintegrating tab: Start 1 tab (25/100 mg) PO three times per day. Increase by 1 tab/day every 1 to 2 days prn. Use 1 tab (25/250 mg) PO three to four times per day when higher levodopa doses are needed. Sustained-release: Start 1 tab (50/200 mg) PO twice per day; separate doses by at least 4 h. Increase prn at intervals of 3 days or more. Typical max dose is 1600 to 2000 mg/day of levodopa, but higher doses have been used. Extended-release caps (Rytari): Start 23.75/95 mg PO three times daily for 3 days. May then increase to 36.25/145 mg three times daily. Max daily dose 97.5/390 mg three times daily. Some patients may require shorter dosing intervals of up to 5 times per day with a max recommended dose of 612.5/2,450 mg per day.

PEDS — Not approved in children.

UNAPPROVED ADULT — Restless legs syndrome: Start ½ tab (25/100 mg) PO at bedtime; increase every 3 to 4 days to max 50/200 mg (two 25/100 tabs) at bedtime. If symptoms recur during the night, then a combination of standard-release (25/100 mg, 1 to 2 tabs at bedtime) and sustained-release (25/100 or 50/200 mg at bedtime) tabs may be used. Dopa-responsive dystonia: Start 1 tab (25/100) PO daily and titrate to max 1000 mg of levodopa daily.

FORMS — Generic/Trade: Tabs (carbidopa-levodopa) 10/100, 25/100, 25/250 mg. Tabs, sustained-release (Sinemet CR, carbidopa-levodopa ER) 25/100, 50/200 mg. Generic only: Orally disintegrating tabs 10/100, 25/100, 25/250 mg. Trade only: Enteral susp (DUOPA): 4.63 mg carbidopa/20 mg levodopa per mL. Caps, extended-release (Rytary): 23.75/95, 36.25/145, 48.75/195, 61.25/245 mg.

NOTES — Motor fluctuations and dyskinesias may occur. The 25/100 mg tabs are preferred as initial therapy, because most patients require at least 70 to 100 mg/day of carbidopa to reduce the risk of N/V. The 10/100 mg tabs have limited clinical utility. Extended-release formulations have a lower bioavailability than conventional preparations. Do not use within 2 weeks of a nonselective MAOI. When used for restless legs syndrome, may precipitate rebound (recurrence of symptoms during the night) or augmentation (earlier daily onset of symptoms). Orally disintegrating tab is placed on top of the tongue and does not require water or swallowing, but is absorbed through the GI tract (not sublingually). Use caution in patients with undiagnosed skin lesions or a history of melanoma. Intense urges (eg, gambling and sexual) have been reported. Consider discontinuing the medication or reducing the dose if these occur. Enteral suspension (DUOPA): Dose is based on the amount of immediate-release carbidopa-levodopa the patient is taking and is administered via enteral feeding tube. Refer to the package insert for full dosing calculation information.

(cont.)

CARBIDOPA-LEVODOPA (*cont.*)

MOA — Levodopa is a dopamine precursor. Carbidopa blocks the peripheral conversion of levodopa to dopamine.

ADVERSE EFFECTS — Serious: Orthostatic hypotension, psychosis, agranulocytosis, leukopenia, hepatotoxicity, thrombocytopenia, pathologic gambling, sudden onset of sleep. Frequent: Dyskinesia, dystonia, orthostatic hypotension, N/V, abdominal cramps, confusion, hallucinations.

PRAMIPEXOLE (*Mirapex, Mirapex ER*) ▶K ♀C ▶? $$$$$
ADULT — Parkinson's disease: immediate-release, start 0.125 mg PO three times per day for one week. Then increase to 0.25 mg three times daily. Increase every 5 to 7 days by 0.25 mg/dose (0.75 mg/day) as needed and tolerated given three times per day. Usual effective range is 1.5 to 4.5 mg/day. When discontinuing reduce dose by 0.75 mg/day until the daily dose is 0.75 mg/day, then reduce the dose by 0.375 mg/day. Extended-release: Start 0.375 mg PO daily. May increase after 5 to 7 days to 0.75 mg daily, then by 0.75 mg/day increments q 5 to 7 days to max 4.5 mg/day. When discontinuing, reduce dose by 0.75 mg/day until the daily dose is 0.75 mg/day, then reduce the dose by 0.375 mg/day. Restless legs syndrome: Start 0.125 mg PO 2 to 3 h before to bedtime. May increase every 4 to 7 days to max 0.5 mg/day given 2 to 3 h before bedtime.
PEDS — Not approved in children.
FORMS — Generic/Trade: Tabs 0.125, 0.25, 0.5, 0.75, 1, 1.5 mg. Tabs, extended-release 0.375, 0.75, 1.5, 2.25, 3, 3.75, 4.5 mg.
NOTES — Decrease dose in renal impairment. Titrate slowly. Taper when discontinuing therapy. May change to extended-release tabs at same daily dose as regular tabs over night. May need to reduce levodpa dose if pramipexole is added to therapy.
MOA — Dopamine agonist (non-ergot).
ADVERSE EFFECTS — Serious: Sleep attacks, orthostatic hypotension, psychosis, impulse control disorders, SIADH. Frequent: Edema, N/V, dizziness, drowsiness, insomnia, constipation, dry mouth, orthostatic hypotension, dyskinesia, dystonia, hallucinations.

ROPINIROLE (*Requip, Requip XL*) ▶L ♀C ▶? $$$
ADULT — Parkinson's disease: Start 0.25 mg PO three times per day, then gradually increase over 4 weeks by 0.25 mg/dose to 1 mg PO three times per day. After this, if needed, the dose can be increased weekly by 1.5 mg/day to 9 mg/day. After this the dose can be increased by 3 mg/day weekly to max 24 mg/day (8 mg three times daily). Extended-release: Start 2 mg PO daily for 1 to 2 weeks, then gradually increase by 2 mg daily at weekly or longer intervals. Max 24 mg/day. Restless legs syndrome: Start 0.25 mg PO 1 to 3 h before bedtime for 2 days, then increase to 0.5 mg/day on days 3 to 7. Increase by 0.5 mg/day at weekly intervals prn to max 4 mg/day given 1 to 3 h before bedtime.
PEDS — Not approved in children.

FORMS — Generic/Trade: Tabs, immediate-release 0.25, 0.5, 1, 2, 3, 4, 5 mg. Tabs, extended-release 2, 4, 6, 8, 12 mg.
NOTES — Retitrate if significant interruption of therapy occurs. For patients with Parkinson's disease and on hemodialysis, start with usual dose and then increase cautiously to max recommended dose of 18 mg/day. Supplemental doses after dialysis are not required.
MOA — Dopamine agonist (non-ergot).
ADVERSE EFFECTS — Serious: Sleep attacks, atrial fibrillation, syncope, orthostatic hypotension, HTN, psychosis, impulse control disorders. Frequent: N/V, dizziness, syncope, drowsiness, fatigue, asthenia, headache, dyspepsia, constipation, abdominal pain, dyskinesia, dystonia, pain, edema, diaphoresis, dry mouth, confusion, hallucinations, visual changes.

ROTIGOTINE (*Neupro*) ▶L – ♀C ▶? $$$$$
ADULT — Early-stage Parkinson's disease: Start 2 mg/24 h patch daily; may increase by 2 mg/24 h at weekly intervals to max 6 mg/24 h. Advanced-stage Parkinson's disease: Start 4 mg/24 h patch daily; may increase by 2 mg/24 h at weekly intervals to max 8 mg/24 h. Restless legs syndrome: Start 1 mg/24 h patch daily; may be increased by 1 mg/24 h at weekly intervals to max 3 mg/24 h.
PEDS — Not approved for use in children.
FORMS — Trade: Transdermal patch 1, 2, 3, 4, 6, 8 mg/24 h.
NOTES — Contains sulfites. Remove prior to MRI or cardioversion to avoid burns. Apply to clean, dry intact skin of the abdomen, thigh, flank, shoulder, or upper arm and hold in place for 20 to 30 seconds. Rotate application sites daily, and wash skin after removal. Taper by 2 mg/24 h every other day when discontinuing.
MOA — Dopamine agonist, non-ergot
ADVERSE EFFECTS — Serious: sleep attacks, orthostatic hypotension, psychosis, syncope, HTN, impulse control disorder. Frequent: N/V, application site reactions, weight gain, fluid retention, dyskinesia, somnolence, dizziness, headache, insomnia, constipation.

STALEVO (**carbidopa + levodopa + entacapone**) ▶L ♀C ▶– $$$$$
ADULT — Parkinson's disease (conversion from carbidopa-levodopa with or without entacapone): Start Stalevo tab that contains the same amount of carbidopa-levodopa as the patient was previously taking, and titrate to desired response. May need to lower the dose of levodopa in patients not already taking entacapone. Max 8 tabs/24 h except for the Stalevo 200 tabs for which it is 6 tabs/24 h.
PEDS — Not approved in children.
FORMS — Trade/generic: Tabs (carbidopa/levodopa/entacapone): Stalevo 50 (12.5/50/200 mg), Stalevo 75 (18.75/75/200 mg), Stalevo 100 (25/100/200 mg), Stalevo 125 (31.25/125/200 mg), Stalevo 150 (37.5/150/200 mg), Stalevo 200 (50/200/200 mg).

(cont.)

STALEVO (*cont.*)

NOTES — Patients who are not currently taking entacapone may benefit from titration of the individual components of this medication before conversion to this fixed-dose preparation. Avoid concomitant use of nonselective MAOIs. Use caution in hepatobiliary dysfunction. Motor fluctuations and dyskinesias may occur.

MOA — Levodopa is a dopamine precursor. Carbidopa blocks the peripheral conversion of levodopa to dopamine. Entacapone blocks the peripheral metabolism of dopamine by inhibiting catechol-o-methyltransferase.

ADVERSE EFFECTS — Serious: Orthostatic hypotension, psychosis, impulse control or compulsive behavior problems, abruptly falling asleep, agranulocytosis, leukopenia, hepatotoxicity, thrombocytopenia, rhabdomyolysis, severe diarrhea, colitis. Frequent: Dyskinesia, hyperkinesia, dystonia, orthostatic hypotension, N/V, abdominal cramps, diarrhea, confusion, hallucinations, urine discoloration.

NEUROLOGY: Parkinsonian Agents—Monoamine Oxidase Inhibitors (MAOIs)

RASAGILINE (*Azilect*) ▶L ♀C ▶? $$$$$

ADULT — Parkinson's disease, monotherapy or as adjunct when not taking levodopa: 1 mg PO every am. Parkinson's disease, adjunctive with levodopa: 0.5 mg PO q am. Max 1 mg/day.

PEDS — Not approved in children.

FORMS — Trade only: Tabs 0.5, 1 mg.

NOTES — Requires an MAOI diet that avoids foods very high in tyramine content. Contraindicated (risk of hypertensive crisis) with meperidine, methadone, tramadol, dextromethorphan, sympathomimetic amines (eg, pseudoephedrine, phenylephrine, ephedrine), antidepressants, other MAOIs, cyclobenzaprine, and general anesthesia. Discontinue at least 14 days before liberalizing diet, starting one of these medications, or proceeding with elective surgery that requires general anesthesia. May need to reduce levodopa dose when used in combination. Reduce dose to 0.5 mg when used with CYP1A2 inhibitors (eg, ciprofloxacin) and in mild hepatic impairment. Do not use in moderate or severe liver disease. Parkinson's disease and drugs used to treat it have been associated with an increased risk of melanoma. Consider periodic skin exams for melanoma.

MOA — Irreversible MAO inhibitor.

ADVERSE EFFECTS — Serious: Hypertensive crisis with food/drug interactions, psychosis, orthostatic hypotension, injury/falls, melanoma, sudden sleep onset, impulse cotrol problems, compulsive behaviors. Frequent: Worsening of levodopa-induced dyskinesias, anorexia, N/V, constipation, abdominal pain, weight loss, hallucinations, arthralgia, dry mouth, rash, ecchymosis, somnolence, paresthesia.

SELEGILINE (*Eldepryl, Zelapar*) ▶LK ♀C ▶? $$$$

ADULT — Parkinsonism (adjunct to levodopa): 5 mg PO every am and every noon; max 10 mg/day. Zelapar ODT: Start 1.25 mg SL every am for at least 6 weeks, then increase prn to max 2.5 mg every am.

PEDS — Not approved in children.

UNAPPROVED ADULT — Parkinsonism (monotherapy): 5 mg PO every am and every noon; max 10 mg/day.

FORMS — Generic/Trade: Caps 5 mg. Tabs 5 mg. Trade only: Orally disintegrating tabs (Zelapar ODT) 1.25 mg.

NOTES — Should not be combined with meperidine or other opioids. Do not exceed max recommended dose; risk of nonselective MAO inhibition at higher doses than recommended. Zelapar should be taken in the morning before food and without water. Intense urges (gambling and sexual for example) have been reported. Consider discontinuing the medication or reducing the dose if these occur. Parkinson's disease and drugs used to treat it have been associated with an increased risk of melanoma. May find that the patient requires less levodopa after a few days on selegiline.

MOA — Selective MAO-B inhibitor.

ADVERSE EFFECTS — Serious: Angina, syncope, mood lability, psychosis, orthostatic hypotension, impulse control disorders. Frequent: N/V, confusion, depression, ataxia, insomnia, orthostatic hypotension, hallucinations, vivid dreams.

NEUROLOGY: Other Agents

ABOBOTULINUM TOXIN A (*DYSPORT*) ▶ ♀C ▶? $$$$$

WARNING — Symptoms of systemic botulism have been reported, particularly in children treated for spasticity due to cerebral palsy.

ADULT — Cervical dystonia: 500 units IM total dose divided among affected muscles. May repeat every 12 weeks or longer. Max dose 1000 units per treatment. Glabellar line (age younger than 65 yo): 50 units IM total dose divided into 10 unit injections at 5 sites (see prescribing information). May repeat every 12 weeks or longer.

PEDS — Lower limb spasticity(ages 2 yo and older): Gastrocnemius, 6 to 9 Units/kg with up to 4 injections per muscle. Soleus, 4 to 6 units/kg with up to 2 injections per muscle. Total dose/session 10 to 15 Units/kg for unilateral injections or 20 to 30 Units/kg for bilateral. Max 15 Units/kg per session for unilateral injections or 30 Units/kg for bilateral.

FORMS — Trade: Vials 300, 500 units for reconstitution.

NOTES — Refer to prescribing information for injection sites and technique. Use caution in peripheral

(cont.)

ABOBOTULINUM TOXIN A (cont.)

motor neuropathic diseases, amyotrophic lateral sclerosis, or neuromuscular junction disorders (eg, myasthenia gravis or Lambert-Eaton syndrome) and monitor closely when given with botulinum toxin due to increased risk of severe dysphagia or respiratory compromise. Contains trace amounts of cow's milk protein: Do not use in patients allergic to milk. Use cautiously with neuromuscular blocking drugs (eg, aminoglycosides and curare-like drugs).
MOA — Acetylcholine release inhibitor and neuromuscular blocking agent
ADVERSE EFFECTS — Serious: dysphagia, respiratory failure, systemic spread of effect, hypersensitivity. Frequent: muscular weakness, dysphagia, dry mouth, injection site discomfort, fatigue, headache, neck pain, musculoskeletal pain, dysphonia, injection site pain, eyelid ptosis and edema.

BETAHISTINE (✱Serc) ▶LK ♀? ▶? $
ADULT — Canada only. Vertigo of Meniere's disease: 8 to 16 mg PO three times per day.
PEDS — Not approved in children.
FORMS — Trade only: Tabs 8, 16 mg.
NOTES — Contraindicated in peptic ulcer disease and pheochromocytoma; use caution in asthmatics.
MOA — Histamine H1-receptor agonist.
ADVERSE EFFECTS — Frequent: Urticaria, pruritus, gastrointestinal upset, nausea, headache.

BOTULINUM TOXIN TYPE B (Myobloc) ▶Not significantly absorbed ♀+ ▶? $$$$$
WARNING — Symptoms of systemic botulism have been reported, particularly in children treated for spasticity due to cerebral palsy.
ADULT — Cervical dystonia: Start 2500 to 5000 units IM in affected muscles. Use lower initial dose if no prior history of botulinum toxin therapy. Benefits usually last for 12 to 16 weeks when a total dose of 5000 to 10,000 units has been administered. Titrate to effective dose. Give treatments at least 3 months apart to decrease the risk of producing neutralizing antibodies.
PEDS — Not approved in children.
FORMS — Trade only: Vials 2500, 5000, and 10,000 units
NOTES — Low systemic concentrations are expected with IM injection; monitor closely for dysphagia. Contraindicated in peripheral motor neuropathic disease (eg, ALS, motor neuropathy), neuromuscular junction disease (eg, myasthenia gravis, Lambert-Eaton syndrome due to an increased risk of systemic effects) and with other drugs that block neuromuscular function (eg, aminoglycosides, curare-like compounds).
MOA — Neuromuscular transmission blockade; inhibits presynaptic acetylcholine release.
ADVERSE EFFECTS — Serious: Systemic botulism, dysphagia, respiratory compromise, hypersensitivity. Frequent: Dry mouth, dyspepsia/nausea, injection site pain, flu-like syndrome, arthralgia, back pain, cough, myasthenia, asthenia, dizziness.

INCOBOTULINUMTOXIN A (Xeomin) ▶not absorbed ♀–C ▶? $$$$$
WARNING — Symptoms of systemic botulism have been reported.
ADULT — Cervical dystonia: Total of 120 units IM divided among the sternocleidomastoid, levator scapulae, splenis capitis, scalenus, and trapezius muscles as indicated. Repeat at intervals of at least 12 weeks with dose individualized according to response. Blepharospasm in patients previously treated with Botox: Start with same dose as Botox used before. If prior Botox dose unknown start with 1.25 to 2.5 units per injection site. Usual number of injections is 6 per eye. Average dose 33 units/eye. Do not exceed initial dose of 35 units/eye. May repeat at intervals of at least 12 weeks. Upper limb spasticity: Dose varies from 5 to 50 units depending on the problem and muscle group involved. Refer to package label for specific dosing.
PEDS — Not approved for use in children or adolescents.
FORMS — Trade only: 50, 100, 200 unit single-use vials.
NOTES — Cannot convert units of Xeomin to other botulinum toxins. The max dose in trials for blepharospasm was 50 units/eye. Toxin effects may become systemic and produce asthenia, muscle weakness, diplopia, ptosis, dysphagia, dysphonia, urinary incontinence, and breathing difficulties.
MOA — Cholinergic neuromuscular blocker. Inhibits presynaptic release of acetylcholine.
ADVERSE EFFECTS — Serious: hypersensitivity. Frequent: dysphagia, neck pain, muscle weakness and pain, injection site pain, dry eye, dry mouth, diarrhea, visual impairment, dypnea, nasopharyngitis, flu-like symptoms..

MANNITOL (Osmitrol, Resectisol) ▶K ♀C ▶? $
ADULT — Intracranial HTN: 0.25 to 2 g/kg IV over 30 to 60 min as a 15, 20, or 25% soln.
PEDS — Not approved in children.
UNAPPROVED ADULT — Increased ICP, head trauma, cerebral edema: 0.25 to 1 g/kg IV push over 20 min. Repeat q 4 to 6 h prn.
UNAPPROVED PEDS — Increased ICP/cerebral edema: 0.25 to 1 g/kg/dose IV push over 20 to 30 min, then 0.25 to 0.5 g/kg/dose IV q 4 to 6 h prn.
NOTES — Monitor fluid and electrolyte balance and cardiac function. Consider holding further doses if serum osmololity > 320 or hypernatremia develops. Filter IV solns with concentrations at least 20%; crystals may be present.
MOA — Osmotic diuretic.
ADVERSE EFFECTS — Serious: Congestive heart failure, pulmonary edema, seizures, electrolyte changes, CNS depression, acute renal failure. Frequent: Headache, dizziness, N/V, polydipsia.

MILNACIPRAN (Savella) ▶KL ♀C ▶? $$$$
ADULT — Fibromyalgia: Start day 1: 12.5 mg PO once, then days 2 to 3: 12.5 mg two times per day. Days 4 to 7: 25 mg two times per day. After that: 50 mg two times per day. Max 200 mg/day.

(cont.)

MILNACIPRAN *(cont.)*

PEDS — Not approved for use in children.

FORMS — Trade only: Tabs 12.5, 25, 50, 100 mg.

NOTES — Reduce dose by 50% for severe renal impairment with CrCl less than 30 mL/min. Taper if discontinued. Do not use with linezolid or methylene blue because of increased risk of serotonin syndrome.

MOA — Selective serotonin/norepinephrine reuptake inhibitor.

ADVERSE EFFECTS — Severe: Worsening of psychiatric symptoms including depression or mania, suicidality, aggression, hostility, anger, serotonin syndrome, hypertension, tachycardia, seizures, hepatotoxicity, abnormal bleeding, hyponatremia. Frequent: Nausea/vomiting, headache, dizziness, insomnia, hot flushes, hyperhidrosis, palpitations, dry mouth.

NIMODIPINE *(Nimotop, Nymalize)* ▶L ♀C ▶– $$$$$

ADULT — Subarachnoid hemorrhage: 60 mg PO every 4 h for 21 days.

PEDS — Not approved in children.

FORMS — Generic only: Caps 30 mg. Trade only: 60 mg/20 mL oral solution (Nymalize)

NOTES — Begin therapy within 96 h. Give 1 h before or 2 h after meals. May give cap contents SL or via NG tube. Reduce dose in hepatic dysfunction.

MOA — Calcium channel blocker.

ADVERSE EFFECTS — Serious: Heart failure, disseminated intravascular coagulation, deep vein thrombosis, neurological deterioration. Frequent: Hypotension, N/V, diarrhea, flushing, edema, headache.

***NUEDEXTA* (dextromethorphan + quinidine)** ▶LK – ♀C ▶? $$$$$

ADULT — Pseudobulbar affect: Start 1 cap PO daily. Increase after 7 days to maintenance dose of 1 cap every 12 h.

PEDS — Not approved for use in children.

FORMS — Trade only: Caps 10 mg dextromethorphan plus 20 mg quinidine.

NOTES — Contraindicated with prolonged QT interval, a history of torsades de pointes, with drugs that prolong the QT interval and metabolized by CYP2D6, or with MAOIs. Contraindicated with complete AV block. Obtain ECG at baseline and at 4 h post-dose to evaluate effect on QT in the presence of CYP3A4 inhibitors, or patients with left ventricular hypertrophy or left ventricular dysfunction. May cause serotonin syndrome if used with serotonergic drugs. Clinical trials were only conducted in patients with PBA secondary to Alzheimer's disease. Response in other subgroups has not been assessed.

MOA — Dextromethorphan: sigma-1 agonist and uncompetitive NMDA antagonist. Quinidine: included to increase DM concentrations by CYP2D6 inhibition.

ADVERSE EFFECTS — Serious: thrombocytopenia, hypersensitivity, lupus-like syndrome, respiratory failure, muscle spasticity, hepatotoxicity, QTc prolongation. Frequent: diarrhea, dizziness, cough, vomiting, asthenia, peripheral edema.

ONABOTULINUM TOXIN TYPE A *(Botox, Botox Cosmetic)*
▶Not absorbed ♀C ▶? $$$$$

WARNING — Symptoms of systemic botulism have been reported, particularly in children treated for spasticity due to cerebral palsy.

ADULT — Moderate to severe glabellar lines in patients no older than age 65 yo: Inject 0.1 mL (4 units) into each of 5 sites. Blepharospasm: 1.25 to 5 units IM into each of several sites in the orbicularis oculi of upper and lower lids every 3 months; use lower doses at initial visit. Strabismus: 1.25 to 5 units depending on diagnosis, injected into extraocular muscles. Cervical dystonia: 15 to 100 units IM (with or without EMG guidance) into affected muscles every 3 months (eg, splenius capitis/cervicis, sternocleidomastoid, levator scapulae, trapezius, semispinalis, scalene, longissimus); usual total dose is 200 to 300 units/treatment. Primary axillary hyperhidrosis: 50 units/axilla intradermally, divided over 10 to 15 sites. Upper limb spasticity: Biceps brachii, 100 to 200 units IM divided into 4 sites (with or without EMG guidance) every 3 months; flexor carpi radialis, 12.5 to 50 units IM in 1 site; flexor carpi ulnaris, 12.5 to 50 units IM in 1 site; flexor digitorum profundus, 30 to 50 units IM in 1 site; flexor digitorum sublimis, 30 to 50 units IM in 1 site. Thumb flexors (adductor pollicis and flexor pollicis longus), 20 units IM into one site. Lower limb spasticity: Gastocnemius medial head, gatrocnemius lateral head, soleus, tibialis posterior, 75 units IM divided into 3 sites. Flexor hallucis longus, flexor digitorum longus, 50 units IM divided into 2 sites. May repeat after 12 weeks or longer. Chronic migraine headache: Dilute to 5 units/0.1 mL then inject 155 units total as a series of 0.1 mL (5 units) IM injections at 7 specific head/neck sites. Refer to prescribing information for locations of injections and amount per site. Repeat every 12 weeks. Botulinum toxin products are not interchangeable. Overactive bladder: 100 units IM into detrusor divided into 20 injections of 0.5 mL each (total volume 10 mL). May repeat no sooner than 12 weeks later if needed. Detrusor overactivity associated with neurological conditions: 200 units IM into detrusor divided into 30 injections of 1 mL each (total volume 30 mL). May repeat no sooner than 12 weeks later if needed. When treating one or more conditions the max dose per 3-month period is 400 units.

PEDS — Not approved in children younger than 12 yo for blepharospasm and strabismus, younger than 16 yo for cervical dystonia, or younger than 18 yo for hyperhidrosis, spasticity, or chronic migraine headache.

UNAPPROVED ADULT — Hemifacial spasm: 1.25 to 2.5 units IM into affected muscles every 3 to 4 months (eg, corrugator, orbicularis oculi, zygomaticus major, buccinator, depressor anguli oris, platysma); usual total dose is 10 to 34 units/treatment.

FORMS — Trade only: 50, 100, 200 unit single-use vials.

(cont.)

ONABOTULINUM TOXIN TYPE A (*cont.*)

NOTES — Clinical benefit occurs within 2 weeks (2 to 3 days for facial injections), peaks at 1 to 6 weeks, and wears off in approximately 3 months. Contraindicated in peripheral motor neuropathic disease (eg, ALS, motor neuropathy) or neuromuscular junction disease (eg, myasthenia gravis, Lambert-Eaton syndrome). The use of lower doses and longer dosing intervals may decrease the risk of producing neutralizing antibodies. Increased risk of dysphagia when more than 100 units are injected into the sternocleidomastoid or with bilateral sternocleidomastoid injections. Potency units of Botox cannot be interchanged with other products. For chronic migraine headache the amount injected varies by muscle site. Refer to prescribing information for specific amounts to inject at each site.

MOA — Neuromuscular transmission blockade; inhibits presynaptic acetylcholine release.

ADVERSE EFFECTS — Severe: Anaphylaxis, dysphagia, arrhythmias, myocardial infarction, systemic botulism, death. Frequent: Rash, urticaria, pruritus, flu-like symptoms, excessive weakness, upper respiratory tract infection, neck pain, headache. Periorbital injections may cause ptosis, dry eyes, superficial keratosis, or lacrimation; injections of facial muscles may cause facial asymmetry.

OXYBATE (*Xyrem, GHB, gamma hydroxybutyrate*) ▶L ♀C ▶? ©III $$$$$

WARNING — CNS depressant with abuse potential; avoid concurrent alcohol or sedative use.

ADULT — Cataplexy or excessive daytime sleepiness in narcolepsy: 2.25 g PO at bedtime. Repeat in 2.5 to 4 h. May increase by 1.5 g/day (0.75 g) at 2-week intervals to effective range of 6 to 9 g/day. Dilute each dose in 60 mL water.

PEDS — Not approved in children.

FORMS — Trade only: Soln 180 mL (500 mg/mL) supplied with measuring device and child-proof dosing cups.

NOTES — Available only through the Xyrem Success Program centralized pharmacy (866-997-3688). Adjust dose in hepatic dysfunction. Prepare doses just prior to bedtime, and use within 24 h. Take at least 2 hours after eating. May need an alarm to signal 2nd dose. Contraindicated with sedative-hypnotics. Do not use with alcohol. Reduce dose when given with divalproex. Product is high in sodium. Use caution if patient is sensitive to salt.

MOA — Unknown. Effect possibly mediated through GABA-B actions are noradrenergic and dopaminergic nerurons.

ADVERSE EFFECTS — Serious: Abuse and dependence, depression, syncope, seizures, CNS and respiratory depression, coma. Frequent: Headache, nausea, dizziness, pain, somnolence, pharyngitis, infection, flu-like symptoms, accidental injury, diarrhea, urinary incontinence, confusion, sleepwalking.

RILUZOLE (*Rilutek*) ▶LK ♀C ▶– $$$$$

ADULT — ALS: 50 mg PO q 12 h.

PEDS — Not approved in children.

FORMS — Generic/Trade: Tabs 50 mg.

NOTES — Take 1 h before or 2 h after meals. Monitor LFTs.

MOA — Glutamate antagonist.

ADVERSE EFFECTS — Serious: Tachycardia, hypertension, hepatotoxicity, neutropenia, interstitial lung disease. Frequent: Asthenia, N/V, diarrhea, abdominal pain, pneumonia, dizziness, paresthesia, drowsiness.

TETRABENAZINE (*Xenazine,* ✱*Nitoman*) ▶L ♀C ▶? ? $$$$$

WARNING — Contraindicated with untreated or inadequately responding depression or suicidality; monitor closely and discontinue at the first signs thereof.

ADULT — Chorea associated with Huntington's disease: Start 12.5 mg PO every am. Increase after 1 week to 12.5 mg PO two times per day. May increase by 12.5 mg/day weekly. For doses greater than 37.5 to 50 mg/day, divide doses three times per day. For doses greater than 50 mg/day, genotype the patient for CYP2D6 activity, titrate by 12.5 mg/day weekly, and divide doses three times per day to max 37.5 mg/dose and 100 mg/day (extensive/intermediate metabolizers) or 25 mg/dose and 50 mg/day (poor metabolizers).

PEDS — Not approved in children.

UNAPPROVED ADULT — Hyperkinetic movement disorders such as tic disorders (including Tourette's syndrome), tardive syndromes, hemiballismus, dystonia, and other choreas (approved dosing in Canada): Start 12.5 mg PO two to three times per day. May increase by 12.5 mg/day every 3 to 5 days to usual dose of 25 mg PO three times per day. Max 200 mg/day, but most patients do not tolerate more than 75 mg/day. Discontinue if there is no benefit after 7 days of treatment at max tolerated dose.

UNAPPROVED PEDS — Limited data suggest that ½ of the adult dose may be used and titrated as tolerated.

FORMS — Generic/Trade: Tabs 12.5, 25 mg.

NOTES — Contraindicated in hepatic impairment, suicidality, untreated/inadequately responding depression, and with MAOIs. Reduce dose by 50% if used with potent CYP2D6 inhibitors. Monitor patient for depression, akathisia, sedation/somnolence, and parkinsonism, which may respond to dose reduction. Retitrate dose if interrupted longer than 5 days. Use caution when combined with antipsychotics and other dopamine–receptor blocking agents. May attenuate the effects of levodopa and antidepressants. Increases QTc by approximately 8 msec.

MOA — Depletes monoamines from storage sites.

ADVERSE EFFECTS — Serious: Parkinsonism, cognitive decline, orthostatic hypotension, depression, suicidality, neuroleptic malignant syndrome. Frequent: Drowsiness, fatigue, weakness, anxiety, insomnia, akathisia, sialorrhea, irritability, agitation, N/V, epigastric pain, confusion, disorientation, dizziness.

OB/GYN

EMERGENCY CONTRACEPTION

Emergency contraception within 72 h of unprotected sex or contraception failure.
Progestin-only method (Causes less nausea and may be more effective. Some available OTC with no age restriction.): Dose is levonorgestrel 1.5 mg tab. Take 1 pill. Many brands and generics available; Aftera, Athentia Next, EContraEZ, Fallback Solo, Her Style, My Way, Next Choice One Dose, Opcicon One-Step, Plan B One-Step, Take Action.
Progestin and estrogen method: Dose goal of 0.5 mg levonorgestrel (or 1 mg norgestrel) plus 100 mcg ethinyl estradiol. Take 1st dose ASAP and repeat 12 h later. If vomiting occurs within 1 h of taking dose, consider repeating that dose with an antiemetic 1 h prior. Dose is defined as 2 pills of Ogestrel, 4 pills of Altavera, Amethia*, Camrese*, Chateal, Cryselle, Daysee*, Elifemme**, Elinest, Enpresse**, Introvale, Jolessa, Kurvelo, Levonest**, Levora, Low-Ogestrel, Marlissa, Myzilra**, Nordette, Portia, Quasense, Seasonale, Seasonique*, Trivora**, or 5 pills of Amathia Lo**, Amethyst, Ashlyna, Aviane, Camresse Lo**, Falmina, Lessina, LoSeasonique***, Lutera, Orsthia, Sronyx.
Anti-progestin: Emergency contraception within 120 h of unprotected sex. Ella (ulipristal 30 mg): Take 1 pill. More info at: www.not-2-late.com.

*Use 0.15 mg levonorgestrel/30 mcg ethinyl estradiol tabs.
**Use 0.125 mg levonorgestrel/30 mcg ethinyl estradiol tabs.
***Use 0.1 mg levonorgestrel/20 mcg ethinyl estradiol tabs.

DRUGS GENERALLY ACCEPTED AS SAFE IN PREGNANCY (SELECTED)

Analgesics	acetaminophen, codeine*, meperidine*, methadone*, oxycodone*
Antimicrobials	azithromycin, cephalosporins, clotrimazole, erythromycins (not estolate), metronidazole, penicillins, permethrin, nitrofurantoin***, nystatin
Antivirals	acyclovir, famciclovir, valacyclovir
CV	hydralazine*, labetalol, methyldopa, nifedipine
Derm	benzoyl peroxide, clindamycin, erythromycin
Endo	insulin, levothyroxine, liothyronine
ENT	chlorpheniramine, diphenhydramine, dextromethorphan, guaifenesin, nasal steroids, nasal cromolyn
GI	antacids*, bisacodyl, cimetidine, docusate, doxylamine, famotidine, lactulose, loperamide, meclizine, metoclopramide, nizatidine, ondansetron, psyllium, ranitidine, simethicone, trimethobenzamide
Heme	Heparin, low molecular wt heparins
Psych	bupropion, buspirone, desipramine, doxepin
Pulmonary	beclomethasone, budesonide, cromolyn, montelukast, prednisone**, short-acting inhaled beta-2 agonists, theophylline

*Except if used long-term or in high dose at term.
**Except 1st trimester.
***Contraindicated at term and during labor and delivery.

ORAL CONTRACEPTIVES*

	Estrogen (mcg)	Progestin (mg)
Monophasic		
Lo Loestrin Fe, Lo Minastrin Fe[c]	10 ethinyl estradiol	1 norethindrone
Beyaz, Gianvi, Loryna, Melamisa, Nikki, *Yaz*	20 ethinyl estradiol	3 drospirenone
Aubra, *Aviane*, Delyla, Falmina, Lessina, Lessina, Lutera, Orsythia, Sronyx, Vienva		0.1 levonorgestrel
Gildess Fe 1/20, Junel 1/20, Junel Fe 1/20, Larin 1/20, Larin Fe 1/20, *Loestrin-21* 1/20, Loestrin Fe 1/20, Loestrin-24 Fe, Lomedia 1/20, Lomedia 24 Fe, Microgestin 1/20, Microgestin Fe 1/20, Minastrin 24 Fe[c], Tarina Fe 1/20		1 norethindrone
Generess Fe[c], Layolis Fe[c]	25 ethinyl estradiol	0.8 norethindrone
Apri, Cyred, Desogen, Emoquette, *Enskyce*, Juleber, *Ortho-Cept*, Reclipsen, Solia	30 ethinyl estradiol	0.15 desogestrel
Ocella, Safyral, Syeda, Yaela, *Yasmin*, Zarah		3 drospirenone
Altavera, Chateal, Kurvelo, Levora, Jolessa, Marlissa, *Nordette*, Portia		0.15 levonorgestrel
Gildess Fe 1.5/30, Junel 1.5/30, Junel 1.5/30 Fe, Larin Fe 1.5/30, *Loestrin 1.5/30, Loestrin Fe 1.5/30*, Microgestin 1.5/30, Microgestin Fe 1.5/30		1.5 norethindrone
Cryselle, Elinest, Low-Ogestrel		0.3 norgestrel
Kelnor 1/35, *Zovia 1/35E*	35 ethinyl estradiol	1 ethynodiol
Balziva, Briellyn, Femcon Fe, Gildagia, *Ovcon 35*, Philith, Vyfemla, Wymzya Fe[c], Zenchent Fe[c]		0.4 norethindrone
Brevicon, *Modicon*, Necon, Nortrel, Wera		0.5 norethindrone
Alyacen 1/35, Cyclafem 1/35, Dasetta 1/35, Necon 1/35, Norinyl 1+35, Nortrel 1/35, Norethin 1/35, *Ortho-Novum 1/35*, Pirmella 1/35		1 norethindrone
Estarylla, Mono-Linyah, MonoNessa, *Ortho-Cyclen*, Previfem, Sprintec		0.25 norgestimate
Zovia 1/50E	50 ethinyl estradiol	1 ethynodiol
Ogestrel		0.5 norgestrel
Necon 1/50, Norinyl 1+50	50 mestranol	1 norethindrone
Progestin only		
Camila, Deblitane, Errin, Heather, Jencycla, Jolivette, Lyza, *Micronor*, Nora-BE, Norlyrox, Nor-QD, Sharobel	None	0.35 norethindrone

(cont.)

ORAL CONTRACEPTIVES* (*continued*)

Biphasic (estrogen and progestin contents vary)		
Azurette, Bekyree, Kariva, Kimidess, *Mircette*, Pimtrea, Viorele	20/10 ethinyl estradiol	0.15/0 desogestrel
Triphasic (estrogen and progestin contents vary)		
Estrostep Fe, Tilia-Fe, Tri-Legest, Tri-Legest Fe	20/30/35 ethinyl estradiol	1 norethindrone
Caziant, Cesia, *Cyclessa*, Velivet	25 ethinyl estradiol	0.1/0.125/0.150 desogestrel
Ortho Tri-Cyclen Lo, Tri-Lo-Marzia, Tri-Lo-Sprintec, TriNessa Lo		0.18/0.215/0.25 norgestimate
Enpresse, Levonest, Myzilra, *Trivora-28*	30/40/30 ethinyl estradiol	0.5/0.75/0.125 levonorgestrel
Alyacen 7/7/7, Cyclafem 7/7/7, Dasetta 7/7/7, Necon 7/7/7, Nortrel 7/7/7, Ortho-Novum 7/7/7, Primella 7/7/7	35 ethinyl estradiol	0.5/0.75/1 norethindrone
Aranelle, *Leena*, *Tri-Norinyl*		0.5/1/0.5 norethindrone
Ortho Tri-Cyclen, Tri-Estarylla, Tri-Linyah, Tri-Previfem, TriNessa, Tri-Sprintec		0.18/0.215/0.25 norgestimate
Quadphasic		
Natazia	3/2/2/1 mg estradiol valerate	0/2/3/0 dienogest
Extended Cycle		
Amethyst	20 ethinyl estradiol	0.09 levonorgestrel
Amethia Lo, Camrese Lo, *LoSeasonique*[††]	20/10 ethinyl estradiol	0.1 levonorgestrel
Quartette[††]	20/25/30/10 ethinyl estradiol	0.15 levonorgestrel
Introvale, Jolessa, Quasense, *Seasonale*, Setlakin	30 ethinyl estradiol	
Amethia, Ashlyna, Camrese, Daysee, Seasonique[††]	30/10 ethinyl estradiol	

Note: Brand names are in *italics*.

***All:** Not recommended in smokers. Increases risk of thromboembolism, CVA, MI, hepatic neoplasia, and gallbladder disease. Nausea, breast tenderness, headache and breakthrough bleeding are common transient side effects. Effectiveness reduced by hepatic enzyme-inducing drugs such as certain anticonvulsants and barbiturates, rifampin, rifabutin, griseofulvin, and protease inhibitors. Coadministration with St. John's wort may decrease efficacy. Vomiting or diarrhea may also increase the risk of contraceptive failure. Consider an additional form of birth control in above circumstances. See product insert for absolute and relative contraindations and instructions on missing doses and initiation of use.

Progestin only: Must be taken at the same time every day. Because much of the literature regarding OC adverse effects pertains mainly to estrogen/progestin combinations, the extent to which progestin-only contraceptives cause these effects is unclear. No significant interaction has been found with broad-spectrum antibiotics. The effect of St. John's wort is unclear. No placebo days, start new pack immediately after finishing current one. Available in 28-day packs. Readers may find the following website useful: www.managingcontraception.com.

[†]Approved for continuous use without a "pill-free" period.

[††]84 active pills and 7 ethinyl estradiol only pills.

[c]Chewable

OB/GYN: Contraceptives—Oral Monophasic

NOTE: Not recommended in women older than 35 yo who smoke or have complex migraine headaches. Increased risk of thromboembolism, CVA, MI, hepatic neoplasia, cervical cancer, and gallbladder disease. Increased risk of breast cancer in current and recent users. Nausea, breast tenderness, and breakthrough bleeding are common, transient side effects. Nighttime dosing may minimize nausea. Effectiveness is reduced by hepatic enzyme-inducing drugs such as certain anticonvulsants and barbiturates, rifampin, rifabutin, griseofulvin, and protease inhibitors. Additionally, products that contain St. John's wort may decrease efficacy. Vomiting or diarrhea may also increase the risk of contraceptive failure. An additional form of birth control may be advisable. Advise patients to take at the same time every day. See PI for instructions on missing doses. Most available in 21- and 28-day packs. Although not approved by the FDA, combined OCPs are used for dysfunctional uterine bleeding, emergency contraception, dysmenorrhea, pelvic pain, and hirsutism (with spironolactone): 1 tab PO daily. Wait 6 weeks postpartum to initiate combination OCPs to decrease the risk of thromboembolism and to support lactation.

AMETHYST (ethinyl estradiol + levonorgestrel) ▶L ♀X ▶– $$$
ADULT — Contraception: 1 tab PO daily.
PEDS — Not approved in children.
FORMS — Generic only: Tabs 20 mcg ethinyl estradiol/90 mcg levonorgestrel.
NOTES — Approved for continuous use without a "pill-free" period. May cause breakthrough bleeding.
MOA — Contraceptive steroid combination.
ADVERSE EFFECTS — Serious: DVT/PE, stroke, MI, hepatic neoplasia, and gallbladder disease. Frequent: Nausea, breast tenderness, and breakthrough bleeding.

AVIANE (ethinyl estradiol + levonorgestrel, *Falmina, Lessina, Orsythia, ✱ Alesse*) ▶L ♀X ▶– $$
ADULT — Contraception: 1 tab PO daily.
PEDS — Not approved in children.
UNAPPROVED ADULT — Emergency contraception: See table.
FORMS — Generic/Trade: Tabs 20 mcg ethinyl estradiol/0.1 mg levonorgestrel.
NOTES — May cause less nausea and breast tenderness and may increase breakthrough bleeding due to lower estrogen content.
MOA — Contraceptive steroid combination.
ADVERSE EFFECTS — Serious: DVT/PE, stroke, MI, hepatic neoplasia, and gallbladder disease. Frequent: Nausea, breast tenderness, and breakthrough bleeding.

BEYAZ (ethinyl estradiol + drospirenone + levomefolate calcium) ▶L ♀X ▶– $$$$
ADULT — Contraception, premenstrual dysphoric disorder, acne, folate supplementation: 1 tab PO daily.
PEDS — Not approved in children.
FORMS — Trade only: Tabs 0.02 mg ethinyl estradiol, 2 mg drospirenone, 0.451 mg levomefolate calcium. 24 active pills followed by 4 inert pills.
NOTES — May cause hyperkalemia due to antimineralocorticoid activity of drospirenone (equal to 25 mg spironolactone). Monitor potassium in patients on ACE inhibitors, ARBs, potassium-sparing diuretics, heparin, aldosterone antagonists, and NSAIDs.
MOA — Contraceptive steroid combination.
ADVERSE EFFECTS — Serious: DVT/PE, stroke, MI, hepatic neoplasia, and gallbladder disease. Frequent: Nausea, HA, breast tenderness, and breakthrough bleeding.

FEMCON FE (ethinyl estradiol + norethindrone + ferrous fumarate) ▶L ♀X ▶– $$$
ADULT — Contraception: 1 tab PO daily.
PEDS — Not approved in children.
FORMS — Generic/Trade: Chewable tabs 35 mcg ethinyl estradiol/0.4 mg norethindrone. Placebo tabs are ferrous fumarate 75 mg.
NOTES — Chewable formulation may be swallowed whole or chewed. If chewed, follow with 8 ounces liquid.
MOA — Contraceptive steroid combination.
ADVERSE EFFECTS — Serious: DVT/PE, stroke, MI, hepatic neoplasia, and gallbladder disease. Frequent: Nausea, breast tenderness, and breakthrough bleeding.

GENERESS FE (ethinyl estradiol + norethindrone + ferrous fumarate) ▶L ♀–X ▶– $$$$
ADULT — Contraception: 1 tab PO daily.
PEDS — Not approved in children
FORMS — Generic/Trade: Tabs 0.8 mg norethindrone and 25 mcg ethinyl estradiol with 4 days 75 mg ferrous fumarate.
MOA — Contraceptive steroid combination
ADVERSE EFFECTS — Serious: DVT/PE, stroke, MI, hepatic neoplasia, and gallbladder disease. Frequent: Nausea, headache, breast tenderness, dysmenorrhea, wt gain.

LO LOESTRIN FE (norethindrone + ethinyl estradiol + ferrous fumarate, *Lo Minastrin Fe*) ▶L ♀–X ▶– $$$$
ADULT — Contraception: 1 tab PO daily.
PEDS — Not approved in children.
FORMS — Trade only: Lo Minastrin Fe is chewable tabs (24) 1 mg norethindrone/10 mcg ethinyl estradiol, tabs (2) 10 mcg ethinyl estradiol and tabs (2) 70 mg ferrous fumarate. Lo Loestrin is same, but not chewable.
MOA — Contraceptive steroid combination.
ADVERSE EFFECTS — Serious: DVT/PE, stroke, MI, hepatic neoplasia and gallbladder disease. Frequent: Nausea, breast tenderness, headache and breakthrough bleeding.

LO/OVRAL-28 (ethinyl estradiol + norgestrel, *Cryselle, Elinest, Low-Ogestrel*) ▶L ♀X ▶– $$
ADULT — Contraception: 1 tab PO daily.
PEDS — Not approved in children.
UNAPPROVED ADULT — Emergency contraception: See table.
FORMS — Generic/Trade: Tabs: 30 mcg ethinyl estradiol/0.3 mg norgestrel.

(cont.)

LO/OVRAL-28 (*cont.*)

MOA — Contraceptive steroid combination.

ADVERSE EFFECTS — Serious: DVT/PE, stroke, MI, hepatic neoplasia, and gallbladder disease. Frequent: Nausea, breast tenderness, and breakthrough bleeding.

LOESTRIN 24 FE (ethinyl estradiol + norethindrone + ferrous fumarate) ▶L ♀X ▶– $$$

ADULT — Contraception: 1 tab PO daily.

PEDS — Not approved in children.

FORMS — Generic/Trade: Tabs 1 mg norethindrone/20 mcg ethinyl estradiol (24 days) with 4 days 75 mg ferrous fumarate.

NOTES — Loestrin 24 Fe 1/20 may cause less nausea and breast tenderness and may increase breakthrough bleeding due to lower estrogen content.

MOA — Contraceptive steroid combination.

ADVERSE EFFECTS — Serious: DVT/PE, stroke, MI, hepatic neoplasia, and gallbladder disease. Frequent: Nausea, breast tenderness, and breakthrough bleeding.

LOESTRIN FE (ethinyl estradiol + norethindrone + ferrous fumarate, *Larin Fe 1/20, Gildess Fe 1/20, Junel Fe 1/20, Microgestin Fe 1/20*) ▶L ♀X ▶– $$$

WARNING — Multiple strengths; see FORMS and write specific product on Rx.

ADULT — Contraception: 1 tab PO daily.

PEDS — Not approved in children.

FORMS — Generic/Trade: Tabs 1 mg norethindrone/20 mcg ethinyl estradiol with 7 days 75 mg ferrous fumarate (1/20); 1.5 mg norethindrone/30 mcg ethinyl estradiol with 7 days 75 mg ferrous fumarate (1.5/30).

NOTES — Loestrin Fe 1/20 may cause less nausea and breast tenderness and may increase breakthrough bleeding due to lower estrogen content. All 28 tabs must be taken.

MOA — Contraceptive steroid combination.

ADVERSE EFFECTS — Serious: DVT/PE, stroke, MI, hepatic neoplasia, and gallbladder disease. Frequent: Nausea, breast tenderness, and breakthrough bleeding.

LOESTRIN (ethinyl estradiol + norethindrone, *Junel,* ✴ *MinEstrin 1/20*) ▶L ♀X ▶– $$$

WARNING — Multiple strengths; see FORMS and write specific product on Rx.

ADULT — Contraception: 1 tab PO daily.

PEDS — Not approved in children.

FORMS — Generic/Trade: Tabs 1 mg norethindrone/20 mcg ethinyl estradiol (Junel 1/20 or Loestrin 1/20). Tabs 1.5 mg norethindrone/30 mcg ethinyl estradiol (Junel 1.5/30, Loestrin 1.5/30 or Microgestin 1.5/30).

NOTES — Loestrin 1/20 may cause less nausea and breast tenderness and may increase breakthrough bleeding due to lower estrogen content.

MOA — Contraceptive steroid combination.

ADVERSE EFFECTS — Serious: DVT/PE, stroke, MI, hepatic neoplasia, and gallbladder disease. Frequent: Nausea, breast tenderness, and breakthrough bleeding.

LOSEASONIQUE (ethinyl estradiol + levonorgestrel, *Amethia Lo, Camrese Lo*) ▶L ♀X ▶– $$$

ADULT — Contraception: 1 tab PO daily.

PEDS — Not approved in children.

FORMS — Generic/Trade: Tabs 20 mcg ethinyl estradiol/0.1 mg levonorgestrel. 84 orange active pills followed by 7 yellow pills with 10 mcg ethinyl estradiol.

NOTES — Decreases menstrual periods from q month to q 3 months; however, intermenstrual bleeding and spotting is more frequent than with 28-day regimens. All 91 tabs must be taken.

MOA — Contraceptive steroid combination.

ADVERSE EFFECTS — Serious: DVT/PE, stroke, MI, hepatic neoplasia, and gallbladder disease. Frequent: Nausea, breast tenderness, and breakthrough bleeding.

MINASTRIN 24 (ethinyl estradiol + norethindrone + ferrous fumarate) ▶L – ♀X ▶– $$$

ADULT — Contraception: 1 tab PO daily.

PEDS — Not approved in children.

FORMS — Trade only. Chewable tab 1 mg norethindrone/20 mcg ethinyl estradiol with 4 tabs of 75 mg ferrous fumarate.

NOTES — Similar to Microgestin Fe 1/20.

MOA — Contraceptive steroid combination.

ADVERSE EFFECTS — Serious: DVT/PE, stroke, MI, HTN, hepatic neoplasia. Frequent: headache, nausea, spotting, breast tenderness, acne, mood swings, and wt gain.

MODICON (ethinyl estradiol + norethindrone, *Brevicon, Necon 0.5/35, Nortrel 0.5/35, Wera*) ▶L ♀X ▶– $$$

ADULT — Contraception: 1 tab PO daily.

PEDS — Not approved in children.

FORMS — Generic/Trade: Tabs 35 mcg ethinyl estradiol/0.5 mg norethindrone.

MOA — Contraceptive steroid combination.

ADVERSE EFFECTS — Serious: DVT/PE, stroke, MI, hepatic neoplasia, and gallbladder disease. Frequent: Nausea, breast tenderness, and breakthrough bleeding.

NORDETTE (ethinyl estradiol + levonorgestrel, *Altavera, Kurvelo, Levora, Marlissa, Portia,* ✴ *MinOvral*) ▶L ♀X ▶– $$$

ADULT — Contraception: 1 tab PO daily.

PEDS — Not approved in children.

UNAPPROVED ADULT — Emergency contraception: See table.

FORMS — Generic/Trade: Tabs 30 mcg ethinyl estradiol/0.15 mg levonorgestrel.

MOA — Contraceptive steroid combination.

ADVERSE EFFECTS — Serious: DVT/PE, stroke, MI, hepatic neoplasia, and gallbladder disease. Frequent: Nausea, breast tenderness, and breakthrough bleeding.

NORETHINDRONE (*Micronor, Camila, Errin, Heather, Jencycla, Jolivette, Nora BE, Nor-QD*) ▶L ♀C ▶+

ADULT — Contraception: 1 tab daily.

FORMS — Generic/Trade: Tabs 0.35 mg.

(cont.)

NORETHINDRONE (*cont.*)

NOTES — Progestin-only pills are often called the "mini-pill."

MOA — Multicausal: Inhibitory cervical mucus, FSH/LH suppression, abnormal ovulation and endometrial changes unfavourable to implantation.

ADVERSE EFFECTS — Frequent: Menstrual irregularity, headache, breast tenderness, nausea, and dizziness.

NORINYL 1+50 (**mestranol + norethindrone**, *Necon 1/50*) ▶L ♀X ▶– $$

ADULT — Contraception: 1 tab PO daily.

PEDS — Not approved in children.

FORMS — Trade only: Tabs 1 mg norethindrone/50 mcg mestranol.

NOTES — 50 mcg estrogen component rarely necessary.

MOA — Contraceptive steroid combination.

ADVERSE EFFECTS — Serious: DVT/PE, stroke, MI, hepatic neoplasia, and gallbladder disease. Frequent: Nausea, breast tenderness, and breakthrough bleeding.

OGESTREL (**ethinyl estradiol + norgestrel**) ▶L ♀X ▶– $$

ADULT — Contraception: 1 tab PO daily.

PEDS — Not approved in children.

UNAPPROVED ADULT — Emergency contraception: See table.

FORMS — Trade only: Tabs: 50 mcg ethinyl estradiol/0.5 mg norgestrel.

NOTES — 50 mcg estrogen component rarely necessary.

MOA — Contraceptive steroid combination.

ADVERSE EFFECTS — Serious: DVT/PE, stroke, MI, hepatic neoplasia, and gallbladder disease. Frequent: Nausea, breast tenderness, and breakthrough bleeding.

ORTHO CYCLEN (**ethinyl estradiol + norgestimate**, *Estarylla, Mono-Linyah, Previfem, Sprintec, ✣ Cyclen*) ▶L ♀X ▶– $$

ADULT — Contraception: 1 tab PO daily.

PEDS — Not approved in children.

FORMS — Generic/Trade: Tabs 35 mcg ethinyl estradiol/0.25 mg norgestimate.

MOA — Contraceptive steroid combination.

ADVERSE EFFECTS — Serious: DVT/PE, stroke, MI, hepatic neoplasia, and gallbladder disease. Frequent: Nausea, breast tenderness, and breakthrough bleeding.

ORTHO-CEPT (**ethinyl estradiol + desogestrel**, *Apri, Desogen, Emoquette, Enskyce, Reclipsen, ✣ Marvelon*) ▶L ♀X ▶– $$$

ADULT — Contraception: 1 tab PO daily.

PEDS — Not approved in children.

FORMS — Generic/Trade: Tabs 30 mcg ethinyl estradiol/0.15 mg desogestrel.

MOA — Contraceptive steroid combination.

ADVERSE EFFECTS — Serious: DVT/PE, stroke, MI, hepatic neoplasia, and gallbladder disease. Frequent: Nausea, breast tenderness, and breakthrough bleeding.

ORTHO-NOVUM 1/35 (**ethinyl estradiol + norethindrone**, *Alyacen 1/35, Cyclafem 1/35, Dasetta 1/35, Necon 1/35, Norinyl 1+35, Nortrel 1/35, Pirmella 1/35*) ▶L ♀X ▶– $$$

ADULT — Contraception: 1 tab PO daily.

PEDS — Not approved in children.

FORMS — Generic/Trade: Tabs 1 mg norethindrone/35 mcg ethinyl estradiol.

MOA — Contraceptive steroid combination.

ADVERSE EFFECTS — Serious: DVT/PE, stroke, MI, hepatic neoplasia, and gallbladder disease. Frequent: Nausea, breast tenderness, and breakthrough bleeding.

OVCON-35 (**ethinyl estradiol + norethindrone**, *Balziva, Briellyn, Gildagia, Philith, Vyfemla, Zenchent*) ▶L ♀X ▶– $$$

ADULT — Contraception: 1 tab PO daily.

PEDS — Not approved in children.

FORMS — Generic/Trade: Tabs 35 mcg ethinyl estradiol/0.4 mg norethindrone.

MOA — Contraceptive steroid combination.

ADVERSE EFFECTS — Serious: DVT/PE, stroke, MI, hepatic neoplasia, and gallbladder disease. Frequent: Nausea, breast tenderness, and breakthrough bleeding.

SAFYRAL (**ethinyl estradiol + drospirenone + levomefolate calcium**) ▶L – ♀C ▶– ©V

ADULT — Contraception and folate supplementation: 1 tab PO daily.

PEDS — Not approved in children.

FORMS — Trade only: Tabs 0.03 mg ethinyl estradiol, 3 mg drospirenone, 0.451 mg levomefolate calcium. 24 active pills are followed by 4 inert pills.

NOTES — May cause hyperkalemia due to antimineralo corticoid activity of drospirenone (equal to 25 mg spironolactone). Monitor potassium in patients on ACE inhibitors, ARBs, potassium-sparing diuretics, heparin, aldosterone antagonists, and NSAIDs. NOTE: Similar to Yasmin.

MOA — Contraceptive steroid combination

ADVERSE EFFECTS — Serious: DVT/PE, stroke, MI, hepatic neoplasia, and gallbladder disease. Frequent: Nausea, headache, breast tenderness, and breakthrough bleeding.

SEASONALE (**ethinyl estradiol + levonorgestrel**, *Introvale, Quasense*) ▶L ♀X ▶– $$$

ADULT — Contraception: 1 tab PO daily.

PEDS — Not approved in children.

UNAPPROVED ADULT — Emergency contraception: See table.

FORMS — Generic/Trade: Tabs 30 mcg ethinyl estradiol/0.15 mg levonorgestrel. 84 pink active pills followed by 7 white placebo pills.

NOTES — Decreases menstrual periods from q month to q 3 months; however, intermenstrual bleeding and spotting are more frequent than with 28-day regimens.

MOA — Contraceptive steroid combination.

ADVERSE EFFECTS — Serious: DVT/PE, stroke, MI, hepatic neoplasia, and gallbladder disease. Frequent: Nausea, breast tenderness, and breakthrough bleeding.

SEASONIQUE (ethinyl estradiol + levonorgestrel, *Amethia, Camrese, Daysee*) ▶L ♀X ▶– $$$
ADULT — Contraception: 1 tab PO daily.
PEDS — Not approved in children.
UNAPPROVED ADULT — Emergency contraception: See table.
FORMS — Generic/Trade: Tabs 30 mcg ethinyl estradiol/0.15 mg levonorgestrel. 84 active pills followed by 7 pills with 10 mcg ethinyl estradiol.
NOTES — Decreases menstrual periods from q month to q 3 months; however, intermenstrual bleeding and spotting is more frequent than with 28-day regimens. All 91 tabs must be taken.
MOA — Contraceptive steroid combination.
ADVERSE EFFECTS — Serious: DVT/PE, stroke, MI, hepatic neoplasia, and gallbladder disease. Frequent: Nausea, breast tenderness, and breakthrough bleeding.

YASMIN (ethinyl estradiol + drospirenone, *Ocella, Syeda, Zarah*) ▶L ♀X ▶– $$$
ADULT — Contraception: 1 tab PO daily.
PEDS — Not approved in children.
FORMS — Generic/Trade: Tabs 30 mcg ethinyl estradiol/3 mg drospirenone.
NOTES — May cause hyperkalemia due to antimineralocorticoid activity of drospirenone (equal to 25 mg spironolactone). Monitor potassium in patients on ACE inhibitors, ARBs, potassium-sparing diuretics, heparin, aldosterone antagonists, and NSAIDs. Safyral also contains levomefolate 0.451 mg in all tabs.
MOA — Contraceptive steroid combination.
ADVERSE EFFECTS — Serious: DVT/PE, stroke, MI, hepatic neoplasia, and gallbladder disease. Frequent: Nausea, breast tenderness, and breakthrough bleeding.

YAZ (ethinyl estradiol + drospirenone, *Gianvi, Loryna, Nikki*) ▶L ♀X ▶– $$$
ADULT — Contraception, premenstrual dysphoric disorder, acne: 1 tab PO daily.
PEDS — Not approved in children.

FORMS — Generic/Trade: Tabs 20 mcg ethinyl estradiol/3 mg drospirenone. 24 active pills are followed by 4 inert pills.
NOTES — May cause hyperkalemia due to antimineralocorticoid activity of drospirenone (equal to 25 mg spironolactone). Monitor potassium in patients on ACE inhibitors, ARBs, potassium-sparing diuretics, heparin, aldosterone antagonists, and NSAIDs.
MOA — Contraceptive steroid combination.
ADVERSE EFFECTS — Serious: DVT/PE, stroke, MI, hepatic neoplasia, and gallbladder disease. Frequent: Nausea, breast tenderness, and breakthrough bleeding.

ZOVIA 1/35 (ethinyl estradiol + ethynodiol, *Kelnor 1/35*) ▶L ♀–X ▶–
WARNING — Multiple strengths; See Forms and write specific product on Rx.
ADULT — Contraception: 1 tab PO daily.
PEDS — Not approved in children.
FORMS — Generic/Trade: Tabs 1 mg ethynodiol/35 mcg ethinyl estradiol. Also available as Zovia 1/50E.
MOA — Contraceptive steroid combination.
ADVERSE EFFECTS — Serious: DVT/PD, stroke, MI, hepatic neoplasia, and gallbladder disease. Frequent: Nausea, breast tenderness, and breakthrough bleeding.

ZOVIA 1/50E (ethinyl estradiol + ethynodiol) ▶L ♀X ▶– $$
WARNING — Multiple strengths; see FORMS and write specific product on Rx.
ADULT — Contraception: 1 tab PO daily.
PEDS — Not approved in children.
FORMS — Trade only: Tabs 1 mg ethynodiol/50 mcg ethinyl estradiol. Also available as Zovia 1/35.
NOTES — 50 mcg estrogen component rarely necessary.
MOA — Contraceptive steroid combination.
ADVERSE EFFECTS — Serious: DVT/PE, stroke, MI, hepatic neoplasia, and gallbladder disease. Frequent: Nausea, breast tenderness, and breakthrough bleeding.

OB/GYN: Contraceptives—Oral Biphasic

NOTE: Not recommended in women older than 35 yo who smoke or have complex migraine headaches. Increased risk of thromboembolism, CVA, MI, hepatic neoplasia, cervical cancer, and gallbladder disease. Nausea, breast tenderness, and breakthrough bleeding are common, transient side effects. Nighttime dosing may minimize nausea. Effectiveness is reduced by hepatic enzyme-inducing drugs such as certain anticonvulsants and barbiturates, rifampin, rifabutin, griseofulvin and protease inhibitors. Additionally, products that contain St. John's wort may decrease efficacy. Vomiting or diarrhea may also increase the risk of contraceptive failure. An additional form of birth control may be advisable. Advise patients to take at the same time every day. See PI for instructions on missing doses. Most available in 21- and 28-day packs. Although not approved by the FDA, combined OCPs are used for dysfunctional uterine bleeding, dysmenorrhea, pelvic pain, and hirsutism (with spironolactone): 1 tab PO daily. Wait 6 weeks postpartum to initiate combination OCPs to decrease the risk of thromboembolism and to support lactation.

AZURETTE (ethinyl estradiol + desogestrel, *Bekyree, Kariva, Kimidess, Pimtrea, Viorele*) ▶L ♀X ▶– $$$
ADULT — Contraception: 1 tab PO daily.
PEDS — Not approved in children.
FORMS — Generic/branded generics only: Tabs 20 mcg ethinyl estradiol/0.15 mg desogestrel (21), 10 mcg ethinyl estradiol (5).

NOTES — May have less breakthrough bleeding. All 28 tabs must be taken.
MOA — Contraceptive steroid combination.
ADVERSE EFFECTS — Serious: DVT/PE, stroke, MI, hepatic neoplasia, and gallbladder disease. Frequent: Nausea, breast tenderness, and breakthrough bleeding.

OB/GYN: Contraceptives—Oral Triphasic

NOTE: Not recommended in women older than 35 yo who smoke. Increased risk of thromboembolism, CVA, MI, hepatic neoplasia, cervical cancer, and gallbladder disease. Nausea, breast tenderness, and breakthrough bleeding are common, transient side effects. Nighttime dosing may minimize nausea. Effectiveness is reduced by hepatic enzyme-inducing drugs such as certain anticonvulsants and barbiturates, rifampin, rifabutin, griseofulvin, and protease inhibitors. Additionally, products that contain St. John's wort may decrease efficacy. Vomiting or diarrhea may also increase the risk of contraceptive failure. An additional form of birth control may be advisable. Advise patients to take at the same time every day. See PI for instructions on missing doses. Most available in 21- and 28-day packs. Although not approved by the FDA, combined OCPs are used for dysfunctional uterine bleeding, emergency contraception, dysmenorrhea, pelvic pain, and hirsutism (with spironolactone): 1 tab PO daily. Wait 6 weeks postpartum to initiate combination OCPs to decrease the risk of thromboembolism and to support lactation.

CYCLESSA (ethinyl estradiol + desogestrel, *Caziant, Velivet*) ▶L ♀X ▶– $$
ADULT — Contraception: 1 tab PO daily.
PEDS — Not approved in children.
FORMS — Generic/Trade: Tabs 25 mcg ethinyl estradiol/0.100 (7), 0.125 (7), 0.150 mg desogestrel (7).
MOA — Contraceptive steroid combination.
ADVERSE EFFECTS — Serious: DVT/PE, stroke, MI, hepatic neoplasia, and gallbladder disease. Frequent: Nausea, breast tenderness, and breakthrough bleeding.

ESTROSTEP FE (ethinyl estradiol + norethindrone + ferrous fumarate, *Tilia Fe-28, Tri-Legest Fe*) ▶L ♀X ▶– $$$
ADULT — Contraception: 1 tab PO daily.
PEDS — Not approved in children.
FORMS — Generic/Trade: Tabs 20, 30, 35 mcg ethinyl estradiol/1 mg norethindrone + "placebo" tabs with 75 mg ferrous fumarate. Packs of 28 only.
NOTES — All 28 tabs must be taken.
MOA — Contraceptive steroid combination.
ADVERSE EFFECTS — Serious: DVT/PE, stroke, MI, hepatic neoplasia, and gallbladder disease. Frequent: Nausea, breast tenderness, and breakthrough bleeding.

ORTHO TRI-CYCLEN LO (ethinyl estradiol + norgestimate) ▶L ♀X ▶– $$$
ADULT — Contraception: 1 tab PO daily.
PEDS — Not approved in children.
FORMS — Generic/Trade: Tabs 25 mcg ethinyl estradiol/0.18 (7), 0.215 (7), 0.25 mg norgestimate (7).
MOA — Contraceptive steroid combination.
ADVERSE EFFECTS — Serious: DVT/PE, stroke, MI, hepatic neoplasia, and gallbladder disease. Frequent: Nausea, breast tenderness, and breakthrough bleeding.

ORTHO TRI-CYCLEN (ethinyl estradiol + norgestimate, *Tri-Estarylla, Tri-Linyah, Tri-Previfem, Tri-Sprintec, ✱ Tri-Cyclen*) ▶L ♀X ▶– $$
ADULT — Contraception, adult acne: 1 tab PO daily.
PEDS — Not approved in children.
FORMS — Generic/Trade: Tabs 35 mcg ethinyl estradiol/0.18 (7), 0.215 (7), 0.25 mg norgestimate (7).
MOA — Contraceptive steroid combination.
ADVERSE EFFECTS — Serious: DVT/PE, stroke, MI, hepatic neoplasia, and gallbladder disease. Frequent: Nausea, breast tenderness, and breakthrough bleeding.

ORTHO-NOVUM 7/7/7 (ethinyl estradiol + norethindrone, *Alyacen 7/7/7, Cyclafem 7/7/7, Dasetta 7/7/7, Necon 7/7/7, Nortrel 7/7/7, Pirmella 7/7/7*) ▶L ♀X ▶– $$
ADULT — Contraception: 1 tab PO daily.
PEDS — Not approved in children.
FORMS — Generic/Trade: Tabs 35 mcg ethinyl estradiol/0.5, 0.75, 1 mg norethindrone.
MOA — Contraceptive steroid combination.
ADVERSE EFFECTS — Serious: DVT/PE, stroke, MI, hepatic neoplasia, and gallbladder disease. Frequent: Nausea, breast tenderness, and breakthrough bleeding.

TRI-LEGEST (ethinyl estradiol + norethindrone) ▶L ♀X ▶– $$$
ADULT — Contraception: 1 tab PO daily.
PEDS — Not approved in children.
FORMS — Trade only: Tabs 20, 30, 35 mcg ethinyl estradiol/1 mg norethindrone.
MOA — Contraceptive steroid combination.
ADVERSE EFFECTS — Serious: DVT/PE, stroke, MI, hepatic neoplasia, and gallbladder disease. Frequent: Nausea, breast tenderness, and breakthrough bleeding.

TRI-NORINYL (ethinyl estradiol + norethindrone, *Aranelle, ✱ Synphasic*) ▶L ♀X ▶– $$
ADULT — Contraception: 1 tab PO daily.
PEDS — Not approved in children.
FORMS — Generic/Trade: Tabs 35 mcg ethinyl estradiol/0.5, 1, 0.5 mg norethindrone.
MOA — Contraceptive steroid combination.
ADVERSE EFFECTS — Serious: DVT/PE, stroke, MI, hepatic neoplasia, and gallbladder disease. Frequent: Nausea, breast tenderness, and breakthrough bleeding.

TRIVORA-28 (ethinyl estradiol + levonorgestrel, *Enpresse, Levonest, Myzilra*) ▶L ♀X ▶– $$
ADULT — Contraception: 1 tab PO daily.
PEDS — Not approved in children.
UNAPPROVED ADULT — Emergency contraception: See table.
FORMS — Generic/Trade: Tabs 30, 40, 30 mcg ethinyl estradiol/0.05, 0.075, 0.125 mg levonorgestrel.
MOA — Contraceptive steroid combination.
ADVERSE EFFECTS — Serious: DVT/PE, stroke, MI, hepatic neoplasia, and gallbladder disease. Frequent: Nausea, breast tenderness, and breakthrough bleeding.

OB/GYN: Contraceptives—Oral Four-Phasic

NATAZIA (estradiol valerate and estradiol valerate + dienogest) ▶L – stomach ♀X ▶–
ADULT — Contraception 1 PO daily, start on day 1 of menstrual cycle. Heavy menstrual bleeding 1 PO daily.
PEDS — Not approved in children.
FORMS — Trade only: Tabs 3 mg estradiol valerate (2), 2 mg estradiol valerate/2 mg dienogest (5), 2 mg estradiol valerate/3 mg dienogest (17), 1 mg estradiol valerate (2), inert (2).
NOTES — Not evaluated in BMI greater than 30. Tablets must be taken as directed on blister pack.
MOA — Contraceptive steroid combination.
ADVERSE EFFECTS — Serious: DVT, MI, hepatic. Frequent: HA, irregular bleeding, breast changes, nausea/vomiting, acne, inc. weight.

QUARTETTE (levonorgestrel + ethinyl estradiol) ▶L ♀–X ▶–
ADULT — Contraception: 1 tab PO daily.
PEDS — Not approved in children.
FORMS — Trade only: 91 tabs per pack. (42) 0.15 mg levonorgestrel/20 mcg ethinyl estradiol, (21) 0.15 mg levonorgestrel/25 mcg ethinyl estradiol, (21) 0.15 levonorgestrel/30 mcg ethinyl estradiol, (7) 10 mcg ethinyl estradiol.
NOTES — All 91 tabs must be taken.
MOA — Contraceptive steroid combination.
ADVERSE EFFECTS — Serious: CVT/PE, stroke, MI, hepatic necrosis, and gallbladder disease. Frequent: nausea, headache, breast tenderness, irregular bleeding.

OB/GYN: Contraceptives—Other

ETONOGESTREL (*Implanon, Nexplanon*) ▶L ♀X ▶+ $$$$$
WARNING — Increased risk of thromboembolism and CVA. Effectiveness may be reduced by hepatic enzyme-inducing drugs such as certain anticonvulsants, barbiturates, griseofulvin, rifampin. Additionally, products that contain St. John's wort may decrease efficacy; an additional form of birth control may be advisable.
ADULT — Contraception: 1 subdermal implant q 3 years. Specific timing for implantation after other contraceptive methods.
PEDS — Not approved in children.
FORMS — Trade only: Single rod implant, 68 mg etonogestrel. Nexplanon also contains 15 mg barium sulfate.
NOTES — Not studied in women greater than 130% of ideal body wt; may be less effective if overweight. Implant should be palpable immediately after insertion.
MOA — Contraceptive progestin.
ADVERSE EFFECTS — Serious: DVT/PE, stroke. Common: HA, weight gain, vaginitis, bleeding irregularities, depression, liver disease.

LEVONORGESTREL (*Plan B, Next Choice*) ▶L ♀X ▶+ – $$
ADULT — Emergency contraception: 1 tab PO ASAP but within 72 h of intercourse. 2nd tab 12 h later.
PEDS — Not approved in children.
UNAPPROVED ADULT — 2 tabs (1.5 mg) PO ASAP but within 72 h of intercourse (lesser efficacy at up to 120 h).
FORMS — OTC Trade Only: Kit contains 2 tabs 0.75 mg. Rx: Generic/Trade: Kit contains 2 tabs 0.75mg.
NOTES — OTC if at least 17 yo; Rx if younger. Nausea uncommon; however, if vomiting occurs within 1 h, initial dose must be given again. Consider adding an antiemetic. Patients should be instructed to then contact their healthcare providers. Can be used at any time during the menstrual cycle.
MOA — Gonadal steroid.

ADVERSE EFFECTS — Serious: None. Frequent: Menstrual changes, nausea, abdominal pain, fatigue.

LEVONORGESTREL—INTRAUTERINE (*Liletta*) ▶L ♀X ▶–
WARNING — Increased risk of perforation if inserted into lactating or postpartum women with fixed retroverted uterus.
ADULT — Contraception: 1 intrauterine system q 3 years
PEDS — Safety and efficacy are expected to be the same for postpubertal adolescents younger than 18 yo as for adults. Use before menarche is not indicated.
FORMS — Trade only: Single plastic, "T" shaped, intrauterine implant, 52 mg levonorgestrel. Releases an average of 15.6 mcg per day levonorgestrel.
MOA — Contraceptive steroid
ADVERSE EFFECTS — Serious: Endometrial perforation, ovarian cysts, PID. Frequent: Vaginal infections, acne, headache, mood swings, dysmenorrhea.

LEVONORGESTREL—INTRAUTERINE (*Mirena*) ▶L – ♀X ▶+
WARNING — Increased risk of perforation if inserted into lactating or postpostpartum women with fixed retroverted uterus.
ADULT — Contraception: 1 intrauterine system q 5 years.
PEDS — Not approved in children.
FORMS — Trade only: Single intrauterine implant. 25 mg levonorgestrel.
MOA — Contraceptive steroid.
ADVERSE EFFECTS — Serious: Endometrial perforation, ovarian cysts, sepsis. Frequent: bleeding irregularities, mood changes, abdominal/pelvic pain, acne and headache.

LEVONORGESTREL—INTRAUTERINE (*Skyla*, ✱*Jaydess*) ▶L ♀–X ▶+
WARNING — Increased risk of perforation if inserted into lactating or postpartum women with fixed retroverted uterus.
ADULT — Contraception: 1 intrauterine system q 3 years.

(cont.)

LEVONORGESTREL—INTRAUTERINE (cont.)

PEDS — Not approved in children.

FORMS — Trade only: Single intrauterine implant, 13.5 mg levonorgestrel.

NOTES — Skyla can only be scanned by MRI under specific conditions.

MOA — Contraceptive steroid

ADVERSE EFFECTS — Serious: Endometrial perforation, ovarian cysts, sepsis. Frequent: bleeding irregularities, vulvovaginitis, abdominal/pelvic pain, acne/seborrhea, ovarian cyst and headache.

LEVONORGESTREL—SINGLE DOSE (Plan B One-Step, Next Choice One-Step, Fallback Solo) ▶L ♀X ▶– $$

ADULT — Emergency contraception: 1 tab PO ASAP but within 72 h of intercourse.

PEDS — Not approved in children.

FORMS — OTC Trade only: Tabs 1.5 mg.

NOTES — OTC if at least 17 yo; Rx if younger. Nausea uncommon; however, if vomiting occurs within 1 h, initial dose must be given again. Consider adding an antiemetic. Patients should be instructed to then contact their healthcare providers. Can be used at any time during the menstrual cycle. Lesser efficacy at up to 120 h.

MOA — Gonadal steroid.

ADVERSE EFFECTS — Serious: None. Frequent: None.

NUVARING (ethinyl estradiol + etonogestrel vaginal ring) ▶L ♀X ▶– $$$

ADULT — Contraception: 1 ring intravaginally for 3 weeks each month.

PEDS — Not approved in children.

FORMS — Trade only: Flexible intravaginal ring, 15 mcg ethinyl estradiol/0.120 mg etonogestrel/day in 1, 3 rings/box.

NOTES — Insert on day 5 of cycle or within 7 days of the last oral contraceptive pill. The ring must remain in place continuously for 3 weeks, including during intercourse. Remove for 1 week, then insert a new ring. May be used continuously for 4 weeks and replaced immediately to skip a withdrawal week. Store at room temperature (59° to 86°F) for up to 4 months. In case of accidental removal, reinsert ASAP after rinsing with cool to lukewarm water. If removal is greater than 3 h during week 1 or 2, use backup method until ring in place for at least 7 days; if during week 3, do not reinsert the used ring, but either insert new ring immediately to start next 21-day cycle or wait no more than 7 days .

MOA — Contraceptive steroid combination.

ADVERSE EFFECTS — Serious: DVT/PE, stroke, MI, hepatic neoplasia, and gallbladder disease. Frequent: Nausea, breast tenderness, breakthrough bleeding, asymptomatic vaginal discharge, galactorrhea.

ORTHO EVRA (ethinyl estradiol + norelgestromin, Xulane, ✷ Evra) ▶L ♀X ▶– $$$$

WARNING — Average estrogen concentration 60% higher than common oral contraceptives (ie, 35 mcg ethinyl estradiol), which may further increase the risk of thromboembolism.

ADULT — Contraception: 1 patch q week for 3 weeks, then 1 week patch-free.

PEDS — Not approved in children.

FORMS — Trade only: Transdermal patch (Xulane) 150 mcg norelgestromin/20 mcg ethinyl estradiol/day in 1, 3 patches/box.

NOTES — May be less effective in women 90 kg or greater (198 lbs). Apply new patch on the same day each week. Do not exceed 7 days between patches. Rotate application sites, avoid the waistline. Do not use earlier than 4 weeks postpartum if not breastfeeding.

MOA — Contraceptive steroid combination.

ADVERSE EFFECTS — Serious: DVT/PE, stroke, MI, hepatic neoplasia, and gallbladder disease. Frequent: Nausea, breast tenderness, breakthrough bleeding.

ULIPRISTAL ACETATE (Ella) ▶L ♀X ▶?

WARNING — Hormonal contraception should not be used within 5 days after using ulipristal acetate. Barrier contraception is recommended until next menstrual cycle.

ADULT — Emergency contraception. 1 tab PO ASAP within 5 days of intercourse.

PEDS — Safety and efficacy are expected to be the same for postpubertal adolescents younger than 18 yo as for adults.

FORMS — Trade only: Tabs 30 mg.

NOTES — If vomiting occurs within 3 h of administration, consider repeating the dose. Can be used at any time during menstrual cycle. Canadian only: Fibristal has different indication and dose.

MOA — Progesterone receptor modulator causes delay of ovulation with possible changes to endometrium to affect implantation.

ADVERSE EFFECTS — Headache, nausea, abdominal pain, acne.

OB/GYN: Estrogens

NOTE: See also Hormone Combinations. Unopposed estrogens increase the risk of endometrial cancer in postmenopausal women. Malignancy should be ruled out in cases of persistent or recurrent abnormal vaginal bleeding. In women with an intact uterus, a progestin should be administered daily throughout the month or for the last 10 to 12 days of the month. Do not use during pregnancy. May increase the risk of DVT/PE, gallbladder disease. Interactions with oral anticoagulants, certain anticonvulsants, rifampin, barbiturates, corticosteroids, and St. John's wort. Estrogens should not be used in the prevention of cardiovascular disease. In the Women's Health Initiative, the use of conjugated estrogens (Premarin) caused an increase in the risk of CVA and PE. Additionally, the combination with medroxyprogesterone increased the risk of breast cancer and MI. Women older than 65 yo with 4 years of therapy had an increased risk of dementia. Estrogens should be prescribed at the lowest effective doses and for the shortest durations. Patients should be counseled regarding the risks/benefits of HRT.

BIEST (estradiol + estriol) ▶L ♀X ▶– $$$

WARNING — For topical dosages: Patient should take precautions to ensure that children and pets do not make contact with skin where topical estrogen has been applied.

UNAPPROVED ADULT — Hormone replacement therapy. Once or twice a day dosing.

FORMS — Must be compounded by a pharmacist. Most common estriol/estradiol ratios 80%/20% or 50%/50%. May be formulated as cream, gel, troche, or capsule.

NOTES — Compounded bioidentical hormones are not FDA approved. These products should be considered to have the same safety issues raised by the Women's Health Initiative as those associated with hormone therapy agents that are FDA approved.

MOA — Gonadal steroid

ADVERSE EFFECTS — Serious: Endometrial cancer, DVT/PE, gallbladder disease, breast cancer, MI, CVA. Frequent: Nausea, breast tenderness.

ESTERIFIED ESTROGENS (*Menest*) ▶L ♀X ▶– $$

ADULT — Moderate to severe menopausal vasomotor symptoms: 1.25 mg PO daily. Atrophic vaginitis: 0.3 to 1.25 mg PO daily. Female hypogonadism: 2.5 to 7.5 mg PO daily in divided doses for 20 days followed by a 10-day rest period. Repeat until bleeding occurs. Bilateral oophorectomy and ovarian failure: 1.25 mg PO daily. Prevention of postmenopausal osteoporosis: 0.3 to 1.25 mg PO daily.

PEDS — Not approved in children.

FORMS — Trade only: Tabs 0.3, 0.625, 1.25, 2.5 mg.

NOTES — Typical hormone replacement regimen consists of a daily estrogen dose with a progestin added either daily or for the last 10 to 12 days of the cycle.

MOA — Gonadal steroid.

ADVERSE EFFECTS — Serious: Endometrial cancer, DVT/PE, gallbladder disease, breast cancer, MI, CVA. Frequent: Nausea, breast tenderness.

ESTRADIOL ▶L ♀X ▶– $

ADULT — Moderate to severe menopausal vasomotor symptoms and atrophic vaginitis, female hypogonadism, bilateral oophorectomy, and ovarian failure: 1 to 2 mg PO daily. Prevention of postmenopausal osteoporosis: 0.5 mg PO daily.

PEDS — Not approved in children.

FORMS — Generic only: Tabs, micronized 0.5, 1, 2 mg, scored.

NOTES — Typical hormone replacement regimen consists of a daily estrogen dose with a progestin added either daily or for the last 10 to 12 days of the cycle.

MOA — Gonadal steroid.

ADVERSE EFFECTS — Serious: Endometrial cancer, DVT/PE, gallbladder disease, breast cancer, MI, CVA. Frequent: Nausea, breast tenderness.

ESTRADIOL ACETATE (*Femtrace*) ▶L ♀X ▶– $$

ADULT — Moderate to severe menopausal vasomotor symptoms: 0.45 to 1.8 mg PO daily.

PEDS — Not approved in children.

FORMS — Trade only: Tabs 0.45, 0.9, 1.8 mg.

NOTES — Typical hormone replacement regimen consists of a daily estrogen dose with a progestin added either daily or for the last 10 to 12 days of the cycle.

MOA — Gonadal steroid.

ADVERSE EFFECTS — Serious: Endometrial cancer, DVT/PE, gallbladder disease, breast cancer, MI, CVA. Frequent: Nausea, breast tenderness.

ESTRADIOL ACETATE VAGINAL RING (*Femring*) ▶L ♀X ▶– $$$

WARNING — A few cases of toxic shock syndrome have been reported. Bowel obstruction.

ADULT — Menopausal vasomotor symptoms or vaginal atrophy: Insert ring into the vagina and replace after 90 days.

PEDS — Not approved in children.

FORMS — Trade only: 0.05 mg/day and 0.1 mg/day.

NOTES — Should the ring fall out or be removed during the 90-day period, rinse in lukewarm water and re-insert. Ring adhesion to vaginal wall has been reported, making removal difficult.

MOA — Gonadal steroid.

ADVERSE EFFECTS — Serious: Toxic shock, bowel obstruction. Frequent: Breast tenderness, breakthrough bleeding.

ESTRADIOL CYPIONATE (*Depo-Estradiol*) ▶L ♀X ▶– – $

WARNING — When estrogen is prescribed for a woman with a uterus, progestin should also be initiated to reduce the risk of endometrial cancer.

ADULT — Moderate to severe menopausal vasomotor symptoms: 1 to 5 mg IM q 3 to 4 weeks. Female hypogonadism: 1.5 to 2 mg IM q month.

PEDS — Not approved in children.

FORMS — Trade only: Injection 5 mg/mL in 5 mL vials.

MOA — Gonadal steroid.

ADVERSE EFFECTS — Serious: Endometrial cancer, DVT/PE, gallbladder disease, breast cancer, MI, CVA. Frequent: Nausea, breast tenderness.

ESTRADIOL GEL (*Divigel, Estrogel, Elestrin*) ▶L ♀X ▶– $$$

WARNING — Patient should take precautions to ensure that children and pets do not make contact with skin where topical estradiol has been applied.

ADULT — Moderate to severe menopausal vasomotor symptoms and atrophic vaginitis: Thinly apply contents of 1 complete pump depression to one entire arm, from wrist to shoulder (Estrogel) or upper arm (Elestrin) or contents of 1 foil packet to left or right upper thigh on alternating days. Allow to dry completely before dressing. Wash both hands thoroughly after application.

PEDS — Not approved in children.

FORMS — Trade only: Gel 0.06% in nonaerosol, metered-dose pump with #64 or #32 1.25 g doses (Estrogel), #100 0.87 g doses (Elestrin). Gel 0.1% in single-dose foil packets of 0.25, 0.5, 1.0 g, carton of 30 (Divigel).

NOTES — Depress the pump 2 times to prime. Concomitant sunscreen may increase absorption. Typical hormone replacement regimen consists of a

(cont.)

ESTRADIOL GEL (cont.)

daily estrogen dose with a progestin added either daily or for the last 10 to 12 days of the cycle.
MOA — Gonadal steroid.
ADVERSE EFFECTS — Serious: Endometrial cancer, DVT/PE, gallbladder disease, breast cancer, MI, CVA. Frequent: Nausea, breast tenderness, rash.

ESTRADIOL TRANSDERMAL PATCH (Alora, Climara, Menostar, Vivelle Dot, Minivelle, ✷Estradot, Oesclim) ▶L ♀X ▶– $$$

ADULT — Moderate to severe menopausal vasomotor symptoms and atrophic vaginitis, female hypogonadism, bilateral oophorectomy, and ovarian failure: Initiate with 0.025 to 0.05 mg/day patch once or twice per week, depending on the product (see FORMS). Prevention of postmenopausal osteoporosis: 0.025 to 0.1 mg/day patch.
PEDS — Not approved in children.
FORMS — Generic/Trade: Transdermal patches doses in mg/day: Climara (once a week) 0.025, 0.0375, 0.05, 0.06, 0.075, 0.1. Trade only: Vivelle Dot (twice per week) 0.025, 0.0375, 0.05, 0.075, 0.1. Alora (twice per week) 0.025, 0.05, 0.075, 0.1. Minivelle (twice per week) 0.0375, 0.05, 0.075, 0.1 mg/day. Menostar (once a week) 0.014 mg.
NOTES — Rotate application sites, avoid the waistline. Transdermal may be preferable for women with high triglycerides and chronic liver disease.
MOA — Gonadal steroid.
ADVERSE EFFECTS — Serious: Endometrial cancer, DVT/PE, gallbladder disease, breast cancer, MI, CVA. Frequent: Nausea, breast tenderness.

ESTRADIOL TRANSDERMAL SPRAY (Evamist) ▶L ♀X ▶– $$$

WARNING — Patient should take precautions to ensure that children and pets do not make contact with skin where topical estradiol has been applied.
ADULT — Moderate to severe menopausal vasomotor symptoms: Initially 1 spray daily to adjacent non-overlapping inner surface of the forearm. Allow to dry for 2 min and do not wash for 30 min. Adjust up to 3 sprays daily based on clinical response.
PEDS — Not approved in children.
FORMS — Trade only: 1.53 mg estradiol per 90 mcL spray, 56 sprays per metered-dose pump.
NOTES — Depress the pump 3 times with the cover on to prime each new applicator. Hold upright and vertical for spraying; rest the plastic cone against the skin. Typical hormone replacement regimen consists of a daily estrogen dose with a progestin added either daily or for the last 10 to 12 days of the cycle.
MOA — Gonadal steroid.
ADVERSE EFFECTS — Serious: Endometrial cancer, DVT/PE, gallbladder disease, breast cancer, MI, CVA. Frequent: Nausea, breast tenderness, nipple discoloration, rash, alopecia, chloasma.

ESTRADIOL VAGINAL RING (Estring) ▶L ♀X ▶– $$$

WARNING — Do not use during pregnancy. Toxic shock syndrome has been reported.

ADULT — Vaginal atrophy and lower urinary tract atrophy: Insert ring into upper third of the vaginal vault and replace after 90 days.
PEDS — Not approved in children.
FORMS — Trade only: 2 mg ring single pack.
NOTES — Should the ring fall out or be removed during the 90-day period, rinse in lukewarm water, and re-insert. Reports of ring adhesion to the vaginal wall making ring removal difficult. Minimal systemic absorption, probable lower risk of adverse effects than systemic estrogens.
MOA — Gonadal steroid.
ADVERSE EFFECTS — Serious: Toxic shock, bowel obstruction, vaginal wall adhesion. Frequent: None.

ESTRADIOL VAGINAL TAB (Vagifem) ▶L ♀X ▶– $$$

WARNING — Do not use during pregnancy.
ADULT — Menopausal atrophic vaginitis: Begin with 1 tab vaginally daily for 2 weeks, maintenance 1 tab vaginally twice per week.
PEDS — Not approved in children.
FORMS — Trade only: Vaginal tab 10 mcg in disposable single-use applicators, 8 or 18/pack.
MOA — Gonadal steroid.
ADVERSE EFFECTS — Serious: None. Frequent: None.

ESTROGEN VAGINAL CREAM (Premarin, Estrace) ▶L ♀X ▶? $$$$

ADULT — Atrophic vaginitis: Premarin: 0.5 to 2 g intravaginally daily for 1 to 2 weeks, then reduce to 0.5 g twice weekly maintenance. Estrace: 1 to 4 g intravaginally daily for 1 to 2 weeks. Gradually reduce to a maintenance dose of 1 g 1 to 3 times per week.
PEDS — Not approved in children.
FORMS — Trade only: Premarin: 0.625 mg conjugated estrogens/g in 30 g with calibrated applicator. Estrace: 0.1 mg estradiol/g in 42.5 g with calibrated applicator. Generic only: Cream 0.625 mg synthetic conjugated estrogens/g in 30 g with calibrated applicator.
NOTES — Possibility of absorption through the vaginal mucosa. Uterine bleeding might be provoked by excessive use in menopausal women. Breast tenderness and vaginal discharge due to mucus hypersecretion may result from excessive estrogenic stimulation. Endometrial withdrawal bleeding may occur if use is discontinued.
MOA — Gonadal steroid.
ADVERSE EFFECTS — Serious: Endometrial cancer, DVT/PE, gallbladder disease. Frequent: Nausea, breast tenderness.

ESTROGENS CONJUGATED (Premarin, C.E.S., Congest) ▶L ♀X ▶– $$$

ADULT — Moderate to severe menopausal vasomotor symptoms, atrophic vaginitis, and urethritis: 0.3 to 1.25 mg PO daily. Female hypogonadism: 0.3 to 0.625 mg PO daily for 3 weeks with 1 week off q month. Bilateral oophorectomy and ovarian failure: 1.25 mg PO daily for 3 weeks with 1 week off q month. Prevention of postmenopausal osteoporosis: 0.625 mg PO daily. Abnormal uterine bleeding: 25 mg IV/IM. Repeat in 6 to 12 h if needed.

(cont.)

ESTROGENS CONJUGATED (cont.)

PEDS — Not approved in children.

UNAPPROVED ADULT — Prevention of postmeno-pausal osteoporosis: 0.3 mg PO daily. Normalizing bleeding time in patients with AV malformations or underlying renal impairment: 30 to 70 mg IV/PO daily until bleeding time normalized.

FORMS — Trade only: Tabs 0.3, 0.45, 0.625, 0.9, 1.25 mg.

MOA — Gonadal steroid.

ADVERSE EFFECTS — Serious: Endometrial cancer, DVT/PE, gallbladder disease, breast cancer, MI, CVA. Frequent: Nausea, breast tenderness.

ESTROGENS SYNTHETIC CONJUGATED B (Enjuvia) ▶L ♀X ▶– $$

ADULT — Moderate to severe menopausal vasomotor symptoms: 0.3 to 1.25 mg PO daily.

PEDS — Not approved in children.

FORMS — Trade only: Tabs 0.3, 0.45, 0.625, 0.9, 1.25 mg.

NOTES — Typical hormone replacement regimen consists of a daily estrogen dose with a progestin either daily or for the last 10 to 12 days of the cycle. The difference between synthetic conjugated estrogens A and B is the additional component of delta-8,9-dehydroestrone sulfate in the B preparation. The clinical significance of this is unknown.

MOA — Gonadal steroid.

ADVERSE EFFECTS — Serious: Endometrial cancer, DVT/PE, gallbladder disease, breast cancer, MI, CVA dementia and angioedema. Frequent: Nausea, breast tenderness.

ESTROPIPATE (Ogen, Ortho-Est) ▶L ♀X ▶– $

ADULT — Moderate to severe menopausal vasomotor symptoms, vulvar and vaginal atrophy: 0.75 to 6 mg PO daily. Female hypogonadism, bilateral oophorectomy, or ovarian failure: 1.5 to 9 mg PO daily. Prevention of osteoporosis: 0.75 mg PO daily.

PEDS — Not approved in children.

FORMS — Generic/Trade: Tabs 0.75, 1.5, 3, 6 mg of estropipate.

NOTES — 6 mg estropipate is 5 mg sodium estrone sulfate.

MOA — Gonadal steroid.

ADVERSE EFFECTS — Serious: Endometrial cancer, DVT/PE, gallbladder disease, breast cancer, MI, CVA. Frequent: Nausea, breast tenderness.

TRIEST (estradiol + estriol + estrone) ▶L ♀X ▶– $$$

WARNING — For topical dosages: Patient should take precautions to ensure that children and pets do not make contact with skin where topical hormone has been applied.

UNAPPROVED ADULT — Hormone replacement therapy. Once or twice a day dosing.

FORMS — Must be compounded by a pharmacist. May be formulated as capsule, cream, gel, troche, or vaginal suppository.

NOTES — Compounded bioidentical hormones are not FDA approved. These products should be considered to have the same safety issues as those associated with hormone therapy agents that are FDA approved.

MOA — Gonadal steroid

ADVERSE EFFECTS — Serious: Endometrial cancer, DVT/PE, gallbladder disease, breast cancer, MI, CVA. Frequent: Nausea, breast tenderness.

OB/GYN: GnRH Agents

NOTE: Anaphylaxis has occurred with synthetic GnRH agents.

CETRORELIX ACETATE (Cetrotide) ▶Plasma ♀X ▶– $$$$$

ADULT — Infertility: Multiple-dose regimen: 0.25 mg SC daily during the early to mid follicular phase. Continue treatment daily until the day of hCG administration. Single-dose regimen: 3 mg SC once usually on stimulation day 7.

PEDS — Not approved in children.

FORMS — Trade only: Injection 0.25 mg and 3 mg vials.

NOTES — Best sites for SC self-injection are on the abdomen around the navel. Storage in original carton: 0.25 mg refrigerated (36° to 46°F); 3 mg room temperature (77°F). Contraindicated with severe renal impairment.

MOA — GnRH analog.

ADVERSE EFFECTS — Serious: Anaphylaxis, ovarian hyperstimulation syndrome. Frequent: Injection site reaction.

GANIRELIX (✱Orgalutran) ▶Plasma ♀X ▶? $$$$$

ADULT — Infertility: 250 mcg SC daily during the early to mid follicular phase. Continue treatment daily until the day of hCG administration.

PEDS — Not approved in children.

FORMS — Generic only: Injection 250 mcg/0.5 mL in prefilled, disposable syringe.

NOTES — Best sites for SC self-injection are on the abdomen around the navel or upper thigh. Store at room temperature (77°F) for up to 3 months. Protect from light. Packaging contains natural rubber latex, which may cause allergic reactions.

MOA — GnRH analog.

ADVERSE EFFECTS — Serious: Anaphylaxis, ovarian hyperstimulation syndrome. Frequent: Injection site reaction.

LUPANETA PACK (leuprolide + norethindrone) ▶L ♀X ▶– $$$$$

ADULT — Endometriosis: Leuprolide 3.75 mg IM injection q month. Norethindrone 5 mg PO daily.

FORMS — Trade only: 3.75 mg leuprolide acetate IM injection + norethindrone acetate 5 mg PO tabs #30 (1 month kit). 11.25 mg leuprolide acetate IM injection and norethindrone acetate 5 mg PO tabs #90 (3-month kit).

NOTES — Do not use longer than 6 months at a time for endometriosis and not more than a total of 12 months.

(cont.)

LUPANETA PACK (cont.)

MOA — Leuprolide: Gonadotropin inhibitor; repeated dosing results in decreased secretion of gonadal steroids. Norethindrone: Induces secretory changes in an estrogen-primed endometrium.

ADVERSE EFFECTS — Serious: Renal calculus, urinary tract infection, depression, bone loss. Frequent: Hot flashes, night sweats, headache, depression, pain, visual changes.

NAFARELIN (Synarel) ▶L ♀X ▶— $$$$$

ADULT — Endometriosis: 200 mcg spray into 1 nostril q am and the other nostril q pm. May be increased to one 200 mcg spray into each nostril two times per day. Duration of treatment: 6 months.

PEDS — Central precocious puberty: 2 sprays into each nostril two times per day for a total of 1600

mcg/day. May be increased to 1800 mcg/day. Allow 30 sec to elapse between sprays.

FORMS — Trade only: Nasal soln 2 mg/mL in 8 mL bottle (200 mcg per spray) approximately 80 sprays/bottle.

NOTES — Ovarian cysts have occurred in the 1st 2 months of therapy. Symptoms of hypoestrogenism may occur. Elevations of phosphorus and eosinophil counts, and decreases in serum calcium and WBC counts have been documented. Consider norethindrone as "add back" therapy to decrease bone loss (see norethindrone).

MOA — GnRH analog.

ADVERSE EFFECTS — Serious: Anaphylaxis. Frequent in Peds: Acne, breast enlargement, vaginal bleeding. Frequent in Adults: Hot flashes, nasal irritation.

OB/GYN: Hormone Combinations

NOTE: See also Estrogens. Unopposed estrogens increase the risk of endometrial cancer in postmenopausal women. Malignancy should be ruled out in cases of persistent or recurrent abnormal vaginal bleeding. Do not use during pregnancy. May increase the risk of DVT/PE, gallbladder disease. Interactions with oral anticoagulants, phenytoin, rifampin, barbiturates, corticosteroids, and St. John's wort. For preparations containing testosterone derivatives, observe women for signs of virilization and lipid abnormalities. In the Women's Health Initiative, the combination of conjugated estrogens and medroxyprogesterone (PremPro) caused an increase in the risk of breast cancer, MI, CVA, and DVT/PE and did not improve overall quality of life. Women older

ACTIVELLA (estradiol + norethindrone, Lopreeza) ▶L ♀X ▶— $$$

ADULT — Moderate to severe menopausal vasomotor symptoms, vulvar and vaginal atrophy, prevention of postmenopausal osteoporosis: 1 tab PO daily.

PEDS — Not approved in children.

FORMS — Trade only: Tabs 1/0.5 mg and 0.5/0.1 mg estradiol/norethindrone acetate in calendar dial pack dispenser.

MOA — Gonadal steroid combination.

ADVERSE EFFECTS — Serious: DVT/PE, gallbladder disease, breast cancer, MI, CVA. Frequent: Nausea, breast tenderness.

ANGELIQ (estradiol + drospirenone) ▶L ♀X ▶— $$$

ADULT — Moderate to severe menopausal vasomotor symptoms, vulvar and vaginal atrophy: 1 tab PO daily.

PEDS — Not approved in children.

FORMS — Trade only: Tabs 1 mg estradiol/0.5 mg drospirenone.

NOTES — May cause hyperkalemia in high-risk patients due to antimineralocorticoid activity of drospirenone. Monitor potassium in patients on ACE inhibitors, ARBs, potassium-sparing diuretics, heparin, aldosterone antagonists, and NSAIDs. Should not be used if renal insufficiency, hepatic dysfunction, or adrenal insufficiency.

MOA — Gonadal steroid combination.

ADVERSE EFFECTS — Serious: DVT/PE, gallbladder disease, breast cancer, MI, CVA. Frequent: Nausea, breast tenderness.

CLIMARA PRO (estradiol + levonorgestrel) ▶L ♀X ▶— $$$

ADULT — Moderate to severe menopausal vasomotor symptoms, prevention of postmenopausal osteoporosis: 1 patch weekly.

PEDS — Not approved in children.

FORMS — Trade only: Transdermal 0.045/0.015 estradiol/levonorgestrel in mg/day, 4 patches/box.

NOTES — Rotate application sites; avoid the waistline.

MOA — Gonadal steroid combination.

ADVERSE EFFECTS — Serious: DVT/PE, gallbladder disease, breast cancer, MI, CVA. Frequent: Nausea, breast tenderness.

COMBIPATCH (estradiol + norethindrone acetate, ✱ Estalis) ▶L ♀X ▶— $$$

ADULT — Moderate to severe menopausal vasomotor symptoms, vulvar and vaginal atrophy, female hypogonadism, bilateral oophorectomy, ovarian failure, and prevention of postmenopausal osteoporosis: 1 patch twice per week.

PEDS — Not approved in children.

FORMS — Trade only: Transdermal patch 0.05 estradiol/0.14 norethindrone and 0.05 estradiol/0.25 norethindrone in mg/day, 8 patches/box.

NOTES — Rotate application sites, avoid the waistline.

MOA — Gonadal steroid combination.

ADVERSE EFFECTS — Serious: Angioedema, DVT/PE, gallbladder disease, breast cancer, MI, CVA. Frequent: HA, back pain, nausea, breast pain, irregular bleeding.

DUAVEE (conjugated estrogens/bazedoxifene) ▶glucuronidation ♀X ▶–
ADULT — Moderate to severe vasomotor symptoms, prevention of postmenopausal osteoporosis: 1 tab daily.
PEDS — Not approved in pediatrics.
FORMS — Trade only: Conjugated estrogens 0.45 mg/bazedoxifene 20 mg tabs.
NOTES — Women using Duavee for prevention of osteoporosis should also use calcium and vitamin D if not getting enough through diet.
MOA — Synthetic estrogen with estrogen agonist/antagonist.
ADVERSE EFFECTS — Serious: Cardiovascular disorder, malignant neoplasms, gallbladder disease, increased triglycerides. Frequent: muscle spasms, nausea, diarrhea, dyspepsia, dizziness, neck pain.

FEMHRT (ethinyl estradiol + norethindrone, *Fyavolv*) ▶L ♀X ▶– $$$
WARNING — Multiple strengths; see FORMS and write specific product on Rx.
ADULT — Moderate to severe menopausal vasomotor symptoms, prevention of postmenopausal osteoporosis: 1 tab PO daily.
PEDS — Not approved in children.
FORMS — Trade only: Tabs 5/1, 2.5/0.5 mcg ethinyl estradiol/mg norethindrone, 28/blister card.
MOA — Gonadal steroid combination.
ADVERSE EFFECTS — Serious: DVT/PE, gallbladder disease, breast cancer, MI, CVA. Frequent: Nausea, breast tenderness.

PREFEST (estradiol + norgestimate) ▶L ♀X ▶– $$$
ADULT — Moderate to severe menopausal vasomotor symptoms, vulvar atrophy, atrophic vaginitis, prevention of postmenopausal osteoporosis: 1 pink tab PO daily for 3 days followed by 1 white tab PO daily for 3 days, sequentially throughout the month.
PEDS — Not approved in children.
FORMS — Generic only: Tabs in 30-day blister packs 1 mg estradiol (15 pink), 1 mg estradiol/0.09 mg norgestimate (15 white).

MOA — Gonadal steroid combination.
ADVERSE EFFECTS — Serious: DVT/PE, gallbladder disease, breast cancer, MI, CVA. Frequent: Nausea, breast tenderness.

PREMPHASE (estrogens conjugated + medroxyprogesterone) ▶L ♀X ▶– $$$
ADULT — Moderate to severe menopausal vasomotor symptoms, vulvar/vaginal atrophy, and prevention of postmenopausal osteoporosis: 0.625 mg conjugated estrogens PO daily on days 1 to 14 and 0.625 mg conjugated estrogens/5 mg medroxyprogesterone PO daily on days 15 to 28.
PEDS — Not approved in children.
FORMS — Trade only: Tabs in 28-day EZ-Dial dispensers: 0.625 mg conjugated estrogens (14), 0.625 mg/5 mg conjugated estrogens/medroxyprogesterone (14).
MOA — Gonadal steroid combination.
ADVERSE EFFECTS — Serious: DVT/PE, gallbladder disease, breast cancer, MI, CVA. Frequent: Nausea, breast tenderness.

PREMPRO (estrogens conjugated + medroxyprogesterone, ✲ *PremPlus*) ▶L ♀X ▶– $$$
WARNING — Multiple strengths; see FORMS and write specific product on Rx.
ADULT — Moderate to severe menopausal vasomotor symptoms, vulvar/vaginal atrophy, and prevention of postmenopausal osteoporosis: 1 PO daily.
PEDS — Not approved in children.
FORMS — Trade only: Tabs in 28-day EZ-Dial dispensers: 0.625 mg/5 mg, 0.625 mg/2.5 mg, 0.45 mg/1.5 mg (Prempro low dose), or 0.3 mg/1.5 mg conjugated estrogens/medroxyprogesterone.
MOA — Gonadal steroid combination.
ADVERSE EFFECTS — Serious: DVT/PE, gallbladder disease, breast cancer, MI, CVA. Frequent: Nausea, breast tenderness.

OB/GYN: Labor Induction/Cervical Ripening

NOTE: Fetal wellbeing should be documented prior to use.

DINOPROSTONE (*PGE2, Prepidil, Cervidil, Prostin E2*) ▶Lung ♀C ▶? $$$$$
ADULT — Cervical ripening: Gel: 1 syringe via catheter placed into cervical canal below the internal os. May be repeated q 6 h to a max of 3 doses. Vaginal insert: Place in posterior fornix. Evacuation of uterine contents after fetal death up to 28 weeks or termination of pregnancy 12th to 20th gestational week: 20 mg intravaginal suppository; repeat at 3 to 5 h intervals until abortion occurs. Do not use for more than 2 days.
PEDS — Not approved in children.
FORMS — Trade only: Gel (Prepidil) 0.5 mg/3 g syringe. Vaginal insert (Cervidil) 10 mg. Vaginal supps (Prostin E2) 20 mg.

NOTES — Patient should remain supine for 15 to 30 min after gel and 2 h after vaginal insert. For hospital use only. Monitor for uterine hyperstimulation and abnormal fetal heart rate. Caution with asthma or glaucoma. Contraindicated in prior C-section or major uterine surgery due to potential for uterine rupture.
MOA — Uterine stimulant.
ADVERSE EFFECTS — Serious: Uterine hyperstimulation, uterine rupture. Frequent: N/V, diarrhea. Rare: disseminated intravascular coagulation (DIC)

MISOPROSTOL—OB (*PGE1, Cytotec*) ▶LK ♀X ▶– $$
WARNING — Contraindicated in desired early or preterm pregnancy due to its abortifacient property. Pregnant women should avoid contact/exposure to

(cont.)

MISOPROSTOL—OB (cont.)

the tabs. Uterine rupture reported with use for labor induction and medical abortion.

UNAPPROVED ADULT — Cervical ripening and labor induction: 25 mcg intravaginally q 3 to 6 h (or 50 mcg q 6 h). First trimester pregnancy failure: 800 mcg intravaginally, repeat on day 3 if expulsion incomplete. Medical abortion less than 63 days' gestation: With mifepristone, see mifepristone; with methotrexate: 800 mcg intravaginally 5 to 7 days after 50 mg/m^2 PO or IM methotrexate. Preop cervical ripening: 400 mcg intravaginally 3 to 4 h before mechanical cervical dilation. Postpartum hemorrhage: 800 mcg PR for 1 dose. Oral dosing has been used but is controversial. Treatment of duodenal ulcers: 100 mcg PO four times per day.

FORMS — Generic/Trade: Oral tabs 100, 200 mcg.

NOTES — Contraindicated with prior C-section. Oral tabs can be inserted into the vagina for labor induction/cervical ripening. Monitor for uterine hyperstimulation and abnormal fetal heart rate. Risk factors for uterine rupture: Prior uterine surgery and 5 or more previous pregnancies.

MOA — Prostaglandin E1 analog, uterine stimulant.

ADVERSE EFFECTS — Serious: Uterine hyperstimulation, uterine rupture. Frequent: diarrhea, abdominal pain.

OXYTOCIN (Pitocin) ▶LK ♀? ▶– $

WARNING — Not approved for elective labor induction, although widely used.

ADULT — Induction/stimulation of labor: 10 units in 1000 mL NS, 1 to 2 milliunits/min IV as a continuous infusion (6 to 12 mL/h). Increase in increments of 1 to 2 milliunits/min q 30 min until a contraction pattern is established, up to a max of 20 milliunits/min. Postpartum bleeding: 10 units IM after delivery of the placenta. 10 to 40 units in 1000 mL NS IV infusion, infuse 20 to 40 milliunits/min.

PEDS — Not approved in children.

UNAPPROVED ADULT — Augmentation of labor: 0.5 to 2 milliunits/min IV as a continuous infusion, increase by 1 to 2 milliunits/min q 30 min until adequate pattern of labor to a max of 40 milliunits/min.

NOTES — Use a pump to accurately control the infusion while patient is under continuous observation. Continuous fetal monitoring is required. Concurrent sympathomimetics may result in postpartum HTN. Anaphylaxis and severe water intoxication have occurred. Caution in patients undergoing a trial of labor after C-section.

MOA — Uterine stimulant.

ADVERSE EFFECTS — Serious: Anaphylaxis, water intoxication. Frequent: N/V.

OB/GYN: Ovulation Stimulants

NOTE: Potentially serious adverse effects include DVT/PE, ovarian hyperstimulation syndrome, adnexal torsion, ovarian enlargement and cysts, and febrile reactions.

CHORIOGONADOTROPIN ALFA (Ovidrel) ▶L ♀X ▶? $$$

ADULT — Specialized dosing for ovulation induction as part of ART administered 1 day following the last dose of the follicle-stimulating agent.

PEDS — Not approved in children.

FORMS — Trade only: Prefilled syringe 250 mcg.

NOTES — Best site for SC self-injection is on the abdomen below the navel. Beware of multiple pregnancy and multiple adverse effects. Store in original package and protect from light. Use immediately after reconstitution.

MOA — Ovulation induction.

ADVERSE EFFECTS — Serious: Arterial thromboembolism, PE, ovarian hyperstimulation syndrome, adnexal torsion, ovarian enlargement & cysts, & febrile reactions. Frequent: Injection site reactions.

CHORIONIC GONADOTROPIN (hCG, Pregnyl) ▶L ♀X ▶? $$$

ADULT — Specialized IM dosing for ovulation induction as part of ART.

PEDS — Not approved in children.

FORMS — Generic/Trade: 10,000 USP Units per vial must be reconstituted with bacteriostatic water for injection.

NOTES — Beware of multiple pregnancy and multiple adverse effects. For IM use only.

MOA — Ovulation induction.

ADVERSE EFFECTS — Serious: Arterial thromboembolism, PE, ovarian hyperstimulation syndrome, ovarian cysts, & ascites. Frequent: Injection site reactions.

CLOMIPHENE CITRATE (Clomid, Serophene) ▶L ♀D ▶? $$$$$

ADULT — Specialized dosing for ovulation induction.

PEDS — Not approved in children.

FORMS — Generic/Trade: Tabs 50 mg, scored.

NOTES — Beware of multiple pregnancy and multiple adverse effects.

MOA — Estrogenic ovulation induction.

ADVERSE EFFECTS — Serious: Blurred vision, ovarian hyperstimulation syndrome, ovarian enlargement & cysts. Frequent: hot flashes, abdominal discomfort.

FOLLITROPIN ALFA (FSH, Gonal-f, Gonal-f RFF vial or redi-ject) ▶L ♀X ▶? $$$$$

ADULT — Specialized dosing for ovulation induction.

PEDS — Not approved in children.

FORMS — Trade only: Powder for injection, 75 international units FSH activity, multidose vial 450, 1050 international units FSH activity. Prefilled, multiple-dose pen, 300 international units, 450 international units, 900 international units FSH activity with single-use disposable needles.

NOTES — Best site for SC self-injection is on the abdomen below the navel. Beware of multiple-gestation pregnancy and multiple adverse effects.

(cont.)

FOLLITROPIN ALFA (*cont.*)

Store in original package and protect from light. Use immediately after reconstitution. Pen may be stored at room temperature for up to 1 month or expiration, whichever is 1st.

MOA — Ovulation induction.

ADVERSE EFFECTS — Serious: Arterial thromboembolism, DVT/PE, ovarian hyperstimulation syndrome, adnexal torsion, ovarian cysts, & febrile reactions. Frequent: Injection site reactions.

FOLLITROPIN BETA (*FSH, Follistim AQ, ✷Puregon*) ▶L ♀X ▶? $$$$$

ADULT — Specialized dosing for ovulation stimulation.

PEDS — Not approved in children.

FORMS — Trade only: AQ Cartridge, for use with the Follistim Pen, 150, 300, 600, 900 international units.

NOTES — Best site for SC self-injection is on the abdomen below the navel. Beware of multiple pregnancy and multiple adverse effects. Store in original package and protect from light. Use powder for injection immediately after reconstitution. Cartridge may be stored for up to 28 days. Store aqueous soln in refrigerator.

MOA — Ovulation induction.

ADVERSE EFFECTS — Serious: Arterial thromboembolism, DVT/PE, ovarian hyperstimulation syndrome, adnexal torsion, ovarian cysts, & febrile reactions. Frequent: Injection site reactions.

GONADOTROPINS (*menotropins, FSH and LH, Menopur, Pergonal, Repronex*) ▶L ♀X ▶– $$$$$

ADULT — Specialized dosing for infertility.

PEDS — Not approved in children.

FORMS — Trade only: Powder for injection, 75 units FSH and 75 units LH activity.

NOTES — Best site for SC self-injection is on the abdomen below the navel. Beware of multiple pregnancy and numerous adverse effects. Use immediately after reconstitution.

MOA — Follicular growth and maturation.

ADVERSE EFFECTS — Serious: Anaphylaxis, arterial thromboembolism, DVT/PE, ovarian hyperstimulation syndrome, adnexal torsion, ovarian cysts, & febrile reactions. Frequent: Injection site reactions.

UROFOLLITROPIN (*Bravelle, FSH, Fertinex*) ▶L ♀X ▶– $$$$$

ADULT — Specialized dosing for infertility and polycystic ovary syndrome.

PEDS — Not approved in children.

FORMS — Trade only: Powder for injection, 75 international units FSH activity.

NOTES — Best site for SC self-injection is on the abdomen below the navel. Beware of multiple pregnancy and numerous adverse effects. Use immediately after reconstitution.

MOA — Ovulation induction.

ADVERSE EFFECTS — Serious: Arterial thromboembolism, DVT/PE, ovarian hyperstimulation syndrome, adnexal torsion, ovarian cysts, & febrile reactions. Frequent: Injection site reactions.

OB/GYN: Progestins

NOTE: Do not use in pregnancy. DVT, PE, cerebrovascular disorders, and retinal thrombosis may occur. Effectiveness may be reduced by hepatic enzyme-inducing drugs such as certain anticonvulsants and barbiturates, rifampin, rifabutin, griseofulvin, and protease inhibitors. The effects of St. John's wort–containing products on progestin-only pills is currently unknown. In the Women's Health Initiative, the combination of conjugated estrogens and medroxyprogesterone (PremPro) caused a statistically significant increase in the risk of breast cancer, MI, CVA, and DVT/PE. Additionally, women older than 65 yo with 4 years of therapy had an increased risk of dementia. Estrogen/progestin combinations should be prescribed at the lowest effective doses and for the shortest durations. Patients should be counseled regarding the risks/benefits of hormone replacement.

MEDROXYPROGESTERONE (*Provera*) ▶L ♀X ▶– $

ADULT — Secondary amenorrhea: 5 to 10 mg PO daily for 5 to 10 days. Abnormal uterine bleeding: 5 to 10 mg PO daily for 5 to 10 days beginning on the 16th or 21st day of the cycle (after estrogen priming). Withdrawal bleeding usually occurs 3 to 7 days after therapy ends. Endometrial hyperplasia: 10 to 30 mg PO daily for 12 to 14 days per month.

PEDS — Not approved in children.

FORMS — Generic/Trade: Tabs 2.5, 5, 10 mg, scored.

NOTES — Breakthrough bleeding/spotting may occur. Amenorrhea usually after 6 months of continuous dosing.

MOA — Gonadal steroid.

ADVERSE EFFECTS — Serious: Thrombophlebitis, cerebrovascular disorders, retinal thrombosis, DVT/PE. Frequent: Breakthrough bleeding.

MEDROXYPROGESTERONE–INJECTABLE (*Depo-Provera, Depo-SubQ Provera 104*) ▶L ♀X ▶+ $

WARNING — Risk of significant bone loss (possibly reversible) increases with duration of use. Long-term use (greater than 2 years) only recommended if other methods of birth control are inadequate or symptoms of endometriosis return after discontinuation. It is unknown if use by younger women will reduce peak bone mass.

ADULT — Contraception/endometriosis: 150 mg IM in deltoid or gluteus maximus or 104 mg SC in anterior thigh or abdomen q 13 weeks. Also used for adjunctive therapy in endometrial and renal carcinoma.

PEDS — Not approved in children.

UNAPPROVED ADULT — Dysfunctional uterine bleeding: 150 mg IM in deltoid or gluteus maximus q 13 weeks.

(cont.)

MEDROXYPROGESTERONE–INJECTABLE (*cont.*)

NOTES — Breakthrough bleeding/spotting may occur. Amenorrhea usually after 6 months. Wt gain is common. To be sure that the patient is not pregnant, give this injection only during the 1st 5 days after the onset of a normal menstrual period or after a negative pregnancy test. May be given immediately post-pregnancy termination as well as postpartum, including breastfeeding women. May be given as often as 11 weeks apart. If the time between injections is greater than 14 weeks, exclude pregnancy before administering. Return to fertility can be variably delayed after last injection, with the median time to pregnancy being 10 months. Bone loss may occur with prolonged administration. Evaluate bone mineral density if considering retreatment for endometriosis.

MOA — Progestational agent that inhibits release of LH.

ADVERSE EFFECTS — Serious: Thromboembolic disorder, increased risk of cancer, jaundice, DVT/PE, bone loss. Frequent: Injection site reactions, breakthrough bleeding, weight gain, headache.

MEGESTROL (*Megace, Megace ES*) ▶L ♀D ▶? $$$$$

ADULT — AIDS anorexia, cachexia, or unexplained weight loss: 800 mg (20 mL) susp PO daily or 625 mg (5 mL) ES daily. Palliative treatment for advanced breast carcinoma: 40 mg (tabs) PO four times per day. Endometrial carcinoma: 40 to 320 mg/day (tabs) in divided doses.

PEDS — Not approved in children.

UNAPPROVED ADULT — Endometrial hyperplasia: 40 to 160 mg PO daily for 3 to 4 months. Cancer-associated or elderly anorexia/cachexia: 80 to 160 mg PO four times per day.

FORMS — Generic/Trade: Tabs 20, 40 mg. Susp 40 mg/mL in 240 mL. Trade only: Megace ES susp 125 mg/mL (150 mL).

NOTES — In HIV-infected women, breakthrough bleeding/spotting may occur.

MOA — Binds to progesterone and glucocorticoid receptors.

ADVERSE EFFECTS — Serious: Thrombophlebitis, cerebrovascular disorders, glucose intollerance, DVT/PE. Frequent: Breakthrough bleeding, weight gain, diarrhea, impotence.

NORETHINDRONE ACETATE (*Aygestin, ✶Norlutate*) ▶L ♀X ▶ $$

ADULT — Amenorrhea, abnormal uterine bleeding: 2.5 to 10 mg PO daily for 5 to 10 days during the 2nd half of the menstrual cycle. Endometriosis: 5 mg PO daily for 2 weeks. Increase by 2.5 mg q 2 weeks to 15 mg/day.

PEDS — Not approved in children.

UNAPPROVED ADULT — "Add back" therapy with GnRH agonists (eg, leuprolide) to decrease bone loss: 5 mg PO daily.

FORMS — Generic/Trade: Tabs 5 mg, scored.

NOTES — Contraceptive doses felt compatible with breastfeeding, but not higher doses.

MOA — Gonadal steroid.

ADVERSE EFFECTS — Serious: Thrombophlebitis, cerebrovascular disorders, retinal thrombosis, DVT/PE. Frequent: Nausea, breast tenderness, breakthrough bleeding.

PROGESTERONE GEL (*Crinone, Prochieve*) ▶Plasma ♀– ▶? $$$

ADULT — Secondary amenorrhea: 45 mg (4%) intravaginally every other day up to 6 doses. If no response, use 90 mg (8%) intravaginally every other day up to 6 doses. Specialized dosing for infertility.

PEDS — Not approved in children.

FORMS — Trade only: 4%, 8% single-use, prefilled applicators.

NOTES — An increase in dose from the 4% gel can only be accomplished using the 8% gel; doubling the volume of 4% does not increase absorption.

MOA — Gonadal steroid.

ADVERSE EFFECTS — Serious: Thrombophlebitis, cerebrovascular disorders, retinal thrombosis, DVT/PE. Frequent: Vaginal discharge.

PROGESTERONE IN OIL ▶L ♀X ▶? $$

WARNING — Contraindicated in peanut allergy since some products contain peanut oil.

ADULT — Amenorrhea, uterine bleeding: 5 to 10 mg IM daily for 6 to 8 days.

PEDS — Not approved in children.

NOTES — Discontinue with thrombotic disorders, sudden or partial loss of vision, proptosis, diplopia or migraine.

MOA — Gonadal steroid.

ADVERSE EFFECTS — Serious: Thrombophlebitis, cerebrovascular disorders, retinal thrombosis, DVT/PE. Frequent: Breakthrough bleeding.

PROGESTERONE MICRONIZED (*Prometrium*) ▶L ♀B ▶+ $$

WARNING — Contraindicated in patients allergic to peanuts because caps contain peanut oil.

ADULT — Hormone therapy to prevent endometrial hyperplasia: 200 mg PO at bedtime 10 to 12 days/month. Secondary amenorrhea: 400 mg PO at bedtime for 10 days.

PEDS — Not approved in children.

UNAPPROVED ADULT — Hormone therapy to prevent endometrial hyperplasia: 100 mg at bedtime daily.

FORMS — Generic/Trade: Caps 100, 200 mg.

NOTES — Breast tenderness, dizziness, headache, and abdominal cramping may occur.

MOA — Gonadal steroid.

ADVERSE EFFECTS — Serious: Thrombophlebitis, cerebrovascular disorders, retinal thrombosis, DVT/PE. Frequent: Breakthrough bleeding.

PROGESTERONE MICRONIZED COMPOUNDED (*Pro-Gest*) ▶L ♀B? ▶? $

WARNING — For topical dosages: Patient should take precautions to ensure that children and pets do not make contact with skin where topical hormone has been applied.

UNAPPROVED ADULT — Hormone replacement therapy. Once or twice a day dosing.

(cont.)

PROGESTERONE MICRONIZED COMPOUNDED (*cont.*)

FORMS — Must be compounded by a pharmacist. May be formulated as capsule, cream, gel, troche, or vaginal suppository.

NOTES — Compounded bioidentical hormones are not FDA approved. These products should be considered to have the same safety issues as those associated with hormone therapy agents that are FDA approved.

MOA — Gonadal steroid

ADVERSE EFFECTS — Serious: Thrombophlebitis, cerebrovascular disorders, retinal thrombosis, DVT/PE. Frequent: Breakthrough bleeding.

PROGESTERONE VAGINAL INSERT (*Endometrin*) ▶Plasma ♀– ▶? $$$$

ADULT — Specialized dosing for infertility.

PEDS — Not approved in children.

FORMS — Trade only: 100 mg vaginal insert.

NOTES — Do not use concomitantly with other vaginal products, such as antifungals, as this may alter absorption.

MOA — Gonadal steroid.

ADVERSE EFFECTS — Serious: Thrombophlebitis, cerebrovascular disorders, retinal thrombosis, DVT/PE. Frequent: Vaginal discharge.

OB/GYN: Selective Estrogen Receptor Modulators

OSPEMIFENE (*Osphena*) ▶L ♀X ▶– $$$$

ADULT — Dyspareunia: 1 tab PO daily with food.

PEDS — Not approved for children.

FORMS — Trade only: Tabs 60 mg.

NOTES — Contraindicated with estrogen-dependent neoplasia, DVT/ PE, abnormal genital bleeding, history of stroke or MI, and pregnancy.

MOA — Tissue selective estrogen agonist/antagonist.

ADVERSE EFFECTS — Severe: Endometrial cancer, stroke, and DVT. Frequent: Hot flush, vaginal discharge, muscle spasm, and sweating.

RALOXIFENE (*Evista*) ▶L ♀X ▶– $$$$

WARNING — Increases the risk of venous thromboembolism and CVA. Do not use during pregnancy.

ADULT — Postmenopausal osteoporosis prevention/treatment, breast cancer prevention: 60 mg PO daily.

PEDS — Not approved in children.

FORMS — Generic/Trade: Tabs 60 mg.

NOTES — Contraindicated with history of venous thromboembolism. Interactions with oral anticoagulants and cholestyramine. May increase risk of DVT/PE. Discontinue use 72 h prior to and during prolonged immobilization because of DVT risk. Does not decrease (and may increase) hot flashes. Leg cramps. Triglyceride levels may increase in women with prior estrogen-associated hypertriglyceridemia (greater than 500 mg/dL).

MOA — Selective Estrogen Receptor Modulator.

ADVERSE EFFECTS — Serious: DVT/PE, hypertriglyceridemia, stroke. Frequent: Hot flashes, leg cramps.

TAMOXIFEN (*Soltamox, Tamone, ✽Tamofen*) ▶L ♀D ▶– $$

WARNING — Uterine malignancies, CVA and pulmonary embolism, sometimes fatal. Visual disturbances, cataracts, hypercalcemia, increased LFTs, bone pain, fertility impairment, hot flashes, menstrual irregularities, endometrial hyperplasia and cancer, alopecia. Do not use during pregnancy.

ADULT — Breast cancer prevention in high-risk women: 20 mg PO daily for 5 years. Breast cancer: 10 to 20 mg PO two times per day for 5 years.

PEDS — Not approved in children.

UNAPPROVED ADULT — Mastalgia: 10 mg PO daily for 4 months. Anovulation: 5 to 40 mg PO two times per day for 4 days.

FORMS — Generic/Trade: Tabs 10, 20 mg. Trade only (Soltamox): Sugar-free soln 10 mg/5 mL (150 mL).

NOTES — Reliable contraception is recommended. Monitor CBCs, LFTs. Regular gynecologic and ophthalmologic examinations. Interacts with oral anticoagulants. Does not decrease hot flashes.

MOA — Selective Estrogen Receptor Modulator.

ADVERSE EFFECTS — Serious: DVT/PE, retinal thrombosis, hepatotoxicity, endometrial cancer,. Frequent: Hot flashes, leg cramps, vaginal discharge.

OB/GYN: Uterotonics

CARBOPROST (*Hemabate, 15-methyl-prostaglandin F2 alpha*) ▶LK ♀C ▶? $$$

ADULT — Refractory postpartum uterine bleeding: 250 mcg deep IM. If necessary, may repeat at 15 to 90 min intervals up to a total dose of 2 mg (8 doses).

PEDS — Not approved in children.

NOTES — Caution with asthma. Transient fever, HTN, nausea, bronchoconstriction, and flushing. May augment oxytocics.

MOA — Uterotonic.

ADVERSE EFFECTS — Serious: Pulmonary edema. Frequent: Fever, flushing, nausea, diarrhea.

METHYLERGONOVINE (*Methergine*) ▶LK ♀C ▶– $$

ADULT — To increase uterine contractions and decrease postpartum bleeding: 0.2 mg IM after

delivery of the placenta, delivery of the anterior shoulder, or during the puerperium. Repeat q 2 to 4 h prn. 0.2 mg PO three to four times per day in the puerperium for a max of 1 week.

PEDS — Not approved in children.

FORMS — Trade only: Tabs 0.2 mg.

NOTES — Contraindicated in pregnancy-induced HTN/preeclampsia. Avoid IV route due to risk of sudden HTN and CVA. If IV absolutely necessary, give slowly over no less than 1 min, monitor BP.

MOA — Uterotonic.

ADVERSE EFFECTS — Serious: CVA, seizure. Frequent: Hypertension, headache, nausea.

OB/GYN: Vaginitis Preparations

NOTE: See also STD/vaginitis table in Antimicrobials section. Many experts recommend 7 days of antifungal therapy for pregnant women with candida vaginitis. Many of these creams and supps are oil-based and may weaken latex condoms and diaphragms. Do not use latex products for 72 h after last dose.

BORIC ACID ▶Not absorbed ♀? ▶– $
PEDS — Not approved in children.
UNAPPROVED ADULT — Resistant vulvovaginal candidiasis: 600 mg suppository intravaginally at bedtime for 2 weeks.
FORMS — No commercial preparation; must be compounded by pharmacist. Vaginal supps 600 mg in gelatin caps.
NOTES — Reported use for azole-resistant non-albicans (C. glabrata) or recurrent albicans failing azole therapy. Do not use if abdominal pain, fever, or foul-smelling vaginal discharge is present. Avoid vaginal intercourse during treatment.
MOA — Antifungal.
ADVERSE EFFECTS — Serious: None. Frequent: Vulvovaginal irritation, erythema, & erosions.

BUTOCONAZOLE (*Gynazole, Mycelex-3*) ▶LK ♀C ▶? $(OTC), $$$(Rx)
ADULT — Local treatment of vulvovaginal candidiasis, nonpregnant patients: Mycelex 3: 1 applicatorful (~5 g) intravaginally at bedtime for 3 days, up to 6 days, if necessary. Pregnant patients: (2nd and 3rd trimesters only) 1 applicatorful (~5 g) intravaginally at bedtime for 6 days. Gynazole-1: 1 applicatorful (~5 g) intravaginally once daily.
PEDS — Not approved in children.
FORMS — OTC: Trade only (Mycelex 3): 2% vaginal cream in 5 g prefilled applicators (3s), 20 g tube with applicators. Rx: Trade only (Gynazole-1): 2% vaginal cream in 5 g prefilled applicator.
NOTES — Do not use if abdominal pain, fever, or foul-smelling vaginal discharge is present. Because small amount may be absorbed from the vagina, use during the 1st trimester only when essential. During pregnancy, use of a vaginal applicator may be contraindicated and manual insertion may be preferred. Vulvar/vaginal burning may occur. Avoid vaginal intercourse during treatment.
MOA — Antifungal.
ADVERSE EFFECTS — Serious: None. Frequent: Vulvovaginal irritation.

CLINDAMYCIN—VAGINAL (*Cleocin, Clindesse, ✳Dalacin*) ▶L ♀– ▶+ $$
ADULT — Bacterial vaginosis: Cleocin: 1 applicatorful (~100 mg clindamycin phosphate in 5 g cream) intravaginally at bedtime for 7 days, or 1 suppository at bedtime for 3 days. Clindesse: 1 applicatorful cream single dose.
PEDS — Not approved in children.
FORMS — Generic/Trade: 2% vaginal cream in 40 g tube with 7 disposable applicators (Cleocin). Vaginal supp (Cleocin Ovules) 100 mg (3) with applicator. 2% vaginal cream in a single-dose prefilled applicator (Clindesse).
NOTES — Clindesse may degrade latex/rubber condoms and diaphragms for 5 days after the last dose

(Cleocin for up to 3 days). Not recommended during pregnancy despite B rating, because it does not prevent the adverse effects of bacterial vaginosis (eg, preterm birth, neonatal infection). Cervicitis, vaginitis, and vulvar irritation may occur. Avoid vaginal intercourse during treatment.
MOA — Antibiotic.
ADVERSE EFFECTS — Serious: Pseudomembranous Colitis. Frequent: Cervicitis, vaginitis, & vulvar irritation.

CLOTRIMAZOLE—VAGINAL (*Mycelex 7, Gyne-Lotrimin, ✳Canesten, Clotrimaderm*) ▶LK ♀B ▶? $
ADULT — Local treatment of vulvovaginal candidiasis: 1 applicatorful 1% cream at bedtime for 7 days. 1 applicatorful 2% cream at bedtime for 3 days. 100 mg suppository intravaginally at bedtime for 7 days. 200 mg suppository at bedtime for 3 days. Topical cream for external symptoms two times per day for 7 days.
PEDS — Not approved in children.
FORMS — OTC Generic/Trade: 1% vaginal cream with applicator (some prefilled). 2% vaginal cream with applicator and 1% topical cream in some combination packs. OTC Trade only (Gyne-Lotrimin): Vaginal supp 100 mg (7), 200 mg (3) with applicators.
NOTES — Do not use if abdominal pain, fever, or foul-smelling vaginal discharge is present. Because small amounts of these drugs may be absorbed from the vagina, use during the 1st trimester only when essential. During pregnancy, use of a vaginal applicator may be contraindicated; manual insertion of tabs may be preferred. Skin rash, lower abdominal cramps, bloating, vulvar irritation may occur. Avoid vaginal intercourse during treatment.
MOA — Antifungal.
ADVERSE EFFECTS — Serious: None. Frequent: Vulvovaginal irritation.

METRONIDAZOLE—VAGINAL (*MetroGel-Vaginal, Nuvessa, Vandazole, ✳Nidagel*) ▶LK ♀B ▶? $$
ADULT — Bacterial vaginosis: 1 applicatorful (approximately 5 g containing approximately 37.5 mg metronidazole) intravaginally at bedtime or two times per day for 5 days (MetroGel, Vandazole). 1 applicatorfull (5 g containing 65 mg metronidazole) administered once intravaginally at bedtime.
PEDS — Not approved in children.
FORMS — Generic/Trade: 0.75% gel in 70 g tube with applicator (MetroGel, Vandazole). Trade only: 1.3% gel in single 5 g pre-filled applicator (Nuvessa).
NOTES — Cure rate same with at bedtime and twice daily dosing. Vaginally applied metronidazole could be absorbed in sufficient amounts to produce systemic effects. Caution in patients with CNS diseases due to rare reports of seizures, neuropathy, and numbness. Do not administer to patients who have taken disulfiram within the last 2 weeks. Interaction with ethanol.

(cont.)

METRONIDAZOLE—VAGINAL (cont.)

Caution with warfarin. Candida cervicitis and vaginitis, and vaginal, perineal, or vulvar itching may occur. Avoid vaginal intercourse during treatment.

MOA — Antibiotic.

ADVERSE EFFECTS — Serious: Seizures. Frequent: Cervicitis, vaginitis, & vulvar irritation.

MICONAZOLE (Monistat, Femizol-M, M-Zole, Micozole, Monazole) ▶LK ♀+ ▶? $

ADULT — Local treatment of vulvovaginal candidiasis: 1 applicatorful 2% cream intravaginally at bedtime for 7 days or 4% cream at bedtime for 3 days. 100 mg suppository intravaginally at bedtime for 7 days, 400 mg at bedtime for 3 days, or 1200 mg for 1 dose. Topical cream for external symptoms two times per day for 7 days.

PEDS — Not approved in children.

FORMS — OTC Generic/Trade: 2% vaginal cream in 45 g with 1 applicator or 7 disposable applicators. Vaginal supp 100 mg (7). OTC Trade only: 400 mg (3), 1200 mg (1) with applicator. Generic/Trade: 4% vaginal cream in 25 g tubes or 3 prefilled applicators. Some in combination packs with 2% miconazole cream for external use.

NOTES — Do not use if abdominal pain, fever, or foul-smelling vaginal discharge is present. Because small amounts of these drugs may be absorbed from the vagina, use during the 1st trimester only when essential. During pregnancy, use of a vaginal applicator may be contraindicated; manual insertion of suppositories may be preferred. Vulvovaginal burning, itching, irritation, and pelvic cramps may occur. Avoid vaginal intercourse during treatment. May increase warfarin effect.

MOA — Antifungal.

ADVERSE EFFECTS — Serious: None. Frequent: Vulvovaginal irritation.

TERCONAZOLE (Terazol) ▶LK ♀C ▶– $$

ADULT — Local treatment of vulvovaginal candidiasis: 1 applicatorful 0.4% cream intravaginally at bedtime for 7 days. 1 applicatorful 0.8% cream intravaginally at bedtime for 3 days. 80 mg suppository intravaginally at bedtime for 3 days.

PEDS — Not approved in children.

FORMS — All forms supplied with applicators: Generic/Trade: Vaginal cream 0.4% (Terazol 7) in 45 g tube, 0.8% (Terazol 3) in 20 g tube. Vaginal supp (Terazol 3) 80 mg (#3).

NOTES — Do not use if abdominal pain, fever, or foul-smelling vaginal discharge is present. Because small amounts of these drugs may be absorbed from the vagina, use during the 1st trimester only when essential. During pregnancy, use of a vaginal applicator may be contraindicated; manual insertion of supps may be preferred. Avoid vaginal intercourse during treatment. Vulvovaginal irritation, burning, and pruritus may occur.

MOA — Antifungal.

ADVERSE EFFECTS — Serious: Anaphylaxis and toxic epidermal necrolysis. Frequent: Vulvovaginal irritation.

TIOCONAZOLE (Monistat 1-Day, Vagistat-1) ▶Not absorbed ♀C ▶– $

ADULT — Local treatment of vulvovaginal candidiasis: 1 applicatorful (~ 4.6 g) intravaginally at bedtime for 1 dose.

PEDS — Not approved in children.

FORMS — OTC Trade only: Vaginal ointment: 6.5% (300 mg) in 4.6 g prefilled single-dose applicator.

NOTES — Do not use if abdominal pain, fever, or foul-smelling vaginal discharge is present. Because small amounts of these drugs may be absorbed from the vagina, use during the first trimester only when essential. During pregnancy, use of a vaginal applicator may be contraindicated. Avoid vaginal intercourse during treatment. Vulvovaginal burning and itching may occur.

MOA — Antifungal.

ADVERSE EFFECTS — Serious: None. Frequent: Vulvovaginal irritation.

OB/GYN: Other OB/GYN Agents

DANAZOL (✿Cyclomen) ▶L ♀X ▶– $$$$$

ADULT — Endometriosis: Start 400 mg PO two times per day, then titrate downward to a dose sufficient to maintain amenorrhea for 3 to 6 months, up to 9 months. Fibrocystic breast disease: 100 to 200 mg PO two times per day for 4 to 6 months.

PEDS — Not approved in children.

UNAPPROVED ADULT — Menorrhagia: 100 to 400 mg PO daily for 3 months. Cyclical mastalgia: 100 to 200 mg PO two times per day for 4 to 6 months.

FORMS — Generic only: Caps 50, 100, 200 mg.

NOTES — Contraindications: Impaired hepatic, renal, or cardiac function. Androgenic effects may not be reversible even after the drug is discontinued. May alter voice. Hepatic dysfunction has occurred. Insulin requirements may increase in diabetics. Prolongation of PT/INR has been reported with concomitant warfarin.

MOA — Androgen.

ADVERSE EFFECTS — Serious: Stroke, intracranial hypertension, hepatic adenoma. Frequent: Acne, edema, hirsutism, deepening voice, emotional lability, depression.

HYDROXYPROGESTERONE CAPROATE (Makena) ▶L + glucuronidation ♀B ▶? $$$$$

WARNING — For singleton pregnancy in women who have history of spontaneous preterm birth. Not intended in multiple gestations or other risk factors for preterm birth.

ADULT — To reduce risk of preterm birth: 250 mg IM once weekly. Begin between gestational age 16 weeks, 0 days and 20 weeks, 6 days. Continue through birth or week 37, whichever occurs 1st.

PEDS — Not approved in children

FORMS — Trade only: 5 mL MDV (250 mg/mL) hydroxyprogesterone caproate in castor oil soln.

(cont.)

HYDROXYPROGESTERONE CAPROATE (cont.)

NOTES — Unique ruling from FDA that compounding pharmacists can continue to make customized hydroxyprogesterone caproate injection.

MOA — unknown

ADVERSE EFFECTS — Serious: Early membrane rupture, cervical incompetence, miscarriage or stillbirth. Common: Injection site pain and swelling, urticaria.

MIFEPRISTONE (Mifeprex) ▶L ♀X ▶? $$$$$

WARNING — Rare cases of sepsis and death have occurred. Surgical intervention may be necessary with incomplete abortions. Patients need to be given info on where such services are available and what do in case of an emergency.

ADULT — Termination of pregnancy, up to 70 days: Day 1: 200 mg PO. Day 2 or 3: 800 mcg misoprostol (unless abortion confirmed). Day 14: Confirmation of pregnancy termination.

PEDS — Not approved in children.

FORMS — Trade only: Tabs 200 mg.

NOTES — Bleeding/spotting and cramping most common side effects. Prolonged heavy bleeding may be a sign of incomplete abortion. Contraindications: Ectopic pregnancy, IUD use, adrenal insufficiency and long-term steroid use, use of anticoagulants, hemorrhagic disorders, and porphyrias. CYP3A4 inducers may increase metabolism and lower levels. Only available through doctor's office.

MOA — Anti-progestational/abortifacient.

ADVERSE EFFECTS — Serious: Sepsis, incomplete abortion. Frequent: Bleeding, spotting, cramping, N/V.

PAROXETINE (Brisdelle) ▶LK ♀X ▶?

ADULT — Moderate to severe vasomotor symptoms associated with menopause: 7.5 mg at bedtime.

PEDS — Not indicated.

FORMS — Trade only: Caps 7.5 mg

NOTES — Paroxetine is a strong inhibitor of CYP2D6 and is contraindicated with thioridazine, pimozide, MAOIs, linezolid, and tryptophan; use caution with barbiturates, cimetidine, phenytoin, tamoxifen, theophylline, TCAs, risperidone, atomoxetine, and warfarin.

MOA — Selective serotonin reuptake inhibitor.

ADVERSE EFFECTS — Serious: Suicidality, serotonin syndrome, abnormal bleeding, narrow angle glaucoma, bone fracture risk. Frequent: headache, fatigue/malaise/lethargy, and nausea/vomiting.

PREMESIS-RX (pyridoxine + folic acid + cyanocobalamin + calcium carbonate) ▶L ♀A ▶+ $$

ADULT — Treatment of pregnancy-induced nausea: 1 tab PO daily.

PEDS — Unapproved in children.

FORMS — Trade only: Tabs 75 mg vitamin B6 (pyridoxine), sustained-release, 12 mcg vitamin B12 (cyanocobalamin), 1 mg folic acid, and 200 mg calcium carbonate.

NOTES — May be taken in conjunction with prenatal vitamins.

MOA — Vitamin combination.

ADVERSE EFFECTS — Serious: None. Frequent: None.

RHO IMMUNE GLOBULIN (HyperRHO S/D, MICRhoGAM, RhoGAM, Rhophylac, WinRho SDF) ▶L ♀C ▶? $$$$$

ADULT — Prevention of hemolytic disease of the newborn if mother Rh– and baby is or might be Rh+: 300 mcg vial IM to mother at 28 weeks' gestation followed by a 2nd dose within 72 h of delivery. Doses more than 1 vial may be needed if large fetal-maternal hemorrhage occurs during delivery (see complete prescribing information to determine dose). Following amniocentesis, miscarriage, abortion, or ectopic pregnancy at least 13 weeks' gestation: 1 vial (300 mcg) IM. Less than 12 weeks' gestation: 1 vial (50 mcg) microdose IM. Immune thrombocytopenic purpura (ITP), nonsplenectomized (WinRho): 250 units/kg/dose (50 mcg/kg/dose) IV for 1 dose if hemoglobin greater than 10 g/dL or 125 to 200 units/kg/dose (25 to 40 mcg/kg/dose) IV for 1 dose if hemoglobin less than 10 g/dL. Additional doses of 125 to 300 units/kg/dose (25 to 60 mcg/kg/dose) IV may be given as determined by patient's response.

PEDS — Immune thrombocytopenic purpura (ITP), nonsplenectomized (WinRho): 250 units/kg/dose (50 mcg/kg/dose) IV for 1 dose if hemoglobin greater than 10 g/dL or 125 to 200 units/kg/dose (25 to 40 mcg/kg/dose) IV for 1 dose if hemoglobin less than 10 g/dL. Additional doses of 125 to 300 units/kg/dose (25 to 60 mcg/kg/dose) IV may be given as determined by patient's response.

UNAPPROVED ADULT — Rh-incompatible transfusion: Specialized dosing.

NOTES — One 300 mcg vial prevents maternal sensitization to the Rh factor if the fetomaternal hemorrhage is less than 15 mL fetal RBCs (30 mL of whole blood). When the fetomaternal hemorrhage exceeds this (as estimated by Kleihauer-Betke testing), administer more than one 300 mcg vial.

MOA — Immune globulin.

ADVERSE EFFECTS — Serious: None. Frequent: Injection site reactions.

ULIPRISTAL ACETATE (✱Fibristal) ▶L ♀X ▶–

ADULT — Canadian indication treatment of moderate-to-severe signs/symptoms of uterine fibroids: 5 mg PO daily for 3 months.

FORMS — Canadian Trade only: Tabs 5 mg.

NOTES — Canadian drug only. Ella Brand product in the US is for a different indication at a different dose.

MOA — Selective progesterone receptor modulator.

ADVERSE EFFECTS — Hot flashes, irregular vaginal bleeding, endometrial thickening, headache.

ONCOLOGY

ONCOLOGY: Alkylating Agents

BENDAMUSTINE (*Treanda*, *Bendeka*, *✦Treanda*)
▶Plasma ♀D ▶– $ varies by therapy
WARNING — Anaphylaxis, bone marrow suppression, nephrotoxicity, Stevens-Johnson syndrome, toxic epidermal necrolysis. Instruct patients to report promptly fever, sore throat, signs of local infection, bleeding from any site, or symptoms suggestive of anemia. Take precautions to avoid extravasation, including monitoring intravenous infusion site during and after administration.
ADULT — Chemotherapy doses vary by indication. CLL, non-Hodgkin's lymphoma.
PEDS — Not approved in children. The effectiveness of bendamustine in pediatric patients has not been established. Bendamustine was evaluated in a single Phase 1/2 trial in pediatric patients with leukemia. The safety profile for bendamustine in pediatric patients was consistent with that seen in adults, and no new safety signals were identified.
UNAPPROVED ADULT — Hodgkin lymphoma, mantle cell lymphoma, multiple myeloma.
FORMS — Treanda: 45 mg/0.5 mL, 180 mg/2 mL IV solution for injection. 25 mg, 100 mg lyophilized powder for IV injection. Bendeka: 100 mg/4 mL IV solution for injection.
NOTES — Reliable contraception is recommended. Monitor CBCs and renal function. Bendamustine liquid formulation is incompatible with closed system transfer devices that contain polycarbonate or acrylonitrile-butadiene-styrene (ABS). The FDA is providing a list of compatible devices and administration sets as of September 2015.
MOA — Alkylating agent.
ADVERSE EFFECTS — Serious: Anaphylaxis, bone marrow suppression, nephrotoxicity, Stevens-Johnson syndrome, toxic epidermal necrolysis. Frequent: Bone marrow suppression, N/V.

BUSULFAN (*Myleran*, *Busulfex*) ▶LK ♀D ▶– $ varies by therapy
WARNING — Secondary malignancies, bone marrow suppression, adrenal insufficiency, hyperuricemia, pulmonary fibrosis, seizures (must initiate prophylactic anticonvulsant therapy prior to use of busulfan), cellular dysplasia, hepatic veno-occlusive disease, fertility impairment, alopecia, tooth hypoplasia. Instruct patients to report promptly fever, sore throat, signs of local infection, bleeding from any site, symptoms suggestive of anemia, or yellow discoloration of the skin or eyes.
ADULT — Chemotherapy doses vary by indication. Tabs: CML. Injection: Conditioning regimen prior to allogeneic hematopoietic progenitor cell transplantation for CML in combination with cyclophosphamide.
PEDS — Chemotherapy doses vary by indication. Tabs: CML. Safety of the injection has not been established.

UNAPPROVED ADULT — High dose in conjunction with stem cell transplant for leukemia and lymphoma. Essential thrombocythemia. Polycythemia vera, refractory.
FORMS — Trade only (Myleran): Tabs 2 mg. Busulfex injection for hospital/oncology clinic use; not intended for outpatient prescribing.
NOTES — Reliable contraception is recommended. Monitor CBCs and LFTs. Hydration and allopurinol to decrease adverse effects of uric acid. Acetaminophen and itraconazole decrease busulfan clearance. Phenytoin increases clearance.
MOA — Alkylating agent.
ADVERSE EFFECTS — Serious: Bone marrow suppression, adrenal insufficiency, seizures, pulmonary fibrosis, hepatic veno-occlusive disease, febrile neutropenia, severe bacterial, viral [e.g., cytomegaloviraemia] and fungal infections, and sepsis), tumor lysis syndrome, thrombotic micro angiopathy (TMA), hyperpigmentation.

CARMUSTINE (*BCNU*, *BiCNU*, *Gliadel*) ▶Plasma ♀D ▶– $ varies by therapy
WARNING — Secondary malignancies, bone marrow suppression, pulmonary fibrosis, nephrotoxicity, hepatotoxicity, ocular nerve fiber-layer infarcts and retinal hemorrhages, fertility impairment, alopecia. Local soft tissue toxicity/extravasation can occur if carmustine is infused too quickly. Infusions should run over at least 2 h. Wafer: Seizures, brain edema and herniation, intracranial infection. Instruct patients to report promptly fever, sore throat, signs of local infection, bleeding from any site, symptoms suggestive of anemia, or yellow discoloration of the skin or eyes.
ADULT — Chemotherapy doses vary by indication. Injection: Glioblastoma, brainstem glioma, medulloblastoma, astrocytoma, ependymoma and metastatic brain tumors, multiple myeloma with prednisone; Hodgkin's disease and non-Hodgkin's lymphomas, in combination regimens. Wafer: Glioblastoma multiforme, adjunct to surgery. High-grade malignant glioma, adjunct to surgery and radiation.
PEDS — Not approved in children.
UNAPPROVED ADULT — Mycosis fungoides, topical soln.
NOTES — Reliable contraception is recommended. Monitor CBCs, PFTs, LFTs, and renal function. May decrease phenytoin and digoxin levels. Cimetidine may increase myelosuppression. Significant absorption to PVC containers will occur. Carmustine must be dispensed in glass or non-PVC containers.
MOA — Alkylating agent.
ADVERSE EFFECTS — Serious: Bone marrow suppression, pulmonary fibrosis, nephrotoxicity, hepatotoxicity, ocular nerve fiber-layer infarcts and retinal hemorrhages. Wafer: Seizures, brain edema and herniation, intracranial infection. Frequent: Bone marrow suppression, N/V.

CHLORAMBUCIL (*Leukeran*) ▶L ♀D ▶— $ varies by therapy
WARNING — Secondary malignancies, bone marrow suppression, seizures, fertility impairment, alopecia. Instruct patients to report promptly fever, sore throat, signs of local infection, bleeding from any site, or symptoms suggestive of anemia.
ADULT — Chemotherapy doses vary by indication. CLL, lymphomas, including indolent lymphoma and Hodgkin's disease.
PEDS — Not approved in children.
UNAPPROVED ADULT — Uveitis and meningoencephalitis associated with Behcet's disease. Idiopathic membranous nephropathy. Ovarian carcinoma.
FORMS — Trade only: Tabs 2 mg.
NOTES — Reliable contraception is recommended. Monitor CBCs. Avoid live vaccines.
MOA — Alkylating agent.
ADVERSE EFFECTS — The most common side effect is bone marrow suppression, anemia, leukopenia, neutropenia, thrombocytopenia, or pancytopenia. Seizures.

CYCLOPHOSPHAMIDE (✱*Procytox*) ▶L ♀D ▶— $ varies by therapy
WARNING — Secondary malignancies, leukopenia, cardiac toxicity, acute hemorrhagic cystitis, hypersensitivity, fertility impairment, alopecia. Instruct patients to report promptly fever, sore throat, signs of local infection, bleeding from any site, symptoms suggestive of anemia, or yellow discoloration of the skin or eyes.
ADULT — Chemotherapy doses vary by indication. Non-Hodgkin's lymphomas, Hodgkin's disease, multiple myeloma, disseminated neuroblastoma, adenocarcinoma of the ovary, retinoblastoma, carcinoma of the breast, CLL, CML, AML, ALL, mycosis fungoides.
PEDS — Chemotherapy doses vary by indication. ALL. "Minimal change" nephrotic syndrome.
UNAPPROVED ADULT — Wegener's granulomatosis, other steroid-resistant vasculitides, severe progressive RA, systemic lupus erythematosus, multiple sclerosis, polyarteritis nodosa. Testicular, and bladder cancer, sarcoma. High risk gestational trophoblastic tumors, Hematopoietic stem cell transplant conditioning, Idiopathic thrombocytopenic purpura, refractory (adults);Pericarditis (recurrent); Small cell lung cancer (SCLC), refractory; Uveitis (adults); Juvenile idiopathic arthritis (refractory); Ovarian germ cell tumors; Pheochromocytoma; Waldenstrom's macroglobulinemia; Wilms tumor; Rheumatoid disorders (severe); Myasthenia gravis; Autoimmune hemolytic anemia; Antibody-induced pure red cell aplasia.
FORMS — Generic only: Tabs 25, 50 mg, capsules 25 mg, 50 mg. Injection for reconstitution, 500 mg, 1 g, 2 g vials for IV use.
NOTES — Reliable contraception is recommended. Monitor CBCs, urine for red cells. Allopurinol may increase myelosuppression. Thiazides may prolong leukopenia. May reduce digoxin levels, reduce fluoroquinolone activity. May increase anticoagulant effects. Coadministration with mesna reduces hemorrhagic cystitis when used in high doses.
MOA — Alkylating agent.
ADVERSE EFFECTS — Serious: Leukopenia, cardiac toxicity, acute hemorrhagic cystitis, hypersensitivity. Frequent: Alopecia, leukopenia.

DACARBAZINE (*DTIC-Dome*) ▶LK ♀C ▶— $ varies by therapy
WARNING — Extravasation associated with severe necrosis. Secondary malignancies, bone marrow suppression, hepatotoxicity, anorexia, N/V, anaphylaxis, alopecia. Instruct patients to report promptly fever, sore throat, signs of local infection, bleeding from any site, symptoms suggestive of anemia, or yellow discoloration of the skin or eyes.
ADULT — Chemotherapy doses vary by indication. Metastatic melanoma. Hodgkin's disease, in combination regimens.
PEDS — Not approved in children.
UNAPPROVED ADULT — Malignant pheochromocytoma, in combination regimens, sarcoma.
NOTES — Monitor CBCs and LFTs.
MOA — Alkylating agent.
ADVERSE EFFECTS — Serious: Bone marrow suppression, hepatotoxicity, anaphylaxis. Frequent: Bone marrow suppression, N/V, anorexia.

IFOSFAMIDE (*Ifex*) ▶L ♀D ▶— $ varies by therapy
WARNING — Secondary malignancies, hemorrhagic cystitis, confusion, coma, bone marrow suppression, hematuria, nephrotoxicity, alopecia. Instruct patients to report promptly fever, sore throat, signs of local infection, bleeding from any site, symptoms suggestive of anemia, or yellow discoloration of the skin or eyes.
ADULT — Chemotherapy doses vary by indication. Germ cell testicular cancer, in combination regimens.
PEDS — Not approved in children.
UNAPPROVED ADULT — Bladder cancer, cervical cancer, ovarian cancer, non-small-cell and small-cell lung cancers, Hodgkin's and non-Hodgkin's lymphomas, ALL, osteosarcoma, and soft tissue sarcomas.
UNAPPROVED PEDS — Ewing's sarcoma, osteosarcoma, soft tissue sarcomas, neuroblastoma.
FORMS — Powder for reconstitution: 1-, 3-g vials. Soln for injection: 50 mg/mL; 20-, 60-mL vials.
NOTES — Reliable contraception is recommended. Monitor CBCs, renal function, and urine for red cells. Coadministration with mesna reduces hemorrhagic cystitis. Requires extensive hydration to minimize bladder toxicity.
MOA — Alkylating agent.
ADVERSE EFFECTS — Serious: Hemorrhagic cystitis, coma, bone marrow suppression, hematuria, nephrotoxicity. Frequent: Bone marrow suppression, CNS, N/V, hematuria, alopecia.

LOMUSTINE (*CCNU, Gleostine*) ▶L ♀D ▶– $ varies by therapy

WARNING — Severe (including fatal) myelosuppression. Serious and fatal adverse events due to overdosage have occurred. Secondary malignancies, hepatotoxicity, nephrotoxicity, pulmonary fibrosis, fertility impairment, alopecia. Instruct patients to report promptly fever, sore throat, signs of local infection, bleeding from any site, symptoms suggestive of anemia, or yellow discoloration of the skin or eyes.

ADULT — Chemotherapy doses vary by indication. Brain tumors. Hodgkin's disease, in combination regimens.

PEDS — Chemotherapy doses vary by indication. Brain tumors. Hodgkin's disease, in combination regimens.

FORMS — Caps 5, 10, 40, 100 mg.

NOTES — Reliable contraception is recommended. Monitor CBCs, LFTs, PFTs, and renal function. Avoid alcohol. Dispense only enough capsules for a single dose. Do not dispense more than one dose at a time. Advise patients that only one dose is taken every six weeks.

MOA — Alkylating agent.

ADVERSE EFFECTS — Serious: Bone marrow suppression, hepatotoxicity, nephrotoxicity, pulmonary fibrosis. Frequent: Bone marrow suppression, N/V.

MECHLORETHAMINE (*Mustargen*) ▶Plasma ♀D ▶– $ varies by therapy

WARNING — Extravasation associated with severe necrosis. Secondary malignancies, bone marrow suppression, amyloidosis, herpes zoster, anaphylaxis, fertility impairment, alopecia. Instruct patients to report promptly fever, sore throat, signs of local infection, bleeding from any site, or symptoms suggestive of anemia.

ADULT — Chemotherapy doses vary by indication. Intravenous: Hodgkin's disease (Stages III and IV), lymphosarcoma, chronic myelocytic or chronic lymphocytic leukemia, polycythemia vera, mycosis fungoides, bronchogenic carcinoma. Intrapleurally, intraperitoneally, or intrapericardially: Metastatic carcinoma resulting in effusion.

PEDS — Not approved in children.

UNAPPROVED ADULT — Cutaneous mycosis fungoides: Topical soln or ointment.

UNAPPROVED PEDS — Hodgkin's disease (Stages III and IV), in combination regimens.

NOTES — Reliable contraception is recommended. Monitor CBCs.

MOA — Alkylating agent.

ADVERSE EFFECTS — Serious: Bone marrow suppression, amyloidosis, herpes zoster, anaphylaxis. Frequent: Bone marrow suppression, N/V.

MECHLORETHAMINE—TOPICAL (*Valchlor*) ▶NA No detectable topical absorption or distribution. ♀D ▶– $$$$$

WARNING — Dermatitis commonly occurs. Secondary malignancies (non-melanoma skin cancers) may occur.

ADULT — Topical treatment of stage 1A and 1B cutaneous T-cell lymphoma in patients who have received prior skin-directed therapy.

FORMS — Trade only: 0.016% topical gel.

MOA — Forms inter- and intra-strand DNA cross links, resulting in inhibition of DNA synthesis.

ADVERSE EFFECTS — Dermatitis, pruritis, skin infections, pancytopenias.

MELPHALAN (*Evomela, Alkeran*) ▶L Plasma ♀D ▶– $ varies by therapy

WARNING — Severe bone marrow suppression with resulting infection or bleeding may occur. Controlled trials comparing intravenous (IV) melphalan to oral melphalan have shown more myelosuppression with the IV formulation. Monitor hematologic laboratory parameters. Hypersensitivity reactions, including anaphylaxis, have occurred in approximately 2% of patients who received the IV formulation of melphalan. Discontinue treatment with Evomela for serious hypersensitivity reactions. Melphalan produces chromosomal aberrations in vitro and in vivo. Evomela should be considered potentially leukemogenic in humans. Fertility impairment, alopecia. Instruct patients to report promptly fever, sore throat, signs of local infection, bleeding from any site, or symptoms suggestive of anemia.

ADULT — Chemotherapy doses vary by indication. Alkeran: Multiple myeloma and nonresectable epithelial ovarian carcinoma. Evomela: use as a high-dose conditioning treatment prior to hematopoietic progenitor (stem) cell transplantation in patients with multiple myeloma. The palliative treatment of patients with multiple myeloma for whom oral therapy is not appropriate.

PEDS — Not approved in children.

UNAPPROVED ADULT — Non-Hodgkin's lymphoma in high doses for stem cell transplant, testicular cancer, amyloidosis, light chain; Hodgkin lymphoma, relapsed/refractory; Autologous hematopoietic stem cell transplantation in adults with hematologic disorders (eg, multiple myeloma) (conditioning regimen).

UNAPPROVED PEDS — Autologous marrow or stem cell transplantation in pediatric neuroblastoma and Ewing sarcoma (conditioning regimen)

FORMS — Alkeran: Tabs 2 mg. Alkeran/generic melphalan: 50 mg solution for IV. (Contains alcohol, propylene glycol.) Evomela: 50 mg per vial, lyophilized powder in a single-dose vial for reconstitution.

NOTES — Reliable contraception is recommended. Monitor CBCs. Avoid live vaccines.

MOA — Alkylating agent.

ADVERSE EFFECTS — Serious: Bone marrow suppression, anaphylaxis. Frequent: Bone marrow suppression, N/V.

PROCARBAZINE (*Matulane*) ▶LK ♀D ▶– $ varies by therapy

WARNING — Secondary malignancies, bone marrow suppression, hemolysis and Heinz-Ehrlich inclusion bodies in erythrocytes, hypersensitivity, fertility impairment, alopecia. Peds: Tremors, convulsions,

(cont.)

PROCARBAZINE *(cont.)*

and coma have occurred. Instruct patients to report promptly fever, sore throat, signs of local infection, bleeding from any site, symptoms suggestive of anemia, black tarry stools, or vomiting of blood.
ADULT — Chemotherapy doses vary by indication. Hodgkin's disease (Stages III and IV), in combination regimens.
PEDS — Chemotherapy doses vary by indication. Hodgkin's disease (Stages III and IV), in combination regimens.
FORMS — Trade only: Caps 50 mg.
NOTES — Reliable contraception is recommended. Monitor CBCs. Renal/hepatic function impairment may predispose toxicity. UA, LFTs, and BUN weekly. May decrease digoxin levels. May increase effects of opioids, sympathomimetics, TCAs. Ingestion of foods with high tyramine content may result in a potentially fatal hypertensive crisis. Alcohol may cause a disulfiram-like reaction.
MOA — Alkylating agent.
ADVERSE EFFECTS — Serious: Bone marrow suppression, hemolysis and Heinz-Ehrlich inclusion bodies in erythrocytes, hypersensitivity. Frequent: Bone marrow suppression, N/V.

STREPTOZOCIN *(Zanosar)* ▶Plasma ♀C ▶– $ varies by therapy
WARNING — Extravasation associated with severe necrosis. Secondary malignancies, nephrotoxicity, N/V, hepatotoxicity, decrease in hematocrit, hypoglycemia, fertility impairment, alopecia.
ADULT — Chemotherapy doses vary by indication. Metastatic islet cell carcinoma of the pancreas.
PEDS — Not approved in children.
NOTES — Hydration important. Monitor renal function, CBCs, and LFTs.
MOA — Alkylating agent.
ADVERSE EFFECTS — Serious: Nephrotoxicity, N/V, hepatotoxicity. Frequent: N/V, hepatotoxicity.

TEMOZOLOMIDE *(Temodar, ✷Temodal)* ▶Plasma ♀D ▶– varies by therapy
WARNING — Secondary malignancies, bone marrow suppression, fertility impairment, alopecia. Instruct patients to report promptly fever, sore throat, signs of local infection, bleeding from any site, or symptoms suggestive of anemia. Cases of interstitial pneumonitis, alveolitis, and pulmonary fibrosis have been reported. Primary cytomegalovirus and fatal reactivation of hepatitis B may occur as opportunistic infections.
ADULT — Chemotherapy doses vary by indication. Anaplastic astrocytoma, glioblastoma multiforme.
PEDS — Not approved in children.
UNAPPROVED ADULT — Metastatic melanoma, renal cell carcinoma, cutaneous T-cell lymphomas, Ewing's sarcoma (recurrent or progressive); neuroendocrine tumors, advanced (carcinoid or islet cell); primary CNS lymphoma, refractory; soft tissue sarcomas, extremity/retroperitoneal/intra-abdominal; soft tissue sarcomas, hemangiopericytoma/solitary fibrous tumor; metastatic CNS lesions.

UNAPPROVED PEDS — Neuroblastoma (pediatric);
FORMS — Generic/Trade: Caps 5, 20, 100, 140, 180, 250 mg. 100 mg IV (reconstituted) solution.
NOTES — Reliable contraception is recommended. Monitor CBCs. Valproic acid decreases clearance.
MOA — Alkylating agent.
ADVERSE EFFECTS — Serious: Bone marrow suppression, erythema multiforme. Frequent: N/V, fatigue, headache. Fatal and severe hepatotoxicty has occurred. Postmarketing experience includes diabetes insipidus and reactivation of infections such as cytomegalovirus and hepatitis B.

THIOTEPA ▶L ♀D ▶– $ varies by therapy
WARNING — Secondary malignancies, bone marrow suppression, hypersensitivity, fertility impairment, alopecia. Instruct patients to report promptly fever, sore throat, signs of local infection, bleeding from any site, symptoms suggestive of anemia, black tarry stools, or vomiting of blood.
ADULT — Chemotherapy doses vary by indication. Adenocarcinoma of the breast or ovary, control of intracavitary malignant effusions, superficial papillary carcinoma of the urinary bladder, Hodgkin's disease, lymphosarcoma.
PEDS — Not approved in children.
NOTES — Reliable contraception is recommended. Monitor CBCs.
MOA — Alkylating agent.
ADVERSE EFFECTS — Serious: Bone marrow suppression, hypersensitivity. Frequent: Bone marrow suppression.

TRABECTEDIN *(Yondelis)* ▶L CYP3A is the predominant CYP enzyme responsible for the hepatic metabolism of trabectedin ♀D Based on its mechanism of action, trabectedin can cause fetal harm when administered during pregnancy ▶–
WARNING — Neutropenic sepsis: Severe, and fatal, neutropenic sepsis may occur. Monitor neutrophil count during treatment. Withhold Yondelis for Grade 2 or greater neutropenia. Rhabdomyolysis may occur; withhold Yondelis for severe or life-threatening increases in creatine phosphokinase level. Hepatotoxicity may occur. Monitor and delay and/or reduce dose if needed. Severe and fatal cardiomyopathy can occur. Withhold Yondelis in patients with left ventricular dysfunction. Embryofetal toxicity: Can cause fetal harm. Advise of potential risk to a fetus and use effective contraception
ADULT — 1.5 mg/m² as a 24-h intravenous infusion, every 3 weeks through a central venous line for the treatment of patients with advanced soft tissue sarcoma (STS), liposarcoma, and leiomyosarcoma subtypes (L-type sarcoma), who have received prior chemotherapy, including an anthracycline regimen.
FORMS — 1 mg sterile lyophilized powder in a single-dose vial.
NOTES — Premedicate with dexamethasone 20 mg IV, 30 min before each infusion. Avoid concomitant strong CYP3A inhibitors and CYP3A inducers.
MOA — Trabectedin is an alkylating drug that binds guanine residues in the minor groove of DNA,

(cont.)

TRABECTEDIN (*cont.*)
forming adducts and resulting in a bending of the DNA helix towards the major groove. Adduct formation triggers a cascade of events that can affect the subsequent activity of DNA binding proteins, including some transcription factors, and DNA repair pathways, resulting in perturbation of the cell cycle and eventual cell death.

ADVERSE EFFECTS — The most common (≥20%) adverse reactions are nausea, fatigue, vomiting, constipation, decreased appetite, diarrhea, peripheral edema, dyspnea, headache. The most common (≥5%) grades 3-4 laboratory abnormalities are: neutropenia, increased ALT, thrombocytopenia, anemia, increased AST, and increased creatine phosphokinase.

ONCOLOGY: Antibiotics

BLEOMYCIN (*✱Blenoxane*) ▶K ♀D ▶– $ varies by therapy
WARNING — Pulmonary fibrosis, skin toxicity, nephro/hepatotoxicity, alopecia, and severe idiosyncratic reaction consisting of hypotension, mental confusion, fever, chills, and wheezing. Because of the possibility of an anaphylactoid reaction, lymphoma patients should be treated with 2 units or less for the 1st 2 doses. If no acute reaction occurs, then the regular dosage schedule may be followed.
ADULT — Chemotherapy doses vary by indication. Squamous cell carcinoma of the head and neck. Carcinoma of the skin, penis, cervix, and vulva. Hodgkin's and non-Hodgkin's lymphoma. Testicular carcinoma. Malignant pleural effusion: Sclerosing agent.
PEDS — Not approved in children.
UNAPPROVED ADULT — Treatment of ovarian germ cell tumors.
NOTES — Reliable contraception is recommended. Frequent chest x-rays. May decrease digoxin and phenytoin levels. Risk of pulmonary toxicity increases with lifetime cumulative dose greater than 400 units.
MOA — Antibiotic.
ADVERSE EFFECTS — Serious: Pulmonary fibrosis, skin toxicity, nephro/hepatotoxicity, severe idiosyncratic reaction: hypotension, mental confusion, fever, chills, and wheezing. Frequent: Pulmonary fibrosis, stomatitis, vomiting, weight loss, alopecia.
DACTINOMYCIN (*Cosmegen*) ▶Not metabolized ♀C ▶– $ varies by therapy
WARNING — Extravasation associated with severe necrosis. Contraindicated with active chickenpox or herpes zoster. Erythema and vesiculation (with radiation), bone marrow suppression, alopecia. Instruct patients to report promptly fever, sore throat, signs of local infection, bleeding from any site, or symptoms suggestive of anemia.
ADULT — Chemotherapy doses vary by indication. Wilms' tumor, rhabdomyosarcoma, metastatic and nonmetastatic choriocarcinoma, nonseminomatous testicular carcinoma, Ewing's sarcoma, sarcoma botryoides. Most in combination regimens.
PEDS — Chemotherapy doses vary by indication. See adult. Contraindicated in infants younger than 6 mo.
NOTES — Monitor CBCs.
MOA — Antibiotic.

ADVERSE EFFECTS — Serious: Erythema and vesiculation (with radiation), bone marrow suppression. Frequent: Bone marrow suppression, N/V, alopecia.
DOXORUBICIN LIPOSOMAL (*Doxil, Lipodox, Lipodox 50, ✱Caelyx, Myocet*) ▶L ♀D ▶+ $ varies by therapy
WARNING — Extravasation associated with severe necrosis. Cardiac toxicity, more frequent in children. Bone marrow suppression, infusion-associated reactions, necrotizing colitis, mucositis, hyperuricemia, palmar-plantar erythrodysesthesia. Secondary malignancies. Instruct patients to report promptly fever, sore throat, signs of local infection, bleeding from any site, or symptoms suggestive of anemia.
ADULT — Chemotherapy doses vary by indication. Advanced HIV-associated Kaposi's sarcoma, multiple myeloma, ovarian carcinoma.
PEDS — Not approved in children.
UNAPPROVED ADULT — Breast cancer, Hodgkin's Lymphoma, non-Hodgkin's lymphoma, soft tissue sarcomas.
NOTES — Heart failure with cumulative doses. Monitor ejection fraction, CBCs, LFTs, uric acid levels, and renal function (toxicity increased with impaired function). Reliable contraception is recommended. Transient urine discoloration (red).
MOA — Antibiotic.
ADVERSE EFFECTS — Serious: Cardiac toxicity, bone marrow suppression, infusion-associated reactions, necrotizing colitis, palmar-plantar erythrodysesthesia, secondary malignancies. Frequent: Cardiac toxicity, bone marrow suppression, hyperuricemia, fatigue, fever, anorexia, N/V, stomatitis, diarrhea, urine discoloration. Very rare cases of secondary oral cancer have been reported in patients with long-term (more than one year) exposure to DOXIL, or those receiving a cumulative DOXIL dose greater than 720 mg/m2.
DOXORUBICIN NON-LIPOSOMAL (*Adriamycin*) ▶L ♀D ▶– $ varies by therapy
WARNING — Extravasation associated with severe necrosis. Cardiac toxicity, more frequent in children. Bone marrow suppression, infusion-associated reactions, necrotizing colitis, mucositis, hyperuricemia, alopecia. Secondary malignancies. Instruct patients to report promptly fever, sore throat, signs of local infection, bleeding from any site, or symptoms suggestive of anemia.
ADULT — Chemotherapy doses vary by indication. ALL, AML, Wilms' tumor, neuroblastoma, soft tissue and bone sarcomas, breast carcinoma, ovarian

(cont.)

DOXORUBICIN NON-LIPOSOMAL (*cont.*)

carcinoma, transitional cell bladder carcinoma, thyroid carcinoma, Hodgkin's and non-Hodgkin's lymphomas, bronchogenic carcinoma, gastric carcinoma.
PEDS — Chemotherapy doses vary by indication: See adult.
UNAPPROVED ADULT — Sarcoma, small-cell lung cancer, multiple myeloma, endometrial carcinoma, uterine sarcoma, thymomas and thymic malignancies, Waldenstrom's macroglobulinemia, head and neck cancer, kidney cancer, liver cancer
FORMS — 2mg/ml solution for injection. 5ml, 10ml, 25ml, 100ml vials.
NOTES — Heart failure with cumulative doses. Monitor ejection fraction, CBCs, LFTs, uric acid levels, and renal function (toxicity increased with impaired function). Reliable contraception is recommended. Transient urine discoloration (red).
MOA — Antibiotic.
ADVERSE EFFECTS — Serious: Cardiac toxicity, bone marrow suppression, secondary malignancies, infusion-associated reactions, necrotizing colitis. Frequent: Cardiac toxicity, bone marrow suppression, secondary malignancies, hyperuricemia, alopecia, urine discoloration.

EPIRUBICIN (*Ellence, ✽Pharmorubicin*) ▶L ♀D ▶– $ varies by therapy
WARNING — Extravasation associated with severe necrosis. Cardiac toxicity, bone marrow suppression, secondary malignancy (AML), hyperuricemia, fertility impairment, alopecia. Instruct patients to report promptly fever, sore throat, signs of local infection, bleeding from any site, or symptoms suggestive of anemia.
ADULT — Chemotherapy doses vary by indication. Adjuvant therapy for primary breast cancer.
PEDS — Not approved in children.
UNAPPROVED ADULT — Neoadjuvant and metastatic breast cancer. Cervical cancer, esophageal cancer, gastric cancer, soft tissue sarcomas, uterine sarcoma.
FORMS — 2 mg/mL soln for IV injection.
NOTES — Reliable contraception is recommended. Monitor CBCs, cardiac, hepatic, and renal function (toxicity increased with impaired function). Cimetidine increase levels. Transient urine discoloration (red).
MOA — Antibiotic.
ADVERSE EFFECTS — Serious: Cardiac toxicity, bone marrow suppression, secondary malignancies. Frequent: Cardiac toxicity, bone marrow suppression, N/V, mucositis, hyperuricemia, alopecia.

IDARUBICIN (*✽Idamycin*) ▶? ♀D ▶– $ varies by therapy
WARNING — Extravasation associated with severe necrosis. Cardiac toxicity, bone marrow suppression, hyperuricemia, alopecia. Instruct patients to report promptly fever, sore throat, signs of local infection, bleeding from any site, or symptoms suggestive of anemia.
ADULT — Chemotherapy doses vary by indication. AML, in combination regimens.

PEDS — Not approved in children.
UNAPPROVED ADULT — ALL, CML.
NOTES — Reliable contraception is recommended. Monitor CBCs, LFTs, cardiac, and renal function (toxicity increased with impaired function).
MOA — Antibiotic.
ADVERSE EFFECTS — Serious: Cardiac toxicity, bone marrow suppression, secondary malignancies. Frequent: Cardiac toxicity, bone marrow suppression, N/V, hyperuricemia, alopecia.

MITOMYCIN (*Mutamycin, Mitomycin-C*) ▶L ♀D ▶– $ varies by therapy
WARNING — Extravasation associated with severe necrosis. Bone marrow suppression, hemolytic uremic syndrome, nephrotoxicity, adult respiratory distress syndrome, alopecia. Instruct patients to report promptly fever, sore throat, signs of local infection, bleeding from any site, or symptoms suggestive of anemia.
ADULT — Chemotherapy doses vary by indication. Disseminated adenocarcinoma of stomach, pancreas, or colorectum, in combination regimens.
PEDS — Not approved in children.
UNAPPROVED ADULT — Superficial bladder cancer, intravesical route; pterygia, adjunct to surgical excision: Ophthalmic soln.
NOTES — Reliable contraception is recommended. Monitor CBCs and renal function.
MOA — Antibiotic.
ADVERSE EFFECTS — Serious: Bone marrow suppression, hemolytic uremic syndrome, nephrotoxicity, adult respiratory distress syndrome. Frequent: Bone marrow suppression, N/V, anorexia.

MITOXANTRONE ▶LK ♀D ▶– $ varies by therapy
WARNING — Secondary malignancies (AML), bone marrow suppression, cardiac toxicity/heart failure, hyperuricemia, increased LFTs. Instruct patients to report promptly fever, sore throat, signs of local infection, bleeding from any site, or symptoms suggestive of anemia.
ADULT — Chemotherapy doses vary by indication. AML, in combination regimens. Symptomatic patients with hormone-refractory prostate cancer. Multiple sclerosis (secondary progressive, progressive relapsing, or worsening relapsing-remitting): 12 mg/m^2 of BSA IV q 3 months.
PEDS — Not approved in children.
UNAPPROVED ADULT — Breast cancer, non-Hodgkin's lymphoma, ALL, CML, ovarian carcinoma. Sclerosing agent for malignant pleural effusions.
NOTES — Reliable contraception is recommended. Monitor CBCs and LFTs. Baseline echocardiogram and repeat echoes prior to each dose are recommended. Transient urine and sclera discoloration (blue-green).
MOA — Antibiotic.
ADVERSE EFFECTS — Serious: Bone marrow suppression, cardiac toxicity, secondary malignancies. Frequent: Bone marrow suppression, N/V, menstrual disorders, stomatitis, urine and sclera discoloration, alopecia.

VALRUBICIN (*Valstar, ✲Valtaxin*) ▸K ♀C ▸– $ varies by therapy
WARNING — Induces complete responses in only 1 in 5 patients. Delaying cystectomy could lead to development of lethal metastatic bladder cancer. Irritable bladder symptoms, alopecia.
ADULT — Chemotherapy doses vary by indication. Bladder cancer, intravesical therapy of BCG-refractory carcinoma in situ.
PEDS — Not approved in children.
NOTES — Reliable contraception is recommended. Transient urine discoloration (red).
MOA — Antibiotic.
ADVERSE EFFECTS — Serious: None. Frequent: Irritable bladder symptoms.

ONCOLOGY: Antimetabolites

AZACITIDINE (✲*Vidaza*) ▸K ♀D ▸– $ varies by therapy
WARNING — Contraindicated with malignant hepatic tumors. Bone marrow suppression. Fertility impairment. Instruct patients to report promptly fever, sore throat, or signs of local infection or bleeding from any site.
ADULT — Chemotherapy doses vary by indication. Myelodysplastic syndrome subtypes.
PEDS — Not approved in children.
NOTES — Reliable contraception is recommended. Men should not father children while on this drug. Monitor CBC, renal and hepatic function.
MOA — Antimetabolite.
ADVERSE EFFECTS — Serious: Bone marrow suppression, hepatotoxicity, renal failure. Frequent: N/V, bone marrow suppression, fever, diarrhea, fatigue, constipation.

BELINOSTAT (*BELEODAQ*) ▸L ♀D ▸?
WARNING — Thrombocytopenia, leukopenia (neutropenia and lymphopenia), and anemia: Monitor blood counts and modify dosage for hematologic toxicities. Infection: Serious and fatal infections (eg, pneumonia and sepsis). Hepatotoxicity: may cause hepatic toxicity and liver function test abnormalities. Monitor liver function tests and omit or modify dosage for hepatic toxicities. Tumor lysis syndrome: Monitor patients with advanced stage disease and/or high tumor burden and take appropriate precautions. Embryo-fetal toxicity: Beleodaq may cause fetal harm when administered to a pregnant woman. Advise women of potential harm to the fetus and to avoid pregnancy while receiving Beleodaq.
ADULT — Treatment of patients with relapsed or refractory peripheral T-cell lymphoma (PTCL). 1000 mg/m^2 once daily on days 1 through 5 of a 21-day cycle.
PEDS — Not approved in children.
FORMS — 500 mg powder for injection.
MOA — Histone deacetylase (HDAC) inhibitor
ADVERSE EFFECTS — Most common: nausea, fatigue, pyrexia, anemia, and vomiting. Thrombocytopenia was reported in 16% of patients with grade 3 or 4 thrombocytopenia in 7% of patients. Serious: pneumonia, pyrexia, infection, anemia, increased creatinine, thrombocytopenia, and multi-organ failure.

CAPECITABINE (✲*Xeloda, Teva-Capecitabine*) ▸L ♀D ▸ – varies by therapy
WARNING — Increased INR and bleeding with warfarin. Contraindicated in severe renal dysfunction (CrCl less than 30 mL/min). Severe diarrhea, fertility impairment, palmar-plantar erythrodysesthesia or chemotherapy-induced acral erythema, cardiac toxicity, hyperbilirubinemia, neutropenia, alopecia, typhlitis. Instruct patients to report promptly fever, sore throat, or signs of local infection or bleeding from any site.
ADULT — Chemotherapy doses vary by indication. Metastatic breast and colorectal cancer.
PEDS — Not approved in children.
UNAPPROVED ADULT — Gastric cancer, esophageal cancer, pancreatic cancer, hepatocellular carcinoma, ovarian cancer, metastatic renal cell cancer, neuroendocrine tumors, metastatic CNS lesions.
FORMS — Generic/Trade: Tabs 150, 500 mg.
NOTES — Reliable contraception is recommended. Antacids containing aluminum hydroxide and magnesium hydroxide increase levels. May increase phenytoin levels. Use in dipyrimidine dehydrogenase (DPD) deficiency varies with the degree of deficiency and mutations of the DPD enzyme.
MOA — Antimetabolite.
ADVERSE EFFECTS — Serious: Bleeding with warfarin, severe diarrhea, palmar-plantar erythrodysesthesia, cardiac toxicity, neutropenia, dehydration and renal failure as well as mucocutaneous and dermatologic toxicity. Frequent: Palmar-plantar erythrodysesthesia, N/V, diarrhea, stomatitis, hyperbilirubinemia.

CLADRIBINE ▸intracellular ♀D ▸– $ varies by therapy
WARNING — Bone marrow suppression, nephrotoxicity, neurotoxicity, fever, fertility impairment, alopecia, headache, rash, infection, prolonged depression of CD4 counts. Instruct patients to report promptly fever, sore throat, or signs of local infection, bleeding from any site, or symptoms suggestive of anemia.
ADULT — Treatment of active hairy cell leukemia. Also known as chlorodeoxyadenosine (2-CDA).
PEDS — Not approved in children.
UNAPPROVED ADULT — Advanced cutaneous T-cell lymphomas, chronic lymphocytic leukemia, non-Hodgkin's lymphomas, AML, autoimmune hemolytic anemia, mycosis fungoides, Sezary syndrome,

(cont.)

CLADRIBINE (*cont.*)

progressive multiple sclerosis, Waldenstrom's macroglobulinemia.

UNAPPROVED PEDS — AML, Langerhans cell histiocytosis.

NOTES — Reliable contraception is recommended. Monitor CBCs and renal function.

MOA — Antimetabolite.

ADVERSE EFFECTS — Serious: Bone marrow suppression, nephrotoxicity, neurotoxicity, fever. Frequent: Bone marrow suppression, fever, N/V, diarrhea, rash.

CLOFARABINE (✱*Clolar*) ▶K ♀D ▶– $ varies by therapy

WARNING — Myelodysplastic syndrome, bone marrow suppression, tumor lysis syndrome, hepatitis, hepatic failure. Instruct patients to report promptly fever, sore throat, signs of local infection, bleeding from any site, or symptoms suggestive of anemia.

ADULT — Not approved in adults.

PEDS — Age 1 to 21 yo: Chemotherapy doses vary by indication. Relapsed or refractory acute lymphoblastic leukemia.

FORMS — 20 mg/20 mL (1 mg/mL) single-use vial.

NOTES — Reliable contraception is recommended. Monitor CBCs, LFTs, and renal function. Dose reduction is recommended with stable, moderate renal impairment.

MOA — Antimetabolite.

ADVERSE EFFECTS — Serious: Myelodysplastic syndrome, bone marrow suppression, serious infections, tumor lysis syndrome, hepatotoxicity. capillary leak, venous occlusive disease, Stevens-Johnson Syndrome (SJS) and toxic epidermal necrolysis (TEN), GI hemorrhage. hemorrhage, enterocolitis, and hyponatremia. Frequent: Bone marrow suppression, N/V, diarrhea.

CYTARABINE (*Cytosar-U, Tarabine, Depo-Cyt, AraC,* ✱*Cytostar*) ▶LK ♀D ▶– $ varies by therapy

WARNING — Bone marrow suppression, hepatotoxicity, N/V/D, hyperuricemia, pancreatitis, peripheral neuropathy, "cytarabine syndrome" (fever, myalgia, bone pain, occasional chest pain, maculopapular rash, conjunctivitis, and malaise), alopecia. Neurotoxicity. Instruct patients to report promptly fever, sore throat, signs of local infection, bleeding from any site, symptoms suggestive of anemia, or yellow discoloration of the skin or eyes.

ADULT — Chemotherapy doses vary by indication. AML. ALL. CML. Prophylaxis and treatment of meningeal leukemia, intrathecal (Cytosar-U, Tarabine). Lymphomatous meningitis, intrathecal.

PEDS — Chemotherapy doses vary by indication. AML. ALL. Chronic myelocytic leukemia. Prophylaxis and treatment of meningeal leukemia, intrathecal (Cytosar-U, Tarabine).

FORMS — Solution for Injection: 20mg/ml and 100mg/ml vials. Powder for injection: 100mg and 500mg vials.

NOTES — Reliable contraception is recommended. Monitor CBCs, LFTs, and renal function. Decreases

digoxin levels. Chemical arachnoiditis can be reduced by coadministration of dexamethasone. Use dexamethasone eye drops with high doses.

MOA — Antimetabolite.

ADVERSE EFFECTS — Serious: Bone marrow suppression, hepatotoxicity, pancreatitis, peripheral neuropathy, "cytarabine syndrome" (fever, myalgia, bone pain, occasional chest pain, maculopapular rash, conjunctivitis, and malaise). Neurotoxicity. Chemical arachnoiditis (N/V, headache, and fever) with Depo-Cyt. Frequent: Bone marrow suppression, N/V, diarrhea, rash.

CYTARABINE LIPOSOMAL (*DepoCyt*) ▶? Systemic exposure following intrathecal administration is negligible. ♀D Conventional cytarabine has been associated with fetal abnormalities. ▶–

WARNING — Chemical arachnoiditis (N/V, headache, and fever) with Depo-Cyt. May be fatal if untreated. Dexamethasone should be administered concomitantly with cytarabine liposomal to diminish chemical arachnoid symptoms.

ADULT — 50 mg intrathecally in varying frequencies for induction, consolidation and maintenance treatment of lymphomatous meningitis.

FORMS — 50 mg/5 mL suspension for intrathecal use.

NOTES — Initiate dexamethasone 4 mg two times per day (oral or IV) for 5 days beginning on the day of cytarabine liposomal administration.

MOA — Sustained release formulation of cytarabine, an antimetabolite which inhibits DNA synthesis and is cell cycle specific for the S-phase of cell division. It's primary action is inhibition of DNA polymerase.

ADVERSE EFFECTS — Peripheral edema, chemical arachnoiditis (without dexamethasone premedication 100%), headache, confusion, fever, fatigue, seizure, dizziness, lethargy, insomnia, memory loss, pain. Dehydration. Nausea /vomiting, constipation, diarrhea, decreased appetite. Weakness, back pain, abnormal gait. Blurred vision.

DECITABINE (*Dacogen*) ▶L ♀D ▶– $ varies by therapy

WARNING — Bone marrow suppression, pulmonary edema. Instruct patients to report promptly fever, sore throat, or signs of local infection, bleeding from any site, or symptoms suggestive of anemia.

ADULT — Myelodysplastic syndromes. Treatment regimen: Option 1: Administer at a dose of 15 mg/m^2 by continuous IV infusion over 3 h repeated q 8 h for 3 days. Repeat cycle q 6 weeks. Option 2: Administer at a dose of 20 mg/m^2 by continuous IV infusion over 1 h repeated daily for 5 days. Repeat cycle q 4 weeks.

PEDS — Not approved in children.

NOTES — Reliable contraception is recommended. Men should not father children during and 2 months after therapy. Monitor CBCs, baseline LFTs.

MOA — Antimetabolite.

ADVERSE EFFECTS — Serious: Bone marrow suppression, pulmonary edema. Frequent: Bone marrow suppression, N/V, fatigue, fever, diarrhea, constipation, hyperglycemia, stomatitis.

FLOXURIDINE (✱*FUDR*) ▶L ♀D ▶– $ varies by therapy
WARNING — Bone marrow suppression, nephrotoxicity, increased LFTs, alopecia. Instruct patients to report promptly fever, sore throat, signs of local infection, bleeding from any site, or symptoms suggestive of anemia.
ADULT — Chemotherapy doses vary by indication. GI adenocarcinoma metastatic to the liver given by intrahepatic arterial pump.
PEDS — Not approved in children.
NOTES — Reliable contraception is recommended. Monitor CBCs, LFTs, and renal function.
MOA — Antimetabolite.
ADVERSE EFFECTS — Serious: Bone marrow suppression. Frequent: Bone marrow suppression, N/V, stomatitis, alopecia.

FLUDARABINE (✱*Fludara*) ▶Serum ♀D ▶– $ varies by therapy
WARNING — Neurotoxicity (agitation, blindness, and coma), progressive multifocal leukoencephalopathy and death, bone marrow suppression, hemolytic anemia, thrombocytopenia, ITP, Evan's syndrome, acquired hemophilia, pulmonary toxicity, fertility impairment, hyperuricemia, alopecia. Instruct patients to report promptly fever, sore throat, signs of local infection, bleeding from any site, or symptoms suggestive of anemia.
ADULT — Chemotherapy doses vary by indication. CLL.
PEDS — Not approved in children.
UNAPPROVED ADULT — Non-Hodgkin's lymphoma, mycosis fungoides, hairy-cell leukemia, Hodgkin's disease.
NOTES — Reliable contraception is recommended. Monitor CBCs and renal function; watch for hemolysis.
MOA — Antimetabolite.
ADVERSE EFFECTS — Serious: Neurotoxicity (agitation, blindness, coma), progressive multifocal leukoencephalopathy and death, bone marrow suppression, hemolytic anemia, pulmonary toxicity. Frequent: Bone marrow suppression, edema, N/V, fever, diarrhea, rash, alopecia.

FLUOROURACIL (*Adrucil, 5-FU*) ▶L ♀D ▶– $ varies by therapy
WARNING — Increased INR and bleeding with warfarin. Bone marrow suppression, angina, fertility impairment, alopecia, diarrhea, mucositis, hand and foot syndrome (palmar/plantar erythrodysesthesia). Instruct patients to report promptly fever, sore throat, signs of local infection, bleeding from any site, or symptoms suggestive of anemia.
ADULT — Chemotherapy doses vary by indication. Colon, rectum, breast, stomach, and pancreatic carcinoma. Dukes' stage C colon cancer with irinotecan or leucovorin after surgical resection.
PEDS — Not approved in children.
UNAPPROVED ADULT — Head and neck, renal cell, prostate, ovarian, esophageal, anal and topical to skin for basal and squamous cell carcinoma.

NOTES — Reliable contraception is recommended. Monitor CBCs.
MOA — Antimetabolite.
ADVERSE EFFECTS — Serious: Bone marrow suppression, bleeding with warfarin, palmar-plantar erythrodysesthesia, angina. Frequent: Bone marrow suppression, N/V, diarrhea, stomatitis, alopecia.

GEMCITABINE (*Gemzar*) ▶intracellular ♀D ▶– $ varies by therapy
WARNING — Bone marrow suppression, fever, rash, increased LFTs, proteinuria, hematuria, alopecia. Instruct patients to report promptly fever, sore throat, signs of local infection, bleeding from any site, or symptoms suggestive of anemia.
ADULT — Chemotherapy doses vary by indication. Adenocarcinoma of the pancreas. Non-small-cell lung cancer, in combination regimens. Metastatic breast cancer, in combination regimens. Advanced ovarian cancer.
PEDS — Not approved in children.
FORMS — 200 mg, 1000, 2000 mg vials of soln for IV use.
NOTES — Reliable contraception is recommended. Monitor CBCs, LFTs and renal function.
MOA — Antimetabolite.
ADVERSE EFFECTS — Serious: Bone marrow suppression. Frequent: Bone marrow suppression, fever, rash, proteinuria, hematuria, increased LFTs.

LONSURF (trifluridine/tipiracil) ▶degraded chemically Trifluridine is mainly eliminated by metabolism via thymidine phosphorylase ♀D ▶–
WARNING — Severe Myelosuppression: Obtain complete blood counts prior to and on Day 15 of each cycle. Reduce dose and/or hold LONSURF as clinically indicated. Embryo-Fetal Toxicity: Fetal harm can occur. Advise women of potential risk to a fetus.
ADULT — 35 mg/m^2 (based on the trifluridine component) orally two times per day on Days 1 through 5 and Days 8 through 12 of each 28-day cycle for the treatment of patients with metastatic colorectal cancer who have been previously treated with fluoropyrimidine-, oxaliplatin- and irinotecan-based chemotherapy, an anti-VEGF biological therapy, and if RAS wild-type, an anti-EGFR therapy.
FORMS — 15 mg trifluridine/6.14 mg tipiracil and 20 mg trifluridine/8.19 mg tipiracil tablets
NOTES — If tablets are stored outside the original bottle, they must be discarded after 30 days.
MOA — Following uptake into cancer cells, trifluridine is incorporated into DNA, interferes with DNA synthesis and inhibits cell proliferation. Inclusion of tipiracil increases trifluridine exposure by inhibiting its metabolism by thymidine phosphorylase.
ADVERSE EFFECTS — The most common adverse reaction (≥10%) are anemia, neutropenia, asthenia/fatigue, nausea, thrombocytopenia, decreased appetite, diarrhea, vomiting, abdominal pain, and pyrexia.

MERCAPTOPURINE (*6-MP, Purixan*) ▸L ♀D ▶– $ varies by therapy
WARNING — Mercaptopurine is mutagenic in animals and humans, carcinogenic in animals, and may increase the patient's risk of neoplasia. Cases of hepatosplenic T-cell lymphoma have been reported in patients treated with mercaptopurine for inflammatory bowel disease. The safety and efficacy of mercaptopurine in patients with inflammatory bowel disease have not been established. Bone marrow suppression, hepatotoxicity, hyperuricemia, alopecia. Instruct patients to report promptly fever, sore throat, signs of local infection, bleeding from any site, symptoms suggestive of anemia, or yellow discoloration of the skin or eyes.
ADULT — Treatment of patients with acute lymphoblastic leukemia (ALL) as part of a combination regimen.
PEDS — Treatment of patients with acute lymphoblastic leukemia (ALL) as part of a combination regimen.
UNAPPROVED ADULT — Inflammatory bowel disease: Start at 50 mg PO daily, titrate to response. Typical dose range 0.5 to 1.5 mg/kg PO daily. Acute promyelocytic leukemia (APL) maintenance (adults); autoimmune hepatitis (children); Crohn's disease (adults); Crohn's disease (children/adolescents); lymphoblastic lymphoma; ulcerative colitis (initial management) (adults); Ulcerative colitis (maintenance therapy) (adults).
UNAPPROVED PEDS — Inflammatory bowel disease: 1.5 mg/kg PO daily. Ulcerative colitis.
FORMS — Generic/Trade: Tabs 50 mg. 20 mg/mL oral susp.
NOTES — Reliable contraception is recommended. Monitor CBCs, LFTs, and renal function. Consider folate supplementation. Allopurinol and trimethoprim/sulfamethoxazole increase toxicity.
MOA — Antimetabolite.
ADVERSE EFFECTS — Serious: Bone marrow suppression, hepatotoxicity, oligospermia. Frequent: Bone marrow suppression, alopecia, rash, diarrhea.

METHOTREXATE—ONCOLOGY (*Rheumatrex, Trexall*) ▸KL – intestinal flora ♀X ▶–
WARNING — Acute renal failure, third-spacing in ascites/pleural effusions/bone marrow suppression/mucositis/hepatotoxicity/pneumonitis.
ADULT — Trophoblastic neoplasms, acute lymphocytic leukemia, meningeal leukemia, breast cancer, head and neck cancer, cutaneous T-cell lymphoma, lung cancer, non-Hodgkin's Lymphoma, osteosarcoma.
PEDS — Acute lymphocytic leukemia, meningeal leukemia, non-Hodgkin's lymphoma, nonmetastatic osteosarcoma.
UNAPPROVED ADULT — Bladder cancer, CNS tumors, acute promyelocytic leukemia, soft tissue sarcomas, acute graft versus host disease prophylaxis.
UNAPPROVED PEDS — Dermatomyositis, juvenile idiopathic arthritis.

FORMS — Injection, powder for reconstitution 1 g. Injection soln: 25 mg/mL. Oral tabs 2.5, 5, 7.5, 10, 15 mg.
MOA — Folate antimetabolite that inhibits DNA synthesis.
ADVERSE EFFECTS — Arachnoiditis, hyperuricemia, mucositis, myelosuppression, renal failure.

NELARABINE (*Arranon*, *✳Atriance*) ▸LK ♀D ▶– $ varies by therapy
WARNING — Peripheral neuropathy, paralysis, demyelination, severe somnolence, convulsions. Bone marrow suppression.
ADULT — Chemotherapy doses vary by indication. ALL, T-cell lymphoblastic lymphoma.
PEDS — Chemotherapy doses vary by indication. ALL, T-cell lymphoblastic lymphoma.
NOTES — Reliable contraception is recommended. Monitor renal function.
MOA — Antimetabolite.
ADVERSE EFFECTS — Serious: Bone marrow suppression, peripheral neuropathy, paralysis, demyelination, convulsions. Frequent: Bone marrow suppression, fatigue, somnolence, N/V/D.

PEMETREXED (*✳Alimta*) ▸K ♀D ▶– $ varies by therapy
WARNING — Bone marrow suppression, rash. Instruct patients to report promptly fever, sore throat, signs of local infection, bleeding from any site, symptoms suggestive of anemia. Dose adjustment is required for patients with hepatic impairment.
ADULT — Chemotherapy doses vary by indication. Malignant pleural mesothelioma, in combination with cisplatin. Nonsquamous non-small-cell lung cancer. Seven days prior to pemetrexed therapy, start supplementation with folic acid 400 to 1000 mcg orally daily until 21 days after last dose and Vitamin B12 1000 mcg IM, q 3 cycles. Give dexamethasone 4 mg orally two times per day for 3 days starting the day before treatment to minimize cutaneous reactions.
PEDS — Not approved in children. No efficacy in pediatric patients has been reported. Pharmacokinetics in pediatric patients are comparable to adults.
UNAPPROVED ADULT — Metastatic bladder cancer, cervical cancer, thymic malignancies.
NOTES — Reliable contraception is recommended. Monitor CBCs and renal function. Do not use in patients with CrCl <45 mL/min. Avoid NSAIDs around the time of administration Drainage of mild or moderate 3rd space fluid collection prior to ALIMTA treatment should be considered, but is probably not necessary. The effect of severe 3rd space fluid on pharmacokinetics is not known.
MOA — Antimetabolite.
ADVERSE EFFECTS — Serious: Bone marrow suppression, severe rash. Frequent: Bone marrow suppression, fatigue, fever, N/V, stomatitis, dyspnea, rash. Cases of esophagitis were reported in clinical trials.

PENTOSTATIN (✱*Nipent*) ▶K ♀D ▶– $ varies by therapy
  WARNING — Bone marrow suppression, nephrotoxicity, hepatotoxicity, CNS toxicity, pulmonary toxicity, severe rash, fertility impairment, alopecia. Instruct patients to report promptly fever, sore throat, signs of local infection, bleeding from any site, symptoms suggestive of anemia, or yellow discoloration of the skin or eyes.
  ADULT — Chemotherapy doses vary by indication. Hairy cell leukemia, refractory to alpha-interferon.
  PEDS — Not approved in children.
  UNAPPROVED ADULT — ALL, CLL, non-Hodgkin's lymphoma, mycosis fungoides.
  NOTES — Reliable contraception is recommended. Monitor CBCs and renal function.
  MOA — Antimetabolite.
  ADVERSE EFFECTS — Serious: Bone marrow suppression, nephrotoxicity, hepatotoxicity, CNS toxicity, pulmonary toxicity, severe rash. Frequent: N/V, fever.

PRALATREXATE (*Folotyn*) ▶+ intracellular ♀D ▶–
  WARNING — Bone marrow suppression, mucositis and hepatotoxicity may require dosage modification. Concomitant administration of drugs that are subject to substantial renal clearance (eg, NSAIDs, trimethoprim-sulfamethoxazole) may result in delayed clearance of pralatrexate. Severe and potentially fatal dermatologic reactions may occur, including toxic epidermal necrolysis (TEN). Skin toxicity may be progressive, with severity increasing with continued treatment. Monitor all dermatologic reactions and discontinue or withhold treatment for severe dermatologic reactions.
  ADULT — 30 mg/m² IV once weekly for 6 out of 7 weeks. Treatment of relapsed/refractory peripheral T-cell lymphoma (PTCL).
  PEDS — Not approved in children.
  UNAPPROVED ADULT — Treatment of relapsed or refractory cutaneous T-cell lymphoma (CTCL).

  NOTES — Folic acid and vitamin B12 supplementation needed to reduce hematologic toxicity and treatment related mucositis. Folic acid 1 to 1.25 mg PO daily should be started within 10 days prior to starting pralatrexate, and continued for 30 days post last pralatrexate dose. Vitamin B12 1000 mcg IM should be administered within 10 weeks prior to starting pralatrexate, and q 8 to 10 weeks thereafter. B12 may be given same day as pralatrexate after the initial dose. Use with caution in patients with renal impairment.
  MOA — Antifolate analog. Inhibits DNA, RNA and protein synthesis by entering cells expressing reduced folate carrier. After polyglutamylation by FPGS (folylpolyglutamate synthetase), competes for DHFR-folate binding site to inhibit DHFR (dihydrofolate reductase).
  ADVERSE EFFECTS — Significant: Edema, fatigue, fever, rash, mucositis, nausea, vomiting, diarrhea, constipation, bone marrow suppression, increased LFTs, back and limb pain, cough, epistaxis, night sweats.

THIOGUANINE (*Tabloid*, ✱*Lanvis*) ▶L ♀D ▶– $ varies by therapy
  WARNING — Bone marrow suppression, hepatotoxicity, hyperuricemia, alopecia. Instruct patients to report promptly fever, sore throat, signs of local infection, bleeding from any site, symptoms suggestive of anemia, or yellow discoloration of the skin or eyes.
  ADULT — Chemotherapy doses vary by indication. Acute nonlymphocytic leukemias.
  PEDS — Chemotherapy doses vary by indication. Acute nonlymphocytic leukemias.
  FORMS — Generic only: Tabs 40 mg, scored.
  NOTES — Reliable contraception is recommended. Monitor CBCs and LFTs.
  MOA — Antimetabolite.
  ADVERSE EFFECTS — Serious: Bone marrow suppression, hepatotoxicity. Frequent: Bone marrow suppression, diarrhea.

ONCOLOGY: Cytoprotective Agents

URIDINE TRIACETATE (*Vistogard*) ▶degraded chemically Metabolized by normal pyrimidine catabolic pathways present in most tissues. ♀B ▶?
  ADULT — Adults: 10 g (1 packet) orally every 6 h for 20 doses, without regard to meals, following a fluorouracil or capecitabine overdose regardless of the presence of symptoms, or for patients who exhibit early-onset, severe or life-threatening toxicity affecting the cardiac or central nervous system, and/or early onset, unusually severe adverse reactions (eg, gastrointestinal toxicity and/or neutropenia) within 96 h following the end of fluorouracil or capecitabine administration.
  PEDS — 6.2 g/m² of body surface area (not to exceed 10 g per dose) orally every 6 hours for 20 doses, without regard to meals following a fluorouracil or

capecitabine overdose regardless of the presence of symptoms, or for patients who exhibit early-onset, severe or life-threatening toxicity affecting the cardiac or central nervous system, and/or early onset, unusually severe adverse reactions (eg, gastrointestinal toxicity and/or neutropenia) within 96 h following the end of fluorouracil or capecitabine administration.
  FORMS — Oral granules: 10-g packets
  NOTES — Vistogard is not recommended for the non-emergent treatment of adverse reactions associated with fluorouracil or capecitabine because it may diminish the efficacy of these drugs. The safety and efficacy of Vistogard initiated more than 96 h following the end of fluorouracil or capecitabine administration have not been established.

(cont.)

URIDINE TRIACETATE (*cont.*)

MOA — Uridine triacetate is an acetylated pro-drug of uridine. Following oral administration, uridine triacetate is deacetylated by nonspecific esterases present throughout the body, yielding uridine in the circulation. Uridine competitively inhibits cell damage and cell death caused by fluorouracil.

ADVERSE EFFECTS — Vomiting, nausea, and diarrhea.

AMIFOSTINE (✱*Ethyol*) ▶Plasma ♀C ▶– $ varies by therapy

WARNING — Hypotension, hypocalcemia, N/V, hypersensitivity.

ADULT — Doses vary by indication. Reduction of renal toxicity with cisplatin. Reduction of xerostomia and mucositis with radiation.

PEDS — Not approved in children.

NOTES — Monitor calcium and BP.

MOA — Cytoprotective.

ADVERSE EFFECTS — Serious: Hypotension, hypocalcemia. Frequent: N/V.

DEFIBROTIDE (*DEFITELIO*) ▶degraded chemically ♀X/X/X ▶–

WARNING — Hemorrhage: Monitor patients for bleeding. Withhold or discontinue Defitelio if significant bleeding occurs. Hypersensitivity Reactions: If severe or life threatening allergic reaction occurs, discontinue Defitelio, treat according to standard of care, and monitor until signs and symptoms resolve

ADULT — 6.25 mg/kg every 6 h given as a 2-h intravenous infusion for the treatment of adult and pediatric patients with hepatic veno-occlusive disease (VOD), also known as sinusoidal obstruction syndrome (SOS), with renal or pulmonary dysfunction following hematopoietic stem-cell transplantation. Treat for a minimum of 21 days. If after 21 days signs and symptoms of VOD have not resolved, continue treatment until resolution.

PEDS — Same as adult above.

FORMS — Injection: 200 mg/2.5 mL (80 mg/mL) in a single-patient-use vial.

NOTES — Concomitant administration with systemic anticoagulant or fibrinolytic therapy is contraindicated.

MOA — Enhances the enzymatic activity of plasmin to hydrolyze fibrin clots. Increases tissue plasminogen activator (t-PA) and thrombomodulin expression, and decreases von Willebrand factor (vWF) and plasminogen activator inhibitor-1 (PAI-1) expression, thereby reducing EC activation and increasing EC-mediated fibrinolysis.

ADVERSE EFFECTS — The most common adverse reactions (incidence ≥10% and independent of causality) with DEFITELIO treatment were hypotension, diarrhea, vomiting, nausea and epistaxis.

DEXRAZOXANE (*Totect*, ✱*Zinecard*) ▶Plasma ♀D ▶– $ varies by therapy

WARNING — Additive bone marrow suppression, secondary malignancies (in pediatric and adult patients), fertility impairment, N/V.

ADULT — Doses vary by indication. Reduction of cardiac toxicity with doxorubicin. Treatment of anthracycline extravasation: Give ASAP within 6 h of extravasation.

PEDS — Not approved in children.

FORMS — Generic/Trade: 250 mg/vial, 500 mg/vial

NOTES — Monitor CBCs.

MOA — Cytoprotective.

ADVERSE EFFECTS — Serious: Additive bone marrow suppression, secondary malignancies. Frequent: N/V.

GLUCARPIDASE (*Voraxaze*) ▶L ♀C ▶?

ADULT — Treatment of toxic plasma methotrexate concentrations (greater than 1 micromole per liter) in patients with delayed methotrexate clearance due to impaired renal function. Given IV 50 units/kg.

PEDS — Treatment of toxic plasma methotrexate concentrations (greater than 1 micromole per liter) in patients with delayed methotrexate clearance due to impaired renal function.

UNAPPROVED ADULT — 2000 units delivered intrathecally as soon as possible after intrathecal methotrexate overdose.

FORMS — 1000 unit powder for injection.

MOA — Glucarpidase is a recombinant enzyme that is able to rapidly decrease serum levels of methotrexate and thus reduce its concentration in most patients to below the threshold for serious toxicity. It lowers systemic methotrexate levels by rapidly causing methotrexate to convert to glutamate and 4-deoxy-4-amino-N 10-methylpteroic acid (DAMPA). Compared with methotrexate, DAMPA is 25 to 100 times less potent an inhibitor of dihydrofolate reductase (DHFR) and is significantly less cytotoxic.

ADVERSE EFFECTS — Antiglucarpidase antibody development (17%). 1-10% incidence: flushing, hypotension, headache, nausea/vomiting, parathesias.

LEUCOVORIN (*Wellcovorin, folinic acid*) ▶Gut ♀C ▶? $ varies by therapy

WARNING — Allergic sensitization.

ADULT — Doses vary by indication. Reduction of toxicity due to folic acid antagonists (ie, methotrexate). Colorectal cancer with 5-FU. Megaloblastic anemias.

PEDS — Not approved in children.

FORMS — Generic only: Tabs 5, 10, 15, 25 mg. Injection for hospital/oncology clinic use; not intended for outpatient prescribing.

NOTES — Monitor methotrexate concentrations and CBCs.

MOA — Folic acid derivative.

ADVERSE EFFECTS — Serious: Bone marrow suppression (with 5-FU). Frequent: Stomatitis, diarrhea (with 5-FU).

LEVOLEUCOVORIN (*Fusilev*) ▶gut ♀C ▶? $ varies by therapy

WARNING — Allergic sensitization.

ADULT — Doses vary by indication. Reduction of toxicity due to high-dose methotrexate for

(cont.)

LEVOLEUCOVORIN (cont.)

osteosarcoma. Indicated for use in combination chemotherapy with 5-fluorouracil in the palliative treatment of patients with advanced metastatic colorectal cancer. Antidote for impaired methotrexate elimination and for inadvertent overdosage of folic acid antagonists.
PEDS — Not approved in children.
FORMS — 50 mg powder for injection.
NOTES — Monitor methotrexate concentrations and CBCs.
MOA — Folic acid derivative. Counter acts the toxic effects of folic acid antogonists such as methotrexate.
ADVERSE EFFECTS — Serious: None. Frequent: Vomiting, stomatitis, nausea.

MESNA (Mesnex, ✷Uromitexan) ▶Plasma ♀B ▶– $ varies by therapy
WARNING — Hypersensitivity, bad taste in the mouth.
ADULT — Doses vary by indication. Reduction of hemorrhagic cystis with ifosfamide.
PEDS — Not approved in children.
UNAPPROVED ADULT — Doses vary by indication. Reduction of hemorrhagic cystis with high-dose cyclophosphamide.
UNAPPROVED PEDS — Doses vary by indication.
FORMS — Trade only: Tabs 400 mg, scored.
NOTES — False positive test urine ketones.
MOA — Cytoprotective.
ADVERSE EFFECTS — Serious: Hypersensitivity. Frequent: Bad taste in mouth.

PALIFERMIN (✷Kepivance) ▶Plasma ♀C ▶? $ varies by therapy
WARNING — Do not administer within 24 hours before, during, or after myelotoxic chemotherapy; may increase the severity and duration of oral mucositis, due to the increased sensitivity of rapidly dividing epithelial cells.
ADULT — Doses vary by indication. Decreases incidence, duration, and severity of severe oral mucositis in patients receiving therapy for hematologic malignancies.
PEDS — Not approved in children. Information on the dosing and safety of palifermin in the pediatric population is limited. However, use of palifermin in pediatric patients age 1 to 16 yo is supported by evidence from adequate and well-controlled studies of palifermin in adults and a phase 1 study that included 27 pediatric patients with acute leukemia undergoing hematopoietic stem cell transplant.
FORMS — 6.25mg vials of powder for reconstitution for IV use.
NOTES — Avoid coadministration of heparin with palifermin, and flush any heparin-maintained IV lines with saline prior to administration of palifermin. Heparin may increase the serum concentration of palifermin.
MOA — Cytoprotective – human keratinocyte growth factor.
ADVERSE EFFECTS — Serious: Fever. Frequent: Rash, erythema, edema, pruritus, oral/perioral dysesthesia, tongue discoloration or thickening, alteration of taste.

ONCOLOGY: Hormones

LEUPROLIDE (Eligard, Lupron Depot, Lupron Depot-Ped) ▶L ♀X ▶– $ varies by therapy
WARNING — Possible increase of diabetes and cardiovascular disease in men receiving leuprolide for prostate cancer. Worsening of symptoms: Increase in bone pain, difficulty urinating. Decreases in bone mineral density. Anaphylaxis, alopecia. Respiratory, thoracic, and mediastinal disorder. Interstitial lung disease. Possible convulsions. Long-term androgen deprivation therapy can lengthen QTc interval.
ADULT — Advanced prostate cancer: Lupron: 1 mg SC daily. Eligard: 7.5 mg SC q month, 22.5 mg SC q 3 months, 30 mg SC q 4 months, or 45 mg SC q 6 months. Lupron depot: 7.5 mg IM q month, 22.5 mg IM q 3 months or 30 mg IM q 4 months. Viadur: 65 mg SC implant q 12 months. Endometriosis or uterine leiomyomata (fibroids): 3.75 mg IM q month or 11.25 mg IM q 3 months for total therapy of 6 months (endometriosis) or 3 months (fibroids). Administer concurrent iron for fibroid-associated anemia.
PEDS — Central precocious puberty: Injection: 50 mcg/kg/day SC. Increase by 10 mcg/kg/day until total down regulation. Depot-Ped: 0.3 mg/kg q 4 weeks IM (minimum dose 7.5 mg). Increase by 3.75 mg q 4 weeks until adequate down regulation.
UNAPPROVED ADULT — Treatment of breast cancer, infertility, menses cessation in patients receiving high-dose chemotherapy, prostatic hyperplasia, premenopausal ovarian ablation in breast cancer, paraphilia/hypersexuality.
NOTES — For prostate cancer, monitor testosterone, prostatic acid phosphatase, and PSA levels. Transient increases in testosterone and estrogen occur. For endometriosis, a fractional dose of the 3-month depot preparation is not equivalent to the same dose of the monthly formulation. Rotate the injection site periodically. Consider norethindrone as "add back" therapy to decrease bone loss (see norethindrone).
MOA — Gonadotropin inhibitor via agonism of luteinizing hormone releasing hormone.
ADVERSE EFFECTS — Serious: Anaphylaxis, urinary obstruction, erythema multiforme, pituitary apoplexy, convulsions. Hepato-biliary disorder: Serious drug-induced liver injury. Frequent: Decrease in bone mineral density, vaginal bleeding, hot flashes, gynecomastia, transient worsening of pain.

ABIRATERONE ACETATE (✱*Zytiga*) ▶L ♀X ▶–

WARNING — Significant increases in hepatic enzymes have been reported; may require dose reduction.

ADULT — Indicated in combination with prednisone for the treatment of patients with metastatic castration-resistant prostate cancer. 1000 mg PO daily in combination with prednisone 5 mg two times per day.

PEDS — Not for use in children.

FORMS — 250 mg tabs.

NOTES — Increased mineralocorticoid levels due to CYP17 inhibition. Avoid concurrent use with CYP3A4 inhibitors and inducers, as well as CYP2D6 substrates. Abiraterone inhibits the hepatic drug-metabolizing enzyme CYP2C8.

MOA — Binds to CYP17 enzyme, resulting in inhibition of the formation of testerone precursors.

ADVERSE EFFECTS — Joint swelling, hypokalemia, hypophosphatemia, hypertriglyceridemia, edema, muscle discomfort, hot flush, diarrhea, urinary tract infection, cough, hypertension, arrhythmia, urinary frequency, nocturia, dyspepsia and upper respiratory tract infection. Non-infectious pneumonitis. Rhabdomyolysis and myopathy. Hepatitis fulminant and acute hepatic failure.

ANASTROZOLE (✱*Arimidex*) ▶L ♀X ▶– $ varies by therapy

WARNING — Patients with estrogen receptor-negative disease and patients who do not respond to tamoxifen therapy rarely respond to anastrozole. Fertility impairment, vaginal bleeding, hot flashes, alopecia, decrease in bone mineral density, trigger finger. Increase in cardiovascular ischemia in women with preexisting ischemic heart disease.

ADULT — Chemotherapy doses vary by indication. Locally advanced or metastatic breast cancer. Adjuvant early breast cancer.

PEDS — Not approved in children.

FORMS — Generic/Trade: Tabs 1 mg.

NOTES — Reliable contraception is recommended. Monitor CBCs. Contraindicated in premenopausal women.

MOA — Aromatase inhibitor.

ADVERSE EFFECTS — Serious: Cardiovascular ischemia. Frequent: Hot flashes, nausea, vasodilatation, mood disturbance, fatigue, arthralgia, myalgia, pharyngitis. Tickling, tingling or numbness.

BICALUTAMIDE (*Casodex*) ▶L ♀X ▶ $ varies by therapy

WARNING — Hypersensitivity, hepatotoxicity, interstitial lung disease, gynecomastia/breast pain, fertility impairment, hot flashes, diarrhea, alopecia. Increased risk for cardiovascular disease and diabetes.

ADULT — Prostate cancer: 50 mg PO daily in combination with an LHRH analog (eg, goserelin or leuprolide). Not indicated in women.

PEDS — Not approved in children.

UNAPPROVED ADULT — Monotherapy for locally advanced prostate cancer at a dose of 150 mg PO daily.

FORMS — Generic/Trade: Tabs 50 mg.

NOTES — Monitor PSA levels, CBC, ECG, serum testosterone, luteinizing hormone, and LFTs. Monitor glucose closely in diabetics. Displaces warfarin, possibly increasing anticoagulant effects. Gynecomastia and breast pain occur. Avoid concomitant use with tolvaptan.

MOA — Anti-androgen.

ADVERSE EFFECTS — Serious: Hypersensitivity, hepatotoxicity, chest pain, hypertension, angioedema, urticaria, interstitial lung disease, photosensitivity. Frequent: Gynecomastia, breast pain, hot flashes, general pain, impotence, anemia.

CYPROTERONE (✱*Androcur*) ▶L ♀X ▶– $ varies by therapy

ADULT — Prostate cancer.

PEDS — Not approved in children.

FORMS — Generic/Trade: Tabs 50 mg.

NOTES — Dose-related hepatotoxicity has occurred, monitor LFTs at initiation and during treatment. Monitor adrenocortical function periodically. May impair carbohydrate metabolism; monitor blood glucose, especially in diabetics.

MOA — Antiandrogen.

ADVERSE EFFECTS — Serious: Hepatotoxicity, thromboembolism, depression. Frequent: Decreased libido, gynecomastia, impotence, abnormal spermatozoa.

DEGARELIX (✱*Firmagon*) ▶LK ♀X ▶– $$$$$

WARNING — QT prolongation.

ADULT — Advanced prostate cancer: Initial dose: 240 mg SC; maintenance: 80 mg SC q 28 days.

PEDS — Not approved in children.

FORMS — Trade only: 80 mg, 120 mg soln for SC injection.

NOTES — Monitor LFTs and PSA. May prolong QT interval. May decrease bone mineral density.

MOA — Gonadotropin-releasing hormone antagonist that suppresses LH and FSH secretion thus lowering serum testosterone.

ADVERSE EFFECTS — Serious: Allergic reactions, hypersensitivity reactions including rash and uticaria, hepatotoxicity, QT prolongation. Frequent: Hot flashes, wt gain, increased LFTs, night sweats.

ENZALUTAMIDE (✱*XTANDI*) ▶L ♀X ▶–

WARNING — Seizure occurred in 0.9% of patients receiving Xtandi. There is no clinical trial experience with Xtandi in patients who have had a seizure, in patients with predisposing factors for seizure, or in patients using concomitant medications that may lower the seizure threshold. Posterior reversible encephalopathy syndrome (PRES) is potentially associated with the use of enzalutamide.

ADULT — First-line treatment of metastatic castration-resistant prostate cancer (mCRPC). 160 mg PO once daily.

PEDS — Not approved in children.

FORMS — 40 mg capsules.

NOTES — Enzalutamide is a strong CYP3A4 inducer and a moderate CYP2C9 and CYP2C19 inducer. At steady state, Xtandi reduced the plasma

(cont.)

ENZALUTAMIDE (*cont.*)

exposure to midazolam (a CYP3A4 substrate), warfarin (a CYP2C9 substrate), and omeprazole (a CYP2C19 substrate) by 86%, 56%, and 70%, respectively. Therefore, concomitant use of Xtandi with narrow therapeutic index drugs that are metabolized by CYP3A4, CYP2C9, or CYP2C19 should be avoided. If coadministration with warfarin (a CYP2C9 substrate) is unavoidable, conduct additional INR monitoring. The concomitant use of strong CYP2C8 inhibitors (gemfibrozil) should be avoided.

MOA — Androgen receptor inhibitor that targets steps in the androgen receptor signaling pathway.

ADVERSE EFFECTS — Asthenia/fatigue, back pain, diarrhea, arthralgia, hot flush, peripheral edema, musculoskeletal pain, headache, upper respiratory infection, muscular weakness, dizziness, insomnia, lower respiratory infection, spinal cord compression and cauda equina syndrome, hematuria, paresthesia, anxiety, and hypertension.

ESTRAMUSTINE (✱*Emcyt*) ▶L ♀X ▶– $ varies by therapy

WARNING — Thrombosis, including MI, glucose intolerance, HTN, fluid retention, increased LFTs, alopecia.

ADULT — Chemotherapy doses vary by indication. Hormone-refractory prostate cancer.

PEDS — Not approved in children.

FORMS — Trade only: Caps 140 mg.

NOTES — Reliable contraception is recommended. Monitor LFTs, glucose, and BP. Milk, milk products, and calcium-rich foods or drugs may impair absorption.

MOA — Alkylating agent.

ADVERSE EFFECTS — Serious: Thrombosis, MI, glucose intolerance, HTN, fluid retention. Frequent: None.

EXEMESTANE (✱*Aromasin*) ▶L ♀D ▶– $ varies by therapy

WARNING — Lymphocytopenia, alopecia, osteoporosis.

ADULT — Chemotherapy doses vary by indication. Breast cancer.

PEDS — Not approved in children.

UNAPPROVED ADULT — Chemotherapy doses vary by indication. Prevention of prostate cancer.

FORMS — Generic/Trade: Tabs 25 mg.

NOTES — Contraindicated in premenopausal women. Reliable contraception is recommended. Monitor CBCs.

MOA — Aromatase inhibitor.

ADVERSE EFFECTS — Serious: Lymphocytopenia. hypersensitivity, urticaria, and pruritis. Frequent: Lymphocytopenia, nausea, hot flashes. Post-marketing Experience: paresthesia, cholestatic hepatitis, and acute generalized exanthematous pustulosis.

FLUTAMIDE (✱*Euflex*) ▶L ♀D ▶– $ varies by therapy

WARNING — Hepatic failure, methemoglobinemia, hemolytic anemia, breast neoplasms, gynecomastia, fertility impairment, photosensitivity, alopecia.

ADULT — Prostate cancer: 250 mg PO q 8 h in combination with an LHRH analog (eg, goserelin or leuprolide). Not indicated in women.

PEDS — Not approved in children.

UNAPPROVED ADULT — Hirsutism in women.

FORMS — Generic only: Caps 125 mg.

NOTES — Monitor LFTs, PSA, methemoglobin levels. Transient urine discoloration (amber or yellow-green). Avoid exposure to sunlight/use sunscreen. Increased INR with warfarin. Gynecomastia and breast pain occur.

MOA — Anti-androgen.

ADVERSE EFFECTS — Serious: Hepatic failure, methemoglobinemia, hemolytic anemia. Frequent: Gynecomastia, urine discoloration, hot flashes, diarrhea, photosensitivity, impotence.

FULVESTRANT (✱*Faslodex*) ▶L ♀D ▶– $ varies by therapy

WARNING — Contraindicated in pregnancy. Hypersensitivity, N/V/D, constipation, abdominal pain, hot flashes. Use with caution in patients with bleeding disorders. Hepatic impairment may require dose adjustment. Elevation of bilirubin, elevation of gamma GT, hepatitis, and liver failure have been reported infrequently (less than 1%). Injection site related neurological events may occur due to proximity of the underlying sciatic nerve.

ADULT — Chemotherapy doses vary by indication. 500 mg IM on days 1, 15, and 29, then 500 mg monthly thereafter. Treatment of metastatic breast cancer in postmenopausal women. Treatment of HR-positive, human epidermal growth factor receptor 2 (HER2)-negative advanced or metastatic breast cancer in combination with palbociclib in women with disease progression after endocrine therapy.

PEDS — Not approved in children.

FORMS — 250 mg/5 mL soln for IM injection.

NOTES — Reliable contraception is recommended. FDA approved only in hormone receptor–positive metastatic breast cancer in postmenopausal women with disease progression following antiestrogen therapy.

MOA — Estrogen receptor antagonist.

ADVERSE EFFECTS — Serious: Hypersensitivity, increased LFTs. Frequent: N/V, diarrhea, abdominal pain, hot flashes, joint disorders.

GOSERELIN (✱*Zoladex*) ▶LK ♀D/X ▶– $ varies by therapy

WARNING — Transient increases in sex hormones, increases in lipids, hypercalcemia, decreases in bone mineral density, vaginal bleeding, fertility impairment, hot flashes, decreased libido, alopecia.

ADULT — Prostate cancer: 3.6 mg implant SC into upper abdominal wall q 28 days, or 10.8 mg implant SC q 12 weeks. Endometriosis: 3.6 mg implant SC q 28 days or 10.8 mg implant q 12 weeks for 6 months. Specialized dosing for breast cancer.

PEDS — Not approved in children.

UNAPPROVED ADULT — Adjuvant prostate cancer. Palliative treatment of breast cancer: 3.6 mg implant SC q 28 days indefinitely. Endometrial

GOSERELIN (*cont.*)

thinning prior to ablation for dysfunctional uterine bleeding: 3.6 mg SC 4 weeks prior to surgery or 3.6 mg SC q 4 weeks for 2 doses with surgery 2 to 4 weeks after last dose.

FORMS — Trade only: Implants 3.6, 10.8 mg.

NOTES — Transient increases in testosterone and estrogen occur. Hypercalcemia may occur in patients with bone metastases. Vaginal bleeding may occur during the 1st 2 months of treatment and should stop spontaneously. Reliable contraception is recommended. Consider norethindrone as "add back" therapy to decrease bone loss (see norethindrone).

MOA — Gonadotropin inhibitor.

ADVERSE EFFECTS — Serious: Hypersensitivity, anaphylaxis, antibody formation, pituitary apoplexy, osteoporosis, decreased bone mineral density, angina, thromboembolism, heart failure, hypercalcemia. Injection site injury resulting in hematoma, hemorrhage, or vascular injury. Frequent: Decrease in bone mineral density, vaginal bleeding, hot flashes, gynecomastia, transient worsening of pain. Observed post-marketing: mood swings, acne, convulsions.

HISTRELIN (*Vantas, Supprelin LA, ✱Vantas*) ▶Not metabolized ♀X ▶– $ varies by therapy

WARNING — Worsening of symptoms, especially during the 1st weeks of therapy: Increase in bone pain, difficulty urinating. Decreases in bone mineral density. Increased risk of cardiovascular disease and diabetes in men with prostate cancer.

ADULT — Palliative treatment of advanced prostate cancer (Vantas): Insert 1 implant SC in the upper arm surgically q 12 months. May repeat if appropriate after 12 months.

PEDS — Central precocious puberty (Supprelin LA), in age older than 2 yo: Insert 1 implant SC in the inner upper arm surgically. May repeat if appropriate after 12 months.

FORMS — Trade only: 50 mg implant.

NOTES — Causes transient increase of testosterone level during the 1st weeks of treatment, which may create or exacerbate symptoms. Patients with metastatic vertebral lesions and/or urinary tract obstruction should be closely observed during the 1st few weeks of therapy. Avoid wetting arm for 24 h after implant insertion and from heavy lifting or strenuous exertion of the involved arm for 7 days after insertion. Measure testosterone levels and PSA periodically. May decrease bone density. Monitor LH, FSH, estradiol or testosterone, height, and bone age in children with central precocious puberty at 1 month post implantation and q 6 months thereafter.

MOA — Gonadotropin releasing hormone agonist

ADVERSE EFFECTS — Serious: Bladder outlet obstruction, hematuria, bone pain, neuropathy, spinal cord compression, seizures. Frequent: Implant site reaction, erectile dysfunction, gynecomastia, hot flashes, testicular atrophy, transient worsening of pain.

LANREOTIDE—ONCOLOGY (*Somatuline Depot*) ▶bile ♀C ▶–

WARNING — Gallbladder: Gallstones may occur; consider periodic monitoring. Glucose metabolism: Hypo- and/or hyperglycemia may occur. Glucose monitoring is recommended and antidiabetic treatment adjusted accordingly. Cardiac function: Decrease in heart rate may occur. Use with caution in at-risk patients.

ADULT — 120 mg administered by deep SC injection q 28 days for treatment of patients with unresectable, well or moderately differentiated, locally advanced or metastatic gastroenteropancreatic neuroendocrine tumors (GEP-NETs).

FORMS — Injection: 60 mg/0.2 mL, 90 mg/0.3 mL, and 120 mg/0.5 mL single-use prefilled syringes.

NOTES — May decrease the bioavailability of cyclosporine.

MOA — Synthetic analog of somatostatin which is a peptide inhibitor of multiple endocrine, neuroendocrine and exocrine mechanisms. Reduces growth hormone secretion and also reduces the levels of insulin-like growth factor 1.

ADVERSE EFFECTS — The most commonly (greater than or equal to 10%) reported adverse reactions: abdominal pain, musculoskeletal pain, vomiting, headache, injection site reaction, hyperglycemia, hypertension, and cholelithiasis.

LETROZOLE (*Femara*) ▶LK ♀D ▶– $$$

WARNING — Fertility impairment, decreases in lymphocytes, increased LFTs, alopecia.

ADULT — 2.5 mg PO daily. Adjuvant treatment of postmenopausal, hormone receptor–positive, early breast cancer. Extended adjuvant treatment of early breast cancer after 5 years of tamoxifen therapy. Advanced breast cancer with disease progression after antiestrogen therapy, hormone receptor–positive or hormone receptorunknown, locally advanced, or metastatic breast cancer.

PEDS — Not approved in children.

UNAPPROVED ADULT — Ovarian (epithelial) cancer, endometrial cancer.

FORMS — Generic/Trade: Tabs 2.5 mg.

NOTES — Reliable contraception is recommended. Monitor CBCs, LFTs, and lipids.

MOA — Aromatase inhibitor.

ADVERSE EFFECTS — Serious: Lymphocytopenia, angioedema, anaphylaxis, toxic epidermal necrolysis, erythema multiforme, and hepatitis. Frequent: Lymphocytopenia, nausea, hot flashes, bone pain, fatigue, dizziness, increased cholesterol, decreased bone mineral density. Possible: carpal tunnel syndrome and trigger finger.

MEDROXYPROGESTERONE-ONCOLOGY (*Provera, Depo-Provera*) ▶L Hydroxylation, conjugation. ♀X Oral product contraindicated in pregnancy. Inadvertent use of Depo-Provera during early pregnancy, in general does not cause increased risk of birth defects. ▶? Oral product not recommended during breast feeding,Injectable product can be

(cont.)

MEDROXYPROGESTERONE-ONCOLOGY (*cont.*)

initiated immediately post-partum in nursing women.

WARNING — Adrenal suppression, loss of bone mineral density with prolonged use, increased risk of invasive breast cancer in postmenopausal women also using conjugated estrogens, increased risk of probable dementia in women 65 or over also using conjugated estrogens, ectopic pregnancy, endometrial cancer, hypertriglyceridemia, ovarian cancer, retinal vascular thrombosis, vaginal bleeding, weight gain.

ADULT — Endometrial carcinoma, recurrent or metastatic. 400mg to 1000mg/week IM. 200mg to 400mg orally daily.

FORMS — Intramuscular suspension 150mg/ml. 2.5mg, 5mg, 10mg tablets.

MOA — Suppress new growth of endometrial tissue, leading to atrophy.

ADVERSE EFFECTS — Most frequent : headache, nervousness, amenorrhea, abdominal pain.

NILUTAMIDE (*Nilandron*, ✲*Anandron®*) ▶L ♀C ▶– $$$$$

WARNING — Interstitial pneumonitis, hepatitis, aplastic anemia (isolated cases), delay in adaptation to the dark, hot flashes, alcohol intolerance, alopecia.

ADULT — Prostate cancer: 300 mg PO daily for 30 days, then 150 mg PO daily. Begin therapy on same day as surgical castration.

PEDS — Not approved in children.

FORMS — Generic/Trade: Tabs 150 mg.

NOTES — Monitor CBCs, LFTs, and chest X-rays. Caution patients who experience delayed adaptation to the dark about driving at night or through tunnels; suggest wearing tinted glasses. May increase phenytoin and theophylline levels. Avoid alcohol.

MOA — Anti-androgen.

ADVERSE EFFECTS — Serious: Interstitial pneumonitis, hepatitis, aplastic anemia. Frequent: Delay in adaptation to the dark, hot flashes, gynecomastia, alcohol intolerance, alopecia.

TOREMIFENE (✲*Fareston*) ▶L ♀D ▶– $ varies by therapy

WARNING — QT prolongation that is dose, and concentration-dependent. Use is contraindicated in the presence of uncorrected hypokalemia or hypomagnesemia. Hypercalcemia and tumor flare, endometrial hyperplasia, thromboembolism, hot flashes, nausea, increased LFTs, vaginal bleeding, fertility impairment, rare myelosuppression, alopecia.

ADULT — Chemotherapy doses vary by indication. Breast cancer.

PEDS — Not approved in children.

UNAPPROVED ADULT — Treatment of soft tissue sarcoma.

FORMS — Trade only: Tabs 60 mg.

NOTES — Avoid concurrent use with strong CYP3A4 inhibitors and QTc-prolonging agents. Reliable contraception is recommended. Monitor CBCs, calcium levels, and LFTs. May increase effects of anticoagulants.

MOA — Selective estrogen receptor modulator.

ADVERSE EFFECTS — Serious: DVT/PE, endometrial cancer, visual disturbances, cataracts, hypercalcemia, tumor flare, hepatotoxicity. Frequent: Hot flashes, vaginal bleeding.

TRIPTORELIN (*Trelstar*) ▶tissues – ? ♀X ▶–

WARNING — Anaphylactic shock, hypersensitivity, and angioedema have been reported. Tumor flare: Transient increase in serum testosterone levels can occur within the 1st few weeks of treatment. This may worsen prostate cancer and result in spinal cord compression and urinary tract obstruction.

ADULT — Palliative treatment of advanced prostate cancer. Administered as a single IM injection: 3.75 mg q 4 weeks. 11.25 mg q 12 weeks. 22.5 mg q 24 weeks.

PEDS — Not indicated in children.

FORMS — Injectable susp: 3.75 mg, 11.25 mg, 22.5 mg.

NOTES — $ - varies by therapy

MOA — Agonist analog of gonadotropin releasing hormone

ADVERSE EFFECTS — Hot flushes, skeletal pain, impotence, and headache, erectile dysfunction, testicular atrophy, convulsions.

TRIPTORELIN (*Trelstar Depot*, ✲*Decapeptyl, Trelstar*) ▶LK ♀X ▶– $ varies by therapy

WARNING — Transient increases in sex hormones, bone pain, neuropathy, hematuria, urethral/bladder outlet obstruction, spinal cord compression, anaphylaxis, hot flashes, impotence, alopecia. Long-term androgen deprivation therapy may prolong QTc interval.

ADULT — Chemotherapy doses vary by indication. Prostate cancer.

PEDS — Not approved in children.

MOA — Gonadotropin inhibitor.

ADVERSE EFFECTS — Serious: Bone pain, neuropathy, hematuria, urethral/bladder outlet obstruction, spinal cord compression, anaphylaxis, convulsions. Frequent: Transient worsening of symptoms, hot flashes, impotence.

ONCOLOGY: Immunomodulators

TEMSIROLIMUS (✲*Torisel*) ▶L ♀C ▶– $ varies by therapy

WARNING — Hypersensitivity, interstitial lung disease, bowel perforation, renal failure, hyperglycemia, bone marrow suppression. Avoid live vaccines. Postmarketing experience: Pancreatitis, cholecystitis,

and cholelithiasis. The levels of temsirolimus may be increased when used with CYP3A4 inhibitors.

ADULT — Chemotherapy doses vary by indication. Advanced renal cell carcinoma.

PEDS — Not approved in children.

(cont.)

TEMSIROLIMUS *(cont.)*

UNAPPROVED ADULT — Relapsed or refractory mantle cell lymphoma.

FORMS — 25 mg/mL soln for injection.

NOTES — Reliable contraception is recommended. Drugs that induce the CYP3A4 system such as phenytoin, phenobarbital, rifampin may decrease concentrations. Inhibitors such as clarithromycin, itraconazole, ketoconazole, and ritonavir may increase concentrations. Avoid live vaccines. Monitor CBC, hepatic, and renal function, glucose and lipid profile. Premedicate with an H1 antagonist 30 minutes prior to infusion to prevent infusion reactions.

MOA — Targeted inhibitor of mTOR (mammalian target of rapamycin) kinase activity, halting the cell cycle at the G1 phase in tumor cells. Also reduces levels of HIF-1 (hypoxia inducible factor) and HIF-2 alpha, and VEGF (vascular endothelial growth factor) thus exhibiting angiogenic activity in renal cell carcinoma.

ADVERSE EFFECTS — Serious: Hypersensitivity, interstitial lung disease, bowel perforation, renal failure, bone marrow suppression. Frequent: Hyperglycemia, hypertriglyceridemia, rash, mucositis, anorexia, N/V.

SIDE EFFECTS — Edema, pain, rash, mucositis, myelosuppression, weakness, hepatic and renal impairment, infection.

ALDESLEUKIN *(interleukin-2, ✦Proleukin)* ▶K ♀C ▶– $ varies by therapy

WARNING — Capillary leak syndrome, resulting in hypotension and reduced organ perfusion. Exacerbation of autoimmune diseases and symptoms of CNS metastases, impaired neutrophil function, hepato/nephrotoxicity, mental status changes, decreased thyroid function, anemia, thrombocytopenia, fertility impairment, alopecia.

ADULT — Chemotherapy doses vary by indication. Renal-cell carcinoma.

PEDS — Not approved in children.

UNAPPROVED ADULT — Kaposi's sarcoma, metastatic melanoma, colorectal cancer, non-Hodgkin's lymphoma.

NOTES — Monitor CBCs, electrolytes, LFTs, renal function, and chest X-rays. Baseline PFTs. Avoid iodinated contrast media. Antihypertensives potentiate hypotension.

MOA — Aldesleukin stimulates a cytokine cascade involving various interferons, interleukins, and tumor necrosis factors, which induces the proliferation and differentiation of B and T-cells, monocytes, macrophages, natural killer cells, and other cytotoxic cells.

ADVERSE EFFECTS — Serious: Capillary leak syndrome, resulting in hypotension and reduced organ perfusion. Exacerbation of autoimmune diseases and of symptoms of CNS metastases, immunosuppression, hepato/nephrotoxicity, decreased thyroid function, anemia, thrombocytopenia. Frequent: Hypotension, tachycardia, mental status changes, anemia, thrombocytopenia, N/V, fever, chills, rigors, pruritus.

BCG VACCINE FOR BLADDER INSTILLATION—ONCOLOGY *(Bacillus of Calmette & Guerin, Pacis, TheraCys, Tice BCG, ✦OncoTICE, ImmuCyst)* ▶Not metabolized ♀C ▶? $ varies by therapy

WARNING — Hypersensitivity, hematuria, urinary frequency, dysuria, bacterial UTI, flu-like syndrome, alopecia.

ADULT — Chemotherapy doses vary by indication. Carcinoma in situ of the urinary bladder, intravesical.

PEDS — Not approved in children.

NOTES — Bone marrow depressants, immunosuppressants and antimicrobial therapy may impair response. Increase fluid intake after treatments.

MOA — BCG is an immunostimulant used to stimulate the immune system to produce immunity against tuberculosis or to mount a local inflammation and immune reaction against superficial cancers from the activation of T-lymphocytes, B-lymphocytes, and natural killer cells.

ADVERSE EFFECTS — Serious: Hypersensitivity, hematuria, urinary frequency, dysuria, bacterial urinary tract infection. Frequent: Flu-like syndrome.

EVEROLIMUS—ONCOLOGY *(Afinitor, Afinitor Disperz)* ▶L ♀D ▶– $$$$$

WARNING — Noninfectious pneumonitis, hyperglycemia, bone marrow suppression. Avoid live vaccines. Angioedema with concomitant use of angiotensin-converting enzyme (ACE) inhibitors, pulmonary hypertension.

ADULT — Chemotherapy doses vary by indication. Advanced renal cell carcinoma. Progressive neuroendocrine tumors of pancreatic origin (PNET) in patients with unresectable, locally advanced, or metastatic disease. Subependymal giant cell astrocytoma (SEGA) associated with tuberous sclerosis. Renal angiomyolipoma associated with tuberous sclerosis complex (TSC), who do not require immediate surgery. Treatment of postmenopausal women with advanced hormone receptor–positive, HER2-negative breast cancer in combination with exemestane, after failure of treatment with letrozole or anastrozole. Treatment of adult patients with progressive, well-differentiated non-functional, neuroendocrine tumors (NET) of gastrointestinal (GI) or lung origin with unresectable, locally advanced or metastatic disease.

PEDS — Everolimus tabs for oral susp (Afinitor Disperz) for the treatment of pediatric and adult patients with tuberous sclerosis complex (TSC) who have subependymal giant cell astrocytoma (SEGA) that requires therapeutic intervention but cannot be curatively resected. Dosing for adult and pediatric patients with SEGA is 4.5 mg/m^2/day, with subsequent dosing based on therapeutic drug monitoring to achieve and maintain everolimus trough levels of 5 to 15 ng/mL.

UNAPPROVED ADULT — Treatment of relapsed or refractory Waldenstrom's macroglobulinemia (WM). Carcinoid tumors (progressive, advanced).

(cont.)

EVEROLIMUS (*cont.*)

FORMS — Afinitor: 2.5, 5, 7.5, and 10 mg tabs. Afinitor Disperz (everolimus tabs for oral susp): 2, 3, and 5 mg tabs for oral susp.

NOTES — Reliable contraception is recommended. Drugs that induce the CYP3A4 system such as phenytoin, phenobarbital, and rifampin may decrease concentrations. Inhibitors such as clarithromycin, itraconazole, ketoconazole, and ritonavir may increase concentrations. Avoid live vaccines. Monitor CBC, hepatic and renal function, glucose and lipid profile. Increased risk of proteinuria when used in combination with cyclosporine.

MOA — m-TOR inhibitor. Reduces protein synthesis and cellular proliferation by binding to the intracellular protein, FK binding protein-12, to form a complex that inhibits activation of m-TOR (mammalian target of rapamycin.)

ADVERSE EFFECTS — Serious: Immunosuppressant properties leading to serious infection, and development of malignancy including lymphoma and skin cancer and advanced RCC. Noninfectious pneumonitis, bone marrow suppression. Acute pancreatitis, impaired wound healing. Frequent: Hyperglycemia, hypertriglyceridemia, rash, mucositis, stomatitis, N/V. Opportunistic infection such as pneumocystis jiroveci pneumonia (PJP) may occur. Postmarketing Experience: cholecystitis, cholelithiasis, arterial thrombotic events and reflex sympathetic dystrophy, gingivitis, angioedema, heart failure.

INTERFERON ALFA-2A (*Roferon-A*) ▶Plasma ♀C ▮– $ varies by therapy

WARNING — GI hemorrhage, CNS reactions, leukopenia, increased LFTs, anemia, neutralizing antibodies, depression/suicidal behavior, alopecia.

ADULT — Discontinued by manufacturer February 2008. Chemotherapy doses vary by indication. Hairy cell leukemia, AIDS-related Kaposi's sarcoma, CML.

PEDS — Not approved in children.

UNAPPROVED ADULT — Superficial bladder tumors, carcinoid tumor, cutaneous T-cell lymphoma, essential thrombocythemia, non-Hodgkin's lymphoma.

NOTES — Reliable contraception is recommended. Monitor CBCs and LFTs. Hydration important. Decreases clearance of theophylline.

MOA — Interferons exert their cellular activities by binding to specific membrane receptors on the cell surface. Once bound to the cell membrane, interferons initiate a complex sequence of intracellular events. In vitro studies demonstrated that these include the induction of certain enzymes, suppression of cell proliferation, immunomodulating activities such as enhancement of the phagocytic activity of macrophages and augmentation of the specific cytotoxicity of lymphocytes for target cells, and inhibition of virus replication in virus-infected cells.

ADVERSE EFFECTS — Serious: Depression/suicidal behavior, GI hemorrhage, CNS reactions, leukopenia, increased LFTs, anemia. Frequent: Rash, N/V, diarrhea, flu-like syndrome.

LENALIDOMIDE (✱*Revlimid*) ▶K ♀X ▮– $ varies by therapy

WARNING — Potential for human birth defects, potential for an increased risk of developing secondary malignancies, bone marrow suppression, DVT, and PE. Instruct patients to report promptly fever, sore throat, signs of local infection, bleeding from any site, or symptoms suggestive of anemia. Increased mortality seen in patients with CLL.

ADULT — Chemotherapy doses vary by indication. Myelodysplastic syndromes in patients with deletion 5q and transfusion-dependent anemia (with or without cytogenetic abnormalities.) Multiple myeloma in combination with dexamethasone in patients who have received at least one prior therapy. Mantle cell lymphoma patients whose disease has relapsed or progressed after two prior therapies, one of which included bortezomib.

PEDS — Not approved in children.

FORMS — Trade only: Caps 5, 10, 15, 25 mg.

NOTES — Analog of thalidomide; can cause birth defects or fetal death. Lenalidomide, a thalidomide analogue, caused limb abnormalities in a developmental monkey study similar to birth defects caused by thalidomide in humans. If lenalidomide is used during pregnancy, it may cause birth defects or death to a developing baby. Pregnancy must be excluded before start of treatment. Prevent pregnancy during treatment by the use of two reliable methods of contraception. Available only through a restricted distribution program. Reliable contraception is mandated; males must use a latex condom. Monitor CBCs. Do not break, chew, or open the caps. Adjust dose for CrCl <60 mL/min.

MOA — Immunomodulator and angiogenesis inhibitor.

ADVERSE EFFECTS — Serious: Potential for birth defects, neutropenia and thrombocytopenia, DVT/PE. Frequent: Bone marrow suppression, diarrhea, pruritus, rash, fatigue. Tasigna prolongs the QT interval. Prior to Tasigna administration and periodically, monitor for hypokalemia or hypomagnesemia and correct deficiencies Obtain ECGs to monitor the QTc at baseline, seven days after initiation, and periodically thereafter, and follow any dose adjustments

PEGINTERFERON ALFA-2B (*Sylatron*) ▶K ♀–C ▮?

WARNING — May cause or aggravate severe depression. Suicide or suicidal ideation.

ADULT — Sylatron brand indicated for adjuvant treatment of melanoma. 6 mcg/kg/week SC for 8 doses, followed by 3 mg/kg/week up to 5 years.

PEDS — No approved oncology indication in children.

FORMS — Powder for injection. 200 mcg, 300 mcg, 600 mcg vials.

NOTES — None

MOA — Inhibits cellular growth, alters the state of cellular differentiation, interferes with oncogene expression, alters cell surface antigen expression, increases phagocytic activity of macrophages, and

(cont.)

PEGINTERFERON ALFA-2B (*cont.*)

augments cytotoxicity of lymphocytes for target cells.

ADVERSE EFFECTS — Serious: Bone marrow suppression, colitis, acute hypersensitivity reactions, hypertriglyceridemia, pulmonary fibrosis. Common: fatigue, fever, headache, depression, rash, anorexia, nausea and vomiting, myalgias.

POMALIDOMIDE (✱*Pomalyst*) ▶L - ♀X ▶– $$$$$

WARNING — Pomalidomide should not be used in pregnant women, because it can cause severe life-threatening birth defects and can cause blood clots.

ADULT — The treatment of multiple myeloma, in combination with dexamethasone, for patients who have received at least 2 prior therapies, including lenalidomide and a proteasome inhibitor, and whose disease did not respond to treatment and progressed within 60 days of the last treatment. 4 mg per day taken orally on days 1 through 21 of repeated 28-day cycles until disease progression.

PEDS — Not approved in children.

FORMS — Capsules: 1, 2, 3, and 4 mg.

NOTES — Avoid concomitant use of strong CYP1A2 inhibitors. If concomitant use cannot be avoided in the presence of strong CYP3A4 or P-gp inhibitors, then pomalidomide dose must be reduced by 50%.

MOA — Inhibits proliferation and induces apoptosis of hematopoietic tumor cells. Inhibits the proliferation of lenalidomide-resistant multiple myeloma cell lines and synergized with dexamethasone in both lenalidomide-sensitive and lenalidomide-resistant cell lines to induce tumor cell apoptosis. Pomalidomide enhanced T cell- and natural killer (NK) cell-mediated immunity and inhibited production of pro-inflammatory cytokines (e.g., TNF-α and IL-6) by monocytes. Pomalidomide demonstrated anti-angiogenic activity in a mouse tumor model and in the in vitro umbilical cord mode

ADVERSE EFFECTS — Severe: embryo-fetal toxicity, venous thromboembolism, angioedema. Common adverse effects include neutropenia, fatigue and weakness, anemia, constipation, diarrhea, thrombocytopenia, upper respiratory tract infections, back pain, and fever.

SIPULEUCEL-T (*Provenge*) ▶?

WARNING — Acute infusion reactions may occur within 1 day of infusion. Cerebrovascular events, including hemorrhagic and ischemic strokes, were observed in clinical trials.

ADULT — Treatment of metastatic hormone-refractory prostate cancer in patients who are symptomatic or minimally symptomatic. Administer a total of 3 doses at 2-week intervals.

PEDS — Not approved in children.

FORMS — Infusion, premixed in preservative-free LR. Greater than 50 million autologous CD54+ cells activated with PAP-GM-CSF (250 mL).

NOTES — No pregnancy or lactation data. Not indicated for use in women. Premedication with oral acetaminophen and diphenhydramine is recommended to minimize infusion reactions.

MOA — Autologous cellular immunotherapy, designed to stimulate a patient's own immune system to respond against the cancer. Each dose of sipuleucel-T is manufactured by obtaining a patient's peripheral blood mononuclear cells, via leukapheresis. Antigen presenting cell precursors are isolated from these cells. To enhance their response against the cancer, these cells are then exposed to a recombinant human fusion protein, PAP-GM-CSF composed of an antigen specific for prostate cancer linked to prostatic acid phosphatase, and granulocyte-macrophage colony stimulating factor. After this process, the final product, sipuleucel-T, is reinfused into the patient to induce T-cell immunity towards the prostate cancer cells.

ADVERSE EFFECTS — Chills, fatigue, fever, back pain, nausea, joint ache and headache.

THALIDOMIDE (✱*Thalomid*) ▶Plasma ♀X ▶? $$$$$

WARNING — Pregnancy category X. Has caused severe, life-threatening human birth defects. Available only through special restricted distribution program. Prescribers and pharmacists must be registered in this program in order to prescribe or dispense. During therapy with thalidomide, patients with a history of seizures or with other risk factors for the development of seizures should be monitored closely for clinical changes that could precipitate acute seizure activity.

ADULT — Chemotherapy doses vary by indication. Multiple myeloma with dexamethasone. Erythema nodosum leprosum: 100 to 400 mg PO at bedtime. Use low end of dose range for initial episodes and if wt less than 50 kg.

PEDS — Not approved in children.

UNAPPROVED ADULT — Graft vs. host reactions after bone marrow transplant, Crohn's disease, Waldenstrom's macroglobulinemia, Langerhans cell histiocytosis, AIDS-related aphthous stomatitis.

UNAPPROVED PEDS — Clinical trials show beneficial effects when combined with dexamethasone in multiple myeloma.

FORMS — Trade only: Caps 50, 100, 150, 200 mg.

MOA — Immunomodulatory agent. Exact mechanism unknown.

ADVERSE EFFECTS — Serious: Birth defects, permanent peripheral neuropathy, bradycardia, Stevens-Johnson syndrome, toxic epidermal necrolysis. Increased risk of venous and arterial thromboembolic events. Frequent: Somnolence, drowsiness, dizziness, orthostatic hypotension, rash, leukopenia including thrombocytopenia.

ONCOLOGY: Mitotic Inhibitors

CABAZITAXEL (*Jevtana*) ▶L ♀–D ▶–
WARNING — Neutropenia, febrile neutropenia: Neutropenic deaths have been reported. Severe hypersensitivity reactions can occur. Mortality related to diarrhea has been reported. Renal failure, including cases with fatal outcomes, has been reported. Patients older than 65 yo were more likely to experience fatal outcomes not related to disease. Should not be given to patients with hepatic impairment. QTc interval prolongation. Interstitial pneumonia/pneumonitis, interstitial lung disease and acute respiratory distress syndrome .
ADULT — Indicated in combination with prednisone for treatment of patients with hormone-refractory metastatic prostate cancer previously treated with a docetaxel-containing treatment regimen. 25 mg/m^2 administered IV q 3 weeks in combination with oral prednisone 10 mg administered daily throughout treatment.
PEDS — Not indicated in children.
FORMS — Single-use vial 60 mg/1.5 mL, supplied with diluent (5.7 mL).
NOTES — Premedication regimen required 30 minutes before each dose: Antihistamine, corticosteroid (dexamethasone 8 mg or equivalent steroid) and H2 antagonist.
MOA — Microtubule inhibitor. Binds to tubulin and promotes its assembly into microtubules while simultaneously inhibiting disassembly. This leads to the stabilization of microtubules, which results in the inhibition of mitotic and interphase cellular functions
ADVERSE EFFECTS — Neutropenia, anemia, leukopenia, thrombocytopenia, diarrhea, fatigue, nausea, vomiting, constipation, asthenia, abdominal pain, hematuria, back pain, anorexia, peripheral neuropathy, pyrexia, dyspnea, dysgeusia, cough, arthralgia, and alopecia.

DOCETAXEL (*Docefrez*, *Taxotere*) ▶L ♀D ▶– $ varies by therapy
WARNING — Severe hypersensitivity with anaphylaxis, bone marrow suppression, fluid retention, neutropenia, rash, erythema of the extremities, nail hypo- or hyperpigmentation, hepatotoxicity, treatment-related mortality, paresthesia/dysesthesia, asthenia, fertility impairment, alopecia. Alopecia may be irreversible. Instruct patients to report promptly fever, sore throat, or signs of local infection. Treatment with docetaxel products may cause alcohol intoxication.
ADULT — Chemotherapy doses vary by indication. Breast cancer, non-small-cell lung cancer. Hormone-refractory, metastatic prostate cancer, advanced gastric adenocarcinoma with cisplatin and fluorouracil, squamous cell carcinoma of the head and neck with cisplatin and fluorouracil.
PEDS — Not approved in children.
UNAPPROVED ADULT — Gastric cancer, melanoma, non-Hodgkin's lymphoma ovarian cancer, pancreatic cancer, prostate cancer, small-cell lung cancer, soft-tissue sarcoma, urothelial cancer, adjuvant and neoadjuvant breast cancer.
FORMS — IV concentrate: 20, 80, 140, 160 mg vials.
NOTES — Reliable contraception is recommended. Monitor CBCs and LFTs. CYP3A4 inhibitors or substrates may lead to significant increases in blood concentrations.
MOA — Mitotic Inhibitor.
ADVERSE EFFECTS — Serious: Hypersensitivity/anaphylaxis, cutaneous events, edema, neutropenia, rash, erythema of the extremities, nail hypo- or hyperpigmentation, hepatotoxicity, paresthesia/dysesthesia. Respiratory: dyspnea, acute pulmonary edema, acute respiratory distress syndrome/pneumonitis, interstitial lung disease, interstitial pneumonia, respiratory failure, and pulmonary fibrosis have rarely been reported and may be associated with fatal outcome. Rare cases of radiation pneumonitis have been reported in patients receiving concomitant radiotherapy Frequent: Rash, N/V, diarrhea, bone marrow suppression. Cases of cystoid macular edema (CME) have been reported in patients treated with docetaxel, as well as with other taxanes.

ERIBULIN (*Halaven*) ▶feces – ♀D ▶–
WARNING — Dose reduction may be required in patients with hepatic impairment or renal impairment.
ADULT — Metastatic breast cancer in patients who have previously received at least two chemotherapeutic regimens for the treatment of metastatic disease. Prior therapy should have included an anthracycline and a taxane in either the adjuvant or metastatic setting. Treatment of patients with unresectable or metastatic liposarcoma who have received a prior anthracycline-containing regimen.
PEDS — Not approved in children.
FORMS — 1 mg/2 mL IV solution for injection.
NOTES — Dose is 1.4 mg/m^2 on days 1 and 8 q 21 days.
MOA — Inhibits formation of mitotic spindles; suppresses microtubule polymerization, but does not affect depolymerization.
ADVERSE EFFECTS — Neutropenia, peripheral neuropathy, QT interval prolongation. Pancreatitis. Fatigue, alopecia, nausea.

IXABEPILONE (*Ixempra*) ▶L ♀D ▶– $ varies by therapy
WARNING — Contraindicated in patients with AST or ALT greater than 2.5 ULN or bilirubin more than 1 times ULN upper limit of normal or higher. Contraindicated in patients with hypersensitivity reactions to products containing Cremophor EL (polyoxyethylated castor oil). Neutropenia. Instruct patients to report promptly fever, sore throat, signs of local infection or anemia. Peripheral neuropathy (sensory and motor) occurs commonly. Dose reductions, delays, or discontinuations may be necessary. Usually occurs during the 1st 3 cycles of treatment.

(cont.)

IXABEPILONE (*cont.*)

ADULT — Chemotherapy doses vary by indication. Metastatic or locally advanced breast cancer.
PEDS — Not approved in children.
FORMS — 15, 45 mg powder for injection.
NOTES — CYP450 inhibitors such as ketoconazole may increase concentration; inducers such as rifampin, phenytoin, or carbamazepine may reduce levels. Patients should receive an H1 and H2 blocker 1h prior to ixabepilone infusion to minimize hypersensitivity reactions. If patients experience such a reaction, they should also receive a corticosteroid prior to the next dose.
MOA — Mitotic Inhibitor.
ADVERSE EFFECTS — Serious: Anaphylaxis, bone marrow suppression, peripheral neuropathy, MI, ventricular dysfunction. Frequent: Bone marrow suppression, peripheral neuropathy, N/V/D, palmar-plantar erythrodysesthesia syndrome, myalgias.

PACLITAXEL (✳*Apo-Paclitaxel*) ▶L ♀D ▶– $ varies by therapy
WARNING — Anaphylaxis, fatal hypersensitivity reactions, bone marrow suppression, cardiac conduction abnormalities, peripheral neuropathy, fertility impairment, alopecia. Contraindicated in patients with hypersensitivity reactions to products containing Cremophor EL (polyoxyethylated castor oil). Instruct patients to report promptly fever, sore throat, signs of local infection or anemia, pneumonitis, cystoid macular edema. Sepsis and neutropenic sepsis have occurred in clinical trials.
ADULT — Chemotherapy doses vary by indication. Breast cancer, AIDS-related Kaposi sarcoma, non-small-cell lung cancer (NSCLC), and ovarian cancer.
PEDS — Not approved in children.
UNAPPROVED ADULT — Advanced head and neck cancer, small-cell lung cancer, adenocarcinoma of the upper GI tract, gastric, esophageal, and colon adenocarcinoma, hormone-refractory prostate cancer, non-Hodgkin's lymphoma, transitional cell carcinoma of the urothelium, adenocarcinoma or unknown primary, adjuvant and neoadjuvant breast cancer, uterine cancer, pancreatic cancer, polycystic kidney disease.
FORMS — 100 mg/16.7 mL, 30 mg/5 mL, 150 mg/25 mL, 300 mg/50 mL soln for injection.
NOTES — Reliable contraception is recommended. Monitor CBCs. Ketoconazole, felodipine, diazepam, and estradiol may increase paclitaxel.
MOA — Mitotic Inhibitor.
ADVERSE EFFECTS — Serious: Anaphylaxis, bone marrow suppression, cardiac conduction abnormalities, peripheral neuropathy. Frequent: Bone marrow suppression, peripheral neuropathy, hypotension, mucositis, N/V, atrioventricular block.

PACLITAXEL PROTEIN BOUND (*Abraxane*) ▶L ♀D ▶–
WARNING — Bone marrow suppression, primarily neutropenia may occur. Hypersensitivity reactions, neuropathy, vision disturbances, pneumonitis, sepsis.

ADULT — 100mg/m2 on Days 1,8, 15 of 21 day cycle for use in combination with carboplatin for the initial treatment of patients with locally advanced or metastatic non-small-cell lung cancer (NSCLC) who are not candidates for curative surgery or radiation therapy. 125mg/m2 on Days 1,8, 15 of 28 day cycle for metastatic adenocarcinoma of the pancreas when used in combination with gemcitabine. 260mg/m2 every 3 weeks for treatment of refractory (metastatic) or relapsed breast cancer after failure of combination therapy.
UNAPPROVED ADULT — Metastatic melanoma, recurrent ovarian, fallopian tube, or primary peritoneal cancer.
FORMS — 100mg vial for IV use.
MOA — Mitotic inhibitor.
ADVERSE EFFECTS — ECG abnormalities, peripheral sensory neuropathy, alopecia, dehydration, nausea, vomiting, diarrhea, anemia, neutropenia, increased LFTs, infection, neuromuscular and skeletal weakness, visual disturbances.

VINBLASTINE (*Velban, VLB*) ▶L ♀D ▶– $ varies by therapy
WARNING — Extravasation associated with severe necrosis. Leukopenia, fertility impairment, bronchospasm, alopecia. Instruct patients to report promptly fever, sore throat, or signs of local infection.
ADULT — Chemotherapy doses vary by indication. Hodgkin's disease, non-Hodgkin's lymphoma, histiocytic lymphoma, mycosis fungoides, advanced testicular carcinoma, Kaposi's sarcoma, Letterer-Siwe disease (histiocytosis X), choriocarcinoma, breast cancer.
PEDS — Not approved in children.
UNAPPROVED ADULT — NSCLC, renal cancer, CML.
NOTES — Reliable contraception is recommended. May decrease phenytoin levels. Erythromycin/drugs that inhibit CYP450 enzymes may increase toxicity.
MOA — Mitotic Inhibitor.
ADVERSE EFFECTS — Serious: Leukopenia, fertility impairment, bronchospasm. Frequent: Leukopenia, alopecia.

VINCRISTINE (*Oncovin, Vincasar, VCR*) ▶L ♀D ▶– $ varies by therapy
WARNING — Extravasation associated with severe necrosis. CNS toxicity, hypersensitivity, bone marrow suppression, hyperuricemia, bronchospasm, fertility impairment, alopecia. Instruct patients to report promptly fever, sore throat, signs of local infection, or anemia.
ADULT — Chemotherapy doses vary by indication. ALL, Hodgkin's disease, non-Hodgkin's lymphomas, rhabdomyosarcoma, neuroblastoma, Wilms' tumor. All in combination regimens.
PEDS — Chemotherapy doses vary by indication. Acute leukemia. Sarcoma, multiple myeloma.
UNAPPROVED ADULT — Idiopathic thrombocytopenic purpura, Kaposi's sarcoma, breast cancer, bladder cancer.

(cont.)

VINCRISTINE (*cont.*)

NOTES — Reliable contraception is recommended. Monitor CBCs. May decrease phenytoin and digoxin levels.

MOA — Mitotic Inhibitor.

ADVERSE EFFECTS — Serious: CNS toxicity, hypersensitivity, bone marrow suppression, uric acid nephropathy, bronchospasm. Frequent: Paresthesias, alopecia.

VINCRISTINE SULFATE LIPOSOME (*Marqibo*) ▶feces ♀–D ▶–

WARNING — For IV Use Only — Fatal if given by other routes. Death has occurred with intrathecal use. Vincristine sulfate liposome injection has different dosage recommendations than vincristine sulfate injection. Verify drug name and dose prior to preparation and administration to avoid overdosage.

ADULT — Treatment of Philadelphia chromosome-negative (Ph–) acute lymphoblastic leukemia (ALL) in 2nd or greater relapse or whose disease has progressed following two or more anti-leukemia therapies. 2.25 mg/m^2 weekly IV.

PEDS — Not approved in children.

FORMS — Marqibo Kit. Contains vincristine sulfate injection 5 mg/5 mL. Vial containing sphingomyelin/cholesterol liposome injection 103 mg/mL. Vial containing sodium phosphate injection.

MOA — Sphingomyelin/cholesterol liposome-encapsulated formulation of vincristine sulfate, an antimitotic agent.

ADVERSE EFFECTS — The most common adverse reactions: constipation, nausea, pyrexia, fatigue, peripheral neuropathy, febrile neutropenia, diarrhea, anemia, decreased appetite, and insomnia.

VINORELBINE (✱*Navelbine*) ▶L ♀D ▶– $ varies by therapy

WARNING — Extravasation associated with severe necrosis. Granulocytopenia, pulmonary toxicity, bronchospasm, peripheral neuropathy, increased LFTs, alopecia. Instruct patients to report promptly fever, sore throat, or signs of local infection.

ADULT — Chemotherapy doses vary by indication. NSCLC, alone or in combination regimens.

PEDS — Not approved in children.

UNAPPROVED ADULT — Breast cancer, cervical carcinoma, desmoid tumors, Kaposi's sarcoma, ovarian cancer, Hodgkin's disease, head and neck cancer.

NOTES — Reliable contraception is recommended. Monitor CBCs. Drugs that inhibit CYP450 enzymes may increase toxicity.

MOA — Mitotic Inhibitor.

ADVERSE EFFECTS — Serious: Granulocytopenia, pulmonary toxicity, bronchospasm, peripheral neuropathy, ileus. Frequent: Granulocytopenia, alopecia, peripheral neuropathy, N/V.

ONCOLOGY: Monoclonal Antibodies

ADO-TRASTUZUMAB EMTANSINE (✱ *Kadcyla*) ▶L ♀–D
Use of effective contraception is necessary during the 7-month washout period when pertuzumab is used in combination with trastuzumab. ▶– $$$$$

WARNING — Hepatotoxicity, cardiac toxicity: may result in left ventricular ejection fraction reductions, embryo-fetal toxicity. Cases of severe hemorrhagic events have been observed.

ADULT — Indicated as a single agent, for the treatment of patients with HER2-positive, metastatic breast cancer who previously received trastuzumab and a taxane, separately or in combination. Patients should have either received prior therapy for metastatic disease, or developed disease recurrence during or within 6 months of completing adjuvant therapy. 3.6 mg/kg given as an IV infusion q 3 weeks.

PEDS — Not approved in children.

FORMS — Lyophilized powder in single-use vials containing 100 mg per vial or 160 mg per vial.

NOTES — Administer Kadcyla as an IV infusion only with a 0.22 micron in-line polyethersulfone (PES) filter. Do not administer as an IV push or bolus. The reconstituted lyophilized vials should be used immediately following reconstitution with sterile water for injection. If not used immediately, the reconstituted Kadcyla vials can be stored for up to 24 h in a refrigerator at 2°C to 8°C (36°F to 46°F);

discard unused Kadcyla after 24 h. Do not freeze. The diluted Kadcyla infusion solution should be used immediately. If not used immediately, the solution may be stored in a refrigerator at 2°C to 8°C (36°F to 46°F) for up to 24 h prior to use. This storage time is additional to the time allowed for the reconstituted vials. Do not freeze or shake.

MOA — HER2-targeted antibody-drug conjugate. The antibody is the humanized anti-HER2 IgG1, trastuzumab. The small molecule cytotoxin, DM1, is a microtubule inhibitor.

ADVERSE EFFECTS — Common: fatigue, nausea, musculoskeletal pain, thrombocytopenia, headache, increased transaminases, and constipation.

ALEMTUZUMAB—ONCOLOGY (*Campath*, ✱*MabCampath*) ▶? ♀C ▶– $$$$$

WARNING — Idiopathic thrombocytopenic purpura, bone marrow suppression, hemolytic anemia, hypersensitivity, and immunosuppression.

ADULT — Chemotherapy doses vary by indication. B-cell chronic lymphocytic leukemia.

PEDS — Not approved in children.

FORMS — 30 mg/mL soln for injection.

NOTES — The Campath Distribution Program was developed to ensure continued access to Campath (alemtuzumab) for appropriate patients. Effective September 4, 2012 Campath was no longer available commercially, but is provided through

(cont.)

ALEMTUZUMAB—ONCOLOGY (*cont.*)

the Campath Distribution Program free of charge. In order to receive Campath, the healthcare provider is required to document and comply with certain requirements.

MOA — The exact mechanism of alemtuzumab is unknown; however, the proposed mechanism involves the binding of alemtuzumab to CD52, a nonmodulating antigen that is present on the surface of essentially all B and T lymphocytes, a majority of monocytes, macrophages, NK cells, and a subpopulation of granulocytes, causing an antibody-dependent lysis of leukemic cells.

ADVERSE EFFECTS — Serious: Idiopathic thrombocytopenic purpura, bone marrow suppression, hemolytic anemia, hypersensitivity, and immunosuppression. Frequent: Hypotension, rigors, fever, shortness of breath, bronchospasm, chills, rash, N/V.

ATEZOLIZUMAB (*Tecentriq*) ▶? ♀X Based on its mechanism of action, Atezolizumab can cause fetal harm. ▶– Because of the potential for serious adverse reactions in breastfed infants, advise a lactating woman not to breastfeed during treatment and for at least 5 months after the last dose.

WARNING — Immune-related pneumonitis: Withhold for moderate and permanently discontinue for severe or life-threatening pneumonitis. Immune-related hepatitis: Monitor for changes in liver function. Withhold for moderate and permanently discontinue for severe or life threatening transaminase or total bilirubin elevation. Immune-related colitis: Withhold for moderate or severe, and permanently discontinue for life-threatening colitis. Immune-related endocrinopathies: Hypophysitis: Withhold for moderate or severe and permanently discontinue for life-threatening hypophysitis. Thyroid Disorders: Monitor for changes in thyroid function. Withhold for symptomatic thyroid disease. Adrenal insufficiency: Withhold for symptomatic adrenal insufficiency. Type 1 diabetes mellitus: Withhold for ≥ Grade 3 hyperglycemia. Immune-related myasthenic syndrome/myasthenia gravis, GuillainBarré or meningoencephalitis: Permanently discontinue for any grade. Ocular inflammatory toxicity: Withhold for moderate and permanently discontinue for severe ocular inflammatory toxicity. Immune-related pancreatitis: Withhold for moderate or severe, and permanently discontinue for life-threatening pancreatitis, or any grade of recurring pancreatitis. Infection: Withhold for severe or life-threatening infection. Infusion reaction: Interrupt or slow the rate of infusion for mild or moderate infusion reactions and discontinue for severe or lifethreatening infusion reactions.

ADULT — 1200 mg administered as an intravenous infusion over 60 minutes every 3 weeks until disease progression or unacceptable toxicity for treatment of patients with locally advanced or metastatic urothelial carcinoma who have disease progression during or following platinum-containing chemotherapy or have disease progression within 12 months of neoadjuvant or adjuvant treatment with platinum-containing chemotherapy. Use in patients with metastatic non-small cell lung cancer (NSCLC) who have progressed during or after treatment with a platinum-based chemotherapy or appropriate targeted therapy.

FORMS — Injection: 1200 mg/20 mL (60 mg/mL) solution in a single-dose vial

MOA — Atezolizumab is a programmed death-ligand 1 (PD-L1) blocking antibody.

ADVERSE EFFECTS — The most common adverse reactions of atezolizumab (greater than or equal to 20% of patients) were fatigue, decreased appetite, nausea, urinary tract infection, pyrexia, and constipation. Grade 3-4 adverse events were seen in 50% of patients. Infection and immune-related adverse events such as pneumonitis, hepatitis, colitis, thyroid disease, adrenal insufficiency, diabetes, pancreatitis, and dermatitis/rash were also seen with atezolizumab.

BEVACIZUMAB (*Avastin*) ▶? ♀D embryo-fetal toxicity ▶– $ varies by therapy

WARNING — CVA, MI, TIA, angina, GI perforation, wound dehiscence, serious hemorrhage, HTN, heart failure, nephrotic syndrome, reversible posterior leukoencephalopathy syndrome (brain capillary leak syndrome), nasal septum perforation. Tracheoesophageal fistula has been reported. Microangiopathic hemolytic anemia (MAHA) in patients on concomitant sunitinib malate. Females of reproductive potential should be informed of increased reproductive failure. Increased risk of venous thromboembolic (VTE) and bleeding events in patients receiving anticoagulation therapy after 1st VTE event while receiving bevacizumab. May cause moderate to severe proteinuria.

ADULT — Chemotherapy doses vary by indication. Metastatic colorectal carcinoma; unresectable, locally advanced, recurrent or metastatic nonsquamous, NSCLC; glioblastoma; metastatic renal cell cancer. Use in combination with fluoropyrimidine-irinotecan or fluoropyrimidine-oxaliplatin based chemotherapy for the treatment of patients with metastatic colorectal cancer (mCRC) whose disease has progressed on a 1st-line bevacizumab-containing regimen; persistent, recurrent, or late-stage cervical cancer in combination with chemotherapy. In combination with paclitaxel, pegylated liposomal doxorubicin, or topotecan for the treatment of patients with platinum-resistant, recurrent epithelial ovarian, fallopian tube, or primary peritoneal cancer.

PEDS — Not approved in children.

UNAPPROVED ADULT — Metastatic breast cancer, recurrent ovarian cancer, recurrent cervical cancer, soft tissue sarcomas, age-related macular degeneration.

FORMS — 100 mg/4 mL, 400 mg/16 mL soln for injection.

(cont.)

BEVACIZUMAB (*cont.*)

NOTES — Monitor BP and UA for protein. Do not use in combination with sunitinib.

MOA — Bevacizumab is a humanized monoclonal antibody which binds the vascular endothelial growth factor (VEGF) preventing the interaction of VEGF to its receptors. In human cancers, VEGF expression is associated with increased microvascular density, tumor growth, metastasis, and poor prognosis.

ADVERSE EFFECTS — Serious: CVA, MI, TIA, angina, GI perforation, wound dehiscence, serious hemorrhage, HTN, heart failure, nephrotic syndrome, reversible posterior leukoencephalopathy syndrome (brain capillary leak syndrome), microangiopathic hemolytic anemia, nasal septum perforation. Osteonecrosis of the jaw without bisphosphonates. necrotizing fasciitis. nonmandibular osteonecrosis and posterior reversible encephalopathy syndrome (PRES). Possible renal injury. Frequent: Headache, HTN, stomatitis, constipation, diarrhea, abdominal pain, N/V, epistaxis, dyspnea, proteinuria.

BLINATUMOMAB (*Blincyto*) ▶? The metabolic pathway of blinatumomab has not been characterized. It is expected to be degraded into small peptides and amino acids via catabolic pathways. ♀C ▶?

WARNING — Cytokine release syndrome (CRS), which may be life-threatening or fatal, occurred in patients receiving Blincyto. Interrupt or discontinue Blincyto as recommended. Neurological toxicities, which may be severe, life-threatening, or fatal, occurred in patients receiving Blincyto. Interrupt or discontinue Blincyto as recommended.

ADULT — For patients weighing at least 45 kg, the recommended dose and schedule for blinatumomab is 9 mcg/day on days 1 to 7 and at 28 mcg/day on days 8 to 28 of the 1st 42-day cycle, and 28 mcg/day on days 1 to 28 in later cycles. For patients < 45kg: Cycle 1: 5mcg/m2/day (up to 9mcg/day) on days 1-7, followed by 15mcg/m2/day (up to 28mcg/day) on days 8 to 28. Cycles 2 through 5: 15mcg/m2/day (up to 28mcg/day) on days 1 to 28. Each treatment cycle consists of 4 weeks of continuous IV infusion followed by a 2 week treatment free interval. Therapy includes 2 induction cycles followed by 3 consolidation cycles. Philadelphia chromosome-negative relapsed or refractory B-cell precursor acute lymphoblastic leukemia (R/R ALL).

UNAPPROVED PEDS — Limited experience in pediatric patients.

FORMS — 35 mcg of lyophilized powder in a single-use vial for reconstitution.

NOTES — Hospitalization is recommended for the 1st 9 days of the 1st cycle and the 1st 2 days of the 2nd cycle. A single cycle of treatment consists of 4 weeks of continuous IV infusion followed by a 2-week treatment-free interval. Premedicate with dexamethasone 20 mg IV 1 h prior to the 1st dose of Blincyto of each cycle, prior to a step dose (eg, cycle 1, day 8), or when restarting an infusion after an interruption of 4 h or more. Administer as a continuous IV infusion at a constant flow rate using an infusion pump.

MOA — Blinatumomab is a bispecific CD19-directed CD3 T-cell engager that activates endogenous T cells when bound to the CD19-expressing target cell. Activation of the immune system results in release of inflammatory cytokines. Blinatumomab mediates the formation of a synapse between the T cell and the tumor cell,upregulation of cell adhesion molecules, production of cytolytic proteins, release of inflammatory cytokines, and proliferation of T cells, which result in redirected lysis of CD19+ cells.

ADVERSE EFFECTS — The most common adverse reactions (≥ 20%) were pyrexia, headache, peripheral edema, febrile neutropenia, nausea, hypokalemia, tremor, rash,and constipation.

BRENTUXIMAB VEDOTIN (*Adcetris*) ▶oxidation – feces ♀D ▶–

WARNING — Peripheral motor neuropathy, infusion reactions, including anaphylaxis (premedication is required), progressive multifocal leukoencephalopathy. Use of brentuximab is contraindicated with bleomycin due to increased risk for pulmonary toxicity.

ADULT — Treatment of Hodgkin's lymphoma after failure of at least 2 prior chemotherapy regimens (in patient ineligible for transplant) or after stem cell transplant failure. Post-autologous hematopoietic stem cell transplantation consolidation treatment of patients with classical Hodgkin lymphoma at high risk of relapse or progression. Systemic anaplastic large cell lymphoma (sALCL) after failure of at least one prior chemotherapy regimen.

PEDS — Not approved in pediatric patients

FORMS — 50 mg powder for injection.

MOA — Antibody drug conjugate directed at CD30.

ADVERSE EFFECTS — Myelosuppression, peripheral sensory neuropathy, fatigue, nausea, pyrexia, rash, cough, upper respiratory infection.

CETUXIMAB (✱*Erbitux*) ▶? ♀C ▶– $ varies by therapy

WARNING — Anaphylaxis, cardiopulmonary arrest/ sudden death, pulmonary toxicity, rash, sepsis, renal failure, pulmonary embolus, hypomagnesemia. Skin rash occurs in 95% of patients, including desquamation, with grades 3/4 in 16%.

ADULT — Chemotherapy doses vary by indication. Indicated for the treatment of patients with K-Ras mutation-negative (wild-type), EGFR-expressing metastatic colorectal cancer as determined by FDA-approved tests. Cetuximab is not indicated for treatment of K-Ras mutation-positive colorectal cancer, or when results of RAS mutation tests are unknown. Indicated for use in combination with FOLFIRI (irinotecan, 5-fluorouracil, leucovorin) for first-line treatment of K-Ras mutation-negative (wild-type), EGFR-expressing metastatic colorectal cancer. Indicated as a single agent in patients who have failed irinotecan or oxaliplatin-based chemotherapy or who are intolerant to irinotecan.

(cont.)

CETUXIMAB (*cont.*)

Treatment of squamous cell cancer of the head and neck.

PEDS — Not approved in children. Safety and effectiveness in children not established. No new safety signals identified in pediatric patients after pharmacokinetic evaluation.

UNAPPROVED ADULT — EGFR-expressing advanced NSCLC.

NOTES — Monitor renal function and electrolytes including magnesium. Caution with known CAD, heart failure, or arrhythmias. Premedication with an H1 antagonist and a 1-h observation period after infusion is recommended due to potential for anaphylaxis. Use is not recommended in patients with codon 12 or 13 K-Ras mutations.

MOA — Cetuximab is a recombinant chimeric monoclonal antibody that binds to and blocks the binding of ligands (eg, epidermal growth factor and tissue growth factor) to the epidermal growth factor receptor (EGFR, HER1, c-ErbB-1) on the surface of normal and tumor cells, resulting in inhibition of cell growth, induction of apoptosis, and decreased vascular endothelial growth factor (VEGF) production.

ADVERSE EFFECTS — Serious: Anaphylaxis, cardiopulmonary arrest/sudden death, pulmonary toxicity, rash, sepsis, renal failure, pulmonary embolus, hypomagnesemia. Use with radiation and cisplatin adds mucosal inflammation. Frequent: Rash, pruritus, nail changes, malaise, diarrhea, abdominal pain, N/V, hypomagnesemia. Dermatologic toxicity: Limit sun exposure. Monitor for inflammatory or infectious sequelae.

DARATUMUMAB (*Darzalex*) ▶? ♀? ▶?

WARNING — Infusion reactions: Interrupt Darzalex infusion for infusion reactions of any severity. Permanently discontinue the infusion in case of life threatening infusion reactions. Interference with cross-matching and red blood cell antibody screening: Type and screen patients prior to starting treatment. Inform blood banks that a patient has received Darzalex.

ADULT — 16 mg/kg IV for treatment of patients with multiple myeloma who have received at least three prior lines of therapy including a proteasome inhibitor (PI) and an immunomodulatory agent or who are double-refractory to a PI and an immunomodulatory agent. Infuse weekly Weeks 1 to 8, every two weeks Weeks 9 to 24, every four weeks Week 25 onwards until disease progression .

FORMS — 100 mg/5 mL vial and 400 mg/20 mL vial.

NOTES — Pre-medicate with corticosteroids, antipyretics and antihistamines.

MOA — Human monoclonal antibody that binds to CD38 and inhibits the growth of CD38 expressing tumor cells by inducing apoptosis directly through Fc mediated cross linking as well as by immune-mediated tumor cell lysis through complement dependent cytotoxicity (CDC), antibody dependent cell mediated cytotoxicity (ADCC) and antibody dependent cellular phagocytosis (ADCP). Myeloid derived suppressor cells (MDSCs) and a subset of regulatory T cells (CD38+Tregs) express CD38 and are susceptible to daratumumab mediated cell lysis.

ADVERSE EFFECTS — Infusion reactions, fatigue, nausea, back pain, pyrexia, cough, and upper respiratory tract infection.

DINUTUXIMAB (*Unituxin*) ▶? ♀D based on mechanism, will cause embryofetal harm ▶–

WARNING — Life-threatening infusion reactions may occur. Causes severe neuropathic pain. IV opioids should be administered prior to, during, and 2 h post dinutuximab infusion.

PEDS — 17.5 mg/m²/day IV for 4 days for up to 5 cycles. Used in combination with GM-CSF, interleukin-2 and 13-cis-retinoic acid for the treatment of pediatric patients with high-risk neuroblastoma who achieve at least a partial response to prior 1st-line multiagent, multimodality therapy.

FORMS — 17.5 mg/5 mL soln for injection.

MOA — Chimeric monoclonal antibody that binds to glycolipid GD2, which is expressed on neuroblastoma cells. It induces cell lysis of GD2 expressing cells through antibody-dependent cell-mediated cytotoxicity and complement dependent cytotoxicity.

ADVERSE EFFECTS — Capillary leak syndrome and hypotension. Infection. Neurological disorders of the eye. Bone marrow suppression. Electrolyte abnormalities. Atypical hemolytic uremic syndrome.

SIDE EFFECTS — Most common side effects (greater than 25%) are pain, pyrexia, thrombocytopenia, lymphopenia, infusion reactions, hypotension, hyponatremia, increased LFTs, anemia, vomiting, diarrhea, hypokalemia, capillary leak syndrome, neutropenia, urticaria, and hypocalcemia.

ELOTUZUMAB (*Empliciti*) ▶? ♀X Not recommended due to use with lenalidomide ▶– Not recommended due to use with lenalidomide

WARNING — Infusion reactions: Premedication is required. Interrupt Empliciti for Grade 2 or higher and permanently discontinue for severe infusion reaction. Infections: Monitor for fever and other signs of infection and treat promptly. Second Primary Malignances (SPM): Higher incidences of SPM were observed in a controlled clinical trial of patients with multiple myeloma receiving Empliciti Hepatotoxicity: Monitor liver function and stop Empliciti if hepatotoxicity is suspected. Interference with determination of complete response: Empliciti can interfere with assays used to monitor M-protein. This interference can impact the determination of complete response.

ADULT — 10 mg/kg intravenously every week for the first two cycles and every 2 weeks, thereafter, until disease progression or unacceptable toxicity, in combination with lenalidomide and dexamethasone for the treatment of patients with multiple myeloma who have received one to three prior therapies.

FORMS — 300 mg or 400 mg lyophilized powder in a single-dose vial for reconstitution.

NOTES — Elotuzumab is taken with lenalidomide 25 mg daily orally on days 1 through 21. Dexamethasone is administered as follows: In weeks

ELOTUZUMAB (*cont.*)

with elotuzumab infusion, dexamethasone is to be administered in divided doses, 8 mg intravenously prior to infusion and 28 mg orally; in weeks without elotuzumab infusion, dexamethasone is to be administered 40 mg orally. Pre-medication with an H1 blocker, H2 blocker, and acetaminophen should be administered prior to elotuzumab infusion

MOA — Elotuzumab is a monoclonal antibody directed against Signaling Lymphocyte Activation Molecule Family 7 (SLAMF7). SLAMF7 is present on myeloma cells and is also present on natural killer cells.

ADVERSE EFFECTS — Most common adverse reactions (20% or higher) are fatigue, diarrhea, pyrexia, constipation, cough, peripheral neuropathy, nasopharyngitis, upper respiratory tract infection, decreased appetite, pneumonia.

IBRITUMOMAB (✱*Zevalin*) ▶L ♀D ▶– $ varies by therapy

WARNING — Contraindicated in patients with allergy to murine proteins. Hypersensitivity. Serious infusion reactions, some fatal, may occur within 24 h of rituximab infusion. Prolonged and severe cytopenias occur in most patients. Severe cutaneous and mucocutaneous reactions, some fatal, reported with Zevalin therapeutic regimen. Do not exceed 32 mCi (1184 MBq) of Y-90 Zevalin.

ADULT — Chemotherapy doses vary by indication. Non-Hodgkin's lymphoma.

PEDS — Not approved in children.

NOTES — Reliable contraception is recommended. Monitor CBCs.

MOA — Ibritumomab tiuxetan contains a monoclonal antibody linked to an active chelator that accounts for its cytotoxic activity. The antibody moiety contains a murine IgG1 kappa monoclonal antibody directed against the CD20 antigen, once bound, the beta emission from the tiuxetan portion induces cellular damage through the formation of free radicals in the target and neighboring cells.

ADVERSE EFFECTS — Serious: Fatal infusion reactions, erythema multiforme, Stevens-Johnson syndrome, toxic epidermal necrolysis, bullous and exfoliative dermatitis, bone marrow suppression, hypersensitivity. Frequent: Bone marrow suppression, N/V, diarrhea.

IPILIMUMAB (✱*Yervoy*) ▶ endogenous – ♀C ▶–

WARNING — Severe and fatal immune-mediated adverse reactions due to T-cell activation and proliferation. Interacts with Vitamin K antagonists and cardiac glycosides. Adverse effects were observed in animal reproduction studies. Drug is known to cross the placenta. Other adverse effects include autoimmune central neuropathy (encephalitis), neurosensory hypoacusis, myositis, polymyositis, ocular myositis, and sarcoidosis.

ADULT — Unresectable or metastatic melanoma. 3 mg/kg q 3 weeks for 4 doses. Adjuvant treatment of patients with cutaneous melanoma with pathologic involvement of regional lymph nodes of more than 1 mm who have undergone complete resection, including total lymphadenectomy at a dose of 10 mg/kg administered intravenously over 90 minutes every 3 weeks for 4 doses followed by 10 mg/kg every 12 weeks for up to 3 years. In the event of toxicity, doses are omitted, not delayed.

PEDS — Not approved in children.

FORMS — 50 mg/10 mL, 200 mg/40 mL IV soln.

NOTES — Scheduled doses will need to be withheld for moderate immune-mediated reactions and symptomatic endocrine disorders. Permanently discontinue drug if cannot complete treatment course within 16 weeks of initial dose. Ipilimumab may increase the levels and side effects of vemurafenib.

MOA — Mab which binds to CTLA-4, allowing for enhanced T-cell activation.

ADVERSE EFFECTS — Fatigue, HA, pruritis, rash, N & V, diarrhea, constipation, abdominal pain.

NECITUMUMAB (*Portrazza*) ▶? ♀X ▶–

WARNING — Cardiopulmonary Arrest: Closely monitor serum electrolytes during and after Portrazza. Hypomagnesemia: Monitor prior to each infusion and for at least 8 weeks following the completion of Portrazza. Withhold Portrazza for Grade 3 or 4 electrolyte abnormalities; subsequent cycles of Portrazza may be administered in these patients once electrolyte abnormalities have improved to Grade ≤2. Replete electrolytes as necessary. Venous and Arterial Thromboembolic Events (VTE and ATE): Discontinue Portrazza for severe VTE or ATE. Dermatologic Toxicities: Monitor for dermatologic toxicities and withhold or discontinue Portrazza for severe toxicity. Limit sun exposure. Infusion-Related Reactions: Monitor for signs and symptoms during and following infusion. Discontinue Portrazza for severe reactions. Increased Toxicity: Non-squamous NSCLC: Increased toxicity and increased mortality.

ADULT — 800 mg as an intravenous infusion over 60 minutes on days 1 and 8 of each 3-week cycle, indicated for use in combination with gemcitabine and cisplatin (GC) for first-line treatment of patients with metastatic squamous non-small cell lung cancer (NSCLC). Necitumumab is not indicated for treatment of non-squamous NSCLC.

FORMS — 800 mg/50 mL (16 mg/mL) solution for injection in a single-dose vial.

NOTES — The geometric mean dose-normalized AUC of gemcitabine was increased by 22% and Cmax increased by 63% compared to administration of gemcitabine and cisplatin alone while exposure to cisplatin was unchanged.

MOA — A recombinant human IgG1 monoclonal antibody that binds to the human epidermal growth factor receptor (EGFR) and blocks the binding of EGFR to its ligands.

ADVERSE EFFECTS — The most common adverse reactions (all grades) observed in necitumumab-treated patients at a rate of greater than or equal to 30% and greater than or equal to 2% higher than GC alone arm were rash and hypomagnesemia. Serious and clinically significant adverse events include hypomagnesemia, venous and

(cont.)

NECITUMUMAB (*cont.*)

arterial thromboembolic events, dermatologic toxicities, infusion reactions, and increased toxicity and increased mortality in patients with non-squamous NSCLC. Death attributed to cardiovascular events or sudden death was reported in 3% of the patients in the necitumumab plus gemcitabine and cisplatin arm. Health care providers should closely monitor serum electrolytes, including serum magnesium, potassium, and calcium, during and after necitumumab administration. Withhold necitumumab for grade 3 or 4 electrolyte abnormalities.

NIVOLUMAB (*Opdivo*) ▶? ♀? Known to cause fetal harm. No category assigned. ▶–

WARNING — Immune-mediated pneumonitis: Withhold for moderate and permanently discontinue for severe or life-threatening pneumonitis. Immune-mediated colitis: Withhold for moderate or severe and permanently discontinue for life-threatening colitis. Immune-mediated hepatitis: Monitor for changes in liver function. Withhold for moderate and permanently discontinue for severe or life-threatening transaminase or total bilirubin elevation. Immune-mediated nephritis and renal dysfunction: Monitor for changes in renal function. Withhold for moderate and permanently discontinue for severe or life-threatening serum creatinine elevation. Immune-mediated hypothyroidism and hyperthyroidism: Monitor for changes in thyroid function. Initiate thyroid hormone replacement as needed. Embryofetal toxicity: Can cause fetal harm. Advise of potential risk to a fetus and use of effective contraception.

ADULT — 240mg administered as a single agent IV q 2 weeks for BRAF V600 wild-type or BRAF V600 mutation-positive unresectable or metastatic melanoma; treatment of unresectable or metastatic melanoma in combination with ipilimumab. (Dose is 1mg/kg every 3 weeks for 4 doses, then 3 mg/kg every 2 weeks.) 240mg IV q 2 weeks for treatment of metastatic NSCLC with progression on or after platinum-based chemotherapy. 240mg IV q 2 weeks for treatment of patients with advanced renal cell carcinoma whose disease progressed on an antiangiogenic therapy. 3mg/kg IV every 2 weeks for treatment of patients with classical Hodgkin lymphoma (cHL) that has relapsed or progressed after autologous hematopoietic stem cell transplantation (HSCT) and post-transplantation brentuximab vedotin (Adcetris®).

FORMS — 40 mg/4 mL and 100 mg/10 mL soln for injection in a single-use vial.

MOA — Human immunoglobulin G4 (IgG4) monoclonal antibody that binds to the PD-1 receptor and blocks its interaction with PD-L1 and PD-L2, releasing PD-1 pathway-mediated inhibition of the immune response, including the anti-tumor immune response. In syngeneic mouse tumor models, blocking PD-1 activity resulted in decreased tumor growth.

ADVERSE EFFECTS — Most common adverse reaction (≥20%) in patients with melanoma was rash. Most common adverse reactions (≥20%) in patients with advanced squamous non-small cell lung cancer were fatigue, dyspnea, musculoskeletal pain, decreased appetite, cough, nausea, and constipation.

OBINUTUZUMAB (✻*Gazyva*) ▶? – ♀C Adverse effects were observed in animals. B-cell counts may be depleted and immunologic function affected in the neonate after birth. ▶?

WARNING — Obinutuzumab is being approved with a boxed warning about hepatitis B virus reactivation. Patients should be assessed for hepatitis B virus and their related reactivation risk. The boxed warning includes another concern: the drug's risk of inducing progressive multifocal leukoencephalopathy.

ADULT — Treatment in combination with chlorambucil of patients with previously untreated chronic lymphocytic leukemia (CLL). Cycle 1: 100 mg intravenously on day 1, 900 mg on day 2, and 1000 mg on days 8 and 15. Cycles 2 to 6: 1000 mg administered IV q 28 days. Treatment in combination with bendamustine chemotherapy followed by treatment with obinutuzumab alone in patients with follicular lymphoma (FL) who failed to respond to a regimen containing rituximab or for patients whose follicular lymphoma relapsed receiving that treatment. Obinutuzumab dosing for FL: 1000 mg administered IV on days 1, 8, and 15 of cycle 1; on day 1 of cycles 2 to 6 (28-day cycles); and then q 2 months for 2 years.

PEDS — Not approved in children.

FORMS — 1000 mg/40 mL (25 mg/mL) single-use vial.

MOA — Obinutuzumab is a monoclonal antibody that targets the CD20 antigen expressed on the surface of pre B- and mature B-lymphocytes. Upon binding to CD20, obinutuzumab mediates B-cell lysis through (1) engagement of immune effector cells, (2) by directly activating intracellular death signaling pathways and/or (3) activation of the complement cascade. The immune effector cell mechanisms include antibody-dependent cellular cytotoxicity and antibody-dependent cellular phagocytosis.

ADVERSE EFFECTS — Infusion-related reactions, neutropenia, thrombocytopenia, anemia, musculoskeletal pain, and pyrexia. Increased risk of thrombocytopenia and hemorrhagic events during the first cycle of infusion with obinutuzumab in combination with chlorambucil.

OFATUMUMAB (✻*Arzerra*) ▶immune system - ♀C ▶?

WARNING — May cause serious infusion reactions. Premedicate with acetaminophen, an antihistamine, and a corticosteroid. May cause prolonged cytopenias. Progressive multifocal leukoencephalopathy (PML) can occur. Risk for reactivation of hepatitis B virus (HBV) infection in patients who once had the virus may occur. Some of the cases

(cont.)

OFATUMUMAB (*cont.*)

of HBV reactivation that have been reported have resulted in fulminant hepatitis, hepatic failure, and death. Intestinal obstruction may occur.

ADULT — 300 mg IV initial dose (dose 1), followed 1 week later by 2000 mg IV weekly for 7 doses (doses 2 through 8), followed 4 weeks later by 2000 mg IV q 4 weeks for 4 doses (doses 9 through 12) for treatment of patients with chronic lymphocytic leukemia (CLL) refractory to fludarabine and alemtuzumab. 300 mg IV initial dose followed by 1000 mg on Day 8, than 1000 mg q 28 days to a maximum of 12 cycles for treatment of untreated CLL in combination with chlorambucil when fludarabine-based therapy is inappropriate. 300 mg IV on day 1 followed by 1000 mg on day 8 and then 7 weeks later and q 8 weeks thereafter for up to a maximum of 2 years for the extended treatment of patients who are in complete or partial response after at least two lines of therapy for recurrent or progressive CLL. In combination with fludarabine and cyclophosphamide for the treatment of patients with relapsed CLL.

PEDS — Not approved for pediatric use.

NOTES — Premedicate 30 min to 2 h prior to ofatumumab infusion with acetaminophen, antihistamine, and corticosteroid. See product labeling for dose reduction guidelines of corticosteroids.

MOA — Binds specifically to both the small and large extracellular loops of the CD20 molecule on B-lymphocytes resulting in complement dependent cell lysis and antibody-dependent cell mediated toxicity.

ADVERSE EFFECTS — Neutropenia, pneumonia, pyrexia, cough, diarrhea, anemia, fatigue, dyspnea, rash, nausea, bronchitis, and upper respiratory tract infections.

OLARATUMAB (*Lartruvo*) ▶? ♀X Embryo-Fetal Toxicity: Can cause fetal harm. Advise females of potential risk to the fetus and to use effective contraception during treatment with LARTRUVO and for 3 months after the last dose. ▶– Advise women not to breastfeed during treatment with LARTRUVO and for 3 months following the last dose.

WARNING — Infusion-Related Reactions: Monitor for signs and symptoms during and following infusion. Discontinue LARTRUVO for Grade 3 or 4 infusion-related reactions. Premedicate with diphenhydramine and dexamethasone intravenously, prior to LARTRUVO on Day 1 of cycle 1.

ADULT — 15 mg/kg administered as an IV infusion over 60 minutes on days 1 and 8 of each 21-day cycle until disease progression or unacceptable toxicity. For the first eight cycles, olaratumab is administered with doxorubicin for treatment of patients with soft tissue sarcoma (STS) not amenable to curative treatment with radiotherapy or surgery and with a histologic subtype for which an anthracycline-containing regimen is appropriate.

FORMS — 500 mg/50 mL (10 mg/mL) solution in a single-dose vial

MOA — Olaratumab is a human IgG1 antibody that binds platelet-derived growth factor receptor alpha (PDGFR-α). PDGFR-α is a receptor tyrosine kinase expressed on cells of mesenchymal origin. Signaling through this receptor plays a role in cell growth, chemotaxis, and mesenchymal stem cell differentiation. The receptor has also been detected on some tumor and stromal cells, including sarcomas, where signaling can contribute to cancer cell proliferation, metastasis, and maintenance of the tumor microenvironment. The interaction between olaratumab and PDGFR-α prevents binding of the receptor by the PDGF-AA and -BB ligands as well as PDGF-AA, -BB, and -CC-induced receptor activation and downstream PDGFR-α pathway signaling. Olaratumab exhibits in vitro and in vivo anti-tumor activity against selected sarcoma cell lines and disrupted the PDGFR-α signaling pathway in in vivo tumor implant models.

ADVERSE EFFECTS — Most common (greater than or equal to 20%): nausea, fatigue, neutropenia, musculoskeletal pain, mucositis, alopecia, vomiting, diarrhea, decreased appetite, abdominal pain, neuropathy, and headache. Infusion-related reactions were seen in 13% of patients. The most common ($\geq$20%) laboratory abnormalities were lymphopenia, neutropenia, thrombocytopenia, hyperglycemia, elevated aPTT, hypokalemia, and hypophosphatemia.

PANITUMUMAB (✲*Vectibix*) ▶Not metabolized ♀C ▶– $ varies by therapy

WARNING — Skin exfoliation, severe dermatologic reactions complicated by sepsis and death. Derm toxicities reported in 90% of patients, 12% severe. Severe infusion reactions. Anaphylaxis.

ADULT — Chemotherapy doses vary by indication. Indicated for patients with wild-type RAS metastatic colorectal carcinoma, either as 1st-line therapy in combination with FOLFOX (fluorouracil, leucovorin, and oxaliplatin) or as monotherapy for patients with disease progression after prior treatment.

PEDS — Not approved in children.

NOTES — Reliable contraception is recommended. Monitor potassium and magnesium. Panitumumab is not indicated for the treatment of RAS mutant metastatic colorectal cancer or for patients in whom the RAS mutation status is unknown.

MOA — Panitumumab is a monoclonal antibody that binds to epidermal growth factor receptor (EGFR) on tumor cells preventing autophosphorylation and activation of receptor-associated kinases, resulting in inhibition of cell growth, induction of apoptosis, decreased proinflammatory cytokine and vascular growth factor production.

ADVERSE EFFECTS — Serious: Infusion-related reactions, anaphylaxis, sepsis, pulmonary fibrosis. Frequent: Hypomagnesemia, acne, pruritus, erythema, rash, skin exfoliation, paronychia, stomatitis, mucositis, diarrhea, photosensitivity.

PEMBROLIZUMAB (✲*Keytruda*) ▶? ♀D ▶–

WARNING — Immune-related adverse reactions: pneumonitis, colitis, hepatitis, hypophysitis,

(cont.)

PEMBROLIZUMAB (*cont.*)

nephritis, hyperthyroidism, hypothyroidism, Type I diabetes mellitus. Embryofetal toxicity. Infusion reactions.

ADULT — 2 mg/kg IV over 30 minutes q 3 weeks. Treatment of patients with unresectable or metastatic melanoma. Treatment of patients with metastatic NSCLC. 200 mg IV over 30 minutes q 3 weeks for treatment of patients with recurrent or metastatic head and neck squamous cell carcinoma (HNSCC) with disease progression on or after platinum-containing chemotherapy.

PEDS — Not approved in children.

UNAPPROVED ADULT — Merkel cell carcinoma.

FORMS — 50 mg powder for injection.

MOA — Monoclonal antibody which inhibits programmed cell death-1 (PD-1) activity by binding to the PD-1 receptor on T-cells to block PD-L1 and PD-L2 ligands from binding. Blocking the PD-1 pathway inhibits the negative immune regulation caused by PD-1 receptor signaling.

ADVERSE EFFECTS — The most common adverse reactions (>20% of patients): fatigue, cough, nausea, pruritis, rash, decreased appetite, constipation, arthralgia, and diarrhea.

PERTUZUMAB (❋*Perjeta*) ▶? – ♀D Use of effective contraception is necessary during the 7-month washout period when pertuzumab is used in combination with trastuzumab. ▶– $$$$$

WARNING — Boxed warning regarding embryo-fetal toxicity and birth defects.

ADULT — Use in combination with trastuzumab and docetaxel for the treatment of patients with HER2-positive metastatic breast cancer who have not received prior anti-HER2 therapy or chemotherapy for metastatic disease. Pertuzumab is now specifically indicated for the neoadjuvant treatment of breast cancer, in combination with trastuzumab and docetaxel, for patients with HER2-positive, locally advanced, inflammatory, or early-stage breast cancer (greater than 2 cm in diameter) that is high risk, as part of a complete early breast cancer regimen also containing fluorouracil, epirubicin, and cyclophosphamide or carboplatin. As part of this regimen, patients will receive trastuzumab after surgery to complete 1 year of treatment. Initial dose: 840 mg IV, followed by 420 mg q 3 weeks thereafter.

PEDS — Not approved in children.

FORMS — Trade only: 420 mg/14 mL single-use vial.

MOA — Recombinant humanized monoclonal antibody that targets the extracellular dimerization domain of HER2, and thereby blocks ligand-dependent heterodimerization of HER2 with other HER family members, including EGFR, HER3 and HER4.

ADVERSE EFFECTS — Most common:diarrhea, alopecia, neutropenia, nausea, fatigue, rash, and peripheral neuropathy. Most severe: left ventricular dysfunction, infusion-associated reactions, hypersensitivity reactions, and anaphylaxis

RAMUCIRUMAB (*Cyramza*) ▶? ♀C ▶?

WARNING — Increased risk of hemorrhage, including severe and sometimes fatal hemorrhagic events. Should be permanently discontinued in patients who experience severe bleeding. Arterial thromboembolic events (ATEs): Serious, sometimes fatal ATEs have been reported in clinical trials. Hypertension: Monitor blood pressure and treat hypertension. Infusion-related reactions: Monitor for signs and symptoms during infusion. Gastrointestinal perforation. Impaired wound healing: Withhold prior to surgery. Clinical deterioration in patients with cirrhosis: New onset or worsening encephalopathy, ascites, or hepatorenal syndrome can occur in patients with Child-Pugh B or C cirrhosis. Reversible posterior leukoencephalopathy syndrome.

ADULT — 8 mg/kg administered as a 60-minute IV infusion q 2 weeks for use as a single agent or in combination with paclitaxel for the treatment of patients with advanced or metastatic, gastric, or gastroesophageal junction (GEJ) adenocarcinoma with disease progression on or after prior treatment with fluoropyrimidine- or platinum-containing chemotherapy. 8 mg/kg q 2 weeks for use in combination with FOLFIRI for the treatment of patients with metastatic colorectal cancer (mCRC) whose disease has progressed on a 1st-line bevacizumab-, oxaliplatin-, and fluoropyrimidine-containing regimen. 10 mg/kg q 3 weeks for use in combination with docetaxel for the treatment of patients with metastatic NSCLC with disease progression on or after platinum-based chemotherapy. Patients with EGFR or ALK genomic tumor aberrations should have disease progression on FDA-approved therapy for these aberrations prior to receiving ramucirumab.

FORMS — 100 mg/10 mL, 500 mg/50 mL soln, single-dose vial.

MOA — Ramucirumab is a recombinant monoclonal antibody of the IgG1 class that binds to vascular endothelial growth factor receptor-2 (VEGFR-2) and blocks the activation of the receptor.

ADVERSE EFFECTS — The most common adverse reactions are hypertension and diarrhea.

TRASTUZUMAB (❋*Herceptin*) ▶Not metabolized ♀B ▶– $ varies by therapy

WARNING — Hypersensitivity, including fatal anaphylaxis, fatal infusion-related reactions, pulmonary events including ARDS and death, ventricular dysfunction, and heart failure. Anemia, leukopenia, diarrhea, alopecia. Boxed warnings are for heart failure, infusion reactions, and pulmonary toxicity.

ADULT — Chemotherapy doses vary by indication. Breast cancer with tumors overexpressing the HER2 NEU protein. HER2-overexpressing metastatic gastric or gastroesophageal junction adenocarcinoma with cisplatin and a fluoropyrimidine.

PEDS — Not approved in children.

FORMS — 440 mg vial, powder for reconstitution.

(cont.)

TRASTUZUMAB (*cont.*)

NOTES — Monitor with ECG, echocardiogram, or MUGA scan. CBCs. Extending adjuvant treatment beyond 1 year is not recommended.

MOA — Trastuzumab is a recombinant DNA-derived humanized monoclonal antibody that selectively binds to the extracellular domain of the human epidermal growth factor receptor 2 protein (HER2). It mediates antibody-dependent cellular cytotoxicity by inhibiting proliferation of cells which overexpress the HER2 protein.

ADVERSE EFFECTS — Serious: Anaphylaxis, fatal infusion-related reactions, ARDS, heart failure, bone marrow suppression. Frequent: Fever, chills, N/V, diarrhea, rash.

ONCOLOGY: Platinum-Containing Agents

CARBOPLATIN (*Paraplatin*) ▶K ♀D ▶– $ varies by therapy

WARNING — Secondary malignancies, bone marrow suppression, increased in patients with renal insufficiency; emesis, anaphylaxis, nephrotoxicity, peripheral neuropathy, increased LFTs, alopecia. Instruct patients to report promptly fever, sore throat, signs of local infection, bleeding from any site, symptoms suggestive of anemia, or yellow discoloration of the skin or eyes.

ADULT — Chemotherapy doses vary by indication. Ovarian carcinoma.

PEDS — Not approved in children.

UNAPPROVED ADULT — Small-cell lung cancer, in combination regimens. Squamous cell carcinoma of the head and neck, advanced endometrial cancer, acute leukemia, seminoma of testicular cancer, NSCLC, adenocarcinoma of unknown primary, cervical cancer, bladder carcinoma, breast cancer, Hodgkin's lymphoma, mesothelioma, melanoma, neuroendocrine tumors, non-Hodgkin's lymphoma, prostate cancer, sarcomas, small-cell lung cancer.

NOTES — Reliable contraception is recommended. Monitor CBCs, LFTs, and renal function. May decrease phenytoin levels.

MOA — Alkylating agent.

ADVERSE EFFECTS — Serious: Bone marrow suppression, peripheral neuropathy, anaphylaxis, nephrotoxicity. Frequent: Bone marrow suppression, N/V, increased LFTs. Possible: alopecia, dehydration, mucositis.

CISPLATIN ▶K ♀D ▶– $ varies by therapy

WARNING — Secondary malignancies, nephrotoxicity, bone marrow suppression, N/V, very highly emetogenic, ototoxicity, anaphylaxis, hepatotoxicity, vascular toxicity, hyperuricemia, electrolyte disturbances, optic neuritis, papilledema and cerebral blindness, neuropathies, muscle cramps, alopecia. Amifostine can be used to reduce renal toxicity in patients with advanced ovarian cancer. Instruct patients to report promptly fever, sore throat, signs of local infection, bleeding from any site, symptoms suggestive of anemia, or yellow discoloration of the skin or eyes. Genetic factors (eg, variants in the thiopurine S-methyltransferase [TPMT] gene) may contribute to cisplatin-induced ototoxicity; although this association has not been consistent across populations and study designs.

ADULT — Chemotherapy doses vary by indication. Metastatic testicular and ovarian tumors, bladder cancer.

PEDS — Not approved in children.

UNAPPROVED ADULT — Esophageal cancer, gastric cancer, non-small-cell lung cancer and small-cell lung cancer, head and neck cancer, endometrial cancer, cervical cancer, neoadjuvant bladder-sparing chemotherapy, sarcoma.

UNAPPROVED PEDS — Germ cell tumors, hepatoblastoma, medulloblastoma, neuroblastoma, osteosarcoma.

FORMS — 50 mg/50 mL, 100 mg/100 mL, 200 mg/200 mL soln for injection.

NOTES — Reliable contraception is recommended. Monitor CBCs, LFTs, renal function, and electrolytes. Audiometry. Aminoglycosides potentiate renal toxicity. Decreases phenytoin levels. Patients older than 65 yo may be more susceptible to nephrotoxicity, bone marrow suppression, and peripheral neuropathy. Verify any dose of cisplatin exceeding 100 mg/m^2 per course of therapy.

MOA — Alkylating agent.

ADVERSE EFFECTS — Serious: Bone marrow suppression, nephrotoxicity, ototoxicity, anaphylaxis, optic neuritis, papilledema and cerebral blindness, peripheral neuropathy. Frequent: Bone marrow suppression, N/V, nephrotoxicity, ototoxicity, hyperuricemia, muscle cramps.

OXALIPLATIN (✱*Eloxatin*) ▶LK ♀D ▶– $ varies by therapy

WARNING — Anaphylactic reactions to oxaliplatin have been reported and may occur within minutes of oxaliplatin administration. Epinephrine, corticosteroids, and antihistamines have been employed to alleviate symptoms. Laryngospasm may occur due to infusion reactions/hypersensitivity. Neuropathy, pulmonary fibrosis, bone marrow suppression including severe neutropenia, cardiovascular toxicity, rhabdomyolysis, transient vision loss, N/V/D, fertility impairment. Instruct patients to report promptly fever, sore throat, signs of local infection, bleeding from any site, or symptoms suggestive of anemia.

ADULT — Chemotherapy doses vary by indication. Colorectal cancer with 5-FU + leucovorin.

PEDS — Not approved in children.

UNAPPROVED ADULT — Esophageal cancer, gastric cancer, non-Hodgkin's lymphoma, ovarian cancer,

(cont.)

OXALIPLATIN (*cont.*)
testicular cancer, hepatobiliary cancer, pancreatic cancer. Biliary adenocarcinoma, advanced; chronic lymphocytic leukemia, refractory; neuroendocrine (carcinoid) tumors; unknown primary cancer.
FORMS — 50, 100, 200 mg vials of soln for injection.

NOTES — Reliable contraception is recommended. Monitor CBCs and renal function.
MOA — Alkylating agent.
ADVERSE EFFECTS — Serious: Bone marrow suppression, anaphylaxis, neuropathy, pulmonary fibrosis. Frequent: N/V, diarrhea. Hypersensitivity reactions may occur.

ONCOLOGY: Radiopharmaceuticals

RADIUM-223 DICHLORIDE FOR INJECTION (*Xofigo*) ▶NA – ♀X ▶–
ADULT — 50 kBq/kg body wt given at 4-week intervals for a total of 6 IV injections. Castration-resistant prostate cancer (CRPC) with symptomatic bone metastases and no known visceral metastatic disease.
PEDS — Not approved in children.
FORMS — Single-use vial at a concentration of 1000 kBq/mL (27 microcurie/mL) at the reference date with a total radioactivity of 6000 kBq/vial (162 microcurie/vial) at the reference date.
MOA — Alpha particle-emitting isotope which mimics calcium and forms complexes with the bone mineral hydroxyapatite at areas of increased bone turnover, such as bone metastases. The high linear energy transfer of alpha emitters leads to a high frequency of double-strand DNA breaks in adjacent cells, resulting in an anti-tumor effect on bone metastases.
ADVERSE EFFECTS — Severe: Bone marrow suppression. Discontinue Xofigo if hematologic values do not recover within 6 to 8 weeks after treatment. Monitor patients with compromised bone marrow reserve closely. Discontinue Xofigo in patients who experience life-threatening complications despite supportive care measures. Frequent: diarrhea, nausea, vomiting, and thrombocytopenia.
SAMARIUM 153 (*Quadramet*) ▶Not metabolized ♀C ▶– $ varies by therapy

WARNING — Bone marrow suppression, flare reactions. Instruct patients to report promptly fever, sore throat, signs of local infection, or anemia.
ADULT — Chemotherapy doses vary by indication. Osteoblastic metastatic bone lesions, relief of pain.
PEDS — Not approved in children.
UNAPPROVED ADULT — Ankylosing spondylitis, Paget's disease, RA.
NOTES — Reliable contraception is recommended. Monitor CBCs. Radioactivity in excreted urine for 12 h after dose.
MOA — Radiopharmaceutical.
ADVERSE EFFECTS — Serious: Bone marrow suppression, flare reactions. Frequent: Bone marrow suppression, N/V.
STRONTIUM-89 (*Metastron*) ▶K ♀D ▶– $ varies by therapy
WARNING — Bone marrow suppression, flare reactions, flushing sensation. Instruct patients to report promptly fever, sore throat, signs of local infection, or anemia.
ADULT — Chemotherapy doses vary by indication. Painful skeletal metastases, relief of bone pain.
PEDS — Not approved in children.
NOTES — Reliable contraception is recommended. Monitor CBCs. Radioactivity in excreted urine for 12 h after dose.
MOA — Radiopharmaceutical.
ADVERSE EFFECTS — Serious: Bone marrow suppression, flare reactions, flushing sensation. Frequent: Bone marrow suppression.

ONCOLOGY: Topoisomerase Inhibitors

ETOPOSIDE (*VP-16, Etopophos, Toposar, ✹Vepesid*) ▶K ♀D ▶– $ varies by therapy
WARNING — Bone marrow suppression, anaphylaxis, hypotension, CNS depression, alopecia. Instruct patients to report promptly fever, sore throat, or signs of local infection.
ADULT — Chemotherapy doses vary by indication. Testicular cancer, small-cell lung cancer, in combination regimens.
PEDS — Not approved in children.
UNAPPROVED ADULT — ALL, AML, Hodgkin's disease, non-Hodgkin's lymphomas, Kaposi's sarcoma, neuroblastoma, choriocarcinoma, rhabdomyosarcoma, hepatocellular carcinoma, epithelial ovarian

cancer, non-small-cell and small-cell lung cancers, testicular cancer, gastric cancer, endometrial cancer, breast cancer, and soft-issue sarcoma.
FORMS — Generic/Trade: Caps 50 mg. Injection for hospital/clinic use; not intended for outpatient prescribing.
NOTES — Reliable contraception is recommended. Monitor CBCs, LFTs, and renal function. May increase INR with warfarin.
MOA — Mitotic inhibitor.
ADVERSE EFFECTS — Serious: Bone marrow suppression, anaphylaxis, hypotension, CNS depression. Frequent: Alopecia, bone marrow suppression, N/V, diarrhea.

IRINOTECAN (*Camptosar*) ▶L ♀D ▶– $ varies by therapy
WARNING — Diarrhea and dehydration (may be life-threatening), bone marrow suppression (worse with radiation), orthostatic hypotension, colitis, hypersensitivity, pancreatitis. Instruct patients to report promptly diarrhea, fever, sore throat, signs of local infection, bleeding from any site, or symptoms suggestive of anemia.
ADULT — Chemotherapy doses vary by indication. Metastatic carcinoma of the colon or rectum, in combination regimens.
PEDS — Not approved in children.
UNAPPROVED ADULT — NSCLC and small-cell lung cancer, ovarian and cervical cancer.
FORMS — 40 mg/2 mL, 100 mg/5 mL, 300 mg/15 mL, 500 mg/25 mL soln for injection.
NOTES — Enzyme-inducing drugs such as phenytoin, phenobarbital, carbamazepine, rifampin, and St. John's wort decrease concentrations and possibly effectiveness. Ketoconazole is contraindicated during therapy. Atazanavir increases concentrations. Reliable contraception is recommended. Monitor CBCs. May want to withhold diuretics during active N/V. Avoid laxatives. Loperamide/fluids/electrolytes for diarrhea. Consider atropine for cholinergic symptoms during the infusion. Patients who are homozygous for the UGT1A1*28 allele are at increased risk for neutropenia. Dosage reductions may be necessary.
MOA — Topoisomerase inhibitor.
ADVERSE EFFECTS — Serious: Severe diarrhea, dehydration, bone marrow suppression, orthostatic hypotension, colitis/ileus, hypersensitivity, pancreatitis. Frequent: Diarrhea, bone marrow suppression, alopecia, N/V, rhinitis, salivation, lacrimation, miosis. Also myocardial ischemic events, elevated serum transaminases, hiccups, and megacolon have occurred.
IRINOTECAN LIPOSOME (*Onivyde*) ▶? Has not been evaluated. ♀D ▶–
WARNING — Fatal neutropenic sepsis occurred in 0.8% of patients receiving Onivyde. Severe or life-threatening neutropenic fever or sepsis occurred in 3% and severe or life-threatening neutropenia occurred in 20% of patients receiving Onivyde in combination with fluorouracil and leucovorin. Withhold Onivyde for absolute neutrophil count below 1500/mm³ or neutropenic fever. Monitor blood cell counts periodically during treatment. Severe diarrhea occurred in 13% of patients receiving Onivyde in combination with fluorouracil and leucovorin. Do not administer Onivyde to patients with bowel obstruction. Withhold Onivyde for diarrhea of Grade 2-4 severity. Severe hypersensitivity reaction: Permanently discontinue Onivyde for severe hypersensitivity reactions. Interstitial lung disease: Fatal ILD has occurred in patients receiving irinotecan HCl. Discontinue Onivyde if ILD is diagnosed.

ADULT — 70 mg/m² IV over 90 minutes, every two weeks in combination with fluorouracil (5FU) and leucovorin for the treatment of patients with metastatic adenocarcinoma of the pancreas whose disease has progressed following gemcitabine-based therapy.
FORMS — 43 mg/10 mL single dose vial
NOTES — Administer loperamide for late diarrhea of any severity. Administer atropine, if not contraindicated, for early diarrhea of any severity.
MOA — A topoisomerase 1 inhibitor encapsulated in a lipid bilayer vesicle or liposome. Topoisomerase 1 relieves torsional strain in DNA by inducing single-strand breaks. Irinotecan and its active metabolite SN-38 bind reversibly to the topoisomerase 1-DNA complex and prevent re-ligation of the single-strand breaks, leading to exposure time-dependent double-strand DNA damage and cell death.
ADVERSE EFFECTS — The most common adverse reactions (≥ 20%): diarrhea, fatigue/asthenia, vomiting, nausea, decreased appetite, stomatitis, and pyrexia. The most common laboratory abnormalities (≥ 10% Grade 3 or 4): lymphopenia and neutropenia.
TENIPOSIDE (✱*Vumon*) ▶K ♀D ▶– $ varies by therapy
WARNING — Bone marrow suppression, anaphylaxis, hypotension, CNS depression, alopecia. Instruct patients to report promptly fever, sore throat, or signs of local infection.
ADULT — Not approved in adult patients.
PEDS — Chemotherapy doses vary by indication. ALL, refractory, in combination regimens.
NOTES — Reliable contraception is recommended. Monitor CBCs, LFTs, and renal function.
MOA — Mitotic Inhibitor.
ADVERSE EFFECTS — Serious: Bone marrow suppression, anaphylaxis, hypotension, CNS depression. Frequent: Mucositis, alopecia, bone marrow suppression, N/V, diarrhea.
TOPOTECAN (✱*Hycamtin*) ▶Plasma ♀D ▶– $ varies by therapy
WARNING — Bone marrow suppression (primary neutropenia), severe bleeding, interstitial lung disease. Instruct patients to report promptly fever, sore throat, signs of local infection, bleeding from any site, or symptoms suggestive of anemia.
ADULT — Chemotherapy doses vary by indication. Ovarian and cervical cancer. Small-cell lung cancer, relapsed.
PEDS — Not approved in children.
FORMS — Trade only: Caps 0.25, 1 mg. Generic/Trade: 4 mg powder for injection.
NOTES — Reliable contraception is recommended. Monitor CBCs.
MOA — Topoisomerase inhibitor.
ADVERSE EFFECTS — Serious: Bone marrow suppression, severe bleeding. Frequent: Bone marrow suppression, N/V, diarrhea, headache.

ONCOLOGY: Tyrosine Kinase Inhibitors

AFATINIB (✸*Giotrif*) ▶feces – ♀D ▶– $$$$$

WARNING — Severe and prolonged diarrhea not responsive to antidiarrheal agents. Bullous and exfoliative skin disorders: Severe bullous, blistering, and exfoliating lesions occurred in 0.15% of patients. Discontinue for life-threatening cutaneous reactions. Interstitial lung disease. Hepatic toxicity. Keratitis.

ADULT — 40 mg orally once daily taken at least 1 h before or 2 h after a meal as a 1st-line treatment of patients with metastatic NSCLC whose tumors have epidermal growth factor receptor (EGFR) exon 19 deletions or exon 21 (L858R) substitution mutations as detected by an FDA-approved test. Metastatic, squamous, NSCLC progressing after platinum-based chemotherapy.

PEDS — Not approved in children.

FORMS — Trade only: 20, 30, 40 mg tabs.

MOA — Afatinib covalently binds to the kinase domains of EGFR (ErbB1), HER2 (ErbB2), and HER4 (ErbB4) and irreversibly inhibits tyrosine kinase autophosphorylation, resulting in downregulation of ErbB signaling.

ADVERSE EFFECTS — Most common adverse reactions (≥20%) are diarrhea, rash/dermatitis acneiform, stomatitis, paronychia, dry skin, decreased appetite, pruritus

ALECTINIB (*Alecensa*) ▶L ♀D Based on mechanism and animal data ▶– Based on mechanism and animal data

WARNING — Hepatotoxicity: Monitor liver laboratory tests every 2 weeks during the first 2 months of treatment, and then periodically during treatment. In case of severe ALT, AST, or bilirubin elevations, withhold, then reduce dose, or permanently discontinue Alecensa. Interstitial Lung Disease (ILD)/Pneumonitis: Occurred in 0.4% of patients. Immediately withhold Alecensa in patients diagnosed with ILD/pneumonitis and permanently discontinue if no other potential causes of ILD/pneumonitis have been identified. Bradycardia: Monitor heart rate and blood pressure regularly. If symptomatic, withhold Alecensa then reduce dose, or permanently discontinue. Severe Myalgia and Creatine Phosphokinase (CPK) Elevation: Occurred in 1.2% and 4.6% of patients, respectively. Assess CPK every 2 weeks during the first month of treatment and in patients reporting unexplained muscle pain, tenderness, or weakness. In case of severe CPK elevations, withhold, then resume or reduce dose.

ADULT — 600 mg orally two times per day for the treatment of patients with anaplastic lymphoma kinase (ALK)-positive, metastatic NSCLC who have progressed on or are intolerant to crizotinib.

FORMS — 150 mg capsules.

NOTES — No pharmacokinetic interactions with alectinib requiring dosage adjustment have been identified.

MOA — Alectinib is a tyrosine kinase inhibitor that targets ALK and RET. In nonclinical studies, alectinib inhibited 232 ALK phosphorylation and ALK-mediated activation of the downstream signaling proteins STAT3 and AKT, 233 and decreased tumor cell viability in multiple cell lines harboring ALK fusions, amplifications, or activating 234 mutations. Th

ADVERSE EFFECTS — The most common adverse reactions (incidence ≥20%) are fatigue, constipation, edema and myalgia.

AXITINIB (✸*Inlyta*) ▶L ♀–D ▶–

ADULT — 5 mg orally two times per day. Advanced renal cell cancer after failure of one prior systemic treatment.

PEDS — Not approved in children.

FORMS — 1, 5 mg oral tabs.

MOA — Tyrosine kinase inhibitor which inhibits VEGF (vascular endothelial growth factor) receptors.

ADVERSE EFFECTS — Hypertension, fatigue, hand-foot syndrome, bicarbonate decreased, hypocalcemia, hyperglycemia, hypothyroidism, hypernatremia, hyperkalemia, hypoalbuminemia, hyponatremia, hypophosphatemia, hypoglycemia, diarrhea, pancytopenia, hemorrhage, increased liver function tests, weakness, increased creatinine, cough.

BOSUTINIB (✸*Bosulif*) ▶L – ♀D ▶–

WARNING — CYP3A inhibitors and inducers: Avoid concurrent use of Bosulif with strong or moderate CYP3A inhibitors and inducers. Proton pump inhibitors: May decrease bosutinib drug levels. Consider short-acting antacids in place of proton pump inhibitors. Fosaprepitant may increase the levels/effects of bosutinib. Bioavailability is 34% when administered with food.

ADULT — Treatment of chronic, accelerated, or blast phase Philadelphia chromosome–positive (Ph+) chronic myelogenous leukemia (CML) in adult patients with resistance or intolerance to prior therapy. 500 mg orally once daily with food.

PEDS — Not approved in children.

FORMS — 100, 500 mg tabs.

NOTES — Consider dose escalation to 600 mg daily in patients who do not reach complete hematologic response by week 8 or complete cytogenetic response by week 12 and do not have Grade 3 or greater adverse reactions.

MOA — Inhibits the Bcr-Abl kinase that promotes CML; it is also an inhibitor of Src-family kinases including Src, Lyn, and Hck.

ADVERSE EFFECTS — Diarrhea, nausea, thrombocytopenia, vomiting, abdominal pain, rash, anemia, pyrexia, and fatigue. Serious adverse reactions reported include anaphylactic shock, myelosuppression, gastrointestinal toxicity (diarrhea), fluid retention, hepatoxicity, increased serum creatinine, renal failure and rash.

CABOZANTINIB (*Cometriq, Cabometyx*) ▶L – ♀D ▶?
$$$$$
WARNING — Hemorrhage: Do not administer cabozanitinib if recent history of severe hemorrhage. GI Perforations and Fistulas: Monitor for symptoms. Discontinue cabozanitinib for fistulas that cannot be adequately managed or perforations. Thrombotic Events: Discontinue cabozanitinib for myocardial infarction, cerebral infarction, or other serious arterial thromboembolic events. Hypertension and Hypertensive Crisis: Monitor blood pressure regularly. Discontinue cabozanitinib for hypertensive crisis or severe hypertension that cannot be controlled with antihypertensive therapy. Diarrhea: May be severe. Interrupt cabozanitinib treatment immediately until diarrhea resolves or decreases to Grade 1. Recommend standard antidiarrheal treatments. Palmar-plantar erythrodysesthesia syndrome (PPES): Interrupt cabozanitinib treatment until PPES resolves or decreases to Grade 1. Reversible posterior leukoencephalopathy syndrome (RPLS): Discontinue cabozanitinib. Embryo-Fetal Toxicity: Can cause fetal harm. Advise females of reproductive potential of the potential risk to a fetus and to use effective contraception
ADULT — Progressive, metastatic medullary thyroid cancer, 140 mg orally daily. (Cometriq). Advanced renal cell carcinoma (RCC) in patients who have received prior antiangiogenic therapy, 60 mg orally daily. (Cabometyx).
FORMS — 20 mg, 40 mg, and 60 mg tablets. (Cabometyx), 20mg, 80mg capsules.
MOA — Inhibits the tyrosine kinase activity of MET, VEGFR-1, -2 and -3, AXL, RET, ROS1, TYRO3, MER, KIT, TRKB, FLT-3, and TIE-2.
ADVERSE EFFECTS — The most commonly reported (≥ 25%) adverse reactions are: diarrhea, fatigue, nausea, decreased appetite, palmar-plantar erythrodysesthesia syndrome (PPES), hypertension, vomiting, weight decreased, and constipation.

CERITINIB (*Zykadia*) ▶L ♀D ▶?
WARNING — Severe or persistent gastrointestinal toxicity: diarrhea, nausea, vomiting, or abdominal pain. Hepatotoxicity. Interstitial lung disease (ILD)/pneumonitis. QT interval prolongation. Hyperglycemia. Bradycardia. Pancreatitis. Embryofetal toxicity.
ADULT — 750 mg PO once daily for treatment of patients with anaplastic lymphoma kinase (ALK)–positive, metastatic NSCLC with disease progression or who are intolerant to crizotinib.
FORMS — 150 mg capsules.
NOTES — Avoid concurrent use with strong CYP3A inhibitors or inducers. If concurrent use of a strong CYP3A inhibitor is unavoidable, reduce the dose of ceritinib. Avoid concurrent use with CYP3A or CYP2C9 substrates with narrow therapeutic indices. A high-fat meal increases AUC by 73%.Avoid concurrent use with proton pump inhibitors.
MOA — Inhibits anaplastic lymphoma kinase (ALK)
ADVERSE EFFECTS — The most common adverse reactions are diarrhea, nausea, elevated

transaminases, vomiting, abdominal pain, fatigue, decreased appetite, and constipation
COBIMETINIB (*Cotellic*) ▶oxidation glucuronidation ♀D ▶–
WARNING — New primary malignancies, cutaneous and non-cutaneous: Monitor patients for new malignancies prior to initiation of therapy, while on therapy, and for up to 6 months following the last dose of Cotellic. Hemorrhage: Major hemorrhagic events can occur with Cotellic. Monitor for signs and symptoms of bleeding. Cardiomyopathy: The risk of cardiomyopathy is increased in patients receiving Cotellic with vemurafenib compared with vemurafenib as a single agent. The safety of Cotellic has not been established in patients with decreased left ventricular ejection fraction (LVEF). Evaluate LVEF before treatment, after one month of treatment, then every 3 months thereafter during treatment with COTELLIC. Severe Dermatologic Reactions: Monitor for severe skin rashes. Interrupt, reduce, or discontinue Cotellic. Serous Retinopathy and Retinal Vein Occlusion: Perform an ophthalmological evaluation at regular intervals and for any visual disturbances. Permanently discontinue COTELLIC for retinal vein occlusion. Hepatotoxicity: Monitor liver laboratory tests during treatment and as clinically indicated. Rhabdomyolysis: Monitor creatine phosphokinase periodically and as clinically indicated for signs and symptoms of rhabdomyolysis. Severe Photosensitivity: Advise patients to avoid sun exposure.
ADULT — 60 mg orally once daily on days 1-21 of an every 28-day cycle for treatment of patients with unresectable or metastatic melanoma with a BRAF V600E or V600K mutation, in combination with vemurafenib. Cobimetinib is not indicated for treatment of patients with wild-type BRAF melanoma.
FORMS — 20 mg tablets.
NOTES — Avoid concomitant administration of COTELLIC with strong or moderate CYP3A inducers or inhibitors.
MOA — A reversible inhibitor of mitogen-activated protein kinase (MAPK)/extracellular signal 306 regulated kinase 1 (MEK1) and MEK2. MEK proteins are upstream regulators of the extracellular signal 307 related kinase (ERK) pathway, which promotes cellular proliferation. BRAF V600E and K mutations result 308 in constitutive activation of the BRAF pathway which includes MEK1 and MEK2.
ADVERSE EFFECTS — Most common adverse reactions for COTELLIC (≥20%) are diarrhea, photosensitivity reaction, nausea, pyrexia, and vomiting. The most common (≥5%) Grade 3-4 laboratory abnormalities are increased GGT, increased CPK, hypophosphatemia, increased ALT, lymphopenia, increased AST, increased alkaline phosphatase, hyponatremia.
CRIZOTINIB (❋*Xalkori*) ▶L – ♀D ▶–
WARNING — Severe fatal pneumonitis, elevations in liver enzymes, QT prolongation. Symptomatic bradycardia may occur. Avoid concurrent use with other

(cont.)

CRIZOTINIB (*cont.*)

agents known to cause bradycardia. Monitor blood pressure and heart rate regularly.

ADULT — 250 mg orally two times per day. Locally advanced or metastatic NSCLC in patients who express an abnormal ALK (anaplastic lymphoma kinase) gene. Metastatic NSCLC whose tumors are ROS1-positive.

PEDS — Not approved in children.

FORMS — 200, 250 mg oral capsules.

NOTES — Avoid use with strong CYP3A4 inhibitors or inducers.

MOA — Multiple tyrosine kinase inhibitor, including ALK.

ADVERSE EFFECTS — Vision disorders, including severe visual loss, myelosuppression, nausea, diarrhea, vomiting, edema, constipation.

DABRAFENIB (✷*Tafinlar*) ▶L – ♀D ▶– $$$$$

WARNING — Advise female patients of reproductive potential to use highly effective contraception during treatment and for 4 weeks after treatment. Counsel patients to use a non-hormonal method of contraception because Tafinlar can render hormonal contraceptives ineffective. New primary cutaneous malignancies: Perform dermatologic evaluations prior to initiation of therapy, q 2 months while on therapy, and for up to 6 months following discontinuation.

ADULT — 150 mg orally two times per day for treatment of patients with unresectable or metastatic melanoma with BRAF V600E mutation. Not indicated for the treatment of patients with wild-type BRAF melanoma. 150 mg orally two times per day in metastatic or unresectable melanoma with BRAF V600E or BRAF V600K mutation in combination with trametinib.

PEDS — Not approved in children.

FORMS — Trade only: 50 mg and 75 mg capsules.

NOTES — Confirmation of the presence of BRAF V600E is needed prior to initiation of dabrafenib because of the risks of potential risk of tumor promotion in patients with BRAF wild-type melanoma.

MOA — Inhibits BRAF kinase V600 mutation-positive melanoma cell growth.

ADVERSE EFFECTS — Frequent: hyperkeratosis, headache, pyrexia, arthralgia, papilloma, alopecia, and palmar-plantar erythrodysesthesia syndrome. Serious: development of new primary skin cancers (cutaneous squamous cell carcinoma, new primary melanomas, and keratoacanthomas), febrile drug reactions requiring hospitalization, hyperglycemia, and uveitis/iritis.

DASATINIB (✷*Sprycel*) ▶L ♀D post-marketing reports of embryo-fetal toxicity ▶– $ varies by therapy

WARNING — Bone marrow suppression, hemorrhage, prolonged QT interval, pleural effusion, congestive heart failure, and myocardial infarction and left ventricular dysfunction. Dasatinib may increase the risk of a rare but serious condition in which there is abnormally high blood pressure in the arteries of the lungs (pulmonary arterial hypertension [PAH]). Symptoms of PAH may include shortness of breath, fatigue, and swelling of the body (eg, the ankles and legs). In reported cases, patients developed PAH after starting dasatinib, including after more than 1 year of treatment. Stevens-Johnson Syndrome.

ADULT — Chemotherapy doses vary by indication. CML, ALL.

PEDS — Not approved in children.

UNAPPROVED ADULT — Post allogeneic stem cell transplant treatment of CML.

FORMS — Trade only: Tabs 20, 50, 70, 100 mg.

NOTES — Reliable contraception is recommended. Monitor LFTs, CBCs, and wt. Monitor for signs and symptoms of fluid retention. Increased by ketoconazole, erythromycin, itraconazole, clarithromycin, ritonavir, atazanavir, indinavir, nelfinavir, saquinavir and telithromycin. Decreased by rifampin, phenytoin, carbamazepine, phenobarbital, and dexamethasone. Increases simvastatin. Antacids should be taken at least 2 h pre- or post-dose. Avoid H2 blockers and PPIs.

MOA — Protein-tyrosine kinase inhibitor that inhibits the Bcr-Abl tyrosine kinase, the constitutive abnormal tyrosine kinase created by the Philadelphia chromosome abnormality in chronic myeloid leukemia, and the SRC family kinases.

ADVERSE EFFECTS — Serious: Bone marrow suppression, hemorrhage, pleural effusion, pulmonary arterial hypertension. Frequent: Bone marrow suppression, N/V, diarrhea, edema.

ERLOTINIB (✷*Tarceva*) ▶L ♀D ▶– $$$$$

WARNING — Interstitial lung disease, acute renal failure, hepatic failure, GI perforations, exfoliative skin disorders, MI, CVA, microangiopathic hemolytic anemia, corneal perforation. Elevated INR and potential bleeding. Patients taking warfarin or other coumarin-derivative anticoagulants should be monitored regularly for changes in prothrombin time or INR.

ADULT — Chemotherapy doses vary by indication. The 1st-line treatment of patients with metastatic NSCLC whose tumors have epidermal growth factor receptor (EGFR) exon 19 deletions or exon 21 substitution mutations as detected by an FDA-approved test. In patients with NSCLC receiving maintenance or second or greater line treatment whose tumors have EGFR exon 19 deletions or exon 21 L858R substitution mutations as detected by an FDA-approved test. Locally advanced, unresectable, or metastatic pancreatic cancer.

PEDS — Not approved in children.

FORMS — Trade only: Tabs 25, 100, 150 mg.

NOTES — Reliable contraception is recommended. Hepato-renal syndrome has been reported; monitor LFTs and SCr. CYP3A4 inhibitors such as ketoconazole increase concentrations. CYP3A4 inducers such as rifampin decrease concentrations. Increases INR in patients on warfarin. Monitor LFTs. Avoid concomitant use of erlotinib with H2 blockers and PPIs.

(cont.)

ERLOTINIB (*cont.*)

MOA — Inhibits the intracellular phosphorylation of tyrosine kinase associated with epidermal growth factor receptor, which is expressed on the surface of normal cells and cancer cells.

ADVERSE EFFECTS — Serious: Pulmonary toxicity, GI bleeding, acute renal failure due to dehydration, hepatic failure, GI perforations, exfoliative skin disorders, MI, CVA, microangiopathic hemolytic anemia, corneal perforation. Decreased tear production. Eye disorders. Frequent: Diarrhea, anorexia, fatigue, stomatitis, rash, infection, pruritus.

GEFITINIB (✱*IRESSA*) ▶L ♀D ▶– $ varies by therapy

WARNING — Pulmonary toxicity, corneal erosion, N/V. Instruct patients to report promptly acute onset of dyspnea, cough, and low-grade fever.

ADULT — 250 mg orally daily for treatment of patients with metastatic NSCLC whose tumors have epidermal growth factor receptor (EGFR) exon 19 deletions or exon 21 (L858R) substitution mutations as detected by an FDA-approved test.

PEDS — Not approved in children.

FORMS — Trade only: Tabs 250 mg.

NOTES — Reliable contraception is recommended. Monitor LFTs. Potent inducers of CYP3A4 (eg, rifampin, phenytoin) decrease concentration; use 500 mg. May increase warfarin effect; monitor INR. Potent inhibitors of CYP3A4 (eg, ketoconazole, itraconazole) increase toxicity. Ranitidine increases concentrations.

MOA — Gefitinib reversibly inhibits the kinase activity of wild-type and certain activating mutations of EGFR, preventing autophosphorylation of tyrosine residues associated with the receptor, thereby inhibiting further downstream signalling and blocking EGFR-dependent proliferation.

ADVERSE EFFECTS — Serious: Pulmonary toxicity, corneal erosion. Frequent: Increased LFTs, diarrhea, rash, acne, dry skin, N/V.

IBRUTINIB (✱*Imbruvica*) ▶L ♀D ▶– $$$$$

WARNING — Renal toxicity: Monitor renal function and maintain hydration. Second primary malignancies: Other malignancies have occurred in patients, including skin cancers, and other carcinomas. Embryo-fetal toxicity: Can cause fetal harm. Advise women of the potential risk to a fetus and to avoid pregnancy while taking the drug. Hemorrhage: Monitor for bleeding. Infections: Monitor patients for fever and infections and evaluate promptly. Myelosuppression: Check complete blood counts monthly.

ADULT — 560 mg taken orally once daily for mantle cell lymphoma. A kinase inhibitor indicated for the treatment of patients with mantle cell lymphoma (MCL) who have received at least one prior therapy. 420 mg orally once daily for chronic lymphocytic leukemia/small lymphocytic lymphoma (CLL/SLL), CLL/SLL with 17p deletion. 420 mg orally once daily for Waldenstrom's macroglobulinemia.

FORMS — Trade only: Caps 140mg.

NOTES — CYP3A Inhibitors: Avoid co-administration with strong and moderate CYP3A inhibitors. If a moderate CYP3A inhibitor must be used, reduce Imbruvica dose. CYP3A Inducers: Avoid co-administration with strong CYP3A inducers. Hepatic Impairment: Avoid use of ibrutinib in patients with baseline hepatic impairment

MOA — Ibrutinib is a small-molecule inhibitor of BTK. Ibrutinib forms a covalent bond with a cysteine residue in the BTK active site, leading to inhibition of BTK enzymatic activity. BTK is a signaling molecule of the B-cell antigen receptor (BCR) and cytokine receptor pathways.

ADVERSE EFFECTS — The most common adverse reactions (≥10%) are thrombocytopenia, peripheral edema, hyperuricemia, diarrhea, neutropenia, anemia, fatigue, musculoskeletal pain, peripheral edema, upper respiratory tract infection, nausea, bruising, dyspnea, constipation, rash, abdominal pain, vomiting and decreased appetite. Interstitial lung disease has been experienced postmarketing.

IMATINIB (✱*Gleevec*) ▶L ♀D ▶– $$$$$

WARNING — Cases of fatal tumor lysis syndrome have been reported. Use caution in patients with high tumor burden or high tumor proliferative rate. Bone marrow suppression, increased LFTs, hemorrhage, erythema multiforme, Stevens-Johnson syndrome, N/V, fluid retention including pulmonary edema, CHF, muscle cramps, GI irritation, hemorrhage. May cause growth retardation in children. Use caution when driving a car or operating machinery.

ADULT — Chemotherapy doses vary by indication. CML, GI stromal tumors (GISTs), Ph+ ALL, aggressive systemic mastocytosis, dermatofibrosarcoma protuberans, hypereosinophilic syndrome, myelodysplastic/myeloproliferative disease associated with platelet-derived growth factor receptor mutations. There are two FDA-approved companion diagnostic tests for patients with aggressive systemic mastocytosis (ASM) and myelodysplastic/myeloproliferative diseases (MDS/MPD).

PEDS — Chemotherapy doses vary by indication. Newly diagnosed pediatric acute lymphoblastic leukemia (ALL) that is Philadelphia chromosome (Ph) positive.

UNAPPROVED ADULT — Treatment of desmoid tumors, post stem cell transplant follow-up treatment in CML, hhordoma, melanoma, advanced or metastatic (C-KIT mutated tumors).

FORMS — Generic/Trade: Tabs 100, 400 mg.

NOTES — Reliable contraception is recommended. Monitor LFTs, CBCs, and wt. Monitor for signs and symptoms of fluid retention. Increased by ketoconazole, erythromycin, itraconazole, clarithromycin. Decreased by phenytoin, carbamazepine, rifampin, phenobarbital, St. John's wort. Increases acetaminophen levels and warfarin effects. Monitor INR. Reduce dose with renal insufficiency.

MOA — Imatinib mesylate is a protein-tyrosine kinase inhibitor that inhibits the Bcr-Abl tyrosine kinase, the constitutive abnormal tyrosine kinase

(cont.)

IMATINIB (*cont.*)

created by the Philadelphia chromosome abnormality in chronic myeloid leukemia.
ADVERSE EFFECTS — Serious: Bone marrow suppression, hepatotoxicity, hemorrhage, erythema multiforme, Stevens-Johnson syndrome, pulmonary edema, cardiac tamponade, CHF, increased intracranial pressure and papilledema, subdural hematoma. Frequent: Bone marrow suppression, N/V, diarrhea, edema, muscle cramps, rash, fatigue. Drug rash with eosinophilia and systemic symptoms (DRESS).

LAPATINIB (✱*Tykerb*) ▶L ♀D ▶– $ varies by therapy
WARNING — Hepatotoxicity has been reported with lapatinib. May be severe or fatal. Decreased LVEF, QT prolongation, hepatotoxicity, interstitial lung disease, pneumonitis, severe diarrhea. Serious cutaneous reactions, including erythema multiforme (EM), Stevens-Johnson syndrome (SJS), and toxic epidermal necrolysis (TEN).
ADULT — Chemotherapy doses vary by indication. Treatment of HER2 overexpressing. Advanced or metastatic breast cancer, in combination with capecitabine, in patients who have received prior therapy including an anthracycline, a taxane, and trastuzumab. Also indicated in combination with letrozole for the treatment of postmenopausal women with hormone receptor–positive metastatic breast cancer that overexpresses the HER2 receptor for whom hormonal therapy is indicated.
PEDS — Not approved in children.
FORMS — Trade only: Tabs 250 mg.
NOTES — Monitor LFTs, CBCs, and wt. Monitor for signs and symptoms of fluid retention. Increased by ketoconazole, erythromycin, itraconazole, clarithromycin. Decreased by phenytoin, carbamazepine, rifampin, phenobarbital, St. John's wort. Increases acetaminophen levels and warfarin effects. Monitor INR. Reduce dose with renal insufficiency. Reliable contraception is recommended. Modify dose for cardiac and other toxicities, severe hepatic impairment, and CYP3A4 drug interactions.
MOA — Lapatinib is a protein-tyrosine kinase inhibitor that inhibits epidermal growth factor receptor and human epidermal receptor type 2 in breast cancer cell lines.
ADVERSE EFFECTS — Serious: Diarrhea, decreased ejection fraction, QT prolongation, hepatotoxicity, interstitial lung disease, pneumonitis. Frequent: N/V, diarrhea, fatigue, plantar-palmar erythrodysesthesia, rash.

LENVATINIB (*Lenvima*) ▶L ♀? No human data. Based on mechanism, can cause fetal harm. ▶–
WARNING — Hypertension, cardiac failure, arterial thrombotic events, hepatotoxicity, proteinuria, renal failure, GI perforation and fistula formation, QT interval prolongation, hypocalcemia, reversible posterior leukoencephalopathy, hemorrhagic events (most frequently epistaxis, but include fatal tumor-related bleeding), impairment of thyroid-stimulating hormone suppression, embryofetal toxicity.
ADULT — 24 mg orally once daily for treatment of refractory differentiated thyroid cancer (DTC), which has progressed despite radioactive iodine therapy. In combination with everolimus, for the treatment of patients with advanced renal cell carcinoma who were previously treated with an anti-angiogenic therapy. The recommended dose and schedule is lenvatinib 18 mg plus everolimus 5 mg taken by mouth once daily.
FORMS — 4 mg and 10 mg capsules.
MOA — Multi-tyrosine kinase inhibitor, including VEGF, FDG, and PDGF, KIT and RET.
ADVERSE EFFECTS — Most common: hypertension, fatigue, diarrhea, arthralgia/myalgia, decreased appetite, nausea, stomatitis, headache, vomiting, proteinuria, palmar-plantar erythrodysesthesia syndrome, abdominal pain, and dysphoria. Serious: cardiac failure, thromboembolic events, hepatotoxicity, renal failure, GI perforation, QTc prolongation, hypocalcemia, reversible posterior leukoencephalopathy syndrome, hemorrhage.

NILOTINIB (✱*Tasigna*) ▶L ♀D ▶– $ varies by therapy
WARNING — Prolonged QT interval and sudden death, bone marrow suppression, intracranial hemorrhage, pneumonia, elevated lipase. Progressive peripheral arterial occlusive disease. Must be administered on an empty stomach. Food increases bioavailability, which may then cause prolonged QTc.
ADULT — Chemotherapy doses vary by indication. Treatment of newly diagnosed adult patients with Philadelphia chromosome–positive chronic myeloid leukemia (Ph+ CML) in chronic phase. Treatment of chronic phase (CP) and accelerated phase (AP) Ph+ CML in adult patients resistant to or intolerant to prior therapy that included imatinib.
PEDS — Not approved in children.
UNAPPROVED ADULT — Refractory gastrointestinal stromal tumor (GIST).
FORMS — Trade only: Caps 150, 200 mg.
NOTES — Contraindicated with hypokalemia, hypomagnesemia, or long QT syndrome. Reliable contraception is recommended. Monitor EKG, LFTs, CBCs, and lipase. Serum levels of nilotinib increased by potent CYP450 inhibitors such as ketoconazole and decreased by CYP450 inducers such as rifampin. Avoid food at least 2 h pre-dose or 1 h post-dose. Food effects: Food increases blood levels of nilotinib.
MOA — Nilotinib is a protein-tyrosine kinase inhibitor that inhibits the Bcr-Abl tyrosine kinase, the constitutive abnormal tyrosine kinase created by the Philadelphia chromosome abnormality in chronic myeloid leukemia.
ADVERSE EFFECTS — Serious: Bone marrow suppression, intracranial hemorrhage, pneumonia. Frequent: Bone marrow suppression, N/V/D, rash, pruritus.

OSIMERTINIB (*Tagrisso*) ▶L ♀D ▶–
WARNING — Interstitial lung disease (ILD)/pneumonitis occurred in 3.3% of patients. Permanently discontinue Tagrisso in patients diagnosed with ILD/pneumonitis. QTc Interval Prolongation: Monitor electrocardiograms and electrolytes in patients who have a history or predisposition for QTc prolongation, or those who are taking medications that are known to prolong the QTc interval. Withhold then restart at a reduced dose or permanently discontinue Tagrisso. Cardiomyopathy occurred in 1.4% of patients. Assess left ventricular ejection fraction (LVEF) before treatment and then every 3 months thereafter.
ADULT — 80 mg orally once daily for metastatic epidermal growth factor receptor (EGFR) T790M mutation-positive NSCLC patients, as detected by an FDA-approved test, who have progressed on or after EGFR tyrosine kinase inhibitor (TKI) therapy.
FORMS — 80 mg and 40 mg tablets.
NOTES — Avoid concurrent administration of osimertinib with strong CYP3A inhibitors if possible. If no alternative exists, the patient should be closely monitored for signs of toxicity. Concomitant use may decrease osimertinib plasma concentrations.
MOA — A kinase inhibitor of the epidermal growth factor receptor (EGFR), which binds irreversibly to certain mutant forms of EGFR (T790M, L858R, and exon 19 deletion) at approximately 9-fold lower concentrations than wild-type.
ADVERSE EFFECTS — Most common adverse reactions (≥25%) were diarrhea, rash, dry skin, and nail toxicity. May cause female fertility impairment.

PAZOPANIB (*✚Votrient*) ▶L + ♀D ▶– $$$$$
WARNING — Severe and fatal hepatotoxicity have occurred. Hepatic toxicity risk is increased in patients over 65 yo. Observe LFTs prior to and during treatment. Prolonged QT intervals and torsades de pointes have been observed. Fatal hemorrhagic events have occurred. Arterial thrombotic events have occurred and can be fatal. Post-marketing experience includes retinal detachment/tear. Interstitial lung disease (ILD)/pneumonitis may occur.
ADULT — 800 mg orally once daily without food. Treatment of advanced renal cell carcinoma. Treatment of advanced soft tissue sarcoma in patients who have received prior chemotherapy.
PEDS — Not indicated in children.
FORMS — Trade only: Tabs 200 mg.
NOTES — Do not coadminister pazopanib with medications that increase gastric pH. Will result in decreased level/effect of pazopanib. There is an increase in the incidence of neutropenia, thrombocytopenia, and palmar-plantar erythrodysesthia (PPES) in patients of East Asian descent.
MOA — Multi-tyrosine kinase inhibitor, including VEGFR-1, VEGFR-2, VEGFR-3, PDGFR-alpha and beta, FGFR-1, FGFR-3, cKIT, Itk, Lck, and c-FMS.
ADVERSE EFFECTS — Diarrhea, hypertension, hair color changes (depigmentation), nausea, anorexia, vomiting, fatigue, tumor pain, skin hypopigmentation, arthralgia and spasms.

PONATINIB (*Iclusig*) ▶L + esterases ♀D ▶? $$$$$
WARNING — Boxed warning: arterial thrombosis and liver toxicity.
ADULT — Chronic myeloid leukemia (CML) and Philadelphia chromosome–positive (Ph+) acute lymphoblastic leukemia (Ph+ ALL) in patients for whom no other tyrosine kinase inhibitor therapy is indicated, or who are T315I positive. 45 mg once daily.
FORMS — Trade only: 15, 45 mg oral tabs.
NOTES — A risk evaluation and mitigation strategy (REMS) is required, due to the risk of serious adverse reactions of vascular occlusions including loss of vision due to blood clots, and occlusion of mesenteric blood vessels, stroke, myocardial infarction, peripheral vascular disease with ischemic necrosis, and other vascular occlusive events.
MOA — Pan-BCR-ABL tyrosine kinase inhibitor with in vitro activity against cells expressing native or mutant BCR-ABL, including T315I.
ADVERSE EFFECTS — Rash, abdominal pain, headache, dry skin, constipation, fatigue, pyrexia, nausea, arthralgia, and hypertension. Pancreatitis, elevation of pancreatic enzymes (lipase in 19%, amylase 7%), and myelosuppression (thrombocytopenia in 42%, neutropenia in 34%, and anemia in 20%). Life-threatening blood clots and blood-vessel narrowing.

REGORAFENIB (*✚Stivarga*) ▶L ♀–D ▶– $
WARNING — Black box warning for hepatotoxicity.
ADULT — Treatment of patients with metastatic colorectal cancer (mCRC) who have been previously treated with fluoropyrimidine-, oxaliplatin-, and irinotecan-based chemotherapy; an anti-VEGF therapy; and, if K-Ras wild-type, an anti-EGFR therapy. Treatment of gastrointestinal stromal tumors (GIST), for use in patients with tumors that cannot be surgically removed and no longer respond to imatinib and sunitinib. 160 mg PO once daily for the first 21 days of each 28-day cycle.
PEDS — Not approved in children.
FORMS — Trade only: 40 mg film-coated tabs.
NOTES — No dose adjustment is needed for patients with mild or moderate hepatic impairment; no dose adjustment is needed for patients with mild, moderate, or severe renal impairment. Regorafenib may increase the levels/effects of BCRP substrates. Avoid concomitant use with strong CYP3A4 inducers and inhibitors.
MOA — Inhibits multiple membrane-bound and intracellular kinases involved in normal cellular functions and in pathologic processes, including those in the RET, VEGFR1, VEGFR2, VEGFR3, KIT, PDGFR-alpha, PDGFR-beta, FGFR1, FGFR2, TIE2, DDR2, Trk2A, Eph2A, RAF-1, BRAF, BRAFV600E, SAPK2, PTK5, and Abl pathways.
ADVERSE EFFECTS —Asthenia/fatigue, decreased appetite and food intake, hand-foot skin reaction, diarrhea, mucositis, wt loss, infection, hypertension and dysphonia. The most serious: hepatotoxicity, hemorrhage, and gastrointestinal perforation. Hypersensitivity reactions have occurred postmarketing.

RUXOLITINIB (✱*Jakavi*) ▶L – ♀C ▶–
ADULT — Treatment of intermediate- or high-risk myelofibrosis. Doses based on platelet count. 10 mg two times per day for polycythemia vera (PV) patients who have had an inadequate response to or are intolerant of hydroxyurea.
PEDS — Not approved in children.
FORMS — 5, 10, 15, 20, 25 mg tabs.
NOTES — Dose modifications are necessary for patients who are on a stable dose of ruxolitinib and then start treatment with a strong CYP3A4 inhibitor or fluconazole.
MOA — Kinase inhibitor which selectively inhibits Janus Associated Kinases, JAK1 and JAK2.
ADVERSE EFFECTS — Dizziness, bruising, increased cholesterol,   hyperlipidemia,pancytopenias, increased liver function tests, reactivation or worsening of hepatitis B infection.

SORAFENIB (✱*Nexavar*) ▶L ♀D ▶– $ varies by therapy
WARNING — Increased risk of bleeding, cardiac ischemia/infarction, GI perforation. Sorafenib in combination with carboplatin and paclitaxel is contraindicated in patients with squamous cell lung cancer. Coadministration of oral neomycin causes a decrease in sorafenib exposure. Stevens-Johnson syndrome and toxic epidermal necrolysis, and drug-induced hepatitis.
ADULT — Chemotherapy doses vary by indication. Advanced renal cell carcinoma. Unresectable hepatocellular carcinoma. Treatment of locally recurrent or metastatic, progressive, differentiated thyroid carcinoma (DTC) refractory to radioactive iodine treatment.
PEDS — Not approved in children.
UNAPPROVED ADULT — Recurrent or metastatic angiosarcoma, imatinib-resistant GIST.
FORMS — Trade only: Tabs 200 mg.
NOTES — Take 1 h before or 2 h after meals for best absorption. Monitor BP. Monitor INR with warfarin. Reliable contraception is recommended. Hepatic impairment may reduce concentrations. Increases docetaxel and doxorubicin.
MOA — Multikinase inhibitor; Angiogenesis inhibitor.
ADVERSE EFFECTS — Serious:Angioedema, hepatitis, hemorrhage, myocardial infarction, bone marrow suppression. Frequent: Hand-foot skin reaction and rash, erythema, HTN, hemorrhage, bone marrow suppression, N/V, diarrhea, increased lipase and amylase, mucositis. Hypokalemia, proteinuria, and nephrotic syndrome seen in clinical trials. Interstitial lung disease-like events and osteonecrosis of the jaw seen post marketing.

SUNITINIB (✱*Sutent*) ▶L ♀D ▶– $ varies by therapy
WARNING — Hepatotoxicity has been observed in clinical trials and post-marketing experience. This hepatotoxicity may be severe, and deaths have been reported. Prolonged QT intervals and torsades de pointes have been observed. Hemorrhagic events including tumor-related hemorrhage have occurred. Decrease in LVEF with possible clinical CHF, adrenal toxicity, serious and fatal GI complications, bone marrow suppression, bleeding, HTN, yellow skin discoloration, depigmentation of hair or skin, thyroid dysfunction. Cases of tumor lysis syndrome, some fatal, have been observed in clinical trials and have been reported in post-marketing experience, primarily in patients with RCC or GIST treated with sunitinib.
ADULT — Chemotherapy doses vary by indication. GI stromal tumors (GIST), advanced renal cell carcinoma. Treatment of progressive, well differentiated pancreatic neuroendocrine tumors (pNET) in patients with unresectable, locally advanced, or metastatic disease.
PEDS — Not approved in children.
UNAPPROVED ADULT — Treatment of advanced thyroid cancer, treatment of pancreatic neuroendocrine tumors, treatment of non-GIST soft tissue sarcomas.
FORMS — Trade only: Caps 12.5, 25, 37.5, 50 mg.
NOTES — Reliable contraception is recommended. CYP3A4 inhibitors such as ketoconazole increase concentrations. CYP3A4 inducers such as rifampin and St. John's wort can decrease concentrations. Increases INR in patients on warfarin. Monitor CBC.
MOA — Inhibits the intracellular phosphorylation of tyrosine kinase associated with epidermal growth factor receptor, which is expressed on the surface of normal cells and cancer cells.
ADVERSE EFFECTS — Serious: CHF, bone marrow suppression, bleeding, thyroid dysfunction. Stevens - Johnson syndrome and Erythema Multiforme, Toxic Epidermal Necrolysis, Necrotizing Fasciitis and Proteinuria. Thrombotic microangiopathy, hemolytic uremic syndrome, and thrombocytopenic purpura along with the risk of renal failure and death. Frequent: Diarrhea, fatigue, anorexia, stomatitis, vomiting, dyspepsia, yellow skin discoloration, depigmentation of hair or skin.

TRAMETINIB (✱*Mekinist*) ▶degraded chemically ♀–D ▶– $$$$$
WARNING — Instruct female patients to use highly effective contraception during treatment and for 4 months after treatment. Trametinib as a single agent is not recommended in patients who have received prior BRAF-inhibitor therapy.
ADULT — 2 mg orally once daily, as a single agent or in combination with dabrafenib, for treatment of patients with unresectable or metastatic melanoma with BRAF V600E or V600K mutation.
PEDS — Not approved in children.
FORMS — Trade only: Tabs 0.5, 1, and 2 mg.
NOTES — Re-assess LVEF after 1 month of treatment, and evaluate approximately q 2 to 3 months thereafter.
MOA — Inhibits BRAF kinase V600 mutation-positive melanoma cell growth via inhibition of MEK1 and MEK2 kinase activity.
ADVERSE EFFECTS — Frequent: rash, diarrhea and lymphedema. Serious: cardiomyopathy, retinal

(cont.)

TRAMETINIB (*cont.*)

pigment epithelial detachment, retinal vein occlusion, interstitial lung disease and serious skin toxicity

VANDETANIB (✻*Caprelsa*) ▶K – ♀? ▶–

WARNING — QT prolongation, torsades de pointes, and sudden death. Intestinal perforation has occurred in clinical trials.

ADULT — Unresectable locally advanced or metastatic medullary thyroid carcinoma.

PEDS — Not approved in children.

FORMS — 100 mg and 300 mg oral capsules.

NOTES — Toxic epidermal necrolysis (TEN) has occurred.

MOA — Tyrosine Kinase Inhibitor

ADVERSE EFFECTS — Diarrhea/colitis, heart failure, acneiform rash, nausea, hypertension, QT prolongation. Drug has prolonged half-life: monitor for cardiac toxicities throughout treatment. Hemorrhage, hypothyroidism, ischemic events, pulmonary toxicity, severe skin reactions, reversible posterior leukoencephalopathy syndrome.

VEMURAFENIB (✻*Zelboraf*) ▶? ♀–D ▶–

WARNING — Cutaneous squamous cell carcinomas were detected in 24% of patients receiving vemurafenib in clinical trials. Noncutaneous squamous cell carcinoma and toxic epidermal necrolysis have occurred. Hypersensitivity reactions, uveitis, severe dermatologic reactions, QT prolongation, and liver enzyme abnormalities. Increased hepatotoxicity associated with concurrent ipilimumab administration. DRESS Syndrome. Progression of pre-existing chronic myelomonocytic leukemia with NRAS mutation. May cause radiation sensitization and recall. Pancreatitis. Nephrotoxicity and creatinine abnormalities may occur during treatment. Continuous creatinine monitoring is required.

ADULT — Treatment of unresectable or metastatic melanoma in patients with the BRAFV600E mutation. Dose is 960 mg orally two times per day.

PEDS — Not approved in pediatric patients.

UNAPPROVED ADULT — Erdheim-Chester disease, refractory. Melanoma, metastatic with BRAFV600K mutation, non-small cell lung cancer, refractory, with BRAF V600 mutation.

FORMS — 240 mg oral tabs.

NOTES — Multiple potentially significant drug interactions may exist. Avoid use with CYP3A4 inhibitors and inducers. Avoid use with P-gp substrates. Do not administer with CYP1A2 substrates.

MOA — BRAF kinase inhibitor, active against BRAFV600E mutated form, thereby blocking cellular proliferation of melanoma cells.

ADVERSE EFFECTS — Arthralgias, rash, alopecia, fatigue, photosensitivity and nausea. Monitor for QTprolongation prior to and following treatment initiation or after dose modification; hypersensitivity, severe dermatologic reactions, ophthalmologic reactions, hepatotoxicity, embryo-fetal toxicity, panniculitis and neutropenia.Acute interstitial nephritis and acute tubular necrosis.

ONCOLOGY: Miscellaneous

PALBOCICLIB (*Ibrance*) ▶L ♀? Adverse events observed in animal reproduction studies. Women of reproductive potential should use effective contraception for at least 2 weeks from last dose. ▶–

WARNING — Neutropenia, infection, pulmonary embolism, embryo-fetal toxicity.

ADULT — 125 mg daily for 21 consecutive days followed by 7 days off treatment with letrozole 2.5 mg daily continuously throughout the 28-day cycle, for the treatment of postmenopausal women with estrogen receptor (ER)–positive, human epidermal growth factor receptor 2 (HER2)–negative advanced breast cancer as initial endocrine-based therapy for metastatic disease. Treatment in combination with fulvestrant for the treatment of women with hormone receptor (HR)–positive, human epidermal growth factor receptor 2 (HER2)–negative advanced or metastatic breast cancer with disease progression following endocrine therapy. The dose is 125 mg daily for 21 consecutive days followed by 7 days off treatment in combination with fulvestrant treatment.

FORMS — 125, 100, and 75 mg capsules.

NOTES — Significant drug interactions with CYP3A inhibitors, inducers, and substrates.

MOA — Inhibitor of cyclin-dependent kinase (CDK) 4 and 6. In vitro palbociclib reduced cellular proliferation of ER-positive breast cancer cell lines by blocking progression of cells from G1 into S phase of the cell cycle.

ADVERSE EFFECTS — Most common adverse reactions (greater than or equal to 10%) were neutropenia, leukopenia, fatigue, anemia, upper respiratory infection, nausea, stomatitis, alopecia, diarrhea, thrombocytopenia, decreased appetite, vomiting, asthenia, peripheral neuropathy, and epistaxis.

ARSENIC TRIOXIDE (✻*Trisenox*) ▶L ♀D ▶– $ varies by therapy

WARNING — APL differentiation syndrome: Fever, dyspnea, wt gain, pulmonary infiltrates and pleural/pericardial effusions, occasionally with impaired myocardial contractility and episodic hypotension, with or without leukocytosis. QT prolongation, AV block, torsades de pointes, N/V/D, hyperglycemia, alopecia.

ADULT — Chemotherapy doses vary by indication. Acute promyelocytic leukemia, refractory.

PEDS — Not approved in children younger than 5 yo. Chemotherapy doses vary by indication. Acute promyelocytic leukemia, refractory.

UNAPPROVED ADULT — Chemotherapy doses vary by indication. CML, ALL.

(cont.)

ARSENIC TRIOXIDE (cont.)

NOTES — Reliable contraception is recommended. Monitor ECG, electrolytes, renal function, CBCs, and PT.

MOA — Unknown.

ADVERSE EFFECTS — Serious: APL differentiation syndrome: fever, dyspnea, weight gain, pulmonary infiltrates and pleural/pericardial effusions, with or w/o leukocytosis. QT prolongation, tachycardia, AV block, torsade de pointes, hyperleukocytosis. Frequent: Hypotension, N/V, diarrhea, hyperglycemia, fever, fatigue, dermatitis, nausea, electrolyte abnormalities.

ASPARAGINASE ERWINIA CHRYSANTHEMI (✱Erwinase) ▶? ♀C ▶?

ADULT — A component of a multi-agent chemotherapeutic regimen for the treatment of patients with acute lymphoblastic leukemia (ALL) who have developed hypersensitivity to E. coli–derived asparaginase. May administer IM or IV.

PEDS — Approved in adults and children with ALL.

FORMS — Powder for injection.

MOA — Catalyzes the deamidation of asparagine to aspartic acid and ammonia, resulting in a reduction in circulating levels of asparagine. The mechanism of action of ERWINAZE is thought to be based on the inability of leukemic cells to synthesize asparagine due to lack of asparagine synthetase activity, resulting in cytotoxicity specific for leukemic cells that depend on an exogenous source of the amino acid asparagine for their protein metabolism and survival.

ADVERSE EFFECTS — Pancreatitis, abnormal transaminases, coagulopathies, hemorrhage, nausea, vomiting and hyperglycemia. Common adverse reactions were similar in severity and incidence to those attributable to E. coli-derived asparaginase.

BEXAROTENE (Targretin) ▶L ♀X ▶– $$$$$

WARNING — Gel: Rash, pruritus, contact dermatitis. Caps: Lipid abnormalities, increased LFTs, pancreatitis, hypothyroidism, leukopenia, cataracts, photosensitivity, alopecia.

ADULT — Chemotherapy doses vary by indication. Cutaneous T-cell lymphoma.

PEDS — Not approved in children.

FORMS — Trade only: 1% gel (60 g). Caps 75 mg.

NOTES — Gel: Do not use with DEET (insect repellant) or occlusive dressings. Caps: Monitor lipids, LFTs, thyroid function tests, CBCs. Multiple drug interactions; consult product insert for info. Reliable contraception is recommended.

MOA — Exact mechanism unknown; binds and activates retinoid X receptor subtypes. These receptors ultimately control cellular proliferation and differentiation.

ADVERSE EFFECTS — Gel- Serious: None. Frequent: Rash, pruritus, contact dermatitis. Caps- Serious: Hyperlipidemia, increased LFTs, pancreatitis, hypothyroidism, leukopenia, cataracts, pseudotumor cerebri. Frequent: Nausea, photosensitivity.

BORTEZOMIB (✱Velcade) ▶L ♀D ▶– $ varies by therapy

WARNING — Peripheral neuropathy, orthostatic hypotension, heart failure, pneumonia, acute respiratory distress syndrome, thrombocytopenia, neutropenia, N/V/D. Instruct patients to report promptly acute onset of dyspnea, cough and low-grade fever, and bleeding from any site. Acute liver failure has been reported rarely. Use with caution in patients with hepatic dysfunction.

ADULT — Chemotherapy doses vary by indication. Multiple myeloma, mantle cell lymphoma. In the US may given IV or SC.

PEDS — Not approved in children.

UNAPPROVED ADULT — Waldenstrom's macroglobulinemia, peripheral T-cell lymphoma, cutaneous T-cell lymphoma, systemic light chain amyloidosis.

FORMS — Single-use 3.5 mg vials.

NOTES — Reliable contraception is recommended. Monitor CBCs.

MOA — Inhibits 26S proteasome.

ADVERSE EFFECTS — Serious: Peripheral neuropathy. Patients with pre-existing peripheral neuropathy should weigh risk/benefit. Thrombocytopenia, neutropenia, orthostatic hypotension, heart failure, pneumonia, acute respiratory distress syndrome, reversible posterior leukoencephalopathy (RPLS). Progressive multifocal leukoencephalopathy. Frequent: Peripheral neuropathy, thrombocytopenia, fatigue, nausea, diarrhea, anorexia, constipation, anemia, rash. Possible: acute febrile neutrophilic dermatosis (Sweet Syndrome).

CARFILZOMIB (Kyprolis) ▶proteolysis – ♀D ▶–

WARNING — Heart failure and ischemia: Monitor for cardiac complications. Pulmonary hypertension. Pulmonary complications. Infusion reactions: Premedicate with dexamethasone to prevent. Thrombocytopenic thrombotic purpura/hemolytic uremic syndrome (TTP/HUS) and posterior reversible encephalopathy syndrome (PRES).

ADULT — Treatment of patients in combination with dexamethasone or with lenalidomide plus dexamethasone for the treatment of patients with relapsed or refractory multiple myeloma who have received one to three lines of therapy. As a single agent for the treatment of patients with relapsed or refractory multiple myeloma who have received one or more lines of therapy. Administered IV over 10 to 30 minutes on 2 consecutive days weekly for 3 weeks, followed by a 12-day rest period (28-day treatment cycle). Dose is 20 mg/m^2 at each dose in cycle 1, and 27 mg/m^2 in subsequent cycles.

PEDS — Not approved in children.

FORMS — Single-use vial: 60 mg sterile lyophilized powder.

MOA — Proteasome inhibitor.

ADVERSE EFFECTS — Most common: fatigue, anemia, nausea, thrombocytopenia, dyspnea, diarrhea, and pyrexia. Most serious: pneumonia, acute renal failure, pyrexia, and congestive heart failure.

IDELALISIB (✷*Zydelig*) ▶L ♀D ▶?
WARNING — Boxed warning alerting patients and healthcare professionals of the following fatal and serious adverse reactions: hepatotoxicity, severe diarrhea or colitis, pneumonitis, and intestinal perforation. Severe cutaneous reactions: Monitor patients for the development of severe cutaneous reactions. Anaphylaxis: Monitor patients for anaphylaxis and discontinue. Neutropenia: Monitor blood counts. Embryo-fetal toxicity: May cause fetal harm. Advise women of potential risk to a fetus and to avoid pregnancy while taking.
ADULT — Treatment of patients with relapsed chronic lymphocytic leukemia (CLL), in combination with rituximab, for whom rituximab alone would be considered appropriate therapy due to other comorbidities. Treatment of patients with relapsed follicular B-cell non-Hodgkin lymphoma (FL) or relapsed small lymphocytic lymphoma (SLL) who have received at least two prior systemic therapies. 150 mg orally two times per day.
PEDS — Not approved in children.
FORMS — 100, 150 mg tabs.
MOA — Idelalisib is an inhibitor of PI3Kδ kinase, which is expressed in normal and malignant B-cells. Idelalisib inhibits several cell signaling pathways, including B-cell receptor (BCR) signaling and the CXCR4 and CXCR5 signaling, which are involved in trafficking and homing of B-cells to the lymph nodes and bone marrow.
ADVERSE EFFECTS — Themost common adverse reactions (incidence ≥20%) are diarrhea, pyrexia, fatigue, nausea, cough, pneumonia, abdominal pain, chills, and rash. The most common laboratory abnormalities (incidence ≥30%) are neutropenia, hypertriglyceridemia, hyperglycemia, ALT elevations, and AST elevations.

IXAZOMIB (*Ninlaro*) ▶L ♀D ▶–
WARNING — Thrombocytopenia: Monitor platelet counts at least monthly during treatment and adjust dosing, as needed. Gastrointestinal Toxicities: Adjust dosing for severe diarrhea, constipation, nausea, and vomiting, as needed. Peripheral Neuropathy: Monitor patients for symptoms of peripheral neuropathy and adjust dosing, as needed. Peripheral Edema: Monitor for fluid retention. Investigate for underlying causes, when appropriate. Adjust dosing, as needed. Cutaneous Reactions: Monitor patients for rash and adjust dosing, as needed. Hepatotoxicity: Monitor hepatic enzymes during treatment.
ADULT — 4 mg orally on Days 1, 8, and 15 of a 28-day cycle. Indicated in combination with lenalidomide and dexamethasone for the treatment of patients with multiple myeloma who have received at least one prior therapy.
FORMS — Capsules: 4 mg, 3 mg, and 2.3 mg
NOTES — Avoid concomitant use with strong CYP3A inducers.

MOA — Ixazomib is a reversible proteasome inhibitor. Ixazomib preferentially binds and inhibits the chymotrypsin-like activity of the beta 5 subunit of the 20S proteasome.
ADVERSE EFFECTS — The most common adverse reactions (≥ 20%) are diarrhea, constipation, thrombocytopenia, peripheral neuropathy, nausea, peripheral edema, vomiting, and back pain.

MITOTANE (✷*Lysodren*) ▶L ♀D ▶– $ varies by therapy
WARNING — Adrenal insufficiency, depression, long-term use may lead to brain damage and functional impairment. Prolonged bleeding time. Instruct patients to report promptly if N/V, loss of appetite, diarrhea, mental depression, skin rash, or darkening of the skin occurs. N/V/D, alopecia.
ADULT — Chemotherapy doses vary by indication. Adrenal cortical carcinoma, inoperable.
PEDS — Not approved in children.
FORMS — Trade only: Tabs 500 mg.
NOTES — Hold after shock or trauma; give systemic steroids. Behavioral and neurological assessments at regular intervals when continuous treatment more than 2 years. May decrease steroid and warfarin effects. Reliable contraception is recommended.
MOA — Unknown.
ADVERSE EFFECTS — Serious: Adrenal insufficiency, depression. Frequent: Anorexia, N/V, diarrhea.

OLAPARIB (*LYNPARZA*) ▶L ♀D ▶–
WARNING — Myelodysplastic syndrome/acute myeloid leukemia occurred in patients exposed to Lynparza, and some cases were fatal. Pneumonitis: Occurred in patients exposed to Lynparza, and some cases were fatal. Embryo-fetal toxicity: Lynparza can cause fetal harm. Advise females of reproductive potential of the potential risk to a fetus and to avoid pregnancy.
ADULT — 400 mg two times per day without regard to food as monotherapy in patients with deleterious or suspected deleterious germline BRCA (gBRCA) mutated (as detected by an FDA-approved test) advanced ovarian cancer who have been treated with three or more prior lines of chemotherapy.
FORMS — 50 mg capsules.
NOTES — AUC of olaparib is significantly altered by concomitant use of CYP3A4 inhibitors or inducers. Dose adjustment will be necessary.
MOA — inhibitor of poly (ADP-ribose) polymerase (PARP) enzymes, including PARP1, PARP2, and PARP3. PARP enzymes are involved in normal cellular homeostasis, such as DNA transcription, cell cycle regulation, and DNA repair.
ADVERSE EFFECTS — Most common adverse reactions (≥20%) in clinical trials were anemia, nausea, fatigue (including asthenia), vomiting, diarrhea, dysgeusia,dyspepsia, headache, decreased appetite,nasopharyngitis/pharyngitis/URI, cough, arthralgia/musculoskeletal pain, myalgia, back pain, dermatitis/rash and abdominal pain/discomfort.

OMACETAXINE MEPESUCCINATE (*Synribo*) ▶esterases ♀D ▶? $$$$$

WARNING — Most severe adverse reactions: myelosuppression, bleeding, hyperglycemia.

ADULT — Treatment of adults with chronic myelogenous leukemia (CML), who progress after treatment with at least 2 tyrosine kinase inhibitors. 1.25 mg/m² SC injected two times per day for 14 consecutive days over a 28-day cycle until a hematologic response occurs and white blood cell counts normalize. The drug is then administered 1.25 mg/m² two times per day for 7 consecutive days over a 28-day cycle as long as the patient continues to clinically benefit.

PEDS — Not approved in children.

FORMS — 3.5 mg powder for injection.

MOA — The mechanism of action of SYNRIBO has not been fully elucidated but includes inhibition of protein synthesis. It acts independently of direct Bcr-Abl binding to reduce protein levels of both the Bcr-Abl oncoprotein and Mcl-1 which inhibits apoptosis.

ADVERSE EFFECTS — Most common: thrombocytopenia; anemia; neutropenia and febrile neutropenia; diarrhea; nausea, weakness, and fatigue; injection-site reaction; and lymphopenia.

PANOBINOSTAT (*Farydak*) ▶L reduction, oxidation, hydrolysis, and glucuronidation ♀D Embryo-fetal toxicity: can cause fetal harm. Advise women of the potential hazard to the fetus and to avoid pregnancy while taking Farydak. ▶–

WARNING — Severe diarrhea occurred in 25% of Farydak-treated patients. Monitor for symptoms, institute antidiarrheal treatment, interrupt Farydak, and then reduce dose or discontinue Farydak. Severe and fatal cardiac ischemic events, severe arrhythmias, and ECG changes have occurred in patients receiving Farydak. Arrhythmias may be exacerbated by electrolyte abnormalities. Obtain ECG and electrolytes at baseline and periodically during treatment as clinically indicated. Hemorrhage: Fatal and serious cases of gastrointestinal and pulmonary hemorrhage. Monitor platelet counts and transfuse as needed. Hepatotoxicity: Monitor hepatic enzymes and adjust dosage if abnormal liver function tests are observed during Farydak therapy.

ADULT — 20 mg, taken orally once every other day for 3 doses per week (on days 1, 3, 5, 8, 10, and 12) of weeks 1 and 2 of each 21-day cycle for 8 cycles in combination with bortezomib and dexamethasone for the treatment of patients with multiple myeloma who have received at least two prior regimens, including bortezomib and an immunomodulatory agent. Consider continuing treatment for an additional 8 cycles for patients with clinical benefit, unless they have unresolved severe or medically significant toxicity.

FORMS — 10, 15, 20 mg capsules.

NOTES — Strong CYP3A4 inhibitors: Reduce Farydak dose. Strong CYP3A4 inducers: Avoid concomitant use with Farydak. Sensitive CYP2D6 substrates: Avoid concomitant use with Farydak. Antiarrhythmic drugs/QT-prolonging drugs: Avoid concomitant use.

MOA — Histone deacetylase inhibitor.

ADVERSE EFFECTS — The most common adverse reactions (incidence of at least 20%) in clinical studies are diarrhea, fatigue, nausea, peripheral edema, decreased appetite, pyrexia, and vomiting. The most common non-hematologic laboratory abnormalities (incidence ≥ 40%) are hypophosphatemia, hypokalemia, hyponatremia, and increased creatinine. The most common hematologic laboratory abnormalities (incidence ≥60%) are thrombocytopenia, lymphopenia, leukopenia, neutropenia, and anemia.

PEGASPARGASE (*Oncaspar*) ▶? ♀C ▶– $ varies by therapy

WARNING — Contraindicated with previous/current pancreatitis. Hypersensitivity, including anaphylaxis. Bone marrow suppression, bleeding, hyperuricemia, hyperglycemia, hepato/nephrotoxicity, CNS toxicity, N/V/D, alopecia.

ADULT — Chemotherapy doses vary by indication. ALL, in combination regimens.

PEDS — Chemotherapy doses vary by indication. ALL, in combination regimens.

NOTES — Monitor CBCs, LFTs, renal function, amylase, glucose, and PT. Bleeding potentiated with warfarin, heparin, dipyridamole, aspirin, or NSAIDs.

MOA — Unknown.

ADVERSE EFFECTS — Serious: Anaphylaxis, bone marrow suppression, bleeding, hyperglycemia, hepato/nephrotoxicity, CNS toxicity. Frequent: N/V, diarrhea, bone marrow suppression, hepatotoxicity, hyperlipidemia.

PORFIMER (✦*Photofrin*) ▶? ♀C ▶– $ varies by therapy

WARNING — Photosensitivity, ocular sensitivity, chest pain, respiratory distress, constipation.

ADULT — Chemotherapy doses vary by indication. Esophageal cancer. Endobronchial non-small-cell lung cancer. High-grade dysplasia in Barrett's esophagus. (All with laser therapy.)

PEDS — Not approved in children.

NOTES — Avoid concurrent photosensitizing drugs.

MOA — Photosensitizer.

ADVERSE EFFECTS — Serious: Photosensitivity, ocular sensitivity, chest pain, respiratory distress. Frequent: Photosensitivity, ocular sensitivity, constipation.

RASBURICASE (*Elitek*, ✦*Fasturtec*) ▶L ♀C ▶– $$$$$

WARNING — May cause serious and fatal hypersensitivity reactions including anaphylaxis, hemolysis (G6PD-deficient patients), methemoglobinemia, interference with uric acid measurements.

ADULT — Uric acid elevation prevention with leukemia, lymphoma, and solid tumor malignancies receiving anticancer therapy: 0.2 mg/kg IV over 30 min daily for up to 5 days.

PEDS — Uric acid elevation prevention in children (1 mo to 17 yo) with leukemia, lymphoma, and solid

(cont.)

RASBURICASE (*cont.*)

tumor malignancies receiving anticancer therapy: 0.2 mg/kg IV over 30 min daily for up to 5 days.

FORMS — 1.5mg, 7.5mg vials.

NOTES — Safety and efficacy have been established only for one 5-day treatment course. Hydrate IV if at risk for tumor lysis syndrome. Screen for G6PD deficiency in high-risk patients.

MOA — Catalyzes enzymatic oxidation of uric acid into an inactive and soluble metabolite.

ADVERSE EFFECTS — Serious: Anaphylaxis, hemolysis, methemoglobinemia, acute renal failure, arrhythmia, cardiac failure, cardiac arrest, cellulitis, cerebrovascular disorder, chest pain, convulsions, dehydration, ileus, infection, intestinal obstruction, hemorrhage, myocardial infarction, paresthesia, pancytopenia, pneumonia, pulmonary edema, pulmonary hypertension, retinal hemorrhage, rigors, thrombosis, and thrombophlebitis. Frequent: Fever, neutropenia with fever, respiratory distress, sepsis, neutropenia, mucositis, vomiting, nausea, headache, abdominal pain, constipation, diarrhea, rash.

ROMIDEPSIN (*Istodax*) ▶L − ♀D ▶−

WARNING — QTc prolongation/ECG changes have been observed. High potential for drug interactions. Avoid concomitant use with CYP3A4 inhibitors and inducers. Pancytopenias.

ADULT — 14 mg/m^2 IV days 1, 8, and 15 of a 28-day cycle. Treatment of cutaneous T-cell lymphoma in patients who have received at least one prior systemic therapy. Refractory peripheral T-cell lymphoma.

PEDS — Not approved in children.

FORMS — 10 mg powder for reconstitution.

MOA — Histone deacetylase inhibitor. Induces arrest in cell cycle at G1 and G2/M phases.

ADVERSE EFFECTS — ST-T wave changes, hypotension, fatigue, fever, pruritis, hyperglycemia, electrolyte changes, nausea, vomiting, anorexia, pancytopenias, transaminitis, weakness, infection.

SONIDEGIB (*Odomzo*) ▶L Primarily metabolized by CYP3A ♀− Sonidegib can cause embryo-fetal death or severe birth defects when administered to a pregnant woman and is embryotoxic, fetotoxic, and teratogenic in animals. ▶− Lactation: Do not breastfeed during treatment with sonidegib and for at least 20 months after the last dose .

WARNING — Sonidegib can cause embryo-fetal death or severe birth defects when administered to a pregnant woman and is embryotoxic, fetotoxic, and teratogenic in animals.

ADULT — 200 mg orally once daily taken on an empty stomach, at least 1 h before or 2 h after a meal for treatment of patients with locally advanced basal cell carcinoma (BCC) that has recurred following surgery or radiation therapy, or those who are not candidates for surgery or radiation therapy.

FORMS — 200 mg capsules.

NOTES — Blood donation: Advise patients not to donate blood or blood products during treatment

with sonidegib and for at least 20 months after the last dose. Musculoskeletal adverse reactions: Obtain serum creatine kinase (CK) and creatinine levels prior to initiating therapy, periodically during treatment, and as clinically indicated. CYP3A inhibitors: Avoid strong CYP3A inhibitors. Avoid long-term (greater than 14 days) use of moderate CYP3A inhibitors. CYP3A inducers: Avoid strong and moderate CYP3A inducers. Avoid acid reducing agents.

MOA — Sonidegib is an inhibitor of the Hedgehog pathway. Sonidegib binds to and inhibits Smoothened, a transmembrane protein involved in Hedgehog signal transduction.

ADVERSE EFFECTS — The most common adverse reactions occurring in ≥10% of patients are muscle spasms, alopecia, dysgeusia, fatigue, nausea, musculoskeletal pain, diarrhea, decreased weight, decreased appetite, myalgia, abdominal pain, headache, pain, vomiting, and pruritus.

TALIMOGENE LAHERPAREPVEC (*Imlygic*) ▶? ♀D ▶−

WARNING — Accidental Exposure to IMLYGIC: Accidental exposure may lead to transmission of IMLYGIC and herpetic infection. Healthcare providers and close contacts should avoid direct contact with injected lesions, dressings, or body fluids of treated patients. Healthcare providers who are immunocompromised or pregnant should not prepare or administer IMLYGIC. If accidental exposure occurs, exposed individuals should clean the affected area. Herpetic Infection: Patients who develop herpetic infections should be advised to follow standard hygienic practices to prevent viral transmission. Injection Site Complications: Consider the risks and benefits before continuing IMLYGIC treatment if persistent infection or delayed healing develops. Immune-Mediated Events: Consider the risks and benefits of IMLYGIC before initiating treatment in patients who have underlying autoimmune disease or before continuing treatment in patients who develop immune-mediated events. Plasmacytoma at Injection Site: Consider the risks and benefits in patients with multiple myeloma or in whom plasmacytoma develops during treatment.

ADULT — Administer IMLYGIC by injection into cutaneous, subcutaneous, and/or nodal lesions. (2) Recommended starting dose is up to a maximum of 4 mL of IMLYGIC at a concentration of 106 (1 million) plaque-forming units (PFU) per mL. Subsequent doses should be administered up to 4 mL of IMLYGIC at a concentration of 108 (100 million) PFU per mL. IMLYGIC is a genetically-modified oncolytic viral therapy indicated for the local treatment of unresectable cutaneous, subcutaneous, and nodal lesions in patients with melanoma recurrent after initial surgery.

FORMS — Injection: 10^6 (1 million) PFU per mL, 10^8 (100 million) PFU per mL in single-use vials

NOTES — Talimogene laherparepvec is administered via direct injection into the recurrent, unresectable melanoma lesions.

(cont.)

TALIMOGENE LAHERPAREPVEC (*cont.*)

MOA — IMLYGIC has been genetically modified to replicate within tumors and to produce the immune stimulatory protein GM-CSF. It is a genetically modified attenuated herpes simplex virus 1 oncolytic virus. IMLYGIC causes lysis of tumors, followed by release of tumor-derived antigens, which together with virally derived GM-CSF may promote an antitumor immune response. However, the exact mechanism of action is unknown.

ADVERSE EFFECTS — The most commonly reported adverse drug reactions (≥ 25%) in IMLYGIC-treated patients were fatigue, chills, pyrexia, nausea, influenza-like illness, and injection site pain.

TRETINOIN—ONCOLOGY (✱*Vesanoid*) ▶L ♀D ▶– $ varies by therapy

WARNING — Retinoic acid-APL (RA-APL) syndrome: Fever, dyspnea, wt gain, pulmonary edema, pulmonary infiltrates and pleural/pericardial effusions, occasionally with impaired myocardial contractility and episodic hypotension, with or without leukocytosis. Reversible hypercholesterolemia/hypertriglyceridemia, increased LFTs, alopecia. Contraindicated in paraben-sensitive patients.

ADULT — Chemotherapy doses vary by indication. Acute promyelocytic leukemia.

PEDS — Not approved in children.

UNAPPROVED PEDS — Acute promyelocytic leukemia. Limited data.

FORMS — Generic/Trade: Caps 10 mg.

NOTES — Reliable contraception is recommended. Monitor CBCs, coags, LFTs, and triglyceride and cholesterol levels. Ketoconazole increases levels.

MOA — Unknown.

ADVERSE EFFECTS — Serious: APL differentiation syndrome: fever, dyspnea, weight gain, pulmonary infiltrates and pleural/pericardial effusions, with or w/o leukocytosis, pseudotumor cerebri. Frequent: Reversible hyperlipidemia, headache, fever.

VENETOCLAX (*VENCLEXTA*) ▶L Venetoclax is predominantly metabolized by CYP3A4/5 ♀X Use in pregnant animals caused post-implantation loss and decreased fetal weight ▶–

WARNING — Tumor Lysis Syndrome (TLS): Anticipate TLS; assess risk in all patients. Premedicate with anti-hyperuricemics and ensure adequate hydration. Employ more intensive measures (intravenous hydration, frequent monitoring, hospitalization) as overall risk increases. Neutropenia: Monitor blood counts and for signs of infection; manage as medically appropriate. Immunization: Do not administer live attenuated vaccines prior to, during, or after VENCLEXTA treatment. Embryo-Fetal Toxicity: May cause embryo-fetal harm. Advise females of reproductive potential of the potential risk to a fetus and to use effective contraception during treatment.

ADULT — Initiate therapy with VENCLEXTA at 20 mg once daily for 7 days, followed by a weekly ramp-up dosing schedule to the recommended daily dose of 400 mg for treatment of patients with chronic lymphocytic leukemia (CLL) with 17p deletion, as detected by an FDA approved test, who have received at least one prior therapy.

FORMS — Tablets: 10 mg, 50 mg, 100 mg

NOTES — Use with strong CYP3A inhibitors at initiation and during ramp up phase is contraindicated. Avoid concomitant use of VENCLEXTA with moderate CYP3A inhibitors, strong or moderate CYP3A inducers, P-glycoprotein inhibitors, or narrow therapeutic index P-gp substrates. If a moderate CYP3A inhibitor or a P-glycoprotein inhibitor must be used, reduce the VENCLEXTA dose by at least 50%. If a strong CYP3A inhibitor must be used after the ramp-up phase, reduce the VENCLEXTA dose by at least 75%. If a narrow therapeutic index P-glycoprotein substrate must be used, it should be taken at least 6 hours before VENCLEXTA.

MOA — Venetoclax is a selective and orally bioavailable small-molecule inhibitor of BCL-2, an anti-apoptotic protein. Overexpression of BCL-2 has been demonstrated in CLL cells where it mediates tumor cell survival and has been associated with resistance to chemotherapeutics. Venetoclax helps restore the process of apoptosis by binding directly to the BCL-2 protein, displacing pro-apoptotic proteins like BIM, triggering mitochondrial outer membrane permeabilization and the activation of caspases. In nonclinical studies, venetoclax has demonstrated cytotoxic activity in tumor cells that overexpress BCL-2.

ADVERSE EFFECTS — The most common adverse reactions (≥20%): neutropenia, diarrhea, nausea, anemia, upper respiratory tract infection, thrombocytopenia, and fatigue.

VISMODEGIB (✱*Erivedge*) ▶oxidation–glucuronidation ♀D ▶–

WARNING — Vismodegib has been approved with a boxed warning stating that use of this drug can result in embryo-fetal death or severe birth defects. Pregnancy status must be verified prior to initiation of treatment, and both male and female patients need to be advised of these risks. Women need to be advised of the need for contraception and men of the potential risk for vismodegib exposure through semen.

ADULT — 150 mg orally once daily for basal cell carcinoma (BCC) that has metastasized or relapsed after treatment with surgery, or for patients who are not candidates for surgery or radiation.

PEDS — Not approved in children.

FORMS — 150 mg capsules.

MOA — Vismodegib is an oral drug that is designed to selectively inhibit abnormal signaling in the Hedgehog pathway, which is an underlying molecular driver of BCC. It binds to and inhibits Smoothened, a transmembrane protein involved in Hedgehog signal transduction.

ADVERSE EFFECTS — Muscle spasms, alopecia, dysgeusia, weight loss, fatigue, nausea, diarrhea, decreased appetite, constipation, arthralgias, vomiting, and ageusia.

VORINOSTAT (✹*Zolinza*) ▶L ♀D ▶– $$$$$
WARNING — PE/DVT, anemia, thrombocytopenia, QT prolongation.
ADULT — Chemotherapy doses vary by indication. Cutaneous T-cell lymphoma.
PEDS — Not approved in children.
FORMS — Trade only: Caps 100 mg.
NOTES — Reliable contraception is recommended. Monitor CBCs, electrolytes, renal function, ECG.
MOA — Unknown.
ADVERSE EFFECTS — Serious: PE/DVT, anemia, thrombocytopenia, QT prolongation. Frequent: N/V/D, hyperglycemia, fatigue, chills.

ZALTRAP (**ziv-aflibercept**) ▶? ♀–C ▶–
WARNING — Severe and sometimes fatal hemorrhages, including gastrointestinal hemorrhages, have been reported in patients receiving ziv-aflibercept. Post-marketing experience includes osteonecrosis of the jaw.
ADULT — Treatment of patients with metastatic colorectal cancer (mCRC) that is resistant to or has progressed following an oxaliplatin-containing regimen. 4 mg/kg administered as a 60-minute IV infusion q 2 weeks in combination with the FOLFIRI regimen.
PEDS — Not approved in children.
FORMS — 100 mg per 4 mL soln, single-use vial 200 mg per 8 mL soln, single-use vial.
MOA — Recombinant fusion protein consisting of vascular endothelial growth factor (VEGF)-binding portions from the extracellular domains of human VEGF receptors 1 and 2 that are fused to the Fc portion of the human IgG1 immunoglobulin. By binding to these endogenous ligands, ziv-aflibercept can inhibit the binding and activation of their cognate receptors. This inhibition can result in decreased neovascularization and decreased vascular permeability.
ADVERSE EFFECTS — Leukopenia, diarrhea, neutropenia, proteinuria, increased AST and ALT, stomatitis, fatigue, thrombocytopenia, hypertension, decreased wt, decreased appetite, epistaxis, abdominal pain, dysphonia, increased serum creatinine, and headache.

OPHTHALMOLOGY

OPHTHALMOLOGY: Antiallergy—Decongestants and Combinations

NOTE: Overuse can cause rebound dilation of blood vessels. Do not administer while wearing soft contact lenses. Wait 10 min after use before inserting contact lenses. On average, each mL of eye drop soln contains approximately 20 gtts. Reserve ointment formulations for bedtime use due to severe vision blurring. Most eye medications can be administered 1 gtt at a time despite common manufacturer recommendations of 1 to 2 gtts concurrently. Even a single gtt is typically more than the eye can hold, and thus a 2nd gtt is wasteful and increases the possibility of systemic toxicity. If 2 gtts of the medication are desired, separate single gtts by at least 5 min.

NAPHAZOLINE (*Albalon, All Clear, Naphcon, Clear Eyes***)** ▶? ♀C ▶? $
ADULT — Ocular vasoconstrictor/decongestant: 1 to 2 gtts four times per day for up to 3 days.
PEDS — Not approved for age younger than 6 yo. Use adult dose for age 6 yo or older.
FORMS — OTC Generic/Trade: Soln 0.012, 0.025% (15, 30 mL). Rx Generic/Trade: 0.1% (15 mL).
NOTES — Avoid in patients with cardiovascular disease, HTN, narrow-angle glaucoma.
MOA — Alpha-adrenergic agonist decongestant.
ADVERSE EFFECTS — Frequent: Blurred vision, cardiovascular stimulation, dizziness, headache, nervousness, nausea, stinging, mucosal irritation, dryness, rebound dilation.

NAPHCON-A (naphazoline + pheniramine) ▶L ♀C ▶? $
ADULT — Ocular decongestant: 1 gtt four times per day prn for up to 3 days.
PEDS — Not approved for age younger than 6 yo. Use adult dose for age 6 yo or older.

FORMS — OTC Trade only: Soln 0.025% + 0.3% (15 mL).
NOTES — Avoid in patients with cardiovascular disease, HTN, narrow-angle glaucoma, age younger than 6 yo.
MOA — Antihistamine, decongestant.
ADVERSE EFFECTS — Frequent: Dry mouth, anticholinergic effects, rebound congestion, pupillary dilation, increase in intraocular pressure.

VASOCON-A (naphazoline + antazoline) ▶L ♀C ▶? $
ADULT — Ocular decongestant: 1 gtt four times per day prn for up to 3 days.
PEDS — Not approved for children younger than 6 yo. Use adult dose for age 6 yo or older.
FORMS — OTC Trade only: Soln 0.05% + 0.5% (15 mL).
NOTES — Avoid in patients with cardiovascular disease, HTN, narrow-angle glaucoma.
MOA — Decongestant, antihistamine.
ADVERSE EFFECTS — Frequent: Dry mouth, anticholinergic effects, rebound congestion.

OPHTHALMOLOGY: Antiallergy—Dual Antihistamine and Mast Cell Stabilizer

NOTE: Wait at least 10 to 15 min after use before inserting contact lenses. On average, each mL of eye drop soln contains approximately 20 gtts. Reserve ointment formulations for bedtime use due to severe vision blurring. Most eye medications can be administered 1 gtt at a time despite common manufacturer recommendations of 1 to 2 gtts concurrently. Even a single gtt is typically more than the eye can hold and thus a 2nd gtt is both wasteful and increases the possibility of systemic toxicity. If 2 gtts of the medication are desired, separate single gtts by at least 5 min.

AZELASTINE—OPHTHALMIC (*Optivar***)** ▶L ♀C ▶? $$$
ADULT — Allergic conjunctivitis: 1 gtt two times per day.
PEDS — Not approved for age younger than 3 yo. Use adult dose for age 3 yo or older.
FORMS — Trade/Generic: Soln 0.05% (6 mL).
MOA — H-1 receptor antagonist, mast cell stabilizer, inhibitor of other mediators of allergic response (eg, leukotrienes).
ADVERSE EFFECTS — Frequent: Burning, stinging, headache, somnolence, bitter taste.

EPINASTINE (*Elestat***)** ▶K ♀C ▶? $$$$
ADULT — Allergic conjunctivitis: 1 gtt two times per day.
PEDS — Not approved for age younger than 2 yo. Use adult dose for age 2 yo or older.
FORMS — Trade only: Soln 0.05% (5 mL).
MOA — H-1 receptor antagonist, mast cell stabilizer.

ADVERSE EFFECTS — Frequent: Burning, pruritus, hyperemia.

KETOTIFEN—OPHTHALMIC (*Alaway, Zaditor***)** ▶minimal absorption ♀C ▶? $
ADULT — Allergic conjunctivitis: 1 gtt in each eye q 8 to 12 h.
PEDS — Not approved in children younger than 3 yo. Use adult dose in children older than 3 yo.
FORMS — OTC Generic/Trade: Soln 0.025% (5 mL, 10 mL).
MOA — H-1-receptor antagonist and mast cell stabilizer.
ADVERSE EFFECTS — Frequent: Stinging, burning, dry eyes, photophobia.

OLOPATADINE—OPHTHALMIC (*Pazeo, Pataday, Patanol***)** ▶K ♀C ▶? $$$$$
ADULT — Allergic conjunctivitis: 1 gtt of 0.1% soln in each eye two times per day (Patanol) or 1 gtt of

(cont.)

OLOPATADINE—OPHTHALMIC (*cont.*)

0.2% soln in each eye daily (Pataday) or 1 gtt of 0.7% soln in each affected eye daily (Pazeo).
PEDS — Not approved for age younger than 3 yo. Use adult dose for age 3 yo or older (Patanol, Pataday) or 2 yo or older (Pazeo).

FORMS — Generic/Trade: Soln 0.1% (5 mL, Patanol). Trade only: Soln 0.2% (2.5 mL, Pataday), soln 0.7% (4 mL, Pazeo).
NOTES — Do not administer while wearing soft contact lenses. Allow 6 to 8 h between doses.
MOA — H-1-receptor antagonist and mast cell stabilizer.
ADVERSE EFFECTS — Ocular: Frequent: Headache.

OPHTHALMOLOGY: Antiallergy—Pure Antihistamines

NOTE: Antihistamines may aggravate dry-eye symptoms. Wait 10 min after use before inserting contact lenses. On average, each mL of eye drop soln contains approximately 20 gtts. Reserve ointment formulations for bedtime use due to severe vision blurring. Most eye medications can be administered 1 gtt at a time despite common manufacturer recommendations of 1 to 2 gtts concurrently. Even a single gtt is typically more than the eye can hold and thus a 2nd gtt is both wasteful and increases the possibility of systemic toxicity. If 2 gtts of the medication are desired, separate single gtts by at least 5 min.

ALCAFTADINE (*Lastacaft*) ▶not absorbed ♀B ▶? $$$
ADULT — Allergic conjunctivitis: 1 gtt in each eye daily.
PEDS — Not approved in children younger than 2 yo. Use adult dosing in children 2 yo or older.
FORMS — Trade: Soln 0.25%, 3 mL.
MOA — H1-receptor blocker.
ADVERSE EFFECTS — Frequent: eye irritation, burning, stinging, reness, pruritis.
BEPOTASTINE (*Bepreve*) ▶L (but minimal absorption) − ♀C ▶? $$$
ADULT — Allergic conjunctivitis: 1 gtt two times per day.
PEDS — Not studied in children younger than 2 yo.

FORMS — Trade only: Soln 1.5% (2.5, 5, 10 mL).
NOTES — Remove contact lenses prior to instillation.
MOA — Direct histamine-1-receptor antagonist.
ADVERSE EFFECTS — Frequent: Mild taste, irritation, headache.
EMEDASTINE (*Emadine*) ▶L ♀B ▶? $$$
ADULT — Allergic conjunctivitis: 1 gtt daily to four times per day.
PEDS — Not approved for age younger than 3 yo. Use adult dose for age 3 yo or older.
FORMS — Trade only: Soln 0.05% (5 mL).
MOA — H-1-receptor antagonist.
ADVERSE EFFECTS — Frequent: Headache.

OPHTHALMOLOGY: Antiallergy—Pure Mast Cell Stabilizers

NOTE: Works best as preventive agent; use continually during at risk season. Wait 10 min after use before inserting contact lenses. On average, each mL of eye drop soln contains approximately 20 gtts. Reserve ointment formulations for bedtime use due to severe vision blurring. Most eye medications can be administered 1 gtt at a time despite common manufacturer recommendations of 1 to 2 gtts concurrently. Even a single gtt is typically more than the eye can hold and thus a 2nd gtt is both wasteful and increases the possibility of systemic toxicity. If 2 gtts of the medication are desired, separate single gtts by at least 5 min.

CROMOLYN—OPHTHALMIC (*Crolom, Opticrom*) ▶LK ♀B ▶? $$
ADULT — Allergic conjunctivitis: 1 to 2 gtts 4 to 6 times per day.
PEDS — Not approved for age younger than 4 yo. Use adult dose for age 4 yo or older.
FORMS — Generic/Trade: Soln 4% (10 mL).
NOTES — Response may take up to 6 weeks.
MOA — Prevents mast cell degranulation and release of histamine, leukotrienes and slow-reacting substance of anaphylaxis.
ADVERSE EFFECTS — Frequent: Conjunctival redness, dryness, irritation, hypersensitivity reactions.
LODOXAMIDE (*Alomide*) ▶K ♀B ▶? $$$
ADULT — Allergic conjunctivitis: 1 to 2 gtts in each eye four times per day for up to 3 months.
PEDS — Not approved for age younger than 2 yo. Use adult dose for age 2 yo or older.

FORMS — Trade only: Soln 0.1% (10 mL).
NOTES — Do not administer while wearing soft contact lenses.
MOA — Mast cell stabilizer.
ADVERSE EFFECTS — Frequent: Blurred vision, eye pain, possible corneal erosion.
NEDOCROMIL—OPHTHALMIC (*Alocril*) ▶L ♀B ▶? $$$
ADULT — Allergic conjunctivitis: 1 to 2 gtts in each eye two times per day.
PEDS — Not approved for age younger than 3 yo. Use adult dosing in children 3 yo or older.
FORMS — Trade only: Soln 2% (5 mL).
NOTES — Soln normally appears slightly yellow.
MOA — Mast cell stabilizer.
ADVERSE EFFECTS — Frequent: Burning, irritation, stinging, conjunctival redness, photophobia.

OPHTHALMOLOGY: Antibacterials—Aminoglycosides

NOTE: On average, each mL of eye drop soln contains approximately 20 gtts. Reserve ointment formulations for bedtime use due to severe vision blurring. Most eye medications can be administered 1 gtt at a time despite common manufacturer recommendations of 1 to 2 gtts concurrently. Even a single gtt is typically more than the eye can hold and thus a 2nd gtt is both wasteful and increases the possibility of systemic toxicity. If 2 gtts of the medication are desired, separate single gtts by at least 5 min.

GENTAMICIN—OPHTHALMIC (*Garamycin, Genoptic, Gentak, ✚Diogent*) ▶K ♀C ▶? $
ADULT — Ocular infections: 1 to 2 gtts q 2 to 4 h or ½ inch ribbon of ointment two to three times per day.
PEDS — Not approved in children.
UNAPPROVED ADULT — Up to 2 gtts q 1 h have been used for severe infections. 1 gtt under nails three times per day has been used for subungual Pseudomonas infection presenting as a green nail.
UNAPPROVED PEDS — Ocular infections: 1 to 2 gtts q 4 h or ½ inch ribbon of ointment two to three times per day.
FORMS — Generic/Trade: Soln 0.3% (5, 15 mL). Oint 0.3% (3.5 g tube).
NOTES — For severe infections, use up to 2 gtts q 1 h.
MOA — Inhibits RNA-dependent bacterial protein synthesis.
ADVERSE EFFECTS — Frequent: Edema, rash, pruritus, ocular irritation.

TOBRAMYCIN—OPHTHALMIC (*Tobrex*) ▶K ♀B ▶– $
ADULT — Ocular infections, mild to moderate: 1 to 2 gtts q 4 h or ½ inch ribbon of ointment two to three times per day. Ocular infections, severe: 2 gtts q 1 h, then taper to q 4 h or ½ inch ribbon of ointment q 3 to 4 h, then taper to two to three times per day.
PEDS — Use adult dose for age 2 mo or older.
UNAPPROVED PEDS — Ocular infections, mild to moderate: 1 to 2 gtts q 4 h or ½ inch ribbon of ointment two to three times per day. Ocular infections, severe: 2 gtts q 1 h, then taper to q 4 h or ½ inch ribbon of ointment q 3 to 4 h, then taper to two to three times per day.
FORMS — Generic/Trade: Soln 0.3% (5 mL). Trade only: Oint 0.3% (3.5 g tube).
MOA — Inhibits RNA-dependent bacterial protein synthesis.
ADVERSE EFFECTS — Frequent: Edema, rash, pruritus, ocular irritation.

OPHTHALMOLOGY: Antibacterials—Fluoroquinolones

NOTE: Avoid the overuse of fluoroquinolones for conjunctivitis. Ocular administration has not been shown to cause arthropathy. On average, each mL of eye drop soln contains approximately 20 gtts. Reserve ointment formulations for bedtime use due to severe vision blurring. Most eye medications can be administered 1 gtt at a time despite common manufacturer recommendations of 1 to 2 gtts concurrently. Even a single gtt is typically more than the eye can hold and thus a 2nd gtt is both wasteful and increases the possibility of systemic toxicity. If 2 gtts of the medication are desired, separate single gtts by at least 5 min.

BESIFLOXACIN (*Besivance*) ▶LK ♀C ▶? $$$
ADULT — Bacterial conjunctivitis: 1 gtt three times per day for 7 days.
PEDS — Not approved for age younger than 1 yo. Use adult dose for age 1 yo or older.
FORMS — Trade: Soln 0.6% (5 mL).
NOTES — Do not wear contacts during use.
MOA — Inhibits DNA-gyrase in susceptible bacteria.
ADVERSE EFFECTS — Frequent: Blurred vision, eye pain, eye irritation, eye pruritus and headache.

CIPROFLOXACIN—OPHTHALMIC (*Ciloxan*) ▶LK ♀C ▶? $$
ADULT — Corneal ulcers/keratitis: 2 gtts q 15 min for 6 h, then 2 gtts q 30 min for 1 day; then 2 gtts q 1 h for 1 day, and 2 gtts q 4 h for 3 to 14 days. Bacterial conjunctivitis: 1 to 2 gtts q 2 h while awake for 2 days, then 1 to 2 gtts q 4 h while awake for 5 days; or ½ inch ribbon ointment three times per day for 2 days, then ½ inch ribbon two times per day for 5 days.
PEDS — Bacterial conjunctivitis: Use adult dose for age 1 yo or older (soln) and age 2 yo or older (ointment). Not approved below these ages.
FORMS — Generic/Trade: Soln 0.3% (2.5, 5, 10 mL). Trade only: Oint 0.3% (3.5 g tube).

NOTES — May cause white precipitate of active drug at site of epithelial defect that may be confused with a worsening infection. Resolves within 2 weeks and does not necessitate discontinuation.
MOA — Inhibits DNA-gyrase in susceptible bacteria.
ADVERSE EFFECTS — Frequent: Headache, eye discomfort, keratopathy, burning sensation. Severe: Hypersensitivity.

LEVOFLOXACIN—OPHTHALMIC (*Iquix, Quixin*) ▶KL ♀C ▶? $$$
ADULT — Bacterial conjunctivitis, Quixin: 1 to 2 gtts q 2 h while awake (up to 8 times per day) on days 1 and 2, then 1 to 2 gtts q 4 h (up to 4 times per day) on days 3 to 7. Corneal ulcers, Iquix: 1 to 2 gtts q 30 min to 2 h while awake and q 4 to 6 h overnight on days 1 to 3, then 1 to 2 gtts q 1 to 4 h while awake on day 4 to completion of therapy.
PEDS — Bacterial conjunctivitis, Quixin: 1 to 2 gtts q 2 h while awake (up to 8 times per day) on days 1 and 2, then 1 to 2 gtts q 4 h (up to 4 times/day) on days 3 to 7 for age older than 1 yo only. Corneal ulcers, Iquix: 1 to 2 gtts q 30 min to 2 h while awake and q 4 to 6 h overnight on days 1 to 3, then 1 to 2 gtts q 1 to 4 h while awake on day 4 to completion of therapy for age older than 6 yo only.

(cont.)

LEVOFLOXACIN—OPHTHALMIC (cont.)

FORMS — Trade/Generic: Soln 0.5% (5 mL).

MOA — Inhibits DNA-gyrase in susceptible bacteria.

ADVERSE EFFECTS — Frequent: Headache, decreased vision, fever, burning, pharyngitis, photophobia. Severe: Hypersensitivity.

MOXIFLOXACIN—OPHTHALMIC (*Vigamox, Moxeza*) ▶LK ♀C ▶? $$$

ADULT — Bacterial conjunctivitis: 1 gtt in each affected eye three times per day for 7 days (Vigamox) or 1 gtt in each affected eye two times per day for 7 days (Moxeza).

PEDS — Use adult dose for age 1 yo or older.

FORMS — Trade only: Soln 0.5% (3 mL, Vigamox and Moxeza).

MOA — Inhibits DNA-gyrase and topoisomerase IV in susceptible bacteria.

ADVERSE EFFECTS — Frequent: Conjunctival irritation, dry eye, ocular discomfort/pain/pruritus, increased lacrimation, keratitis, conjunctivitis.

OFLOXACIN—OPHTHALMIC (*Ocuflox*) ▶LK ♀C ▶? $$

ADULT — Corneal ulcers/keratitis: 1 to 2 gtts q 30 min while awake and 1 to 2 gtts 4 to 6 h after retiring for 2 days, then 1 to 2 gtts q 1 h while awake for 5 days, then 1 to 2 gtts four times per day for 3 days. Bacterial conjunctivitis: 1 to 2 gtts q 2 to 4 h for 2 days, then 1 to 2 gtts four times per day for 5 days.

PEDS — Bacterial conjunctivitis: Use adult dose for age 1 yo or older, not approved age younger than 1 yo.

FORMS — Generic/Trade: Soln 0.3% (5, 10 mL).

MOA — Inhibits DNA-gyrase in susceptible bacteria.

ADVERSE EFFECTS — Frequent: Ocular burning, eye discomfort. Severe: Chemical conjunctivitis/keratitis, ocular/facial edema, hypersensitivity reaction.

OPHTHALMOLOGY: Antibacterials—Other

NOTE: On average, each mL of eye drop soln contains approximately 20 gtts. Reserve ointment formulations for bedtime use due to severe vision blurring. Most eye medications can be administered 1 gtt at a time despite common manufacturer recommendations of 1 to 2 gtts concurrently. Even a single gtt is typically more than the eye can hold and thus a 2nd gtt is both wasteful and increases the possibility of systemic toxicity. If 2 gtts of the medication are desired, separate single gtts by at least 5 min.

AZITHROMYCIN—OPHTHALMIC (*AzaSite*) ▶L ♀B ▶? $$$

ADULT — Ocular infections: 1 gtt two times per day for 2 days, then 1 gtt daily for 5 more days.

PEDS — Not approved in children younger than 1 yo. Use adult dose for age 1 yo or older.

FORMS — Trade only: Soln 1% (2.5 mL).

MOA — Inhibits RNA-dependent protein synthesis.

ADVERSE EFFECTS — Frequent: Eye irritation.

BACITRACIN—OPHTHALMIC (*AK Tracin*) ▶minimal absorption ♀C ▶? $

ADULT — Ocular infections: ¼ to ½ inch ribbon of ointment q 3 to 4 h or two to four times per day for 7 to 10 days.

PEDS — Not approved in children.

UNAPPROVED PEDS — Ocular infections: ¼ to ½ inch ribbon of ointment q 3 to 4 h or two to four times per day for 7 to 10 days.

FORMS — Generic/Trade: Oint 500 units/g (3.5 g tube).

MOA — Inhibits bacterial cell wall synthesis.

ADVERSE EFFECTS — Frequent: Edema of face, pain, rash, pruritus.

ERYTHROMYCIN—OPHTHALMIC (*Ilotycin, AK-Mycin*) ▶L ♀B ▶+ $

ADULT — Ocular infections, corneal ulceration: ½ inch ribbon of ointment q 3 to 4 h or 2 to 6 times per day. For chlamydial infections: ½ inch ribbon of ointment two times per day for 2 months or two times per day for the first 5 days of each month for 6 months.

PEDS — Ophthalmia neonatorum prophylaxis: ½ inch ribbon to both eyes within 1 h of birth.

FORMS — Generic only: Oint 0.5% (1, 3.5 g tube).

MOA — Inhibits RNA-dependent protein synthesis.

ADVERSE EFFECTS — Frequent: None.

FUSIDIC ACID—OPHTHALMIC (*✱Fucithalmic*) ▶L ♀? ▶? $

ADULT — Canada only. Eye infections: 1 gtt in both eyes q 12 h for 7 days for age 2 yo or older.

PEDS — Not approved in children younger than 2 yo. Use adult dose for age 2 yo or older.

FORMS — Canada trade only: gtts 1%. Multidose tubes of 3, 5 g. Single-dose, preservative-free tubes of 0.2 g in a box of 12.

MOA — Antibacterial, interferes with bacterial protein synthesis.

ADVERSE EFFECTS — Frequent: Stinging, irritation. Severe: Hypersensitivity.

NEOSPORIN OINTMENT—OPHTHALMIC (neomycin—ophthalmic + bacitracin—ophthalmic + polymyxin—ophthalmic) ▶KL ♀C ▶? $

ADULT — Ocular infections: ½ inch ribbon of ointment q 3 to 4 h for 7 to 10 days or ½ inch ribbon two to three times per day for mild to moderate infection.

PEDS — Not approved in children.

UNAPPROVED PEDS — ½ inch ribbon of ointment q 3 to 4 h for 7 to 10 days.

FORMS — Generic only: Oint. (3.5 g tube).

NOTES — Contact dermatitis can occur after prolonged use.

MOA — Inhibits RNA-dependent protein synthesis and interferes with cell wall membranes.

ADVERSE EFFECTS — Frequent: Topical hypersensitivity, contact dermatitis.

NEOSPORIN SOLUTION—OPHTHALMIC (neomycin—ophthalmic + polymyxin—ophthalmic + gramicidin) ▶KL ♀C ▶? $$
ADULT — Ocular infections: 1 to 2 gtts q 4 to 6 h for 7 to 10 days.
PEDS — Not approved in children.
UNAPPROVED PEDS — 1 to 2 gtts q 4 to 6 h for 7 to 10 days.
FORMS — Generic/Trade: Soln (10 mL).
NOTES — Contact dermatitis can occur after prolonged use.
MOA — Inhibits RNA-dependent protein synthesis and interferes with cell wall membranes.
ADVERSE EFFECTS — Frequent: Topical hypersensitivity, contact dermatitis, eye irritation, burning, stinging, edema, pruritus, failure to heal.

POLYSPORIN—OPHTHALMIC (polymyxin—ophthalmic + bacitracin—ophthalmic) ▶K ♀C ▶? $$
ADULT — Ocular infections: ½ inch ribbon of ointment q 3 to 4 h for 7 to 10 days or ½ inch ribbon two to three times per day for mild to moderate infection.
PEDS — Not approved in children.
UNAPPROVED PEDS — Ocular infections: ½ inch ribbon of ointment q 3 to 4 h for 7 to 10 days.
FORMS — Generic only: Oint (3.5 g tube).
MOA — Inhibits synthesis of and interferes with bacterial cell wall membranes.
ADVERSE EFFECTS — Frequent: None.

POLYTRIM—OPHTHALMIC (polymyxin—ophthalmic + trimethoprim—ophthalmic) ▶KL ♀C ▶? $
ADULT — Ocular infections: 1 to 2 gtts q 4 to 6 h (up to 6 gtts per day) for 7 to 10 days.
PEDS — Not approved age younger than 2 mo. Use adult dose for age 2 mo or older.
FORMS — Generic/Trade: Soln (10 mL).
MOA — Interferes with bacterial cell wall membranes, folate reduction.
ADVERSE EFFECTS — Frequent: None.

SULFACETAMIDE—OPHTHALMIC (*Bleph-10, Sulf-10*) ▶K ♀C ▶– $
ADULT — Ocular infections, corneal ulceration: 1 to 2 gtts q 2 to 3 h initially, then taper by decreasing frequency as condition allows over 7 to 10 days or ½ inch ribbon of ointment q 3 to 4 h initially, then taper 7 to 10 days. Trachoma: 2 gtts q 2 h with systemic antibiotic such as doxycycline or azithromycin.
PEDS — Not approved age younger than 2 mo. Use adult dose for age 2 mo or older.
FORMS — Generic/Trade: Soln 10% (15 mL), Oint 10% (3.5 g tube). Generic only: Soln 30% (15 mL).
NOTES — Ointment may be used as an adjunct to soln. Caution in sulfa-allergic patients.
MOA — Inhibits bacterial folic acid synthesis.
ADVERSE EFFECTS — Frequent: Irritation, stinging, burning. Severe: Stevens-Johnson syndrome, toxic epidermal necrolysis, hypersensitivity.

OPHTHALMOLOGY: Antiviral Agents

GANCICLOVIR—OPHTHALMIC (*Zirgan*) ▶minimal absorption ♀C ▶? $$$$
ADULT — Herpetic keratitis: 1 gtt five times per day (approximately q 3 h) until ulcer heals, then 1 gtt three times per day for 7 days.
PEDS — Not approved in children younger than 2 yo. Use adult dosing for age 2 yo and older.
FORMS — Trade only: Gel 0.15% (5g).
NOTES — Do not wear contact lenses.
MOA — Inhibits DNA replication.
ADVERSE EFFECTS — Frequent: Blurred vision, eye irritation, punctate keratitis, conjunctival hyperemia.

TRIFLURIDINE (*Viroptic*) ▶minimal absorption ♀C ▶– $$$
ADULT — Herpetic keratitis: 1 gtt q 2 h to maximum 9 gtts per days. After re-epithelialization, decrease dose to 1 gtt q 4 to 6 h while awake for 7 to 14 days. Max of 21 days of treatment.
PEDS — Not approved age younger than 6 yo. Use adult dose for age 6 yo or older.
FORMS — Generic/Trade: Soln 1% (7.5 mL).
NOTES — Avoid continuous use more than 21 days; may cause keratitis and conjunctival scarring. Urge frequent use of topical lubricants (ie, tear substitutes) to minimize surface damage.
MOA — Inhibits viral DNA replication as thymidine analog.
ADVERSE EFFECTS — Frequent: Burning, stinging.

OPHTHALMOLOGY: Corticosteroid and Antibacterial Combinations

NOTE: Recommend that only ophthalmologists or optometrists prescribe due to infection, cataract, corneal/scleral perforation, and glaucoma risk from prolonged use. Monitor intraocular pressure. Gradually taper when discontinuing. Shake suspensions well before using. On average, each mL of eye drop soln contains approximately 20 gtts. Reserve ointment formulations for bedtime use due to severe vision blurring. Most eye medications can be administered 1 gtt at a time despite common manufacturer recommendations of 1 to 2 gtts concurrently. Even a single gtt is typically more than the eye can hold and thus a 2nd gtt is both wasteful and increases the possibility of systemic toxicity. If 2 gtts of the medication are desired, separate single gtts by at least 5 min.

BLEPHAMIDE (prednisolone—ophthalmic + sulfacetamide—ophthalmic) ▶KL ♀C ▶? $
ADULT — Steroid-responsive inflammatory condition with bacterial infection or risk of bacterial infection: Start 1 to 2 gtts q 1 h during the day and q 2 h during the night, then 1 gtt q 4 h and at bedtime; or ½ inch ribbon to lower conjunctival sac three to four times/day and 1 to 2 times at night.

(cont.)

BLEPHAMIDE (cont.)

PEDS — Not approved in children younger than 6 yo.

FORMS — Generic/Trade: Soln/Susp (5, 10 mL). Trade only: Oint (3.5 g tube).

MOA — Inhibits bacterial folic acid synthesis, anti-inflammatory.

ADVERSE EFFECTS — Frequent: Insomnia, nervousness, increased appetite, indigestion, local irritation, burning, stinging. Severe: Cataracts, secondary ocular infections, glaucoma, Stevens-Johnson syndrome, toxic epidermal necrolysis, hypersensitivity.

CORTISPORIN—OPHTHALMIC (neomycin—ophthalmic + polymyxin—ophthalmic + hydrocortisone—ophthalmic) ▶LK ♀C ▶? $

ADULT — Steroid-responsive inflammatory condition with bacterial infection or risk of bacterial infection: 1 to 2 gtts or ½ inch ribbon of ointment q 3 to 4 h or more frequently prn.

PEDS — Not approved in children.

UNAPPROVED PEDS — 1 to 2 gtts or ½ inch ribbon of ointment q 3 to 4 h.

FORMS — Generic only: Susp (7.5 mL). Oint (3.5 g tube).

MOA — Inhibits RNA-dependent protein synthesis, interferes with bacterial cell wall membranes, anti-inflammatory.

ADVERSE EFFECTS — Frequent: None. Severe: Cataracts, secondary ocular infections, glaucoma, Stevens-Johnson syndrome, toxic epidermal necrolysis, hypersensitivity.

FML-S LIQUIFILM (prednisolone—ophthalmic + sulfacetamide—ophthalmic) ▶KL ♀C ▶? $$

ADULT — Steroid-responsive inflammatory condition with bacterial infection or risk of bacterial infection: Start 1 to 2 gtts q 1 h during the day and q 2 h during the night, then 1 gtt q 4 to 8 h.

PEDS — Not approved in children.

FORMS — Trade only: Susp (10 mL).

MOA — Anti-inflammatory.

ADVERSE EFFECTS — Frequent: Insomnia, nervousness, increased appetite, indigestion, local irritation, burning, stinging. Severe: Cataracts, secondary ocular infections, glaucoma, Stevens-Johnson syndrome, toxic epidermal necrolysis, hypersensitivity.

MAXITROL (dexamethasone—ophthalmic + neomycin—ophthalmic + polymyxin—ophthalmic) ▶KL ♀C ▶? $

ADULT — Steroid-responsive inflammatory condition with bacterial infection or risk of bacterial infection: Ointment: Place a small amount (about ½ inch) in the affected eye 3 to 4 times per day or apply at bedtime as an adjunct with gtts. Susp: Instill 1 to 2 gtts into affected eye(s) 4 to 6 times daily; in severe disease, gtts may be used hourly and tapered to discontinuation.

PEDS — Not approved in children.

FORMS — Generic/Trade: Susp (5 mL). Oint (3.5 g tube).

MOA — Inhibits RNA-dependent protein synthesis, interferes with bacterial cell wall membranes, anti-inflammatory.

ADVERSE EFFECTS — Frequent: None. Severe: Cataracts, secondary ocular infections, glaucoma, Stevens-Johnson syndrome, toxic epidermal necrolysis, hypersensitivity.

PRED G (prednisolone—ophthalmic + gentamicin—ophthalmic) ▶KL ♀C ▶? $$

ADULT — Steroid-responsive inflammatory condition with bacterial infection or risk of bacterial infection: Start 1 to 2 gtts q 1 h during the day and q 2 h during the night, then 1 gtt 2 to 4 times daily or ½ inch ribbon of ointment 1 to 3 times per day.

PEDS — Not approved in children.

FORMS — Trade only: Susp (2, 5, 10 mL). Oint (3.5 g tube).

MOA — Inhibits RNA-dependent protein synthesis, anti-inflammatory.

ADVERSE EFFECTS — Frequent: None. Severe: Cataracts, secondary ocular infections, glaucoma, Stevens-Johnson syndrome, toxic epidermal necrolysis, hypersensitivity.

TOBRADEX (tobramycin—ophthalmic + dexamethasone—ophthalmic) ▶L ♀C ▶? $$$

ADULT — Steroid-responsive inflammatory condition with bacterial infection or risk of bacterial infection: 1 to 2 gtts q 2 h for 1 to 2 days, then 1 to 2 gtts q 4 to 6 h; or ½ inch ribbon of ointment three to four times per day.

PEDS — 1 to 2 gtts q 2 h for 1 to 2 days, then 1 to 2 gtts q 4 to 6 h; or ½ inch ribbon of ointment three to four times per day for age 2 yo or older.

FORMS — Trade/Generic: Susp (tobramycin 0.3%/dexamethasone 0.1%, 2.5, 5, 10 mL). Trade: Oint (tobramycin 0.3%/dexamethasone 0.1%, 3.5 g tube).

MOA — Inhibits RNA-dependent protein synthesis, anti-inflammatory.

ADVERSE EFFECTS — Frequent: Eyelid itching, swelling, conjunctival erythema. Severe: Cataracts, secondary ocular infections, glaucoma.

TOBRADEX ST (tobramycin—ophthalmic + dexamethasone—ophthalmic) ▶L ♀C ▶? $$$

ADULT — Steroid-responsive inflammatory condition with bacterial infection or risk of bacterial infection: 1 gtt q 2 h for 1 to 2 days, then 1 gtt q 4 to 6 h.

PEDS — Not approved in children younger than 2 yo. Use adult dose in children 2 yo or older.

FORMS — Trade only: Tobramycin 0.3%/dexamethasone 0.05% susp (2.5, 5, 10 mL).

MOA — Inhibits RNA-dependent protein synthesis, anti-inflammatory.

ADVERSE EFFECTS — Frequent: Eyelid itching, swelling, conjunctival erythema. Severe: Cataracts, secondary ocular infections, glaucoma.

VASOCIDIN (prednisolone—ophthalmic + sulfacetamide—ophthalmic) ▶KL ♀C ▶? $

ADULT — Steroid-responsive inflammatory condition with bacterial infection or risk of bacterial infection: Start 1 to 2 gtts q 1 h during the day and q 2 h

(cont.)

VASOCIDIN (*cont.*)

during the night, then 1 gtt q 4 to 8 h; or ½ inch ribbon (ointment) three to four times per day initially, then one to two times per day thereafter.

PEDS — Not approved in children.

FORMS — Generic only: Soln (5, 10 mL).

MOA — Inhibits bacterial folic acid synthesis, anti-inflammatory.

ADVERSE EFFECTS — Frequent: Insomnia, nervousness, increased appetite, indigestion, local irritation, burning, stinging. Severe: Cataracts, secondary ocular infections, Stevens-Johnson syndrome, toxic epidermal necrolysis, hypersensitivity.

ZYLET (loteprednol + tobramycin—ophthalmic) ▶LK ♀C ▶? $$$

ADULT — Steroid-responsive inflammatory condition with bacterial infection or risk of bacterial infection: 1 to 2 gtts q 1 to 2 h for 1 to 2 days then 1 to 2 gtts q 4 to 6 h.

PEDS — Steroid-responsive inflammatory condition with bacterial infection or risk of bacterial infection: 1 to 2 gtts q 1 to 2 h for 1 to 2 days then 1 to 2 gtts q 4 to 6 h.

FORMS — Trade only: Susp 0.5% loteprednol + 0.3% tobramycin (2.5, 5, 10 mL).

NOTES — Prescribe a maximum of 20 mL initially, then reevaluate.

MOA — Anti-inflammatory (loteprednol) and inhibits RNA-dependent bacterial protein synthesis (tobramycin).

ADVERSE EFFECTS — Frequent: Injection, superficial punctate keratitis, ocular burning and stinging, headache. Severe: Cataracts, secondary ocular infections, glaucoma.

OPHTHALMOLOGY: Corticosteroids

NOTE: Recommend that only ophthalmologists or optometrists prescribe due to infection, cataract, corneal/scleral perforation, and glaucoma risk. Monitor intraocular pressure. Gradually taper when discontinuing. Shake susp well before using. On average, each mL of eye drop soln contains approximately 20 gtts. Reserve ointment formulations for bedtime use due to severe vision blurring. Most eye medications can be administered 1 gtt at a time despite common manufacturer recommendations of 1 to 2 gtts concurrently. Even a single gtt is typically more than the eye can hold and thus a 2nd gtt is both wasteful and increases the possibility of systemic toxicity. If 2 gtts of the medication are desired, separate single gtts by at least 5 min.

DIFLUPREDNATE (*Durezol*) ▶not absorbed ♀C ▶? $$$$

ADULT — Inflammation and pain associated with ocular surgery: 1 gtt in each affected eye four times per day, beginning 24 h after surgery for 2 weeks, then 1 gtt in each affected eye 2 times per day for 1 week, then taper based on response. Endogenous anterior uveitis: 1 gtt in each affected eye 4 times daily for 14 days followed by tapering as indicated.

PEDS — Not approved in children. Limited efficacy and safety data in children 0 to 3 yo indicated similar effects as seen with prednisolone acetate susp.

FORMS — Trade only: Ophthalmic emulsion 0.05% (2.5, 5 mL).

NOTES — If used for more than 10 days, monitor IOP.

MOA — Anti-inflammatory.

ADVERSE EFFECTS — Frequent: Corneal edema, ciliary and conjunctival hyperemia, pain, photophobia, posterior capsule opacification, blepharitis. Severe: Cataracts, secondary ocular infections, glaucoma.

FLUOCINOLONE—OPHTHALMIC (*Retisert*) ▶not absorbed ♀C ▶? $$$$$

PEDS — Not approved in children younger than 12 yo.

FORMS — Implantable tablet 0.59 mg only available from manufacturer.

NOTES — Releases 0.6 mcg/day decreasing over about 1 month, then 0.3 to 0.4 mcg/day over about 30 months. Within 34 weeks 60% require medication to control intraocular pressure and within 2 years nearly all phakic eyes develop cataracts.

MOA — Anti-inflammatory

ADVERSE EFFECTS — Frequent: headache, eye pain, procedural complications including implant expulsion, injury, migration of implant, wound dehiscence. Severe: cataracts, secondary ocular infections, glaucoma.

FLUOROMETHOLONE (*FML, FML Forte, Flarex*) ▶L ♀C ▶? $$

ADULT — 1 to 2 gtts q 1 to 2 h or ½ inch ribbon of ointment q 4 h for 1 to 2 days, then 1 to 2 gtts two to four times per day or ½ inch of ointment one to three times per day.

PEDS — Not approved age younger than 2 yo. Use adult dose for age 2 yo or older.

FORMS — Trade only: Susp 0.1% (5, 10, 15 mL), 0.25% (2, 5, 10, 15 mL). Oint 0.1% (3.5 g tube).

NOTES — Fluorometholone acetate (Flarex) is more potent than fluorometholone (FML, FML Forte). Use caution in glaucoma.

MOA — Anti-inflammatory.

ADVERSE EFFECTS — Frequent: Burning, blurred vision. Severe: Cataracts, secondary ocular infections, glaucoma.

LOTEPREDNOL (*Alrex, Lotemax*) ▶L ♀C ▶? $$$

ADULT — 1 to 2 gtts four times per day, may increase to 1 gtt q 1 h during 1st weeks of therapy prn. Postop inflammation: 1 to 2 gtts four times per day or ½ inch four times daily beginning 24 h after surgery.

PEDS — Not approved in children.

FORMS — Trade only: Susp 0.2% (Alrex 5, 10 mL), 0.5% (Lotemax 2.5, 5, 10, 15 mL). Oint 0.5% 3.5 g, Gel drop 0.5% (Lotemax 10 mL).

MOA — Anti-inflammatory.

ADVERSE EFFECTS — Frequent: Headache, rhinitis, pharyngitis, blurring of vision, chemosis, dry eyes, pruritus. Severe: Cataracts, secondary ocular infections, glaucoma.

PREDNISOLONE—OPHTHALMIC (*Pred Forte, Pred Mild, Inflamase Forte, Econopred Plus*) ▶L ♀C ▶? $$
ADULT — Soln: 1 to 2 gtts (up to q 1 h during day and q 2 h at night), when response observed, then 1 gtt q 4 h, then 1 gtt three to four times per day. Susp: 1 to 2 gtts two to four times per day.
PEDS — Not approved in children.
FORMS — Generic/Trade: Soln, Susp 1% (5, 10, 15 mL). Trade only (Pred Mild): Susp 0.12% (5, 10 mL), Susp (Pred Forte) 1% (1 mL).
NOTES — Prednisolone acetate (Pred Mild, Pred Forte) is more potent than prednisolone sodium phosphate (AK-Pred, Inflamase Forte).
MOA — Anti-inflammatory.
ADVERSE EFFECTS — Frequent: Insomnia, nervousness, indigestion, increased appetite, hirsutism, diabetes mellitus. Severe: Cataracts, secondary ocular infections, glaucoma.

RIMEXOLONE (*Vexol*) ▶L ♀C ▶? $$
ADULT — Postop inflammation: 1 to 2 gtts four times per day for 2 weeks. Uveitis: 1 to 2 gtts q 1 h while awake for 1 week, then 1 gtt q 2 h while awake for 1 week, then taper.
PEDS — Not approved in children.
FORMS — Trade only: Susp 1% (5, 10 mL).
NOTES — Prolonged use associated with corneal/scleral perforation and cataracts.
MOA — Anti-inflammatory.
ADVERSE EFFECTS — Frequent: Blurred vision. Severe: Cataracts, secondary ocular infections, glaucoma.

TRIAMCINOLONE–VITREOUS (*Triesence*) ▶L ♀D ▶? ?
ADULT — Administered intravitreally.
PEDS — Not approved in children.
NOTES — Do not use in patients with systemic fungal infections.
MOA — Anti-inflammatory
ADVERSE EFFECTS — Severe: cataracts, secondary ocular infections, glaucoma

OPHTHALMOLOGY: Glaucoma Agents—Beta-Blockers

NOTE: May be absorbed and cause side effects and drug interactions associated with systemic beta-blocker therapy. Use caution in cardiac conditions and asthma. Advise patients to apply gentle pressure over nasolacrimal duct for 5 min after instillation to minimize systemic absorption. On average, each mL of eye drop soln contains approximately 20 gtts. Reserve ointment formulations for bedtime use due to severe vision blurring. Most eye medications can be administered 1 gtt at a time despite common manufacturer recommendations of 1 to 2 gtts concurrently. Even a single gtt is typically more than the eye can hold and thus a 2nd gtt is both wasteful and increases the possibility of systemic toxicity. If 2 gtts of the medication are desired, separate single gtts by at least 5 min.

BETAXOLOL—OPHTHALMIC (*Betoptic, Betoptic S*) ▶LK ♀C ▶? $$
ADULT — Chronic open-angle glaucoma or ocular HTN: 1 to 2 gtts two times per day.
PEDS — Chronic open-angle glaucoma or ocular HTN: 1 to 2 gtts two times per day.
FORMS — Trade only: Susp 0.25% (10, 15 mL). Generic only: Soln 0.5% (5, 10, 15 mL).
NOTES — Selective beta-1-blocking agent. Shake susp before use.
MOA — Inhibits beta-1 receptors to decrease aqueous fluid production.
ADVERSE EFFECTS — Frequent: Dizziness, erythema, conjunctival hyperemia, anisocoria, keratitis, corneal staining, eye pain, vision disturbances.

CARTEOLOL—OPHTHALMIC (*Ocupress*) ▶KL ♀C ▶? $
ADULT — Chronic open-angle glaucoma or ocular HTN: 1 gtt two times per day.
PEDS — Not approved in children.
FORMS — Generic only: Soln 1% (5, 10, 15 mL).
NOTES — Nonselective beta-blocker but has intrinsic sympathomimetic activity.
MOA — Inhibits beta receptors to decrease aqueous fluid production.
ADVERSE EFFECTS — Frequent: Conjunctival hyperemia.

LEVOBUNOLOL (*Betagan*) ▶? ♀C ▶– $$
ADULT — Chronic open-angle glaucoma or ocular HTN: 1 to 2 gtts (0.5%) one to two times per day or 1 to 2 gtts (0.25%) two times per day.

PEDS — Not approved in children.
FORMS — Generic/Trade: Soln 0.25% (5, 10 mL), 0.5% (5, 10, 15 mL).
NOTES — Nonselective beta-blocker.
MOA — Inhibits beta receptors to decrease aqueous fluid production.
ADVERSE EFFECTS — Frequent: Stinging, burning eyes.

METIPRANOLOL (*Optipranolol*) ▶? ♀C ▶? $
ADULT — Chronic open-angle glaucoma or ocular HTN: 1 gtt two times per day.
PEDS — Not approved in children.
FORMS — Generic/Trade: Soln 0.3% (5, 10 mL).
NOTES — Nonselective beta-blocker.
MOA — Nonselectively inhibits beta receptors to decrease aqueous fluid production.
ADVERSE EFFECTS — Frequent: Transient, local discomfort.

TIMOLOL—OPHTHALMIC (*Betimol, Timoptic, Timoptic XE, Istalol, Timoptic Ocudose*) ▶LK ♀C ▶+ $$
ADULT — Chronic open-angle glaucoma or ocular HTN: 1 gtt (0.25 or 0.5%) two times per day or 1 gtt of gel-forming soln (0.25 or 0.5% Timoptic XE) daily or 1 gtt (0.5% Istalol soln) daily.
PEDS — Chronic open-angle glaucoma or ocular HTN: 1 gtt (0.25 or 0.5%) of gel-forming soln daily.
FORMS — Generic/Trade: Soln 0.25, 0.5% (5, 10, 15 mL). Preservative-free soln (Timoptic Ocudose) 0.25% (0.2 mL). Gel-forming soln (Timoptic XE) 0.25, 0.5% (5 mL).

(cont.)

TIMOLOL—OPHTHALMIC (cont.)

NOTES — Administer other eye meds at least 10 min before Timoptic XE. Greatest effect if Timoptic XE is administered in the morning. Nonselective beta-blocker.

MOA — Inhibits beta receptors to decrease aqueous fluid production.
ADVERSE EFFECTS — Frequent: Conjunctival hyperemia.

OPHTHALMOLOGY: Glaucoma Agents—Carbonic Anhydrase Inhibitors

NOTE: Sulfonamide derivatives; verify absence of sulfa allergy before prescribing. On average, each mL of eye drop soln contains approximately 20 gtts. Reserve ointment formulations for bedtime use due to severe vision blurring. Most eye medications can be administered 1 gtt at a time despite common manufacturer recommendations of 1 to 2 gtts concurrently. Even a single gtt is typically more than the eye can hold and thus a 2nd gtt is both wasteful and increases the possibility of systemic toxicity. If 2 gtts of the medication are desired, separate single gtts by at least 5 min.

ACETAZOLAMIDE (Diamox, Diamox Sequels) ▶LK ♀C ▶+ $$
ADULT — Glaucoma: 250 mg PO up to four times per day (immediate-release) or 500 mg PO up to two times per day (sustained-release). Max 1 g/day. Acute glaucoma: 250 mg IV q 4 h or 500 mg IV initially with 125 to 250 mg q 4 h, followed by oral therapy. Mountain sickness prophylaxis: 125 to 250 mg PO two to three times per day, beginning 1 to 2 days prior to ascent and continuing at least 5 days at higher altitude. Edema: Rarely used, start 250 to 375 mg IV/PO q am given intermittently (every other day or 2 consecutive days followed by none for 1 to 2 days) to avoid loss of diuretic effect.
PEDS — Diuretic: 5 mg/kg PO/IV q am.
UNAPPROVED ADULT — Urinary alkalinization: 5 mg/kg IV, may repeat two or three times daily prn to maintain an alkaline diuresis.
UNAPPROVED PEDS — Glaucoma: 8 to 30 mg/kg/day PO, divided three times per day. Acute glaucoma: 5 to 10 mg/kg IV q 6 h.
FORMS — Generic only: Tabs 125, 250 mg. Generic/Trade: Caps, extended-release 500 mg.
NOTES — A susp (250 mg/5 mL) can be made by crushing and mixing tabs in flavored syrup. The susp is stable for 7 days at room temperature. 1 tab may be softened in 2 teaspoons of hot water, then added to 2 teaspoons of honey or syrup, and swallowed at once. Use cautiously in sulfa allergy. Prompt descent is necessary if severe forms of high-altitude sickness occur (eg, pulmonary or cerebral edema). Test the drug for tolerance/allergies 1 to 2 weeks before initial dosing prior to ascent.
MOA — Inhibition of carbonic anhydrase.
ADVERSE EFFECTS — Serious: Metabolic acidosis, electrolyte imbalance, sulfonamide hypersensitivity (rare). Frequent: Nausea, diarrhea, drowsiness, numbness, tingling, altered taste, loss of appetite, tinnitus.

BRINZOLAMIDE (Azopt) ▶LK ♀C ▶? $$$
ADULT — Chronic open-angle glaucoma or ocular HTN: 1 gtt three times per day.
PEDS — Not approved in children.
FORMS — Trade only: Susp 1% (10, 15 mL).
NOTES — Do not administer while wearing soft contact lenses. Wait 10 min after use before inserting contact lenses.
MOA — Inhibition of carbonic anhydrase to decrease aqueous fluid production.
ADVERSE EFFECTS — Frequent: Dermatitis, taste disturbances, transient blurred vision.

DORZOLAMIDE (Trusopt) ▶KL ♀C ▶– $$$
ADULT — Chronic open-angle glaucoma or ocular HTN: 1 gtt three times per day.
PEDS — Chronic open-angle glaucoma or ocular HTN: 1 gtt three times per day.
FORMS — Generic/Trade: Soln 2% (10 mL).
NOTES — Do not administer while wearing soft contact lenses. Keep bottle tightly capped to avoid crystal formation. Wait 10 min after use before inserting contact lenses.
MOA — Inhibition of carbonic anhydrase to decrease aqueous fluid production.
ADVERSE EFFECTS — Frequent: Bitter taste, ocular burning and stinging. Severe: Corneal edema in patients with low endothelial cell counts, Stevens-Johnson syndrome, and toxic epidermal necrolysis.

METHAZOLAMIDE ▶LK ♀C ▶? $$
ADULT — Glaucoma: 100 to 200 mg PO initially, then 100 mg PO q 12 h until desired response. Maintenance dose: 25 to 50 mg PO (up to three times per day).
PEDS — Not approved in children.
FORMS — Generic only: Tabs 25, 50 mg.
NOTES — Mostly metabolized in the liver thus less chance of renal calculi than with acetazolamide.
MOA — Inhibition of carbonic anhydrase to decrease aqueous fluid production.
ADVERSE EFFECTS — Frequent: Malaise, anorexia, diarrhea, metallic taste, polyuria, muscular weakness.

OPHTHALMOLOGY: Glaucoma Agents—Combinations and Other

NOTE: On average, each mL of eye drop soln contains approximately 20 gtts. Reserve ointment formulations for bedtime use due to severe vision blurring. Most eye medications can be administered 1 gtt at a time despite common manufacturer recommendations of 1 to 2 gtts concurrently. Even a single gtt is typically more than the eye can hold and thus a 2nd gtt is both wasteful and increases the possibility of systemic toxicity. If 2 gtts of the medication are desired, separate single gtts by at least 5 min.

COMBIGAN (brimonidine + timolol—ophthalmic) ▶LK ♀C ▶− $$$
ADULT — Chronic open-angle glaucoma or ocular HTN: 1 gtt twice a day.
PEDS — Contraindicated in age younger than 2 yo. Use adult dosing in 2 yo or older.
FORMS — Trade only: Soln brimonidine 0.2% + timolol 0.5% (5, 10 mL).
NOTES — Do not administer while wearing soft contact lenses. Wait 10 min after use before inserting contact lenses. Contraindicated with MAOIs. See beta-blocker warnings.
MOA — Stimulation of alpha-2 receptors and inhibition of beta-1 receptors to decrease aqueous fluid production.
ADVERSE EFFECTS — Ocular: Frequent: Headache, drowsiness, fatigue, xerostomia, hyperemia, burning, stinging, blurring, foreign body sensation, hypersensitivity.

COSOPT (dorzolamide + timolol—ophthalmic) ▶LK ♀D ▶− $$$
ADULT — Chronic open-angle glaucoma or ocular HTN: 1 gtt two times per day.
PEDS — Not approved in children younger than 2 yo. Children older than 2 yo, use adult dose.
FORMS — Generic/Trade: Soln dorzolamide 2% + timolol 0.5% (5, 10 mL). Trade only: Soln, preservative-free dorzolamide 2% + timolol 0.5% (30 single-use containers).
NOTES — Do not administer while wearing soft contact lenses. Wait 10 min after use before inserting contact lenses. Not recommended if severe renal or hepatic dysfunction. Use caution in sulfa allergy. See beta-blocker warnings.
MOA — Inhibition of carbonic anhydrase and beta-1 receptors to decrease aqueous fluid production.
ADVERSE EFFECTS — Ocular: Frequent: Bitter taste, burning, stinging in eyes, allergic reaction, conjunctivitis, lid reactions. Severe: Corneal edema in patients with low endothelial cell counts, Stevens-Johnson syndrome, and toxic epidermal necrolysis.

SIMBRINZA (brinzolamide + brimonidine) ▶LK − ♀C ▶? $$$$
ADULT — Open-angle glaucoma, ocular hypertension: 1 gtt in each affected eye three times per day.
PEDS — Contraindicated in younger than 2 yo.
FORMS — Trade: Brinzolamide 1% and brimonidine 0.2% 8 mL.
MOA — See components.
ADVERSE EFFECTS — See components.

OPHTHALMOLOGY: Glaucoma Agents—Miotics

NOTE: Observe for cholinergic systemic effects (eg, salivation, lacrimation, urination, diarrhea, GI upset, excessive sweating). On average, each mL of eye drop soln contains approximately 20 gtts. Reserve ointment formulations for bedtime use due to severe vision blurring. Most eye medications can be administered 1 gtt at a time despite common manufacturer recommendations of 1 to 2 gtts concurrently. Even a single gtt is typically more than the eye can hold and thus a 2nd gtt is both wasteful and increases the possibility of systemic toxicity. If 2 gtts of the medication are desired, separate single gtts by at least 5 min.

ACETYLCHOLINE (*Miochol-E*) ▶acetylcholinesterases ♀? ▶? $$
ADULT — Intraoperative miosis or pressure lowering: 0.5 mL to 2 mL injected intraocularly.
PEDS — Not approved in children.
MOA — Stimulates cholinergic receptors to increase aqueous fluid outflow.
ADVERSE EFFECTS — Frequent: Blurred vision, miosis, headache.

CARBACHOL (*Isopto Carbachol, Miostat*) ▶? ♀C ▶? $$
ADULT — Glaucoma: 1 gtt three times per day. Intraoperative miosis or pressure lowering: 0.5 mL injected intraocularly.
PEDS — Not approved in children.
FORMS — Trade only: Soln (Isopto Carbachol) 1.5, 3% (15 mL). Intraocular soln (Miostat) 0.01%.
NOTES — Vial stopper contains latex.
MOA — Inhibits acetylcholinesterase resulting in cholineric stimulation to increase aqueous fluid outflow.

ADVERSE EFFECTS — Frequent: Blurred vision, miosis, headache.

ECHOTHIOPHATE IODIDE (*Phospholine Iodide*) ▶? ♀C ▶? $$$
ADULT — Glaucoma: 1 gtt two times per day.
PEDS — Accommodative esotropia: 1 gtt daily (0.06%) or 1 gtt every other day (0.125%).
FORMS — Trade only: Soln 0.125% (5 mL).
NOTES — Use lowest effective dose strength. Use extreme caution if asthma, spastic GI diseases, GI ulcers, bradycardia, hypotension, recent MI, epilepsy, Parkinson's disease, history of retinal detachment. Stop 3 weeks before general anesthesia as may cause prolonged succinylcholine paralysis. Discontinue if cardiac effects noted.
MOA — Inhibits acetylcholinesterase resulting in cholineric stimulation to increase aqueous fluid outflow.
ADVERSE EFFECTS — Frequent: Blurred vision, miosis, headache. Infrequent: Iris cysts, cataracts, ocular surface scarring.

PILOCARPINE—OPHTHALMIC (*Isopto Carpine, ✲Diocarpine, Akarpine*) ▶plasma ♀C ▶? $

ADULT — Reduction of IOP with open-angle glaucoma, acute angle-closure glaucoma, prevention of postoperative elevated IOP associated with laser surgery, induction of miosis: 1 gtt up to four times per day.

PEDS — Glaucoma: 1 gtt up to four times per day.

FORMS — Generic/Trade: Soln 0.5% (15 mL), 1% (2 mL, 15 mL), 2% (2 mL, 15 mL), 4% (2 mL, 15 mL), 6% (15 mL).

NOTES — Do not administer while wearing soft contact lenses. Wait at least 15 min after use before inserting contact lenses. Causes miosis. May cause blurred vision and difficulty with night vision.

MOA — Stimulates cholinergic receptors to increase aqueous fluid outflow.

ADVERSE EFFECTS — Ocular: Frequent: Blurred vision, miosis.

OPHTHALMOLOGY: Glaucoma Agents—Prostaglandin Analogs

NOTE: Do not administer while wearing soft contact lenses. Wait 10 min after use before inserting contact lenses. May aggravate intraocular inflammation. On average, each mL of eye drop soln contains approximately 20 gtts. Reserve ointment formulations for bedtime use due to severe vision blurring. Most eye medications can be administered 1 gtt at a time despite common manufacturer recommendations of 1 to 2 gtts concurrently. Even a single gtt is typically more than the eye can hold and thus a 2nd gtt is both wasteful and increases the possibility of systemic toxicity. If 2 gtts of the medication are desired, separate single gtts by at least 5 min.

BIMATOPROST (*Lumigan, Latisse*) ▶LK ♀C ▶? $$$$

ADULT — Chronic open-angle glaucoma or ocular HTN: 1 gtt in each affected eye at bedtime. Hypotrichosis of the eyelashes (Latisse): Apply at bedtime to the skin of the upper eyelid margin at the base of the eyelashes.

PEDS — Not approved in children.

FORMS — Generic only: Soln 0.03% 2.5, 5, 7.5 mL. Trade only: Soln 0.01% (Lumigan), 2.5, 5, 7.5 mL. Soln 0.03% (Latisse) 3 mL with 70 disposable applicators, 5 mL with 140 disposable applicators.

NOTES — Concurrent administration of bimatoprost for hypotrichosis and IOP-lowering prostaglandin analogs in ocular hypertensive patients may decrease the IOP-lowering effect. Monitor closely for changes in IOP. May cause discoloration of soft contact lenses.

MOA — Prostaglandin F-2 analog increases aqueous fluid outflow.

ADVERSE EFFECTS — Ocular: Frequent: Blurred vision, burning, stinging, ocular hyperemia, increased pigmentation of iris and eyelid skin, growth of eyelashes, periorbital erythema, ocular pruritus. Severe: hypersensitivity reactions.

LATANOPROST (*Xalatan*) ▶LK ♀C ▶? $

ADULT — Chronic open-angle glaucoma or ocular HTN: 1 gtt at bedtime.

PEDS — Not approved in children.

FORMS — Generic/Trade: Soln 0.005% (2.5 mL).

MOA — Prostaglandin F-2 analog increases aqueous fluid outflow.

ADVERSE EFFECTS — Ocular: Frequent: Blurred vision, burning, stinging, ocular hyperemia, increased pigmentation of iris and eyelid skin, growth of eyelashes, ocular pruritus, headache, dizziness.

TAFLUPROST (*Zioptan*) ▶L ♀C ▶? $$$

ADULT — Chronic open-angle glaucoma or ocular HTN: 1 gtt in each affected eye q pm.

PEDS — Not approved in children.

FORMS — Trade: Soln 0.0015%

NOTES — Can cause pigmentation of iris, periorbital tissue, and eyelashes. Discard 30 days after opening foil pouch.

MOA — Prostaglandin analog.

ADVERSE EFFECTS — Frequent: conjunctival hyperemia. Severe: uveitis and iritis, respiratory symptoms such as asthma exacerbation.

TRAVOPROST (*Travatan Z*) ▶L ♀C ▶? $$$$

ADULT — Chronic open-angle glaucoma or ocular HTN: 1 gtt at bedtime.

PEDS — Not approved in children.

FORMS — Trade only: Benzalkonium chloride-free (Travatan Z) 0.004% (2.5, 5 mL). Generic only: Travoprost 0.004% (2.5 mL, 5 mL).

NOTES — Wait 10 min after use before inserting contact lenses. Avoid if prior or current intraocular inflammation.

MOA — Prostaglandin F-2 analog increases aqueous fluid outflow.

ADVERSE EFFECTS — Ocular: Frequent: Conjunctival hyperemia, ocular hyperemia, increased pigmentation of iris and eyelid skin, growth of eyelashes, decreased visual acuity, eye discomfort, foreign body sensation, pain, and pruritus. Severe: Contraindicated in pregnancy, pigmentation changes.

OPHTHALMOLOGY: Glaucoma Agents—Sympathomimetics

NOTE: Do not administer while wearing soft contact lenses. Wait 10 min after use before inserting contact lenses. On average, each mL of eye drop soln contains approximately 20 gtts. Reserve ointment formulations for bedtime use due to severe vision blurring. Most eye medications can be administered 1 gtt at a time despite common manufacturer recommendations of 1 to 2 gtts concurrently. Even a single gtt is typically more than the eye can hold and thus a 2nd gtt is both wasteful and increases the possibility of systemic toxicity. If 2 gtts of the medication are desired, separate single gtts by at least 5 min.

APRACLONIDINE (*Iopidine*) ▸KL ♀C ▶? $$$$
ADULT — Perioperative IOP elevation: 1 gtt (1%) 1 h prior to surgery, then 1 gtt immediately after surgery.
PEDS — Not approved in children.
FORMS — Generic/Trade: Soln 0.5% (5, 10 mL). Trade only: Soln 1% (0.1 mL).
NOTES — Rapid tachyphylaxis may occur. Do not use long term.
MOA — Alpha-2-agonist decreases aqueous fluid production.
ADVERSE EFFECTS — Frequent: Decreases night vision, distance vision alterations, lethargy, xerostomia, burning and itching eyes.

BRIMONIDINE (*Alphagan P, ✱Alphagan*) ▸L ♀B ▶? $$
ADULT — Chronic open-angle glaucoma or ocular HTN: 1 gtt three times per day.
PEDS — Glaucoma: 1 gtt three times per day for age older than 2 yo.
FORMS — Trade only: Soln 0.1% (5, 10, 15 mL). Generic/Trade: Soln 0.15% (5, 10, 15 mL). Generic only: Soln 0.2% (5, 10, 15 mL).
NOTES — Contraindicated in patients receiving MAOIs. Twice daily dosing may have similar efficacy.
MOA — Alpha-2-agonist decreases aqueous fluid production.
ADVERSE EFFECTS — Frequent: Headache, drowsiness, fatigue, xerostomia, hyperemia, burning, stinging, blurring, foreign body sensation.

OPHTHALMOLOGY: Macular Degeneration

PEGAPTANIB (*Macugen*) ▸minimal absorption ♀B ▶? $$$$$
ADULT — "Wet" macular degeneration: 0.3 mg intravitreal injection q 6 weeks.
PEDS — Not approved in children.
MOA — Selective antagonist of vascular endothelial growth factor.
ADVERSE EFFECTS — Ocular: Chamber inflammation, blurred vision, cataracts, corneal edema, reduced visual acuity, visual changes. Injection-related adverse events include: Endophthalmitis, retinal detachment, iatrogenic traumatic cataract, subconjunctival hemorrhage, and increased intraocular pressure. Severe: Anaphylaxis/anaphylactoid, angioedema.

RANIBIZUMAB (*Lucentis*) ▸intravitreal ♀C ▶? $$$$$
ADULT — Treatment of neovascular (wet) macular degeneration: 0.5 mg intravitreal injection q 28 days. If monthly injections not feasible, can administer q 3 months or 3 monthly doses followed by less frequent dosing with regular assessment, but these regimens are less effective. Macular edema following retinal vein occlusion, diabetic retinopathy in patients with diabetic macula edema: 0.5 mg intravitreal injection q 28 days.
PEDS — Not approved in children.
NOTES — Increased CVA risk noted with higher doses (0.5 mg) and with prior CVA.
MOA — Binds to the receptor of VEGF-A.
ADVERSE EFFECTS — Severe: Stroke. Frequent: Eye pain, vitreous floaters, intraocular inflammation, blurred vision. Injection-related adverse events include: Endophthalmitis, retinal detachment, iatrogenic traumatic cataract, subconjunctival hemorrhage, and increased intraocular pressure.

VERTEPORFIN (*Visudyne*) ▸L plasma ♀C ▶– $$$$$
ADULT — Treatment of exudative age-related macular degeneration: 6 mg/m^2 IV over 10 min; laser light therapy 15 min after start of infusion.
PEDS — Not approved in children.
NOTES — Severe risk of photosensitivity for 5 days; must avoid exposure to sunlight.
MOA — Laser-induced free radicals cause occlusion of abnormal vessels.
ADVERSE EFFECTS — Frequent: Injection-site irritation, blurred vision, visual field defects, decreased visual acuity (sometimes severe).

OPHTHALMOLOGY: Mydriatics and Cycloplegics

NOTE: Use caution in infants. On average, each mL of eye drop soln contains approximately 20 gtts. Reserve ointment formulations for bedtime use due to severe vision blurring. Most eye medications can be administered 1 gtt at a time despite common manufacturer recommendations of 1 to 2 gtts concurrently. Even a single gtt is typically more than the eye can hold and thus a 2nd gtt is both wasteful and increases the possibility of systemic toxicity. If 2 gtts of the medication are desired, separate single gtts by at least 5 min.

ATROPINE—OPHTHALMIC (*Isopto Atropine, Atropine Care*) ▸L ♀C ▶+ $
ADULT — Uveitis: 1 to 2 gtts of 0.5% or 1% soln daily to four times per day, or ⅛ to ¼ inch ribbon (1% ointment) daily (up to three times per day). Refraction: 1 to 2 gtts of 1% soln 1 h before procedure or ⅛ to ¼ inch ribbon one to three times per day.
PEDS — Uveitis: 1 to 2 gtts of 0.5% soln one to three times per day) or ⅛ to ¼ inch ribbon one to three times per day. Refraction: 1 to 2 gtts (0.5%) two times per day for 1 to 3 days before procedure or ⅛ inch ribbon (1% ointment) for 1 to 3 days before procedure.
UNAPPROVED PEDS — Amblyopia: 1 gtt in good eye daily.
FORMS — Generic/Trade: Soln 1% (2, 5, 15 mL). Generic only: Oint 1% (3.5 g tube).
NOTES — Cycloplegia may last up to 5 to 10 days and mydriasis may last up to 7 to 14 days. Each drop of a 1% soln contains 0.5 mg atropine. Treat atropine overdose with physostigmine 0.25 mg q 15 min until symptoms resolve.

(cont.)

ATROPINE—OPHTHALMIC (cont.)

MOA — Anticholinergic blockage of ciliary body and iris muscles to produce loss of accommodation and pupil dilation.

ADVERSE EFFECTS — Frequent: Dry, hot skin, impaired GI motility, dry throat, xerostomia, dry eyes, blurred vision, especially reading vision, photophobia.

CYCLOPENTOLATE (AK-Pentolate, Cyclogyl, Pentolair) ▶? ♀C ▶? $

ADULT — Refraction: 1 to 2 gtts (1% or 2%), repeat in 5 to 10 min prn. Give 45 min before procedure.

PEDS — May cause CNS disturbances in children. Refraction: 1 to 2 gtts (0.5%, 1%, or 2%), repeat in 5 to 10 min prn. Give 45 min before procedure.

FORMS — Generic/Trade: Soln 1% (2, 15 mL). Trade only (Cyclogyl): 0.5% (15 mL), 1% (5 mL), 2% (2, 5, 15 mL).

NOTES — Cycloplegia may last 6 to 24 h; mydriasis may last 1 day.

MOA — Anticholinergic blockage of ciliary body and iris muscles to produce loss of accommodation and pupil dilation.

ADVERSE EFFECTS — Frequent: Tachycardia, CNS effects, blurred vision, especially reading vision, increased sensitivity to light, photophobia.

HOMATROPINE—OPHTHALMIC (Isopto Homatropine) ▶? ♀C ▶? $

ADULT — Refraction: 1 to 2 gtts (2%) or 1 gtt (5%) immediately before procedure, repeat q 5 to 10 min prn. Max 3 doses. Uveitis: 1 to 2 gtts (2 to 5%) two to three times per day or as often as q 3 to 4 h.

PEDS — Refraction: 1 gtt (2%) immediately before procedure, repeat q 10 min prn. Uveitis: 1 gtt (2%) two to three times per day.

FORMS — Trade only: Soln 2% (5 mL), 5% (15 mL). Generic/Trade: Soln 5% (5 mL).

NOTES — Cycloplegia and mydriasis last 1 to 3 days.

MOA — Anticholinergic blockage of ciliary body and iris muscles to produce loss of accommodation and pupil dilation.

ADVERSE EFFECTS — Ocular: Frequent: Blurred vision, especially reading vision, photophobia.

PHENYLEPHRINE—OPHTHALMIC ▶plasma L ♀C ▶? $

ADULT — Ophthalmologic exams: 1 to 2 gtts (2.5%, 10%) before procedure. Ocular surgery: 1 to 2 gtts (2.5%, 10%) before surgery.

PEDS — Not routinely used in children.

UNAPPROVED PEDS — Ophthalmologic exams: 1 gtt (2.5%) before procedure. Ocular surgery: 1 gtt (2.5%) before surgery.

FORMS — Rx Generic: Soln 2.5% (2, 3, 5, 15 mL), 10% (5 mL).

NOTES — Overuse can cause rebound dilation of blood vessels. No cycloplegia; mydriasis may last up to 5 h. Systemic absorption, especially with 10% soln, may be associated with sympathetic stimulation (eg, increased BP).

MOA — Alpha-adrenergic and (weak) beta-adrenergic agonist to stimulate iris dilator and cause mydriasis.

ADVERSE EFFECTS — Frequent: Reflex bradycardia, excitability, restlessness, photophobia.

TROPICAMIDE (Mydriacyl, Tropicacyl) ▶? ♀C ▶? $

ADULT — Dilated eye exam: 1 to 2 gtts (0.5%) in eye(s) 15 to 20 min before exam, repeat q 30 min prn.

PEDS — Not approved in children.

FORMS — Generic/Trade: Soln 0.5% (15 mL), 1% (3, 15 mL). Generic only: Soln 1% (2 mL).

NOTES — Mydriasis may last 6 h and has weak cycloplegic effects.

MOA — Anticholinergic blockage of iris sphincter muscle to produce pupil dilation.

ADVERSE EFFECTS — Frequent: Tachycardia, CNS effects, blurred vision, photophobia, possible increased intraocular pressure.

OPHTHALMOLOGY: Non-Steroidal Anti-Inflammatories

NOTE: On average, each mL of eye drop soln contains approximately 20 gtts. Reserve ointment formulations for bedtime use due to severe vision blurring. Most eye medications can be administered 1 gtt at a time despite common manufacturer recommendations of 1 to 2 gtts concurrently. Even a single gtt is typically more than the eye can hold and thus a 2nd gtt is both wasteful and increases the possibility of systemic toxicity. If 2 gtts of the medication are desired, separate single gtts by at least 5 min.

BROMFENAC—OPHTHALMIC (Bromday, Prolensa) ▶minimal absorption ♀C, D (3rd trimester) ▶? $$$$$

ADULT — Postop inflammation and pain following cataract surgery: 1 gtt once daily beginning 1 day prior to surgery and continuing for 14 days after surgery (Bromday, Prolensa) or twice daily (generic).

PEDS — Not approved in children.

FORMS — Trade only: Soln 0.09% (Bromday) 1.7, 3.4 mL (two 1.7 mL twin packs). Soln 0.07% (Prolensa) 1.6, 3 mL. Generic only: Soln 0.09% (twice-daily soln 2.5, 5 mL).

NOTES — Not for use with soft contact lenses. Contains sodium sulfite and may cause allergic reactions.

MOA — Blocks prostaglandin synthesis by inhibiting cyclooxygenase.

ADVERSE EFFECTS — Frequent: Abnormal eye sensation, conjunctival hyperemia, eye irritation, pain, pruritus, redness, headache, iritis. Severe: Keratitis, corneal thinning, erosion, ulceration, perforation.

DICLOFENAC—OPHTHALMIC (Voltaren, ✱Voltaren Ophtha) ▶L ♀C ▶? $$$

ADULT — Postop inflammation following cataract surgery: 1 gtt four times per day for 1 to 2 weeks. Ocular photophobia and pain associated with corneal refractive surgery: 1 to 2 gtts to operative eye(s) 1 h prior to surgery and 1 to 2 gtts within 15

(cont.)

DICLOFENAC—OPHTHALMIC (*cont.*)

min after surgery, then 1 gtt four times per day prn for no more than 3 days.

PEDS — Not approved in children.

FORMS — Generic/Trade: Soln 0.1% (2.5, 5 mL).

NOTES — Contraindicated for use with soft contact lenses.

MOA — Blocks prostaglandin synthesis by inhibiting cyclooxygenase.

ADVERSE EFFECTS — Frequent: Lacrimation, keratitis, eye pain, increased intraocular pressure, burning, stinging. Severe: Keratitis, corneal thinning, erosion, ulceration, perforation.

FLURBIPROFEN—OPHTHALMIC (*Ocufen*) ▶L ♀C ▶? $

ADULT — Inhibition of intraoperative miosis: 1 gtt q 30 min beginning 2 h prior to surgery (total of 4 gtts).

PEDS — Not approved in children.

UNAPPROVED ADULT — Treatment of cystoid macular edema, inflammation after glaucoma or cataract laser surgery, uveitis syndromes.

FORMS — Generic/Trade: Soln 0.03% (2.5 mL).

MOA — Blocks prostaglandin synthesis by inhibiting cyclooxygenase.

ADVERSE EFFECTS — Frequent: Transient stinging/burning. Severe: Keratitis, corneal thinning, erosion, ulceration, perforation.

KETOROLAC—OPHTHALMIC (*Acular, Acular LS, Acuvail*) ▶L ♀C ▶? $$$$

ADULT — Allergic conjunctivitis: 1 gtt (0.5%) four times per day (Acular). Postop inflammation following cataract surgery: 1 gtt (0.5%) four times per day beginning 24 h after surgery for 1 to 2 weeks (Acular). 1 gtt in each affected eye twice daily (Acuvail). Postop corneal refractive surgery: 1 gtt (0.4%) prn for up to 4 days (Acular LS).

PEDS — Not approved age younger than 3 yo. Use adult dose for age 3 yo or older.

FORMS — Generic/Trade: Soln (Acular LS) 0.4% (5 mL). Trade only: Acular 0.5% (3, 5, 10 mL), preservative-free Acuvail 0.45% unit dose (0.4 mL).

NOTES — Do not administer while wearing soft contact lenses. Wait 10 min after use before inserting contact lenses. Avoid use in late pregnancy.

MOA — Blocks prostaglandin synthesis by inhibiting cyclooxygenase.

ADVERSE EFFECTS — Frequent: Transient stinging/burning. Severe: Keratitis, corneal thinning, erosion, ulceration, ulcerative keratitis, perforation.

NEPAFENAC (*Nevanac, Ilevro*) ▶minimal absorption ♀C D in 3rd trimester ▶? $$$$

ADULT — Postop inflammation following cataract surgery: 1 gtt three times per day beginning 24 h before cataract surgery and continued for 2 weeks after surgery.

PEDS — Not approved in children.

FORMS — Trade only: Susp 0.1% (Nevanac-3 mL). Susp 0.3% (Ilevro-1.7 mL).

NOTES — Not for use with contact lenses. Caution if previous allergy to aspirin or other NSAIDs.

MOA — A prodrug that is converted by ocular tissues to amfenac, which blocks prostaglandin synthesis by inhibiting cyclooxygenase.

ADVERSE EFFECTS — Frequent: Abnormal eye sensation, conjunctival hyperemia, eye irritation, pain, photophobia, dry eye, pruritus, redness, headache, iritis. Severe: Increased bleeding time, keratitis, corneal thinning, erosion, ulceration, perforation.

OPHTHALMOLOGY: Other Ophthalmologic Agents

AFLIBERCEPT (*Eylea*) ▶minimal absorption – ♀C ▶– $$$$$

ADULT — Wet macular degeneration, macular edema after central retinal vein occlusion: 2 mg (0.05 mL) intravitreal injection q 4 weeks for 3 doses, then 2 mg (0.05 mL) intravitreal injection q 8 weeks. Diabetic retinopathy with diabetic macular edema: 2 mg (0.05 mL) intravitreal injection q 4 weeks for 5 doses, then 2 mg (0.05 mL) intravitreal injection q 8 weeks. Macular edema following retinal vein occlusion: 2 mg (0.05 mL) intravitreal injection q 4 weeks.

PEDS — Not approved for use in children.

FORMS — Sterile powder for reconstitution.

NOTES — Endophthalmitis and retinal detachments may occur. Can increase IOC. Potential risk of arterial thromboembolic events following intravitreal use. Women of child-bearing potential should use effective contraception prior to the initial dose, during treatment, and for at least 3 months after the last dose.

MOA — Inhibits binding and activation of vascular endothelial growth factor-A (VEGF-A) and placental growth factor (PIGF) receptors

ADVERSE EFFECTS — Frequent: conjunctival hemorrhage, eye pain, cataract, vitreous detachment, vitreous floaters, and increased IOP. Severe: Endophthalmitis, retinal detachments, arterial thromboembolic events.

ARTIFICIAL TEARS (*Tears Naturale, Hypotears, Refresh Tears, GenTeal, Systane*) ▶minimal absorption ♀A ▶+ $

ADULT — Ophthalmic lubricant: 1 to 2 gtts prn.

PEDS — Ophthalmic lubricant: 1 to 2 gtts prn.

FORMS — OTC Generic/Trade: Soln (15, 30 mL, among others).

MOA — Lubricant.

ADVERSE EFFECTS — Frequent: Mild stinging, temporary blurred vision.

CYCLOSPORINE—OPHTHALMIC (*Restasis*) ▶minimal absorption ♀C ▶? $$$$

ADULT — Keratoconjunctivitis sicca (chronic dry eye disease): 1 gtt in each eye q 12 h.

(cont.)

CYCLOSPORINE—OPHTHALMIC (*cont.*)
PEDS — Not approved in children.
FORMS — Trade only: Emulsion 0.05% (0.4 mL single-use vials).
NOTES — Wait 10 min after use before inserting contact lenses. May take 1 month to note clinical improvement.
MOA — Immunomodulator and anti-inflammatory.
ADVERSE EFFECTS — Frequent: Ocular burning.

CYSTEAMINE (*Cystaran*) ▶minimal absorption - ♀C ▶? $$$$$
ADULT — Corneal cysteine crystal accumulation: 1 gtt in each eye q waking h.
PEDS — Not approved in children.
FORMS — Trade: 0.44% soln, 15mL.
NOTES — Insert contact lenses 15 min after administration.
MOA — converts cystine to cysteine and cysteine-cysteamine mixed disulfides thereby reducing corneal cystine crystal accumulation
ADVERSE EFFECTS — Frequent: sensitivity to light, erythema/itching/irritation of eyes, headache, visual field defects.

FLUORESCEIN (*Fluor-I-Strip, Fluor-I-Strip AT, Ful-Glo*) ▶minimal absorption ♀? ▶? $
ADULT — Following ocular anesthetic: Apply enough stain to bulbar conjunctiva to assess integrity of cornea.
PEDS — Following ocular anesthetic: Apply enough stain to bulbar conjunctiva to assess integrity of cornea.
FORMS — Trade only (Fluor-I-Strip AT): Fluorescein 1 mg in sterile ophthalmic strip; (Fluor-I-Strip): Fluorescein 9 mg in sterile ophthalmic strip.
NOTES — Do not use with soft contact lenses.
MOA — Dye
ADVERSE EFFECTS — Frequent: local irritation.

HYDROXYPROPYL CELLULOSE (*Lacrisert*) ▶minimal absorption ♀+ ▶+ $$$
ADULT — Moderate to severe dry eyes: 1 insert in each eye daily. Some patients may require twice daily use.
PEDS — Not approved in children.
FORMS — Trade only: Ocular insert 5 mg.
NOTES — Do not use with soft contact lenses.
MOA — Lubricant.
ADVERSE EFFECTS — Frequent: Blurred vision, ocular discomfort, matting of eyelashes.

LIDOCAINE—OPHTHALMIC ▶L ♀B ▶? $
ADULT — Do not prescribe for unsupervised use. Corneal toxicity may occur with repeated use. Local anesthetic: 2 gtts before procedure, repeat prn.
PEDS — Not approved in children.
FORMS — Generic only: Gel 3.5% (5 mL).
MOA — Ester-type local anesthetic that prevents nerve impulse initiation and potentiation through blockage of sodium ion channels.
ADVERSE EFFECTS — Ocular: Frequent: Hyperemia, corneal epithelial changes, headache, and burning.

LIFITEGRAST (*Xiidra*) ▶minimal absorption ♀? ?/?/? ▶?
ADULT — Dry eye disease: 1 gtt in each eye q12h.
PEDS — Not approved for use in children.
FORMS — Rx, Trade: Ophthalmic solution: single-use containers .
MOA — Inhibits T-cell adhesion by binding to integrin lymphocyte function-associated antigen-1.
ADVERSE EFFECTS — Frequent: eye irritation, dysgeuia, decreased visual acuity.

OCRIPLASMIN (*Jetrea*) ▶minimal absorption - ♀C ▶? $$$$$
ADULT — Symptomatic vitreomacular adhesion: 0.125 mg (0.1 mL) intravitreal injection as a single dose.
PEDS — Not approved in children.
FORMS — Sterile solution of 0.5mg in 0.2ml. Dilution required with 0.2ml of normal saline (0.5mg/0.4ml). Final concentration 0.125mg/0.1ml
MOA — Proteolytic enzyme
ADVERSE EFFECTS — Severe: decreased vision, intravitreal injection procedure effects, lens sublxation, retinal breaks

OMIDRIA **(phenylephrine—ophthalmic irrigation + ketorolac—ophthalmic irrigation)** ▶minimal absorption ♀C ▶? $$$$$
ADULT — Cataract surgery, intraocular lens replacement: Dilute 4 mL in 500 mL ophthalmic irrigating soln. Irrigate prn during procedure.
PEDS — Not approved in children younger than 18 yo.
FORMS — Trade: Sterile soln concentrate (phenylephrine 1% + ketorolac 0.3%), 4 mL.
MOA — Alpha-1 adrenergic receptor agonist (phenylephrine) + inhibition of cyclooxygenase (ketorolac).
ADVERSE EFFECTS — Frequent: eye irritation, posterior capsule opacification, increased intraocular pressure, anterior chamber inflammation.

PETROLATUM (*Lacri-lube, Dry Eyes, Refresh PM, ✱DuoLube*) ▶minimal absorption ♀A ▶+ $
ADULT — Ophthalmic lubricant: Apply ¼ to ½ inch ointment to inside of lower lid prn.
PEDS — Ophthalmic lubricant: Apply ¼ to ½ inch ointment to inside of lower lid prn.
FORMS — OTC Trade only: Oint (3.5, 7 g) tube.
MOA — Lubricates dry eyes.
ADVERSE EFFECTS — Frequent: Blurred vision.

PROPARACAINE (*Ophthaine, Ophthetic, ✱Alcaine*) ▶L ♀C ▶? $
ADULT — Do not prescribe for unsupervised use. Corneal toxicity may occur with repeated use. Local anesthetic: 1 to 2 gtts before procedure. Repeat q 5 to 10 min for 1 to 3 doses (suture or foreign body removal) or for 5 to 7 doses (ocular surgery).
PEDS — Not approved in children.
FORMS — Generic/Trade: Soln 0.5% (15 mL).
MOA — Amide-type local anesthetic that prevents nerve impulse initiation and potentiation through blockage of sodium ion channels.
ADVERSE EFFECTS — Ocular: Frequent: Burning, stinging.

TETRACAINE—OPHTHALMIC (*Pontocaine*) ▶plasma ♀C ▶? $
ADULT — Do not prescribe for unsupervised use. Corneal toxicity may occur with repeated use. Local anesthetic: 1 to 2 gtts before procedure.
PEDS — Not approved in children.
FORMS — Generic only: Soln 0.5% (15 mL), unit-dose vials (0.7, 2 mL).
MOA — Ester-type local anesthetic that prevents nerve impulse initiation and potentiation through blockage of sodium ion channels.
ADVERSE EFFECTS — Ocular: Frequent: Burning, stinging, angioedema, contact dermatitis, chemosis, lacrimation, photophobia, transient stinging.

TRYPAN BLUE (*Vision Blue, Membrane Blue*) ▶Not absorbed ♀C ▶? $$
ADULT — Aid during ophthalmic surgery by staining anterior cap: Inject into anterior chamber of eye.
PEDS — Not approved in children.
FORMS — Trade only: 0.06% (Vision Blue) Ophthalmic soln (0.5 mL), 0.15% (Membrane Blue) Ophthalmic soln (0.5 mL).
MOA — Acid di-azo group dye.
ADVERSE EFFECTS — Inadvertent staining of posterior lens capsule and vitreous face.

PSYCHIATRY

BODY MASS INDEX

BMI	Class	4' 10"	5' 0"	5' 4"	5' 8"	6' 0"	6' 4"
< 19	Underweight	< 91	< 97	< 110	< 125	< 140	< 156
19–24	Healthy weight	91–119	97–127	110–144	125–163	140–183	156–204
25–29	Overweight	120–143	128–152	145–173	164–196	184–220	205–245
30–40	Obese	144–191	153–204	174–233	197–262	221–293	246–328
> 40	Very Obese	> 191	> 204	174–233	> 262	> 293	> 328

*BMI = kg/m^2 = (wt in pounds)(703)/(height in inches)^2. Anorectants appropriate if BMI ≥30 (with comorbidities ≥27); surgery an option if BMI > 40 (with comorbidities 35–40). www.nhlbi.nih.gov

PSYCHIATRY: Antidepressants—Heterocyclic Compounds

NOTE: Gradually taper when discontinuing cyclic antidepressants to avoid withdrawal symptoms. Seizures, orthostatic hypotension, arrhythmias, and anticholinergic side effects may occur. Do not use with MAOIs. Avoid use during treatment with linezolid or IV methylene blue. Antidepressants increase the risk of suicidal thinking and behavior in children, adolescents, and young adults; carefully weigh the risks and benefits before starting and monitor patients closely. Antidepressants have been associated with acute narrow angle glaucoma.

AMITRIPTYLINE ▶L ♀C ▶– $$
ADULT — Depression: Start 50 to 100 mg PO at bedtime; gradually increase by 25 to 50 mg/day to usual effective dose of 50 to 300 mg/day.
PEDS — Depression, adolescents: Use adult dosing. Not approved in children younger than 12 yo.
UNAPPROVED ADULT — Migraine prophylaxis and/or chronic pain: 10 to 100 mg/day. Fibromyalgia: 25 to 50 mg/day.
UNAPPROVED PEDS — Depression, age younger than 12 yo: Start 1 mg/kg/day PO divided three times per day for 3 days, then increase to 1.5 mg/kg/day. Max 5 mg/kg/day.
FORMS — Generic: Tabs 10, 25, 50, 75, 100, 150 mg. Elavil brand name no longer available.
NOTES — Tricyclic, tertiary amine; primarily inhibits serotonin reuptake. Demethylated to nortriptyline, which primarily inhibits norepinephrine reuptake. Usual therapeutic range is 150 to 300 ng/mL (amitriptyline + nortriptyline).
MOA — Serotonin/norepinephrine reuptake inhibitor.
ADVERSE EFFECTS — Serious: Atrial/ventricular arrhythmias, seizures, MI, CHF, stroke. Frequent: Drowsiness, dry mouth, constipation, nausea, orthostatic hypotension, dizziness, confusion, urinary retention, sexual dysfunction.
AMOXAPINE ▶L ♀C ▶– $$$
ADULT — Rarely used; other drugs preferred. Depression: Start 50 mg PO two to three times per day; increase to 100 mg two to three times per day after 1 week. Usual effective dose is 150 to 400 mg/day. Max 600 mg/day.
PEDS — Not approved in children younger than 16 yo.

FORMS — Generic only: Tabs 25, 50, 100, 150 mg.
NOTES — Tetracyclic; primarily inhibits norepinephrine reuptake. Dose 300 mg/day or less may be given once daily at bedtime.
MOA — Norepinephrine/serotonin reuptake inhibitor. Active metabolite is a partial dopamine receptor antagonist.
ADVERSE EFFECTS — Serious: Atrial/ventricular arrhythmias, seizures, MI, CHF, stroke, neuroleptic malignant syndrome, tardive dyskinesia. Frequent: Drowsiness, dry mouth, constipation, nausea, orthostatic hypotension, dizziness, confusion, urinary retention, sexual dysfunction, extrapyramidal side effects.
CLOMIPRAMINE (*Anafranil*) ▶L ♀C ▶+ $$$
ADULT — OCD: Start 25 mg PO at bedtime; gradually increase to 100 mg/day over first 2 weeks in divided doses with meals. May increase to usual effective dose of 150 to 250 mg/day. May give one daily dose at bedtime after titration. Max 250 mg/day.
PEDS — OCD, age 10 yo or older: Start 25 mg PO at bedtime, then increase gradually over 2 weeks to 3 mg/kg/day or 100 mg/day whichever is smaller in divided doses with meals. May then titrate over several weeks to daily max of 3 mg/kg/day or 200 mg, whichever is smaller. May give one daily dose at bedtime once titrated. Not approved for age younger than 10 yo.
UNAPPROVED ADULT — Depression: 100 to 250 mg/day. Panic disorder: 12.5 to 150 mg/day. Chronic pain: 100 to 250 mg/day.
FORMS — Generic/Trade: Caps 25, 50, 75 mg.

(cont.)

CLOMIPRAMINE (*cont.*)

NOTES — Tricyclic, tertiary amine; primarily inhibits serotonin reuptake.

MOA — Serotonin/norepinephrine reuptake inhibitor.

ADVERSE EFFECTS — Serious: Atrial/ventricular arrhythmias, seizures, MI, CHF, stroke, serotonin syndrome, mania. Frequent: Drowsiness, dry mouth, constipation, nausea, orthostatic hypotension, dizziness, confusion, urinary retention, sexual dysfunction, weight gain.

DESIPRAMINE (*Norpramin*) ▶L ♀?/?/? ▶+ $$

ADULT — Depression: Start 25 to 100 mg PO given once daily or in divided doses. Gradually increase to usual effective dose of 100 to 200 mg/day, max 300 mg/day.

PEDS — Depression, adolescents: Usual dose 25 to 100 mg PO daily. Start at lower doses and titrate. Max 150 mg/day. Not approved in children.

FORMS — Generic/Trade: Tabs 10, 25, 50, 75, 100, 150 mg.

NOTES — Tricyclic, secondary amine; primarily inhibits norepinephrine reuptake. Usual therapeutic range is 125 to 300 ng/mL. May cause fewer anticholinergic side effects than tertiary amines. Use lower doses in adolescents or elderly.

MOA — Norepinephrine/serotonin reuptake inhibitor.

ADVERSE EFFECTS — Serious: Atrial/ventricular arrhythmias, seizures, MI, CHF, stroke, serotonin syndrome, mania. Frequent: Drowsiness, dry mouth, constipation, nausea, orthostatic hypotension, dizziness, confusion, urinary retention, sexual dysfunction.

DOXEPIN (*Silenor*) ▶L ♀C ▶– $$

ADULT — Depression and/or anxiety: Start 75 mg PO at bedtime. Gradually increase to usual effective dose of 75 to 150 mg/day, max 300 mg/day. Doses above 150 mg/day should be divided. Insomnia (Silenor): 6 mg PO 30 min before bedtime, 3 mg in age 65 yo or older.

PEDS — Adolescents: Use adult dosing. Not approved in children younger than 12 yo.

UNAPPROVED ADULT — Chronic pain: 50 to 300 mg/day. Pruritus: Start 10 to 25 mg at bedtime. Usual effective dose is 10 to 100 mg/day.

FORMS — Generic only: Caps 10, 25, 50, 75, 100, 150 mg. Oral concentrate 10 mg/mL. Trade only: Tabs 3, 6 mg (Silenor).

NOTES — Tricyclic, tertiary amine; primarily inhibits norepinephrine reuptake. Do not mix oral concentrate with carbonated beverages. Some patients with mild symptoms may respond to 25 to 50 mg/day. Brand name Sinequan no longer available.

MOA — Norepinephrine/serotonin reuptake inhibitor.

ADVERSE EFFECTS — Serious: Atrial/ventricular arrhythmias, seizures, MI, CHF, stroke, sleep-driving. Frequent: Drowsiness, dry mouth, constipation, nausea, orthostatic hypotension, dizziness, confusion, urinary retention, sexual dysfunction.

IMIPRAMINE (*Tofranil, Tofranil PM*) ▶L ♀?/?/? ▶– $$$

ADULT — Depression: Hospitalized patients, start 100 mg/day PO in divided doses. Gradually increase to 200 mg/day as required. May increase to 250 to 300 mg/day after two weeks. Outpatients, start 75 mg/day in divided doses and may increase to 150 mg/day. Usual maintenance 50 to 150 mg/day. Geriatric patients, start 30 to 40 mg/day and increase as needed and tolerated to max 100 mg/day.

PEDS — Enuresis, age 6 yo or older: 25 mg/day PO given 1 h before bedtime. May increase after one week to 50 mg/day for 6 to 12 yo or 75 mg/day if older than 12 yo. Max 75 mg/day. Depression, adolescents, start 30 to 40 mg/day in divided doses. May increase to 100 mg/day if needed. Max 100 mg/day.

UNAPPROVED ADULT — Panic disorder: Start 10 mg PO at bedtime, titrate to usual effective dose of 50 to 300 mg/day. Enuresis: 25 to 75 mg PO at bedtime.

UNAPPROVED PEDS — Depression, children: Start 1.5 mg/kg/day PO divided three times per day; increase by 1 to 1.5 mg/kg/day every 3 to 4 days to max 5 mg/kg/day.

FORMS — Generic/Trade: Tabs 10, 25, 50 mg. Caps 75, 100, 125, 150 mg (as pamoate salt).

NOTES — Tricyclic, tertiary amine; inhibits serotonin and norepinephrine reuptake. Demethylated to desipramine, which primarily inhibits norepinephrine reuptake.

MOA — Serotonin/norepinephrine reuptake inhibitor.

ADVERSE EFFECTS — Serious: Atrial/ventricular arrhythmias, seizures, MI, CHF, orthostatic hypotension, stroke, agranulocytosis. Frequent: Drowsiness, dry mouth, constipation, nausea, dizziness, confusion, urinary retention, sexual dysfunction.

MAPROTILINE ▶KL ♀B ▶? $$$

ADULT — Rarely used; other drugs preferred. Depression: Start 25 mg PO daily, then gradually increase by 25 mg every 2 weeks to max 225 mg/day. Usual effective dose is 150 to 225 mg/day. Max 200 mg/day for chronic use.

PEDS — Not approved in children.

FORMS — Generic only: Tabs 25, 50, 75 mg.

NOTES — Tetracyclic—primarily inhibits norepinephrine reuptake.

MOA — Norepinephrine reuptake inhibitor

ADVERSE EFFECTS — Serious: atrial/ventricular arrhythmias, seizures, MI, CHF, stroke, mania. Frequent: drowsiness, dry mouth, constipation, nausea, orthostatic hypotension, dizziness, confusion, urinary retention, sexual dysfunction

NORTRIPTYLINE (*Pamelor*) ▶L ♀?/?/? ▶+ $$$

ADULT — Depression: Usual dose 25 mg PO three to four times daily. Start at lower doses and increase as required. Max 150 mg/day. Elderly: 30 to 50 mg/day in one or divided doses. Once titrated total daily dose may be given once daily.

(cont.)

NORTRIPTYLINE (*cont.*)

PEDS — Depression, adolescents: 30 to 50 mg PO daily in divided doses or once daily. Not approved in children.

UNAPPROVED ADULT — Panic disorder: Start 25 mg PO at bedtime, titrate to usual effective dose of 50 to 150 mg/day. Smoking cessation: Start 25 mg PO daily 14 days prior to quit date. Titrate to 75 mg/day as tolerated. Continue for 6 weeks or more after quit date. Chronic pain: Start 10 to 25 mg PO every am or at bedtime. Max 150 mg/day.

UNAPPROVED PEDS — Depression, age 6 to 12 yo: 1 to 3 mg/kg/day PO divided three to four times per day or 10 to 20 mg/day PO divided three to four times per day.

FORMS — Generic/Trade: Caps 10, 25, 50, 75 mg. Oral soln 10 mg/5 mL.

NOTES — Tricyclic, secondary amine; primarily inhibits norepinephrine reuptake. Usual therapeutic range is 50 to 150 ng/mL. May cause fewer anticholinergic side effects than tertiary amines. May be used in combination with nicotine replacement for smoking cessation.

MOA — Norepinephrine/serotonin reuptake inhibitor.

ADVERSE EFFECTS — Serious: Atrial/ventricular arrhythmias, seizures, MI, CHF, stroke, serotonin syndrome, mania. Frequent: Drowsiness, dry mouth, constipation, nausea, orthostatic hypotension, dizziness, confusion, urinary retention, sexual dysfunction.

PROTRIPTYLINE (*Vivactil*) ▶L ♀?/?/? ▶+ $$$$

ADULT — Depression: 15 to 40 mg/day PO divided three to four times per day. Max dose is 60 mg/day.

PEDS — Not approved in children.

FORMS — Generic/Trade: Tabs 5, 10 mg.

NOTES — Tricyclic, secondary amine; primarily inhibits norepinephrine reuptake. May cause fewer anticholinergic side effects than tertiary amines. Dose increases should be made in the morning.

MOA — Serotonin/norepinephrine reuptake inhibitor.

ADVERSE EFFECTS — Serious: Atrial/ventricular arrhythmias, seizures, MI, CHF, stroke. Frequent: Drowsiness, dry mouth, constipation, nausea, orthostatic hypotension, dizziness, confusion, urinary retention, sexual dysfunction.

TRIMIPRAMINE (*Surmontil*) ▶L ♀C ▶? $$$

ADULT — Depression: Outpatients, start 75 mg/day in divided doses, may then increase to 150 mg/day. Usual maintenance range 50 to 150 mg/day, max 200 mg/day. Once titrated may give entire dose at bedtime. Hospitalized patients, start 100 mg/day in divided doses. May gradually increase over a few days to 200 mg/day. Max 250 to 300 mg/day. Elderly, start 50 mg/day. May gradually increase to 100 mg/day.

PEDS — Depression, adolescents: start 50 mg/day. May gradually increase to 100 mg/day. Not approved in children.

FORMS — Generic/Trade: Caps 25, 50, 100 mg.

NOTES — Tricyclic, tertiary amine—primarily inhibits serotonin reuptake.

MOA — Serotonin/norepinephrine reuptake inhibitor

ADVERSE EFFECTS — Serious: atrial/ventricular arrhythmias, seizures, MI, CHF, stroke, mania, serotonin syndrome. Frequent: drowsiness, dry mouth, constipation, nausea, orthostatic hypotension, dizziness, confusion, urinary retention, sexual dysfunction

---

PSYCHIATRY: Antidepressants—Monoamine Oxidase Inhibitors (MAOIs)

NOTE: May interfere with sleep; avoid at-bedtime dosing. Must be on tyramine-free diet throughout treatment, and for 2 weeks after discontinuation. Numerous drug interactions; risk of hypertensive crisis and serotonin syndrome with many medications, including OTC. Allow at least 2 weeks washout when converting from an MAOI to an SSRI (6 weeks after fluoxetine), TCA, or other antidepressant. Contraindicated with carbamazepine or oxcarbazepine. Antidepressants increase the risk of suicidal thinking and behavior in children, adolescents, and young adults; carefully weigh the risks and benefits before starting and monitor patients closely.

ISOCARBOXAZID (*Marplan*) ▶L ♀C ▶? $$$

WARNING — Antidepressans including isocarboxazid may be associated with the development of suicidal thinking and behavior among children, adolescents,and young adults.

ADULT — Depression: Start 10 mg PO two times per day; increase by 10 mg every 2 to 4 days to 40 mg/day. Max 60 mg/day divided two to four times per day.

PEDS — Not approved in children younger than 16 yo.

FORMS — Trade only: Tabs 10 mg.

NOTES — Requires MAOI diet. Contraindicated with other antidepressants, sympathomimetics, meperidine, and dextromethorphan. Reserve use as 2nd- or 3rd-line agent.

MOA — Irreversible, nonselective monoamine oxidase inhibitor.

ADVERSE EFFECTS — Serious: Hypertensive crisis with food/drug interactions, serotonin syndrome, seizures, suicidality, hepatotoxicity, agranulocytosis. Frequent: Dizziness, dry mouth, constipation, urinary retention, headache, confusion, blurred vision, weight gain.

MOCLOBEMIDE ▶L ♀C ▶– $$

ADULT — Canada only. Depression: Start 300 mg/day PO divided two times per day after meals. May increase after 1 week to max 600 mg/day.

PEDS — Not approved in children.

FORMS — Generic/Trade: Tabs 150, 300 mg. Generic only: Tabs 100 mg.

(cont.)

MOCLOBEMIDE (*cont.*)

NOTES — No dietary restrictions. Do not use with TCAs; use caution with conventional MAOIs, other antidepressants, epinephrine, thioridazine, sympathomimetics, dextromethorphan, meperidine, and other opiates. Reduce dose in severe hepatic dysfunction.

MOA — Short-acting, reversible MAOI (preferentially affects MAO-A).

ADVERSE EFFECTS — Serious: Hypertensive crisis with drug or food interactions (theoretical risk), hypotension, bradycardia. Frequent: Sleep disturbance, tremor.

PHENELZINE (*Nardil*) ▶L Primarily monoamine oxidase ♀?/?/? ▶? $$$

WARNING — Antidepressants including phenelzine have been associated with the development of suicidal thinking and behavior in children, adolescents, and young adults.

ADULT — Depression: Start 15 mg PO three times per day. Usual effective dose is 60 to 90 mg/day in divided doses.

PEDS — Not approved in children younger than 16 yo.

FORMS — Trade only: Tabs 15 mg.

NOTES — Requires MAOI diet. May increase insulin sensitivity. Contraindicated with meperidine, dextromethorphan, sympathomimetics, or other antidepressants. Multiple serious drug interactions.

MOA — Irreversible, nonselective monoamine oxidase inhibitor.

ADVERSE EFFECTS — Serious: Hypertensive crisis with food/drug interactions, serotonin syndrome, suicidality, mania, hepatotoxicity, agranulocytosis. Frequent: Dizziness, dry mouth, constipation, urinary retention, headache, confusion, blurred vision, weight gain.

SELEGILINE—TRANSDERMAL (*Emsam*) ▶L ♀C ▶? $$$$$

ADULT — Depression: Start 6 mg/24 h patch q 24 h. Adjust dose in 2-week intervals or more to max 12 mg/24 h.

PEDS — Not approved in children.

FORMS — Trade only: Transdermal patch 6 mg/day, 9 mg/24 h, 12 mg/24 h.

NOTES — MAOI diet is required for doses 9 mg/day or higher. Intense urges (eg, gambling and sexual) have been reported. Consider discontinuing the medication or reducing the dose if these occur.

MOA — Irreversible inhibitor of MAO-B; also inhibits MAO-A when doses at least 9 mg/day are used.

ADVERSE EFFECTS — Serious: Hypertensive crisis with food/drug interactions, serotonin syndrome, orthostatic hypotension, mania/hypomania, impulse control disorders. Frequent: Application site reactions, headache, insomnia, dry mouth.

TRANYLCYPROMINE (*Parnate*) ▶L ♀?/?/? ▶– $$

WARNING — Antidepressants including tranylcypromine have been associated with the development of suicidal thinking and behaviors.

ADULT — Depression: Start 10 mg PO every am; increase by 10 mg/day at 1- to 3-week intervals to usual effective dose of 30 mg/day divided two times per day. Max 60 mg/day.

PEDS — Not approved in children younger than 16 yo.

FORMS — Generic/Trade: Tabs 10 mg.

NOTES — Requires MAOI diet. Contraindicated with sympathomimetics, other antidepressants, meperidine, and dextromethorphan. Multiple drug interactions.

MOA — Reversible, nonselective monoamine oxidase inhibitor.

ADVERSE EFFECTS — Serious: Hypertensive crisis with food/drug interactions, serotonin syndrome, suicidality, mania, seizures, hepatotoxicity, agranulocytosis. Frequent: Dizziness, dry mouth, constipation, urinary retention, headache, confusion, blurred vision, weight gain.

PSYCHIATRY: Antidepressants—Selective Serotonin Reuptake Inhibitors (SSRIs)

NOTE: Gradually taper when discontinuing SSRIs to avoid withdrawal symptoms. Observe patients for worsening depression or the emergence of suicidality, anxiety, agitation, panic attacks, insomnia, irritability, hostility, impulsivity, akathisia, mania, or hypomania, particularly early in therapy or after increases in dose. Antidepressants increase the risk of suicidal thinking and behavior in children, adolescents, and young adults; carefully weigh the risks and benefits before starting treatment and then monitor patients closely. Use of SSRIs during the 3rd trimester of pregnancy has been associated with neonatal complications including respiratory (including persistent pulmonary HTN), GI, and feeding problems, as well as seizures and withdrawal symptoms. Balance these risks against those of withdrawal and depression for the mother. Paroxetine should be avoided throughout pregnancy. Increased risk of abnormal bleeding; use caution when combined with NSAIDs or aspirin. SSRIs have been associated with serotonin syndrome and neuroleptic malignant syndrome. Use cautiously and observe closely for serotonin syndrome if SSRI is used with a triptan or other serotonergic drugs. SSRIs and SNRIs have been associated with hyponatremia, which is often associated with SIADH. The elderly and those taking diuretics may be at increased risk. Avoid use with MAOIs used for psychiatric conditions or during active treatment with linezolid or IV methylene blue. Antidepressants have been associated with acute narrow-angle glaucoma. Antidepressants including some SSRIs and depression itself have been associated with an increased risk of bone fractures. The mechanism is unclear. However, this is not a consistent finding among studies. Monitor bone health in susceptible populations.

CITALOPRAM (*Celexa*) ▶LK ♀C Use in 3rd trimester associated with complications at birth. ▶– $$$
ADULT — Depression: Start 20 mg PO daily. May increase after 1 or more weeks to max 40 mg PO daily or 20 mg daily if older than 60 yo.
PEDS — Not approved in children.
FORMS — Generic/Trade: Tabs 10, 20, 40 mg. Generic only: Orally disintegrating tabs 10, 20, 40 mg, oral soln 10 mg/5 mL.
NOTES — Do not use with MAOIs or tryptophan.
MOA — Selective serotonin reuptake inhibitor.
ADVERSE EFFECTS — Serious: Suicidality, mania, serotonin syndrome, neuroleptic malignant syndrome, abnormal bleeding, withdrawal reactions, increased QTc interval, Torsade de Pointes. Frequent: N/V, diarrhea, insomnia, drowsiness, headache, sexual dysfunction, dry mouth, anorexia, anxiety, nervousness.

ESCITALOPRAM (*Lexapro*, ✲*Cipralex*) ▶LK ♀C Use in 3rd trimester associated with complications at birth. ▶– $$$$
ADULT — Depression, generalized anxiety disorder: Start 10 mg PO daily; may increase to max 20 mg PO daily after 1st week.
PEDS — Depression, Age 12 yo and older: Start 10 mg PO daily. May increase to max 20 mg/day after at least 3 weeks.
UNAPPROVED ADULT — Social anxiety disorder: 5 to 20 mg PO daily.
FORMS — Generic/Trade: Tabs 5, 10, 20 mg. Oral soln 1 mg/mL.
NOTES — Do not use with MAOIs. Doses greater than 20 mg daily have not been shown to be superior to 10 mg daily. Escitalopram is the active isomer of citalopram. Reduce max dose to 10 mg/day with hepatic impairment.
MOA — Selective serotonin reuptake inhibitor.
ADVERSE EFFECTS — Serious: Suicidality, mania, serotonin syndrome, abnormal bleeding, withdrawal reactions. Frequent: Insomnia, ejaculatory disorders, nausea, sweating, fatigue, somnolence.

FLUOXETINE (*Prozac, Prozac Weekly, Sarafem, Selfemra*) ▶L ♀C ▶– $$$
ADULT — Depression, OCD: Start 20 mg PO every am; usual effective dose is 20 to 40 mg/day (depression) or 20 to 60 mg/day (OCD), max 80 mg/day. Depression, maintenance: 20 to 40 mg/day (immediate-release) or 90 mg PO once a week (Prozac Weekly) starting 7 days after last immediate-release dose. Bulimia: 60 mg PO daily in the morning; may need to titrate slowly to this dose over several days for some patieints. Panic disorder: Start 10 mg PO every am; titrate to 20 mg/day after 1 week, max 60 mg/day. Premenstrual dysphoric disorder (Sarafem): 20 mg PO daily, given either throughout the menstrual cycle or for 14 days prior to menses; max 80 mg/day. Doses greater than 20 mg/day can be divided two times per day (in morning and at noon). Bipolar I depression, olanzapine + fluoxetine given separately: Start 5 mg olanzapine + 20 mg fluoxetine daily in the evening. Increase to usual range of 5 to 12.5 mg olanzapine + 20 to 50 mg fluoxetine as tolerated. See also Symbyax combination product entry. Treatment-resistant depression, olanzapine + fluoxetine given separately: Start 5 mg olanzapine + 20 fluoxetine daily in the evening. Increase to usual range of 5 to 20 mg olanzapine + 20 to 50 mg fluoxetine as tolerated. See also Symbyax combination product entry.
PEDS — Depression, age 8 to 17 yo: 10 to 20 mg PO q am (10 mg for smaller children), max 20 mg/day. OCD, age 7 to 17 yo: Start 10 mg PO q am, max 60 mg/day (30 mg/day for smaller children). Bipolar I depression (ages 10 to 17 yo) start 2.5 mg olanzapine plus 20 mg fluoxetine PO daily in the evening. Increase as needed and tolerated. Doses above 12 mg olanzapine and 50 mg of fluoxetine have not been studied.
UNAPPROVED ADULT — Hot flashes: 20 mg PO daily. Posttraumatic stress disorder: 20 to 80 mg PO daily. Social anxiety disorder: 10 to 60 mg PO daily.
FORMS — Generic: Tabs 10, 20, 60 mg. Generic/Trade: Caps 10, 20, 40 mg. Generic: Oral soln 20 mg/5 mL. Trade: Tabs (Sarafem and Selfemra) 10, 15, 20 mg. Generic/Trade: Caps, delayed-release (Prozac Weekly and generics) 90 mg.
NOTES — Half-life of parent is 1 to 3 days and for active metabolite norfluoxetine is 6 to 14 days. Do not use with thioridazine, pimozide, MAOIs, or tryptophan; use caution with lithium, phenytoin, TCAs, and warfarin. Pregnancy exposure has been associated with premature delivery, low birth wt, and lower Apgar scores. Decrease dose with liver disease. Increases risk of mania with bipolar disorder.
MOA — Selective serotonin reuptake inhibitor.
ADVERSE EFFECTS — Serious: Suicidality, mania, serotonin syndrome, neuroleptic malignant syndrome, SIADH, abnormal bleeding, withdrawal reactions, hypoglycemia. Frequent: N/V, diarrhea, insomnia, drowsiness, headache, sexual dysfunction, dry mouth, anorexia, anxiety, nervousness.

FLUVOXAMINE (*Luvox, Luvox CR*) ▶L ♀C Use in 3rd trimester associated with complications at birth. ▶– $$$$
ADULT — OCD: Immediate-release: Start 50 mg PO at bedtime, then increase by 50 mg/day every 4 to 7 days to usual effective dose of 100 to 300 mg/day divided two times per day. Max 300 mg/day. Controlled-release: Start 100 mg PO at bedtime and increase by 50 mg/day weekly as tolerated to max 300 mg/day.
PEDS — OCD (children age 8 yo or older): Immediate-release: Start 25 mg PO at bedtime; increase by 25 mg/day every 4 to 7 days to usual effective dose of 50 to 200 mg/day divided two times per day. Max 200 mg/day (8 to 11 yo) or 300 mg/day (older than 11 yo). Therapeutic effect may be seen with lower doses in girls.
FORMS — Generic/Trade: Tabs 25, 50, 100 mg. Caps, extended-release 100, 150 mg.
NOTES — Do not use with thioridazine, alosetron, tizanidine, tryptophan, or MAOIs; use caution with

(cont.)

FLUVOXAMINE (*cont.*)

benzodiazepines, theophylline, TCAs, and warfarin. Luvox brand not currently on US market.

MOA — Selective serotonin reuptake inhibitor.

ADVERSE EFFECTS — Serious: Suicidality, mania, serotonin syndrome, neuroleptic malignant syndrome, SIADH, hypnatremia, seizures, abnormal bleeding, withdrawal reactions. Frequent: N/V, diarrhea, insomnia, drowsiness, headache, sexual dysfunction, dry mouth, anorexia, anxiety, nervousness.

PAROXETINE (*Paxil, Paxil CR, Pexeva*) ▶LK ♀D ▶? $$$

ADULT — Depression: Start 20 mg PO every am; increase by 10 mg/day at intervals of 1 week or more to usual effective dose of 20 to 50 mg/day, max 50 mg/day. Depression, controlled-release tabs: Start 25 mg PO every am; may increase by 12.5 mg/day at intervals of 1 week or more to usual effective dose of 25 to 62.5 mg/day; max 62.5 mg/day. OCD: Start 20 mg PO every am; increase by 10 mg/day at intervals of 1 week or more to usual recommended dose of 40 mg/day; max 60 mg/day. Panic disorder: Start 10 mg PO every am; increase by 10 mg/day at intervals of 1 week or more to target dose of 40 mg/day; max 60 mg/day. Panic disorder, controlled-release tabs: Start 12.5 mg/day; increase by 12.5 mg/day at intervals of 1 week or more to usual effective dose of 12.5 to 75 mg/day; max 75 mg/day. Social anxiety disorder: Start 20 mg PO every am (which is the usual effective dose); max 60 mg/day. Social anxiety disorder, controlled-release tabs: Start 12.5 mg PO every am; may increase at intervals of 1 week or more by 12.5 mg/day to max 37.5 mg/day. Generalized anxiety disorder: Start 20 mg PO every am (which is the usual effective dose); doses higher than 20 mg/day have not been shown to be more effective. Max 50 mg/day in trials. Posttraumatic stress disorder: Start 20 mg PO every am; doses higher than 20 mg/day have not been shown to be more effective. Max 50 mg/day in clincal trials. Premenstrual dysphoric disorder (PMDD), continuous dosing: Start 12.5 mg PO every am (controlled-release tabs); may increase dose after 1 week to max 25 mg every am. PMDD, intermittent dosing (given for 2 weeks prior to menses): Start 12.5 mg PO every am (controlled-release tabs), max 25 mg/day.

PEDS — Not recommended for use in children or adolescents due to increased risk of suicidality.

UNAPPROVED ADULT — Hot flashes related to menopause or breast cancer: 20 mg PO daily (tabs), or 12.5 to 25 mg PO daily (controlled-release tabs). Avoid combining with tamoxifen.

FORMS — Generic/Trade: Tabs 10, 20, 30, 40 mg. Oral susp 10 mg/5 mL. Controlled-release tabs 12.5, 25 mg. Trade only: (Paxil CR) 37.5 mg.

NOTES — Doses should usually be given in the morning. Start at 10 mg/day and do not exceed 40 mg/day in elderly or debilitated patients or those with renal or hepatic impairment.

Paroxetine is an inhibitor of CYP2D6, and is contraindicated with thioridazine, pimozide, MAOIs, linezolid, and tryptophan; use caution with barbiturates, cimetidine, phenytoin, theophylline, TCAs, risperidone, atomoxetine, and warfarin. Taper gradually after long-term use; reduce by 10 mg/day every week to 20 mg/day; continue for 1 week at this dose, and then stop. If withdrawal symptoms develop, restart at prior dose and taper more slowly. Pexeva is paroxetine mesylate and is a generic equivalent for paroxetine HCl. Paroxetine may reduce the efficacy of tamoxifen. Avoid the combination.

MOA — Selective serotonin reuptake inhibitor.

ADVERSE EFFECTS — Serious: Suicidality, serotonin syndrome, SIADH, hyponatremia, abnormal bleeding, withdrawal reactions, akathisia, mania. Frequent: Asthenia, nausea, diarrhea, constipation, insomnia, drowsiness, sexual dysfunction, dry mouth, anorexia, nervousness, sweating, dizziness, tremor.

SERTRALINE (*Zoloft*) ▶LK ♀C Use in 3rd trimester associated with complications at birth. ▶+ $$$

ADULT — Depression, OCD: Start 50 mg PO daily; may increase after 1 week. Usual effective dose is 50 to 200 mg/day, max 200 mg/day. Panic disorder, posttraumatic stress disorder, social anxiety disorder: Start 25 mg PO daily; may increase after 1 week to 50 mg PO daily. Usual effective dose is 50 to 200 mg/day; max 200 mg/day. PMDD, continuous dosing: Start 50 mg PO daily; max 150 mg/day. PMDD, intermittent dosing (given for 14 days prior to menses): Start 50 mg PO daily for 3 days, then increase to max 100 mg/day.

PEDS — OCD, age 6 to 12 yo: Start 25 mg PO daily, max 200 mg/day. OCD, age 13 yo or older: Use adult dosing.

UNAPPROVED PEDS — Major depressive disorder: Start 25 mg PO daily; usual effective dose is 50 to 200 mg/day.

FORMS — Generic/Trade: Tabs 25, 50, 100 mg. Oral concentrate 20 mg/mL (60 mL).

NOTES — Do not use with tryptophan, or MAOIs; use caution with cimetidine, warfarin, pimozide, or TCAs. Must dilute oral concentrate before administration. Administration during pregnancy has been associated with premature delivery, low birth wt, and lower Apgar scores.

MOA — Selective serotonin reuptake inhibitor.

ADVERSE EFFECTS — Serious: Suicidality, mania, serotonin syndrome, neuroleptic malignant syndrome, SIADH, hyponatremia, abnormal bleeding, withdrawal symptoms. Frequent: N/V, diarrhea, insomnia, drowsiness, headache, sexual dysfunction, dry mouth, anorexia, anxiety, nervousness.

VORTIOXETINE (*Trintellix*▪*Trintellix*) ▶L ♀C ▶? $$$$$

ADULT — Depression: Start 10 mg PO daily. Increase to recommended dose of 20 mg daily as tolerated. Max 20 mg/day. May consider 5 mg/day inititial dose for those not tolerating higher doses.

PEDS — Not approved for use in children.

(cont.)

VORTIOXETINE (*cont.*)

FORMS — Trade only: Tabs 5, 10, 15, 20 mg.

NOTES — Reduce dose by half when using with strong CYP2D6 inhibitors such as bupropion, fluoxetine, and paroxetine, or in CYP2D6 poor metabolizers.

MOA — Serotonin reuptake inhibitor, 5-HT3 antagonist, 5-HT1 agonist

ADVERSE EFFECTS — Serious: serotonin syndrome, hyponatremia, bleeding, suicidal thoughts and behaviors, activation of mania. Frequent: nausea, vomiting, constipation.

PSYCHIATRY: Antidepressants—Serotonin-Norepinephrine Reuptake Inhibitors (SNRIs)

NOTE: Monitor for the emergence of anxiety, agitation, panic attacks, insomnia, irritability, hostility, impulsivity, akathisia, mania, or hypomania, and for worsening depression or the emergence of suicidality, particularly early in therapy or after increases in dose. Antidepressants increase the risk of suicidal thinking and behavior in children, adolescents, and young adults; carefully weigh the risks and benefits before starting treatment, and then monitor closely. Antidepressants have been associated with acute narrow angle glaucoma. SSRIs and SNRIs have been associated with hyponatremia, which is often associated with SIADH. The elderly and those taking diuretics may be at increased risk. Do not use with MAOIs. SNRIs have been associated with serotonin syndrome and neuroleptic malignant syndrome when used alone and especially in combination with other serotonergic drugs.

DESVENLAFAXINE (*Pristiq, Khedezla*) ▶LK ♀C ▶? $$$$

ADULT — Depression: 50 mg PO daily.

PEDS — Not approved for use in children.

FORMS — Trade/generic: extended-release tabs 25, 50, 100 mg

NOTES — There is no evidence that doses greater than 50 mg/day offer additional benefit. Reduce dose to 25 mg/day or 50 mg PO every other day in severe renal impairment (CrCl <30 mL/min). Caution in cardiovascular, cerebrovascular, or lipid disorders.

MOA — Selective inhibitor of serotonin and norepinephrine reuptake.

ADVERSE EFFECTS — Serious: Hypersensitivity, suicidality, serotonin syndrome, neuroleptic malignant syndrome, hypertension, hyperlipidemia, abnormal bleeding, hyponatremia, mania, seizures, narrow angle glaucoma, acute pancreatitis. Frequent: Nausea, vomiting, dry mouth, constipation, diarrhea, fatigue, decreased appetite, insomnia, hyperhidrosis, headache, dizziness.

DULOXETINE (*Cymbalta*) ▶L ♀C ▶? $$$$

ADULT — Depression: Start: 20 mg PO twice daily or 60 mg/day given once daily or divided twice daily. May start 30 mg PO once daily in some patients to improve tolerability. Increase as tolerated to 60 mg/day given once daily or divided twice daily. Max 120 mg/day. Doses of 120 mg/day have been used but have not been shown to be more effective than 60 mg/day. Generalized anxiety disorder: Start 30 to 60 mg PO daily, max 120 mg/day. Elderly: Start 30 mg PO daily for 2 weeks. Then increase to target dose of 60 mg/day, max 120 mg/day. Doses above 60 mg/day have not been shown to be more effective. Diabetic peripheral neuropathic pain: 60 mg PO daily. Fibromyalgia: Start 30 mg PO daily for one week then increase to 60 mg/day if needed and tolerated. Max 60 mg/day. Chronic musculoskeletal pain: Start 30 mg PO once daily for 1 week. Then increase to 60 mg once daily. Max 60 mg/day.

PEDS — Generalized anxiety disorder (age 7 to 17 yo):Start 30 mg PO once daily. May increase after 2 weeks to 60 mg once daily. Recommended range is 30 mg to 60 mg daily, but may increase by 30 mg/day to max 120 mg/day if needed and tolerated.

UNAPPROVED ADULT — Chemotherapy-induced peripheral neuropathy: start 20 to 30 mg PO daily. May increase if tolerated after one week to 60 mg/day.

FORMS — Generic/Trade: Caps 20, 30, 60 mg.

NOTES — Avoid in renal insufficiency (CrCl <30 mL/min), hepatic insufficiency, or substantial alcohol use. Do not use with thioridazine, MAOIs, or potent inhibitors of CYP1A2; use caution with inhibitors of CYP2D6. Small BP increases have been observed.

MOA — Serotonin and norepinephrine reuptake inhibitor; also a weak inhibitor of dopamine reuptake.

ADVERSE EFFECTS — Serious: Suicidality, mania, hypertension, seizures, hepatitis, cholestatic jaundice, serotonin syndrome, abnormal bleeding, orthostatic hypotension, hyponatremia. Frequent: N/V, dry mouth, constipation, decreased appetite, fatigue, somnolence, insomnia, sweating, dizziness, headache.

LEVOMILNACIPRAN (*Fetzima*) ▶KL ♀C ▶? $$$$$

ADULT — Major depressive disorder: Start 20 mg PO once daily. Increase after 2 days to 40 mg PO once daily. May increase in increments of 40 mg/day at intervals of 2 or more days to max of 120 mg/day based on response.

PEDS — Not approved for use in children or adolescents.

FORMS — Trade only: Caps 20, 40, 80, 120 mg.

NOTES — Reduce max dose to 80 mg/day for moderate renal insufficiency and 40 mg/day for severe.

MOA — Serotonin-norepinephrine reuptake inhibitor

ADVERSE EFFECTS — Serious: suicidal thoughts and behaviors, hypertension, serotonin syndrome, bleeding, mania/hypomania, hypersensitivity, angle closure glaucoma. Frequent: nausea, constipation,

(cont.)

LEVOMILNACIPRAN (*cont.*)

vomiting, hyperhidrosis, tachycardia, palpitations, erectile dysfunction.

VENLAFAXINE (*Effexor XR*) ▶LK ♀C ▶? $$$$

ADULT — Depression: Start 37.5 to 75 mg PO daily (Effexor XR) or 75 mg/day divided two to three times per day (immediate-release tabs). Increase in 75 mg increments every 4 days to usual effective dose of 150 to 225 mg/day, max 225 mg/day (Effexor XR) or 375 mg/day (Effexor). Generalized anxiety disorder: Start 37.5 to 75 mg PO daily (Effexor XR); increase in 75 mg increments every 4 days to max 225 mg/day. Social anxiety disorder: 75 mg PO daily (Effexor XR). Panic disorder: Start 37.5 mg PO daily (Effexor XR), may titrate by 75 mg/day at weekly intervals to max 225 mg/day. Give with food.

PEDS — Not approved in children.

UNAPPROVED ADULT — Hot flashes (primarily in cancer patients): 37.5 to 75 mg/day of the extended-release form. Chemotherapy-induced peripheral neuropathy: Start 50 mg PO immediate-release tab on day 1 followed by venlafaxine XR 37.5 mg PO twice daily thereafter.

FORMS — Generic/Trade: Caps, extended-release 37.5, 75, 150 mg. Tabs 25, 37.5, 50, 75, 100 mg. Generic only: Tabs, extended-release 37.5, 75, 150, 225 mg.

NOTES — Decrease dose in renal or hepatic impairment. Monitor for increases in BP. Do not give with MAOIs; use caution with cimetidine and haloperidol. Use caution and monitor for serotonin syndrome if used with triptans. Gradually taper when discontinuing therapy to avoid withdrawal symptoms after prolonged use. Hostility, suicidal ideation, and self-harm have been reported when used in children. Mydriasis and increased intraocular pressure can occur; use caution in glaucoma.

MOA — Serotonin and norepinephrine reuptake inhibitor; also a weak inhibitor of dopamine reuptake.

ADVERSE EFFECTS — Serious: Suicidality, mania/hypomania, seizures, hypertension, withdrawal symptoms, serotonin syndrome, neuroleptic malignant syndrome, interstitial lung disease and eosinophilic pneumonia, toxic epidermal necrolysis. Frequent: Drowsiness, dizziness, sexual dysfunction, anorexia, N/V, asthenia, nervousness, insomnia, diaphoresis, constipation, dry mouth, abnormal vision.

PSYCHIATRY: Antidepressants—Other

NOTE: Monitor for the emergence of anxiety, agitation, panic attacks, insomnia, irritability, hostility, impulsivity, akathisia, mania, or hypomania, and for worsening depression or the emergence of suicidality, particularly early in therapy or after increases in dose. Antidepressants increase the risk of suicidal thinking and behavior in children, adolescents, and young adults; carefully weigh the risks and benefits before starting treatment, and then monitor closely. Avoid use with MAOIs. Antidepressants have been associated with acute narrow angle glaucoma.

BUPROPION (*Wellbutrin, Wellbutrin SR, Wellbutrin XL, Aplenzin, Zyban, Buproban, Forfivo XL*) ▶LK ♀C ▶– $$

WARNING — Neuropsychiatric reactions including depression, mania, psychosis, hallucinations, delusions, homicidal ideation, hostility, agitation, aggression, anxiety, and suicidality have occurred when bupropion is used for smoking cessation. Observe for these reactions.

ADULT — Depression: Start 100 mg PO two times per day (immediate-release tabs); can increase to 100 mg three times per day after 4 to 7 days. May increase gradually to 450 mg/day in divided doses if no response after several weeks. Usual effective dose is 300 to 450 mg/day, max 150 mg/dose and 450 mg/day. Depression, sustained-release tabs (Wellbutrin SR): Start 150 mg PO every morning; may increase to 150 mg two times per day after 3 days, max 400 mg/day. Give the last dose no later than 5 pm. Depression, extended-release tabs (Wellbutrin XL): Start 150 mg PO every morning; may increase to 300 every morning after 4 days, max 450 mg every morning. Depression, extended-release (Aplenzin): Start 174 mg PO every morning; increase to target dose of 348 mg/day after 4 days or more. Extended-release (Forfivo XL): 450 mg PO once daily. Do not use to initiate therapy. If standard tabs tolerated and patient requires more than 300 mg/day, may use 450 mg PO daily, max 450 mg/day. Seasonal affective disorder, extended-release tabs (Wellbutrin XL): Start 150 mg PO every morning in autumn; may increase after 1 week to target dose of 300 mg every morning, max 300 mg/day. In the spring, decrease to 150 mg/day for 2 weeks and then discontinue. Extended-release (Aplenzin): Start 174 mg PO each morning. Increase to 348 mg/day after 7 days. Smoking cessation (Zyban, Buproban): Start 150 mg PO every morning for 3 days, then increase to 150 mg PO two times per day for 7 to 12 weeks. Allow 8 h between doses, with the last dose given no later than 5 pm. Max 150 mg PO two times per day. Target quit date should be after at least 1 week of therapy. Stop if there is no progress toward abstinence by the 7th week. Write "dispense behavioral modification kit" on first script.

PEDS — Not approved in children.

UNAPPROVED ADULT — ADHD: Immediate-release: Start 100 mg PO twice daily for 3 days, then increase to 100 mg PO three times daily as tolerated. Sustained-release: Start 150 mg PO each morning

BUPROPION (*cont.*)

for 3 days, then increase to 150 mg PO twice daily as tolerated. Extended-release (XL): Start 150 mg PO each morning for 3 days then increase to 300 mg PO each morning as tolerated. Target range for all is 300 mg to 450 mg per day as tolerated.
UNAPPROVED PEDS — ADHD: 1.4 to 5.7 mg/kg/day PO.
FORMS — Generic/Trade (for depression, bupropion HCl): Tabs 75, 100 mg. Sustained-release tabs 100, 150, 200 mg. Extended-release tabs 150, 300 mg (Wellbutrin XL). Generic/Trade (Smoking cessation): Sustained-release tabs 150 mg (Zyban, Buproban). Trade only: Extended-release (Aplenzin, bupropion hydrobromide) tabs 174, 348, 522 mg. Extended-release (Forfivo XL) tab 450 mg.
NOTES — Weak inhibitor of dopamine reuptake. Do not use with MAOIs. Seizures occur in 0.4% of patients taking 300 to 450 mg/day. Contraindicated in seizure disorders, eating disorders, or with abrupt alcohol or sedative withdrawal. Wellbutrin SR, Zyban, and Buproban are all the same formulation. Equivalent doses: 174 HBr = 150 mg HCl, 348 mg HBr = 300 mg HCl, 522 mg HBr = 450 mg HCl. Consider dose reductions for hepatic and renal impairment. Has been associated with false-positive urine test results for amphetamines when using immunoassay procedures. Bupropion has been associated with hypertensive reactions when used with drugs that increase dopamine and/or norepinephrine. Inappropriate inhalation or injection of Zyban tablets has been reported and has resulted in seizures and death.
MOA — Norepinephrine and dopamine reuptake inhibitor.
ADVERSE EFFECTS — Serious: Suicidality, seizures, psychosis, HTN, Stevens-Johnson syndrome, rhabdomyolysis, hallucinations, parkinsonism. Frequent: Headache, tremor, agitation, insomnia, diaphoresis, weight loss, dry mouth, nausea, constipation, dizziness.

MIRTAZAPINE (*Remeron, Remeron SolTab*) ▶LK ♀C ▶? $$

ADULT — Depression: Start 15 mg PO at bedtime, increase after 1 to 2 weeks to usual effective dose of 15 to 45 mg/day.
PEDS — Not approved in children.
UNAPPROVED ADULT — Antipsychotic-induced akathisia: 15 mg PO once daily in the morning.
FORMS — Generic/Trade: Tabs 15, 30, 45 mg. Tabs, orally disintegrating (SolTab) 15, 30, 45 mg. Generic only: Tabs 7.5 mg.
NOTES — 0.1% risk of agranulocytosis. May cause drowsiness, increased appetite, and wt gain. Do not use with MAOIs.
MOA — Presynaptic alpha-2 receptor antagonist; 5-HT2A, 5-HT-2C, and 5-HT-3 receptor antagonist; enhances norepinephrine and serotonin release.

ADVERSE EFFECTS — Serious: Suicidality, mania, agranulocytosis, dyslipidemia, serotonin syndrome, hyponatremia, akathisia. Frequent: Drowsiness, increased appetite, weight gain, dizziness, dry mouth, constipation.

NEFAZODONE ▶L ♀C ▶? $$$

WARNING — Rare reports of life-threatening liver failure. Discontinue if signs or symptoms of liver dysfunction develop. Brand name product withdrawn from the market in the US and Canada.
ADULT — Depression: Start 100 mg PO two times per day. Increase by 100 to 200 mg/day at 1-week intervals or longer to usual effective dose of 150 to 300 mg PO two times per day, max 600 mg/day. Start 50 mg PO two times per day in elderly or debilitated patients.
PEDS — Not approved in children.
FORMS — Generic only: Tabs 50, 100, 150, 200, 250 mg.
NOTES — Do not use with MAOIs, pimozide, or triazolam; use caution with alprazolam. Many other drug interactions.
MOA — Serotonin reuptake inhibitor and 5-HT2 receptor antagonist.
ADVERSE EFFECTS — Serious: Suicidality, hepatotoxicity, liver failure. Frequent: N/V, dry mouth, constipation, drowsiness, dizziness, asthenia.

TRAZODONE (*Oleptro*) ▶L ♀C ▶- $

ADULT — Depression: Start 50 to 150 mg/day PO in divided doses, increase by 50 mg/day every 3 to 4 days. Usual effective dose is 400 to 600 mg/day. Extended release: Start 150 mg PO at bedtime. May increase by 75 mg/day every 3 days to max 375 mg/day.
PEDS — Not approved in children.
UNAPPROVED ADULT — Insomnia: 50 to 100 mg PO at bedtime, max 150 mg/day.
FORMS — Trade only: Extended-release tabs (Oleptro) 150, 300 mg. Generic only: Tabs 50, 100, 150, 300 mg.
NOTES — May cause priapism. Rarely used as monotherapy for depression; most often used as a sleep aid and adjunct to another antidepressant. Use caution with CYP3A4 inhibitors or inducers. Brand name Desyrel no longer available. Oleptro can be split along score line, but not crushed.
MOA — Serotonin reuptake inhibitor and 5-HT2A receptor antagonist.
ADVERSE EFFECTS — Serious: Orthostatic hypotension, priapism, syncope. Frequent: Drowsiness, dizziness, nervousness, headache, tremor, fatigue, dry mouth, blurred vision.

TRYPTOPHAN ▶K ♀? ▶? $$

ADULT — Canada only. Adjunct to antidepressant treatment for affective disorders: 8 to 12 g/day in 3 to 4 divided doses.
PEDS — Not indicated.
FORMS — Trade only: L-tryptophan tabs 250, 500, 750, 1000 mg.

(cont.)

TRYPTOPHAN (*cont.*)

NOTES — Caution in diabetics; may worsen glycemic control.

MOA — An essential amino acid that increases serotonin synthesis in the CNS.

ADVERSE EFFECTS — Serious: Serotonin syndrome. Frequent: Drowsiness, dizziness, nausea, dry mouth.

VILAZODONE (*Viibryd*) ▶L ♀C Rated C by ACOG ▶?

WARNING — Reduce max dose to 20mg/day when used with strong inhibitors of CYP3A4.

ADULT — Major depressive disorder: Start 10 mg PO once daily for 7 days. Then increase to 20 mg/day for another 7 days. Then may increase to 40 mg/day if needed..

PEDS — Not approved for use in children.

FORMS — Trade only: Tabs 10, 20, 40 mg.

NOTES — Give this medication with food. Bioavailability is reduced up to 50% if taken on empty stomach. Metabolized primarily by CYP3A4. Refer to package insert for dosing with strong CYP3A4 inhibitors or inducers.

MOA — Inhibition of serotonin reuptake and 5-HT1A partial agonist

ADVERSE EFFECTS — Severe: serotonin syndrome, bleeding, seizures, mania, hyponatremia. Frequent: nausea, diarrhea, vomiting, dry mouth, insomnia, dizziness.

PSYCHIATRY: Antimanic (Bipolar) Agents

LAMOTRIGINE—PSYCHIATRY (*Lamictal, Lamictal CD, Lamictal ODT, Lamictal XR*) ▶LK ♀C Possible risk of cleft palate or lip. ▶– $$$$

WARNING — Potentially life-threatening rashes (eg, Stevens-Johnson syndrome, toxic epidermal necrolysis) have been reported in 0.3% of adults and 0.8% of children, usually within 2 to 8 weeks of initiation; discontinue at first sign of rash. Drug reaction with eosinophilia and systemic symptoms (DRESS) has also been reported. Drug interaction with valproate; see adjusted dosing guidelines. Increased risk of suicidal ideation or behaviors with antiepileptic drugs. Monitor closely for signs of depression, anxiety, hostility, and hypomania/mania. Symptoms may develop within 1 week of initiation and risk continues through at least 24 weeks.

ADULT — Bipolar disorder (maintenance): Start 25 mg PO daily for 2 weeks, 50 mg PO daily if on carbamazepine or other enzyme-inducing drugs, or 25 mg PO every other day if on valproate. Increase for weeks 3 to 4 to 50 mg/day, 50 mg twice per day if on enzyme-inducing drugs, or 25 mg/day if on valproate, then adjust over weeks 5 to 7 to target dose of 200 mg/day, up to 400 mg/day divided twice per day if on enzyme-inducing drugs, or 100 mg/day if on valproate. See Neurology section for epilepsy dosing.

PEDS — Not approved in children.

FORMS — Generic/Trade: Chewable dispersible tabs (Lamictal CD) 5, 25 mg. Tabs 25, 100, 150, 200 mg. Extended-release tabs (XR) 25, 50, 100, 200, 250, 300 mg. Orally disintegrating tabs (ODT) 25, 50, 100, 200 mg. Trade only: Chewable dispersible tabs 2 mg.

NOTES — Drug interactions with valproate and enzyme-inducing antiepileptic drugs (ie, carbamazepine, phenobarbital, phenytoin, primidone); may need to adjust dose if these drugs are added or discontinued. May increase carbamazepine toxicity. Preliminary evidence suggests that exposure during the 1st trimester of pregnancy is associated with a risk for cleft palate and/or cleft lip.

Please report all fetal exposure to the Lamotrigine Pregnancy Registry (800-336-2176) and the North American Antiepileptic Drug Pregnancy Registry (888-233-2334). The extended-release product has not been FDA approved for use in bipolar disorder. Lamotrigine has not been shown to be effective for acute mania or mixed episodes of bipolar disorder. Chewable dispersable tablets available only through the manufacturer. Significant interaction with estrogen-containing oral contraceptives. See prescribing information for alterations in initiation and maintenence doses.

MOA — Unknown in bipolar.

ADVERSE EFFECTS — Serious: Rash (including Stevens-Johnson syndrome and toxic epidermal necrolysis), hypersensitivity reactions, drug reaction with eosinophilia and systemic symptoms (DRESS), blood dyscrasias, multiorgan failure, aseptic meningitis. Frequent: N/V, insomnia, back pain, fatigue, rhinitis, abdominal pain, dry mouth, constipation, exacerbation of cough, pharyngitis.

LITHIUM (*Lithobid, ✲Lithane*) ▶K ♀D ▶– $

WARNING — Lithium toxicity can occur at therapeutic levels.

ADULT — Acute mania: Start 300 to 600 mg PO two to three times per day. Starting at the lower dose may improve tolerability. Usual effective dose is 900 to 1800 mg/day. Steady state is achieved in 5 days. Bipolar maintenance: Usually 900 to 1200 mg/day in divided doses titrated to therapeutic trough level of 0.6 to 1.2 mEq/L.

PEDS — Age 12 yo or older: Use adult dosing.

UNAPPROVED PEDS — Mania (age younger than 12 yo): Start 15 to 60 mg/kg/day PO divided three to four times per day. Adjust weekly to achieve therapeutic levels.

FORMS — Generic/Trade: Caps 300 mg; Extended-release tabs 300, 450 mg. Generic only: Caps 150, 600 mg; Tabs 300 mg; Syrup 300 mg/5 mL.

NOTES — Steady-state levels occur in 5 days (later in elderly or renally impaired patients). Usual therapeutic trough levels are 1.0 to 1.5 mEq/L (acute

(cont.)

LITHIUM (*cont.*)

mania) or 0.6 to 1.2 mEq/L (maintenance). 300 mg = 8 mEq or mmol. A dose increase of 300 mg/day will increase the level by approx 0.2 mEq/L. Monitor renal and thyroid function, avoid dehydration or salt restriction, and watch closely for polydipsia or polyuria. Diuretics, ACE inhibitors, angiotensin receptor blockers, and NSAIDs may increase lithium levels (aspirin and sulindac OK). Dose-related side effects (eg, tremor, GI upset) may improve by dividing doses three to four times per day or using extended-release tabs. Monitor renal function and electrolytes. Brand name Eskalith no longer available.
MOA — Unknown, may increase synthesis and release of serotonin and inhibit its reuptake.
ADVERSE EFFECTS — Serious: Seizures, ventricular arrhythmias, leukocytosis, hypothyroidism, renal failure, nephrogenic diabetes insipidus, coma, drug-induced parkinsonism. Frequent: Tremor, N/V, diarrhea, cramps, polyuria, polydipsia, rash, fatigue.

TOPIRAMATE—PSYCHIATRY (*Topamax*) ▶K ♀D ▶? $$$$$
WARNING — Risk of suicidal ideation or behaviors with antiepileptic drugs. Monitor closely for signs of depression, anxiety, hostility, and hypomania/mania. Symptoms may develop within 1 week of initiation and risk continues through at least 24 weeks.
ADULT — See entry in Neurology section.
PEDS — Not approved for psychiatric use in children; see Neurology section.
UNAPPROVED ADULT — Bipolar disorder: Start 25 to 50 mg/day PO; titrate prn to max 400 mg/day divided twice daily. Alcohol dependence: Start 25 mg/day PO; titrate weekly to max 150 mg twice daily.
FORMS — Generic/Trade: Tabs 25, 50, 100, 200 mg. Sprinkle caps 15, 25 mg.
NOTES — Give ½ usual adult dose to patients with renal impairment (CrCl less than 70 mL/min). Cognitive symptoms, confusion, renal stones, glaucoma, and wt loss may occur. Risk of oligohidrosis and hyperthermia, particularly in children; use caution in warm ambient temperatures and/or with vigorous physical activity. Hyperchloremic, nonanion gap metabolic acidosis may occur; monitor serum bicarbonate and reduce dose or taper off if this occurs. Report fetal exposure to North American Antiepileptic Drug Pregnancy Registry (888-233-2334). May increase the risk of hyperammonemia if used with valproic acid.
MOA — Unknown, but may modulate sodium channels and enhance GABA action. Weak carbonic anhydrase inhibitor.
ADVERSE EFFECTS — Serious: Angle closure glaucoma, visual field defects, nephrolithiasis, oligohidrosis, hyperthermia, metabolic acidosis, bleeding. Frequent: Sedation, ataxia, psychomotor slowing, cognitive symptoms, confusion, diplopia, nystagmus, dizziness, depression, nervousness, weight loss, paresthesia.

VALPROIC ACID —PSYCHIATRY (*Depakote, Depakote ER, Stavzor, divalproex, ✦Epival*) ▶L ♀D ▶+ $$$$
WARNING — Fatal hepatic failure reported, especially in children younger than 2 yo with comorbidities and on multiple anticonvulsants. Monitor LFTs during 1st 6 months of treatement and periodically thereafter. Should not be used in children under 2 yo. Life-threatening pancreatitis reported; evaluate for abdominal pain, N/V, and/or anorexia and discontinue if pancreatitis occurs. May be more teratogenic than other anticonvulsants and is associated with neural tube defects, lower IQ in offspring, and other malformations. Hepatic failure and clotting disorders have also occured when used during pregnancy. Use during pregnancy only when no other options and provide effective contraception.
ADULT — Mania: Start 250 mg PO three times per day (Depakote or Stavzor) or 25 mg/kg once daily (Depakote ER); titrate to therapeutic level and effect. Max 60 mg/kg/day.
PEDS — Not approved for mania in children.
UNAPPROVED PEDS — Bipolar disorder, manic or mixed phase (age older than 2 yo): Start 125 to 250 mg PO two times per day or 15 mg/kg/day in divided doses. Titrate to therapeutic trough level of 45 to 125 mcg/mL, max 60 mg/kg/day.
FORMS — Generic only: Syrup (valproic acid) 250 mg/5 mL. Generic/Trade: Delayed-release tabs (Depakote) 125, 250, 500 mg. Extended-release tabs (Depakote ER) 250, 500 mg. Delayed-release sprinkle caps (Depakote) 125 mg. Trade only (Stavzor): Delayed-release caps 125, 250, 500 mg.
NOTES — Contraindicated in urea cycle disorders or hepatic dysfunction and in patients with genetic mutations in mitochondrial DNA polymerase gamma. Reduce dose in the elderly. In clinical trials Depakote was dosed to response at trough serum concentrations between 50 and 125 mcg/mL while Depakote ER was dosed to a range of 85 to 125 mcg/mL. Many drug interactions. Hyperammonemia (risk increased by concurrent topiramate), GI irritation, or thrombocytopenia may occur. Depakote ER is approximately 10% less bioavailable than Depakote. Divalproex sodium is released over 8 to 12 h with Depakote (1 to 4 doses daily), and 18 to 24 h with Depakote ER (1 dose/day).
MOA — Anticonvulsant; may increase GABA levels and modulate sodium channels.
ADVERSE EFFECTS — Serious: Hepatotoxicity, anaphylaxis, polycystic ovarian syndrome, bone marrow suppression, thrombocytopenia, pancreatitis, Stevens-Johnson syndrome, hyperammonemia, drug-induced parkinsonism. Frequent: N/V, diarrhea, dyspepsia, weight gain, CNS depression, drowsiness, dizziness, tremor, alopecia, rash, nystagmus.

PSYCHIATRY: Antipsychotics—First Generation (Typical)

ANTIPSYCHOTIC RELATIVE ADVERSE EFFECTS[a]

Generation	Antipyschotic	Anti-choline-rgic	Seda-tion	Hypot-ension	EPS	Weight Gain	Diabetes/ Hyper-glycemia	Dyslipid-emia
1st	chlorpromazine	+++	+++	++	++	+++	+++	+++
1st	fluphenazine	++	+	+	++++	+	+	+
1st	haloperidol	+	+	+	++++	+	+	+
1st	loxapine	++	+	+	++	++	++	?
1st	molindone	++	++	+	++	+	?	?
1st	perphenazine	++	++	+	++	++	++	?
1st	pimozide	+	+	+	+++	+	+	?
1st	thioridazine	++++	+++	+++	+	++	++	?
1st	thiothixene	+	++	++	+++	++	++	?
1st	trifluoperazine	++	+	+	+++	++	++	?
2nd	aripiprazole	++	+	0	0	0/+	0/+	0
2nd	asenapine	+	+	++	++	++	++	0
2nd	brexipiprazole	+	+	0/+	+	+	?	?
2nd	cariprazine	+	+	+	++	+	?	?
2nd	clozapine	++++	+++	+++	0	++++	++++	++++
2nd	lurasidone	+	+	+	+	+	+	0
2nd	iloperidone	++	+	+++	+	++	++	++
2nd	olanzapine	+++	++	+	0[b]	++++	++++	++++
2nd	paliperidone	+	+	++	++	+++	+++	+
2nd	risperidone	+	++	+	+[b]	+++	+++	+
2nd	quetiapine	+	+++	++	0	+++	+++	+++
2nd	ziprasidone	+	+	0	0	0/+	0	0

Crismon M, Argo T, Bickley P. Schizophrenia. In: DiPiro J, Talbert R, Yee G, et al. ed. Pharmacotherapy.
A pathophysiologic approach, 9th ed. New York: McGraw Hill Education, 2014 and Jibson M. Second generation antipsychotic medications: pharmacology, administration, and comparative side effects. UpToDate, 2015 (www.uptodate.com), and Muench J, Hamer A. Adverse effects of antipsychotic medications, *Am Fam Physician* 2010;81(5):617-22.
[a]Risk of specific adverse effects is graded from 0 (absent) to ++++ (high). ? = Limited or inconsistent comparative data.
[b]Extrapyramidal symptoms (EPS) are dose-related and are more likely for risperidone greater than 6 to 8 mg/day, olanzapine greater than 20 mg/day. Akathisia risk remains unclear and may not be reflected in these ratings. There are limited comparative data for aripiprazole iloperidone, paliperidone, and asenapine relative to other 2nd-generation antipsychotics.

NOTE: Antipsychotic potency is determined by affinity for D2 receptors. Extrapyramidal side effects (EPS) including tardive dyskinesia and dystonia may occur with antipsychotics. Use cautiously in patients with Parkinson's disease. High-potency agents are more likely to cause EPS and hyperprolactinemia. Can be given at bedtime, but may be divided initially to decrease side effects and daytime sedation. Antipsychotics have been associated with an increased risk of venous thromboembolism, especially early in therapy. Assess for other risk factors and monitor carefully. Off-label use for dementia-related psychosis in the elderly has been associated with increased mortality. Newborns exposed during the 3rd trimester are at increased risk for abnormal muscle movements (EPS) and withdrawal symptoms.

CHLORPROMAZINE ▶LK ♀C Per ACOG Guidelines ▷– $$$
ADULT — Psychotic disorders: 10 to 25 mg PO two to four times per day or 25 to 50 mg IM, can repeat in 1 h. Severe acute psychosis may require 400 mg IM every 4 to 6 h up to max 2000 mg/day IM. Intractable hiccups: 25 to 50 mg PO/IM three to four times per day. Persistent hiccups may require 25 to 50 mg in 0.5 to 1 liter NS by slow IV infusion.

(cont.)

CHLORPROMAZINE (*cont.*)

PEDS — Severe behavioral problems/psychotic disorders, age 6 mo to 12 yo: 0.5 mg/kg PO every 4 to 6 h prn or 1 mg/kg PR every 6 to 8 h prn or 0.5 mg/kg IM every 6 to 8 h prn.

FORMS — Generic only: Tabs 10, 25, 50, 100, 200 mg.

NOTES — Monitor for hypotension with IM or IV use. Brand name Thorazine no longer available.

MOA — Low-potency dopamine antagonist.

ADVERSE EFFECTS — Serious: Seizures, neuroleptic malignant syndrome, extrapyramidal side effects, tardive dyskinesia, QT prolongation, jaundice. Frequent: Drowsiness, nausea, dry mouth, constipation, urinary retention, hypotension, headache, hyperprolactinemia.

FLUPENTHIXOL (✱*Fluanxol, Fluanxol Depot*) ▶? ♀? ▶– $$

ADULT — Canada only. Schizophrenia/psychosis: Tabs, initial dose: 3 mg PO daily in divided doses, maintenance 3 to 12 mg daily in divided doses. IM initial dose 5 to 20 mg IM q 2 to 4 weeks, maintenance 20 to 40 mg q 2 to 4 weeks. Higher doses may be necessary in some patients.

PEDS — Not approved in children.

FORMS — Trade only: Tabs 0.5, 3 mg.

NOTES — Relatively nonsedating antipsychotic.

MOA — High-potency dopamine receptor antagonist.

ADVERSE EFFECTS — Serious: NMS, tardive dyskinesia. Frequent: Extrapyramidal reactions, restlessness, agitation.

FLUPHENAZINE (✱*Modecate*) ▶LK ♀C ▶? $$$

ADULT — Psychotic disorders: Start 0.5 to 10 mg/day PO divided every 6 to 8 h. Usual effective dose 1 to 20 mg/day. Max dose is 40 mg/day PO or 1.25 to 10 mg/day IM divided every 6 to 8 h. Max dose is 10 mg/day IM. May use long-acting formulations (enanthate/decanoate) when patients are stabilized on a fixed daily dose. Approximate conversion ratio: 12.5 to 25 mg IM/SC (depot) every 3 to 6 weeks is equivalent to 10 to 20 mg/day PO.

PEDS — Not approved in children.

FORMS — Generic/Trade: Tabs 1, 2.5, 5, 10 mg. Elixir 2.5 mg/5 mL. Oral concentrate 5 mg/mL.

NOTES — Do not mix oral concentrate with coffee, tea, cola, or apple juice. Brand name Prolixin no longer available.

MOA — High-potency dopamine antagonist.

ADVERSE EFFECTS — Serious: Seizures, neuroleptic malignant syndrome, agranulocytosis, aplastic anemia, extrapyramidal side effects, tardive dyskinesia, QT prolongation. Frequent: Drowsiness, nausea, dry mouth, constipation, urinary retention, hypotension, headache, hyperprolactinemia.

HALOPERIDOL (*Haldol*) ▶LK ♀C ▶– $$

ADULT — Psychotic disorders and Tourette syndrome: 0.5 to 5 mg PO two to three times per day. Usual effective dose is 6 to 20 mg/day, max dose is 100 mg/day PO or 2 to 5 mg IM every 1 to 8 h prn to max 20 mg/day IM. May use long-acting (depot) formulation when patients are stabilized on a fixed daily

dose. Approximate conversion ratio: 100 to 200 mg IM (depot) q 4 weeks is equivalent to 10 mg/day PO haloperidol.

PEDS — Psychotic disorders age 3 to 12 yo: 0.05 to 0.15 mg/kg/day PO divided two to three times per day. Tourette syndrome or nonpsychotic behavior disorders, age 3 to 12 yo: 0.05 to 0.075 mg/kg/day PO divided two to three times per day. Increase dose by 0.5 mg every week to max dose of 6 mg/day. Not approved for IM administration in children.

UNAPPROVED ADULT — Acute psychosis and combative behavior: 5 to 10 mg IV/IM, repeat prn in 10 to 30 min. IV route associated with QT prolongation, torsades de pointes, and sudden death; use ECG monitoring.

UNAPPROVED PEDS — Psychosis, age 6 to 12 yo: 1 to 3 mg/dose IM (as lactate) q 4 to 8 h, max 0.15 mg/kg/day.

FORMS — Generic only: Tabs 0.5, 1, 2, 5, 10, 20 mg. Oral concentrate 2 mg/mL.

NOTES — Therapeutic range is 2 to 15 ng/mL.

MOA — High-potency dopamine antagonist.

ADVERSE EFFECTS — Serious: Seizures, neuroleptic malignant syndrome, extrapyramidal side effects, tardive dyskinesia, QT prolongation, sudden death, jaundice, rhabdomyolysis. Frequent: Drowsiness, nausea, dry mouth, constipation, urinary retention, hypotension, headache, hyperprolactinemia.

LOXAPINE (*Adasuve*, ✱*Loxapac*) ▶LK ♀C ▶– $$$$

WARNING — Adasuve (inhaled loxapine) has been associated with severe bronchoconstriction and respiratory distress or arrest. It can only be administered in a healthcare facility that has the ability to manage these emergencies by advanced airway management, intubation, and mechanical ventilation, and that is enrolled in the Adasuve REMS program. Information on enrollment can be obtained by calling 888-970-7367 or at www.adasuverems.com. All patients should be screened for asthma, COPD, or other pulmonary diseases prior to administration.

ADULT — Psychotic disorders: Start 10 mg PO two times per day, usual effective dose is 60 to 100 mg/day divided two to four times per day. Max dose is 250 mg/day. Acute agitation with schizophrenia or bipolar I disorder (Adasuve): 10 mg inhaled once. No more than one dose per 24 h.

PEDS — Not approved in children.

FORMS — Generic only: Caps 5, 10, 25, 50 mg. Trade (Adasuve): 10 mg single-use inhaler.

MOA — Mid-potency dopamine antagonist.

ADVERSE EFFECTS — Serious: Seizures, neuroleptic malignant syndrome, extrapyramidal side effects, tardive dyskinesia, QT prolongation, jaundice. Frequent: Drowsiness, nausea, dry mouth, constipation, urinary retention, hypotension, headache, hyperprolactinemia.

METHOTRIMEPRAZINE ▶L ♀? ▶? $

ADULT — Canada only. Anxiety/analgesia: 6 to 25 mg PO per day given three times per day. Sedation: 10 to 25 mg bedtime. Psychoses/intense pain: Start 50

(cont.)

METHOTRIMEPRAZINE (cont.)

to 75 mg PO per day given in 2 to 3 doses, max 1000 mg/day. Postop pain: 20 to 40 mg PO or 10 to 25 mg IM q 8 h. Anesthesia premedication: 10 to 25 mg IM or 20 to 40 mg PO q 8 h with last dose of 25 to 50 mg IM 1 h before surgery. Limit therapy to less than 30 days.

PEDS — Canada only. 0.25 mg/kg/day given in 2 to 3 doses, max 40 mg/day for child age younger than 12 yo.

FORMS — Canada only: Generic/Trade: Tabs 2, 5, 25, 50 mg.

MOA — Mid-potency dopamine antagonist.

ADVERSE EFFECTS — Serious: QT interval prolongation, neuroleptic malignant syndrome, tardive dyskinesia, orthostatic hypotension, agranulocytosis, jaundice. Frequent: Drowsiness, dry mouth, nausea, constipation, urinary retention, tachycardia, weight gain.

PERPHENAZINE ▶LK ♀C ▶? $$$

ADULT — Psychotic disorders: Start 4 to 8 mg PO three times per day or 8 to 16 mg PO two to four times per day (hospitalized patients), max PO dose is 64 mg/day. Can give 5 to 10 mg IM every 6 h, max IM dose is 30 mg/day.

PEDS — Not approved in children.

FORMS — Generic only: Tabs 2, 4, 8, 16 mg.

NOTES — Do not mix oral concentrate with coffee, tea, cola, or apple juice.

MOA — High-potency dopamine antagonist.

ADVERSE EFFECTS — Serious: Seizures, neuroleptic malignant syndrome, extrapyramidal side effects, tardive dyskinesia, QT prolongation, jaundice. Frequent: Drowsiness, nausea, dry mouth, constipation, urinary retention, hypotension, headache, hyperprolactinemia.

PIMOZIDE (Orap) ▶L ♀C ▶– $$$

ADULT — Tourette syndrome: Start 1 to 2 mg/day PO in divided doses, increase every 2 days to usual effective dose of 1 to 10 mg/day. Max dose is 0.2 mg/kg/day or 10 mg/day whichever is lower.

PEDS — Tourette syndrome, older than 12 yo: 0.05 mg/kg PO at bedtime, increase every 3 days to max 0.2 mg/kg/day up to 10 mg/day.

FORMS — Trade only: Tabs 1, 2 mg.

NOTES — QT prolongation may occur. Monitor ECG at baseline and periodically throughout therapy. Contraindicated with macrolide antibiotics, nefazodone, sertraline, citalopram, and escitalopram. Use caution with inhibitors of CYP3A4 and CYP2D6, and contraindicated with strong inhibitors of these enzymes. Consider CYP2D6 genotyping for doses > 0.05 mg/kg in children or 4 mg in adults. Reduce dose in poor metabolizers.

MOA — High-potency dopamine antagonist.

ADVERSE EFFECTS — Serious: Seizures, neuroleptic malignant syndrome, extrapyramidal side effects, tardive dyskinesia, QT prolongation, jaundice. Frequent: Drowsiness, nausea, dry mouth, constipation, urinary retention, hypotension, headache, hyperprolactinemia.

THIORIDAZINE ▶LK ♀C ▶? $$

WARNING — Can cause QTc prolongation, torsades de pointes–type arrhythmias, and sudden death.

ADULT — Psychotic disorders: Start 50 to 100 mg PO three times per day, usual effective dose is 200 to 800 mg/day divided two to four times per day. Max dose is 800 mg/day.

PEDS — Behavioral disorders, 2 to 12 yo: 10 to 25 mg PO two to three times per day, max dose is 3 mg/kg/day.

FORMS — Generic only: Tabs 10, 15, 25, 50, 100 mg.

NOTES — Not recommended as 1st-line therapy. Contraindicated in patients with a history of cardiac arrhythmias, congenital long QT syndrome, or those taking fluvoxamine, propranolol, pindolol, drugs that inhibit CYP2D6 (eg, fluoxetine, paroxetine), and other drugs that prolong the QTc interval. Only use for patients with schizophrenia who do not respond to other antipsychotics. Monitor baseline ECG and potassium. Pigmentary retinopathy with doses greater than 800 mg/day. Brand name Mellaril no longer available.

MOA — Low-potency dopamine antagonist.

ADVERSE EFFECTS — Serious: Seizures, neuroleptic malignant syndrome, extrapyramidal side effects, tardive dyskinesia, QT prolongation, jaundice. Frequent: Drowsiness, nausea, dry mouth, constipation, urinary retention, hypotension, headache, hyperprolactinemia.

THIOTHIXENE ▶LK ♀C ▶? $$$

ADULT — Psychotic disorders: Start 2 mg PO three times per day. Usual effective dose is 20 to 30 mg/day, max dose is 60 mg/day.

PEDS — Adolescents: Adult dosing. Not approved in children younger than 12 yo.

FORMS — Generic/Trade: Caps 1, 2, 5, 10 mg.

NOTES — Brand name Navane no longer available.

MOA — High-potency dopamine antagonist.

ADVERSE EFFECTS — Serious: Seizures, neuroleptic malignant syndrome, orthostatic hypotension, hyperglycemia, dysphagia, jaundice, dystonia. Frequent: Headache, anxiety, insomnia, N/V, lightheadedness, somnolence, akathisia, constipation, weight gain.

TRIFLUOPERAZINE ▶LK ♀C ▶– $$$

ADULT — Psychotic disorders: Start 2 to 5 mg PO two times per day. Usual effective dose is 15 to 20 mg/day; some patients may require 40 mg/day or more. Anxiety: 1 to 2 mg PO two times per day for up to 12 weeks. Max dose is 6 mg/day.

PEDS — Psychotic disorders, age 6 to 12 yo: 1 mg PO one to two times per day, gradually increase to max dose of 15 mg/day.

FORMS — Generic only: Tabs 1, 2, 5, 10 mg.

NOTES — Dilute oral concentrate just before giving.

MOA — High-potency dopamine antagonist.

ADVERSE EFFECTS — Serious: Seizures, neuroleptic malignant syndrome, extrapyramidal side effects, tardive dyskinesia, QT prolongation, jaundice. Frequent: Drowsiness, nausea, dry mouth, constipation, urinary retention, hypotension, headache, hyperprolactinemia.

ZUCLOPENTHIXOL (*✲Clopixol, Clopixol Depot, Clopixol Accuphase*) ▶L ♀? ▶? $$$$
ADULT — Canada only. Antipsychotic. Tabs: Start 10 to 50 mg PO daily, maintenance 20 to 60 mg daily. Injectable: Accuphase (acetate) 50 to 150 mg IM every 2 to 3 days; Depot (decanoate) 150 to 300 mg IM every 2 to 4 weeks.

PEDS — Not approved in children.
FORMS — Trade, Canada only: Tabs 10, 20 mg (Clopixol).
MOA — Low-potency dopamine antagonist.
ADVERSE EFFECTS — Serious: NMS, tardive dyskinesia. Frequent: Extrapyramidal reactions, drowsiness, dizziness.

PSYCHIATRY: Antipsychotics—Second Generation (Atypical)

NOTE: Tardive dyskinesia, neuroleptic malignant syndrome, drug-induced parkinsonism, dystonia, and other extrapyramidal side effects may occur with antipsychotic medications. Atypical antipsychotics have been associated with wt gain, dyslipidemia, hyperglycemia, and diabetes mellitus; monitor closely. Off-label use for dementia-related psychosis in the elderly has been associated with increased mortality. Antipsychotics have been associated with an increased risk of venous thromboembolism, particularly early in therapy; assess for other risk factors and monitor carefully. Antipsychotics when used for schizophrenia or bipolar disorder have been associated with an increased risk of suicidal thinking and behavior. Monitor closely. Antipsychotics may increase prolactin levels through dopamine receptor antagonism. Consider obtaining prolactin levels if symptoms of excess appear.

ARIPIPRAZOLE (*Abilify, Abilify Maintena, Aristada*) ▶L ♀C ▶? $$$$$
ADULT — Schizophrenia: Start 10 to 15 mg PO daily. Max 30 mg daily; however, doses greater than 15 mg/day have not been shown to be more effective. Schizophrenia, maintenance (Maintena): Start 400 mg IM monthly. May reduce to 300 mg IM monthly if adverse reactions to higher dose. Schizophrenia, maintenance (Aristada): Establish tolerability with PO aripiprazole first. May start with 441 mg, 662 mg, or 882 mg IM monthly based on oral dose. The 882 mg dose may also be given every 6 weeks. The 441 mg dose can be substituted for the 10 mg/day oral dose, 662 mg for 15 mg/day, and 882 mg for 20 mg/day. In conjunction with the first IM Aristada dose, give oral aripiprazole for 21 consecutive days. See package insert for missed doses. Bipolar disorder (acute manic or mixed episodes): start 15 mg PO daily or 10 to 15 mg PO daily if used with lithium or valproate. Agitation associated with schizophrenia or bipolar disorder: 9.75 mg IM recommended. May consider 5.25 to 15 mg if indicated. May repeat after 2 h up to max 30 mg/day. Major depressive disorder, adjunctive therapy: Start 2 to 5 mg PO daily. May increase by 5 mg/day at intervals 1 week or more to max of 15 mg/day.
PEDS — Schizophrenia, 13 to 17 yo: Start 2 mg PO daily. May increase to 5 mg/day after 2 days, and to target dose of 10 mg/day after 2 more days. Max 30 mg/day; however, doses greater than 10 mg/day have not been shown to be more effective. Bipolar disorder (acute manic or mixed episodes, monotherapy or adjunctive to lithium or valproate), 10 to 17 yo: Start 2 mg PO daily. May increase to 5 mg/day after 2 days, and to target dose of 10 mg/day after 2 more days. Increase by 5 mg/day to max 30 mg/day. Irritability associated with autism: Start 2 mg PO daily. Increase to 5 mg/day prn at weekly intervals up to max 15 mg/day. Tourette's disorder (age 6 to 18 yo): For weight less than 50 kg, start 2 mg PO daily and increase to 5 mg/day after 2 days. Then increase weekly as needed to max 10 mg/day.

For weight 50 kg or greater start 2 mg PO daily, then increase to 5 mg/day for 5 days, then increase to target dose of 10 mg/day on day 8. May increase as needed by 5 mg/day at weekly intervals to max 20 mg/day.
FORMS — Generic/Trade: Tabs 2, 5, 10, 15, 20, 30 mg. Generic only: Orally disintegrating tabs 10, 15 mg. Trade only: Susp, extended-release for injection (Abilify Maintena) 300 mg and 400 mg/vial. Pre-filled susp, extended-release injection (Abilify Maintena) 300 mg and 400 mg/syringe. Generic only: oral solution 1 mg/mL.
NOTES — Low EPS and tardive dyskinesia risk. Increase dose when used with CYP3A4 inducers such as carbamazepine. Decrease usual dose by at least half when used with CYP3A4 or CYP2D6 inhibitors such as ketoconazole, fluoxetine, or paroxetine. Increase dose by ½ to 20 to 30 mg/day when used with CYP3A4 inducers such as carbamazepine. Reduce when inducer is stopped. Establish tolerability to oral aripiprazole prior to initiating long-acting IM formulation. Continue oral aripiprazole for 14 days after 1st dose of long-acting IM form and then discontinue. Avoid use of CYP3A4 inducers for more than 14 days with long-acting IM form. Dose adjustments required when used with CYP2D6 or 3A4 inhibitors. See PI.
MOA — Dopamine-2 partial agonist, serotonin-1A partial agonist, serotoin-2A antagonist.
ADVERSE EFFECTS — Serious: Seizures, neuroleptic malignant syndrome, orthostatic hypotension, hyperglycemia, dysphagia, jaundice, suicidal thinking/behavior, pathologic gambling, impaired impulse control. Frequent: Headache, anxiety, insomnia, N/V, lightheadedness, somnolence, akathisia, constipation, weight gain.

ASENAPINE (*Saphris*) ▶L ♀C ?/?/?R withdrawal and EPS in neonates exposed in 3rd trimester. ▶–
WARNING — Antipsychotics when used for schizophrenia or bipolar disorder have been associated with an increased risk of suicidal thinking and behavior. Monitor closely.

(cont.)

ASENAPINE (cont.)

ADULT — Schizophrenia: Initial and maintenance: Start 5 mg SL two times per day. Max 20 mg/day; however, may not be more effective than lower dose. Bipolar disorder, acute manic or mixed episodes: Start 5 mg SL two times per day (adjunctive) or 10 mg sublingual two times per day (monotherapy). Max 20 mg/day.

PEDS — Bipolar disorder, acute manic and mixed episodes, age 10 to 17 yo:Start 2.5 mg PO twice daily. After 3 days may increase to 5 mg twice daily, and from 5 to 10 mg twice daily after 3 more days. Max 20 mg/day. Dystonic reactions more common if dose is titrated more rapidly than recommended.

FORMS — Trade: SL tabs 5, 10 mg.

NOTES — Must be used sublingually and not chewed or crushed.

MOA — Serotonin and dopamine receptor antagonist.

ADVERSE EFFECTS — Serious: Neuroleptic malignant syndrome, tardive dyskinesia, hyperglycemia/diabetes, syncope, orthostatic hypotension, leukopenia, neutropenia, agranulocytosis, seizures, dysphagia/choking. Frequent: Akathisia, EPS, oral hypoesthesia, somnolence, dizziness, weight gain.

BREXPIPRAZOLE (Rexulti) ▶L ♀? ?/?/?R Withdrawal and extrapyramidal symptoms for neonate at birth ▶?

ADULT — Major depressive disorder, adjunctive: Start 0.5 mg to 1 mg PO daily. Increase weekly by 1 mg/day to max 3 mg/day. Schizophrenia: Start 1 mg PO daily for days 1 to 4, then increase to 2 mg once daily for days 5-7. Then increase to max 4 mg/day as needed and tolerated. Reduce dose with hepatic or severe renal impairment.

PEDS — Not approved for use for children or adolescents.

FORMS — Trade only: Tabs 0.25, 0.5, 1, 2, 3, 4 mg.

NOTES — Reduce dose for moderate to severe hepatic impairment or severe renal impairment to max of 2 mg/day for major depressive disorder of 3 mg/day for schizophrenia.

MOA — Partial agonist at serotonin 5-HT1A and dopamine D2, and antagonist at serotonin 5-HT2A receptors.

ADVERSE EFFECTS — Serious: Neuroleptic malignant syndrome, tardive dyskinesia, hyperglycemia and diabetes, seizures, suicidality. Frequent: constipation or diarrhea, fatigue, weight gain, extrapyramidal reactions including akathisia, somnolence, tremor, dizziness.

CARIPRAZINE (Vraylar) ▶L ♀? ?/?/?R Neonates who have been exposed in the third trimester are at increased risk for extrapyramidal or withdrawal reactions at delivery. ▶?

ADULT — Schizophrenia: Start 1.5 mg PO once daily. The dose can be increased to 3 mg/day on day 2. May increase by 1.5 mg/day to 3 mg/day as needed and tolerated to max 6 mg/day. Bipolar I disorder, acute manic or mixed episodes: Start 1.5 mg PO once daily. May increase to 3 mg/day on day 2. May increase by 1.5 mg/day to 3 mg/day to recommended range of 3-6 mg/day, max 6 mg/day.

PEDS — Not approved for use in children or adolescents.

FORMS — Trade only: Caps 1.5 , 3, 4.5, 6 mg.

NOTES — Reduce the dose of cariprazine by half or more if used in the presence of strong CYP3A4 inhibitors. See package insert for details. Avoid use in patients with severe hepatic impairment.

MOA — Partial agonist of central dopamine D2 and serotonin 1A receptors, and antagonist at serotonin 2A receptors.

ADVERSE EFFECTS — Serious: neuroleptic malignant syndrome, hyperglycemia, diabetes, stroke, dyslipidemia, orthostatic hypotension, syncope, leukopenia, neutropenia, seizures, dysphagia. Frequent: weight gain, extrapyramidal symptoms including akathisia, nausea, vomiting, somnolence, restlessness.

CLOZAPINE (Clozaril, FazaClo ODT, Versacloz) ▶L ♀B ▶– $$$$$

WARNING — Risk of agranulocytosis is 1 to 2%. As of October 2015 a single national registry was established by the FDA. All patients enrolled in manufacturer-based registries were transitioned to the new site. Newly started patients are enrolled at the new site. Patients, prescribers, and pharmacies must be registered at www.clozapinerems.com. The absolute neutrophil count (ANC) will be the only lab reported and is caluclated as the WBC x % neutrophils based on the complete blood count with differential. The ANC required for initiation of therapy has been lowered to 1500/mcL. For patients with benign ethnic neutropenia (BEN), the reqired level is at least 1000/mcL. Monitoring frequencies for patients not experiencing neutropenia remain weekly for the first 6 months of therapy, then every 2 weeks up to 12 months, and then monthly thereafter. For patients experiencing mild to severe neutropenia the monitoring frequencies are increased. See prescribing information for more details. Clozapine should be stopped if the ANC goes below 1000/mcL in the general population and below 500/mcL in those with BEN and it is felt to be due to the clozapine. Risk of myocarditis (particularly during the 1st month), seizures, orthostatic hypotension, and cardiopulmonary arrest. Antipsychotics when used for schizophrenia or bipolar disorder have been associated with an increased risk of suicidal thinking and behavior. Monitor closely.

ADULT — Severe, medically refractory schizophrenia or schizophrenia/schizoaffective disorder with suicidal behavior: Start 12.5 mg PO one to two times per day. Titrate by 25 to 50 mg increments over two weeks to achieve a target dose of 300 to 450 mg/day divided two times per day. May then increase the dose every 1 to 2 weeks by up to 100 mg/day to max 900 mg/day. Retitrate if stopped for more than 2 days. Must monitor ANC per package insert and report to www.clozapinerems.com.

(cont.)

CLOZAPINE (cont.)

PEDS — Not approved in children.

FORMS — Generic/Trade: Tabs 25, 100 mg. Orally disintegrating tabs 12.5, 25, 100, 150, 200 mg. Generic only: Tabs 50, 200 mg. Trade only: Susp (Versacloz): 50 mg/mL.

NOTES — It is necessary to begin with low doses to avoid orthostatic hypotension, bradycardia, and syncope. Patients rechallenged with clozapine after an episode of neutropenia are at increased risk of agranulocytosis. Guidelines for monitoring can be found in the package insert or at www.clozpinerems.com. Much lower risk of EPS and tardive dyskinesia than other neuroleptics. May be effective for treatment-resistant patients who have not responded to conventional agents. May cause significant wt gain, dyslipidemia, hyperglycemia, or new-onset DM; monitor wt, fasting blood glucose, and triglycerides before initiation and at regular intervals during treatment. Excessive sedation or respiratory depression may occur when used with CNS depressants, particularly benzodiazepines. If an orally disintegrating tab is split, then discard the remaining portion.

MOA — Dopamine receptor antagonist; 5-HT2A receptor antagonist.

ADVERSE EFFECTS — Serious: Agranulocytosis, leukopenia, seizures, hyperglycemia, diabetes, dyslipidemia, neuroleptic malignant syndrome, hepatotoxicity, QT prolongation, orthostatic hypotension, syncope, cardiopulmonary arrest, myocarditis, cardiomyopathy. Frequent: Drowsiness, weight gain, N/V, dry mouth, constipation, tachycardia, hypersalivation.

ILOPERIDONE (*Fanapt*) ▶L ♀? ?/?/?R Withdrawal reactions and EPS in neonates exposed during third trimester. ▶– ?

ADULT — Schizophrenia: Start 1 mg PO two times per day. Increase by no more than 2 mg twice daily to usual effective range of 6 to 12 mg PO two times per day. Max 24 mg/day. Retitrate if stopped for more than 3 days.

PEDS — Not approved in children.

FORMS — Trade: Tabs 1, 2, 4, 6, 8, 10, 12 mg.

NOTES — Dose must be titrated slowly to avoid orthostatic hypotension. Retitrate the dose if off the drug more than 3 days. Reduce dose by 50% if given with strong inhibitors of CYP2D6 or CYP3A4 such as fluoxetine or paroxetine or for poor metabolizers of CYP2D6. Avoid use with other drugs that prolong the QT interval. Fanapt is not recommended for patients with severe hepatic impairment.

MOA — Receptor antagonist; D2 and 5-HT2A receptor antagonist.

ADVERSE EFFECTS — Serious: Neuroleptic malignant syndrome, QTc prolongation, ventricular arrhythmias, tardive dyskinesia, hyperglycemia/diabetes, lipid abnormalities, seizures, orthostatic hypotension, anaphylaxis, angioedema. Frequent: Dizziness, dry mouth, fatigue, nasal congestion, somnolence, tachycardia, weight gain.

LURASIDONE (*Latuda*) ▶K – ♀B ▶?

ADULT — Schizophrenia: Start 40 mg PO daily. Effective dose range 40 to 160 mg/day, max 160 mg/day. Reduce starting dose to 20 mg PO daily if moderate to severe renal or hepatic insufficiency or use with moderate CYP3A4 inhibitors, max 80 mg/day unless severe hepatic insufficiency which is 40 mg/day. Depression associated with bipolar I disorder (monotherapy or adjunctive with lithium or valproate): Start 20 mg PO daily. Usual range 20 to 120 mg/day. Doses greater than 20 to 60 mg/day did not provide further efficacy as monotherapy in clinical trials.

PEDS — Not approved for use in children.

FORMS — Trade only: Tabs 20, 40, 60, 80, 120 mg.

NOTES — Take with a meal of at least 350 Cal. Do not use with strong CYP3A4 inhibitors or inducers. Reduce dose if used with moderate inhibitors. Avoid with grapefruit juice.

MOA — Dopamine-2/serotonin 2A antagonist

ADVERSE EFFECTS — Serious: Neuroleptic malignant syndrome, hyperglycemia, diabetes, tardive dyskinesia, hyperlipidemia, hyperprolactinemia, leukopenia, neutropenia, agranulocytosis, orthostatic hypotension, syncope. Frequent: Parkinsonism, akathisia, somnolence, nausea, agitation.

OLANZAPINE (*Zyprexa, Zyprexa Zydis, Zyprexa Relprevv*) ▶L ♀C ▶– $$$$$

ADULT — Agitation in acute bipolar mania or schizophrenia: Start 10 mg IM (may use 5 to 7.5 mg if warranted or 2.5 to 5 mg in elderly or debilitated patients); may repeat in 2 h and again in 4 h if warranted. Max 30 mg/day. Schizophrenia, oral therapy: Start 5 to 10 mg PO daily. Target dose is 10 mg/day. Max 20mg/day; however, doses above 10 mg/day have not been shown to be more effective. Reduce to 5 mg in debilitated patients or those predisposed to hypotension. Schizophrenia, extended-release injection: Dose based on prior oral dose and ranges from 150 to 300 mg deep IM (gluteal) every 2 weeks or 300 to 405 mg q 4 weeks. See prescribing information. Bipolar disorder, maintenance treatment or monotherapy for acute manic or mixed episodes: Start 10 to 15 mg PO daily. Increase by 5 mg/day at intervals of 24 h or more if needed. Usual effective dose range 5 to 20 mg/day, max 20 mg/day. Bipolar disorder, adjunctive therapy for acute mixed or manic episodes: Start 10 mg PO daily; usual effective dose is 5 to 20 mg/day, max 20 mg/day. Bipolar depression, olanzapine + fluoxetine given separately: Start 5 mg olanzapine + 20 mg fluoxetine daily in the evening. Increase to usual range of 5 to 12.5 mg olanzapine plus 20 to 50 mg fluoxetine as tolerated. See also Symbyax combination product entry. Treatment-resistant depression, olanzapine + fluoxetine: Start 5 mg olanzapine + 20 mg fluoxetine daily in the evening. Increase to usual range of 5 to 20 mg olanzapine plus 20 to 50 mg fluoxetine as tolerated. See also Symbyax combination product entry.

(cont.)

OLANZAPINE (*cont.*)

PEDS — Schizophrenia and bipolar manic or mixed episodes (13 to 17 yo): Start 2.5 to 5 mg PO once daily. Increase by 2.5 or 5 mg/day to target of 10 mg/day. Max 20 mg/day. Bipolar depression, olanzapine + fluoxetine given separately : Start 2.5 mg olanzapine + 20 mg fluoxetine PO daily in the evening. May increase if needed to max 12.5 mg olanzapine + 50 mg fluoxetine. See also Symbyax combination product entry.

UNAPPROVED ADULT — Augmentation of SSRI therapy for OCD: Start 2.5 to 5 mg PO daily, max 20 mg/day. Posttraumatic stress disorder, adjunctive therapy: Start 5 mg PO daily, max 20 mg/day.

UNAPPROVED PEDS — Bipolar disorder, manic or mixed phase: Start 2.5 mg PO daily; increase by 2.5 mg/day every 3 days to max 20 mg/day.

FORMS — Generic/Trade: Tabs 2.5, 5, 7.5, 10, 15, 20 mg. Tabs, orally disintegrating (Zyprexa Zydis) 5, 10, 15, 20 mg. Trade only: Long-acting injection (Zyprexa Relprevv) 210, 300, 405 mg/vial.

NOTES — May cause significant wt gain, dyslipidemia, hyperglycemia, or new-onset diabetes; monitor wt, fasting blood glucose, and triglycerides before initiation and at regular intervals during treatment. Monitor for orthostatic hypotension, particularly when given IM. IM injection can also be associated with bradycardia and hypoventilation, especially if used with other drugs that have these effects. Use lower initial doses of the combination of olanzapine plus fluoxetine in patients predisposed to hypotension or those with liver disease. Use caution with benzodiazepines. Use of Zyprexa Relprevv requires registration in the Zyprexa Relprevv Patient Care Program 1-877-772-9390.

MOA — Dopamine receptor antagonist; 5-HT2A receptor antagonist.

ADVERSE EFFECTS — Serious: Seizures, orthostatic hypotension, syncope, hyperglycemia, diabetes, dyslipidemia, neuroleptic malignant syndrome, extrapyramidal side effects, QT prolongation, hepatitis, suicidal thinking/behavior, drug reaction with eosinophilia and systemic symptoms (DRESS). Frequent: Drowsiness, weight gain, nausea, dry mouth, constipation, dizziness.

PALIPERIDONE (*Invega Trinza, Invega, Invega Sustenna*) ▶KL ♀C ▶– $$$$$

ADULT — Schizophrenia and schizoaffective disorder (adjunctive and monotherapy): Start 6 mg PO every am. 3 mg/day may be sufficient in some. Max 12 mg/day. Extended-release injection: Schizophrenia (Invega Sustenna): Start 234 mg IM (deltoid) and then 156 mg IM 1 week later. Recommended monthly dose 117 mg IM (deltoid or gluteal) or within range of 39 to 234 mg based on response. Patient must be able to tolerate oral paliperidone or risperidone prior to starting Sustenna. Schizophrenia (Invega Trinza):Use only after tolerability to Invega Sustenna has been established for at least 4 months. The dose of Trinza is given IM every 3 months based on the prior dose of Sustenna. For Sustenna 78 mg use Trinza 273 mg, Sustenna 117 mg use Trinza 410 mg, Sustenna 156 mg use Trinza 546 mg, and Sustenna 234 mg use Trinza 819 mg. Adjust dose at intervals of 3 months. Schizoaffective disorder (Invega Sustenna): Start 234 mg IM (deltoid) and then 156 mg on day 8. Usual range 78 to 234 mg, max 234 mg.

PEDS — Schizophrenia, adolescents (12 to 17 yo): Start 3 mg PO once daily. Max 6 mg/day (weight less than 51 kg) or 12 mg/day (51 kg and greater). Not approved in children under 12 yo.

FORMS — Generic/Trade: Extended-release tabs 1.5, 3, 6, 9 mg.Trade only: Depot formulation (Sustenna): 39, 78, 117, 156, 234 mg. Depot formulation (Trinza) 273, 410, 546, 819 mg.

NOTES — Active metabolite of risperidone. For CrCl 50 to 79 mL/min, start 3 mg/day with a max of 6 mg/day. For CrCl 10 to 50 mL/min, start 1.5 mg/day with a max of 3 mg/day. Refer to PI for instructions if injections of the long-acting forms are missed.

MOA — Dopamine receptor antagonist; 5-HT2A receptor antagonist.

ADVERSE EFFECTS — Serious: Orthostatic hypotension, syncope, QT prolongation, neuroleptic malignant syndrome, tardive dyskinesia, hyperglycemia, diabetes, stroke, extrapyramidal symptoms, suicidal thinking/behavior. Frequent: Drowsiness, salivary hypersecretion, tachycardia, akathisia, dystonia, hypertonia, parkinsonism, weight gain, dyspepsia, dizziness, headache, anxiety.

PIMAVANSERIN (*Nuplazid*) ▶L ♀?/?/? ▶?

ADULT — Hallucinations and delusions due to Parkinson's disease: Initiate and maintain 34 mg PO once daily.

PEDS — Not approved for use in children or adolescents.

FORMS — Trade only: tabs 17 mg

NOTES — Reduce dose in the presence of CYP3A4 inibitors to 17 mg/day. May need to increase the dose if on CYP3A4 inducers. Prolongs QTc. Avoid in patients with severe renal impairment. Avod use in patients with hepatic impairment.

MOA — Inverse agonist and antagonist at 5-HT2A and 5-HT2C receptors

ADVERSE EFFECTS — Serious: QTc prolongation, hallucinations. Frequent: peripheral edema, confusional state, urinary tract infection, nausea.

QUETIAPINE (*Seroquel, Seroquel XR*) ▶LK ♀C ▶– $$$$

ADULT — Schizophrenia: Start 25 mg PO two times per day (regular tabs); increase by 25 to 50 mg two to three times per day on days 2 and 3, and then to target dose of 300 to 400 mg/day divided two to three times per day on day 4. Usual effective dose is 150 to 750 mg/day, max 750 mg/day initial therapy or 800 mg/day maintenance. Schizophrenia, extended-release tabs: Start 300 mg PO daily in evening, increase by up to 300 mg/day at intervals of more than 1 day to usual effective range of 400 to 800 mg/day. Max 800 mg/day. Acute bipolar mania, monotherapy or adjunctive: Start 50 mg PO two times per day on day 1, then

(cont.)

QUETIAPINE (*cont.*)

increase to no higher than 100 mg two times per day on day 2, 150 mg two times per day on day 3, and 200 mg two times per day on day 4. May increase prn to 300 mg two times per day on day 5 and 400 mg two times per day thereafter. Usual effective dose is 400 to 800 mg/day. Max 800 mg/day. Bipolar disorder, acute manic or mixed, monotherapy or adjunctive, extended-release: Start 300 mg PO in evening on day 1, 600 mg day 2, and 400 to 800 mg/day thereafter. Max 800 mg/day. Bipolar depression, adjunctive, regular and extended release: 50 mg, 100 mg, 200 mg and 300 mg once daily at bedtime for days 1 to 4 respectively, and 300mg/day thereafter. Max 300 mg/day. Bipolar maintenance: Use dose required to maintain remission of symptoms. Major depressive disorder, adjunctive to antidepressants, extended release: Start 50 mg evening of days 1 and 2, may increase to 150 mg on day 3. Max 300 mg/day.

PEDS — Schizophrenia (13 to 17 yo): Start 25 mg PO twice daily on day 1, 50 mg twice daily on day 2, 100 mg twice daily on day 3, 150 mg twice daily on day 4, and 200 mg twice daily on day 5. May give three times daily if better tolerated. Recommended range 400 to 800 mg/day. Max 800 mg/day. Schizophrenia (13 to 17 yo), extended release: 50 mg PO day 1, 100 mg day 2, 200 mg day 3, 300 mg day 4, 400 mg day 5. Usual effective dose 400 mg to 800 mg/day. Max 800 mg/day. Bipolar acute mania (10 to 17 yo): Start 50 mg/day PO day 1, 100 mg on day 2, 200 mg/day on day 3, 300 mgday on day 4, 400 mg/day on day 5, all divided twice daily. May give three times daily if better tolerated. Recommended range 400 to 600 mg/day. Max 600 mg/day. Bipolar acute mania (10 to 17 yo), extended-release: 50 mg PO day 1, 100 mg day 2, 200 mg day 3, 300 mg day 4, 400 mg day 5. Recommended range 400 to 600 mg/day. Max 600 mg/day.

UNAPPROVED ADULT — Augmentation of SSRI therapy for OCD: Start 25 mg PO two times per day, max 300 mg/day. Adjunctive for posttraumatic stress disorder: Start 25 mg daily, max 300 mg/day.

UNAPPROVED PEDS — Bipolar disorder (manic or mixed phase): Start 12.5 mg PO two times per day (children) or 25 mg PO two times per day (adolescents); max 150 mg PO three times per day.

FORMS — Generic/Trade: Tabs 25, 50, 100, 200, 300, 400 mg. Trade only: Extended-release tabs 50, 150, 200, 300, 400 mg.

NOTES — Eye exam for cataracts recommended every 6 months. Low risk of EPS and tardive dyskinesia. May cause significant wt gain, dyslipidemia, hyperglycemia, or new-onset DM; monitor wt, fasting blood glucose, and triglycerides before initiation and at regular intervals during treatment. Use lower doses and slower titration in elderly patients or hepatic dysfunction. Extended-release tabs should be taken without food or after light meal.

MOA — Dopamine receptor antagonist; 5-HT2A receptor antagonist.

ADVERSE EFFECTS — Serious: Seizures, orthostatic hypotension, syncope, hyperglycemia, diabetes, dyslipidemia, neuroleptic malignant syndrome, QT prolongation, suicidal thinking/behavior, drug reaction with eosinophilia and systemic symptoms (DRESS). Frequent: Drowsiness, weight gain, nausea, dry mouth, constipation, dizziness.

RISPERIDONE (*Risperdal, Risperdal Consta, Risperdal M-Tab*) ▶LK ♀C ▶– $$$$

ADULT — Schizophrenia: Start 2 mg/day PO given once daily or divided two times per day; increase by 1 to 2 mg/day at intervals of 24 h or more. Start 0.5 mg/dose and titrate by no more than 0.5 mg two times per day in elderly, debilitated, hypotensive, or renally or hepatically impaired patients; increases to doses greater than 1.5 mg two times per day should occur at intervals of 1 week or more. Usual effective dose is 4 to 8 mg/day given once daily or divided two times per day; max 16 mg/day; however, doses greater than 6 mg/day have not been shown to be more effective. Schizophrenia (long-acting injection, Consta): Start 25 mg IM every 2 weeks while continuing oral dose for 3 weeks. May increase q 4 weeks to max 50 mg every 2 weeks. Bipolar mania or mixed episodes, monotherapy or adjunctive: Start 2 to 3 mg PO daily; may adjust by 1 mg/day at 24 h intervals to max 6 mg/day.

PEDS — Schizophrenia (13 to 17 yo): Start 0.5 mg PO daily; increase by 0.5 to 1 mg/day at intervals of 24 h or more to target dose of 3 mg/day. Max 6 mg/day; however, doses greater than 3 mg/day have not been shown to be more effective. Twice daily dosing can be used if somnolence is a problem. Bipolar mania, or mixed episodes, monotherapy (10 to 17 yo): Start 0.5 mg PO daily; increase by 0.5 to 1 mg/day at intervals of 24 h or more to recommended dose of 1 to 2.5 mg/day. Max 6 mg/day. Autistic disorder irritability (age 5 to 16 yo): Start 0.25 mg (for wt less than 20 kg) or 0.5 mg (wt 20 kg or greater) PO daily. May increase after 4 days to target dose of 0.5 mg/day (for wt less than 20 kg) or 1.0 mg/day (wt 20 kg or greater). Maintain at least 14 days. May then increase if needed at 14-day intervals or more by increments of 0.25 mg/day (for wt less than 20 kg) or 0.5 mg/day (wt 20 kg or greater). Usual effective range 0.5 to 3 mg/day.

UNAPPROVED ADULT — Augmentation of SSRI therapy for OCD: Start 1 mg/day PO, max 6 mg/day. Adjunctive therapy for posttraumatic stress disorder: Start 0.5 mg PO at bedtime, max 3 mg/day.

UNAPPROVED PEDS — Psychotic disorders, mania, aggression: 0.5 to 1.5 mg/day PO.

FORMS — Generic/Trade: Tabs 0.25, 0.5, 1, 2, 3, 4 mg. Oral soln 1 mg/mL (30 mL). Orally disintegrating tabs 0.5, 1, 2, 3, 4 mg. Generic only: Orally disintegrating tabs 0.25 mg. Trade only: IM injection (Risperdal Consta) 12.5, 25, 37.5, 50 mg.

NOTES — Has a greater tendency to produce extrapyramidal side effects (EPS) than other atypical antipsychotics. EPS reported in neonates following use in 3rd trimester of pregnancy. May cause wt

(cont.)

RISPERIDONE (*cont.*)

gain, hyperglycemia, or new-onset diabetes; monitor closely. Patients with Parkinson's disease and dementia have increased sensitivity to side effects such as EPS, confusion, falls, and neuroleptic malignant syndrome. Soln is compatible with water, coffee, orange juice, and low-fat milk; is not compatible with cola or tea. Place orally disintegrating tabs on tongue and do not chew. Establish tolerability with oral form before starting long-acting injection. Alternate injections between buttocks. May also give in deltoid.

MOA — Dopamine receptor antagonist; 5-HT2A receptor antagonist.

ADVERSE EFFECTS — Serious: Seizures, orthostatic hypotension, syncope, hyperglycemia, diabetes, neuroleptic malignant syndrome, tardive dyskinesia, extrapyramidal symptoms, QT prolongation, stroke, transient ischemic attack, suicidal thinking/behavior, dysphagia. Frequent: Drowsiness, insomnia, weight gain, N/V, dyspepsia, dry mouth, constipation, dizziness, orthostatic hypotension, agitation, anxiety, akathisia, tachycardia.

ZIPRASIDONE (*Geodon, ✷Zeldox*) ▶L ♀C ▶– $$$$$

WARNING — May prolong QTc. Avoid with drugs that prolong QTc or in those with long QT syndrome or cardiac arrhythmias.

ADULT — Schizophrenia: Start 20 mg PO two times per day with food; may increase at greater than 2-day intervals to max 80 mg PO two times per day. Acute agitation in schizophrenia: 10 to 20 mg IM. May repeat 10 mg dose every 2 h or 20 mg dose every 4 h, to max 40 mg/day. Bipolar I disorder, monotherapy for acute manic or mixed episodes and adjunctive for maintenance: Start 40 mg PO two times per day with food; may increase to 60 to 80 mg two times per day on day 2. Usual effective dose is 40 to 80 mg two times per day. Must be taken with a meal of at least 500 Cal for adequate absorption.

PEDS — Not approved in children.

FORMS — Trade/Generic: Caps 20, 40, 60, 80 mg. Trade only: 20 mg/mL injection.

NOTES — Drug interactions with carbamazepine and ketoconazole.

MOA — Dopamine receptor antagonist; 5-HT2A receptor antagonist.

ADVERSE EFFECTS — Serious: Seizures, orthostatic hypotension, syncope, hyperglycemia, diabetes, dyslipidemia, neuroleptic malignant syndrome, tardive dyskinesia, extrapyramidal side effects, QT prolongation, suicidal thinking/behavior, drug reaction with eosinophilia and systemic symptoms (DRESS) and other serious cutaneous reactions. Frequent: Drowsiness, weight gain, nausea, dry mouth, constipation, dizziness.

PSYCHIATRY: Anxiolytics/Hypnotics—Barbiturates

BUTABARBITAL (*Butisol*) ▶LK ♀D ▶? ©III $$$

ADULT — Rarely used; other drugs preferred. Sedative: 15 to 30 mg PO three to four times per day. Hypnotic: 50 to 100 mg PO at bedtime for up to 2 weeks.

PEDS — Preop sedation: 2 to 6 mg/kg PO before procedure, max 100 mg.

FORMS — Trade only: Tabs 30, 50 mg. Elixir 30 mg/5 mL.

MOA — Nonselective CNS depressant

ADVERSE EFFECTS — Serious: Respiratory depression, blood dyscrasias, anemia, thrombocytopenia, Stevens-Johnson syndrome, angioedema, dependence, withdrawal reactions, "sleep driving".

Frequent: drowsiness, fatigue, N/V bradycardia, paradoxical CNS excitation

SECOBARBITAL (*Seconal*) ▶LK ♀D ▶+ ©II $

ADULT — Rarely used; other drugs preferred. Hypnotic: 100 mg PO at bedtime for up to 2 weeks.

PEDS — Pre-anesthetic: 2 to 6 mg/kg PO up to 100 mg.

FORMS — Trade only: Caps 100 mg.

MOA — Nonselective CNS depressant

ADVERSE EFFECTS — Serious: Respiratory depression, blood dyscrasias, anemia, thrombocytopenia, Stevens-Johnson syndrome, angioedema, dependence, withdrawal reactions. Frequent: drowsiness, fatigue, N/V bradycardia, paradoxical CNS excitation

PSYCHIATRY: Anxiolytics/Hypnotics—Benzodiazepines—Short Half-Life (< 12 h)

ALPRAZOLAM (*Xanax, Xanax XR, Niravam*) ▶LK ♀D ▶–
©IV $

ADULT — Anxiety: Start 0.25 to 0.5 mg PO three times per day, may increase every 3 to 4 days to max dose of 4 mg/day. Use 0.25 mg PO two times per day in elderly or debilitated patients. Panic disorder: Start 0.5 mg PO three times per day (or 0.5 to 1 mg PO daily of Xanax XR), may increase by up to 1 mg/day every 3 to 4 days to usual effective dose of 5 to 6 mg/day (3 to 6 mg/day for Xanax XR), max dose is 10 mg/day.

PEDS — Not approved in children.

FORMS — Generic/Trade: Tabs 0.25, 0.5, 1, 2 mg. Tabs, extended-release 0.5, 1, 2, 3 mg. Orally disintegrating tabs (Niravam) 0.25, 0.5, 1, 2 mg. Generic only: Oral concentrate (Intensol) 1 mg/mL.

NOTES — Half-life 12 h, but need to give three times per day. Divide administration time evenly during waking hours to avoid interdose symptoms. Do not give with antifungals (ie, ketoconazole, itraconazole); use caution with macrolides, oral contraceptives, TCAs, cimetidine, antidepressants,

ALPRAZOLAM (*cont.*)

anticonvulsants, paroxetine, sertraline, and others that inhibit CYP3A4.

MOA — Enhances actions of GABA.

ADVERSE EFFECTS — Serious: Respiratory depression, dependence, withdrawal reactions, seizures. Frequent: Sedation, fatigue, ataxia, memory impairment, depression, confusion, nausea, constipation, dry mouth, rash.

OXAZEPAM ▶LK ♀D ▶– ©IV $$$

ADULT — Anxiety: 10 to 30 mg PO three to four times per day. Acute alcohol withdrawal: 15 to 30 mg PO three to four times per day.

PEDS — Not approved in children younger than 6 yo.

UNAPPROVED ADULT — Restless legs syndrome: Start 10 mg PO at bedtime. Max 40 mg at bedtime.

FORMS — Generic/Trade: Caps 10, 15, 30 mg. Trade only: Tabs 15 mg.

NOTES — Half-life 8 h. Brand name discontinued.

MOA — Enhances actions of GABA.

ADVERSE EFFECTS — Serious: Respiratory depression, dependence, withdrawal reactions, seizures. Frequent: Sedation, fatigue, ataxia, memory

impairment, depression, confusion, nausea, constipation, dry mouth, rash.

TRIAZOLAM (*Halcion*) ▶LK ♀X ▶– ©IV $

ADULT — Insomnia: 0.125 to 0.25 mg PO at bedtime for 7 to 10 days, max dose is 0.5 mg/day, but should be used only in exceptional patients. Start 0.125 mg/day in elderly or debilitated patients.

PEDS — Not approved in children.

UNAPPROVED ADULT — Restless legs syndrome: Start 0.125 mg PO at bedtime. Max 0.5 mg at bedtime.

FORMS — Generic/Trade: Tabs 0.25 mg. Generic only: Tabs 0.125 mg.

NOTES — Half-life 2 to 3 h. Anterograde amnesia may occur. Do not use with protease inhibitors, ketoconazole, itraconazole, or nefazodone; use caution with macrolides, cimetidine, and other CYP3A4 inhibitors.

MOA — Enhances actions of GABA.

ADVERSE EFFECTS — Serious: Respiratory depression, dependence, withdrawal reactions, seizures. Frequent: Sedation, fatigue, ataxia, memory impairment, depression, confusion, nausea, constipation, dry mouth, rash.

PSYCHIATRY: Anxiolytics/Hypnotics—Benzodiazepines—Medium Half-Life (10 to 15 h)

NOTE: To avoid withdrawal, gradually taper when discontinuing after prolonged use. Sedative-hypnotics have been associated with complex sleep behaviors including sleep driving. Use caution and discuss with patients.

ESTAZOLAM (*ProSom*) ▶LK ♀X ▶– ©IV $$

ADULT — Insomnia: 1 to 2 mg PO at bedtime for up to 12 weeks. Reduce dose to 0.5 mg in elderly, small, or debilitated patients.

PEDS — Not approved in children.

FORMS — Generic/Trade: Tabs 1, 2 mg.

NOTES — For short-term treatment of insomnia. Avoid with ketoconazole or itraconazole; caution with less potent inhibitors of CYP3A4. Brand name ProSom no longer available.

MOA — Enhances actions of GABA.

ADVERSE EFFECTS — Serious: Respiratory depression, dependence, withdrawal reactions, seizures. Frequent: Sedation, fatigue, ataxia, memory impairment, depression, confusion, nausea, constipation, dry mouth, rash.

LORAZEPAM (*Ativan*) ▶LK ♀D Per ACOG guidelines ▶– ©IV $

ADULT — Anxiety: Start 0.5 to 1 mg PO two to three times per day, usual effective dose is 2 to 6 mg/day. Max dose is 10 mg/day PO. Anxiolytic/sedation: 0.04 to 0.05 mg/kg IV/IM; usual dose 2 mg, max 4 mg. Insomnia: 2 to 4 mg PO at bedtime. Status epilepticus: 4 mg IV over 2 min. May repeat in 10 to 15 min.

PEDS — Not approved in children.

UNAPPROVED ADULT — Alcohol withdrawal: 1 to 2 mg PO/IM/IV every 2 to 4 h prn or 2 mg PO/IM/IV every 6 h for 24 h then 1 mg every 6 h for 8 doses. Chemotherapy-induced N/V: 1 to 2 mg PO/SL/IV/IM every 6 h.

UNAPPROVED PEDS — Status epilepticus: 0.05 to 0.1 mg/kg IV over 2 to 5 min. May repeat 0.05 mg/kg

for 1 dose in 10 to 15 min. Do not exceed 4 mg as single dose. Anxiolytic/sedation: 0.05 mg/kg/dose every 4 to 8 h PO/IV, max 2 mg/dose. Chemotherapy-induced N/V: 0.05 mg/kg PO/IV every 8 to 12 h prn, max 3 mg/dose; or 0.02 to 0.05 mg/kg IV every 6 h prn, max 2 mg/dose.

FORMS — Generic/Trade: Tabs 0.5, 1, 2 mg. Generic only: Oral concentrate 2 mg/mL.

NOTES — Half-life 10 to 20 h. No active metabolites. For short-term treatment of insomnia.

MOA — Enhances actions of GABA.

ADVERSE EFFECTS — Serious: Cardiovascular collapse, hypotension, apnea (parenteral), respiratory depression, dependence, withdrawal syndrome. Frequent: Drowsiness, dizziness, ataxia, headache, confusion, memory problems, depression, paradoxical CNS stimulation.

NITRAZEPAM (*✱Mogadan*) ▶L ♀C ▶– $

ADULT — Canada only. Insomnia: 5 to 10 mg PO at bedtime.

PEDS — Canada only. Myoclonic seizures: 0.3 to 1 mg/kg/day in 3 divided doses.

FORMS — Generic/Trade: Tabs 5, 10 mg.

NOTES — Use lower doses in elderly/debilitated patients.

MOA — Benzodiazepine with an intermediate half life.

ADVERSE EFFECTS — Serious: Dependence. Frequent: Dizziness, drowsiness, fatigue.

TEMAZEPAM (*Restoril*) ▶LK ♀X ▶– ©IV $

ADULT — Insomnia: 7.5 to 30 mg PO at bedtime (usual dose 15 mg) for 7 to 10 days.

(cont.)

TEMAZEPAM (*cont.*)

PEDS — Not approved in children.
FORMS — Generic/Trade: Caps 7.5, 15, 22.5, 30 mg.
NOTES — Half-life 8 to 25 h. For short-term treatment of insomnia.

MOA — Enhances actions of GABA.
ADVERSE EFFECTS — Serious: Respiratory depression, dependence, withdrawal reactions, seizures. Frequent: Sedation, fatigue, ataxia, memory impairment, depression, confusion, nausea, constipation, dry mouth, rash.

PSYCHIATRY: Anxiolytics/Hypnotics—Benzodiazepines—Long Half-Life (25-100 h)

NOTE: To avoid withdrawal, gradually taper when discontinuing after prolonged use. Use cautiously in the elderly; may accumulate and lead to side effects, psychomotor impairment. Sedative-hypnotics have been associated with complex sleep behaviors including sleep driving. Use caution and discuss with patients.

BROMAZEPAM (✱*Lectopam*) ▶L ♀D ▶– $

ADULT — Canada only. 6 to 18 mg/day PO in equally divided doses.
PEDS — Not approved in children.
FORMS — Generic/Trade: Tabs 1.5, 3, 6 mg.
NOTES — Do not exceed 3 mg/day initially in the elderly or debilitated. Gradually taper when discontinuing after prolonged use. Half-life approximately 20 h in adults but increased in elderly. Cimetidine may prolong elimination.
MOA — Benzodiazepine; enhances actions of GABA.
ADVERSE EFFECTS — Serious: Respiratory depression, dependence, withdrawal reactions. Frequent: Sedation, ataxia, depression, confusion, tinnitus, N/V.

CHLORDIAZEPOXIDE ▶LK ♀D ▶– ©IV $$

ADULT — Anxiety: 5 to 25 mg PO three to four times per day. Acute alcohol withdrawal: 50 to 100 mg PO, repeat every 3 to 4 h prn up to 300 mg/day.
PEDS — Anxiety, age older than 6 yo: 5 to 10 mg PO two to four times per day.
UNAPPROVED ADULT — Acute alcohol withdrawal: 25 to 100 mg PO. May repeat hourly based on symptom scores from a validated instrument such as the CIWA scale.
FORMS — Generic/Trade: Caps 5, 10, 25 mg.
NOTES — Half-life 5 to 30 h. Trade product Librium no longer available.
MOA — Enhances actions of GABA.
ADVERSE EFFECTS — Serious: Respiratory depression, dependence, withdrawal reactions, seizures. Frequent: Sedation, fatigue, ataxia, memory impairment, depression, confusion, nausea, constipation, dry mouth, rash.

CLONAZEPAM (*Klonopin, Klonopin Wafer,* ✱*Rivotril, Clonapam*) ▶LK ♀X/?/? Category D per ACOG guidelines ▶– ©IV $

ADULT — Panic disorder: 0.25 mg PO two times per day, increase by 0.125 to 0.25 mg every 3 days as needed to target dose of 1 mg/day. Max 4 mg/day; however, doses greater than 1 mg/day have not been shown to be more effective for most patients. Akinetic, Lennox-Gastaut syndrome, or myoclonic seizures: Start 0.5 mg PO three times per day. Increase by 0.5 to 1 mg every 3 days prn. Max 20 mg/day.
PEDS — Akinetic or myoclonic seizures, Lennox-Gastaut syndrome (petit mal variant), or absence seizures (10 yo or younger or 30 kg or less): start 0.01 to 0.03 mg/kg/day PO divided two to three times per day. Increase by 0.25 to 0.5 mg every 3 days prn. Max 0.1 to 0.2 mg/kg/day divided three times per day.
UNAPPROVED ADULT — Neuralgias: 2 to 4 mg PO daily. Restless legs syndrome: Start 0.25 mg PO at bedtime. Max 2 mg at bedtime. REM sleep behavior disorder: 1 to 2 mg PO at bedtime.
FORMS — Generic/Trade: Tabs 0.5, 1, 2 mg. Orally disintegrating tabs (approved for panic disorder only) 0.125, 0.25, 0.5, 1, 2 mg.
NOTES — Half-life 18 to 50 h. Usual therapeutic range is 20 to 80 ng/mL. Contraindicated in hepatic failure or acute narrow-angle glaucoma.
MOA — Enhances actions of GABA.
ADVERSE EFFECTS — Serious: Respiratory depression, CNS depression, dependence, withdrawal reactions, seizures. Frequent: Sedation, fatigue, ataxia, memory impairment, depression, confusion, nausea, constipation, dry mouth, rash.

CLORAZEPATE (*Tranxene*) ▶LK ♀D ▶– ©IV $$$$

ADULT — Anxiety: Start 7.5 to 15 mg PO at bedtime or two to three times per day; usual effective dose is 15 to 60 mg/day. Partial seizures, adjunctive: 13 yo and older, start 7.5 mg PO three times daily. May increase by no more than 7.5 mg per week to max 90 mg/day. Acute alcohol withdrawal: 60 to 90 mg/day on 1st day divided two to three times per day, gradually reduce dose to 7.5 to 15 mg/day over 5 days. Max dose is 90 mg/day.
PEDS — Partial seizures, adjunctive, age 9 to 12 yo: Start 7.5 mg PO twice daily. May increase by no more than 7.5 mg per week to max of 60 mg/day.
FORMS — Generic/Trade: Tabs 3.75, 7.5, 15 mg.
NOTES — Half-life 40 to 50 h.
MOA — Enhances actions of GABA.
ADVERSE EFFECTS — Serious: Respiratory depression, dependence, withdrawal reactions, seizures. Frequent: Sedation, fatigue, ataxia, memory impairment, depression, confusion, nausea, constipation, dry mouth, rash.

DIAZEPAM (*Valium, Diastat, Diastat AcuDial, Diazemuls*) ▶LK ♀D ▶– ©IV $

ADULT — Status epilepticus: 5 to 10 mg IV. Repeat every 10 to 15 min prn to max 30 mg. Epilepsy, adjunctive therapy: 2 to 10 mg PO two to four times per day. Increased seizure activity: 0.2 to 0.5 mg/kg

DIAZEPAM (*cont.*)

PR (rectal gel) to max 20 mg/day. Skeletal muscle spasm, spasticity related to cerebral palsy, paraplegia, athetosis, "stiff man syndrome": 2 to 10 mg PO/PR three to four times per day. 5 to 10 mg IM/IV initially, then 5 to 10 mg every 3 to 4 h prn. Decrease dose in elderly. Anxiety: 2 to 10 mg PO two to four times per day or 2 to 20 mg IM/IV, repeat dose in 3 to 4 h prn. Alcohol withdrawal: 10 mg PO three to four times per day for 24 h then 5 mg PO three to four times per day prn.

PEDS — Skeletal muscle spasm: 0.04 to 0.2 mg/kg/dose IV/IM every 2 to 4 h. Max dose 0.6 mg/kg within 8 h. Status epilepticus, age 1 mo to 5 yo: 0.2 to 0.5 mg IV slowly every 2 to 5 min to max 5 mg. Status epilepticus, age older than 5 yo: 1 mg IV slowly every 2 to 5 min to max 10 mg. Repeat q 2 to 4 h prn. Epilepsy, adjunctive therapy, muscle spasm, and anxiety disorders, age older than 6 mo: 1 to 2.5 mg PO three to four times per day; gradually increase as tolerated and needed. Increased seizure activity (rectal gel, age older than 2 yo): 0.5 mg/kg PR (2 to 5 yo), 0.3 mg/kg PR (6 to 11 yo), or 0.2 mg/kg PR (age older than 12 yo). Max 20 mg. May repeat in 4 to 12 h prn.

UNAPPROVED ADULT — Loading dose strategy for alcohol withdrawal: 10 to 20 mg PO or 10 mg slow IV in closely monitored setting, then repeat similar or lower doses every 1 to 2 h prn until sedated. Further doses should be unnecessary due to long half-life. Restless legs syndrome: 0.5 to 4 mg PO at bedtime.

FORMS — Generic/Trade: Tabs 2, 5, 10 mg. Rectal gel 2.5 mg ($$$$$). Generic only: Oral soln 5 mg/5 mL. Oral concentrate (Intensol) 5 mg/mL. Rectal gel 10, 20 mg ($$$$$). Trade only: Rectal gel (Diastat AcuDial-$$$$$) 10, 20 mg syringes. Available doses from 10 mg AcuDial syringe 5, 7.5, 10 mg. Available doses from 20 mg AcuDial syringe 12.5, 15, 17.5, 20 mg.

NOTES — Half-life 20 to 80 h. Respiratory and CNS depression may occur. Caution in liver disease. Abuse potential. Long half-life may increase the risk of adverse effects in the elderly. Cimetidine, oral contraceptives, disulfiram, fluoxetine, isoniazid, ketoconazole, metoprolol, propranolol, and valproic acid may increase diazepam concentrations. Diazepam may increase digoxin and phenytoin concentrations. Rifampin may increase the metabolism of diazepam. Avoid combination with protease inhibitors. Diastat AcuDial is for home use and allows dosing from 5 to 20 mg in 2.5 mg increments.

MOA — Enhances actions of GABA, skeletal muscle relaxant.

ADVERSE EFFECTS — Serious: Respiratory depression, oversedation, dependence, withdrawal reactions, cardiovascular collapse (parenteral), vascular impairment or venous thrombosis (IV only), seizures. Frequent: Sedation, ataxia, CNS stimulation, depression, N/V, constipation or diarrhea, confusion, tinnitus, blurred vision.

FLURAZEPAM ▶LK ♀X ▶– ©IV $

ADULT — Insomnia: 15 to 30 mg PO at bedtime.

PEDS — Not approved in children age younger than 15 yo.

FORMS — Generic/Trade: Caps 15, 30 mg.

NOTES — Half-life 70 to 90 h. For short-term treatment of insomnia. Brand name discontinued.

MOA — Enhances actions of GABA.

ADVERSE EFFECTS — Serious: Respiratory depression, dependence, withdrawal reactions, seizures. Frequent: Sedation, fatigue, ataxia, memory impairment, depression, confusion, nausea, constipation, dry mouth, rash.

QUAZEPAM (*Doral*) ▶L ♀C ▶? ©IV

ADULT — Insomnia: Start 7.5 mg PO at bedtime. May increase to max 15 mg if needed.

PEDS — Not approved for use by children or adolescents.

FORMS — Trade: Tabs 15 mg.

MOA — Enhances actions of GABA.

ADVERSE EFFECTS — Serious: Resiratory depression, dependence, withdrawal reactions including seizures, worsening depression. Frequent: Sedation, fatigue, ataxia, memory impairment, confusion, nausea.

PSYCHIATRY: Anxiolytics/Hypnotics—Other

NOTE: Sedative-hypnotics have been associated with complex sleep behaviors including sleep driving. Use caution and discuss with patients.

BUSPIRONE ▶K ♀B ▶– $$$

ADULT — Anxiety: Start 15 mg "dividose" daily (7.5 mg PO two times per day), increase by 5 mg/day q 2 to 3 days to usual effective dose of 30 mg/day, max dose is 60 mg/day.

PEDS — Not approved in children.

FORMS — Generic/Trade: Tabs 5, 10 mg. Dividose tabs 15, 30 mg (scored to be easily bisected or trisected). Generic only: Tabs 7.5 mg.

NOTES — Slower onset than benzodiazepines; optimum effect requires 3 to 4 weeks of therapy. Do not use with MAOIs; caution with itraconazole, cimetidine, nefazodone, erythromycin, and other CYP3A4 inhibitors. Brand name no longer available.

MOA — Serotonin 5-HT1A partial agonist.

ADVERSE EFFECTS — Serious: Parkinsonism, akathisia, dystonia, restless legs syndrome. Frequent: Drowsiness, dizziness, nausea, headache, nervousness.

ESZOPICLONE (*Lunesta*) ▶L ♀C ▶? ©IV $$$$$

ADULT — Insomnia: 2 mg PO at bedtime prn, max 3 mg. Elderly: 1 mg PO at bedtime prn, max 2 mg.

(cont.)

ESZOPICLONE (*cont.*)

PEDS — Not approved for children.

FORMS — Generic/Trade: Tabs 1, 2, 3 mg.

NOTES — Half-life is approximately 6 h. Take immediately before bedtime.

MOA — Binds to GABA-A receptors.

ADVERSE EFFECTS — Serious: chest pain. Frequent: Headache, unpleasant taste, dry mouth, dizziness, nervousness, dyspepsia, sleepdriving and other complex sleep behaviors.

RAMELTEON (*Rozerem*) ▶L ♀C ▶? $$$$

ADULT — Insomnia: 8 mg PO at bedtime.

PEDS — Not approved for children.

FORMS — Trade only: Tabs 8 mg.

NOTES — Do not take with/after high-fat meal. No evidence of dependence or abuse liability. Inhibitors of CYP1A2, CYP3A4, and CYP2C9 may increase serum level and effect. Avoid with severe liver disease. May decrease testosterone and increase prolactin.

MOA — Melatonin receptor agonist.

ADVERSE EFFECTS — Serious: None. Frequent: Headache, somnolence, fatigue, dizziness.

SUVOREXANT (*Belsomra*) ▶L ♀C ▶? ©IV

ADULT — Insomnia: Start 10 mg PO once nightly 30 minutes before bedtime. May increase if needed to max 20 mg once nightly.

PEDS — Not approved for use in children and adolescents.

FORMS — Trade: Tabs 5, 10, 15, 20 mg.

NOTES — Reduce dose in the presence of moderate CYP3A4 inhibitors to 5 mg once nightly and not to exceed 10 mg. Avoid with strong CYP3A4 inhibitors. Ensure at least 7 hours remains before planned awakening when taken.

MOA — Orexin receptor antagonist

ADVERSE EFFECTS — Serious: daytime sleepiness, impaired alertness and motor coordination, abnormal thinking and behavior, depression/suicidal ideation, sleep paralysis, cataplexy-like symptoms. Frequent: somnolence

TASIMELTEON (*Hetlioz*) ▶L ♀C ▶?

ADULT — Non 24-h sleep/wake disorder: 20 mg before bedtime. Take on empty stomach.

PEDS — Not approved for use in children and adolescents.

FORMS — Trade only: Caps 20 mg.

NOTES — Full effect may not be seen for weeks or months. Avoid use with strong CYP1A2 inhibitors or CYP3A4 inducers.

MOA — Agonist of melatonin MT1 and MT2 receptors.

ADVERSE EFFECTS — Serious: none. Frequent: headache, somnolence, increased ALT, nightmares, abnormal dreams, upper respiratory infections, urinary tract infection.

ZALEPLON (*Sonata*) ▶L ♀C ▶– ©IV $$$$

ADULT — Insomnia: 5 to 10 mg PO at bedtime prn, max 20 mg.

PEDS — Not approved in children.

FORMS — Generic/Trade: Caps 5, 10 mg.

NOTES — Half-life is approximately 1 h. Useful if problems with sleep initiation or morning grogginess. For short-term treatment of insomnia. Take immediately before bedtime or after going to bed and experiencing difficulty falling asleep. Use 5 mg dose in patients with mild to moderate hepatic impairment, elderly patients, and in patients taking cimetidine. Possible drug interactions with rifampin, phenytoin, carbamazepine, and phenobarbital. Do not use for benzodiazepine or alcohol withdrawal.

MOA — Selective GABA-benzodiazepine omega-1 agonist.

ADVERSE EFFECTS — Serious: Rebound insomnia, nightmares, seizures, sleepdriving, anaphylactic reactions. Frequent: Drowsiness, abdominal pain, chest pain, headache, asthenia, fatigue, photosensitivity.

ZOLPIDEM (*Ambien, Ambien CR, ZolpiMist, Intermezzo, Edluar, ✦Sublinox*) ▶L ♀C ▶+ ©IV $$$$

ADULT — Insomnia: Standard tabs: Women 5 mg and men 5 to 10 mg PO at bedtime. May increase the 5 mg dose to 10 mg if needed. Age older than 65 yo or debilitated: 5 mg PO at bedtime. Oral spray: Women 5 mg and men 5 to 10 mg PO at bedtime. May increase the 5 mg dose to 10 mg if needed. Age older than 65 yo or debilitated: 5 mg PO at bedtime. Controlled-release tabs: Women 6.25 mg and men 6.25 to 12.5 mg PO at bedtime. May increase the 6.25 mg dose to 12.5 mg if needed. Age older than 65 yo or debilitated: 6.25 mg PO at bedtime. SL tabs (Edluar): Women 5 mg and men 5 to 10 mg SL at bedtime. May increase the 5 mg dose to 10 mg if needed. Age older than 65 yo or debilitated: 5 mg SL at bedtime. Middle of the night awakening: SL tabs (Intermezzo): Women 1.75 mg and men 3.5 mg SL once nightly with at least 4 h of sleep remaining.

PEDS — Not approved in children.

FORMS — Generic/Trade: Tabs 5, 10 mg. Controlled-release tabs 6.25, 12.5 mg. SL tabs 1.75, 3.5 mg (Intermezzo). Trade only: Oral spray 5 mg/actuation (ZolpiMist); SL tabs 5, 10 mg (Edluar).

NOTES — Half-life is 2.5 h. Ambien regular-release is for short-term treatment of insomnia characterized by problems with sleep initiation. CR is useful for problems with sleep initiation and maintenance, and has been studied for up to 24 weeks. Do not use for benzodiazepine or alcohol withdrawal. Oral spray is sprayed into the mouth over the tongue. Device must be primed with 5 pumps prior to 1st use or if not used for 14 days. Oral ulcers, blisters, and mucosal inflammation have been observed with the use of Intermezzo SL tabs.

MOA — Selective GABA-benzodiazepine omega-1 agonist.

ADVERSE EFFECTS — Serious: Sleepdriving, abnormal thinking, behavioral changes, depression, suicidal ideation, hallucinations, anaphylaxis. Frequent: Drowsiness, dizziness, nausea, headache, nervousness, decreased daytime recall.

ZOPICLONE (✱*Imovane*) ▸L ♀D ▸– $

ADULT — Canada only. Short-term treatment of insomnia: 5 to 7.5 mg PO at bedtime. In elderly or debilitated, use 3.75 mg at bedtime initially, and increase prn to 5 to 7.5 mg at bedtime. Max 7.5 mg at bedtime.

PEDS — Not approved in children.

FORMS — Generic/Trade: Tabs 5, 7.5 mg. Generic only: Tabs 3.75 mg.

NOTES — Treatment should usually not exceed 7 to 10 days without reevaluation.

MOA — Short-acting hypnotic; structurally unrelated to benzodiazepines but shares a similar pharmacological profile to many of the benzodiazepines.

ADVERSE EFFECTS — Frequent: Taste alteration (bitter taste), anterograde amnesia, confusion, N/V, anorexia.

PSYCHIATRY: Combination Drugs

LIMBITROL (chlordiazepoxide + amitriptyline) ▸LK ♀D ▸– ©IV $$$

ADULT — Rarely used; other drugs preferred. Depression/anxiety: 1 tab PO three to four times per day, may increase up to 6 tabs/day.

PEDS — Not approved in children younger than 12 yo.

FORMS — Generic/Trade: Tabs 5/12.5, 10/25 mg chlordiazepoxide/amitriptyline.

MOA — Antidepressant-benzodiazepine combination.

ADVERSE EFFECTS — Serious: Seizures, arrhythmias, hypotension, agranulocytosis, dependence, withdrawal reactions, respiratory depression. Frequent: Drowsiness, dizziness, dry mouth, constipation, urinary retention, confusion, memory problems.

SYMBYAX (olanzapine + fluoxetine) ▸LK ♀C ▸– $$$$$

WARNING — Observe patients started on SSRIs for worsening depression or emergence of suicidal thoughts or behaviors in children, adolescents, and young adults, especially early in therapy or after increases in dose. Monitor for emergence of anxiety, agitation, panic attacks, insomnia, irritability, hostility, impulsivity, akathisia, mania, and hypomania. Carefully weigh risks and benefits before starting and then monitor such individuals closely. The use of atypical antipsychotics to treat behavioral problems in patients with dementia has been associated with higher mortality rates. Atypical antipsychotics have been associated with wt gain, dyslipidemia, hyperglycemia, and DM; monitor closely.

ADULT — Bipolar type 1 with depression and treatment-resistant depression: Start 6 mg olanzapine/25 mg fluoxetine PO at bedtime. Max 18/75 mg/day.

PEDS — Depression associated with bipolar disorder type I (10 to 17 yo): Start 3 mg olanzapine/25 mg fluoxetine PO at bedtime. Max 12/50 mg/day.

FORMS — Generic/Trade: Caps (olanzapine/fluoxetine) 3/25, 6/25, 6/50, 12/25, 12/50 mg.

NOTES — Efficacy beyond 8 weeks not established. Monitor wt, fasting glucose, and triglycerides before initiation and periodically during treatment. Contraindicated with thioridazine; do not use with thioridazine, tryptophan, or MAOIs; caution with lithium, phenytoin, TCAs, aspirin, NSAIDs, and warfarin. Do not use during active therapy with linezolid or IV methylene blue. Pregnancy exposure to fluoxetine associated with premature delivery, low birth wt, and lower Apgar scores. Decrease dose with liver disease or patients predisposed to hypotension.

MOA — Olanzapine: Dopamine antagonist, serotonin 2A antagonist. Fluoxetine: Inhibits serotonin reuptake.

ADVERSE EFFECTS — Serious: Serotonin syndrome, neuroleptic malignant syndrome, hyponatremia, SIADH, seizures, hypotension, hyperglycemia/diabetes, QT prolongation, hepatitis, abnormal bleeding, drug reaction with eosinophilia and systemic symptoms (DRESS). Frequent: Asthenia, edema, increased appetite, peripheral edema, pharyngitis, somnolence, abnormal thinking, tremor, weight gain.

PSYCHIATRY: Drug Dependence Therapy

ACAMPROSATE (*Campral*) ▸K ♀C ▸? $$$$$

ADULT — Maintenance of abstinence from alcohol: 666 mg (2 tabs) PO three times per day. Start after alcohol withdrawal and when patient is abstinent.

PEDS — Not approved in children.

FORMS — Generic/Trade: Tabs, delayed-release 333 mg.

NOTES — Reduce dose to 333 mg if CrCl 30 to 50 mL/min. Contraindicated if CrCl <30 mL/min.

MOA — Unknown. Structural analogue of GABA and may restore balance to that system.

ADVERSE EFFECTS — Serious: Depression, suicidality. Frequent: Asthenia, diarrhea, anxiety, insomnia.

BUPRENORPHINE + NALOXONE (Bunavail, Suboxone, Zubsolv) ▸L ♀C ▸– ©III $$$$$

ADULT — Treatment of opioid dependence: Induction (Suboxone SL film): Day 1 start with 2 mg/0.5 mg SL or 4 mg/1 mg SL and titrate upward in increments of 2 or 4 mg of buprenorphine at approximately 2-h intervals to 8 mg/2 mg total dose. Day 2 a dose of up to 16 mg/4 mg is recommended. Maintenance (SL tabs and film): Target dose 16 mg/4 mg SL daily. Can individualize to range of 4 to 24 mg of buprenorphine daily. Induction (Zubsolv): Day 1 start with 1.4 mg/0.36 mg and titrate upward in increments of 1 or 2 of these tablets every 1.5-2 h to

(cont.)

BUPRENORPHINE + NALOXONE (cont.)

a dose of 5.7 mg/1.4 mg. Some patients may tolerate three of the tablets as the second dose depending upon recent narcotic exposure. Day 2 a dose of 11.4 mg/2.9 mg is recommended. Maintenance (Zubsolv): 11.4 mg/2.8 mg SL daily. Can individualize to range of 2.8/0.72 to 17.1/4.2 mg SL daily.

PEDS — Not approved in children.

FORMS — Generic only: SL tabs 2/0.5 mg and 8/2 mg buprenorphine/naloxone. Trade only: SL film 2/0.5, 4/1, 8/2, 12/3 mg buprenorphine/naloxone, SL tabs (Zubsolv) 1.4/0.36, 5.7/1.4 mg.

NOTES — Titrate in 2 to 4 mg increments/decrements to maintain therapy compliance and prevent withdrawal. Prescribers must complete training and apply for special DEA number. See www.suboxone.com. Zubsolv 5.7/1.4 mg tab is equivalent to Suboxone 8/2 mg tab. During induction, therapy should be started when objective signs of moderate withdrawal appear. Avoid in severe hepatic impairment, and carefully consider whether appropriate or not with moderate impairment. See package insert for more information. For patients dependent on methadone or other long-acting opioids sublingual buprenorphine monotherapy (without naloxone) is recommended for induction on days 1 and 2.

MOA — Partial opiate agonist/antagonist.

ADVERSE EFFECTS — Serious: Respiratory/CNS depression, hepatitis, dependence. Frequent: Headache, N/V, constipation, abdominal pain, sweating.

BUPRENORPHINE (Subutex, Probuphine) ▶L ♀C ▶– ©III

WARNING — Probuphine: Implants may protrude, migrate, be expelled, or cause nerve damage with insertion and removal. Use is only through the Probuphine REMS program. All providers must undergo training and be certified to perform insertions and removals.

ADULT — Treatment of opioid dependence - Induction (Subutex): 8 mg SL on day 1, and 16 mg on day 2. Maintenance dose 16 mg daily, but may individualize in a range of 4 to 24 mg daily. Treatment of opioid maintenance (Probuphine): Use only if stable on 8 mg/day or less of a transmucosal form. Four implants in the inner aspect of one arm and left in place for 6 months and then removed. May repeat at 6 months in the other arm one time only. Must undergo special training and be registered to prescribe for this indication.

PEDS — Not approved for use in children or adolescents.

FORMS — Trade and generic: SL tabs 2 and 8 mg. Trade only: Implants (Probuphine): 74.2 mg (= 80 mg buprenorphine HCl)

NOTES — Buprenorphine (Subutex) is preferred for induction for patients dependent upon long-acting opioids such as methadone. Induction should not be started unless signs and symptoms of withdrawal have begun. The combination of burprenorphine/naloxone is preferred for maintenance treatment.

Prescribers must complete training and be certified. See www.suboxone.com. Patients treated with Probuphine can return to SL forms when implants are removed.

MOA — Opioid agonist/antagonist

ADVERSE EFFECTS — Serious: Respiratory depression, bradycardia, hypotension, hepatitis, hypersensitivity. Frequent: sedation, dizziness, nausea, headache, constipation.

DISULFIRAM (Antabuse) ▶L ♀C ▶? $$

WARNING — Never give to an intoxicated patient.

ADULT — Maintenance of abstinence from alcohol: 125 to 500 mg PO daily.

PEDS — Not approved in children.

FORMS — Generic/Trade: Tabs 250, 500 mg.

NOTES — Patient must abstain from any alcohol for at least 12 h before using. Disulfiram-alcohol reaction may occur for up to 2 weeks after discontinuing disulfiram. Metronidazole and alcohol in any form (eg, cough syrups, tonics) contraindicated. Hepatotoxicity.

MOA — Inhibits aldehyde dehydrogenase.

ADVERSE EFFECTS — Serious: Angina, MI, hypotension, tachycardia, heart failure, syncope, seizures. Frequent: Rash, drowsiness, headache, impotence, rash, optic neuropathy.

NALTREXONE (ReVia, Depade, Vivitrol) ▶LK ♀C ▶? $$$$

WARNING — Naltrexone has been associated with hepatotoxicity. Monitor for signs and symptoms.

ADULT — Alcohol dependence: 50 mg PO daily. Extended-release injectable susp: 380 mg IM every 4 weeks or monthly. Opioid dependence following detoxification: Start 25 mg PO daily, increase to 50 mg PO daily if no signs of withdrawal. Extended-release injectable susp: 380 mg IM every 4 weeks or monthly.

PEDS — Not approved in children.

FORMS — Generic/Trade: Tabs 50 mg. Trade only (Vivitrol): Extended-release injectable susp kits 380 mg.

NOTES — Avoid if recent (past 7 to 10 days) ingestion of opioids. Conflicting evidence of efficacy for chronic, severe alcoholism. Extended-release injectable suspension (Vivitrol) should be given in the gluteal muscle and use alternate side each month.

MOA — Opiate antagonist.

ADVERSE EFFECTS — Serious: Suicidal ideation, paranoia, depression, hepatotoxicity. Frequent: Insomnia, nervousness, headache, dizziness, N/V.

NICOTINE GUM (Nicorette, Nicorette DS) ▶LK ♀C ▶– $$$$

ADULT — Smoking cessation: Gradually taper 1 piece (2 mg) every 1 to 2 h for 6 weeks, 1 piece (2 mg) every 2 to 4 h for 3 weeks, then 1 piece (2 mg) every 4 to 8 h for 3 weeks. Max 30 pieces/day of 2 mg gum or 24 pieces/day of 4 mg gum. Use 4 mg pieces (Nicorette DS) for high cigarette use (more than 24 cigarettes/day).

PEDS — Not approved in children.

FORMS — OTC/Generic/Trade: Gum 2, 4 mg.

(cont.)

NICOTINE GUM (*cont.*)

NOTES — Chew slowly and park between cheek and gum periodically. May cause N/V, hiccups. Coffee, juices, wine, and soft drinks may reduce absorption. Avoid eating/drinking for 15 min before/during gum use. Available in original, orange, or mint flavor. Do not use beyond 6 months.

MOA — Nicotine receptor agonist.

ADVERSE EFFECTS — Serious: Atrial and ventricular arrhythmias. Frequent: Local reactions, burning, stinging, headache, insomnia, nausea, diarrhea, tachycardia, chest pain, hypertension.

NICOTINE INHALATION SYSTEM (*Nicotrol Inhaler, ✷Nicorette Inhaler*) ▶LK ♀D ▶– $$$$$

ADULT — Smoking cessation: 6 to 16 cartridges/day for 12 weeks.

PEDS — Not approved in children.

FORMS — Trade only: Oral inhaler 10 mg/cartridge (4 mg nicotine delivered), 42 cartridges/box.

MOA — Nicotine receptor agonist.

ADVERSE EFFECTS — Serious: Atrial and ventricular arrhythmias. Frequent: Local reactions, burning, stinging, headache, insomnia, nausea, diarrhea, tachycardia, chest pain, hypertension.

NICOTINE LOZENGE (*Commit, Nicorette*)   ▶LK ♀D ▶– $$$$$

ADULT — Smoking cessation: In those who smoke within 30 min of waking use 4 mg lozenge; others use 2 mg. Take 1 to 2 lozenges every 1 to 2 h for 6 weeks, then every 2 to 4 h in week 7 to 9, then every 4 to 8 h in week 10 to 12. Length of therapy 12 weeks.

PEDS — Not approved in children.

FORMS — OTC Generic/Trade: Lozenge 2, 4 mg.

NOTES — Allow lozenge to dissolve and do not chew. Do not eat or drink within 15 min before use. Avoid concurrent use with other sources of nicotine.

MOA — Nicotine receptor agonist.

ADVERSE EFFECTS — Serious: Atrial and ventricular arrhythmias. Frequent: Local reactions, headache, insomnia, nausea, diarrhea, tachycardia, chest pain, hypertension.

NICOTINE NASAL SPRAY (*Nicotrol NS*) ▶LK ♀D ▶– $$$$$

ADULT — Smoking cessation: 1 to 2 doses each h; each dose is 2 sprays, 1 in each nostril (1 spray contains 0.5 mg nicotine). Minimum recommended: 8 doses/day, max 40 doses/day.

PEDS — Not approved in children.

FORMS — Trade only: Nasal soln 10 mg/mL (0.5 mg/ inhalation); 10 mL bottles.

MOA — Nicotine receptor agonist.

ADVERSE EFFECTS — Serious: Atrial and ventricular arrhythmias. Frequent: Local reactions, burning, stinging, headache, insomnia, nausea, diarrhea, tachycardia, chest pain, hypertension.

NICOTINE PATCHES (*Habitrol, NicoDerm CQ, Nicotrol*) ▶LK ♀D ▶– $$$$

ADULT — Smoking cessation: Start 1 patch (14 to 22 mg) daily and taper after 6 weeks. Total duration of therapy is 12 weeks.

PEDS — Not approved in children.

FORMS — OTC/Rx/Generic/Trade: Patches 11, 22 mg/24 h. 7, 14, 21 mg/24 h (Habitrol and NicoDerm). OTC/Trade: 15 mg/16 h (Nicotrol).

NOTES — FDA revised warning about continued smoking in 2014 to advise patients that if they relapse and smoke they can still use nicotine replacement products to curb use. Dispose of patches safely; can be toxic to children, pets. Remove opaque NicoDerm CQ patch prior to MRI procedures to avoid possible burns.

MOA — Nicotine receptor agonist.

ADVERSE EFFECTS — Serious: Atrial and ventricular arrhythmias, peptic ulcer formation. Frequent: Local reactions, burning, stinging, headache, insomnia, nausea, diarrhea, tachycardia, chest pain, hypertension.

VARENICLINE (*Chantix, ✷Champix*) ▶K ♀C ▶? $$$$

WARNING — Has been associated with the development of suicidal ideation, changes in behavior, depressed mood, and attempted/completed suicides, both during treatment and after withdrawal. Unclear safety in serious psychiatric conditions.

ADULT — Smoking cessation: Start 0.5 mg PO daily for days 1 to 3, then 0.5 mg two times per day days 4 to 7, then 1 mg two times per day thereafter. Take after meals with full glass of water. Start 1 week prior to cessation and continue for 12 weeks or patient may start the drug and stop smoking between days 8 and 35 of treatment.

PEDS — Not approved in children.

FORMS — Trade only: Tabs 0.5, 1 mg.

NOTES — For severe renal dysfunction, reduce max dose to 0.5 mg two times per day. For renal failure on hemodialysis may use 0.5 mg once daily if tolerated. May worsen underlying neuropsychiatric symptoms in patients with pre-existing psychiatric conditions. May potentiate the intoxicating effects of alcohol. Advise patients to reduce intake until they know if it impacts their tolerance of alcohol.

MOA — Nicotinic acetylcholine receptor agonist.

ADVERSE EFFECTS — Serious: Depression, suicidal thoughts, aggression, erratic behavior, MI, stroke, angina, seizures, somnambulism. Frequent: N/V, drowsiness, dreaming disturbances, insomnia, headache, abnormal dreams, constipation.

PSYCHIATRY: Stimulants/ADHD/Anorexiants

NOTE: Sudden cardiac death has been reported with stimulants and atomoxetine at usual ADHD doses; carefully assess prior to treatment and avoid if cardiac conditions or structural abnormalities. Amphetamines are associated with high abuse potential and dependence with prolonged administration. Stimulants may also cause or worsen underlying psychosis or induce a manic or mixed episode in bipolar disorder. Problems with visual accommodation have also been reported with stimulants. Stimulants have been associated with rhabodomyolysis.

ADDERALL XR (dextroamphetamine + amphetamine Adderall) ▶L ♀C ▶– ©II $$$$
ADULT — Narcolepsy, immediate-release: Start 10 mg PO every am, increase by 10 mg every week; max dose is 60 mg/day divided two to three times per day at 4 to 6 h intervals. ADHD, extended-release caps (Adderall XR): 20 mg PO daily.
PEDS — ADHD, immediate-release tabs: Start 2.5 mg (3 to 5 yo) or 5 mg (age 6 yo or older) PO one to two times per day, increase by 2.5 mg (3 to 5 yo) to 5 mg (6 yo and older) each week, max 40 mg/day. ADHD, extended-release caps (Adderall XR): If age 6 to 12 yo, start 5 to 10 mg PO daily to a max of 30 mg/day. If 13 to 17 yo, start 10 mg PO daily to a max of 20 mg/day. Not recommended age younger than 3 yo. Narcolepsy, immediate-release: Age 6 to 12 yo: Start 5 mg PO daily, increase by 5 mg each week. Age older than 12 yo: Start 10 mg PO every am, increase by 10 mg each week, max dose is 60 mg/day divided two to three times per day at 4 to 6 h intervals.
FORMS — Generic/Trade: Tabs 5, 7.5, 10, 12.5, 15, 20, 30 mg. Caps, extended-release (Adderall XR) 5, 10, 15, 20, 25, 30 mg.
NOTES — Caps may be opened and the beads sprinkled on applesauce; do not chew beads. Adderall XR should be given upon awakening. Avoid evening doses. Monitor growth and use drug holidays when appropriate. May increase pulse and BP. May exacerbate bipolar or psychotic conditions.
MOA — CNS stimulant, increases norepinephrine and dopamine.
ADVERSE EFFECTS — Serious: Sudden death, seizures, psychosis, manic or mixed episodes of bipolar disorder, hypertension, priapism, Raynaud's phenomenon, vasculopathy, rhabodmyolysis. Frequent: Appetite suppression, weight loss, insomnia, nervousness, N/V, dizziness, palpitations, tachycardia, headache, bruxism.

AMPHETAMINE (**Adzenys XR, Dyanavel XR**) ▶LK ♀?
Limited data in humans. Premature delivery and low birth weight have been observed. Adzenys is C. ▶– ©II
ADULT — ADHD: Dyanavel XR, start 2.5 mg to 5 mg PO once daily. May increase every 4-7 days by 2.5 mg to 10 mg per day to max 20 mg/day. Adzenys, 12.5 mg dissolved on the tongue once daily in the morning.
PEDS — ADHD: Dyanavel XR, 6 yo and older: Start 2.5 mg to 5 mg once daily. May increase every 4-7 days by 2.5 mg to 10 mg per day to max 20 mg/day. Adzenys XR: Start 6.3 mg dissolved on the tongue once daily in the morning. Increase at weekly intervals by 3.1 mg to 6.3 mg to max of 18.8 mg daily for ages 6-12 yo and 12.5 mg daily for ages 13-17 yo.
FORMS — Trade: Dyanavel XR, extended-release susp 2.5 mg/mL. Adzenys XR : orally disintegrating extended-release tabs 3.1, 6.3, 9.4, 12.5, 15.7, 18.8 mg.
NOTES — Pre-treatment screen for cardiac disease and risk for substance abuse. For Adzenys the whole tablet should be placed on the tongue and allowed to disintegrate without or chewing. Do not use concurrently or within 14 days of using a monoamine oxidase inhibitor. Dyanavel XR can be taken with or without food.
MOA — Blocks the reuptake of norepinephrine and dopamine and increase their release into the synapse.
ADVERSE EFFECTS — Serious: Sudden death, stroke, myocardial infarction, hypertension, psychosis, mania, peripheral vasculopathy, abuse and dependence. Frequent: epistaxis, allergic rhinitis, abdominal pain, insomnia, appetite and growth suppression, restlessness, irritability, palpitations, tachycardia, dry mouth.

ARMODAFINIL (**Nuvigil**) ▶L ♀C ▶? ©IV $$$$$
ADULT — Obstructive sleep apnea/hypopnea syndrome and narcolepsy: 150 to 250 mg PO every am. Inconsistent evidence for improved efficacy of 250 mg/day dose. Shift work sleep disorder: 150 mg PO 1 h prior to start of shift.
PEDS — Not approved in children.
FORMS — Trade only: Tabs 50, 150, 200, 250 mg.
NOTES — Weak inducer for substrates of CYP3A4/5 (eg, carbamazepine, cyclosporine), which may require dose adjustments. May inhibit metabolism of substrates of CYP2C19 (eg, omeprazole, diazepam, phenytoin). May reduce efficacy of oral contraceptives; consider alternatives during treatment. Reduce dose with severe liver impairment.
MOA — R-enantiomer of modafinil. Wake promoting agent – CNS stimulant.
ADVERSE EFFECTS — Serious: Rash, Stevens-Johnson syndrome, multi-organ hypersensitivity reactions, mania, psychosis, suicidal ideation, aggression. Frequent: Headache, nausea, dizziness, insomnia.

ATOMOXETINE (**Strattera**) ▶K ♀C ▶? $$$$$
WARNING — Severe liver injury and failure have been reported; discontinue if jaundice or elevated LFTs. Increases risk of suicidal thinking and behavior in children and adolescents; carefully weigh risks/benefits before starting and then monitor such individuals closely for worsening depression or emergence of suicidal thoughts or behaviors, especially early in therapy or after increases in dose. Monitor for emergence of anxiety, agitation, panic attacks, insomnia, irritability, hostility, impulsivity, akathisia, mania, and hypomania.
ADULT — ADHD: Start 40 mg PO daily, then increase after more than 3 days to target of 80 mg/day divided one to two times per day. May increase after another 2 to 4 weeks to max dose 100 mg/day.
PEDS — ADHD (6 to 17 yo): Children/adolescents wt 70 kg or less: Start 0.5 mg/kg daily, then increase after more than 3 days to target dose of 1.2 mg/kg/day divided one to two times per day. Max dose 1.4 mg/kg or 100 mg/day, whichever is less. If wt greater than 70 kg, use adult dose.
FORMS — Trade only: Caps 10, 18, 25, 40, 60, 80, 100 mg.

(cont.)

ATOMOXETINE (*cont.*)

NOTES — For patients taking strong CYP2D6 inhibitors (eg, paroxetine or fluoxetine), or known to be poor metabolizers use same starting dose but only increase if well tolerated at 4 weeks and symptoms unimproved. Reduce target dose to 50% usual for moderate heaptic insufficiency or 25% for severe. Caution when coadministered with oral or parenteral albuterol or other beta-2 agonists, as increases in heart rate and BP may occur. May be stopped without tapering. Monitor growth. Give "Patient Medication Guide" when dispensed. Does not appear to exacerbate tics.

MOA — Selective norepinephrine reuptake inhibitor.

ADVERSE EFFECTS — Serious: Sudden death, increased blood pressure and heart rate, liver injury and failure, psychosis, suicidal ideation, mania, aggression, priapism, rhabdomyolysis. Frequent: N/V, dyspepsia, fatigue, decreased appetite, weight loss, dizziness, mood swings, constipation, dry mouth, insomnia, sexual dysfunction, urinary hesitancy/retention, hot flushes, dysuria, dysmenorrhea.

BENZPHETAMINE ▶K ♀X ▶? ☺III $$$

WARNING — Chronic overuse/abuse can lead to marked tolerance and psychic dependence; caution with prolonged use.

ADULT — Obesity (short-term): Start with 25 to 50 mg once daily in the morning and increase if needed to 1 to 3 times daily.

PEDS — Not approved for children younger than 12 yo.

FORMS — Generic/Trade: Tabs 50 mg.

NOTES — Tolerance to anorectic effect develops within week and cross-tolerance to other drugs in class common.

MOA — CNS stimulant, increases dopamine and norepinephrine.

ADVERSE EFFECTS — Serious: Seizures, psychosis, hypertension, dependence. Frequent: Appetite suppression, weight loss, insomnia, nervousness, N/V, dizziness, palpitations, tachycardia, headache.

CAFFEINE (*NoDoz, Vivarin, Caffedrine, Stay Awake, Quick-Pep, Cafcit*) ▶L ♀B/C ▶? $

ADULT — Fatigue: 100 to 200 mg PO every 3 to 4 h prn.

PEDS — Not approved in children younger than 12 yo, except apnea of prematurity in infants between 28 and less than 33 weeks gestational age (Cafcit): Load 20 mg/kg IV over 30 min. Maintenance 5 mg/kg PO q 24 h. Monitor for necrotizing enterocolitis.

FORMS — OTC Generic/Trade: Tabs/Caps 200 mg. Oral soln caffeine citrate (Cafcit) 20 mg/mL. OTC Trade only: Tabs, extended-release 200 mg. Lozenges 75 mg.

NOTES — 2 mg caffeine citrate = 1 mg caffeine base.

MOA — CNS and cardiovascular stimulant.

ADVERSE EFFECTS — Serious: Arrhythmias, delirium, seizures, necrotizing enterocolitis. Frequent: Tremor, anxiety, twitches, headache, insomnia, N/V.

CLONIDINE—PSYCHIATRY (*Kapvay, Catapres, Catapres TTS*) ▶LK ♀C ▶? Present in human milk $$$$$

ADULT — ADHD (Kapvay, monotherapy or adjunctive): Start 0.1 mg PO daily at bedtime. Increase by 0.1 mg/day at weekly intervals to max 0.4 mg/day given twice daily. If split doses are not equal give the largest dose at bedtime. Taper if discontinued.

PEDS — ADHD (Kapvay, monotherapy or adjunctive, 6 to 17 yo): Start 0.1 mg PO daily at bedtime. Increase by 0.1 mg/day at weekly intervals to max 0.4 mg/day given twice daily. If split doses are not equal give the largest dose at bedtime. Taper if discontinued.

UNAPPROVED ADULT — Tourette syndrome: 3 to 5 mcg/kg/day PO divided two to four times per day. Opioid withdrawal, adjunct: 0.1 to 0.3 mg PO three to four times per day or 0.1 to 0.2 mg PO q 4 h prn. Smoking cessation: Start 0.1 mg PO two times per day, increase 0.1 mg/day at weekly intervals to 0.75 mg/day as tolerated; transdermal (Catapres TTS): 0.1 to 0.2 mg/24 h patch once a week for 2 to 3 weeks after cessation.

UNAPPROVED PEDS — Tourette syndrome: 3 to 5 mcg/kg/day PO divided two to four times per day.

FORMS — Generic/Trade: Extended-release tabs 0.1 mg. Tabs, immediate-release, 0.1, 0.2, 0.3 mg. Transdermal weekly patch 0.1 mg/day (TTS-1), 0.2 mg/day (TTS-2), 0.3 mg/day (TTS-3).

NOTES — Do not interchange with other clonidine products on a mg/mg basis.

MOA — Centrally acting alpha-2 agonist

ADVERSE EFFECTS — Serious: Hypotension, bradycardia, rebound hypertension, cardiac conduction abnormalities. Frequent: somnolence, fatigue, irritability, insomnia, nightmares, constipation, dry mouth.

DEXMETHYLPHENIDATE (*Focalin, Focalin XR*) ▶LK ♀C ▶? ☺II $$$

ADULT — ADHD (not already on stimulants): Start 10 mg PO every am (extended-release) or 2.5 mg PO two times per day (immediate-release). Max 20 mg/day for immediate release and 40 mg/day for extended-release. If taking racemic methylphenidate, use conversion of 2.5 mg for each 5 mg of methylphenidate.

PEDS — ADHD (age 6 yo or older and not already on stimulants): Start 5 mg PO every am (extended-release) or 2.5 mg PO two times per day (immediate-release), max 20 mg/day (immediate-release) or 30 mg/day (extended-release). If already on racemic methylphenidate, use conversion of 2.5 mg for each 5 mg of methylphenidate.

FORMS — Generic/Trade: Tabs, immediate-release 2.5, 5, 10 mg. Extended-release caps ($$$$$) 5, 10, 15, 20, 30, 40 mg. Trade only: Extended-release caps (Focalin XR-$$$$$) 25, 35 mg.

NOTES — Avoid evening doses. Monitor growth and use drug holidays when appropriate. May increase pulse and BP. 2.5 mg is equivalent to 5

(cont.)

DEXMETHYLPHENIDATE (cont.)

mg racemic methylphenidate. Focalin XR caps may be opened and sprinkled on applesauce, but beads must not be chewed. May exacerbate bipolar or psychotic conditions. Avoid in patients allergic to methylphenidate.

MOA — CNS stimulant, increases norepinephrine and dopamine.

ADVERSE EFFECTS — Serious: Sudden death, seizures, psychosis, hypertension, priapism, peripheral vasculopathy, Raynaud's phenomenon, rhabdomyolysis. Frequent: Appetite suppression, weight loss, insomnia, nervousness, N/V, dizziness, palpitations, tachycardia, headache.

DEXTROAMPHETAMINE (Dexedrine Spansules, ProCentra, Zenzedi) ▶L ♀C ▶– ⊚II $$$$$

ADULT — Narcolepsy: Start 10 mg PO every am, increase by 10 mg/day each week, max 60 mg/day divided daily (sustained-release) or two to three times per day at 4- to 6-h intervals.

PEDS — Narcolepsy: Age 6 to 12 yo: Start 5 mg PO every am, increase by 5 mg/day every week. Age older than 12 yo: Start 10 mg PO every am, increase by 10 mg/day every week, max 60 mg/day divided daily (sustained-release) or two to three times per day at 4- to 6-h intervals. ADHD: Age 3 to 5 yo: Start 2.5 mg PO daily, increase by 2.5 mg every week. Age 6 yo or older: Start 5 mg PO one to two times per day, increase by 5 mg every week, usual max 40 mg/day divided one to three times per day at 4- to 6-h intervals. Not recommended for patients younger than 3 yo. Extended-release caps not recommended for age younger than 6 yo.

FORMS — Generic/Trade: Caps, extended-release 5, 10, 15 mg. Tabs 5, 10 mg. Oral soln 5 mg/5 mL. Trade only: Tabs 2.5, 7.5 mg (Zenzedi).

NOTES — Avoid evening doses. Monitor growth and use drug holidays when appropriate. May exacerbate bipolar or psychotic conditions.

MOA — CNS stimulant, increases norepinephrine and dopamine.

ADVERSE EFFECTS — Serious: Sudden death, seizures, psychosis, hypertension, priapism, peripheral vasculopathy, Raynaud's phenomenon, rhabdomyolysis. Frequent: Appetite suppression, weight loss, insomnia, nervousness, N/V, dizziness, palpitations, tachycardia, headache.

DIETHYLPROPION (Tenuate, Tenuate Dospan) ▶K ♀B ▶? ⊚IV $

WARNING — Chronic overuse/abuse can lead to marked tolerance and psychic dependence; caution with prolonged use.

ADULT — Obesity (short term): 25 mg PO three times per day 1 h before meals and mid evening if needed or 75 mg sustained-release daily at midmorning.

PEDS — Not approved for children younger than 12 yo.

FORMS — Generic/Trade: Tabs 25 mg; Tabs, extended-release 75 mg.

NOTES — Tolerance to anorectic effect develops within week and cross-tolerance to other drugs in class common.

MOA — CNS stimulant, increases dopamine and norepinephrine.

ADVERSE EFFECTS — Serious: Seizures, psychosis, hypertension, dependence. Frequent: Appetite suppression, weight loss, insomnia, nervousness, N/V, dizziness, palpitations, tachycardia, headache.

GUANFACINE—PSYCHIATRY (Intuniv) ▶LK – ♀B ▶?

ADULT — ADHD: Start 1 mg PO once daily in the morning or evening. Increase by 1 mg/week to max 7 mg/day.

PEDS — ADHD (6 y and older): Start 1 mg PO once daily in the morning or evening. Increase by 1 mg/week to target range based on weight: 25 to 33.9 kg 2 to 3 mg/day, 34 to 41.4 kg 2 to 4 mg/day, 41.5 to 49.4 3 to 5 mg/day, 49.5 to 58.4 kg 3 to 6 mg/day, 58.5 to 91 kg 4 to 7 mg/day, and > 91 kg 5 to 7 mg/day.

FORMS — Generic/Trade: Tabs, extended-release 1, 2, 3, 4 mg.

NOTES — Taper when discontinuing. Use cautiously with strong CYP3A4 inhibitors or inducers. Refer to package label for dosing in various clinical scenarios. Immediate-release tabs not indicated for ADHD and should not be substituted on a mg per mg basis with Intuniv.

MOA — Selective alpha-2A adrenergic agonist.

ADVERSE EFFECTS — Serious: Hypotension, bradycardia, syncope. Frequent: Somnolence/sedation, abdominal pain, dizziness, hypotension, dry mouth, constipation, headache.

LISDEXAMFETAMINE (Vyvanse) ▶L ♀C ▶– ⊚II $$$$

ADULT — ADHD: Start 30 mg PO every am. May increase weekly by 10 to 20 mg/day to max 70 mg/day. Binge eating disorder, mild to moderate: Start 30 mg PO once daily. May increase weekly by 20 mg/day to suggested range of 50 mg to 70 mg daily. Max 70 mg/day.

PEDS — ADHD, children and adolescents ages 6 yo and older: Start 30 mg PO every am. May increase weekly by 10 to 20 mg/day to max 70 mg/day.

FORMS — Trade: Caps 20, 30, 40, 50, 60, 70 mg.

NOTES — May open cap and place contents in water for administration. Avoid evening doses. Monitor growth and use drug holidays when appropriate. Reduce max dose to 50 mg/day with moderate renal insufficiency (CrCl 15 to <30 mL/min) and 30 mg/day in severe (CrCl <15 mL/min).

MOA — Prodrug of dextroamphetamine. CNS stimulant, increases norepinephrine and dopamine.

ADVERSE EFFECTS — Serious: Sudden death, seizures, psychosis, hypertension, priapism, peripheral vasculopathy, Raynaud's phenomonon, rhabdomyolysis. Frequent: Appetite suppression, weight loss, insomnia, nervousness, N/V, dizziness, palpitations, tachycardia, headache, irritability, dry mouth, bruxism.

METHYLPHENIDATE (*Quillichew ER, Aptensio XR, Ritalin, Ritalin LA, Methylin, Methylin ER, Metadate ER, Metadate CD, Concerta, Daytrana, Quillivant XR, ✦Biphentin*) ▶LK ♀C ▶? ©II $$

ADULT — ADHD: 5 to 10 mg PO two to three times per day (immediate-release) or 20 mg PO every am (extended-release), max 60 mg/day. Extended-release (Concerta) 18 to 36 mg PO every am, max 72 mg/day. Extended-release, chewable (Quillichew ER): Start 20 mg PO (chewed) once daily in the morning. May increase at weekly intervals by 10 mg, 15 mg, or 20 mg daily based on efficacy and tolerability. Max 60 mg/day. Extended-release (Aptensio XR): Start 10 mg PO once daily in the morning. May increase by 10 mg/day at weekly intervals to max 60 mg/day. Sustained-release suspension (Quillivant XR) 6 yo and older: Start 20 mg PO in the morning. May increase weekly by 10 to 20 mg daily to max 60 mg/day. Avoid evening doses. Monitor growth and use drug holidays when appropriate. Narcolepsy (Ritalin): 10 mg PO two to three times per day before meals. Usual effective dose is 20 to 30 mg/day, max 60 mg/day.

PEDS — ADHD, age 6 yo or older: Start 5 mg PO two times per day before breakfast and lunch, increase gradually by 5 to 10 mg/day at weekly intervals to max 60 mg/day. Extended-release: Start 20 mg PO daily, max 60 mg daily. Extended-release, chewable (Quillichew ER): Start 20 mg PO (chewed) once daily in the morning. Increase or decrease at weekly intervals by 10 mg, 15 mg, or 20 mg daily based on efficacy and tolerability. Max 60 mg/day. Concerta (extended-release): Start 18 mg PO every am; titrate in 9 to 18 mg increments at weekly intervals to max 54 mg/day (age 6 to 12 yo) or 72 mg/day (13 to 17 yo). Consult product labeling for dose conversion from other methylphenidate regimens. Discontinue after 1 month if no improvement observed. Transdermal patch, age 6 to 17 yo: Start 10 mg/9 h, may increase at weekly intervals to max dose of 30 mg/9 h. Apply 2 h prior to desired onset and remove 9 h later. Effect may last up to 12 h after application. Must alternate sites daily. Sustained-release suspension (Quillivant XR), 6 yo and older: Start 20 mg PO in the morning. May increase weekly by 10 to 20 mg daily to max 60 mg/day. Extended-release caps (Aptensio XR), age 12 to 17 yo: Start 10 mg PO daily in the morning. May increase by 10 mg/day at weekly intervals to max 60 mg/day. Narcolepsy, ages 6 yo and older, (Ritalin): Start 5 mg PO twice daily before breakfast and lunch. May iucrease by 5 to 10 mg/day at weekly intervals to max 60 mg/day. Avoid doses later in the day if possible. Max 60 mg/day.

FORMS — Trade only: Tabs, extended-release 10, 20 mg (Methylin ER, Metadate ER). Tabs, extended-release, chewable 20, 30 mg. Transdermal patch (Daytrana) 10 mg/9 h, 15 mg/9 h, 20 mg/9 h, 30 mg/9 h. Susp, extended-release 5 mg/mL (Quillivant XR). Generic/Trade: Tabs, chewable 2.5, 5, 10 mg (Methylin). Tabs, 5, 10, 20 mg (Ritalin). Tabs, extended-release 18, 27, 36, 54 mg (Concerta). Caps, extended-release 10, 20, 30, 40, 50, 60 mg (Metadate CD), may be sprinkled on food. Caps, extended-release 10, 20, 30, 40 mg (Ritalin LA). Caps, extended-release (Aptensio XR) 10, 15, 20, 30, 40, 50, 60 mg. Oral soln 5 mg/5 mL, 10 mg/5 mL. Generic only: Tabs 5, 10, 20 mg. Tabs, extended-release 10, 20 mg.

NOTES — Avoid evening doses. Avoid use with severe anxiety, tension, or agitation. Monitor growth and use drug holidays when appropriate. May increase pulse and BP. Ritalin LA may be opened and sprinkled on applesauce. Avoid alcohol ingestion with Ritalin LA , Concerta, and Metadate CD as it may change release patterns. Apply transdermal patch to hip below beltline to avoid rubbing it off. Chemical leukoderma (loss of skin pigmentation) has been reported with Daytrana patches. This can occur locally or at sites distant from the application site. Discontinue if this occurs. May exacerbate bipolar, psychotic, or seizure conditions. Quillichew ER is scored and the 20 mg and 30 mg tablets may be broken in half to give 10 mg or 15 mg doses.

MOA — CNS stimulant, increases norepinephrine and dopamine.

ADVERSE EFFECTS — Serious: Sudden death, seizures, psychosis, hypertension, priapism, peripheral valsculopathy, Raynaud's phenomenon, rhabdomyolysis, contact sensitization and leukoderma (Daytrana). Frequent: Appetite suppression, weight loss, insomnia, nervousness, N/V, dizziness, palpitations, tachycardia, headache.

MODAFINIL (*Provigil, ✦Alertec*) ▶L ♀C ▶? ©IV $$$$$

WARNING — Associated with serious, life-threatening rashes in adults and children; discontinue immediately if unexplained rash.

ADULT — Narcolepsy and sleep apnea/hypopnea: 200 mg PO q am. Shift work sleep disorder: 200 mg PO 1 h before shift.

PEDS — Not approved in children younger than 16 yo.

FORMS — Generic/Trade: Tabs 100, 200 mg.

NOTES — May increase levels of diazepam, phenytoin, TCAs, warfarin, or propranolol; may decrease levels of cyclosporine, oral contraceptives, or theophylline. Reduce dose in severe liver impairment.

MOA — Wake-promoting agent; CNS stimulant.

ADVERSE EFFECTS — Serious: Rash, Stevens-Johnson syndrome, multi-organ hypersensitivity, leukopenia, psychosis, mania, suicidal ideation, aggression. Frequent: Insomnia, nausea, headache, nervousness, anxiety.

PHENTERMINE (*Adipex-P, Suprenza*) ▶KL ♀C ▶– ©IV $

WARNING — Chronic overuse/abuse can lead to marked tolerance and psychic dependence; caution with prolonged use.

ADULT — Obesity: 15 to 37.5 mg PO before or 1 to 2 h after breakfast. Alternatively, 18.75 mg PO two times daily. Avoid late evening dosing.

PEDS — Not approved in children younger than 16 yo.

(cont.)

PHENTERMINE (*cont.*)

FORMS — Generic/Trade: Caps 15, 30, 37.5 mg. Tabs 37.5 mg. Trade only: Orally disintegrating tabs (Suprenza) 15, 30, 37.5 mg. Generic only: Caps, extended-release 15, 30 mg.

NOTES — Indicated for short-term (8 to 12 weeks) use only. Contraindicated for use during or within 14 days of MAOIs (hypertensive crisis). Brand name Ionamin discontinued.

MOA — CNS stimulant, increases norepinephrine and dopamine.

ADVERSE EFFECTS — Serious: Seizures, psychosis, hypertension. Frequent: Appetite suppression, weight loss, insomnia, nervousness, N/V, dizziness, palpitations, tachycardia, headache.

PULMONARY

INHALER COLORS (Body then cap—Generics may differ)

Inhaler	Colors
Advair Diskus	purple
Advair HFA	purple/light purple
Aerobid-M	grey/green
Aerospan	purple/grey
Alvesco 80 mcg 160 mcg	brown/red red/red
Anoro Ellipta	grey/red
Arcapta Neohaler	white/red
Arnuity Ellipta	grey/red
Asmanex HFA	blue/red
Asmanex Twisthaler 110 mcg 220 mcg	white/grey white/pink
Atrovent HFA	clear/green
Bevespi Aerosphere	grey/orange
Breo Ellipta	grey/blue
Combivent Respimat	grey/orange
Dulera	blue
Flovent Diskus	orange
Flovent HFA	orange/peach
Foradil Aerolizer	blue
Incruse Ellipta	white/green
ProAir HFA	red/white
Proair Respiclick	red/white
Proventil HFA	yellow/orange
Pulmicort Flexhaler	white/brown

(cont.)

INHALER COLORS (Body then cap—Generics may differ) (*continued*)

Inhaler	Colors
QVAR 40 mcg 80 mcg	beige/grey mauve/grey
Seebri Neohaler	white/amber
Serevent Diskus	green
Spiriva	grey
Spiriva Respimat 1.25 mcg 2.5 mcg	grey/blue grey/green
Stiolto Respimat	grey/green
Striverdi Respimat	grey/yellow
Symbicort	red/grey
Tudorza Pressair	white/green
Utibron Neohaler	white/yellow
Ventolin HFA	light blue/navy
Xopenex HFA	blue/red

INHALED STEROIDS: ESTIMATED COMPARATIVE DAILY DOSES*

Adults and Children older than 12 yo				
Drug	**Form**	**Low dose**	**Medium dose**	**High dose**
beclomethasone HFA MDI	40 mcg/puff 80 mcg/puff	2–6 puffs/day 1–3 puffs/day	6–12 puffs/day 3–6 puffs/day	> 12 puffs/day > 6 puffs/day
budesonide DPI	90 mcg/dose 180 mcg/dose	2–6 inhalations/day 1–3 inhalations/day	6–13 inhalations/day 3–7 inhalations/day	> 13 inhalations/day > 7 inhalations/day
budesonide	soln for nebs	—	—	—
flunisolide HFA MDI	80 mcg/puff	4 puffs/day	5–8 puffs/day	> 8 puffs/day
fluticasone HFA MDI	44 mcg/puff 110 mcg/puff 220 mcg/puff	2–6 puffs/day 1–2 puffs/day 1 puff/day	6–10 puffs/day 2–4 puffs/day 1–2 puffs/day	> 10 puffs/day > 4 puffs/day > 2 puffs/day
fluticasone DPI	50 mcg/dose 100 mcg/dose 250 mcg/dose	2–6 inhalations/day 1–3 inhalations/day 1 inhalation/day	6–10 inhalations/day 3–5 inhalations/day 2 inhalations/day	> 10 inhalations/day > 5 inhalations/day > 2 inhalations/day
mometasone DPI	220 mcg/dose	1 inhalation/day	2 inhalations/day	> 2 inhalations/day

(cont.)

INHALED STEROIDS: ESTIMATED COMPARATIVE DAILY DOSES* (*continued*)

CHILDREN (age 5 to 11 yo)				
Drug	Form	Low dose	Medium dose	High dose
beclomethasone HFA MDI	40 mcg/puff 80 mcg/puff	2–4 puffs/day 1–2 puffs/day	4–8 puffs/day 2–4 puffs/day	> 8 puffs/day > 4 puffs/day
budesonide DPI	90 mcg/dose 180 mcg/dose	2–4 inhalations/day 1–2 inhalations/day	4–9 inhalations/day 2–4 inhalations/day	> 9 inhalations/day > 4 inhalations/day
budesonide	soln for nebs	0.5 mg 0.25–0.5 mg (0–4 yo)	1 mg > 0.5–1 mg (0–4 yo)	2 mg > 1 mg (0–4 yo)
flunisolide HFA MDI	80 mcg/puff	2 puffs/day	4 puffs/day	≥ 8 puffs/day
fluticasone HFA MDI (0–11 yo)	44 mcg/puff 110 mcg/puff 220 mcg/puff	2–4 puffs/day 1–2 puff/day n/a	4–8 puffs/day 2–3 puffs/day 1–2 puffs/day	> 8 puffs/day > 4 puffs/day > 2 puffs/day
fluticasone DPI	50 mcg/dose 100 mcg/dose 250 mcg/dose	2–4 inhalations/day 1–2 inhalations/day n/a	4–8 inhalations/day 2–4 inhalations/day 1 inhalation/day	> 8 inhalations/day > 4 inhalations/day > 1 inhalation/day
mometasone DPI	220 mcg/dose	n/a	n/a	n/a

*HFA = Hydrofluoroalkane (propellant). MDI = metered dose inhaler. DPI = dry powder inhaler.
Reference: http://www.nhlbi.nih.gov/guidelines/asthma/asthsumm.pdf

PREDICTED PEAK EXPIRATORY FLOW (liters/min)

Age (yo)	Women (height in inches)					Men (height in inches)					Child (height in inches)
	55"	60"	65"	70"	75"	60"	65"	70"	75"	80"	
20	390	423	460	496	529	554	602	649	693	740	44" – 160
30	380	413	448	483	516	532	577	622	664	710	46" – 187
40	370	402	436	470	502	509	552	596	636	680	48" – 214
50	360	391	424	457	488	486	527	569	607	649	50" – 240
60	350	380	412	445	475	463	502	542	578	618	52"– 267
70	340	369	400	432	461	440	477	515	550	587	54" – 293

Am Rev Resp Dis 1963;88:644.

PULMONARY: Beta Agonists—Short-Acting

NOTE: Palpitations, tachycardia, tremor, lightheadedness, nervousness, headache, and nausea may occur; these effects may be more pronounced with systemic administration. Hypokalemia can occur from the transient shift of potassium into cells, rarely leading to adverse cardiovascular effects; monitor accordingly. Potential for tolerance with continued use of short-acting beta-agonists.

ALBUTEROL (*ProAir RespiClick, AccuNeb, Ventolin HFA, Proventil HFA, ProAir HFA, VoSpire ER, ✷Airomir, salbutamol, Apo-Salvent*) ▶L ♀C ▶? $$
ADULT — Acute asthma: MDI: 2 puffs q 4 to 6 h prn. Soln for inhalation: 2.5 mg nebulized three to four times per day. Dilute 0.5 mL 0.5% soln with 2.5 mL NS. Deliver over 5 to 15 min. One 3 mL unit dose (0.083%) nebulized three to four times per day. Prevention of exercise-induced bronchospasm: MDI: 2 puffs 10 to 30 min before exercise. Chronic

(cont.)

ALBUTEROL (cont.)

asthma: 2 to 4 mg PO three to four times per day or extended-release 4 to 8 mg PO q 12 h up to 16 mg PO q 12 h.

PEDS — Acute asthma: MDI: Age 4 yo or older: 1 to 2 puffs q 4 to 6 h prn. Soln for inhalation (0.5%): 2 to 12 yo: 0.1 to 0.15 mg/kg/dose not to exceed 2.5 mg three to four times per day, diluted with NS to 3 mL. Chronic asthma: Tabs, syrup 6 to 12 yo: 2 to 4 mg PO three to four times per day, max dose 24 mg/day in divided doses or extended-release 4 mg PO q 12 h. Syrup 2 to 5 yo: 0.1 to 0.2 mg/kg/dose PO three times per day up to 4 mg three times per day. Prevention of exercise-induced bronchospasm age 4 yo or older: 2 puffs 10 to 30 min before exercise.

UNAPPROVED ADULT — COPD: MDI, soln for inhalation: Use asthma dose. Acute asthma: MDI, soln for inhalation: Dose same as approved dose q 20 min for 3 doses or until improvement. Continuous nebulization: 10 to 15 mg/h until improvement. Emergency hyperkalemia: 10 to 20 mg via MDI or soln for inhalation.

UNAPPROVED PEDS — Acute asthma: Soln for inhalation: 0.15 mg/kg (minimum dose is 2.5 mg) q 20 min for 3 doses then 0.15 to 0.3 mg/kg up to 10 mg q 1 to 4 h prn, or 0.5 mg/kg/h continuous nebulization. MDI: 4 to 8 puffs q 20 min for 3 doses then q 1 to 4 h prn. Soln for inhalation (0.5%): Age younger than 2 yo: 0.05 to 0.15 mg/kg/dose q 4 to 6 h. Syrup, age younger than 2 yo: 0.3 mg/kg/24 h PO divided three times per day, max dose 12 mg/24 h. Prevention of exercise-induced bronchospasm: MDI: Age 4 yo or older 2 puffs 10 to 30 min before exercise.

FORMS — Trade only: MDI 90 mcg/actuation, 200 metered doses/canister. "HFA" inhalers use hydrofluoroalkane propellant instead of CFCs but are otherwise equivalent. "RespiClick" is a breath-actuated DPI. Generic/Trade: Soln for inhalation 0.021% (AccuNeb), 0.042% (AccuNeb), and 0.083% in 3 mL vials, 0.5% (5 mg/mL) in 20 mL with dropper. Tabs, extended-release 4, 8 mg (VoSpire ER). Generic only: Syrup 2 mg/5 mL. Tabs, immediate-release 2, 4 mg.

NOTES — Do not crush or chew extended-release tabs. Use with caution in patients on MAOIs or cyclic antidepressants: May increase cardiovascular side effects.

MOA — Short-acting beta agonist bronchodilator.

ADVERSE EFFECTS — Serious: Hypersensitivity, paradoxical bronchospasm. Frequent: Palpitations, tachycardia, hypokalemia, tremor, lightheadedness, nervousness, headache, and nausea.

LEVALBUTEROL (Xopenex Concentrate, Xopenex, Xopenex HFA) ▶L ♀C ▶? $$$

ADULT — Acute asthma: MDI 2 puffs q 4 to 6 h prn. Soln for inhalation: 0.63 to 1.25 mg nebulized q 6 to 8 h.

PEDS — Acute asthma: MDI age 4 yo or older: 2 puffs q 4 to 6 h prn. Soln for inhalation age 12 yo or older: Use adult dose. For age 6 to 11 yo: 0.31 mg nebulized three times per day.

FORMS — Generic/Trade: Soln for inhalation 0.31, 0.63, 1.25 mg in 3 mL and 1.25 mg in 0.5 mL unit-dose vials. Trade only: HFA MDI 45 mcg/actuation, 15 g 200/canister. "HFA" inhalers use hydrofluoroalkane propellant.

NOTES — R-isomer of albuterol. Dyspepsia may occur. Use with caution in patients on MAOIs or cyclic antidepressants; may increase cardiovascular side effects.

MOA — Short-acting beta agonist bronchodilator.

ADVERSE EFFECTS — Serious: Hypersensitivity, paradoxical bronchospasm, arrhythmias. Frequent: Palpitations, tachycardia, hypokalemia, tremor, lightheadedness, nervousness, headache, and nausea.

METAPROTERENOL (✶Orciprenaline) ▶L ♀C ▶? $$

ADULT — Acute asthma: MDI: 2 to 3 puffs q 3 to 4 h; max dose 12 puffs/day. Soln for inhalation: 0.2 to 0.3 mL of the 5% soln in 2.5 mL NS. 20 mg PO three to four times per day.

PEDS — Acute asthma: Soln for inhalation: 0.1 to 0.3 mL of the 5% soln in 2.5 mL NS for age older than 6 yo. Tabs or syrup: 1.3 to 2.6 mg/kg/day PO in divided doses three to four times per day for age 2 to 5 yo. 10 mg PO three to four times per day for age 6 to 9 yo or wt less than 60 lbs, 20 mg PO three to four times per day for age older than 9 yo or wt 60 lbs or greater.

UNAPPROVED PEDS — Acute asthma: MDI: 2 to 3 puffs q 3 to 4 h (up to 12 puffs/day) for age older than 6 yo. Soln for inhalation: 0.1 to 0.3 mL of the 5% soln in 2.5 mL NS q 4 to 6 h prn or q 20 min until improvement. Tabs or syrup, age younger than 2 yo: 0.4 mg/kg/dose PO three to four times per day.

FORMS — Trade only: MDI 0.65 mg/actuation, 14 g 200/canister. Generic/Trade: Soln for inhalation 0.4%, 0.6% in 2.5 mL unit-dose vials. Generic only: Syrup 10 mg/5 mL. Tabs 10, 20 mg.

MOA — Short-acting beta agonist bronchodilator.

ADVERSE EFFECTS — Serious: Hypersensitivity, paradoxical bronchospasm. Frequent: Palpitations, tachycardia, hypokalemia, tremor, lightheadedness, nervousness, headache, and nausea.

TERBUTALINE (✶Bricanyl Turbuhaler) ▶L ♀B ▶– $$$

ADULT — Asthma: 2.5 to 5 mg PO q 6 h while awake. Max dose 15 mg/24 h. Acute asthma: 0.25 mg SC into lateral deltoid area; may repeat once within 15 to 30 min. Max dose 0.5 mg/4 h.

PEDS — Not approved in children.

UNAPPROVED ADULT — Preterm labor: 0.25 mg SC q 30 min up to 1 mg in 4 h. Infusion: 2.5 to 10 mcg/min IV, gradually increased to effective max doses of 17.5 to 30 mcg/min.

UNAPPROVED PEDS — Asthma: 0.05 mg/kg/dose PO three times per day, increase to max of 0.15 mg/kg/dose three times per day, max 5 mg/day for age 12 yo or younger, use adult dose for age older than 12 yo up to max 7.5 mg/ 24 h. Acute asthma: 0.01 mg/kg SC q 20 min for 3 doses then q 2 to 6 h prn.

FORMS — Generic only: Tabs 2.5, 5 mg. Injectable 1 mg/1 mL.

MOA — Short-acting beta agonist bronchodilator; tocolytic.

PULMONARY: Beta Agonists—Long-Acting

NOTE: Long-acting beta-agonists may increase the risk of asthma-related death. Use only as a 2nd agent if inadequate control with an optimal dose of inhaled corticosteroids. Do not use for rescue therapy. Palpitations, tachycardia, tremor, lightheadedness, nervousness, headache, and nausea may occur. Decreases in serum potassium can occur, rarely leading to adverse cardiovascular effects; monitor accordingly.

ARFORMOTEROL (*Brovana*) ▶L ♀C ▶? $$$$$
ADULT — COPD: 15 mcg nebulized two times per day.
PEDS — Not approved in children.
FORMS — Trade only: Soln for inhalation 15 mcg in 2 mL vial.
NOTES — Not for acute COPD exacerbations.
MOA — Long-acting beta agonist bronchodilator.
ADVERSE EFFECTS — Serious: Hypersensitivity, paradoxical bronchospasm. Frequent: Palpitations, tachycardia, hypokalemia, tremor, lightheadedness, nervousness, headache, and nausea.

FORMOTEROL (*Foradil Aerolizer, Perforomist, ✲Oxeze Turbuhaler*) ▶L ♀C ▶? $$$
ADULT — Chronic asthma, COPD: 1 puff two times per day. Prevention of exercise-induced bronchospasm: 1 puff 15 min prior to exercise. COPD: 20 mcg nebulized q 12 h.
PEDS — Chronic asthma, age 5 yo or older: 1 puff two times per day. Prevention of exercise-induced bronchospasm age 12 yo or older: Use adult dose.
FORMS — Trade only: DPI 12 mcg, 12, 60 blisters/pack (Foradil). To be used only with Aerolizer device. Soln for inhalation: 20 mcg in 2 mL vial (Perforomist). Canada only (Oxeze): DPI 6, 12 mcg 60 blisters/pack.
NOTES — For asthma, must use in combination with inhaled steroid. Do not use additional doses for exercise if on maintenance.
MOA — Long-acting beta agonist bronchodilator.
ADVERSE EFFECTS — Serious: Hypersensitivity, paradoxical bronchospasm. Frequent: Palpitations, tachycardia, hypokalemia, tremor, insomnia, lightheadedness, nervousness, headache, and nausea.

INDACATEROL (*Arcapta Neohaler, ✲Onbrez Breezhaler*) ▶L – ♀C ▶?
ADULT — COPD: DPI: 75 mcg inhaled once daily.
PEDS — Not approved for children.
FORMS — Trade only: DPI: 75 mcg caps for inhalation, 30 blisters. To be used only with Neohaler device. Contains lactose.

MOA — Long-acting beta agonist bronchodilator.
ADVERSE EFFECTS — Serious: Hypersensitivity. Frequent: Palpitations, tachycardia, hypokalemia, tremor, lightheadedness, nervousness, headache, pharyngitis, and nausea.

OLODATEROL (*Striverdi Respimat*) ▶LK ♀C ▶?
ADULT — COPD: 2 inhalations once daily.
PEDS — Not approved for children.
FORMS — Trade only: Carton with canister containing 28 or 60 metered actuations for use with provided Striverdi Respimat device. Each actuation delivers 2.5 mcg olodaterol.
NOTES — Not for acute COPD exacerbations.
MOA — Long-acting beta agonist bronchodilator
ADVERSE EFFECTS — Serious: Paradoxical bronchospasm, angioedema. Frequent: Palpitations, tachycardia, tremor, nasopharyngitis.

SALMETEROL (*Serevent Diskus, ✲Serevent Diskhaler disk*) ▶L ♀C ▶? $$$$
ADULT — Chronic asthma/COPD: 1 inhalation two times per day. Prevention of exercise-induced bronchospasm: 1 inhalation 30 min before exercise.
PEDS — Chronic asthma age 4 yo or older: 1 inhalation two times per day. Prevention of exercise-induced bronchospasm: 1 inhalation 30 min before exercise.
FORMS — Trade only: DPI (Diskus): 50 mcg, 60 blisters.
NOTES — For asthma, must use in combination with inhaled steroid. Do not use additional doses for exercise if on maintenance. Concomitant ketoconazole increases levels and prolongs QT interval. Do not use with strong CYP3A4 inhibitors such as ritonavir, itraconazole, clarithromycin, nefazodone, etc.
MOA — Long-acting beta agonist bronchodilator.
ADVERSE EFFECTS — Serious: Hypersensitivity. Frequent: Palpitations, tachycardia, hypokalemia, tremor, lightheadedness, nervousness, headache, pharyngitis, and nausea.

PULMONARY: Combinations

***ADVAIR HFA* (fluticasone—inhaled + salmeterol, ✲ *Advair, Advair Diskus*)** ▶L ♀C ▶? $$$$$
WARNING — Long-acting beta-agonists may increase the risk of asthma-related death; use as an adjunct only if inadequate control with an optimal dose of inhaled corticosteroids. Avoid in significantly worsening or acute asthma. Do not use for rescue therapy. Do not stop abruptly.
ADULT — Chronic asthma: DPI: 1 inhalation two times per day (all strengths). MDI: 2 puffs two times per day (all strengths). COPD maintenance: DPI: 1 inhalation two times per day (250/50 only).

PEDS — Chronic asthma: DPI: 1 inhalation two times per day (100/50 only) for age 4 to 11 yo. Use adult dose for 12 yo or older.
UNAPPROVED ADULT — COPD: 500/50, 1 inhalation two times per day.
FORMS — Trade only: DPI: 100/50, 250/50, 500/50 mcg fluticasone/salmeterol per actuation; 60 doses/DPI. Trade only (Advair HFA): MDI 45/21, 115/21, 230/21 mcg fluticasone/salmeterol per actuation; 120 doses/canister.
NOTES — See individual components for additional information. Ritonavir and other CYP3A4 inhibitors

(cont.)

ADVAIR HFA (*cont.*)

such as ketoconazole significantly increase both salmeterol and fluticasone concentrations, resulting in prolongation of QT interval (salmeterol) and systemic effects, including adrenal suppression (fluticasone). Very rare anaphylactic reaction in patients with severe milk protein allergy. Increased risk of pneumonia in COPD.
MOA — Anti-inflammatory/long-acting beta agonist bronchodilator combination.
ADVERSE EFFECTS — Serious: Hypersensitivity, anaphylaxis, paradoxical bronchospasm, Churg-Strauss syndrome. Frequent: Thrush, dysphonia, pharyngitis, palpitations, tachycardia, tremor, lightheadedness, nervousness, headache, nausea.

BEVESPI AEROSPHERE (glycopyrrolate—inhaled + formoterol) ▶KL ♀C ▶?
WARNING — Not approved for acute bronchospasm or treatment of asthma.
ADULT — COPD: Two inhalations twice daily.
PEDS — Not approved for use in children.
FORMS — Trade only: MDI: 9/4.8 mcg glycopyrrolate/formoterol per inhalation. 120 inhalations (10.7 g) per canister.
MOA — Anticholinergic/long-acting beta-2 agonist combination.
ADVERSE EFFECTS — Common: nasopharyngitis, couch. Severe: paradoxical bronchospasm, hypersensitivity reactions.

BREO ELLIPTA (fluticasone—inhaled + vilanterol, ✱ Breo Ellipta) ▶L – ♀C ▶? $$$$$
WARNING — Long-acting beta-agonists may increase the risk of asthma-related death; use as an adjunct only if inadequate control with an optimal dose of inhaled corticosteroids. Avoid in significantly worsening or acute asthma. Do not use for rescue therapy. Do not stop abruptly.
ADULT — Chronic asthma, COPD: 1 inhalation once daily. 200/25 mcg fluticasone/vilanterol strength only approved for asthma.
PEDS — Not approved in children
FORMS — Trade only: DPI: 100/25 mcg, 200/25 mcg fluticasone/vilanterol per actuation; 30 doses/DPI.
NOTES — See individual components for additional information. Ritonavir and other CYP3A4 inhibitors such as ketoconazole significantly increase both vilanterol and fluticasone concentrations, resulting in prolongation of QT interval (vilanterol) and systemic effects, including adrenal suppression (fluticasone). Very rare anaphylactic reaction in patients with severe milk protein allergy. Increased risk of pneumonia in COPD.
MOA — Anti-inflammatory/long-acting beta agonist bronchodilator combination.
ADVERSE EFFECTS — Serious: Hypersensitivity, anaphylaxis, paradoxical bronchospasm, Churg-Strauss syndrome. Frequent: Thrush, dysphonia, pharyngitis, palpitations, tachycardia, tremor, lightheadedness, nervousness, headache, nausea.

COMBIVENT RESPIMAT (albuterol—inhaled + ipratropium—inhaled, ✱ Combivent Respimat) ▶L ♀C ▶? $$$$
ADULT — COPD: Respimat: 1 puff four times per day. Max dose 6 inhalations/24 h.
PEDS — Not approved in children.
FORMS — Trade only: Respimat: 100 mcg albuterol/20 mcg ipratropium per inhalation, 120/canister.
MOA — Short-acting beta agonist/anticholinergic bronchodilator combination.
ADVERSE EFFECTS — Serious: Paradoxical bronchospasm. Frequent: Palpitations, tachycardia, tremor, lightheadedness, nervousness, headache, and nausea.

DULERA (mometasone—inhaled + formoterol, ✱ Zenhale) ▶L – ♀C ▶? $$$$$
WARNING — Long-acting beta-agonists may increase the risk of asthma-related death; use as an adjunct only if inadequate control with an optimal dose of inhaled corticosteroids. Avoid in significantly worsening or acute asthma. Do not use for rescue therapy. Do not stop abruptly.
ADULT — Chronic asthma: 2 inhalations two times per day (all strengths).
PEDS — Chronic asthma: Use adult dose for 12 yo or older.
UNAPPROVED ADULT — COPD: 2 puffs two times per day (all strengths).
FORMS — Trade only: MDI 100/5, 200/5 mcg mometasone/formoterol per actuation; 120 doses/canister.
NOTES — See individual components for additional information. Ritonavir and other CYP3A4 inhibitors such as ketoconazole significantly increase mometasone concentration resulting in systemic effects including adrenal suppression. Canister comes with 124 doses; patient must prime before first use and after more than 5 days of disuse by spraying 4 doses in air away from face, shaking canister after each spray.
MOA — Anti-inflammatory/long-acting beta agonist bronchodilator combination.
ADVERSE EFFECTS — Serious: Hypersensitivity, anaphylaxis, paradoxical bronchospasm, Churg-Strauss syndrome. Frequent: Thrush, dysphonia, pharyngitis, palpitations, tachycardia, tremor, lightheadedness, nervousness, headache, nausea.

DUONEB (albuterol—inhaled + ipratropium—inhaled, ✱ Combivent inhalation soln) ▶L ♀C ▶? $$$$$
ADULT — COPD: 1 unit dose nebulized four times per day; may add 2 doses/day prn to max of 6 doses/day.
PEDS — Not approved in children.
FORMS — Generic/Trade: Unit dose: 2.5 mg albuterol/0.5 mg ipratropium per 3 mL vial, premixed; 30, 60 vials/carton.
NOTES — Refer to components; 3.0 mg albuterol is equivalent to 2.5 mg albuterol base.
MOA — Short-acting beta agonist/anticholinergic bronchodilator combination.

(cont.)

DUONEB (*cont.*)

ADVERSE EFFECTS — Serious: None. Frequent: Palpitations, tachycardia, tremor, lightheadedness, nervousness, headache, nausea, dry mouth, blurred vision.

✲ DUOVENT UDV (ipratropium--inhaled + fenoterol) ▶L ♀? ▶? $$$$$

ADULT — Canada only. Bronchospasm associated with asthma/COPD: 1 vial (via nebulizer) q 6 h prn.

PEDS — Canada only. Children age 12 yo or older: 1 vial (via nebulizer) q 6 h prn.

FORMS — Canada trade only: Unit dose vial (for nebulization) 0.5 mg ipratropium, 1.25 mg fenoterol in 4 mL of saline.

MOA — Anticholinergic and short-acting beta agonist bronchodilator.

ADVERSE EFFECTS — Serious: Hypokalemia, bronchospasm. Frequent: Dry mouth or throat, tremor.

STIOLTO RESPIMAT (tiotropium + olodaterol) ▶KL ♀C ▶?

WARNING — Not approved to treat asthma or acute bronchoconstriction.

ADULT — COPD: 2 inhalations once per day using Respimat device.

PEDS — Not approved for use in children.

FORMS — Trade only: Inhalation spray: equivalent of 2.5/2.5 mcg tiotropium/olodaterol per inhalation. Canisters contain 60 inhalations each. For use with Respimat device only.

MOA — Anticholinergic/long-acting beta-2 agonist combination.

ADVERSE EFFECTS — Serious: paradoxical bronchospasm, hypersensitivity reactions. Common: cough, nasophyringeal irritation.

SYMBICORT (budesonide—inhaled + formoterol, ✲ Symbicort Turbuhaler) ▶L ♀C ▶? $$$$

WARNING — Long-acting beta-agonists may increase the risk of asthma-related death; use as an adjunct only if inadequate control with an optimal dose of inhaled corticosteroids. Avoid in significantly worsening or acute asthma. Do not use for rescue therapy. Do not stop abruptly.

ADULT — Chronic asthma, 2 puffs two times per day (both strengths). COPD: 2 puffs two times per day (160/4.5).

PEDS — Chronic asthma: age 12 yo or older: Use adult dose.

FORMS — Trade only: MDI: 80/4.5, 160/4.5 mcg budesonide/formoterol per actuation; 120 doses/canister.

NOTES — See individual components for additional information. Ritonavir and other CYP3A4 inhibitors such as ketoconazole significantly increase budesonide concentrations, resulting in systemic effects, including adrenal suppression.

MOA — Anti-inflammatory/long-acting beta agonist bronchodilator combination.

ADVERSE EFFECTS — Serious: Hypersensitivity, anaphylaxis, paradoxical bronchospasm, Churg-Strauss syndrome. Frequent: Thrush, dysphonia, pharyngitis, palpitations, tachycardia, tremor, lightheadedness, nervousness, headache, nausea.

UTIBRON NEOHALER (indacaterol + glycopyrrolate—inhaled) ▶L ♀C ▶?

WARNING — Not approved for acute bronchospasm or treatment of asthma.

ADULT — COPD: Inhale powder contents of one cap twice daily using Neohaler device.

PEDS — Not approved for use in children.

FORMS — Trade only: caps: 27.6 mcg/15.6 mcg indacaterol/glycopyrrolate in blister packs in boxes of 6 or 60 caps for use with Neohaler device.

MOA — Long-acting beta-2 agonist and anticholinergic combination.

ADVERSE EFFECTS — Common: nasopharyngitis, hypertension. Severe: paradoxical bronchospasm, hypersensitivity reactions.

PULMONARY: Inhaled Steroids

NOTE: See Endocrine—Corticosteroids when oral steroids necessary. Beware of adrenal suppression when changing from systemic to inhaled steroids. Inhaled steroids are not for treatment of acute asthma; higher doses may be needed for severe asthma and exacerbations. Adjust to lowest effective dose for maintenance. Use of a DPI and a spacing device and rinsing the mouth with water after each use may decrease the incidence of thrush and dysphonia. Pharyngitis and cough may occur with all products. Use with caution in patients with active or quiescent TB; untreated systemic fungal, bacterial, viral, or parasitic infections; or ocular HSV. Inhaled steroids produce small, transient reductions in growth velocity in children. Prolonged use may lead to decreases in bone mineral density and osteoporosis, thereby increasing fracture risk.

BECLOMETHASONE—INHALED (✲QVAR) ▶L ♀C ▶? $$$

ADULT — Chronic asthma: 40 mcg: 1 to 4 puffs two times per day. 80 mcg: 1 to 2 puffs two times per day.

PEDS — Chronic asthma in 5 to 11 yo: 40 mcg 1 to 2 puffs two times per day.

UNAPPROVED ADULT — Chronic asthma: NHLBI dosing schedule (puffs/day divided two times per day): Low dose: 2 to 6 puffs of 40 mcg or 1 to 3 puffs of 80 mcg. Medium dose: 6 to 12 puffs of 40 mcg or 3 to 6 puffs of 80 mcg. High dose: More than 12 puffs of 40 mcg or more than 6 puffs 80 mcg.

UNAPPROVED PEDS — Chronic asthma (5 to 11 yo): NHLBI dosing schedule (puffs/day divided two times per day): Low dose: 2 to 4 puffs of 40 mcg or 1 to 2 puffs of 80 mcg. Medium dose: 4 to 8 puffs of 40 mcg or 2 to 4 puffs of 80 mcg. High dose: More than 8 puffs of 40 mcg or more than 4 puffs of 80 mcg.

FORMS — Trade only: HFA MDI: 40, 80 mcg/actuation, 7.3 g 100 actuations/canister.

MOA — Steroidal anti-inflammatory.

(cont.)

BECLOMETHASONE—INHALED (*cont.*)

ADVERSE EFFECTS — Serious: Adrenal suppression (high dose), hypersensitivity, bronchospasm. Frequent: Thrush, dysphonia.

BUDESONIDE—INHALED (*Pulmicort Respules, Pulmicort Flexhaler*, ✣*Pulmicort Turbuhaler*) ▶L ♀B ▶? $$$$

ADULT — Chronic asthma: DPI: 1 to 2 puffs daily to two times per day up to 4 puffs two times per day.

PEDS — Chronic asthma, 6 to 12 yo: DPI: 1 to 2 puffs daily to two times per day. 12 mo to 8 yo: Susp for inhalation (Respules): 0.5 mg to 1 mg daily or divided two times per day.

UNAPPROVED ADULT — Chronic asthma: NHLBI dosing schedule (puffs/day daily or divided two times per day): DPI: Low dose is in the range of 1 to 3 puffs of 180 mcg or 2 to 6 puffs of 90 mcg. Medium dose is in the range of 3 to 7 puffs of 180 mcg or 6 to 13 puffs of 90 mcg. High dose more than 7 puffs of 180 mcg or more than 13 puffs of 90 mcg.

UNAPPROVED PEDS — Chronic asthma (5 to 11 yo): NHLBI dosing schedule (puffs/day daily or divided two times per day): DPI: Low dose: 1 to 2 puffs of 180 mcg or 2 to 4 puffs of 90 mcg. Medium dose: 2 to 4 puffs of 180 mcg or 4 to 9 puffs of 90 mcg. High dose more than 4 puffs of 180 mcg or more than 9 puffs of 90 mcg. Susp for inhalation (daily or divided two times per day): Low dose is in the range of 0.25 to 0.5 mg for age 4 yo or younger and about 0.5 mg for age 5 to 11 yo. Medium dose more than 0.5 to 1 mg for age 4 yo or younger and 1 mg for age 5 to 11 yo. High dose more than 1 mg for age 4 yo or younger and 2 mg for age 5 to 11 yo. Some doses may be outside the package labeling.

FORMS — Trade only: DPI (Flexhaler) 90, 180 mcg powder/actuation 60, 120 doses/canister, repsectively. Generic/Trade: Respules 0.25, 0.5, 1 mg/2 mL unit dose.

NOTES — Respules should be delivered via a jet nebulizer with a mouthpiece or face mask. CYP3A4 inhibitors such as ketoconazole, erythromycin, or ritonavir may significantly increase systemic concentrations, possibly causing adrenal suppression. Flexhaler contains trace amounts of milk proteins; caution with severe milk protein hypersensitivity.

MOA — Steroidal anti-inflammatory.

ADVERSE EFFECTS — Serious: Adrenal suppression (high dose), hypersensitivity, bronchospasm. Frequent: Thrush, dysphonia, headache, nausea.

CICLESONIDE—INHALED (*Alvesco*) ▶L ♀C ▶? $$$$

ADULT — Chronic asthma: MDI: 80 mcg/puff: 1 to 4 puffs two times per day. 160 mcg/puff: 1 to 2 puffs two times per day.

PEDS — Chronic asthma, age 12 yo or older: Use adult dose.

FORMS — Trade only: 80 mcg/actuation, 60 per canister. 160 mcg/actuation, 60, 120 per canister.

NOTES — CYP3A4 inhibitors such as ketoconazole may significantly increase systemic concentrations, possibly causing adrenal suppression.

MOA — Steroidal anti-inflammatory.

ADVERSE EFFECTS — Serious: Adrenal suppression (high dose), hypersensitivity, bronchospasm. Frequent: Thrush, dysphonia, headache, nausea.

FLUNISOLIDE—INHALED (*Aerospan*) ▶L ♀C ▶? $$$

ADULT — Chronic asthma: MDI: 2 puffs two times per day up to 4 puffs two times per day.

PEDS — Chronic asthma, age: 6 to 15 yo: MDI: 2 puffs two times per day.

UNAPPROVED ADULT — Chronic asthma: NHLBI dosing schedule (puffs/day divided two times per day): Low dose: 2 to 4 puffs. Medium dose: 4 to 8 puffs. High dose: More than 8 puffs.

UNAPPROVED PEDS — Chronic asthma (5 to 11 yo): NHLBI dosing schedule (puffs/day divided two times per day): Low dose: 2 to 3 puffs. Medium dose: 4 to 5 puffs. High dose: More than 5 puffs (8 puffs or more for 80 mcg HFA).

FORMS — Trade only: MDI: 250 mcg/actuation, 100 metered doses/canister. AeroBid-M (AeroBid + menthol flavor). Aerospan HFA MDI: 80 mcg/actuation, 60, 120 metered doses/canister.

MOA — Steroidal anti-inflammatory.

ADVERSE EFFECTS — Serious: Adrenal suppression (high dose), bronchospasm. Frequent: Thrush, dysphonia.

FLUTICASONE FUROATE (*Flovent Diskus, Flovent HFA, Arnuity Ellipta*, ✣*Flovent Diskus, Flovent HFA, Arnuity Ellipta*) ▶L ♀C ▶?

ADULT — Chronic asthma: 1 inhalation once daily.

PEDS — Chronic asthma, age 12 yo or over: Use adult dose.

FORMS — Trade only: Foil strip with 30 blisters each containing 100 or 200 mcg fluticasone furoate for use with Ellipta DPI device.

NOTES — Ritonavir, ketoconazole, and other strong CYP3A4 inhibitors can increase systemic adverse effects including adrenal suppression.

MOA — Steroidal anti-inflammatory.

ADVERSE EFFECTS — Serious: adrenal suppression, anaphylaxis. Frequent: thrush, headache.

FLUTICASONE—INHALED (*Arnuity Ellipta, Flovent HFA, Flovent Diskus*, ✣*Arnuity Ellipta, Flovent HFA, Flovent Diskus*) ▶L ♀C ▶? $$$$

ADULT — Chronic asthma: MDI: 2 puffs two times per day up to 4 puffs two times per day. Max dose 880 mcg two times per day.

PEDS — Chronic asthma: 2 puffs two times per day of 44 mcg/puff for age 4 to 11 yo. Use adult dose for age 12 yo or older.

UNAPPROVED ADULT — Chronic asthma: NHLBI dosing schedule (puffs/day divided two times per day): Low dose: 2 to 6 puffs of 44 mcg MDI. Medium dose: 2 to 4 puffs of 110 mcg MDI or 2 puffs of 220 mcg MDI. High dose: More than 4 puffs 110 mcg MDI or more than 2 puffs 220 mcg MDI.

UNAPPROVED PEDS — Chronic asthma, age 11 yo or younger: NHLBI dosing schedule (puffs/day divided two times per day): Low dose: 2 to 4 puffs of 44 mcg MDI. Medium dose: 4 to 8 puffs of 44 mcg MDI. 2 to 3 puffs of 110 mcg MDI. 1 to 2 puffs of 220 mcg MDI. High dose: 4 puffs or more 110 mcg MDI. 2 puffs or more 220 mcg MDI.

(cont.)

FLUTICASONE—INHALED (*cont.***)**

FORMS — Trade only: HFA MDI: 44, 110, 220 mcg/actuation 120/canister. DPI (Diskus): 50, 100, 250 mcg/actuation delivering 44, 88, 220 mcg respectively.

NOTES — Ritonavir and other CYP3A4 inhibitors such as ketoconazole significantly increase fluticasone concentrations, resulting in systemic effects, including adrenal suppression. Increased risk of pneumonia in COPD.

MOA — Steroidal anti-inflammatory.

ADVERSE EFFECTS — Serious: Adrenal suppression (high dose), anaphylaxis, Churg-Strauss syndrome, bronchospasm. Frequent: Thrush, dysphonia, pharyngitis, headache.

MOMETASONE—INHALED (*Asmanex HFA, Asmanex Twisthaler, *✽*Asmanex Twisthaler***)** ▶L ♀C ▶? $$$$

ADULT — Chronic asthma: 1 to 2 puffs q pm or 1 puff two times per day. If prior oral corticosteroid therapy: 2 puffs two times per day.

PEDS — Chronic asthma: Age 12 yo or older: Use adult dose.

UNAPPROVED ADULT — Chronic asthma: NHLBI dosing schedule (puffs/day divided two times per day): Low dose: 1 puff. Medium dose: 2 puffs. High dose: More than 2 puffs.

FORMS — Trade only: DPI: 110 mcg/actuation with #30 dosage units, 220 mcg/actuation with #30, 60, 120 dosage units.

NOTES — CYP3A4 inhibitors such as ketoconazole may significantly increase concentrations.

MOA — Steroidal anti-inflammatory.

ADVERSE EFFECTS — Serious: Adrenal suppression (high dose). Frequent: Thrush, dysphonia.

PULMONARY: Leukotriene Inhibitors

NOTE: Not for treatment of acute asthma. Abrupt substitution for corticosteroids may precipitate Churg-Strauss syndrome. Postmarket cases of agitation, aggression, anxiousness, dream abnormalities and hallucinations, depression, insomnia, irritability, restlessness, suicidal thinking and behavior (including suicide), and tremor have been reported.

MONTELUKAST (*Singulair***)** ▶L ♀B ▶? $$$$

ADULT — Chronic asthma, allergic rhinitis: 10 mg PO daily. Administer in evening for asthma. Prevention of exercise-induced bronchoconstriction: 10 mg PO 2 h before exercise.

PEDS — Chronic asthma, allergic rhinitis: Give 4 mg (chew tab or oral granules) PO daily for age 2 to 5 yo, give 5 mg PO daily for age 6 to 14 yo. Asthma, age 12 to 23 mo: 4 mg (oral granules) PO daily. Allergic rhinitis, age 6 to 23 mo: 4 mg (oral granules) PO daily. Prevention of exercise-induced bronchoconstriction: Age 6 yo or older: Use adult dose.

FORMS — Generic/Trade only: Tabs 10 mg. Oral granules 4 mg packet, 30/box. Chewable tabs (cherry flavored) 4, 5 mg.

NOTES — Chewable tabs contain phenylalanine. Oral granules may be placed directly into the mouth or mixed with a spoonful of breastmilk, baby formula, applesauce, carrots, rice, or ice cream. If mixed with food, must be taken within 15 min. Do not mix with other liquids. Levels decreased by phenobarbital and rifampin. Dyspepsia may occur. Do not take an additional dose for exercise-induced bronchospasm if already taking other doses chronically.

MOA — Leukotriene receptor antagonist.

ADVERSE EFFECTS — Serious: Churg-Strauss syndrome, hepatitis, anaphylaxis, angioedema, erythema nodosum, suicidal thinking, pancreatitis. Frequent: Headache, dyspepsia.

ZAFIRLUKAST (*✽AccolateA***)** ▶L ♀B ▶− $$$$

WARNING — Hepatic failure has been reported.

ADULT — Chronic asthma: 20 mg PO two times per day, 1 h before meals or 2 h after meals.

PEDS — Chronic asthma, age 5 to 11 yo: 10 mg PO two times per day, 1 h before meals or 2 h after meals. Use adult dose for age 12 yo or older.

UNAPPROVED ADULT — Allergic rhinitis: 20 mg PO two times per day, 1 h before meals or 2 h after meals.

FORMS — Trade only: Tabs 10, 20 mg.

NOTES — Potentiates warfarin and theophylline. Levels decreased by erythromycin and increased by high-dose aspirin. Nausea may occur. If liver dysfunction is suspected, discontinue drug and manage accordingly. Consider monitoring LFTs.

MOA — Leukotriene receptor antagonist.

ADVERSE EFFECTS — Serious: Churg-Strauss syndrome, hypersensitivity, hepatotoxicity, anaphylaxis, angioedema. Frequent: Headache, dyspepsia.

ZILEUTON (*Zyflo, Zyflo CR***)** ▶L ♀C ▶? $$$$$

WARNING — Contraindicated in active liver disease.

ADULT — Chronic asthma: 1200 mg PO two times per day.

PEDS — Chronic asthma, age 12 yo or older: Use adult dose.

FORMS — Trade only: Tabs, extended-release 600 mg.

NOTES — Monitor LFTs for elevation. Potentiates warfarin, theophylline, and propranolol. Dyspepsia and nausea may occur.

MOA — Leukotriene formation inhibitor.

ADVERSE EFFECTS — Serious: Hepatotoxicity, leukopenia. Frequent: Headache, dyspepsia.

PULMONARY: Other Pulmonary Medications

ACETYLCYSTEINE—INHALED (*Mucomyst*) ▶L ♀B ▶? $

ADULT — Mucolytic nebulization: 3 to 5 mL of the 20% soln or 6 to 10 mL of the 10% soln three to four times per day. Instillation, direct or via tracheostomy: 1 to 2 mL of a 10 to 20% soln q 1 to 4 h; via percutaneous intratracheal catheter: 1 to 2 mL of the 20% soln or 2 to 4 mL of the 10% soln q 1 to 4 h.

PEDS — Mucolytic nebulization: Use adult dosing.

FORMS — Generic/Trade: Soln for inhalation 10, 20% in 4, 10, 30 mL vials.

NOTES — Increased volume of liquefied bronchial secretions may occur; maintain an open airway. Watch for bronchospasm in asthmatics. Stomatitis, N/V, fever, and rhinorrhea may occur. A slightly disagreeable odor may occur and should soon disappear. A face mask may cause stickiness on the face after nebulization; wash with water. The 20% soln may be diluted with NaCl or sterile water.

MOA — Mucolytic.

ADVERSE EFFECTS — Serious: Bronchospasm (asthmatics), anaphylaxis. Frequent: Stomatitis, N/V, fever, and rhinorrhea.

ACLIDINIUM (*Tudorza Pressair*, ✷*Tudorza Genuair*) ▶L — ♀C ▶? $$$$$

ADULT — COPD: Pressair: 400 mcg two times per day.

PEDS — Not approved in children.

FORMS — Trade only: Sealed aluminum pouches 400 mcg per actuation. To be used with Pressair device only. Packages of 60 with Pressair device.

NOTES — Not for acute bronchospasm. Use with caution in narrow-angle glaucoma, myasthenia gravis, BPH, or bladder-neck obstruction. Paradoxical bronchospasm may occur. Eye pain or blurred vision may occur if powder enters eyes. Avoid if severe lactose allergy.

MOA — Long-acting anticholinergic bronchodilator.

ADVERSE EFFECTS — Serious: anaphylaxis, paradoxical bronchospasm. Common: headache, nasopharyngitis, cough.

ALPHA-1 PROTEINASE INHIBITOR (*alpha-1 antitrypsin, Aralast NP, Prolastin-C, Zemaira, Glassia*, ✷*Prolastin-C*) ▶Plasma ♀C ▶? $

WARNING — Possible transmission of viruses and Creutzfeldt-Jakob disease.

ADULT — Congenital alpha-1 proteinase inhibitor deficiency with emphysema: 60 mg/kg IV once per week.

PEDS — Not approved in children.

NOTES — Contraindicated in selected IgA deficiencies with known antibody to IgA. Hepatitis B vaccine recommended in preparation for Prolastin use.

MOA — Alpha-1 proteinase inhibitor.

ADVERSE EFFECTS — Serious: Anaphylaxis, increased LFTs. Frequent: Headache, somnolence, flu-like symptoms.

AMINOPHYLLINE ▶L ♀C ▶? $

ADULT — Acute asthma: Loading dose if currently not receiving theophylline: 6 mg/kg IV over 20 to 30 min. Maintenance IV infusion: Dose 0.5 to 0.7 mg/

kg/h, mix 1 g in 250 mL D5W (4 mg/mL) set at rate 11 mL/h delivers 0.7 mg/kg/h for wt 70 kg patient. In patients with cor pulmonale, heart failure, liver failure, use 0.25 mg/kg/h. If currently on theophylline, each 0.6 mg/kg aminophylline will increase the serum theophylline concentration by approximately 1 mcg/mL. Maintenance: 200 mg PO two to four times per day.

PEDS — Acute asthma: Loading dose if currently not receiving theophylline: 6 mg/kg IV over 20 to 30 min. Maintenance oral route age older than 1 yo: 3 to 4 mg/kg/dose PO q 6 h. Maintenance IV route for age older than 6 mo: 0.8 to 1 mg/kg/h IV infusion.

UNAPPROVED PEDS — Neonatal apnea of prematurity: Loading dose 5 to 6 mg/kg IV/PO, maintenance: 1 to 2 mg/kg/dose q 6 to 8 h IV/PO.

NOTES — Aminophylline is 79% theophylline. Administer IV infusion no faster than 25 mg/min. Multiple drug interactions (especially ketoconazole, rifampin, carbamazepine, isoniazid, phenytoin, macrolides, zafirlukast, and cimetidine). Review meds before initiating treatment. Irritability, nausea, palpitations, and tachycardia may occur. Overdose may be life-threatening.

MOA — Bronchodilator.

ADVERSE EFFECTS — Serious: Arrhythmias, seizures. Frequent: Irritability, nausea, palpitations, tachycardia.

BERACTANT (✷*Survanta*) ▶Lung ♀? ▶? $$$$$

PEDS — RDS (hyaline membrane disease) in premature infants: Specialized dosing.

MOA — Lung surfactant.

ADVERSE EFFECTS — Serious: Bradycardia, nosocomial sepsis. Frequent: Bradycardia, oxygen desaturation.

CALFACTANT (*Infasurf*) ▶Lung ♀? ▶? $$$$$

PEDS — RDS (hyaline membrane disease) in premature infants: Specialized dosing.

FORMS — Trade only: Oral susp: 35 mg/mL in 3, 6 mL vials. Preservative-free.

MOA — Lung surfactant.

ADVERSE EFFECTS — Serious: Bradycardia, cyanosis. Frequent: Cyanosis, bradycardia, airway obstruction.

CROMOLYN—INHALED (✷*Nu-Cromolyn, PMS-Sodium Cromoglycate*) ▶LK ♀B ▶? $

ADULT — Chronic asthma: MDI: 2 to 4 puffs four times per day. Soln for inhalation: 20 mg four times per day. Prevention of exercise-induced bronchospasm: MDI: 2 puffs 10 to 15 min prior to exercise. Soln for nebulization: 20 mg 10 to 15 min prior. Mastocytosis: 200 mg PO four times per day, 30 min before meals and at bedtime.

PEDS — Chronic asthma for age older than 5 yo using MDI: 2 puffs four times per day; for age older than 2 yo using soln for nebulization 20 mg four times per day. Prevention of exercise-induced bronchospasm for age older than 5 yo using MDI: 2 puffs 10 to 15 min prior to exercise. Using soln for nebulization

(cont.)

CROMOLYN—INHALED (*cont.***)**

for age older than 2 yo: 20 mg 10 to 15 min prior. Mastocytosis: Age 2 to 12 yo: 100 mg PO four times per day 30 min before meals and at bedtime.

FORMS — Generic only: Soln for nebs: 20 mg/2 mL. Generic/Trade: Oral concentrate 100 mg/5 mL in individual amps.

NOTES — Not for treatment of acute asthma. Pharyngitis may occur. Directions for oral concentrate: 1) Break open and squeeze liquid contents of ampule(s) into a glass of water. 2) Stir soln. 3) Drink all of the liquid.

MOA — Mast cell stabilizer.

ADVERSE EFFECTS — Serious: Paradoxical bronchospasm, anaphylaxis. Frequent: Cough, pharyngitis.

DORNASE ALFA (✿*Pulmozyme***) ▶L ♀B ▶? $$$$$**

ADULT — Cystic fibrosis: 2.5 mg nebulized one to two times per day.

PEDS — Cystic fibrosis age 6 yo or older: 2.5 mg nebulized one to two times per day.

UNAPPROVED PEDS — Has been used in a small number of children as young as 3 mo with similar efficacy and side effects.

FORMS — Trade only: Soln for inhalation: 1 mg/mL in 2.5 mL vials.

NOTES — Voice alteration, pharyngitis, laryngitis, and rash may occur. Do not dilute or mix with other drugs.

MOA — Mucolytic.

ADVERSE EFFECTS — Serious: None. Frequent: Voice alteration, pharyngitis, laryngitis, and rash.

DOXAPRAM (*Dopram***) ▶L ♀B ▶? $$$**

ADULT — Acute hypercapnia due to COPD: 1 to 2 mg/min IV, max 3 mg/min. Max infusion time: 2 h.

PEDS — Not approved in children.

UNAPPROVED PEDS — Apnea of prematurity unresponsive to methylxanthines: Load 2.5 to 3 mg/kg over 15 min, then 1 mg/kg/h titrated to lowest effective dose. Max: 2.5 mg/kg/h. Contains benzyl alcohol; caution in neonates.

NOTES — Monitor arterial blood gases at baseline and q 30 min during infusion. Do not use with mechanical ventilation. Contraindicated with seizure disorder, severe HTN, CVA, head injury, CAD, and severe heart failure.

MOA — Respiratory stimulant.

ADVERSE EFFECTS — Serious: None. Frequent: Hypertension, N/V, diarrhea, cough, dyspnea, tachypnea, tachycardia, arrhythmias, seizure, fever, and sweating.

EPINEPHRINE RACEMIC (*S-2***, ✿***Vaponefrin***) ▶Plasma ♀C ▶– $**

ADULT — See Cardiovascular section.

PEDS — Severe croup: Soln for inhalation: 0.05 mL/kg/dose diluted to 3 mL with NS over 15 min prn not to exceed q 1 to 2 h dosing. Max dose 0.5 mL.

FORMS — Trade only: Soln for inhalation: 2.25% epinephrine in 15, 30 mL.

NOTES — Cardiac arrhythmias and HTN may occur.

MOA — Bronchodilator.

ADVERSE EFFECTS — Serious: Arrhythmias, cerebral hemorrhage, hypertension. Frequent: Palpitations, tachycardia, tremor, lightheadedness, nervousness, headache, and nausea.

GLYCOPYRROLATE—INHALED (*Seebri Neohaler***) ▶KL ♀C ▶?**

WARNING — Not for treatment of acute symptoms.

ADULT — COPD: Inhale powder contents of one cap twice daily using Neohaler device.

PEDS — Not approved for use in children.

FORMS — Trade only: caps: 15.6 mcg glycopyrrolate in blister packs in boxes of 60 caps for use with Neohaler device.

MOA — Long-acting anticholinergic

ADVERSE EFFECTS — Common: URI, nasopharyngitis. Serious: paradoxical bronchospasm, hypersensitivity reactions.

IPRATROPIUM—INHALED (✿*Atrovent HFA, Gen-Ipratropium***) ▶Lung ♀B ▶? $$$$**

ADULT — COPD: MDI (Atrovent, Atrovent HFA): 2 puffs four times per day; may use additional inhalations not to exceed 12 puffs/day. Soln for inhalation: 500 mcg nebulized three to four times per day.

PEDS — Not approved in children younger than 12 yo.

UNAPPROVED PEDS — Acute asthma: MDI (Atrovent, Atrovent HFA): 1 to 2 puffs three to four times per day for age 12 yo or younger. Soln for inhalation: Give 250 mcg/dose three to four times per day for age 12 yo or younger: Give 250 to 500 mcg/dose three to four times per day for age older than 12 yo. Acute asthma: Age 2 to 18 yo: 500 mcg nebulized with 2nd and 3rd doses of albuterol.

FORMS — Trade only: Atrovent HFA MDI: 17 mcg/actuation, 200/canister. Generic/Trade: Soln for nebulization: 0.02% (500 mcg/vial) in unit dose vials.

NOTES — Atrovent MDI is contraindicated with soy or peanut allergy; HFA not contraindicated. Caution with glaucoma, myasthenia gravis, BPH, or bladder-neck obstruction. Cough, dry mouth, and blurred vision may occur.

MOA — Short-acting anticholinergic bronchodilator.

ADVERSE EFFECTS — Serious: Anaphylaxis, angioedema. Frequent: Dry mouth, blurred vision.

KETOTIFEN (✿*Zaditen***) ▶L ♀C ▶– $$**

ADULT — Not approved.

PEDS — Canada only. Chronic asthma: 6 mo to 3 yo: 0.05 mg/kg PO two times per day. Children older than 3 yo: 1 mg PO two times per day.

FORMS — Generic/Trade: Tabs 1 mg. Syrup 1 mg/5 mL.

NOTES — Several weeks may be necessary before therapeutic effect. Full clinical effectiveness is generally reached after 10 weeks.

MOA — Non-bronchodilator antihistamine.

ADVERSE EFFECTS — Serious: Seizures, thrombocytopenia. Frequent: Drowsiness, weight gain.

METHACHOLINE (✿*Provocholine, Methacholine Omega***) ▶Plasma ♀C ▶? $$**

WARNING — Life-threatening bronchoconstriction can result; have resuscitation capability available.

(cont.)

METHACHOLINE (*cont.*)

ADULT — Diagnosis of bronchial airway hyperreactivity in nonwheezing patients with suspected asthma: 5 breaths each of ascending serial concentrations, 0.025 mg/mL to 25 mg/mL, via nebulization. The procedure ends when there is more than 20% reduction in the FEV1 compared with baseline.

PEDS — Diagnosis of bronchial airway hyperreactivity: Use adult dose.

NOTES — Avoid with epilepsy, bradycardia, peptic ulcer disease, thyroid disease, urinary tract obstruction, or other conditions that could be adversely affected by a cholinergic agent. Hold beta-blockers. Do not inhale powder.

MOA — Bronchoconstrictor.

ADVERSE EFFECTS — Serious: Respiratory/cardiac arrest, syncope. Frequent: Wheezing.

NINTEDANIB (*✽Ofev*) ▶L ♀D ▶?

WARNING — May cause elevated liver enzymes that necessitate temporary dose reduction or discontinuation. Check at baseline, monthly for 3 months, then q 3 months or as clinically indicated. If AST or ALT are 3 to 5 times the upper limit of normal without signs of severe liver damage, decrease dose to 100 mg twice daily. May increase back to 150 mg twice daily if enzymes return to baseline. AST or ALT above 5 times the upper limit of normal or with signs of severe liver damage should result in discontinuation. Diarrhea, nausea, and vomiting are common and, if severe, may necessitate dose reduction or discontinuation.

ADULT — Idiopathic pulmonary fibrosis: 150 mg twice daily 12 h apart with food. If not tolerated (liver enzymes, diarrhea, nausea, vomiting), may decrease to 100 mg twice daily 12 h apart with food.

PEDS — Not approved in children.

FORMS — Trade only: Caps: 100, 150 mg.

NOTES — Substrate of P-glycoprotein and CYP3A4. Use with caution if coadministered with a drug (erythromycin, ketoconazole) that inhibits these enzymes. Enzyme inducers (rifampin, carbamazepine, phenytoin, St. John's wort) can significantly decrease exposure. Smoking can also decrease exposure.

MOA — Kinase inhibitor

ADVERSE EFFECTS — Serious: Elevated liver enzymes. arterial thromboebolism, bleeding, gastrointestinal perforation. Frequent: Diarrhea, nausea, vomiting, abdominal pain, decreased appetite. Diarrhea, nausea, and vomiting can be severe.

OMALIZUMAB (*✽Xolair*) ▶Plasma, L ♀B ▶? $$$$$

WARNING — Anaphylaxis may occur; monitor closely and be prepared to treat. Anaphylaxis most commonly occurs within 1 h of administration; 78% of cases occur within 12 h.

ADULT — Moderate to severe asthma with perennial allergy when symptoms not controlled by inhaled steroids: 150 to 375 mg SC q 2 to 4 weeks, based on pretreatment serum total IgE level and body wt.

PEDS — Moderate to severe asthma with perennial allergy: Age 12 yo or older: Use adult dose.

NOTES — Not for treatment of acute asthma. Divide doses greater than 150 mg over more than 1 injection site. Monitor for signs of anaphylaxis including bronchospasm, hypotension, syncope, urticaria, angioedema.

MOA — Monoclonal antibody that inhibits IgE binding to mast cells and basophils.

ADVERSE EFFECTS — Serious: Anaphylaxis, malignancy. Frequent: Injection site reactions.

PIRFENIDONE (*✽Esbriet*) ▶LK ♀C ▶?

WARNING — May cause elevated liver enzymes that necessitate temporary dose reduction or discontinuation. Check at baseline, monthly for the 1st 6 months, and q 3 months thereafter. If AST or ALT are 3 to 5 times the upper limit of normal with no symptoms of liver disease and normal bilirubin, may continue at current dose or decrease dose as clinically indicated. If elevated bilirubin, symptoms of liver disease, or AST or ALT are above 5 times the upper limit of normal, discontinue and do not rechallenge. Other adverse effects (nausea, rash, diarrhea) may also require a temporary or permanent dose reduction or discontinuation.

ADULT — Idiopathic pulmonary fibrosis: 267 mg three times a day for 7 days, then 534 mg three times a day for 7 days, then 801 mg three times a day thereafter. Should be taken with meals.

FORMS — Trade only: Caps 267 mg.

NOTES — Metabolized by CYP1A2, CYP2C9, CYP2C19, CYP2D6, and CYP2E1. Strong (fluvoxamine, enoxacin) or moderate (ciprofloxacin 750 mg twice daily) CYP1A2 inhibitors require lower doses of pirfenidone to be used. Agents or combinations of agents that are moderate or strong inhibitors of CYP1A2 and one or more of the other isoenzymes should be discontinued before starting pirfenidone. Smoking decreases exposure to pirfenidone. Patients who miss 14 or more consecutive days of treatment should be restarted at the lowest dose and retitrated.

MOA — Pyridone; mechanism of action has not been established.

ADVERSE EFFECTS — Serious: Elevated liver enzymes, photosensitivity. Frequent: Nausea, rash, abdominal pain, diarrhea, fatigue, dyspepsia, vomiting, anorexia, GERD.

PORACTANT (*Curosurf*) ▶Lung ♀? ▶? $$$$$

PEDS — RDS (hyaline membrane disease) in premature infants: Specialized dosing.

MOA — Lung surfactant.

ADVERSE EFFECTS — Serious: Bradycardia, hypotension. Frequent: Bradycardia, hypotension, oxygen desaturation.

RESLIZUMAB (*Cinqair*) ▶plasma ♀− Potential effects on a fetus are likely to be greater during the second and third trimester of pregnancy. No evidence of harm in animal models. ▶? Human IgG antibodies are known to be present in breast milk.

WARNING — Anaphylaxis may occur; monitor closely and be prepared to treat. In clinical trials, all cases of anaphylaxis occured during or within 20 minutes after infusion.

(cont.)

RESLIZUMAB (cont.)

ADULT — Severe asthma with an eosinophilic pheno-type: 3 mg/kg IV infusion over 20-50 minutes every 4 weeks.

PEDS — Not approved for usd in children.

FORMS — Trade only: 100 mg/10 mL single-use vials.

MOA — Monoclonal IgG4 kappa antibody that antag-onizes interleukin 5

ADVERSE EFFECTS — Serious: anaphylaxis, malig-nancy. Common: oropharyngeal pain.

ROFLUMILAST (Daliresp, ✚Daxas) ▶L – ♀C ▶– $$$$$

ADULT — Severe COPD due to chronic bronchitis: 500 mcg PO daily with or without food.

PEDS — Not approved for use in children.

FORMS — Trade only: Tabs 500 mcg.

NOTES — Contraindicated in moderate-to-severe liver disease. Inhibitors of CYP3A4 or dual CYP3A4 and 1A2 (erythromycin, ketoconazole, cimetidine) may increase concentrations. Not recommended for use with strong CYP inducers (rifampin, carbam-azepine, phenobarbital, phenytoin). Not for relief of acute bronchospasm. Main effect is decreased exacerbations.

MOA — Phosphodiesterase-4 inhibitor. Exact mecha-nism in COPD is unknown but believed to be related to the increase in intracellular cyclic AMP in lung cells.

ADVERSE EFFECTS — Serious: psychiatric events including suicidality, depression, anxiety. Frequent: diarrhea, weight loss, nausea, headache, insomnia.

THEOPHYLLINE (Elixophyllin, Uniphyl, Theo-24, T-Phyl, ✚Theo-Dur, Theolair) ▶L ♀C ▶+ $

ADULT — Chronic asthma: 5 to 13 mg/kg/day PO in divided doses. Max dose 900 mg/day.

PEDS — Chronic asthma: Initial: Age older than 1 yo and wt less than 45 kg: 12 to 14 mg/kg/day PO divided q 4 to 6 h to max of 300 mg/24 h. Maintenance: 16 to 20 mg/kg/day PO divided q 4 to 6 h to max of 600 mg/24 h. For age older than 1 yo and wt 45 kg or more: Initial: 300 mg/24 h PO divided q 6 to 8 h. Maintenance: 400 to 600 mg/24 h PO divided q 6 to 8 h. Infants age 6 to 52 weeks: [(0.2 × age in weeks) + 5] × kg = 24 h dose in mg PO divided q 6 to 8 h.

UNAPPROVED ADULT — COPD: 10 mg/kg/day PO in divided doses.

UNAPPROVED PEDS — Apnea and bradycardia of prematurity: 3 to 6 mg/kg/day PO divided q 6 to 8 h. Maintain serum concentrations 3 to 5 mcg/mL.

FORMS — Generic/Trade: Elixir 80 mg/15 mL. Trade only: Caps Theo-24: 100, 200, 300, 400 mg. T-Phyl: 12 h SR tabs 200 mg. Theolair: Tabs 125, 250 mg. Generic only: 12 h tabs 100, 200, 300, 450 mg, 12 h caps 125, 200, 300 mg.

NOTES — Multiple drug interactions (especially ketoconazole, rifampin, carbamazepine, isoniazid, phenytoin, macrolides, zafirlukast, and cimetidine). Review meds before initiating treatment. Overdose may be life-threatening.

MOA — Bronchodilator.

ADVERSE EFFECTS — Serious: Arrhythmias, sei-zures. Frequent: Irritability, nausea, palpitations, tachycardia.

TIOTROPIUM (Spiriva HandiHaler, Spiriva Respimat, ✚Spiriva, Spiriva Respimat) ▶K ♀C ▶– $$$$

WARNING — QT prolongation has been reported.

ADULT — COPD: HandiHaler: 18 mcg inhaled daily. Respimat: 2 inhalations of 2.5 mcg/inhalation once daily. Asthma: Respimat: age 12 yo old or older: 2 inhalations of 1.25 mcg/inhalation once daily.

PEDS — Asthma: Respimat: age 12 yo old or older: 2 inhalations of 1.25 mcg/inhalation once daily. Not approved in children under 12 yo.

FORMS — Trade only: HandiHaler: caps for oral inha-lation 18 mcg to be used with HandiHaler device only. Packages of 5, 30, 90 caps with HandiHaler device. Respimat: canister containing 1.25 or 2.5 mcg tiotropium/inhalation to be used with Respimat device only, 60 actuations/canister.

NOTES — Not for acute bronchospasm. Administer at the same time each day. Use with caution in narrow-angle glaucoma, myasthenia gravis, BPH, or bladder-neck obstruction. Avoid touching opened cap. Glaucoma, eye pain, or blurred vision may occur if powder enters eyes. May increase dosing interval in patients with CrCl less than 50 mL/min. Avoid if severe lactose allergy.

MOA — Long-acting anticholinergic bronchodilator.

ADVERSE EFFECTS — Serious: Anaphylaxis, angio-edema, paradoxical bronchospasm, QT prolonga-tion. Frequent: Dry mouth, cough.

UMECLIDINIUM (✚Incruse Ellipta) ▶L ♀C ▶?

ADULT — COPD: 1 inhalation once daily.

PEDS — Not approved in children.

FORMS — Trade only: Foil blister strip with 30 blis-ters each containing 62.5 mcg for use with Ellipta device.

NOTES — Not for acute bronchospasm. Administer at the same time each day. Use with caution in narrow-angle glaucoma, myasthenia gravis, BPH, or bladder-neck obstruction. Avoid if severe lactose allergy.

MOA — Long-acting anticholinergic bronchodilator

ADVERSE EFFECTS — Serious: Paradoxical broncho-spasm, angioedema. Common: Nasopharyngitis, URI, cough.

RHEUMATOLOGY

**INITIAL TREATMENT OF RHEUMATOID ARTHRITIS (RA):
AMERICAN COLLEGE OF RHEUMATOLOGY RECOMMENDATIONS**

Disease Activity Treatment-experience	Treatment Options
Early disease (duration <6 months)	
Low and DMARD-naive	Single DMARD (MTX 1st-line)[1]
Moderate or high and DMARD-naive	Consider single DMARD[1, 4]
Moderate or high on single DMARD	Combination DMARD[2, 4] *or* TNF-blocker ± MTX[4] *or* Non-TNF biologic[3] ± MTX[4]
Established disease (duration ≥6 months)	
Low and DMARD-naive	Single DMARD (MTX 1st-line) preferred over TNF-blocker
Moderate to high and DMARD-naive	Consider single DMARD (MTX 1st-line); see guideline for more options[4]
Moderate or high on single DMARD	Combination DMARD[4] *or* Add TNF-blocker ± MTX[4] *or* Non-TNF biologic[3] ± MTX[4] *or* Tofacinitib ± MTX[4]
Moderate or high on TNF-blocker without DMARD	Add one or two DMARDs[4] see guideline for more options
Moderate or high on DMARD, TNF-blocker, or non-TNF biologic[3]	Consider ≤10 mg/day prednisone equivalent for <3 months; see guideline for more options

Adapted from: *Arthritis Rheumatol.* 2016 Jan;68(1): 1–26. Available online at: http://www.rheumatology.org.
DMARD = disease-modifying anti-rheumatic drug; HCQ = hydroxychloroquine; LEF = leflunomide;
MTX = methotrexate; SSZ = sulfasalazine; TNF = tumor necrosis factor.
Treatment target is low disease activity or remission, giving each regimen for at least 3 months before therapy escalation.
[1]Single DMARD: HCQ, LEF, MTX, or SSZ.
[2]DMARD combination: MTX + SSZ; MTX + HCQ; SSZ+ HCQ; MTX + SSZ + HCQ; combinations + LEF.
[3]Non-TNF biologics: abatacept, rituximab, tocilizumab.
[4]Consider adding ≤10 mg/day prednisone for patients with moderate or high disease activity when starting
a DMARD or in patients with DMARD or biologic failure. Also consider corticosteroid to manage disease flares, using the lowest possible
dose for the shortest possible duration (<3 months).

RHEUMATOLOGY: Biologic Response Modifiers—TNF-Blockers

NOTE: TNF-blockers increase the risk of serious infections (e.g., TB, sepsis, invasive fungal and opportunistic infections); discontinue if serious infection. Screen for HBV and latent TB (treat if present) before using a TNF-blocker; monitor for active TB during treatment. Hold TNF-blockers for at least 1 week before and after surgery. Other adverse events include lymphoma and other malignancies in children and adolescents; new onset/exacerbation of demyelinating disorders and heart failure (avoid if NYHA Class III/IV heart failure), a lupus-like syndrome, and serious hypersensitivity reactions including anaphylaxis. Increased risk of HBV reactivation; refer to AGA guideline (www.gastro.org) for prevention and treatment. Avoid live vaccines. Do not coadminister other biologic response modifiers (e.g., abatacept, anakinra, tofacitinib). Refer to ACR RA guidelines (www.rheumatology.org) for advice on TB screening, vaccines, and other safety issues.

ADALIMUMAB (*Humira*) ▶proteolysis ♀O/?/?/R Increased fetal exposure after 20th week. ▶? Caution advised, but no known risks. $$$$$

WARNING — Increased risk of serious infections (e.g., TB, sepsis, invasive fungal and opportunistic infections); discontinue if a serious infection. Test for latent TB (and treat if present) before using a TNF-blocker; monitor for active TB during treatment. Lymphoma and other malignancies reported in children and adolescents; hepatosplenic T-cell lymphoma reported in adolescents and young adults with inflammatory bowel disease.

ADULT — RA, psoriatic arthritis, ankylosing spondylitis: 40 mg SC q 2 weeks, alone or in combination with methotrexate or other DMARD. May increase frequency to q week if not receiving methotrexate. Plaque psoriasis, non-infectious uveitis: 80 mg SC on day 1, 40 mg SC on day 8, then 40 mg SC q 2 weeks. Crohn's disease, ulcerative colitis: 160 mg SC on day 1, 80 mg SC on day 15, then 40 mg SC q 2 weeks starting on day 29. Only continue treatment in ulcerative colitis patients with evidence of clinical remission by week 8. Hidradenitis suppurativa: 160 mg SC on day 1, 80 mg on day 15, then 40 mg q week starting on day 29. Can give day 1 regimen as four 40 mg injections on day 1 or two 40 mg injections per day for 2 days. Inject SC into thigh or abdomen, rotating injection sites.

PEDS — Polyarticular JIA, age 2 yo or older: Give SC q 2 weeks at a dose of 10 mg for wt 10 to less than 15 kg; 20 mg for wt 15 to less than 30 kg; 40 mg for wt 30 kg or greater. Crohn's disease, age 6 yo or older: For wt 17 kg to less than 40 kg: 80 mg SC (two 40 mg injections) on day 1, then 40 mg SC 2 weeks later. Maintain with 20 mg SC q 2 weeks. For wt 40 kg and greater: 160 mg SC on day 1, then 80 mg SC (two 40 mg injections) 2 weeks later. Maintain with 40 mg SC q 2 weeks. Can give day 1 regimen as four 40 mg injections on day 1 or two 40 mg injections per day for 2 days. Inject SC into thigh or abdomen, rotating injection sites.

FORMS — Trade only: Single-use injection pen or syringe (2 per pack): 40 mg/0.8 mL. Crohn's disease/ulcerative colitis/hidradenitis suppurativa starter pack: Six 40 mg pens. Psoriasis/uveitis starter pack: Four 40 mg pens. Pediatric single-use syringe (2 per pack): 10 mg/0.2 mL, 20 mg/0.4 mL. Pediatric Crohn's disease starter pack: Three or six 40 mg/0.8 mL syringes.

NOTES — Do not coadminister other biologic DMARDs. Onset of response in RA in 2 to 4 weeks; effects may last up to 4 months after discontinuation. Infants with in utero adalimumab exposure may have altered immunity due to active placental transfer of the drug, esp in the 3rd trimester; the safety of administering live vaccines to infants with in utero adalimumab exposure is unclear. Leave Humira at room temperature for 15 to 30 min before injecting to reduce injection pain. Refrigerate Humira for storage and protect from light; may keep at room temperature for up to 14 days; dispose of Humira kept at room temperature for >14 days.

MOA — Human IgG1 monoclonal antibody against TNF-α. Blockade of TNF inhibits production of pro-inflammatory cytokines.

ADVERSE EFFECTS — Serious: Increased risk of serious infections, including sepsis, TB, opportunistic, and invasive fungal infections. Reactivation of hepatitis B infection. Increased risk of malignancies, esp lymphoma, in young people. New onset and exacerbation of heart failure and demyelinating disorders. Hematologic cytopenias. Serious hypersensitivity reactions. Increased transaminases. Autoantibodies and lupus-like syndrome. Frequent: Injection site reactions.

CERTOLIZUMAB (*Cimzia*) ▶K proteolysis ♀B Increased fetal exposure after 20th week. R ▶? $$$$$

WARNING — Increased risk of serious infections (e.g., TB, sepsis, invasive fungal and opportunistic infections); discontinue if a serious infection. Test for latent TB (and treat if present) before using a TNF-blocker; monitor for active TB during treatment. Lymphoma and other malignancies reported with TNF-blockers in children and adolescents, but certolizumab not indicated for children.

ADULT — Crohn's disease: 400 mg SC at 0, 2, and 4 weeks. Maintain with 400 mg SC q 4 weeks if response. RA, psoriatic arthritis: 400 mg SC at 0, 2, and 4 weeks. Maintain with 200 mg SC q 2 weeks; can consider 400 mg SC q 4 weeks. Ankylosing spondylitis: 400 mg at 0, 2 and 4 weeks, then 200 mg q 2 weeks or 400 mg q 4 weeks. Divide 400 mg dose into 2 separate 200 mg SC injections at different sites on thigh or abdomen. Rotate injection sites.

PEDS — Not approved for use in children.

FORMS — Trade only: Packs of 2 vials for reconstitution or 2 prefilled syringes, 200 mg/1 mL each. Starter pack of 6 syringes.

NOTES — Do not coadminister rituximab or natalizumab. Onset of response in RA in 2 to 4 weeks. Effects may last up to 5 months after discontinuation. Store in refrigerator and protect from light. Leave syringe at room temperature for about 30 minutes before injecting to reduce injection pain.

MOA — Fab antibody fragment against human TNF-α that is PEG-conjugated. Blockade of TNF inhibits production of pro-inflammatory cytokines.

ADVERSE EFFECTS — Serious: Increased risk of serious infections, including sepsis, TB, opportunistic, and invasive fungal infections. Reactivation of hepatitis B infection. Increased risk of malignancies, esp lymphoma, in young people. New onset and exacerbation of heart failure and demyelinating disorders. Hematologic cytopenias. Serious hypersensitivity reactions. Autoantibodies and lupus-like syndrome. Frequent: Rash, UTI, upper respiratory infection.

ETANERCEPTETANERCEPT-SZZS (*Enbrel, Erelzi*) ▸proteolysis ♀B Increased fetal exposure after 20th week. R ▶? $$$$$

WARNING — Increased risk of serious infections (e.g., TB, sepsis, invasive fungal and opportunistic infections); discontinue if a serious infection. Test for latent TB (and treat if present) before using a TNF-blocker; monitor for active TB during treatment. Lymphoma and other malignancies reported in children and adolescents.

ADULT — RA, psoriatic arthritis, ankylosing spondylitis: 50 mg SC q week. Can use alone or with methotrexate for RA and psoriatic arthritis. Plaque psoriasis: 50 mg SC twice per week for 3 months, then 50 mg SC q week. Initial doses of 25 or 50 mg SC q week can also be used. Inject into thigh, abdomen, or outer upper arm. Rotate injection sites.

PEDS — JIA, age 2 yo or older: 0.8 mg/kg SC q week for wt less than 63 kg; 50 mg SC q week for wt of 63 kg or greater. Inject into thigh, abdomen, or outer upper arm. Rotate injection sites. Use 50 mg autoinjector only if wt is 63 kg or greater. Multi-dose vial recommended for mg/kg doses.

UNAPPROVED PEDS — Plaque psoriasis, age 4 to 17 yo: 0.8 mg/kg (max dose 50 mg) SC q week. Inject into thigh, abdomen, or outer upper arm. Rotate injection sites.

FORMS — Trade only (Enbrel): Single-use prefilled syringe or autoinjector 50 mg/1 mL. Single-use prefilled syringe 25 mg/0.5 mL. Multidose vial 25 mg. Etanercept-szzs (Erelzi) is not available yet.

NOTES — Etanercept biosimilar (Erelzi; etanerceptszzs) and Enbrel are not interchangeable. Warn latex-sensitive patients that Enbrel needle cover contains latex. Refrigerate and protect from light; leave at room temperature for 15 to 30 minutes before injecting. In the US, autoinjector or syringes can be stored at room temperature for up to 14 days; discard after 14 days at room temperature.

MOA — Fusion protein of human p75 TNF-α receptor linked to Fc portion of human IgG1. Blockade of TNF inhibits production of pro-inflammatory cytokines. Etanercept-szzs is biosimilar to etanercept.

ADVERSE EFFECTS — Serious: Increased risk of serious infections, including sepsis, TB, opportunistic, and invasive fungal infections. Reactivation of hepatitis B infection. Increased risk of malignancies, esp. lymphoma, in young people. New onset and exacerbation of heart failure and demyelinating disorders. Hematologic cytopenias. Serious hypersensitivity reactions. Autoantibodies and lupus-like syndrome. Frequent: Infections; injection site reactions.

GOLIMUMAB (*Simponi, Simponi Aria*) ▸? ♀B Increased fetal exposure after 20th week. ▶– $$$$$

WARNING — Increased risk of serious infections (e.g., TB, sepsis, invasive fungal and opportunistic infections); discontinue if a serious infection. Test for latent TB (and treat if present) before using a TNF-blocker; monitor for active TB during treatment. Lymphoma and other malignancies reported in children and adolescents with TNF-blockers, but golimumab not indicated in children.

ADULT — RA, psoriatic arthritis, ankylosing spondylitis: 50 mg SC q month. IV regimen (Simponi Aria) for RA: 2 mg/kg IV infused over 30 minutes at weeks 0 and 4, then q 8 weeks. Use IV/SC golimumab with methotrexate to treat RA. Ulcerative colitis: 200 mg SC at week 0, 100 mg SC at week 2, then 100 mg SC q 4 weeks. Give SC injection in thigh, abdomen, or upper outer arm. Rotate injection sites. Give at separate sites if a dose requires more than 1 injection.

PEDS — Not approved for use in children.

FORMS — Trade only: Single-dose autoinjector or prefilled syringe: 50 mg/0.5 mL, 100 mg/1 mL.

NOTES — Do not use with other biologics to treat RA, psoriatic arthritis, or ankylosing spondylitis. Warn latex-sensitive patients that needle cover contains latex. Refrigerate for storage; leave at room temperature for 30 minutes before injection. Clinical response to golimumab is usually achieved within 14 to 16 weeks.

MOA — Monoclonal antibody against human TNF-α. Blockade of TNF inhibits production of pro-inflammatory cytokines.

ADVERSE EFFECTS — Serious: Increased risk of serious infections, including sepsis, TB, opportunistic, and invasive fungal infections. Reactivation of hepatitis B infection. Increased risk of malignancies, esp lymphoma, in young people. New onset and exacerbation of heart failure and demyelinating disorders. Hematologic cytopenias. Serious hypersensitivity reactions. Increased transaminases. Autoantibodies and lupus-like syndrome. Frequent: upper respiratory infections, nasopharyngitis, injection site reactions.

INFLIXIMABINFLIXIMAB-DYYB (*Remicade, Inflectra*) ▸proteolysis ♀B Increased fetal exposure after 20th week. ▶? $$$$$

WARNING — Increased risk of serious infections (e.g., TB, sepsis, invasive fungal and opportunistic infections); discontinue if a serious infection. Test for latent TB (and treat if present) before using a TNF-blocker; monitor for active TB during treatment. Lymphoma and other malignancies reported in children and adolescents; hepatosplenic T-cell lymphoma reported in adolescents and young adults with inflammatory bowel disease.

ADULT — RA, with methotrexate: 3 mg/kg IV at weeks 0, 2, and 6. Maintain with 3 mg/kg IV q 8 weeks. For incomplete response, can increase dose to max of 10 mg/kg or reduce dosing interval to as short as q 4 weeks. Ankylosing spondylitis: 5 mg/kg IV at weeks 0, 2, and 6. Maintain with 5 mg/kg IV q 6 weeks. Plaque psoriasis, psoriatic arthritis: 5 mg/kg IV at weeks 0, 2, and 6. Maintain with 5 mg/kg IV q 8 weeks. Crohn's disease, moderate to severe or fistulizing; ulcerative colitis: 5 mg/kg IV at weeks 0, 2, and 6. Maintain with 5 mg/kg IV q 8 weeks. For Crohn's disease: Consider discontinuing if no response by week 14; consider increasing to

(cont.)

INFLIXIMABINFLIXIMAB-DYYB (*cont.*)

10 mg/kg in patients who respond and then lose response. Infuse IV over 2 h or more.

PEDS — Ulcerative colitis, Crohn's disease, age 6 yo or older: 5 mg/kg IV infusion at weeks 0, 2, and 6. Maintain with 5 mg/kg IV q 8 weeks. Infuse IV over 2 h or more.

UNAPPROVED PEDS — JIA, with methotrexate, age 4 yo or older: 3 to 6 mg/kg IV at weeks 0, 2, and 6. Maintain with 3 to 6 mg/kg IV q 8 weeks. Infuse IV over 2 h or more.

FORMS — Infliximab-dyyb (Inflectra) is not available yet.

NOTES — Infliximab biosimilar (Inflectra; infliximab-dyyb) and Remicade are not interchangeable. Consider antihistamines, acetaminophen, and/ or corticosteroids to prevent infusion reactions. Three cases of toxic optic neuropathy reported. Hepatotoxicity (rare); discontinue if LFTs more than 5 times upper limit of normal. For infants exposed to infliximab in utero, live vaccines should not be administered for at least 6 months after birth in order to avoid the risk of life-threatening secondary infection.

MOA — Chimeric mouse-human monoclonal antibody against human TNF. Blockade of TNF inhibits production of pro-inflammatory cytokines. Infliximab-dyyb is biosimilar to infliximab.

ADVERSE EFFECTS — Serious: Increased risk of serious infections, including sepsis, TB, opportunistic, and invasive fungal infections. Reactivation of hepatitis B infection. Increased risk of malignancies, esp lymphoma, in young people. New onset and exacerbation of heart failure and demyelinating disorders. Hematologic cytopenias. Serious hypersensitivity reactions. Increased transaminases. Autoantibodies and lupus-like syndrome. Hepatotoxicity. Optic neuropathy (rare). Frequent: Upper respiratory infections, sinusitis, pharyngitis, infusion-related reactions, headache, abdominal pain.

RHEUMATOLOGY: Biologic Response Modifiers—Other

ABATACEPT (❋*Orencia*) ▶serum ♀?/?/?. R ▶– $$$$$

ADULT — RA, moderate to severe. IV regimen: Infuse IV over 30 minutes at weight-based dose of 500 mg for wt less than 60 kg, 750 mg for 60 to 100 kg, 1000 mg for greater than 100 kg. Give additional IV doses at weeks 2 and 4, then q 4 weeks. SC regimen: 125 mg SC once weekly after optional initial IV dose. Give 1st SC dose within 1 day of initial IV dose. For patients transitioning from IV regimen, give first SC dose when the next IV dose is due. Give SC injection in thigh or abdomen, or by caregiver in outer area of upper arm. Rotate injection sites.

PEDS — JIA, moderate to severe, age 6 yo or older: 10 mg/kg IV infused over 30 minutes. Give additional IV doses at weeks 2 and 4, and q 4 weeks thereafter. Use adult dose if weight 75 kg or greater (max 1000 mg per IV dose).

FORMS — Trade only: Prefilled single-dose syringe or autoinjector 125 mg/1 mL.

NOTES — Do not coadminister TNF-blockers, other biologic DMARDs, or tofacitinib. May increase risk of infection in patients at risk for recurrent infections; discontinue if serious infection. Test for latent TB (treat if present) before use. Can reactivate HBV infection; screen for at baseline and refer to AGA guideline (www.gastro.org) for management. Do not give live vaccines during or for 3 months after treatment. Bring immunizations up to date before starting abatacept. Adverse events more frequent in patients with COPD; monitor for exacerbations and pulmonary infections. Maltose in IV abatacept can falsely increase blood glucose readings on the day of infusion with glucose monitoring systems that use test strips containing glucose dehydrogenase pyrroloquinoline quinone (GDH-PQQ). Store in the refrigerator and protect from light. Leave at room temperature for 30 to 60 mins before injecting to reduce injection pain.

MOA — Soluble fusion protein composed of extracellular domain of T-lymphocyte-associated antigen 4 linked to Fc portion of human IgG1. A selective costimulation modulator that inhibits T-cell activation.

ADVERSE EFFECTS — Serious: Increased risk of infection. More frequent respiratory adverse events in patients with COPD. Hypersensitivity (reported with IV infusion). Frequent: Headache, nausea, pharyngitis, upper respiratory infection.

ANAKINRA (*Kineret*) ▶K ♀B ▶? $$$$$

ADULT — RA: 100 mg SC daily, alone or in combination with other DMARDs, except TNF-blockers. Neonatal-onset multisystem inflammatory disease: 1 to 2 mg/kg SC daily, titrated in 0.5 to 1 mg/kg increments to max of 8 mg/kg/day. Inject SC into thigh, abdomen, outer upper arm, or upper outer area of buttocks. Rotate injection sites.

PEDS — Neonatal-onset multisystem inflammatory disease: 1 to 2 mg/kg SC daily, titrated in 0.5 to 1 mg/kg increments to max of 8 mg/kg/day. Inject SC into thigh, abdomen, outer upper arm, or upper outer area of buttocks. Rotate injection sites.

UNAPPROVED ADULT — Refractory acute gout: 100 mg SC daily for 3 days.

UNAPPROVED PEDS — JIA: Initial dose of 1 to 2 mg/ kg (max 100 mg) SC once daily. Inject SC into thigh, abdomen, outer upper arm, or upper outer area of buttocks.

FORMS — Trade only: Prefilled graduated syringe 100 mg/0.67 mL.

NOTES — Contraindicated if hypersensitivity to E. coli-derived proteins. Increased incidence of serious infections. Do not use in active infection or with TNF-blockers, other biologic DMARDs, or tofacitinib.

(cont.)

ANAKINRA (*cont.*)

Can cause neutropenia; monitor neutrophil counts q month for 3 months, then q 3 months for up to 1 year. Avoid live vaccines. Graduated syringes can provide doses between 20 and 100 mg. Store in refrigerator and protect from light. Leave at room temperature for 30 minutes before injecting to reduce injection pain. Dosage adjustment for CrCl <30 mL/min: Consider giving every other day.

MOA — Recombinant interleukin-1 receptor antagonist (IL-1 ra).

ADVERSE EFFECTS — Serious: Increased risk of serious infection; neutropenia,hypersensitivity reactions. Frequent: Injection site reaction.

CANAKINUMAB (*Ilaris*) ▶? ♀?/?/? Increased fetal exposure expected after 20th week. ▶? $$$$$

ADULT — Cryopyrin-associated periodic syndromes (familial cold autoinflammatory syndrome, Muckle-Wells syndrome): 150 mg SC q 8 weeks.

PEDS — Systemic JIA, age 2 yo or older and wt 7.5 kg or greater: 4 mg/kg up to 300 mg SC q 4 weeks. Cryopyrin-associated periodic syndromes (familial cold autoinflammatory syndrome, Muckle-Wells syndrome), age 4 yo or older: 150 mg SC q 8 weeks for wt greater than 40 kg; 2 mg/kg SC q 8 weeks, increasing to 3 mg/kg q 8 weeks if inadequate response for wt 15 to 40 kg.

NOTES — Increased risk of serious infections; do not use during treatment of active infection or coadminister a TNF-blocker. May increase the risk of TB; screen for active/latent TB (and treat if present) before use. Avoid live vaccines. Monitor for macrophage activation syndrome, especially in systemic JIA.

MOA — Recombinant monoclonal antibody against interleukin-1 beta, a pro-inflammatory cytokine.

ADVERSE EFFECTS — Serious: Increased risk of serious infections, including upper respiratory and opportunistic infections, and possibly TB. Possible increased risk of malignancy due to immunosuppression. Frequent: nasopharyngitis, diarrhea, influenza, headache, nausea, abdominal pain, injection site reactions. Decreased WBC, increased transaminases and slightly increased bilirubin.

RITUXIMAB (*Rituxan*) ▶? ♀C ▶— $$$$$

WARNING — Life-threatening infusion reactions, especially with first infusion. Monitor closely. Discontinue if severe reaction and treat grade 3 and 4 infusion reactions. Can cause life-threatening mucocutaneous reactions and progressive multifocal leukoencephalopathy; discontinue if these occur. Can cause life-threatening HBV reactivation. Screen for HBV infection before use. Monitor for HBV reactivation during and after treatment; discontinue rituximab and concomitant chemotherapy if it occurs and refer to AGA guideline (www.gastro.org) for management. Can cause tumor lysis syndrome in NHL; use IV hydration and anti-hyperuricemic drugs in high-risk patients.

ADULT — RA, in combination with methotrexate: 1000 mg IV infusion weekly for 2 doses q 24

weeks. Premedicate with acetaminophen and antihistamine. Give methylprednisolone 100 mg IV 30 minutes before infusion. Granulomatosis with polyangiitis (Wegener's), microscopic polyangiitis, in combination with corticosteroids: 375 mg/m² q week for 4 weeks. Chemotherapy doses vary by indication. Non-Hodgkin's lymphoma (NHL). A 90-minute infusion can be used starting at Cycle 2 for patients with NHL who did not experience a grade 3 or 4 infusion-related adverse reaction during Cycle 1. Do not use faster infusion in patients with clinically significant cardiovascular disease and high circulating lymphocyte counts (greater than 5000/mcL). Chronic lymphocytic leukemia (CLL), previously untreated and previously treated CD20-positive CLL, in combination with fludarabine and cyclophosphamide (FC).

PEDS — Not approved for use in children.

UNAPPROVED ADULT — Immune thrombocytopenic purpura (ITP), thrombotic thrombocytopenic purpura (TTP), multiple sclerosis, Hodgkin's lymphoma, systemic autoimmune diseases other than RA, steroid-refractory chronic graft-versus-host disease.

UNAPPROVED PEDS — Autoimmune hemolytic anemia.

NOTES — Can cause serious bacterial, fungal, and new or reactivated viral infections. If serious infection occurs, discontinue rituximab and treat infection. Monitor CBC q 2 to 4 months in patients with RA or granulomatosis/microscopic polyangiitis. Avoid live vaccines. Do not coadminister TNF-blockers, tofacitinib, or other biologic response modifiers in RA. Give non-live vaccines at least 4 weeks before rituximab in RA/polyangiitis patients.

MOA — Chimeric murine-human monoclonal antibody that binds to the CD20 antigen on the surface of B-cell precursors and mature B-lymphocytes.

ADVERSE EFFECTS — Serious: Life-threatening infusion reactions, hepatitis, hepatic failure, tumor lysis syndrome in non-Hodgkin's lymphoma (NHL), severe mucocutaneous reactions, progressive multifocal leukoencephalopathy, HBV reactivation, cardiac arrhythmias during or after infusion, nephrotoxicity in NHL, bowel obstruction and perforation (rituximab with chemotherapy), hypersensitivity, bone marrow suppression, infection. Frequent: Bone marrow suppression, infection, infusion reactions.

SECUKINUMAB (*Cosentyx*) ▶proteolysis ♀B ▶? $$$$$

ADULT — Plaque psoriasis, moderate to severe: 300 mg SC weekly for 5 weeks (weeks 0 to 4), then 300 mg SC q 4 weeks. A dose of 150 mg may be adequate for some patients. Each 300 mg dose is 2 injections of 150 mg SC at different sites. Psoriatic arthritis (± methotrexate), ankylosing spondylitis: 150 mg SC weekly for 5 weeks, then 150 mg q 4 weeks; can also give 150 mg SC q 4 weeks without loading regimen. Consider 300 mg dose for continued active psoriatic arthritis. Give SC injection in thigh, abdomen, or upper outer arm.

PEDS — Safety and efficacy not established in children.

(cont.)

SECUKINUMAB (*cont.*)

FORMS — Trade only: 150 mg/mL prefilled syringe or pen. 150 mg vial for reconstitution by healthcare provider.

NOTES — Dose-dependent risk of infection; caution advised if history of serious or recurrent infections; hold during treatment for serious infection. Screen for TB before use; monitor for TB during using. Do not use if active TB; start treatment for latent TB before secukinumab. Can exacerbate inflammatory bowel disease (IBD); may increase risk of new-onset IBD; monitor for signs and symptoms of IBD. Can cause anaphylaxis. Cap of pen/prefilled syringe contains latex. Avoid live vaccines; non-live vaccines are acceptable. Store in refrigerator and protect from light. Allow soln to reach room temperature (15 to 30 minutes) before giving a dose.

MOA — Recombinant monoclonal IgG1 antibody that is an interleukin-17A antagonist; inhibits release of pro-inflammatory cytokines.

ADVERSE EFFECTS — Serious: Increased risk of infections, including serious infections; new onset or exacerbation of inflammatory bowel disease; anaphylaxis and urticariua. Frequent: Nasopharyngitis, diarrhea, upper respiratory tract infections.

SILTUXIMAB (*Sylvant*) ▶unknown ♀C ▶– $$$$$

ADULT — Multicentric Castleman's disease, HIV-negative and herpesvirus-8 negative: 11 mg/kg infused IV over 1 h q 3 weeks until treatment failure. Can cause serious infusion reactions; administer in a facility with resuscitation equipment, drugs, and personnel trained to provide resuscitation. Discontinue if signs/symptoms of anaphylaxis. Stop infusion if mild/moderate infusion reaction; consider restarting at a slower rate if reaction resolves. Consider giving antihistamines, corticosteroids, and acetaminophen. Discontinue if infusion is not tolerated after these interventions.

PEDS — Safety and efficacy not established in children.

NOTES — Monitor hematologic indices before each dose for the first year and q 3 doses thereafter. Consider delaying treatment if ANC <1 × 10⁹/L, platelet count <75 × 10⁹/L, or Hg >17 g/L. May mask signs and symptoms of inflammation; monitor for infection and hold if severe infection develops. Discontinue if severe infusion/allergic reaction, anaphylaxis, or cytokine release syndrome. Avoid live vaccines. May cause GI perforation; use cautiously in at-risk patients. May increase CYP450 activity; monitor INR with warfarin, cyclosporine levels, and use oral contraceptives with caution.

MOA — Mouse-human monoclonal antibody that binds to human interleukin-6 (IL-6).

ADVERSE EFFECTS — Serious: Infusion reactions (back/chest pain, N/V, flushing, erythema, palpitations). Anaphylaxis. May cause GI perforation. Frequent: pruritus, weight gain, rash, hyperuricemia, upper respiratory infection.

TOCILIZUMAB (*Actemra*) ▶? ♀C ▶– $$$$$

WARNING — Increased risk of serious infections (e.g., TB, sepsis, invasive fungal and opportunistic infections); monitor and discontinue if a serious infection. Test for latent TB (and treat if present) before use; monitor for active TB during treatment.

ADULT — RA, moderate to severe with inadequate response to DMARD: 162 mg SC q 2 weeks titrated to q week based on clinical response for wt less than 100 kg; 162 mg SC q week for wt 100 kg or greater. IV regimen: 4 mg/kg IV q 4 weeks, increasing to 8 mg/kg (max 800 mg) IV q 4 weeks based on clinical response. Infuse over 1 h. Can be used alone or with other non-biologic DMARDs. See product labeling for dosage adjustments for elevated liver enzymes, low ANC, or low platelet count.

PEDS — Polyarticular JIA, age 2 yo or older: 10 mg/kg IV q 4 weeks for wt less than 30 kg; 8 mg/kg IV q 4 weeks for wt 30 kg or greater. Infuse over 1 h. Can be used alone or with methotrexate. Systemic JIA, age 2 yo or older: 12 mg/kg q 2 weeks for wt less than 30 kg; 8 mg/kg q 2 weeks for wt 30 kg or greater. Infuse over 1 hour. Can be used alone or with methotrexate. See product labeling for managing elevated liver enzymes, low ANC, or low platelet count.

FORMS — Trade only: 162 mg/0.9 mL prefilled single-use syringe.

NOTES — Can cause neutropenia, thrombocytopenia, and increased AST/ALT. Do not start tocilizumab if baseline ANC <2000, platelet count <100,000, or ALT/AST >1.5 times upper limit of normal. In adults with RA, monitor neutrophils, platelets, AST/ALT after 4 to 8 weeks of treatment, then q 3 months. For children, monitor neutrophils, platelets, ALT/AST at 2nd dose, then q 4 to 8 weeks for polyarticular JIA and q 2 to 4 weeks for systemic JIA. Can cause hyperlipidemia; monitor lipids after 4 to 8 weeks of treatment, then q 6 months. Monitor for signs of infection; do not give during active infection. May increase risk of GI perforation (esp. RA patients with history of diverticulitis). Avoid live vaccines. Not for use in active liver disease or impaired liver function.

MOA — Monoclonal antibody that is an interleukin-6 receptor antagonist.

ADVERSE EFFECTS — Serious: Neutropenia, thrombocytopenia, serious infections (TB, bacterial, viral, invasive fungal, opportunistic), anaphylaxis (rare). Reactivation of viral infections like herpes zoster. GI perforation, primarily as complication of diverticulitis in RA patients. May increase risk of malignancy. Possible risk of demyelinating disorders like multiple sclerosis. Frequent: upper respiratory tract infection, nasopharyngitis, headache, HTN, increased ALT, injection site reactions.

TOFACITINIB (*Xeljanz, Xeljanz XR*) ▶LK ♀C ▶– $$$$$

WARNING — Increased risk of serious infections (e.g., TB, sepsis, invasive fungal and opportunistic infections); monitor and hold during serious infection until controlled. Test for latent TB (and treat if present) before use; monitor for active TB

(cont.)

TOFACITINIB (*cont.*)

during treatment. Lymphoma and other malignancies reported. Increased rate of Epstein Barr Virus–associated post-transplant lymphoproliferative disorder in renal transplant patients treated with both tofacitinib and immunosuppressive drugs.

ADULT — RA: 5 mg PO two times per day or Xeljanz XR 11 mg PO once daily. Reduce to 5 mg PO once daily if given with fluconazole, strong CYP3A4 inhibitor, or combination of moderate CYP3A4 inhibitor and strong CYP2C19 inhibitor (see P450 isozyme table). Dosage adjustments for lymphopenia, neutropenia, and anemia in product labeling. Do not crush, split, or chew Xeljanz XR. Indicated for moderate to severe RA with inadequate response or intolerance to methotrexate. For use as monotherapy or in combination with methotrexate or another nonbiologic DMARD.

PEDS — Not approved in children.

FORMS — Trade only: Tabs 5 mg. Extended-release tabs 11 mg.

NOTES — Can cause lymphopenia, neutropenia, anemia, increased LFTs, hyperlipidemia, and may increase risk of GI perforation (esp. if history of diverticulitis). Increased risk of viral reactivation, esp. herpes zoster in Japan. Do not start tofacitinib if baseline ANC <1000, absolute lymphocyte count <500, or Hg <9 mg/dL. Monitor lymphocyte count at baseline and q 3 months. Monitor ANC and hemoglobin at baseline, after 4 to 8 weeks of treatment, then q 3 months. Monitor LFTs routinely. Monitor lipids after 4 to 8 weeks of treatment. Refer to product labeling for dosage adjustments for lymphopenia, neutropenia, or anemia. Do not coadminister biologic DMARDs or potent immunosuppressants like cyclosporine or azathioprine. Avoid live vaccines. Do not coadminister strong CYP3A4 inducers (carbamazepine, phenobarbital, phenytoin, rifampin, rifapentine, St. John's wort). Dosage reduction for moderate/severe renal impairment or moderate hepatic impairment: 5 mg PO once daily.

MOA — Janus kinase (JAK) inhibitor. JAKs activate Signal Transducers and Activators of Transcription (STATs) in an intracellular cytokine signaling pathway. Inhibition of JAK 1 and 3 by tofacitinib blocks production of inflammatory mediators and suppresses STAT1-dependent genes in joint tissue.

ADVERSE EFFECTS — Serious: Serious infections, including TB and reactivation of viral infections like herpes zoster. May increase risk of lymphoma, other malignancies, and non-melanoma skin cancers. Increased rate of Epstein Barr Virus-associated post-transplant lymphoproliferative disorder in renal transplant patients treated with both tofacitinib and immunosuppressive drugs. May increase risk of GI perforation (esp if history of diverticulitis). Lymphocytopenia, neutropenia, anemia, hyperlipidemia, and increased LFTs. Frequent: Upper respiratory tract infections, headache, diarrhea, nasopharyngitis.

RHEUMATOLOGY: Disease-Modifying Antirheumatic Drugs (DMARDs)

AZATHIOPRINE (*Azasan, Imuran, AZA*) ▶LK ♀D ▶– $$$

WARNING — Chronic immunosuppression with azathioprine increases the risk of neoplasia, including lymphoma and skin malignancies. May cause marrow suppression or GI hypersensitivity reaction characterized by severe N/V.

ADULT — Severe RA: Initial dose 1 mg/kg (50 to 100 mg) PO daily or divided two times per day. Increase by 0.5 mg/kg/day at 6 to 8 weeks; if no serious toxicity and if initial response is unsatisfactory, can then increase thereafter at 4-week intervals. Max dose 2.5 mg/kg/day. In patients with clinical response, use the lowest effective dose for maintenance therapy. Prevention of rejection after renal transplant: Individualized dosing with initial dose of 3 to 5 mg/kg IV/PO daily; usual maintenance dose of 1 to 3 mg/kg PO daily.

PEDS — Not approved in children.

UNAPPROVED ADULT — Crohn's disease: 50 to 100 mg PO daily or 2 to 3 mg/kg/day PO. Myasthenia gravis, multiple sclerosis: 2 to 3 mg/kg/day PO. Behcet's syndrome: 2.5 mg/kg/day PO. Vasculitis: 2 mg/kg/day PO. Ulcerative colitis: 1.5 to 2.5 mg/kg/day PO. Lupus nephritis: 2 mg/kg/day PO.

UNAPPROVED PEDS — Prevention of rejection after renal transplant: Individualized dosing with usual doses ranging from 1 to 3 mg/kg/day PO.

FORMS — Generic/Trade (Imuran-$$$$$): Tabs 50 mg, scored. Trade only (Azasan-$$$$$): 75, 100 mg, scored.

NOTES — Monitor CBC q 1 to 2 weeks with dose changes, then q 1 to 3 months. Can cause severe myelosuppression in TPMT-deficient patients; consider TPMT testing, esp. if cytopenia does not respond to azathioprine dosage reduction. Dosage adjustments based on TPMT testing available at www.pharmgkb.org. Azathioprine toxicity increased by ACE inhibitors, allopurinol, febuxostat, and methotrexate. Reduce azathioprine dose by 66% to 75% if allopurinol coadministered; substantially greater dosage reduction required in TPMT-deficient patients. Azathioprine may decrease the activity of anticoagulants, cyclosporine, and neuromuscular blockers.

MOA — Immunosuppressant. Metabolized to 6-mercaptopruine.

ADVERSE EFFECTS — Serious: Bone marrow depression. Increased risk of serious infections. Increased risk of malignancy. GI hypersensitivity. Progressive multifocal leukencephalopathy. Frequent: Malaise, skin rash.

HYDROXYCHLOROQUINE (*Plaquenil, HCQ*) ▶K ♀C ▶+ $

WARNING — Clinicians should be knowledgeable about hydroxychloroquine product labeling before prescribing.

ADULT — Doses as hydroxychloroquine sulfate. RA: 400 to 600 mg PO daily to start. After clinical response, decrease to 200 to 400 mg PO daily. Discontinue if no objective improvement within 6 months. SLE: 400 mg PO one to two times per day to

(cont.)

HYDROXYCHLOROQUINE (cont.)

start. Decrease to 200 to 400 PO daily for prolonged maintenance. Malaria prophylaxis, chloroquine-sensitive areas: 400 mg PO q week from 1 to 2 weeks before exposure until 4 weeks after. Malaria treatment, chloroquine-sensitive areas: 800 mg PO once, then 400 mg at 6, 24, and 48 h (total dose of 2 g). Take with food or milk to improve GI tolerability.

PEDS — Doses as hydroxychloroquine base (200 mg hydroxychloroquine sulfate = 155 mg base). Malaria prophylaxis, chloroquine-sensitive areas: 5 mg/kg to max of 310 mg base PO q week from 1 to 2 weeks before exposure until 4 weeks after. Malaria treatment, chloroquine-sensitive areas: 10 mg/kg base PO once, then 5 mg/kg base at 6, 24, and 48 h. Take with food or milk to improve GI tolerability.

UNAPPROVED PEDS — JIA or SLE: 3 to 5 mg/kg/day, up to a max of 400 mg/day PO daily or divided two times per day. Max dose 7 mg/kg/day. Take with food or milk to improve GI tolerability.

FORMS — Generic/Trade: Tabs 200 mg hydroxychloroquine sulfate (200 mg sulfate equivalent to 155 mg base), scored.

NOTES — May exacerbate psoriasis or porphyria. Retinopathy (rare, but irreversible; risk related to dose and duration of use). Per American Academy of Ophthalmology, get baseline fundus exam in 1st year of use to detect preexisting maculopathy; add visual field and spectral-domain optical coherence tomography if maculopathy present. Begin annual screening after 5 years of use, or sooner if risk factors (dose >5 mg/kg/day real weight; renal disease; coadministration of tamoxifen; macular disease). Asian patients need wider screening patterns to detect extra-macular damage. See www.aao.org for details. Can cause anorexia, N/V. May increase digoxin and metoprolol levels.

MOA — Unclear in the treatment of RA.

ADVERSE EFFECTS — Serious: Retinopathy (rare but irreversible; risk related to dose and duration of use), angioedema, bronchospasm, exacerbation of psoriasis or porphyria. Frequent: Anorexia, N/V.

LEFLUNOMIDE (Arava, LEF) ▶LK ♀X/X/X. R ▶– $$$$$

WARNING — Hepatotoxicity, interstitial lung disease. Rare reports of lymphoma, pancytopenia, agranulocytosis, thrombocytopenia, Stevens-Johnson syndrome, cutaneous necrotizing vasculitis, and severe HTN. For women with childbearing potential, exclude pregnancy before starting and provide reliable contraception.

ADULT — RA. Optional loading dose: 100 mg PO daily for 3 days. Not for patients at risk of hepatotoxicity (e.g., taking methotrexate) or myelosuppression (e.g., taking an immunosuppressant). Maintenance dose: 10 to 20 mg PO daily.

PEDS — Not approved in children.

UNAPPROVED ADULT — Psoriatic arthritis: Optional loading dose: 100 mg PO daily for 3 days. Maintenance: 10 to 20 mg PO daily.

FORMS — Generic/Trade: Tabs 10, 20 mg. Trade only: Tabs 100 mg.

NOTES — Leflunomide half-life is 18 to 19 days, an important consideration for pregnancy, drug interactions, and vaccine administration. Omitting the loading dose may reduce risk of hematologic and hepatic toxicity. Avoid leflunomide in hepatic or renal insufficiency, severe immunodeficiency, bone marrow dysplasia, or severe infections. Consider interruption of therapy if serious infection occurs and administer cholestyramine (see below). Monitor LFTs, CBC, and creatinine monthly until stable, then q 1 to 2 months. Avoid in men wishing to father children. Avoid live vaccines. May increase INR with warfarin; check INR within 1 to 2 days of initiation, then weekly for 2 to 3 weeks and adjust the dose accordingly. Rifampin increases and cholestyramine decreases leflunomide levels. Accelerated elimination procedure: Give charcoal or cholestyramine in cases of overdose, serious adverse event, or a woman becomes or wants to become pregnant. Initiate procedure as soon as pregnancy is detected. Cholestyramine: 8 g PO three times per day for up to 11 days. Activated charcoal susp: 50 g PO or NG q 6 h for 24 h. Administration on consecutive days is not necessary unless rapid elimination desired. Repeat cholestyramie and/or charcoal if 2 teriflunomide levels taken at least 14 days apart are 0.02 mg/L or greater.

MOA — Immunosuppressant that inhibits pyrimidine synthesis.

ADVERSE EFFECTS — Serious: Lymphoma, pancytopenia, Stevens-Johnson Syndrome, hepatotoxicity, interstitial lung disease, cutaneous necrotizing vasculitis. Frequent: Diarrhea.

METHOTREXATE—RHEUMATOLOGY (Otrexup, Rasuvo, Rheumatrex, Trexall, MTX) ▶LK ♀X ▶– $$

WARNING — Deaths have occurred from hepatotoxicity, pulmonary disease, intestinal perforation, and marrow suppression. According to the manufacturer, use is restricted to patients with severe, recalcitrant, disabling rheumatic disease unresponsive to other therapy. Contraindicated in pregnancy due to risk of fetal harm. After discontinuation of methotrexate, men should wait at least 3 months and women at least 1 ovulatory cycle before attempting to conceive. Use with extreme caution in renal insufficiency. Folate deficiency may increase toxicity. The ACR recommends supplementation with 1 mg/day of folic acid.

ADULT — Severe RA: Initial dose of 7.5 mg PO/SC once weekly. Alternative regimen: 2.5 mg PO q 12 h for 3 doses given as a course once weekly. May increase dose gradually to max of 20 mg/week. After clinical response, reduce to lowest effective dose. Severe psoriasis: 10 to 25 mg PO/SC/IV/IM once weekly until response, then decrease to lowest effective dose. Max usual dose is 30 mg/week. Supplement with 1 mg/day of folic acid. When converting between PO and SC administration, consider that SC administration has higher bioavailability. Give SC injection in abdomen or thigh.

PEDS — Severe JIA: 10 mg/m^2 PO/SC q week. When converting between PO and SC administration,

(cont.)

METHOTREXATE—RHEUMATOLOGY (*cont.*)
consider that SC administration has higher bio-availability. Give SC injection in abdomen or thigh. UNAPPROVED ADULT — Polymyalgia rheumatica: 7.5 to 10 mg PO q week with folic acid 7.5 mg/week. Early ectopic pregnancy: 50 mg/m^2 IM single dose.
FORMS — Trade only (Trexall): Tabs 5, 7.5, 10, 15 mg. Dose Pak (Rheumatrex) 2.5 mg (# 8, 12, 16, 20, 24). Generic/Trade: Tabs 2.5 mg, scored. Trade only: Single-dose SC auto-injectors. Otrexup: 7.5, 10, 12.5, 15, 17.5, 20, 22.5, 25 mg/0.4 mL. Rasuvo: 7.5, 10, 12.5, 15, 17.5, 20, 22.5, 25, 27.5, 30 mg (volume ranges from 0.15 to 0.6 mL).
NOTES — Contraindicated in pregnant and lactating women, alcoholism, liver disease, immunodeficiency, blood dyscrasias. Monitor CBC q month, liver and renal function q 1 to 3 months. Beware of medication errors in which intended weekly doses of methotrexate are given daily. Can cause dizziness and fatigue which can impair driving ability.
MOA — Immunosuppressant, antimetabolite.
ADVERSE EFFECTS — Serious: Hepatotoxicity, pulmonary disease, lymphoma, bone marrow suppression, intestinal perforation. Frequent: Increased LFTs, diarrhea, stomatitis, bone marrow suppression.

SULFASALAZINE—RHEUMATOLOGY (*Azulfidine, Azulfidine EN-tabs, ✲Salazopyrin EN-tabs*) ▶L ♀B ▶? $$
WARNING — Beware of hypersensitivity, marrow suppression, renal and liver damage, central nervous system effects, irreversible neuromuscular and CNS changes, fibrosing alveolitis.

ADULT — RA: 500 mg PO two times per day after meals to start. Increase to 1 g PO two times per day.
PEDS — JIA, age 6 yo or older, EN-tabs: Initial dose of 10 mg/kg/day, increasing to 30 to 50 mg/kg/day (max 2 g/day) PO divided two times per day. Safety and efficacy not established for age younger than 2 yo.
UNAPPROVED ADULT — Ankylosing spondylitis with peripheral arthritis: 500 mg PO once daily for 1st week, 500 mg PO two times per day for 2nd week, then slowly titrated to max of 3 g/day. Psoriasis: Initial dose of 500 mg PO two times per day increased up to 3 to 4 g/day as tolerated. Psoriatic arthritis: 1 g PO two times per day.
FORMS — Generic/Trade: Tabs 500 mg, scored. Enteric-coated, delayed-release (EN-tabs) 500 mg.
NOTES — Avoid with hepatic or renal dysfunction, intestinal or urinary obstruction, porphyria, or sulfonamide or salicylate sensitivity. Monitor CBC q 2 to 4 weeks for 3 months, then q 3 months. Monitor LFTs and renal function. Oligospermia and infertility, and photosensitivity may occur. May decrease folic acid, digoxin, cyclosporine, and iron levels. May turn body fluids, contact lenses, or skin orange-yellow. Enteric-coated (Azulfidine EN, Salazopyrin EN) tabs may cause fewer GI adverse effects. Supplement with folic acid during pregnancy. Reports of bloody stools or diarrhea in breastfed infants of mothers taking sulfasalazine.
ADVERSE EFFECTS — Serious: Agranulocytosis, hemolytic anemia, nephro/hepatotoxicity, hepatic failure, drug rash and other severe skin reactions, hypersensitivity, anaphylaxis, angioedema, neural tube defect, reversible male infertility. Frequent: Nausea, dyspepsia, rash.

RHEUMATOLOGY: Gout-Related—Xanthine Oxidase Inhibitors

ALLOPURINOL (*Aloprim, Zyloprim*) ▶K ♀C ▶+ $
ADULT — Prevention of recurrent gout: 100 mg PO daily initially, titrating weekly in 100 mg increments to target serum uric acid <6 mg/dL. Usual dose is 200 to 300 mg/day for mild gout, 400 to 600 mg/day for moderate gout. Maximum dose is 800 mg/day. Divide doses greater than 300 mg/day. Prevention of recurrent urinary calcium oxalate stones: Initial dose of 100 mg PO daily; usual dose is 200 to 300 mg/day. Titrate dose based on 24-h urinary urate levels. Prevention of tumor lysis syndrome in patients unable to tolerate PO: 200 to 400 mg/m^2/day IV as single infusion or in equally divided infusions q 6 to 12 h. Max 600 mg/day. Initiate 24 to 48 h before chemotherapy. To improve tolerability, take PO allopurinol after meals.
PEDS — Prevention of tumor lysis syndrome: 150 mg PO daily for age younger than 6 yo; 300 mg PO daily for age 6 to 10 yo. Evaluate response after 48 h and adjust dose. Prevention of tumor lysis syndrome in patients unable to tolerate PO: Initial dose of 200 mg/m^2/day IV as single infusion or in equally divided infusions q 6 to 12 h. Initiate 24 to 48 h before chemotherapy. To improve tolerability, take PO allopurinol after meals.

UNAPPROVED ADULT — Prevention of gout, American College of Rheumatology recommendation: Initial dose of 100 mg PO daily, titrating upward q 2 to 5 weeks to achieve target serum urate level for individual patient (usually <6 mg/dL, but may be <5 mg/dL). Initial dose is 50 mg/day for CrCl <30 mL/min.
UNAPPROVED PEDS — Prevention of tumor lysis syndrome: 50 to 100 mg/m^2/dose PO q 8 h (max 300 mg/m^2/day) or 10 mg/kg/day PO divided q 8 h (max 800 mg/day). Prevention of tumor lysis syndrome in patients unable to tolerate PO: 200 to 400 mg/m^2/day IV in 1 to 3 divided doses (max 600 mg/day).
FORMS — Generic/Trade (Zyloprim-$$$$): Tabs 100, 300 mg.
NOTES — Sudden changes in serum urate may precipitate acute gout; consider prophylactic NSAIDs or colchicine during titration of allopurinol. Risk of allopurinol hypersensitivity syndrome increased by renal impairment; risk of rash increased by amoxicillin/ampicillin. Discontinue if rash or allergic symptoms; do not restart after severe rash. Increased risk of severe skin reactions in patients with HLA-B*58:01; avoid in patients known to have this genotype. Consider HLA-testing in Koreans with stage 3 or worse chronic kidney disease, Han Chinese, and Thai. Increased INR with warfarin. Reduce azathioprine or

(cont.)

ALLOPURINOL (*cont.*)

mercaptopurine dose by 66% to 75% and monitor CBC; substantially greater dosage reduction required in TPMT-deficient patients. Ensure hydration before IV administration. Dosage reduction of PO/IV allopurinol for renal insufficiency: 200 mg/day for CrCl 10 to 20 mL/min; 100 mg/day for CrCl 3 to 10 mL/min; 100 mg/day at extended intervals for CrCl <3 mL/min.

MOA — Inhibits xanthine oxidase, decreasing uric acid production.

ADVERSE EFFECTS — Serious: Hepatotoxicity, hypersensitivity reaction, severe rash, renal failure, mobilization gout, bone marrow depression. Frequent: Headache, peripheral neuropathy, rash, neuritis, somnolence, N/V, diarrhea, dyspepsia, abdominal pain, fever, myopathy.

FEBUXOSTAT (*Uloric*) ▶LK ♀C ▶? $$$$$

ADULT — Hyperuricemia with gout: Start 40 mg PO daily. After 2 weeks, if uric acid greater than 6 mg/dL may increase to 80 mg daily.

PEDS — Not approved in children.

FORMS — Trade only: Tabs 40, 80 mg.

NOTES — May precipitate acute gout; consider using NSAIDs or colchicine prophylactically for up to 6 months. Monitor LFTs at baseline and periodically, transaminase elevations reported. Do not use with azathioprine, mercaptopurine, or theophylline. May increase risk of thromboembolic events, monitor for cardiovascular events (MI, CVA). Caution in severe renal or hepatic impairment.

MOA — Inhibits xanthine oxidase, decreasing uric acid production.

ADVERSE EFFECTS — Serious: Thromboembolism, anaphylaxis, Stevens Johnson syndrome, rhabdomyolysis. aggressive psychotic behavior, interstitial nephritis, hepatic failure. Frequent: Transaminase elevations, nausea, arthralgia, rash, gout flare.

RHEUMATOLOGY: Gout-Related—Other

COLCHICINE: DOSAGE REDUCTIONS FOR COADMINISTRATION WITH INHIBITORS OF COLCHICINE METABOLISM

Usual colchicine dose	Colchicine dosage reduction for...		
	Strong CYP3A4 inhibitors[a]	Moderate CYP3A4 inhibitors[b]	P-glycoprotein inhibitors[c]
Prevention of gout flares: 0.6 mg PO two times per day	0.3 mg PO once daily	0.3 mg PO two times per day or 0.6 mg PO once daily	0.3 mg PO once daily
Prevention of gout flares: 0.6 mg PO once daily	0.3 mg PO once every other day	0.3 mg PO once daily	0.3 mg PO once every other day
Treatment of gout flares: 1.2 mg PO followed by 0.6 mg 1 hour later[d]	0.6 mg PO followed by 0.3 mg 1 hour later[d]	1.2 mg PO in a single dose[d]	0.6 mg PO in a single dose[d]
Familial Mediterranean Fever: Up to 1.2 to 2.4 mg/day PO	Up to 0.6 mg/day PO (can give as 0.3 mg two times per day)	Up to 1.2 mg/day PO (can give as 0.6 mg two times per day)	Up to 0.6 mg/day PO (can give as 0.3 mg two times per day)

Notes: Do not give colchicine to patients with renal or hepatic impairment who are taking a strong CYP3A4 or P-glycoprotein inhibitor. Do not treat gout flares with colchicine in patients already receiving it for prevention of gout flares and also receiving a CYP3A4 inhibitor. Dosage reductions of colchicine are recommended for patients who are currently taking or discontinued a CYP3A4 or P-glycoprotein inhibitor within the past 14 days. This table may not list all possible CYP3A4 and P-glycoprotein inhibitors that increase the risk of colchicine toxicity.

[a]**Strong CYP3A4 inhibitors**: atazanavir, clarithromycin, cobicistat (alone or in combination products), conivaptan, darunavir-ritonavir, fosamprenavir-ritonavir, indinavir, itraconazole, ketoconazole, lopinavir-ritonavir, nefazodone, nelfinavir, posaconazole, ritonavir, saquinavir-ritonavir, telithromycin, tipranavir-ritonavir, voriconazole.

[b]**Moderate CYP3A4 inhibitors**: aprepitant, ciprofloxacin, crizotinib, diltiazem, dronedarone, erythromycin, fluconazole, fosamprenavir (unboosted), grapefruit juice, imatinib, isavuconazole, netupitant (in Akynzeo) verapamil.

[c]**P-glycoprotein inhibitors**: cyclosporine, ranolazine.

[d]For colchicine treatment of gout flares, do not repeat earlier than 3 days.

(colchicine + probenecid) ▶KL ♀C ▶? $

ADULT — Chronic gouty arthritis: Start 1 tab PO daily for 1 week, then 1 tab PO two times per day.

PEDS — Not approved in children.

FORMS — Generic only: Tabs 0.5 mg colchicine + 500 mg probenecid.

NOTES — Maintain alkaline urine. Probenecid ineffective if CrCl <30 mL/min.

MOA — Combination product that reduces the inflammatory response to deposited crystals, diminishes phagocytosis and inhibits tubular reabsorption of uric acid.

ADVERSE EFFECTS — Serious: Peripheral neuritis, hepatotoxicity, renal failure, bone marrow depression with aplastic anemia, thrombocytopenia, purpura, myopathy, hypersensitivity, nephrotic syndrome, hemolytic anemia, mobilization gout. Frequent: Diarrhea, N/V, abdominal pain, dermatoses, hair loss, headache, anorexia, urinary frequency, sore gums, dizziness.

COLCHICINE (*Colcrys, Mitigare*) ▶L ♀C ▶? $$$$$

ADULT — Treatment of gout flares: 1.2 mg PO at signs of attack then 0.6 mg 1 h later. Do not repeat this regimen for 3 days. In patients already receiving colchicine for prevention of gout flares, give this regimen and resume prophylactic dose 12 h later. Prevention of gout flares: 0.6 mg PO one or two times per day. Max dose of 1.2 mg/day. Familial Mediterranean fever: 1.2 to 2.4 mg PO daily or divided two times per day, with dose titrated up or down in 0.3 mg/day increments. See table for colchicine dose reduction when given with strong/moderate CYP3A4 inhibitors or P-glycoprotein inhibitors.

PEDS — Familial Mediterranean fever: 0.3 to 1.8 mg PO daily or divided two times per day for age 4 to 6 yo; 0.9 to 1.8 mg daily or divided two times per day for age 6 to 12 yo; use adult dosage for age 12 yo or older. Prevention of gout flares, older than 16 yo: 0.6 mg PO one or two times per day. Max dose of 1.2 mg/day.

UNAPPROVED ADULT — Primary biliary cirrhosis: 0.6 mg PO two times per day. Acute pericarditis: 0.6 mg PO once daily for wt 70 kg or less; 0.6 mg PO two times per day for wt greater than 70 kg. Treat for 3 months in combination with ibuprofen or aspirin.

FORMS — Generic/Trade: Tabs 0.6 mg (Colcrys). Caps 0.6 mg (Mitigare).

NOTES — Coadministration of colchicine and P-glycoprotein or strong CYP3A4 inhibitors (including all HIV protease inhibitors, except unboosted fosamprenavir) is contraindicated in renal or hepatic impairment. Dosage reductions required for coadministration with strong or moderate CYP3A4 inhibitors or P-glycoprotein inhibitors (see table). Most effective when initiated on the 1st day of gouty arthritis. Do not treat gout flares with colchicine in patients with renal impairment who are already receiving colchicine for prevention of gout flares. Dosage adjustment for renal dysfunction.

Treatment of gout flares: Usual dose given no more frequently than q 2 weeks for CrCl <30 mL/min; 0.6 mg PO single dose given no more frequently than q 2 weeks for dialysis. Prevention of gout flares: 0.3 mg PO once daily initially with any dosage increase closely monitored for CrCl <30 mL/min; 0.3 mg PO two times per week with close monitoring for dialysis. Familial Mediterranean fever: 0.3 mg PO once daily initially with close monitoring for any dosage increase for CrCl <30 mL/min or dialysis.

MOA — Reduces the inflammatory response to deposited crystals, and diminishes phagocytosis.

ADVERSE EFFECTS — Serious: Peripheral neuritis, hepatotoxicity, renal failure, bone marrow depression, leukocytopenia, granulocytopenia, aplastic anemia, thrombocytopenia, purpura, myopathy, rhabdomyolysis, hypersensitivity. Frequent: Diarrhea, N/V, abdominal pain, dermatoses, hair loss.

LESINURAD (*Zurampic*) ▶L ♀?/?/? ▶? $$$$$

WARNING — Risk of acute renal failure increased with lesinurad monotherapy; use with xanthine oxidase inhibitor.

ADULT — Gout, added to allopurinol or febuxostat: 200 mg PO q morning with food and water, at the same time as xanthine oxidase inhibitor. Tell patients to drink at least 2 L of fluid daily. Not for monotherapy due to increased risk of acute renal failure. Not for use with allopurinol doses less than 300 mg/day (less than 200 mg/day if CrCl less than 60 mL/min). Provide gout flare prophylaxis when starting lesinurad.

PEDS — Safety and efficacy not established in children.

FORMS — Trade only: Tab 200 mg.

NOTES — Increased risk of renal adverse events: Monitor renal function at baseline and periodically, esp if CrCl is <60 mL/min or SrCr increases 1.5- to 2-fold over baseline; discontinue if CrCl is persistantly <45 mL/min or SrCr increase is >2-fold over baseline. Hold if sx of uric acid nephropathy. Contraindicated if CrCl <30 mL/min, ESRD, dialysis, kidney transplant recipient; tumor lysis syndrome; Lesch-Nyhan syndrome. Possible increase in major CVD events; causality unclear. Metabolized by CYP2C9; caution advised for CYP2C9 poor metabolizers or coadministration of moderate CYP2C9 inhibitors (e.g. amiodarone, fliuconazole). Weak CYP3A4 inducer; monitor for reduced efficacy of amlodipine, and sensitive CYP3A4 substrates. Use in renal/hepatic impairment: Not for CrCl <45 mL/min or severe hepatic impairment (Child-Pugh C).

MOA — Increases urinary uric acid excretion by inhibiting uric acid transporter 1 (URAT1) and organic anion transporter 4 (OAT4).

ADVERSE EFFECTS — Serious: Acute renal failure, esp with monotherapy; possible risk of acute uric acid nephropathy; possible increase in major CVD events. Frequent: Headache, influenza, SrCr increase, GERD.

PEGLOTICASE (*Krystexxa*) ▶? ♀C ▶? $$$$$
WARNING — Anaphylaxis and infusion reactions reported. Premedicate with antihistamines and corticosteroids and administer in a healthcare setting. Anaphylaxis and infusion reactions more common if loss of therapeutic response. Monitor uric acid levels before infusion and discontinue if greater than 6 mg/dL, especially if two consecutive levels greater than 6.
ADULT — Chronic gout (refractory): 8 mg IV infusion q 2 weeks. Administer over 120 minutes or longer.
NOTES — Gout flares frequent upon initiation. Recommend gout flare prophylaxis with NSAID or colchicine to start 1 week prior to therapy and continue for 6 months. Discontinue urate-lowering therapy. Contraindicated in G6PD deficiency due to risk of hemolysis and methemoglobinemia; screen those at high risk including those of African and Mediterranean ancestry.
MOA — Recombinant uricase which causes oxidation of uric acid
ADVERSE EFFECTS — Serious: anaphylaxis, delayed-type hypersensitivity, heart failure exacerbation, chest pain. Frequent: infusion reactions, gout flare, nausea, vomiting, constipation, bruising, nasopharyngitis.

PROBENECID ▶KL ♀B ▶? $
ADULT — Gout: 250 mg PO two times per day for 7 days, then 500 mg PO two times per day. May increase by 500 mg/day q 4 weeks not to exceed 2 g/day. Adjunct to penicillin: 2 g/day PO in divided doses.
PEDS — Adjunct to penicillin: In children 2 to 14 yo, use 25 mg/kg PO for initial dose, then 40 mg/kg/day divided four times per day. For wt greater than 50 kg, use adult dose. Contraindicated in children age younger than 2 yo.
FORMS — Generic only: Tabs 500 mg.
NOTES — Decrease dose if GI intolerance occurs. Maintain alkaline urine. Begin therapy 2 to 3 weeks after acute gouty attack subsides. Ineffective if CrCl <30 mL/min. Not recommended in combination with penicillin if renal impairment.
MOA — Inhibits tubular reabsorption of uric acid.
ADVERSE EFFECTS — Serious: Hepatotoxicity, nephrotic syndrome, hemolytic anemia, hypersensitivity, mobilization gout. Frequent: Headache, anorexia, N/V, urinary frequency, sore gums, dizziness.

RHEUMATOLOGY: Other

APREMILAST (*Otezla*) ▶L ♀C ▶? $$$$$
ADULT — Psoriatic arthritis, moderate to severe plaque psoriasis: Give PO 10 mg in am on day 1, 10 mg two times per day on day 2, 10 mg in am and 20 mg in pm on day 3, 20 mg two times per day on day 4, 20 mg in am and 30 mg in pm on day 5, 30 mg two times per day on day 6 and thereafter. Do not crush, split, or chew tabs.
PEDS — Safety and efficacy not established in children.
FORMS — Trade only: Tabs 30 mg. Two-week starter pack of 10, 20, and 30 mg tabs.
NOTES — May cause or worsen depression; monitor symptoms. May cause weight loss; monitor weight. Do not coadminister strong CYP450 inducers (eg, carbamazepine phenobarbital, phenytoin, rifampin, St. John's wort). Dosage adjustment for CrCl less than 30 mL/min: Give PO 10 mg PO q am for 3 days, then 20 mg q am for 2 days, then 30 mg q am thereafter.
MOA — Phosphodiesterase 4 inhibitor that down-regulates the inflammatory response.
ADVERSE EFFECTS — Serious: May cause or worsen depression. Weight loss (up to 10% of body weight). Frequent: Diarrhea, nausea, headache, weight loss.

BELIMUMAB (*Benlysta*) ▶? – ♀C ▶? $$$$$
ADULT — Systemic lupus erythematosus (SLE): 10 mg/kg IV infusion q 2 weeks for 1st 3 doses, then 10 mg/kg IV infusion q 4 weeks. Infuse over 1 h. Slow or hold infusion if symptoms of infusion reaction. Consider premedication to prevent reactions.
PEDS — Not approved in children.
NOTES — Use for autoantibody-positive SLE in patients on standard therapy. Do not give live vaccines during therapy. More deaths reported with belimumab than placebo during clinical trials. Use with caution in patients with chronic infections and consider stopping therapy if new serious infection develops; reports of serious or fatal infections. Reports of progressive multifocal leukoencephalopathy. Suicide and depression reported. Do not combine with biologic therapies or IV cyclophosphamide.
MOA — Human 1gG1 monoclonal antibody that is a B-lymphocyte stimulator-specific inhibitor (inhibits survival of B cells and the autoimmune response).
ADVERSE EFFECTS — Serious: Progressive multifocal leukoencephalopathy; acute hypersensitivity including anaphylaxis; non-acute hypersensitivity or infusion reactions. Frequent: nausea, diarrhea, itching, nasopharyngitis, pharyngitis, bronchitis, insomnia, pain in extremity, depression, migraine.

HYALURONATE (*Euflexxa, Gel-One, Hyalgan, Monovisc, Orthovisc, Supartz, ✱Neovisc, Neovisc [Single Dose])* ▶proteolysis ♀? ▶? $$$$$
WARNING — Do not inject extra-articularly; avoid the synovial tissues and cap. Do not use disinfectants containing benzalkonium chloride for skin preparation.
ADULT — OA (knee): Give by intra-articular injection with strict aseptic technique. Euflexxa: 2 mL q week for 3 weeks. Gel-One: 3 mL single-dose. Hyalgan: 2 mL q week for 3 to 5 weeks. Monovisc: 4 mL single-dose. Neovisc (Canada): 2 mL q week for 3 to 5 weeks. Neovisc single-dose (Canada): 6

(cont.)

HYALURONATE (*cont.*)

mL single-dose. Orthovisc: 2 mL q week for 3 or 4 weeks. Supartz: 2.5 mL q week for 3 to 5 weeks. Can inject local anesthetic SC before hyaluronate, but do not mix with hyaluronate.

PEDS — Not approved in children.

FORMS — Trade only: Euflexxa: 2 mL (10 mg/mL) prefilled syringe. Gel-One: 3 mL (10 mg/mL) prefilled syringe. Hyalgan: 2 mL (10 mg/mL) vial, prefilled syringe. Monovisc: 4 mL (22 mg/mL) prefilled syringe. Neovisc (Canada): 2 mL (10 mg/mL) prefilled syringe. Neovisc single-dose (Canada): 6 mL (10 mg/mL) prefilled syringe. Orthovisc: 2 mL (15 mg/mL) prefilled syringe. Supartz: 2.5 mL (10 mg/mL) prefilled syringe.

NOTES — For those who have failed conservative therapy. Caution in allergy to eggs, avian proteins, or feathers (except Euflexxa and Monovisc). Caution in cinnamon allergy for Gel-One. Remove synovial fluid or effusion before each injection. Knee pain and swelling most common side effects. Tell patients to avoid strenuous activity or prolonged weight bearing for 48 h after injection.

MOA — Improves viscoelasticity of synovial fluid. Euflexxia and Monovisc are derived from bacteria. Gel-one (cross-linked with cinnamic acid), Hyalgan, Neovisc (no avian protein), and Orthovisc are derived from rooster combs.

ADVERSE EFFECTS — Serious: Anaphylactic or anaphylactoid reactions; pseudoseptic reactions; joint infections. Frequent: Injection site pain; joint pain or swelling; local skin reactions.

HYLAN G-F 20 (***Synvisc, Synvisc-One***) ▶proteolysis ♀? ▶? $$$$$

WARNING — Do not inject extra-articularly; avoid the synovial tissues and cap. Do not use disinfectants containing benzalkonium chloride for skin preparation.

ADULT — OA (knee): Give by intra-articular injection with strict aseptic technique. Synvisc: 2 mL q week for 3 weeks. Synvisc-One: 6 mL single-dose. Can inject local anesthetic SC before hylan G-F 20, but do not mix with it.

PEDS — Not approved in children.

FORMS — Trade only: Synvisc: 2 mL (8 mg/mL) prefilled syringe; 3/pack. Synvisc-One: 6 mL (8 mg/mL) prefilled syringe.

NOTES — For those who have failed conservative therapy. Caution in allergy to eggs, avian proteins, or feathers. Remove synovial fluid or effusion before each injection. Knee pain and swelling most common side effects. Tell patients to avoid strenuous activity or prolonged weight bearing for 48 h after injection.

MOA — Cross-linked hyaluronate derivative (hylan A and B polymers derived from chicken combs); improves viscoelasticity of synovial fluid.

ADVERSE EFFECTS — Serious: Anaphylactic and anaphylactoid reactions; pseudoseptic reactions; joint infections. Frequent: Injection site pain; joint pain or swelling; local skin reactions.

TOXICOLOGY

ANTIDOTES

Toxin	Antidote/Treatment
acetaminophen	N-acetylcysteine
TCAs	sodium bicarbonate
arsenic, mercury	dimercaprol (BAL)
benzodiazepine	flumazenil
beta-blockers	glucagon
calcium channel blockers	calcium chloride, glucagon
cyanide	Cyanokit (hydroxocobalamin)
dabigatran	idarucizumab
digoxin	dig immune Fab
ethylene glycol	fomepizole
heparin	protamine
iron	deferoxamine
lead	BAL, EDTA, succimer
local anesthetics	intralipid
methanol	fomepizole
methemoglobin	methylene blue
opioids/opiates	naloxone
organophosphates	atropine + pralidoxime
warfarin	vitamin K, FFP

ACETYLCYSTEINE (***N-acetylcysteine, Mucomyst, Acetadote, ✦Parvolex***) ▶L ♀B ▸? $$$$
ADULT — Acetaminophen toxicity: Mucomyst: Loading dose 140 mg/kg PO or NG, then 70 mg/kg q 4 h for 17 doses. May be mixed in water or soft drink diluted to a 5% soln. Acetadote (IV): Loading dose 150 mg/kg in 200 mL of D5W infused over 60 min; maintenance dose 50 mg/kg in 500 mL of D5W infused over 4 h followed by 100 mg/kg in 1000 mL of D5W infused over 16 h.
PEDS — Acetaminophen toxicity: Same as adult dosing.
UNAPPROVED ADULT — Prevention of contrast-induced nephropathy: 600 to 1200 mg PO two times per day for 2 doses before procedure and 2 doses after procedure.
FORMS — Generic/Trade: Soln 10, 20%. IV (Acetadote).
NOTES — May be diluted with water or soft drink to a 5% soln; use diluted soln within 1 h. Repeat loading dose if vomited within 1 h. Critical ingestion-treatment interval for maximal protection against severe hepatic injury is between 0 and 8 h. Efficacy diminishes after 8 h and treatment initiation between 15 and 24 h post-ingestion yields limited efficacy. However, treatment should not be withheld, because the reported time of ingestion may not be correct. Anaphylactoid reactions usually occur 30 to 60 min after initiating infusion. Stop infusion, administer antihistamine or epinephrine, restart infusion slowly. If anaphylactoid reactions return or severity increases, then stop treatment.
MOA — Directly combines with the toxic acetaminophen metabolite as a glutathione substitute. Antioxidant believed to attenuate ischemic renal failure.
ADVERSE EFFECTS — Serious: Hypersensitivity, anaphylaxis, angioedema, bronchoconstriction, chest tightness. Frequent: Nausea, vomiting, disagreeable odor, generalized urticaria, rash, stomatitis, fever, rhinorrhea, drowsiness, clamminess, pruritus, tachycardia, hypertension, hypotension.

CHARCOAL (***activated charcoal, Actidose-Aqua, CharcoAid, EZ-Char, ✦Charcodate***) ▶Not absorbed ♀+ ▸+ $
ADULT — Gut decontamination: 25 to 100 g (1 to 2 g/kg or 10 times the amount of poison ingested) PO or NG as soon as possible. May repeat q 1 to 4 h prn at

(cont.)

CHARCOAL (*cont.*)

doses equivalent to 12.5 g/h. When sorbitol is coadministered, use only with the first dose if repeated doses are to be given.

PEDS — Gut decontamination: 1 g/kg for age younger than 1 yo; 10 to 25 g or 1 to 2 g/kg for age 1 to 12 yo PO or NG as soon as possible. Repeat doses in children have not been established, but half the initial dose is recommended. Repeat q 2 to 6 h prn. When sorbitol is coadministered, use only with the first dose if repeated doses are to be given.

FORMS — OTC/Generic/Trade: Powder 15, 30, 40, 120, 240 g. Soln 12.5 g/60 mL, 15 g/75 mL, 15 g/120 mL, 25 g/120 mL, 30 g/120 mL, 50 g/240 mL. Susp 15 g/120 mL, 25 g/120 mL, 30 g/150 mL, 50 g/240 mL. Granules 15 g/120 mL.

NOTES — Some products may contain sorbitol to improve taste and reduce GI transit time. Chocolate milk/powder may enhance palatability for pediatric use. Not usually effective for toxic alcohols (methanol, ethylene glycol, isopropanol), heavy metals (lead, iron, bromide), arsenic, lithium, potassium, hydrocarbons, and caustic ingestions (acids, alkalis). Mix powder with 8 ounces water. Greatest effect when administered within 1 h of ingestion.

MOA — Adsorbs substances therefore inhibiting GI absorption.

ADVERSE EFFECTS — Serious: Bronchiolitis obliterans, aspiration. Frequent: Vomiting, constipation, diarrhea, black stools, hypokalemia, hypernatremia.

DEFERIPRONE (✳*Ferriprox*) ▶glucuronidation — ♀D ▶– ©V $$$$$

WARNING — Ferriprox can cause agranulocytosis; neutropenia may precede this development. Measure the ANC before starting and monitor weekly. Interrupt Ferriprox if infection develops and monitor the ANC more frequently.

ADULT — Transfusional iron overload due to thalassemia syndromes when current chelation therapy is inadequate: 25 mg/kg, orally, three times per day for a total of 75 mg/kg/day. Max dose is 33 mg/kg three times per day for a total of 99 mg/kg/day.

PEDS — Not approved.

FORMS — 500 mg film-coated tabs with a functional score. Oral solution 100 mg/mL

NOTES — Contraindicated with pre-existing agranulocytosis or neutropenia. Advise patients taking Ferriprox to report immediately any symptoms indicative of infection. Inform patients that their urine might show a reddish/brown discoloration due to the excretion of the iron-deferiprone complex.

MOA — Binds with ferric ions(iron III) to form neutral 3:1 (deferiprone:iron) and has a lower affinity for copper, aluminum and zinc.

ADVERSE EFFECTS — Serious: agranulocytosis. Common: chromaturia, nausea, vomiting, abdominal pain, LFT increase, arthralgia and neutropenia.

DEFEROXAMINE (*Desferal*) ▶K ♀C ▶? $$$$$

ADULT — Chronic iron overload: 500 to 1000 mg IM daily and 2 g IV infusion (no faster than 15 mg/kg/h) with each unit of blood or 1 to 2 g SC daily (20 to 40 mg/kg/day) over 8 to 24 h via continuous infusion pump. Acute iron toxicity: IV infusion up to 15 mg/kg/h.

PEDS — Acute iron toxicity: IV infusion up to 15 mg/kg/h.

NOTES — Contraindicated in renal failure/anuria unless undergoing dialysis.

MOA — Chelates iron in serum, ferritin, and hemosiderin.

ADVERSE EFFECTS — Serious: Cataracts, neurotoxicity-related hearing loss, hypersensitivity, hypotension, ARDS. Frequent: Visual changes (decreased acuity; impaired peripheral, night, and color vision), red urine, generalized erythema, dysuria, abdominal pain, leg cramps, tachycardia, fever, skin rash.

DIMERCAPROL (*BAL in oil*) ▶KL ♀C ▶? $$$$$

ADULT — Contraindicated in peanut allergy. Mild arsenic or gold toxicity: 2.5 mg/kg IM four times per day for 2 days, then two times per day for 1 day, then daily for 10 days. Severe arsenic or gold toxicity: 3 mg/kg IM q 4 h for 2 days, then four times per day for 1 day, then two times per day for 10 days. Mercury toxicity: 5 mg/kg IM initially, then 2.5 mg/kg daily to two times per day for 10 days. Begin therapy within 1 to 2 h of toxicity. Acute lead encephalopathy: 4 mg/kg IM initially, then q 4 h. May reduce dose to 3 mg/kg IM for less severe toxicity. Deep IM injection needed. When used in combination regimen with IV calcium edetate, BAL should be given 4 hours prior to calcium edetate.

PEDS — Not approved in children.

UNAPPROVED PEDS — Same as adult dosing.

MOA — Chelates arsenic, gold, and mercury to promote fecal and urinary excretion of the complex.

ADVERSE EFFECTS — Contraindicated in peanut allergy. Serious: Hemolytic anemia, HTN, tachycardia, hypersensitivity. Frequent: N/V, headache, perioral burning sensation, feeling of constriction or pain (in throat, chest or hands), conjunctivitis, blepharospasm, rhinorrhea, salivation, burning penis sensation, sweating, abdominal pain, injection-site irritation, painful sterile abscess, anxiety, weakness.

DUODOTE (atropine + pralidoxime) ▶K ♀C ▶? $

ADULT — Organophosphate insecticide/nerve agent poisoning, mild symptoms: 1 injection in thigh. Severe symptoms: 3 injections in rapid succession (may administer through clothes).

PEDS — Not approved in children.

FORMS — Each auto-injector dose delivers atropine 2.1 mg + pralidoxime 600 mg.

MOA — Atropine is to reverse muscarinic toxicity. Pralidoxime reactives acetylcholinesterase deactivated by organophosphate nerve agents or insecticide.

ADVERSE EFFECTS — Serious: Hyperthermia, anticholinergic syndrome, myocardial ischemia. Frequent: Anticholinergic syndrome, hypertension, diplopia, dizziness.

EDETATE (*EDTA, Endrate, versenate*) ▶K ♀C ▶– $$$
WARNING — Rapid IV infusions may elevate intracranial pressure in lead encephalopathy. Contraindicated in active renal disease, anuria, and hepatitis.
ADULT — Use calcium disodium form only for lead indications. Noncalcium form (eg, Endrate) is not interchangeable and is rarely used anymore. Lead toxicity in combination with dimercaprol or succimer:(administer first dose 4 h after first dose of dimercaprol or succimer) 1000 to 1500 mg/m^2/day IM (divided into equal doses q 8 to 12 h) or IV (infuse total dose over 8 to 12 h) for 5 days. Interrupt therapy for 2 to 4 days, then repeat same regimen. Two courses of therapy are usually necessary. Acute lead encephalopathy in combination with dimercaprol: (administer first dose 4 h after first dose of dimercaprol) 1000 to 1500 mg/m^2/day IV over 8 to 12 h for 5 days or divide into 2 to 4 IV doses for 5 days. Interrupt therapy for 2 to 4 days, then repeat same regimen. Two courses of therapy are usually necessary. Lead nephropathy: 500 mg/m^2/dose q 24 h for 5 doses (if creatinine 2 to 3 mg/dL), q 48 h for 3 doses (if creatinine 3 to 4 mg/dL), or once per week (if creatinine greater than 4 mg/dL). May repeat at 1-month intervals.
PEDS — Specialized dosing for lead toxicity; same as adult dosing also using calcium form.
FORMS — Calcium disodium formulation used for lead poisoning; other form without calcium (ie, Endrate) is not interchangeable and rarely used anymore.
MOA — Chelates heavy metals to form complexes that undergo urinary excretion.
ADVERSE EFFECTS — Serious: Arrhythmia, renal toxicity (proteinuria, hematuria, acute tubular necrosis), hypersensitivity, transient bone marrow suppression. Frequent: Hypotension, tremor, headache, numbness, tingling, cheilosis, vomiting, anorexia, thirst, glycosuria, pain at injection site, hypercalcemia, zinc deficiency, nasal congestion, rash, increased serum transaminases, fever, chills, fatigue, malaise, myalgia, arthralgia.

ETHANOL (*alcohol*) ▶L ♀D ▶+ $
PEDS — Not approved in children.
UNAPPROVED ADULT — Specialized dosing for methanol, ethylene glycol toxicity if fomepizole is unavailable or delayed: 1000 mg/kg (10 mL/kg) of 10% ethanol (100 mg/mL) IV over 1 to 2 h then 100 mg/kg/h (1 mL/kg/h) to keep ethanol level approximately 100 mg/dL.
MOA — Prevents formation of toxic methanol metabolite formic acid by saturating alcohol dehydrogenase.
ADVERSE EFFECTS — Serious: Multiple reports of serious adverse effects with chronic use. Frequent: Acute intoxication, dehydration, numerous others with chronic use.

FAT EMULSION (*Intralipid, Nutrilipid*) ▶L ♀C ▶? $$$$$
WARNING — Deaths have occurred in preterm infants after infusion of IV fat emulsions. Autopsy results showed intravascular fat accumulation in the lungs. Strict adherence to total daily dose and administration rate is mandatory. Premature and small for gestational age infants have poor clearance of IV fat emulsion. Monitor infant's ability to eliminate fat (ie, triglycerides or plasma-free fatty acid levels). Antidote dose intralipid interferes with many laboratory tests.
ADULT — Calorie and essential fatty acids source: As part of TPN, fat emulsion should be no more than 60% of total calories; when correcting essential fatty acid deficiency, 8 to 10% of caloric intake should be supplied by lipids. Initial infusion rate 1 mL/min IV (10% fat emulsion) or 0.5 mL/min (20% fat emulsion) IV for 1st 15 to 30 min. If tolerated, increase rate. If using 10% fat emulsion, infuse no more than 500 mL 1st day and increase the next day. Max daily dose 2.5 g/kg. If using 20% fat emulsion, infuse up to 250 mL (Liposyn II) or up to 500 mL (Intralipid) 1st day and increase the next day. Max daily dose 2.5 g/kg.
PEDS — Calorie and essential fatty acids source: As part of TPN, fat emulsion should be no more than 60% of total calories; when correcting essential fatty acid deficiency, 8 to 10% of caloric intake should be supplied by lipids. Initial infusion rate 0.1 mL/min IV (10% fat emulsion) or 0.05 mL/min (20% fat emulsion) for 1st 10 to 15 min. If tolerated, increase rate up to 1 mL/kg/h (10% fat emulsion) or 0.5 mL/kg/h (20% fat emulsion). Max daily dose 3 g/kg. For premature infants, start at 0.5 g/kg/day and increase based on infant's ability to eliminate fat. Max infusion rate 1 g fat/kg in 4 h.
UNAPPROVED ADULT — Local anesthetic toxicity: Bolus of 1.5 mL/kg of 20% intralipid over 1 minute, may repeat once in 5 min prn, followed by infusion at a rate of 0.25 mL/kg/min for 20 to 60 min until hemodynamics improve. Max of 10 mL/kg over first 30 min.
NOTES — Do not use in patients with severe egg allergy; contains egg yolk phospholipids. Use caution in severe liver disease, pulmonary disease, anemia, blood coagulation disorders, when there is the danger of fat embolism, or in jaundiced or premature infants. Monitor CBC, blood coagulation, LFTs, plasma lipid profile and platelet count.
MOA — Treats or prevents nutritional deficiency by providing essential fatty acids. Acts as lipid sink to reduce toxicity of drugs with a high lipid partition coefficient.
ADVERSE EFFECTS — Serious: Intravascular fat accumulation in lungs (preterm infants), sepsis, hepatomegaly (long-term use). Frequent: Thrombophlebitis, hypertriglyceridemia, brown pigmentation (long-term use).

FLUMAZENIL ▶LK ♀C ▶? $$$$
WARNING — Do not administer in chronic benzodiazepine use or acute overdose with TCAs due to seizure risk.
ADULT — Benzodiazepine sedation reversal: 0.2 mg IV over 15 sec, then 0.2 mg q 1 min prn up to 1 mg

(cont.)

FLUMAZENIL (*cont.*)

total dose. Usual dose is 0.6 to 1 mg. Benzodiazepine overdose reversal: 0.2 mg IV over 30 sec, then 0.3 to 0.5 mg q 30 sec prn up to 3 mg total dose.

PEDS — Benzodiazepine sedation reversal: 0.01 mg/kg up to 0.2 mg IV over 15 sec; repeat q 1 min to max 4 additional doses.

UNAPPROVED PEDS — Benzodiazepine overdose reversal: 0.01 mg/kg IV. Benzodiazepine sedation reversal: 0.01 mg/kg IV initially (max 0.2 mg), then 0.005 to 0.01 mg/kg (max 0.2 mg) q 1 min to max total dose 1 mg. May repeat doses in 20 min, max 3 mg in 1 h.

NOTES — Onset of action 1 to 3 min, peak effect 6 to 10 min. For IV use only, preferably through an IV infusion line into a large vein. Local irritation may occur following extravasation.

MOA — Benzodiazepine receptor antagonist.

ADVERSE EFFECTS — Serious: Seizures, arrhythmia, chest pain. Frequent: Injection-site irritation, sweating, hot flashes, flushing, hypotension, hypertension, bradycardia, tachycardia, dizziness, agitation, dry mouth, tremor, insomnia, dyspnea, hyperventilation, emotional lability, confusion, dysphonia, glossitis, N/V, hiccups, visual changes, paresthesia, abnormal hearing, rigors, shivering.

FOMEPIZOLE (*Antizol*) ▶L ♀C ▶? $$$$$

ADULT — Ethylene glycol or methanol toxicity: 15 mg/kg IV (load), then 10 mg/kg IV q 12 h for 4 doses, then 15 mg/kg IV q 12 h until ethylene glycol or methanol level is below 20 mg/dL. Administer doses as slow IV infusions over 30 min. Increase frequency to q 4 h during hemodialysis.

PEDS — Not approved in children.

MOA — Inhibits alcohol dehydrogenase.

ADVERSE EFFECTS — Serious: Hypersensitivity, seizure, shock, hypotension, disseminated intravascular coagulation, multiorgan system failure. Frequent: Injection-site irritation, rash, eosinophilia, tachycardia, sinus bradycardia/tachycardia, phlebitis, phlebosclerosis, lightheadedness, nystagmus, agitation, flushing, anxiety, feeling of decreased environmental awareness, abdominal pain, diarrhea, dyspepsia, anorexia, heartburn, increases serum transaminases, anemia, pharyngitis, lymphangitis, hiccups, speech/visual disturbance, abnormal smell, blurred vision, N/V.

HYDROXOCOBALAMIN (*Cyanokit*) ▶K ♀C ▶? $$$$$

ADULT — Cyanide poisoning: 5 g IV over 15 min; may repeat prn.

PEDS — Not approved in children.

MOA — Binds cyanide to form cyanocobalamin

ADVERSE EFFECTS — Serious: Anaphylaxis, allergy, hypertension. Frequent: None.

IPECAC SYRUP ▶Gut ♀C ▶? $

ADULT — Induced emesis: 15 to 30 mL PO, then 3 to 4 glasses of water.

PEDS — AAP no longer recommends home ipecac for poisoning. Induced emesis, age younger than 1 yo: 5 to 10 mL, then ½ to 1 glass of water (controversial in children younger than 1 yo). Induced emesis,

age 1 to 12 yo: 15 mL, then 1 to 2 glasses of water. May repeat dose (15 mL) if vomiting does not occur within 20 to 30 min.

FORMS — OTC Generic only: Syrup 30 mL.

NOTES — Many believe ipecac to be contraindicated in infants age younger than 6 mo. Do not use if any potential for altered mental status (eg, seizure, neurotoxicity), strychnine, beta-blocker, calcium channel blocker, clonidine, digitalis glycoside, corrosive, petroleum distillate ingestions, or if at risk for GI bleeding (coagulopathy).

MOA — Locally irritates the GI mucosa and stimulates the chemoreceptor trigger zone in the central medullary to produce vomiting.

ADVERSE EFFECTS — Serious: Cardiomyopathy (after prolonged use). Frequent: Diarrhea, coughing, choking, drowsiness, dyspepsia.

METHYLENE BLUE (*Urolene blue*) ▶K ♀C ▶? $

ADULT — Methemoglobinemia: 1 to 2 mg/kg IV over 5 min. Dysuria: 65 to 130 mg PO three times per day after meals with liberal water.

PEDS — Not approved in children.

UNAPPROVED PEDS — Methemoglobinemia: 1 to 2 mg/kg/dose IV over 5 min; may repeat in 1 h prn.

FORMS — Trade only: Tabs 65 mg.

NOTES — Avoid in G6PD deficiency. May turn urine, stool, skin, contact lenses, and undergarments blue-green. Can interact with serotonergic drugs due to its MAOI properties (eg, SSRIs, SNRIs, clomipramine). Generally avoid coadministration with serotonergic drugs; monitor for signs/symptoms of serotonin syndrome if coadministration is unavoidable.

MOA — Converts methemoglobin to hemoglobin by reducing the ferric iron form of oxidized hemoglobin to ferrous form. Converts methemoglobin (Fe^{3+}) to hemoglobin (Fe^{2+}) by enhancing the activity of NADPH-methemoglobin reductase. Also genitourinary antiseptic and germicidal agent.

ADVERSE EFFECTS — Serious: Hypersensitivity, hemolytic anemia, cyanosis, cardiovascular abnormalities. Frequent: Photosensitivity, N/V, diarrhea, fever, bladder irritation, blue-green urine and/or stool.

PENICILLAMINE (*Cuprimine, Depen*) ▶K ♀D ▶– $$$$$

WARNING — Fatal drug-related adverse events have occurred; caution if penicillin allergy.

ADULT — Wilson's disease, copper toxicity: 750 mg to 1.5 g/day PO for 3 months based on 24 h urinary copper excretion, max 2 g/day. May start 250 mg/day PO in patients unable to tolerate. Reduce cystine excretion in cystinuria, severe, active rheumatoid arthritis unresponsive to conventional therapy: see package insert for specialized dosing.

PEDS — Wilson's disease, copper toxicity: 750 mg to 1.5 g/day PO for 3 months based on 24 h urinary copper excretion, max 2 g/day. May start 250 mg/day PO in patients unable to tolerate. Reduce cystine excretion in cystinuria, severe, active rheumatoid arthritis unresponsive to conventional therapy: see package insert for specialized dosing.

(cont.)

PENICILLAMINE (*cont.*)
FORMS — Trade only: Caps 125, 250 mg; Tabs 250 mg.
NOTES — Patients may require supplemental pyridoxine 25 to 50 mg/day PO. Promotes excretion of heavy metals in urine.
MOA — Chelates excess copper.
ADVERSE EFFECTS — Serious: Proteinuria, hematuria, aplastic anemia, hepatotoxicity, pancreatitis, agranulocytosis, production of insulin antibodies, thrombocytopenia, sideroblastic anemia, leukopenia, autoimmune syndromes (Goodpasture's syndrome, myasthenia gravis, pemphigus vulgaris, drug-induced lupus), hypoglycemia, hypersensitivity. Frequent: Increased serum transaminases, oral ulcers, metallic taste, rash, fever, tinnitus, neuropathy, muscle weakness, anorexia, epigastric pain.

PHYSOSTIGMINE (*Antilirium*) ▶LK ♀D ▶? $
WARNING — Discontinue if excessive salivation, emesis, frequent urination, or diarrhea. Rapid administration can cause bradycardia, hypersalivation, respiratory difficulties, and seizures. Atropine should be available as an antagonist.
ADULT — Life-threatening anticholinergic toxicity: 2 mg IV/IM, administer IV no faster than 1 mg/min. May repeat q 10 to 30 min for severe toxicity.
PEDS — Life-threatening anticholinergic toxicity: 0.02 mg/kg IM/IV injection, administer IV no faster than 0.5 mg/min. May repeat q 15 to 30 min until a therapeutic effect or max 2 mg dose.
UNAPPROVED ADULT — Postanesthesia reversal of neuromuscular blockade: 0.5 to 1 mg IV/IM, administer IV no faster than 1 mg/min. May repeat q 10 to 30 min prn.
FORMS — Generic/Trade: 1 mg/mL in 2 mL ampules.
MOA — Reversible cholinesterase inhibitor, acts as substrate for acetylcholinesterase and increases acetylcholine.
ADVERSE EFFECTS — Serious: cardiac arrest, bradycardia, hypersalivation leading to respiratory problems or convulsions. Frequent: salivation, N/V, miosis, sweating, lacrimation, bronchospasm, abdominal pain

PRALIDOXIME (*Protopam, 2-PAM*) ▶K ♀C ▶? $$$$
ADULT — Organophosphate toxicity: 1 to 2 g IV infusion over 15 to 30 min or slow IV injection over 5 min or longer (max rate 200 mg/min). May repeat dose after 1 h if muscle weakness persists.
PEDS — Not approved in children.
UNAPPROVED ADULT — 20 to 40 mg/kg/dose IV infusion over 15 to 30 min.

UNAPPROVED PEDS — 25 mg/kg load then 10 to 20 mg/kg/h or 25 to 50 mg/kg load followed by repeat dose in 1 to 2 h then q 10 to 12 h.
NOTES — Administer within 36 h of exposure when possible. Rapid administration may worsen cholinergic symptoms. Give in conjunction with atropine. IM or SC may be used if IV access is not available.
MOA — Reactivates cholinesterase (primarily peripherally).
ADVERSE EFFECTS — Serious: Myasthenia gravis exacerbation. Frequent: Pain at injection site, transient increase in serum transaminases, increased CK, dizziness, visual changes (blurred, diplopia, decreased accommodation), headache, drowsiness, nausea, tachycardia, increased blood pressure, hyperventilation, muscular weakness.

PRUSSIAN BLUE (*Radiogardase*) ▶Fecal ♀C ▶+ $$$$$
ADULT — Internal contamination with radioactive cesium/thallium: 3 g PO three times per day.
PEDS — Internal contamination with radioactive cesium/thallium, 2 to 12 yo: 1 g PO three times per day.
FORMS — Trade only: Caps 500 mg.
MOA — Enhances excretion of cesium and thallium through ion exchange, adsorption, and mechanical trapping.
ADVERSE EFFECTS — Serious: Hypokalemia. Frequent: Constipation.

SUCCIMER (*Chemet*) ▶K ♀C ▶? $$$$$
PEDS — Lead toxicity 1 yo or older: Start 10 mg/kg PO or 350 mg/m^2 q 8 h for 5 days, then reduce the frequency to q 12 h for 2 weeks. Not approved in children younger than 1 yo.
FORMS — Trade only: Caps 100 mg.
NOTES — Manufacturer recommends doses of 100 mg (wt 8 to 15 kg), 200 mg (wt 16 to 23 kg), 300 mg (wt 24 to 34 kg), 400 mg (wt 35 to 44 kg), and 500 mg (wt 45 kg or greater). Can open cap and sprinkle medicated beads over food, or give them in a spoon and follow with fruit drink. Indicated for blood lead levels greater than 45 mcg/dL. Allow at least 4 weeks between edetate disodium and succimer treatment.
MOA — Chelates lead to increase urinary excretion.
ADVERSE EFFECTS — Serious: Hypersensitivity, arrhythmia. Frequent: Rash, increased serum transaminases (transient), N/V, anorexia, hemorrhoids, loose stools, metallic taste, body pain, abdominal cramps, fever, flu-like syndrome, drowsiness, dizziness, paresthesia, sensorimotor neuropathy, headache, moniliasis.

UROLOGY

UROLOGY: Benign Prostatic Hyperplasia

ALFUZOSIN (*UroXatral,* ✸*Xatral*) ▸KL ♀B ▸– $
WARNING — Postural hypotension with or without symptoms may develop within a few hours after administration. Postural hypotension is more common in patients taking blood pressure–reducing agents. Avoid in moderate or severe hepatic insufficiency. Avoid coadministration with potent CYP3A4 inhibitors.
ADULT — BPH: 10 mg PO daily after the same meal each day.
PEDS — Not approved in children.
UNAPPROVED ADULT — Promotes spontaneous passage of ureteral calculi: 10 mg PO daily usually combined with an NSAID, antiemetic, and opioid of choice.
FORMS — Generic/Trade: Tabs, extended-release 10 mg.
NOTES — Caution in congenital or acquired QT prolongation and severe renal insufficiency. Intraoperative floppy iris syndrome has been observed during cataract surgery, but stopping alpha blocker therapy prior to cataract surgery does not appear to be helpful. Should not be used concomitantly with other alpha blockers.
MOA — Selective alpha-1 receptor antagonist that increases urinary flow rate.
ADVERSE EFFECTS — Serious: Postural hypotension, chest pain, priapism, angioedema, hepatocellular and cholestatic liver disease. Frequent: Dizziness, headache.

DUTASTERIDE (*Avodart*) ▸L ♀X Capsules should not be touched by a woman who is pregnant or may become pregnant due to transdermal absorption resulting in fetal exposure. ▸– $$
WARNING — May increase risk of high-grade prostate cancer. Patients should not donate blood until 6 months after last dose of dutasteride. Use caution when prescribed concomitantly with CYP3A4 inhibitors.
ADULT — BPH: 0.5 mg PO daily with/without tamsulosin 0.4 mg PO daily.
PEDS — Not approved in children.
FORMS — Generic/Trade: Caps 0.5 mg.
NOTES — 6 months of therapy may be needed to assess effectiveness. Pregnant or potentially pregnant women should not handle caps due to fetal risk from absorption. Caution in hepatic insufficiency. Dutasteride will decrease PSA by 50%; new baseline PSA should be established after 3 to 6 months and monitored periodically thereafter. Any confirmed increase in PSA on dutasteride may indicate presence of prostate cancer. To interpret an isolated PSA in a man treated with dutasteride for 3 months or longer, the PSA should be doubled for comparison with normal values for untreated men.

The free:total PSA remains constant on dutasteride. Cap should be swallowed whole and not chewed or opened to avoid oropharyngeal irritation.
MOA — 5-alpha reductase inhibitor that decreases conversion of testosterone into dihydrotestosterone.
ADVERSE EFFECTS — Serious: Angioedema, breast enlargement and tenderness. Frequent: Impotence, decreased libido, ejaculatory dysfunction.

FINASTERIDE (*Proscar, Propecia*) ▸L ♀X ▸– $
WARNING — Contraindicated in women who are pregnant or may become pregnant.
ADULT — Proscar: 5 mg PO daily alone or in combination with doxazosin to reduce the risk of symptomatic progression of BPH. Propecia: Androgenetic alopecia in men: 1 mg PO daily.
PEDS — Not approved in children.
UNAPPROVED ADULT — Cancer prevention in "at-risk" men older than 55 yo: 5 mg daily. Androgenetic alopecia in postmenopausal women (no evidence of efficacy): 1 mg PO daily.
FORMS — Generic/Trade: Tabs 1 mg (Propecia), 5 mg (Proscar).
NOTES — Therapy for 6 to 12 months may be needed to assess effectiveness for BPH and at least 3 months for alopecia. Pregnant or potentially pregnant women should not handle crushed tabs because of possible absorption and fetal risk. Use with caution in hepatic insufficiency. Monitor PSA before therapy; finasteride will decrease PSA by 50% in patients with BPH, even with prostate cancer. Does not appear to alter detection of prostate cancer. Any confirmed increase in PSA from the nadir while on finasteride may signal the presence of prostate cancer. May increase risk of high-grade prostate cancer.
MOA — 5-alpha reductase inhibitor that decreases conversion of testosterone into dihydrotestosterone.
ADVERSE EFFECTS — Serious: Hypersensitivity, angioedema, breast cancer (long-term treatment), depression. Frequent: Impotence, decreased libido, decreased ejaculatory volume, testicular pain, rash, pruritus.

JALYN (dutasteride + tamsulosin, *Combodart, Duodart*) ▸LK - ♀X ▸– $$$$
WARNING — May increase risk of high grade prostate cancer. Caution when using with PDE-5 inhibitors; can increase risk of hypotension. Should not be used in combination with strong inhibitors of CYP3A4. Caution when used in combination with moderate CYP3A4 inhibitors, with strong or moderate CYP2D6 inhibitors, and in patients known to be poor metabolizers through CYP2D6. Patients should not donate blood until 6 months after stopping this combination. Has not been adequately studied in patients with severe hepatic and/or renal impairment.

(cont.)

JALYN (cont.)

ADULT — BPH: 0.5 mg dutasteride + 0.4 mg tamsulosin daily 30 minutes after the same meal each day.

PEDS — Not approved in children.

FORMS — Trade only: Caps 0.5 mg dutasteride + 0.4 mg tamsulosin.

NOTES — Refer to components.

MOA — Combination 5-alpha reductase inhibitor and selective alpha-1 antagonist.

ADVERSE EFFECTS — Serious: Angioedema, arrhythmia, orthostatic hypotension, chest pain, syncope, priapism, floppy iris syndrome. Frequent: impotence, breast enlargement and pain, decreased libido, dizziness, ejaculatory dysfunction.

SILODOSIN (*RAPAFLO*) ▶LK ♀–B ▶– $$$$

ADULT — BPH: 8 mg daily with a meal.

PEDS — Not approved in children.

FORMS — Trade: Caps 8 mg.

NOTES — Dizziness, headache, abnormal ejaculation. Alpha-blockers are generally considered to be 1st-line treatment in men with more than minimal obstructive urinary symptoms. Intraoperative floppy iris syndrome with cataract surgery reported. Avoid administration with strong inhibitors of CYP3A4 (ketoconazole, clarithromycin, itraconazole, ritonavir).

MOA — Selective alpha-1 receptor antagonist that increases urinary flow rate.

ADVERSE EFFECTS — Serious: orthostatic hypotension. Frequent: dizziness, headache, nasal congestion, diarrhea, abnormal ejaculation.

TAMSULOSIN (*Flomax*) ▶LK ♀B ▶– $$$$

ADULT — BPH: 0.4 mg PO daily 30 min after the same meal each day. If an adequate response is not seen after 2 to 4 weeks, may increase dose to 0.8 mg PO daily. If therapy is interrupted for several days, restart at the 0.4 mg dose.

PEDS — Not approved in children.

UNAPPROVED ADULT — Promotes spontaneous passage of ureteral calculi: 0.4 mg PO daily usually combined with an NSAID, antiemetic, and opioid of choice.

FORMS — Generic/Trade: Caps 0.4 mg.

NOTES — Dizziness, headache, abnormal ejaculation. Alpha-blockers are generally considered to be 1st-line treatment in men with more than minimal obstructive urinary symptoms. Caution in serious sulfa allergy: Rare allergic reactions reported. Intraoperative floppy iris syndrome with cataract surgery reported. Caution with strong inhibitors of CYP450 2D6 (fluoxetine) or 3A4 (ketoconazole).

MOA — Selective alpha-1 receptor antagonist that increases urinary flow rate.

ADVERSE EFFECTS — Serious: Arrhythmia, orthostatic hypotension, chest pain. Frequent: Dizziness, headache, fatigue, somnolence, edema, dyspnea, asthenia, diarrhea, dyspepsia, dry mouth, nausea, palpitations, blurred vision, abnormal ejaculation.

UROLOGY: Bladder Agents—Anticholinergics and Combinations

B&O SUPPRETTES (belladonna + opium) ▶L ♀C ▶? ©II $$$$

WARNING — Contraindications include glaucoma, severe renal or hepatic disease, asthma, respiratory depression, acute alcoholism, delirium tremens, premature labor. Use with caution in older patients.

ADULT — Bladder or ureteral spasm: 1 suppository PR once or twice daily, max 4 doses/day.

PEDS — Not approved in children younger than 12 yo.

FORMS — Trade only: Supps 30 mg opium with 16.2 mg belladonna extract (15A), 60 mg opium with 16.2 mg belladonna extract (16A).

NOTES — Store at room temperature. Contraindicated in narrow-angle glaucoma, obstructive conditions (eg, pyloric, duodenal or other intestinal obstructive lesions, ileus, achalasia, and obstructive uropathies).

MOA — Belladonna: Inhibits the muscarinic action of acetylcholine to decrease motility in the urinary tract. Opium: Opioid agonist analgesic.

ADVERSE EFFECTS — Serious: Hypersensitivity, respiratory coma, bradycardia, hallucinations. Frequent: Dizziness, drowsiness, sedation, N/V, lightheadedness, euphoria, constipation, dry mouth, blurred vision, urinary retention, decreased sweating.

DARIFENACIN (*Enablex*) ▶LK ♀C ▶– $$$$$

ADULT — Overactive bladder with symptoms of urinary urgency, frequency, and urge incontinence: 7.5 mg PO daily. May increase to max dose 15 mg PO daily as early as 2 weeks after starting therapy. Max dose 7.5 mg PO daily with moderate liver impairment or when coadministered with potent CYP3A4 inhibitors (ketoconazole, itraconazole, ritonavir, nelfinavir, clarithromycin, and nefazodone).

PEDS — Not approved in children.

FORMS — Generic/Trade: Tabs, extended-release 7.5, 15 mg.

NOTES — Contraindicated with uncontrolled narrow-angle glaucoma, urinary and gastric retention, or bladder outlet obstruction. Avoid use in severe hepatic impairment. May increase concentration of medications metabolized by CYP2D6. Use with caution in patients with myasthenia gravis or with decreased GI motility.

MOA — Muscarinic receptor antagonist, inhibiting detrusor muscle contractions.

ADVERSE EFFECTS — Serious: Hypersensitivity, angioedema, hallucinations. Frequent: Dry mouth, constipation, blurred vision, dyspepsia.

FESOTERODINE (*Toviaz*) ▶Plasma ♀C ▶– $$$$

ADULT — Overactive bladder: 4 mg PO daily. Increase to 8 mg if needed. Do not exceed 4 mg daily with renal insufficiency (CrCl <30 mL/min) or specific coadministered drugs (see Notes).

PEDS — Not approved in children.

FORMS — Trade only: Tabs, extended-release 4, 8 mg.

(cont.)

FESOTERODINE (*cont.***)**

NOTES — Contraindicated with urinary or gastric retention, or uncontrolled glaucoma. 4 mg daily max dose in renal dysfunction or with concomitant use of CYP3A4 inhibitors (eg, erythromycin, ketoconazole, itraconazole).

MOA — Muscarinic receptor antagonist to decrease bladder spasm.

ADVERSE EFFECTS — Serious: QT prolongation, angioedema. Frequent: Dry mouth, constipation, headache, vertigo/dizziness, abdominal pain.

FLAVOXATE (*Urispas***)** ▶K ♀B ▶? $$$$

ADULT — Symptomatic relief of dysuria, urgency, nocturia, suprapubic pain, frequency and incontinence as may occur in cystitis, prostatitis, urethritis, urethrocystitis/urethrotrigonitis: 100 or 200 mg PO three to four times per day. Reduce dose when improved.

PEDS — Not approved in children younger than 12 yo.

FORMS — Generic/Trade: Tabs 100 mg.

NOTES — May cause dizziness, drowsiness, blurred vision, dry mouth, N/V, urinary retention. Contraindicated in glaucoma, obstructive conditions (eg, pyloric, duodenal or other intestinal obstructive lesions, ileus, achalasia, GI hemorrhage, and obstructive uropathies of the lower urinary tract).

MOA — Anticholinergic that directly counteracts urinary smooth muscle contraction.

ADVERSE EFFECTS — Serious: Increased ocular pressure, eosinophilia, leukopenia, hyperpyrexia. Frequent: N/V, dry mouth, nervousness, vertigo, headache, drowsiness, mental confusion, fever, blurred vision, rash, dysuria, tachycardia, disturbed eye accommodation.

OXYBUTYNIN (*Ditropan, Ditropan XL, Gelnique, Oxytrol, ✦Oxybutyn, Uromax***)** ▶LK ♀B ▶? $$

WARNING — Use caution in frail elderly, patients with hepatic or renal impairment, and patients with myasthenia gravis. May aggravate symptoms of hyperthyroidism, coronary artery disease, heart failure, arrhythmias, hiatal hernia, tachycardia, hypertension, and BPH. Potent CYP3A4 inhibitors increase concentration of oxybutynin 3 to 4 fold.

ADULT — Bladder instability associated with voiding in patients with uninhibited neurogenic and reflex neurogenic bladder: 2.5 to 5 mg PO two to three times per day, max 5 mg PO four times per day. Extended-release tabs: 5 to 10 mg PO daily same time each day, increase 5 mg/day q week to 30 mg/day. Oxytrol: 1 patch twice per week on intact skin on abdomen, hip, or buttocks. Do not reuse same site within 7 days. Gelnique: Apply contents of 1 sachet once daily to intact skin on abdomen, upper arms/shoulders, or thighs. Rotate application sites.

PEDS — Bladder instability associated with voiding in patients with uninhibited neurogenic and reflex neurogenic bladder older than 5 yo: Usual dose is 5 mg PO twice per day, max dose 5 mg PO three times per day. Extended-release, older than 6 yo: 5 mg PO daily, max 20 mg/day. Transdermal patch and Gelnique not approved in children.

UNAPPROVED ADULT — Case reports of use for hyperhidrosis.

UNAPPROVED PEDS — Bladder instability for age younger than 6 yo: 0.2 mg/kg/dose PO two to four times per day.

FORMS — Generic/Trade: Tabs, 5 mg. Syrup 5 mg/5 mL. Tabs, extended-release 5, 10, 15 mg. Trade only: OTC Transdermal patch (Oxytrol) 3.9 mg/day. Gelnique 3, 10% gel, 1 g unit dose.

NOTES — May cause dizziness, drowsiness, blurred vision, dry mouth, urinary retention. Contraindicated with uncontrolled narrow-angle glaucoma, urinary retention, obstructive GU or GI disease, unstable cardiovascular status, and myasthenia gravis. Use with caution in patients with Parkinson's disease or autonomic neuropathy. Transdermal patch causes less dry mouth than oral form; avoid dose reduction by cutting. Wash hands immediately after applying Gelnique.

MOA — Anticholinergic that exerts direct antispasmodic effects and inhibits muscarinic effects on smooth muscle.

ADVERSE EFFECTS — Serious: Heat stroke, hallucinations, QT prolongation, angioedema. Frequent: Somnolence, headache, dizziness, agitation, confusion, dry mouth, constipation, diarrhea, nausea, dyspepsia, blurred vision, dry eyes, asthenia, pain, rhinitis, urinary tract infection, application site reaction.

PROSED/DS (*methenamine + phenyl salicylate + methylene blue + benzoic acid + hyoscyamine***)** ▶KL ♀C ▶? $$

WARNING — A careful risk/benefit evaluation should be performed when the following medical problems exist: glaucoma, urinary bladder neck obstruction, pyloric or duodenal obstruction, or cardiospasm. Rapid pulse, flushing, shortness of breath, trouble breathing, or difficulty voiding may occur.

ADULT — Discomfort of lower urinary tract caused by hypermotility resulting from inflammation or diagnostic procedures and in the treatment of cystitis, urethritis, and trigonitis caused by organisms that maintain or produce an acid urine and are susceptible to formaldehyde: 1 tab PO four times per day with liberal fluids.

PEDS — Not approved in children.

UNAPPROVED PEDS — Bladder spasm in children 12 yo or older: Individualized dosing by physician.

FORMS — Trade only: Tabs (methenamine 81.6 mg/phenyl salicylate 36.2 mg/methylene blue 10.8 mg/benzoic acid 9.0 mg/hyoscyamine sulfate 0.12 mg).

NOTES — May cause dizziness, drowsiness, blurred vision, dry mouth, N/V, urinary retention. May turn urine/contact lenses blue.

MOA — Combination product that decreases bladder spasm and has mild antiseptic and analgesic activity.

ADVERSE EFFECTS — Serious: Respiratory depression. Frequent: Blue urine, rash, dry mouth, flushing, urinary retention, tachycardia, dizziness, blurred vision.

SOLIFENACIN (*VESIcare*) ▶LK ♀C ▶– $$$$
ADULT — Overactive bladder with symptoms of urinary urgency, frequency, or urge incontinence: 5 mg PO daily. Max dose: 10 mg PO daily (5 mg PO daily if CrCl <30 mL/min, moderate hepatic impairment, or concurrent ketoconazole or other potent CYP3A4 inhibitors).
PEDS — Not approved in children.
FORMS — Trade only: Tabs 5, 10 mg.
NOTES — Contraindicated with uncontrolled narrow-angle glaucoma, urinary and gastric retention. Avoid use in severe hepatic impairment. Hallucinations have been reported.
MOA — Muscarinic receptor antagonist, inhibiting detrusor muscle contractions.
ADVERSE EFFECTS — Serious: Fecal impaction, intestinal obstruction, angioedema, hallucinations, QT prolongation, torsade de pointes. Frequent: Dry mouth, constipation, blurred vision.

TOLTERODINE (*Detrol, Detrol LA*) ▶L ♀C ▶– $$$$$
WARNING — Use caution in patients with clinically significant bladder outlet obstruction, GI obstructive disorders, and patients being treated for narrow-angle glaucoma. Use caution in patients with known history of QT prolongation or who are taking class IA or III antiarrhythmic medications.
ADULT — Overactive bladder: 2 mg PO two times per day (Detrol) or 4 mg PO daily (Detrol LA). Decrease dose to 1 mg PO two times per day (Detrol) or 2 mg PO daily (Detrol LA) if adverse symptoms, hepatic insufficiency, or specific coadministered drugs (see Notes).
PEDS — Not approved in children.
FORMS — Generic/Trade: Tabs 1, 2 mg. Caps, extended-release 2, 4 mg.
NOTES — Contraindicated with urinary or gastric retention or uncontrolled narrow-angle glaucoma. High doses may prolong the QT interval. Decrease dose to 1 mg PO two times per day or 2 mg PO daily (Detrol LA) in severe hepatic or renal dysfunction (CrCl 10 to 30 mL/min) or with concomitant use of CYP3A4 inhibitors (eg, erythromycin, ketoconazole, itraconazole). Do not use if CrCl <10 mL/min.
MOA — Muscarinic receptor antagonist to decrease bladder spasm.
ADVERSE EFFECTS — Serious: Angioedema, QT prolongation. Frequent: Dry mouth, constipation, headache, vertigo/dizziness, abdominal pain.

TROSPIUM (*Sanctura, Sanctura XR, ✱Trosec*) ▶LK ♀C ▶? $$$$
ADULT — Overactive bladder with urge incontinence: 20 mg PO two times per day; give 20 mg at bedtime if CrCl <30 mL/min. If age 75 yo or older, may taper down to 20 mg daily. Extended-release: 60 mg PO q am, 1 h before food; this form not recommended with CrCl <30 mL/min.
PEDS — Not approved in children.
FORMS — Generic only: Tabs 20 mg. Caps, extended-release 60 mg.
NOTES — Contraindicated with uncontrolled narrow-angle glaucoma, urinary retention, gastroparesis.

May cause heat stroke due to decreased sweating. Take on an empty stomach. Improvement in signs and symptoms may be seen in a week.
MOA — Acetylcholine antagonist that reduces bladder smooth muscle tone and spasms.
ADVERSE EFFECTS — Serious: Supraventricular tachycardia, Stevens-Johnson syndrome, anaphylaxis, angioedema, hypertensive crisis, rhabdomyolysis, hallucinations, delirium, heat stroke. Frequent: Dry mouth, constipation, headache, dizziness, blurred vision.

URISED (**methenamine + phenyl salicylate + atropine + hyoscyamine + benzoic acid + methylene blue**) ▶K ♀C ▶? $
ADULT — Dysuria: 2 Tabs PO four times per day.
PEDS — Dysuria, age 6 yo or older: Reduce dose based on age and wt. Not recommended for children younger than 6 yo.
FORMS — Trade only: Tabs (methenamine 40.8 mg/phenyl salicylate 18.1 mg/atropine 0.03 mg/hyoscyamine 0.03 mg/4.5 mg benzoic acid/5.4 mg methylene blue).
NOTES — Take with food to minimize GI upset. May precipitate urate crystals in urine. Avoid use with sulfonamides. May turn urine/contact lenses blue.
MOA — Combination product that decreases bladder spasm and has mild antiseptic and analgesic activity.
ADVERSE EFFECTS — Serious: Respiratory depression. Frequent: Blue urine, rash, dry mouth, flushing, urinary retention, tachycardia, dizziness, blurred vision.

UTA (**methenamine + sodium phosphate + phenyl salicylate + methylene blue + hyoscyamine**) ▶KL ♀C ▶? $
WARNING — A careful risk/benefit analysis should be performed when the following medical problems exist: cardiac disease, GI obstructive disease, glaucoma, myasthenia gravis, or bladder outlet obstruction.
ADULT — Treatment of irritative voiding/relief of inflammation, hypermotility, and pain with lower UTI/relief of urinary tract symptoms caused by diagnostic procedures: 1 cap PO four times per day with liberal fluids.
PEDS — Not recommended for age younger than 6 yo. Dosing must be individualized by physician for age older than 6 yo.
FORMS — Trade only: Caps (methenamine 120 mg/sodium phosphate 40.8 mg/phenyl salicylate 36 mg/methylene blue 10 mg/hyoscyamine 0.12 mg).
NOTES — May turn urine/feces blue to blue-green. Take 2 h apart from ketoconazole. May decrease absorption of thiazide diuretics. Antacids and antidiarrheals may decrease effectiveness of methenamine.
MOA — Methenamine degrades in acidic environment releasing formaldehyde which is bactericidal/static. Methylene blue is a weak antiseptic. Hyoscyamine is a parasympatholytic that relaxes smooth muscle resulting in antispasmodic action.

(cont.)

UTA (*cont.*)

Sodium phosphate is an acidifier that helps maintain pH for degradation of methenamine.

ADVERSE EFFECTS — Serious: respiratory depression. Frequent: blue to blue-green urine/feces, tachycardia, blurred vision, dizziness, urinary retention, dry mouth, N/V.

UTIRA-C (methenamine + sodium phosphate + phenyl salicylate + methylene blue + hyoscyamine) ►KL ♀C ▶? $$

WARNING — A careful risk/benefit analysis should be performed when the following medical problems exist: cardiac disease, GI obstructive disease, glaucoma, myasthenia gravis, or bladder outlet obstruction.

ADULT — Treatment of irritative voiding/relief of inflammation, hypermotility, and pain with lower UTI/relief of urinary tract symptoms caused by diagnostic procedures: 1 cap PO four times per day with liberal fluids.

PEDS — Not recommended age younger than 6 yo. Dosing must be individualized by physician for age older than 6 yo.

FORMS — Trade only: Tabs (methenamine 81.6 mg/ sodium phosphate 40.8 mg/phenyl salicylate 36.2 mg/methylene blue 10.8 mg/hyoscyamine 0.12 mg).

NOTES — May turn urine/feces blue to blue-green. Take 2 h apart from ketoconazole. May decrease absorption of thiazide diuretics. Antacids and antidiarrheals may decrease effectiveness of methenamine.

MOA — Combination product that decreases bladder spasms and has mild antiseptic and analgesic activity.

ADVERSE EFFECTS — Serious: Respiratory depression. Frequent: Blue to blue-green urine/feces, tachycardia, blurred vision, dizziness, urinary retention, dry mouth, N/V.

UROLOGY: Bladder Agents—Other

BETHANECHOL (*Urecholine, Duvoid, ✻Myotonachol*) ►L ♀C ▶? $$$$

ADULT — Urinary retention: 10 to 50 mg PO three to four times per day or 2.5 to 5 mg SC three to four times per day. Take 1 h before or 2 h after meals to avoid N/V. Determine the minimum effective dose by giving 5 to 10 mg PO initially and repeat at hourly intervals until response or to a maximum of 50 mg. The minimum effective dose may also be determined by injecting 2.5 mg SC, then repeating the same dose at 15 to 30 minute intervals until satisfactory response is obtained or a maximum of 4 doses is given.

PEDS — Not approved in children.

UNAPPROVED PEDS — Urinary retention/abdominal distention: 0.6 mg/kg/day PO divided q 6 to 8 h or 0.12 to 0.2 mg/kg/day SC divided q 6 to 8 h.

FORMS — Generic/Trade: Tabs 5, 10, 25, 50 mg.

NOTES — May cause drowsiness, lightheadedness, and fainting. Not for obstructive urinary retention. Avoid with cardiac disease, hyperthyroidism, parkinsonism, peptic ulcer disease, epilepsy, latent or active bronchial asthma, pronounced bradycardia or hypotension, vasomotor instability.

MOA — Cholinergic agent that stimulates the parasympathetic nervous system to increase the strength of detrusor muscle contraction.

ADVERSE EFFECTS — Serious: Hypersensitivity, hypotension with tachycardia, bronchoconstriction/ asthma attack, seizures. Frequent: Flushing, sense of warmth, sweating, abdominal pain, nausea, belching, diarrhea, salivation, borborygmi, lacrimation, myosis, urinary urgency, headache, malaise.

DIMETHYL SULFOXIDE (*DMSO, Rimso-50*) ►KL ♀C ▶? $$$

ADULT — Interstitial cystitis: Instill 50 mL soln into bladder by catheter and allow to remain for 15 min; expelled by spontaneous voiding. Repeat q 2 weeks until symptomatic relief is obtained; thereafter, may increase time intervals between treatments.

PEDS — Not approved in children.

NOTES — Apply analgesic lubricant gel to urethra prior to inserting the catheter to avoid spasm. May administer oral analgesics or supps containing belladonna and opium prior to instillation to reduce spasms. May give anesthesia in patients with severe interstitial cystitis and very sensitive bladders during the 1st, 2nd, and 3rd treatment. May cause lens opacities and changes in refractive index; perform eye exams before and periodically during treatment. May cause a hypersensitivity reaction by liberating histamine. Monitor liver and renal function tests and CBC q 6 months. May be harmful in patients with urinary tract malignancy; can cause DMSO-induced vasodilation. Peripheral neuropathy may occur when used with sulindac. Garlic-like taste may occur within a few min of administration; odor on breath and skin may be present and remain for up to 72 h.

MOA — Has broad pharmacological properties: anti-inflammatory, antifungal activity cryoprotective effects for living cells and tissues, dissolution of collagen, nerve blockade, diuresis, cholinesterase inhibition, vasodilation, and muscle relaxation.

ADVERSE EFFECTS — Serious: Hypersensitivity, transient chemical cystitis. Frequent: Sedation, N/V, headache, dizziness, garlic-like breath, burning on urination, diarrhea, transient disturbance of color perception, photophobia, burning or aching eyes, weight loss/gain, flu syndrome, discomfort during administration.

MIRABEGRON (*Myrbetriq*) ►LK – ♀C ▶?

ADULT — Overactive bladder with symptoms of urge incontinence, urgency, and urinary frequency: 25 mg PO daily. May increase to 50 mg unless severe renal impairment (CrCl <30 mL/min) or moderate hepatic impairment (Child-Pugh Class B). Not recommended in ESRD or Child-Pugh Class C liver disease.

(cont.)

MIRABEGRON (*cont.*)

PEDS — Not approved in children.

FORMS — Trade only: Extended-release tabs 25, 50 mg.

NOTES — Do not chew, crush, or split tablets. May increase blood pressure; not recommended in patients with severe uncontrolled hypertension. Moderate CYP2D6 inhibitor; may increase concentrations of CYP2D6 substrates such as metoprolol.

MOA — Beta-3 adrenergic agonist.

ADVERSE EFFECTS — Common: Hyppertension, nasopharyngitis, urinary tract infection, headache.

PENTOSAN (*Elmiron*) ▶LK ♀B ▶? $$$$$

WARNING — Use caution in patients with heparin-induced thrombocytopenia or hepatic insufficiency.

ADULT — Interstitial cystitis: 100 mg PO three times per day 1 h before or 2 h after a meal.

PEDS — Not approved in children.

FORMS — Trade only: Caps 100 mg.

NOTES — Pain relief usually occurs at 2 to 4 months and decreased urinary frequency takes 6 months. Reassess after 3 months of use; if improvement has not occurred and limiting adverse effects are not present, may continue for another 3 months. Clinical value and risks of continued treatment in patients whose pain has not improved by 6 months are not known. May increase risk of bleeding, especially with NSAID use. Use with caution in hepatic or splenic dysfunction.

MOA — Heparin-like molecule that adheres to bladder wall mucosa and exerts anticoagulant and fibrinolytic effects and is thought to prevent irritation by buffering cell permeability and preventing irritating solutes in the urine from reaching the cells.

ADVERSE EFFECTS — Serious: Thrombocytopenia, bleeding. Frequent: Alopecia, headache, rash, nausea, abdominal pain.

PHENAZOPYRIDINE (*Pyridium, Azo-Standard, Urogesic, Prodium, Pyridiate, Urodol, Baridium, UTI Relief, Azourinary Pain Relief, Uristat, Azo-Gesic, Azo-Septic, Phenazo, Re-Azo, Uricalm*) ▶K ♀B ▶? $

WARNING — May cause yellowish tinge to skin or sclera.

ADULT — Dysuria: 200 mg PO three times per day after meals for 2 days.

PEDS — Dysuria in children 6 to 12 yo: 12 mg/kg/day PO divided three times per day for 2 days.

FORMS — OTC Generic/Trade: Tabs 95, 97.2 mg. Rx Generic/Trade: Tabs 100, 200 mg.

NOTES — May turn urine/contact lenses orange. Contraindicated with hepatitis or renal insufficiency.

MOA — Produces a topical analgesic effect on the urinary mucosa.

ADVERSE EFFECTS — Serious: Hypersensitivity, hemolytic anemia, methemoglobinemia, nephrotoxicity, hepatotoxicity. Frequent: Headache, rash, pruritus, dyspepsia, contact lens staining, urine discoloration, yellowish tinge on sclera or skin.

UROQUID-ACID NO. 2 (**methenamine + sodium phosphate**) ▶K ♀C ▶? $

WARNING — Contraindicated in patients with renal insufficiency, severe hepatic disease, severe dehydration, or hyperphosphatemia.

ADULT — Chronic/recurrent UTIs: Initial: 2 tabs PO four times per day with full glass of water. Maintenance: 2 to 4 tabs PO daily, in divided doses with full glass of water.

PEDS — Not approved in children.

FORMS — Trade only: Tabs methenamine mandelate 500 mg/sodium acid phosphate 500 mg.

NOTES — 83 mg sodium/tab. Thiazide diuretics, carbonic anhydrase inhibitors, antacids, and urinary alkalinizing agents may decrease effectiveness. Caution with concurrent salicylates, may increase levels. Do not use if renal insufficiency, high blood phosphorus levels, or severe dehydration.

MOA — Antibacterial/urinary acidifier. Works by concentrating in the urine as formaldehyde.

ADVERSE EFFECTS — Serious: Hematuria. Frequent: N/D/V, rash, headache, dizziness.

SIDE EFFECTS — Dysuria, painful or difficult urination, bone or joint pain, confusion, weakness, muscle cramps, numbness, tingling pain or weakness in hands or feet, shortness of breath, fast or irregular heart beat, swelling of lower extremities, weight gain, low urine output, increased thirst.

UROLOGY: Erectile Dysfunction

ALPROSTADIL (*Muse, Caverject, Caverject Impulse, Edex, Prostin VR Pediatric, prostaglandin E1,* ✦*Prostin VR*) ▶L ♀– ▶– $$$$

ADULT — Erectile dysfunction: 1.25 to 2.5 mcg intracavernosal injection over 5 to 10 sec initially using a ½ in, 27 or 30 gauge needle. If no response, may give next higher dose after 1 h, max 2 doses/day. May increase by 2.5 mcg and then 5 to 10 mcg incrementally on separate occasions. Dose range is 1 to 40 mcg. Alternative: 125 to 250 mcg intraurethral pellet (Muse). Increase or decrease dose on separate occasions until erection achieved. Max intraurethral dose 2 pellets/24 h. The lowest possible dose to produce an acceptable erection should be used.

PEDS — Temporary maintenance of patent ductus arteriosus in neonates: Start 0.1 mcg/kg/min IV infusion. Reduce dose to minimal amount that maintains therapeutic response. Max dose 0.4 mcg/kg/min.

UNAPPROVED ADULT — Erectile dysfunction intracorporeal injection: Specially formulated mixtures of alprostadil, papaverine, and phentolamine. 0.10 to 0.50 mL injection.

FORMS — Trade only: Syringe system (Edex) 10, 20, 40 mcg; (Caverject) 5, 10, 20, 40 mcg; (Caverject Impulse) 10, 20 mcg. Pellet (Muse) 125, 250, 500, 1000 mcg. Intracorporeal injection of locally compounded combination agents (many variations):

(cont.)

ALPROSTADIL (*cont.*)

"Bi-mix" can be 30 mg/mL papaverine + 0.5 to 1 mg/mL phentolamine, or 30 mg/mL papaverine + 20 mcg/mL alprostadil in 10 mL vials. "Tri-mix" can be 30 mg/mL papaverine + 1 mg/mL phentolamine + 10 mcg/mL alprostadil in 5, 10, or 20 mL vials.

NOTES — Contraindicated in patients at risk for priapism, with penile fibrosis (Peyronie's disease), with penile implants, in women or children, in men for whom sexual activity is inadvisable, and for intercourse with a pregnant woman. Onset of effect is 5 to 20 min.

MOA — Relaxes trabecular smooth muscles and dilates cavernosal arteries to produce erection. Relaxes smooth muscle of the ductus arteriosus.

ADVERSE EFFECTS — Serious: Priapism, hypotension. Frequent: Penile and testicular pain, urethral discomfort (pain, burning, bleeding/spotting).

AVANAFIL (*Stendra*) ▶L – ♀C ▷? $$$$

ADULT — Erectile dysfunction: 100 mg PO 30 minutes prior to sexual activity. Max 1 dose/day. Use lower dose (50 mg) if taking certain coadministered drugs (see Notes).

PEDS — Not approved in children.

FORMS — Trade only (Stendra): Tabs 50, 100, 200 mg.

NOTES — For patients taking strong CYP3A4 inhibitors (ketoconazole, ritonavir, atazanavir, clarithromycin, indinavir, itraconazole, nefazodone, nelfinavir, saquinavir, and telithromycin), do not use. For patients taking moderate CYP3A4 inhibitors (erythromycin, amprenavir, aprepitant, diltiazem, fluconazole, fosamprenavir, and verapamil), use 50 mg dose. For patients taking alpha-blocker, start at 50 mg. Do not initiate alpha-blocker and avanafil at same time. Not recommended for patients within 6 months of MI, CVA, life-threatening arrhythmia, or coronary revascularization, resting BP less than 90/50 or greater than 170/100, or unstable angina, angina with sexual intercourse, or NYHA Class II or greater heart failure. Avanafil can potentiate the effects of alcohol.

MOA — Selectively inhibits phosphodiesterase-5 resulting in enhanced relaxation of penile arteries & corpus cavernosal smooth muscle; enhances erectile function by increasing penile blood flow. Relaxes pulmonary vascular smooth muscle cells resulting in vasodilation of the pulmonary vascular bed.

ADVERSE EFFECTS — Serious: Priapism, hypotension, syncope, vision loss (nonarteritic ischemic optic neuropathy). Frequent: Headache, flushing, nasal congestion.

SILDENAFIL—UROLOGY (*Viagra*) ▶LK ♀B ▷– $$$$

ADULT — Erectile dysfunction: 50 mg PO approximately 1 h (range 0.5 to 4 h) before sexual activity. Usual effective dose range: 25 to 100 mg. Max 1 dose/day. Use lower dose (25 mg) if older than 65 yo, hepatic/renal impairment, or certain coadministered drugs (see Notes).

PEDS — Not approved in children.

UNAPPROVED ADULT — Antidepressant-associated sexual dysfunction: Same dosing as for approved indications.

FORMS — Trade only (Viagra): Tabs 25, 50, 100 mg. Unscored tab but can be cut in half.

NOTES — Drug interactions with cimetidine, erythromycin, ketoconazole, itraconazole, saquinavir, ritonavir, and other CYP3A4 inhibitors; use 25 mg dose. Do not exceed 25 mg/48 h with ritonavir. Doses greater than 25 mg should not be taken less than 4 h after an alpha-blocker. Caution if CVA, MI, or other cardiovascular event within last 6 months. Do not use with itraconazole, ketoconazole, ritonavir, or pulmonary veno-occlusive disease. Coadministration with CYP3A4 inducers (ie, bosentan; barbiturates, carbamazepine, phenytoin, efavirenz, nevirapine, rifampin, rifabutin) may change levels of either medication; adjust doses as needed. Use caution with CVA, MI, or life-threatening arrhythmia in last 6 months; unstable angina; BP greater than 170/110; or retinitis pigmentosa. Contraindicated in patients taking nitrates within prior/subsequent 24 h. Caution with alpha-blockers due to potential for symptomatic hypotension. There have been a few reports of sudden vision loss due to nonarteritic ischemic optic neuropathy (NAION). Patients with prior NAION are at higher risk. Sudden hearing loss, with or without tinnitus, vertigo, or dizziness, has been reported. Transient global amnesia has also been reported.

MOA — Selectively inhibits phosphodiesterase-5 resulting in enhanced relaxation of penile arteries & corpus cavernosal smooth muscle; enhances erectile function by increasing penile blood flow. Relaxes pulmonary vascular smooth muscle cells resulting in vasodilation of the pulmonary vascular bed.

ADVERSE EFFECTS — Serious: MI, CVA, hypotension, syncope, cerebral thrombosis, retinal hemorrhage, vision loss (nonarteritic ischemic optic neuropathy). Frequent: Headache, flushing, dyspepsia, abnormal vision.

TADALAFIL—UROLOGY (*Cialis*) ▶L ♀B ▷– $$$$

WARNING — Contraindicated with nitrates. Caution with alpha-blockers due to potential for symptomatic hypotension. There have been a few reports of sudden vision loss due to nonarteritic ischemic optic neuropathy (NAION). Patients with prior NAION are at higher risk. Retinal artery occlusion has been reported. Sudden hearing loss, with or without tinnitus, vertigo, or dizziness, has been reported. Transient global amnesia has been reported. Use caution with daily use in patients with mild to moderate hepatic impairment; daily use is not recommended in severe hepatic impairment.

ADULT — Erectile dysfunction: 2.5 to 5 mg PO daily without regard to timing of sexual activity. As-needed dosing: 10 mg PO prn prior to sexual activity. Optimal timing of administration unclear, but should be at least 30 to 45 min before sexual activity. May increase to 20 mg or decrease to 5 mg. Max 1 dose/day. Start 5 mg (max 1 dose/day) if CrCl

(cont.)

TADALAFIL *(cont.)*

31 to 50 mL/min. Max 5 mg/day if CrCl <30 mL/min on dialysis. Max 10 mg/day if mild to moderate hepatic impairment; avoid in severe hepatic impairment. Max 10 mg once in 72 h if concurrent potent CYP3A4 inhibitors. BPH with or without erectile dysfunction: 5 mg PO daily. Caution with ritonavir; see prescribing information for specific dose adjustments.

PEDS — Not approved in children.

FORMS — Trade only (Cialis): Tabs 2.5, 5, 10, 20 mg.

NOTES — If nitrates needed, give at least 48 h after the last tadalafil dose. Improves erectile function for up to 36 h. Not FDA-approved for women. Not recommended if MI in prior 90 days, angina during sexual activity, NYHA Class II or greater heart failure in prior 6 months, hypotension (less than 90/50), HTN (greater than 170/100), or CVA in prior 6 months. Rare reports of prolonged erections. Do not use with ketoconazole or itraconazole. CYP3A4 inducers (rifampin) decrease exposure to tadalafil.

MOA — Selectively inhibits phosphodiesterase-5 resulting in enhanced relaxation of penile arteries & corpus cavernosal smooth muscle; enhances erectile function by increasing penile blood flow.

ADVERSE EFFECTS — Serious: Priapism, hypotension, myocardial infarction, vision loss (nonarteritic ischemic optic neuropathy), retinal artery occlusion. Frequent: Headache, flushing, dyspepsia, back pain.

VARDENAFIL (*Levitra, Staxyn*) ▶LK ♀B ▶– $$$$$

WARNING — Contraindicated with nitrates (time interval for safe administration unknown). Caution with alpha-blockers due to potential for symptomatic hypotension. There have been a few reports of sudden vision loss due to nonarteritic ischemic optic neuropathy (NAION). Patients with prior NAION are at higher risk. Sudden hearing loss, with or without tinnitus, vertigo, or dizziness, has been reported. Seizures and seizure recurrence have been reported.

ADULT — Erectile dysfunction: 10 mg PO 1 h before sexual activity. Usual effective dose range: 5 to 20 mg. Max 1 dose/day. Use lower dose (5 mg) if age 65 yo or older or moderate hepatic impairment (max 10 mg); 2.5 mg when coadministered with certain drugs (see Notes). Not FDA-approved in women.

PEDS — Not approved in children.

FORMS — Trade only: Tabs 2.5, 5, 10, 20 mg. Orally disintegrating tabs, 10 mg (Staxyn).

NOTES — See the following parenthetical vardenafil dose adjustments when taken with ritonavir (max 2.5 mg/72 h); indinavir, saquinavir, atazanavir, clarithromycin, ketoconazole 400 mg daily, or itraconazole 400 mg daily (max 2.5 mg/24 h); ketoconazole 200 mg daily, itraconazole 200 mg daily, or erythromycin (max 5 mg/24 h). Avoid with alpha-blockers and antiarrhythmics, and in congenital QT prolongation. Caution if CVA, MI, or other cardiovascular event within last 6 months; unstable angina; severe liver impairment; ESRD, or retinitis pigmentosa.

MOA — Selectively inhibits phosphodiesterase-5 resulting in enhanced relaxation of penile arteries & corpus cavernosal smooth muscle; enhances erectile function by increasing penile blood flow.

ADVERSE EFFECTS — Serious: Hypotension, syncope, myocardial infarction, priapism, vision loss (nonarteritic ischemic optic neuropathy), seizures, transient global amnesia. Frequent: Headache, flushing, rhinitis, dyspepsia.

UROLOGY: Nephrolithiasis

ACETOHYDROXAMIC ACID (*Lithostat*) ▶K ♀X ▶? $$$$

WARNING — Contraindicated in (1) patients whose physical state and disease are amenable to definitive surgery and appropriate antimicrobials, (2) patients whose urine is infected with non-urease-producing organisms, (3) patients whose UTIs can be controlled with culture-specific oral antibiotics, (4) patients with poor renal function (creatinine greater than 2.5 and/or creatinine clearance less than 20 mL/min), (5) patients without a satisfactory method of contraception, and (6) pregnant patients.

ADULT — Chronic UTI, adjunctive therapy: 250 mg PO three to four times per day for a total dose of 10 to 15 mg/kg/day. Max dose is 1.5 g/day. Decrease dose in patients with renal impairment (serum creatinine greater than 1.8) to no more than 1 g/day. Recommended starting dose is 12 mg/kg/day administered at 6 to 8 hour intervals on an empty stomach.

PEDS — Adjunctive therapy in chronic urea-splitting UTI (eg, Proteus): 10 mg/kg/day PO divided two to three times per day.

FORMS — Trade only: Tabs 250 mg.

NOTES — Do not use if CrCl <20 mL/min. Administer on an empty stomach.

MOA — Inhibits urease and the production of ammonia by urea-splitting urinary organisms (eg, Proteus).

ADVERSE EFFECTS — Serious: Bone marrow suppression, hemolytic anemia. Frequent: Headache, rash, malaise, nervousness, anxiety, depression, vomiting, anorexia, phlebitis.

CELLULOSE SODIUM PHOSPHATE (*Calcibind*) ▶Fecal ♀C ▶+ $$$$

WARNING — Avoid in heart failure or ascites due to high sodium content.

ADULT — Absorptive hypercalciuria Type 1 (age older than 16 yo): Initial dose with urinary calcium greater than 300 mg/day (on moderate calcium-restricted diet): 5 g with each meal. Decrease dose to 5 g with supper, 2.5 g with each remaining meal when calcium declines to less than 150 mg/day. Initial dose with urinary calcium 200 to 300 mg/day (controlled calcium-restricted diet): 5 g with supper, 2.5 g with

(cont.)

CELLULOSE SODIUM PHOSPHATE (cont.)

each remaining meal. Mix with water, soft drink, or fruit juice. Ingest within 30 min of meal.

PEDS — Do not use if younger than 16 yo.

FORMS — Trade only: Bulk powder 300 mg.

NOTES — Give concomitant supplement of 1.5 g magnesium gluconate with 15 g/day. 1 g magnesium gluconate with 10 g/day. Take magnesium supplement at least 1 h before or after each dose to avoid binding. May cause hyperparathyroidism. Long-term use may cause hypomagnesemia, hyperoxaluria, hypomagnesuria, depletion of trace metals (copper, zinc, iron); monitor calcium, magnesium, trace metals, and CBC q 3 to 6 months; monitor parathyroid hormone once between the 1st 2 weeks and 3 months, then q 3 to 6 months thereafter. Adjust or stop treatment if PTH rises above normal. Stop when inadequate hypocalciuric response (urinary calcium <30 mg/5 g of cellulose sodium phosphate) occurs while patient is on moderate calcium restriction. Avoid vitamin C supplementation since metabolized to oxalate. Mix in a full glass (8 ounces) of water, soft drink, or fruit juice; rinse glass with a little more liquid and drink that also. Take with meals.

MOA — Nonabsorbable ion-exchange resin. Binds to divalent cations. Used to prevent formation of calcium-containing kidney stones

ADVERSE EFFECTS — Serious: Hyperoxaluria, convulsions. Frequent: Diarrhea, dyspepsia, altered taste, hypomagnesemia, hyperparathyroidism, drowsiness, anorexia, mood changes, muscle spasms, nausea/vomiting, trembling, tiredness, weakness, abdominal pain.

CITRATE (Polycitra-K, Urocit-K, Bicitra, Oracit, Polycitra, Polycitra-LC) ▶K ♀C ▶? $$$

ADULT — Prevention of calcium and urate kidney stones: 1 packet in water/juice PO three to four times per day with meals. 15 to 30 mL PO soln three to four times per day with meals. Tabs 10 to 20 mEq PO three to four times per day with meals. Max 100 mEq/day. Severe hypocitraturia (urinary citrate less than 150 mg/day): Start at 60 mEq/day either 30 mEq twice a day or 20 mEq three times a day with meals or within 30 minutes after meals or bedtime snack. Mild or moderate hypocitraturia (urinary citrate greater than 150 mEq/day): Start with 30 mEq/day, either 10 mEq three times a day or 15 mEq twice a day with meals or within 30 minutes after meal or bedtime snack.

PEDS — Urinary alkalinization: 5 to 15 mL PO four times per day with meals.

FORMS — Generic/Trade: Polycitra-K packet 3300 mg potassium citrate/ea, Polycitra-K oral soln (1100 mg potassium citrate/5 mL, 480 mL). Oracit oral soln (490 mg sodium citrate/5 mL, 15, 30, 480 mL). Bicitra oral soln (500 mg sodium citrate/5 mL, 480 mL). Urocit-K wax (potassium citrate): Tabs 5, 10 mEq. Polycitra-LC oral soln (550 mg potassium citrate/500 mg sodium citrate per 5 mL, 480 mL). Polycitra oral syrup (550 mg potassium citrate/500 mg sodium citrate per 5 mL, 480 mL).

NOTES — Contraindicated in renal insufficiency, PUD, UTI, and hyperkalemia.

MOA — Increases urinary-free bases thereby increasing pH.

ADVERSE EFFECTS — Serious: Hyperkalemia. Frequent: N/V, diarrhea, dyspepsia.

APPENDIX

	ADULT EMERGENCY DRUGS (selected)
ALLERGY	diphenhydramine (Benadryl): 25 to 50 mg IV/IM/PO epinephrine: 0.1 to 0.5 mg IM/SC (1:1000 solution) repeat in 20 min. If hypotension consider 0.01 to 0.1 mg IV push (1:10,000) methylprednisolone (Solu-Medrol): 125 mg IV/IM.
HYPERTENSION	esmolol (Brevibloc): 500 mcg/kg IV over 1 minute, then titrate 50 to 200 mcg/kg/min nicardipine (Cardene): Start 5 mg/h IV titrate by 2.5 mg/h every 5 to 15 min to a max of 15 mg/h labetalol: Start 20 mg slow IV, then 40 to 80 mg IV q10 min prn up to 300 mg total cumulative dose. nitroglycerin: Start 10 to 20 mcg/min IV infusion, then titrate prn up to 100 mcg/min. nitroprusside (Nitropress): Start 0.3 mcg/kg/min IV infusion, then titrate prn up to 10 mcg/kg/min.
DYSRHYTHMIAS/ARREST	adenosine (Adenocard): PSVT (not A-fib): 6 mg rapid IV & flush, preferably through a central line or proximal IV. If no response after 1-2 minutes, then 12 mg. A third dose of 12mg may be given prn. amiodarone: V-fib or pulseless V-tach: 300 mg IV/IO; may repeat 150 mg just once. Life-threatening ventricular arrhythmia: Load 150 mg IV over 10 min, then 1 mg/min × 6 h, then 0.5 mg/min × 18 h. procainamide: 100 mg IV every 10 min or 20 mg/min until QRS widens 50%, dysrhythma suppressed, hypotension or 17 mh/kg or 1000mg delivered. atropine: 0.5 to 1 mg IV, repeat q 3-5 minutes prn to maximum of 3 mg. diltiazem (Cardizem): Rapid A-fib: bolus 0.25 mg/kg or 20 mg IV over 2 min. May repeat 0.35 mg/kg or 25 mg 15 min after 1st dose. Infusion 5-15 mg/h. epinephrine: 1 mg IV/IO q 3-5 minutes for cardiac arrest. [1:10,000 solution]. lidocaine (Xylocaine): Load 1 mg/kg IV, then 0.5 mg/kg q 8-10 min prn to max 3 mg/kg. Maintenance 2 g in 250 mL D5W (8 mg/mL) at 1 to 4 mg/min drip (7-30 mL/h).
PRESSORS	dobutamine: 2 to 20 mcg/kg/min. 70 kg: 5 mcg/kg/min with 1 mg/mL concentration (eg, 250 mg in 250 mL D5W) = 21 mL/h. dopamine: Pressor: Start at 5 mcg/kg/min, increase prn by 5 to 10 mcg/kg/min increments at 10 min intervals, max 50 mcg/kg/min. 70 kg: 5 mcg/kg/min with 1600 mcg/mL concentration (eg, 400 mg in 250 mL D5W) = 13 mL/h. Doses in mcg/kg/min: 2-4 = (traditional renal dose, apparently < 2 ineffective) dopaminergic receptors; 5-10= (cardiac dose) dopaminergic and beta1 receptors; >10 = dopaminergic, beta1, and alpha1 receptors. norepinephrine (Levophed): 4 mg in 500 mL D5W (8 mcg/mL), start 8 to 12 mcg/min (1 to 1.5 mL/h), usual dose once BP is stabilized 2 to 4 mcg/min. 22.5 mL/h = 3 mcg/min. phenylephrine: 20 mg in 250 mL D5W (80 mcg/mL), start 100 to 180 mcg/min (75 to 135 mL/h), usual dose once BP is stabilized 40 to 60 mcg/min (30 to 45 mL/h). epinephrine: infusion 0.1 to 0.5 ucg/kg/minute; push dose 5 to 20 ucg IV once

(cont.)

ADULT EMERGENCY DRUGS (selected)	
INTUBATION	etomidate (Amidate): 0.3 mg/kg IV. methohexital (Brevital): 1 to 1.5 mg/kg IV. propofol (Diprivan): 2.0 to 2.5 mg/kg IV. rocuronium (Zemuron): 0.6 to 1.2 mg/kg IV. succinylcholine (Anectine, Quelicin): 0.6 to 1.1 mg/kg IV. Peds (<5 yo): 2 mg/kg IV. ketamine: 1 to 2 mg/kg IV over 1 to 2 min
SEIZURES	diazepam (Valium): 5 to 10 mg IV, or 0.2 to 0.5 mg/kg rectal gel up to 20 mg PR. fosphenytoin (Cerebyx): Load 15 to 20 mg "phenytoin equivalents" (PE)/ kg IV, no faster than 100 to 150 mg PE/min. lorazepam (Ativan): Status epilepticus: 4 mg IV over 2 min, may repeat in 10-15 min. Anxiolytic/sedation: 0.04 to 0.05 mg/kg IV/IM; usual dose 2 mg, max 4 mg. phenobarbital: Status epilepticus: 15 to 20 mg/kg IV load; may give additional 5 mg/kg doses q 15-30 mins to max total dose of 30 mg/kg. phenytoin (Dilantin): 15 to 20 mg/kg IV, no faster than 50 mg/min.

CARDIAC DYSRHYTHMIA PROTOCOLS (for adults and adolescents)

Chest compressions ~100/min. Ventilations 8-10/min if intubated; otherwise 30:2 compression/ventilation ratio. Use IO line if IV access delayed. Drugs that can be administered down ET tube (use 2–2.5 × usual dose): epinephrine, atropine, lidocaine, naloxone, vasopressin*.

V-Fib, Pulseless V-Tach

Compression. airway, oxygen until defibrillator ready

Defibrillate 360 J (old monophasic), 120–200 J (biphasic), or with AED

Resume CPR × 2 min (5 cycles)

Repeat defibrillation if no response

Vasopressor during CPR:
• Epinephrine 1 mg IV/IO q 3–5 minutes, or
• Vasopressin* 40 units IV to replace 1st or 2nd dose of epinephrine

Rhythm/pulse check every ~2 minutes

Consider antiarrhythmic during CPR:
• Amiodarone 300 mg IV/IO; may repeat 150 mg just once
• Lidocaine 1.0–1.5 mg/kg IV/IO, then repeat 0.5–0.75 mg/kg to max 3 mg/kg at 5 to 10 minute intervals
• Magnesium sulfate 1–2 g IV/IO over 5 to 20 minutes if suspect torsades de pointes

Asystole or Pulseless Electrical Activity (PEA)

Compressions, airway, oxygen

Vasopressor (when IV/IO access):
• Epinephrine 1 mg IV/IO q 3–5 min

Rhythm/pulse check every ~2 minutes

Consider 6 H's: hypovolemia, hypoxia, H+acidosis, hyper/ hypokalemia, hypoglycemia, hypothermia

Consider 5 T's: Toxins, tamponade, tension pneumothorax, thrombosis (coronary or pulmonary), trauma

Bradycardia, <50 bpm and Inadequate Perfusion

Airway, oxygen, IV

Prepare for transcutaneous pacing; don't delay if advanced heart block

Consider atropine 0.5 mg IV; may repeat q 3–5 min to max 3 mg

Consider epinephrine (2–10 mcg/min) or dopamine(2–10mcg/kg/min)

Prepare for transvenous pacing

Tachycardia with Pulses

Airway, oxygen, IV

If unstable and heart rate >150 bpm, then synchronized cardioversion
Doses: Narrow Regular Sync 50-100J, Narrow Irregular Sync 120-200 J Biphasic or 200 J Monophasic, Wide Regular Sync 100J, Wide Irregular Defibrillation Dose (not synchronized)

If stable narrow-QRS (<120 ms):
• Regular: Attempt vagal maneuvers, If no success, adenosine 6 mg IV, can be followed by 2 additional 12 mg boluses if needed
• Irregular: Control rate with diltiazem or beta blocker (caution in CHF or severe obstructive disease). Amiodarone 150 mg indicated for patients with low EF or signs of CHF.

(cont.)

CARDIAC DYSRHYTHMIA PROTOCOLS (for adults and adolescents) (*continued*)

If stable wide-QRS (>120 ms):
• Regular and suspect V-tach (older patient, hx of MI, prior VT): Amiodarone 150 mg IV over 10 min; repeat prn to max 2.2 g/24 h.
Prepare for elective synchronized cardioversion.
• Regular and suspect SVT with aberrancy: Adenosine as per narrow-QRS above. If unsure if V-tach or SVT with aberrancy, adenosine still considered safe *
• Irregular and known to be A-fib with aberrancy: Control rate with diltiazem or beta blocker (caution in CHF/severe obstructive pulmonary disease).
• Irregular and A-fib with pre-excitation (WPW) (e.g. polymorphic, rate >200): Avoid amiodarone, adenosine, digoxin, or nondihydropyridine calcium channel antagonists as they are contraindicated **; use procainamide, consider ibutilide, others
• Irregular and torsades de pointes: magnesium 1–2 g IV load over 5–60 min, then infusion.

bpm=beats per minute; CPR=cardiopulmonary resuscitation; ET=endotracheal; IO=intraosseous; J=Joules; ms=milliseconds; WPW=Wolff-Parkinson-White. Sources: Circulation 2005; 112, suppl IV;
*Marill KA et al. Adenosine is safe and effective for differentiating wide-complex supraventricular tachycardia from ventricular tachycardia. Crit Care Med 2009 Sep 37:2512
**2014 AHA/ACC/HRS Guideline for the Management of Patients With Atrial Fibrillation: Executive Summary. Circulation.2014; 130: 2071-2104

INDEX

NOTE: Information in tables is denoted with a "*t*" after the page number. Entries in bold indicate page number of main drug monograph.

M

Stay Connected with Tarascon Publishing!

Monthly Dose eNewsletter
—Tarascon's Monthly eNewsletter

Stay up-to-date and subscribe today at: www.tarascon.com

Written specifically with Tarascon customers in mind, the Tarascon Monthly Dose will provide you with new drug information, tips and tricks, updates on our print, mobile and online products as well as some extra topics that are interesting and entertaining.

Sign up to receive the Tarascon Monthly Dose Today! Simply register at www.tarascon.com.

You can also stay up-to-date with Tarascon news, new product releases, and relevant medical news and information on Facebook, Twitter page, and our Blog.

STAY CONNECTED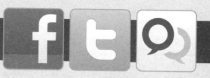

Facebook: www.facebook.com/tarascon
Twitter: @JBL_Medicine
Blog: blogs.jblearning.com/medicine